PEDIATRICS
Just the Facts

D1558515

Thomas P. Green, MD

Professor and Chairman
Department of Pediatrics
Children's Memorial Hospital
Northwestern University Feinberg School of Medicine

Wayne H. Franklin, MD, MPH

Associate Professor
Department of Pediatrics
Division of Cardiology
Children's Memorial Hospital
Northwestern University Feinberg School of Medicine

Robert R. Tanz, MD

Professor of Pediatrics
Northwestern University Feinberg School of Medicine
Attending Physician
Division of General Academic Pediatrics
Children's Memorial Hospital

McGraw-Hill
Medical Publishing Division

New York   Chicago   San Francisco   Lisbon   London   Madrid
Mexico City   Milan   New Delhi   San Juan   Seoul
Singapore   Sydney   Toronto

PEDIATRICS
Just the Facts

1 2 3 4 5 6 7 8 9 0   QPD/QPD   0 9 8 7 6 5 4

ISBN 0-07-141642-0

This book was set in Times New Roman by International Typesetting and Composition.
The editors were James Shanahan and Michelle Watt.
The production supervisor was Catherine Saggese.
Project management was provided by International Typesetting and Composition.
Quebecor Dubuque was printer and binder.

This book is printed on acid-free paper.

> **NOTICE**
>
> Medicine is an ever-changing science. As new research and clinical experience broaden our knowledge, changes in treatment and drug therapy are required. The authors and the publisher of this work have checked with sources believed to be reliable in their efforts to provide information that is complete and generally in accord with the standards accepted at the time of publication. However, in view of the possibility of human error or changes in medical sciences, neither the authors nor the publisher nor any other party who has been involved in the preparation or publication of this work warrants that the information contained herein is in every respect accurate or complete, and they disclaim all responsibility for any errors or omissions or for the results obtained from use of the information contained in this work. Readers are encouraged to confirm the information contained herein with other sources. For example and in particular, readers are advised to check the product information sheet included in the package of each drug they plan to administer to be certain that the information contained in this work is accurate and that changes have not been made in the recommended dose or in the contraindications for administration. This recommendation is of particular importance in connection with new or infrequently used drugs.

Library of Congress Cataloging-in-Publication Data

Pediatrics : just the facts / edited by Thomas Green, Wayne Franklin, Robert R. Tanz.
      p. ; cm.
   Includes bibliographical references and index.
   ISBN 0-07-141642-0
   1. Pediatrics—Handbooks, manuals, etc.   I. Green, Thomas, MD.
   II. Frankin, Wayne H.   III. Tanz, Robert R.
   [DNLM: 1. Pediatrics—Handbooks. WS 39 P37195 2004]
   RJ48.P44 2004
   618.92—dc22

                                                                              2004044843

CONTENTS

CONTRIBUTORS

Maria Luiza C. Albuquerque, MD, Associate Professor, Department of Pediatrics, Division of Critical Care Medicine, Children's Memorial Hospital, Northwestern University Feinberg School of Medicine

Adolfo Ariza, MD, Research Assistant Professor, Department of Pediatrics, Child Health Research, Children's Memorial Insititute for Education and Research, Northwestern University Feinberg School of Medicine

Ruba Azzam, MD, Fellow, Department of Pediatrics, Division of Gastroenterology, Hepatology and Nutrition, Children's Memorial Hospital, Northwestern University Feinberg of Medicine

Alexander Bassuk, MD, Fellow, Department of Pediatrics, Division of Neurology, Children's Memorial Hospital, Northwestern University Feinberg School of Medicine

Barbara W. Bayldon, MD, Assistant Professor, Department of Pediatrics; Division of General Academic Pediatrics; Children's Memorial Hospital; Northwestern University Feinberg School of Medicine

Catherine M. Bendel, MD, Assistant Professor, Department of Pediatrics, Division of Neonatology; University of Minnesota/Fairview University Medical Center

Susan P. Berger, PhD, Assistant Professor, Department of Pediatrics; Division of General Academic Pediatrics; Northwestern University Feinberg School of Medicine; Children's Memorial Hospital

Wendy J. Brickman, MD, Assistant Professor, Department of Pediatrics, Division of Endocrinology, Children's Memorial Hospital, Northwestern University Feinberg School of Medicine

Deborah L. Brown, MD, Assistant Professor, Department of Pediatrics, University of Texas Health Science Center at Houston

Jeffrey B. Brown, MD, Assistant Professor, Department of Pediatrics, Division of Gastroenterology, Hepatology and Nutrition, Children's Memorial Hospital, Northwestern University Feinberg of Medicine

Barbara K. Burton, MD, Professor, Department of Pediatrics, Division of Genetics, Children's Memorial Hospital, Northwestern University Feinberg School of Medicine

Sarah L. Chamlin, MD, Assistant Professor, Department of Pediatrics, Division of Dermatology, Children's Memorial Hospital, Northwestern University Feinberg School of Medicine

Joel Charrow, MD, Professor, Department of Pediatrics, Division of Genetics, Children's Memorial Hospital, Northwestern University Feinberg School of Medicine

Colleen Cicchetti, PhD, Instructor, Department of Psychiatry and Behavioral Science, Child and Adolescent Medicine, Children's Memorial Hospital, Northwestern University Feinberg School of Medicine

Susan L. Cohn, MD, Professor, Department of Pediatrics, Division of Hematology/Oncology, Children's Memorial Hospital, Northwestern University Feinberg School of Medicine

Kelly Coyne, RN, MSN, CPNP, Pediatric Nurse Practitioner, Division of Hematology/Oncology/Transplantation, Children's Memorial Hospital

Charles S. Czerepak, DMD, MS, Assistant Professor, Departemnt of Surgery, Children's Memorial Hospital, Northwestern University Feinberg School of Medicine

Jennifer A. Daru, MD, Instructor Clinical, Department of Pediatrics, Children's Memorial Hospital, Northwestern University Feinberg School of Medicine

Barbara J. Deal, MD, Professor, Department of Pediatrics, Division of Cardiology, Children's Memorial Hospital, Northwestern University Feinberg School of Medicine

Ruth B. Deddish, MD, Associate Professor, Department of Pediatrics, Division of Neonatology, Children's Memorial Hospital, Northwestern University Feinberg School of Medicine

Isabelle G. DePlaen, MD, Assistant Professor, Department of Pediatrics, Division of Neonatology, Children's Memorial Hospital, Northwestern University Feinberg School of Medicine

Marissa deUngria, MD, Instructor, Department of Pediatrics, Division of Neonatology, Children's Memorial Hospital, Northwestern University Feinberg School of Medicine

Kimberley J. Dilley, MD, Attending Physician, Division of Hematology/Oncology; Children's Memorial Hospital; Northwestern University Feinberg School of Medicine

Maria L.V. Dizon, MD, Instructor, Department of Pediatrics, Division of Neonatology, Children's Memorial Hospital, Northwestern University Feinberg School of Medicine

Maria L. Dowell, M.D., Formerly: Fellow, Division of Pulmonary Medicine, Department of Pediatrics, Children's Memorial Hospital, Northwestern University Feinberg School of Medicine

Cynthia Etzler Budek, RN, MS, CPNP, Pediatric Nurse Practitioner, Children's Memorial Hospital

Richard Evans III, MD, MPH, Professor Emeritus, Department of Pediatrics, Division of Allergy, Children's Memorial Hospital, Northwestern University Feinberg School of Medicine

Wayne H. Franklin, MD, MPH, Associate Professor, Department of Pediatrics, Division of Cardiology, Children's Memorial Hospital, Northwestern University Feinberg School of Medicine

Robert Garofalo, MD, MPH, Assistant Professor, Department of Pediatrics and Department of Preventive Medicine; Division of General Academic Pediatrics; Northwestern University Feinberg School of Medicine; Children's Memorial Hospital

Mark E. Gerber, MD, Assistant Professor, Department of Otolaryngology, Division of Otolaryngology, Children's Memorial Hospital, Northwestern University Feinberg School of Medicine

Mariana Glusman, MD, Instructor, Department of Pediatrics; Division of General Academic Pediatrics; Children's Memorial Hospital; Northwestern University Feinberg School of Medicine

Stewart Goldman, MD, Associate Professor, Department of Pediatrics, Division of Hematology/Oncology, Children's Memorial Hospital, Northwestern University Feinberg School of Medicine

Joshua L. Goldstein, MD, Assistant Professor, Department of Pediatrics, Division of Neurology, Children's Memorial Hospital, Northwestern University Feinberg School of Medicine

Denise M. Goodman, MD, MSc, Associate Professor, Department of Pediatrics, Division of Critical Care Medicine, Children's Memorial Hospital, Northwestern University Feinberg School of Medicine

Yasmin Gosiengfiao, MD, Fellow, Department of Pediatrics, Division of Hematology/Oncology, Children's Memorial Hospital, Northwestern University Feinberg School of Medicine

Thomas P. Green, MD, Professor and Chairman, Department of Pediatrics, Children's Memorial Hospital, Northwestern University Feinberg School of Medicine

Reema L. Habiby, MD, Assistant Professor, Department of Pediatrics, Division of Endocrinology, Children's Memorial Hospital, Northwestern University Feinberg School of Medicine

Corinda M. Hankins, MD, Formerly: Fellow, Department of Pediatrics, Division of Pulmonary Medicine, Children's Memorial Hospital, Northwestern University Feinberg School of Medicine; Currently: Private Practice, Hood River, Oregon

Maureen Haugen, RN, CPNP, Pediatric Nurse Practiction, Department of Pediatrics, Division of Hematology/Oncology, Children's Memorial Hospital, Northwestern University Feinberg School of Medicine

Denise T. Ibrahim, MD, Formerly: Fellow; Department of Orthopedic Surgery, Division of Orthopedics, Children's Memorial Hospital, Northwestern University Feinberg School of Medicine; Currently: private Practice, Southwest Orthopedics, Evergreen Park, Illinois

Preeti Jaggi, MD, Fellow, Department of Pediatrics; Division of Infectious Diseases, Children's Memorial Hospital, Northwestern University Feinberg School of Medicine

Ronald J. Kallen, MD, Associate Professor, Clinical Department of Pediatrics, Division of Kidney Diseases, Children's Memorial Hospital, Northwestern University Feinberg School of Medicine

Howard M. Katzenstein, MD, Clinical Associate Professor, Department of Pediatrics, Division of Hematology/Oncology, Children's Health Care of Atlanta at Egleston, Emory University School of Medicine

Rae-Ellen W. Kavey, MD, MPH, Professor, Department of Pediatrics, Division of Cardiology, Children's Memorial Hospital, Northwestern University Feinberg School of Medicine

Kent R. Kelley, MD, Assistant Professor, Department of Pediatrics, Division of Neurology, Children's Memorial Hospital, Northwestern University Feinberg School of Medicine

Janine Y. Khan, MD, Assistant Professor, Department of Pediatrics, Division of Neonatology, Children's Memorial Hospital, Northwestern University Feinberg School of Medicine

Jennifer S. Kim, MD, Fellow, Department of Pediatrics, Division of Allergy, Children's Memorial Hospital, Northwestern University Feinberg School of Medicine

Marisa S. Klein-Gitelman, MD, Assistant Professor, Department of Pediatrics, Division of Immunology/Rheumatology, Children's Memorial Hospital, Northwestern University Feinberg School of Medicine

Morris Kletzel, MD, Professor, Department of Pediatrics, Division of Hematology/Oncology, Children's Memorial Hospital, Northwestern University Feinberg School of Medicine

Rohit Kohli, MD, Fellow, Department of Pediatrics, Division of Gastroenterology, Hepatology and Nutrition, Children's Memorial Hospital, Northwestern University Feinberg of Medicine

Kristen Koridek, BS, RRT, Department of Pediatrics, Division of Allergy, Children's Memorial Hospital, Northwestern University Feinberg School of Medicine

Praveen Kumar, MD, Assistant Professor, Department of Pediatrics, Division of Neonatology, Children's Memorial Hospital, Northwestern University Feinberg School of Medicine

Rajesh Kumar, MD, MPH, Assistant Professor, Department of Pediatrics, Division of Allergy, Children's Memorial Hospital, Northwestern University Feinberg School of Medicine

Oren J. Lakser, MD, Assistant Professor, Department of Pediatrics,; Division of Pulmonary Medicine, Children's Memorial Hospital, Northwestern University Feinberg School of Medicine

Jerome C. Lane, MD, Assistant Professor, Department of Pediatrics, Division of Kidney Diseases, Children's Memorial Hospital, Northwestern University Feinberg School of Medicine

Craig B. Langman, MD, Professor, Department of Pediatrics, Division of Kidney Diseases, Children's Memorial Hospital, Northwestern University Feinberg School of Medicine

Janice B. Lasky, MD, Assistant Professor, Department of Ophthalmology, Division of Ophthalmology, Children's Memorial Hospital, Northwestern University Feinberg School of Medicine

Linda C. Laux, MD, Assistant Professor, Department of Pediatrics, Division of Neurology, Children's Memorial Hospital, Northwestern University Feinberg School of Medicine

John Lavigne, PhD, Professor, Department of Psychiatry and Behavioral Science and Department of Pediatrics, Child and Adolescent Psychiatry, Children's Memorial Hospital, Northwestern University Feinberg School of Medicine

Steven O. Lestrud, MD, Instructor, Department of Pediatrics, Division of Critical Care Medicine, Children's Memorial Hospital, Northwestern University Feinberg School of Medicine

B U.K. Li, MD, Professor, Department of Pediatrics, Division of Gastroenterology, Hepatology and Nutrition, Children's Memorial Hospital, Northwestern University Feinberg of Medicine

Laurie MacDonald, MD, Formerly: Fellow; Department of Pediatrics, Division of Hematology/Oncology, Children's Memorial Hospital, Northwestern University Feinberg School of Medicine; Currently: Private Practice, Forsyth Pediatrics, Kernersville, North Carolina

Anthony J. Mancini, MD, Associate Professor, Department of Pediatarics, Division of Dermatology, Children's Memorial Hospital, Northwestern University Feinberg School of Medicine

Lisa A. Martin MD, MPH, Assistant Professor of Pediatrics, Loyola University, Stritch School of Medicine, Maywood, IL

Suzan S. Mazor, MD, Instructor, Department of Pediatrics, Division of Emergency Medicine, Children's Memorial Hospital, Northwestern University Feinberg School of Medicine

Susanna A. McColley, MD, Associate Professor, Department of Pediatrics, Division of Pulmonary Medicine, Children's Memorial Hospital, Northwestern University Feinberg School of Medicine

Kathleen McKenna, MD, Department of Psychiatry and Behavioral Science and Department of Pediatrics, Child and Adolescent Psychiatry, Children's Memorial Hospital, Northwestern University Feinberg School of Medicine

Wes McRae, MD, Assistant Professor, Department of Pediatrics, Division of Neurology, Children's Memorial Hospital, Northwestern University Feinberg School of Medicine

Karen K.L. Mestan, MD, Instructor, Department of Pediatrics, Division of Neonatology, Children's Memorial Hospital, Northwestern University Feinberg School of Medicine

Marilyn B. Mets, MD, Professor, Department of Ophthalmology, Division of Ophthalmology, Children's Memorial Hospital, Northwestern University Feinberg School of Medicine

Michael L. Miller, MD, Associate Professor, Department of Pediatrics, Division of Immunology/Rheumatology, Children's Memorial Hospital, Northwestern University Feinberg School of Medicine

Elaine R. Morgan, MD, Associate Professor, Department of Pediatrics, Division of Hematology/Oncology, Children's Memorial Hospital, Northwestern University Feinberg School of Medicine

Jill Nelson, MD, Fellow, Department of Pediatrics, Division of Dermatology, Children's Memorial Hospital, Northwestern University Feinberg School of Medicine

Mary A. Nevin, MD, Fellow, Department of Pediatrics, Division of Pulmonary Medicine, Children's Memorial Hospital, Northwestern University Feinberg School of Medicine

Kelly Newhall, MD, Fellow, Department of Pediatrics, Division of Allergy, Children's Memorial Hospital, Northwestern University Feinberg School of Medicine

Zehava L. Noah, MD, Associate Professor, Department of Pediatrics, Division of Critical Care Medicine, Children's Memorial Hospital, Northwestern University Feinberg School of Medicine

Lauren M. Pachman, MD, Professor, Department of Pediatrics, Division of Immunology/Rheumatology, Children's Memorial Hospital, Northwestern University Feinberg School of Medicine

Elfriede Pahl, MD, Professor, Department of Pediatrics, Division of Cardiology, Children's Memorial Hospital, Northwestern University Feinberg School of Medicine

Amy S. Paller, MD, Professor, Department of Pediatrics, Division of Dermatology, Children's Memorial Hospital, Northwestern University Feinberg School of Medicine

Jonathan M. Pochyly, PhD, Instructor, Department of Psychiatry and Behavioral Sicence, Child and Adolescent Psychiatry, Children's Memorial Hospital, Northwestern University Feinberg School of Medicine

Jacqueline A. Pongracic, MD, Associate Professor, Department of Pediatrics, Division of Allergy, Children's Memorial Hospital, Northwestern University Feinberg School of Medicine

Nicolas F.M. Porta, MD, Assistant Professor, Department of Pediatrics, Division of Neonatology, Children's Memorial Hospital, Northwestern University Feinberg School of Medicine

Elizabeth C. Powell, MD, MPH, Associate Professor, Department of Pediatrics, Division of Emergency Medicine, Children's Memorial Hospital, Northwestern University Feinberg School of Medicine

Sally L. Reynolds, MD, Associate Professor, Department of Pediatrics, Division of Emergency Medicine, Children's Memorial Hospital, Northwestern University Feinberg School of Medicine

David G. Ritacco, MD, PhD, Assistant Professor, Department of Pediatrics, Division of Neurology, Children's Memorial Hospital, Northwestern University Feinberg School of Medicine

Ranna A. Rozenfeld, MD, Assistant Professor, Department of Pediatrics, Division of Critical Care Medicine, Children's Memorial Hospital, Northwestern University Feinberg School of Medicine

Sandra M. Sanguino, MD, MPH, Assistant Professor, Department of Pediatrics; Division of General Academic Pediatrics; Children's Memorial Hospital; Northwestern University Feinberg School of Medicine

John F. Sarwark, MD, Professor, Department of Orthopedic Surgery, Division of Orthopedics, Children's Memorial Hospital, Northwestern University Feinberg School of Medicine

Robert L. Satcher, MD, PhD, Assistant Professor, Department of Orthopedic Surgery, Division of Orthopedics, Children's Memorial Hsopital, Northwestern University Feinberg School of Medicine

H. William Schnaper, MD, Professor, Department of Pediatrics, Division of Kidney Diseases, Children's Memorial Hospital, Northwestern University Feinberg School of Medicine

Timothy A. Sentongo, MD, Assistant Professor, Department of Pediatrics, Division of Gastroenterology, Hepatology and Nutrition, Children's Memorial Hospital, Northwestern University Feinberg of Medicine

Malika D. Shah, MD, Fellow, Instructor, Department of Pediatrics, Division of Neonatology, Children's Memorial Hospital, Northwestern University Feinberg School of Medicine

Raed Shatnawi, Fellow, Department of Ophthalmology, Children's Memorial Hospital, Northwestern University Feinberg School of Medicine

Stephen H. Sheldon, DO, Associate Professor, Department of Pediatrics, Division of Pulmonary Medicine, Children's Memorial Hospital, Northwestern University Feinberg School of Medicine

Horace E. Smith, MD, Instructor, Clinical, Department of Pediatrics, Division of Hematology/Oncology, Children's Memorial Hospital, Northwestern University Feinberg School of Medicine

David M. Steinhorn, MD, Associate Professor, Department of Pediatrics, Division of Critical Care Medicine, Children's Memorial Hospital, Northwestern University Feinberg School of Medicine

Lisa M. Sullivan MD, Fellow, Division of Allergy, Rush Medical Center, Chicago, IL

Shikha S. Sundaram, MD, Fellow, Department of Pediatrics, Division of Gastroenterology, Hepatology and Nutrition, Children's Memorial Hospital, Northwestern University Feinberg of Medicine

Bhanu Sunku, MD, Fellow, Department of Pediatrics, Division of Gastroenterology, Hepatology and Nutrition, Children's Memorial Hospital, Northwestern University Feinberg of Medicine

Charles N. Swisher, MD, Associate Professor, Department of Pediatrics, Division of Neurology, Children's Memorial Hospital, Northwestern University Feinberg School of Medicine

Robert R. Tanz, MD, Professor of Pediatrics, Director, Diagnostic and Consultation Services, Department of Pediatrics, Children's Memorial Hospital, Northwestern University Feinberg School of Medicine

Alexis A. Thompson, MD, MPH, Associate Professor, Department of Pediatrics, Division of Hematology/Oncology, Children's Memorial Hospital, Northwestern University Feinberg School of Medicine

Jacquie Toia, RN, MS, ND, CPNP, Pediatric Nurse Practitioner, Department of Pediatrics, Division of Hematology/Oncology, Children's Memorial Hospital, Northwestern University Feinberg School of Medicine

Rebecca Unger, MD, Assistant Professor, Clinical, Department of Pediatrics, Northwestern University Feinberg School of Medicine

Annette M. Wagner, MD, Assistant Professor, Department of Pediatrics, Division of Dermatology, Children's Memorial Hospital, Northwestern University Feinberg School of Medicine

Mark S. Wainwright, MD, PhD, Assistant Professor, Department of Pediatrics, Division of Neurology, Children's Memorial Hospital, Northwestern University Feinberg School of Medicine

Heather J. Walter, MD, Associate Professor, Department of Psychiatry and Behavioral Science, Child and Adolescent Psychiatry, Children's Memorial Hospital, Northwestern University Feinberg School of Medicine

David O. Walterhouse, MD, Associate Professor, Department of Pediatrics, Division of Hematology/Oncology, Children's Memorial Hospital, Northwestern University Feinberg School of Medicine

Kendra M. Ward, MD, Fellow, Department of Pediatrics, Division of Cardiology, Children's Memorial Hospital, Northwestern University Feinberg School of Medicine

Constance M. Weil, PhD, Assistant Professor, Department of Psychiatry and Behavioral Science, Child and Adolescent Psychiatry, Children's Memorial Hospital, Northwestern University Feinberg School of Medicine

Joanna L. Weinstein, MD, Instructor, Department of Pediatrics, Division of Hematology/Oncology, Children's Memorial Hospital, Northwestern University Feinberg School of Medicine

Gretchen Wieck, MD, Previously: Fellow, Department of Pediatrics, Division of Neurology, Children's Memorial Hospital, Northwestern University Feinberg School of Medicine; Currently: Private Practice, Chicago, Illinois

Gwendolyn M. Wright, MD, Instructor, Department of Pediatrics; Division of General Academic Pediatrics; Children's Memorial Hospital; Northwestern University Feinberg School of Medicine

Peter Zage, MD, Fellow, Department of Pediatrics, Division of Hematology/ Oncology, Children's Memorial Hospital, Northwestern University Feinberg School of Medicine

Donald L. Zimmerman, MD, Professor, Department of Pediatrics, Division of Endocrinology, Children's Memorial Hospital, Northwestern University Feinberg School of Medicine

PREFACE

In *Just the Facts in Pediatrics*, we have attempted to create a book that will fulfill the needs of several groups of medical professionals. Medical students, residents, and specialty fellows, as well as pediatricians, nurses, practitioners, and other child health providers require rapid access to a broad base of pediatric knowledge to develop complete differential diagnoses and comprehensive treatment plans. Additionally, recertifying pediatricians are seeking a concise, but comprehensive pediatric knowledge base for review and self-study.

We hope that the content and the format are helpful in meeting these needs. The organization of the book was designed to make the process of finding information as straightforward and as intuitive as possible. In addition, a separate section on common office problems and pediatric emergencies was added to facilitate access to readers interested in specific information in those common situations.

We want to express our gratitude and appreciation to the individuals whose work and commitment made this project possible. First, we relied almost exclusively on the physician faculty of Children's Memorial Hospital as section editors and authors. Their collective expertise, displayed in their chapters, reflects on their love of children and the science of pediatrics, as well as the collective pride we feel for this great institution. Our editors at McGraw Hill, Jim Shanahan and Michelle Watt were understanding, supportive, expert, and, above all, patient. Finally, Diana Vires brought her skills, persistence, and always positive demeanor to pull us through to the finish.

We welcome your comments and suggestions so that future editions are more accurate and helpful to all that are committed to the health of children.

1 GROWTH AND NORMAL NUTRITION

Lisa A. Martin

GROWTH PARAMETERS

- Monitoring a child's growth is a key part of a nutritional assessment. Growth parameters should be measured and plotted at each health care visit. Growth charts for age and sex were updated in 2000 and can be found on the Centers for Disease Control and Prevention, (CDC) website (www.cdc.gov/growthcharts).
- During infancy (birth to 2 years), recumbent length should be measured. After a child can stand independently (between the ages of 2 and 3 years), height may be measured while the child is not wearing shoes. A child whose height is less than the 5th percentile for age and sex has short stature, which may be a result of malnutrition, chronic illness, or delayed skeletal maturation.
- An infant's weight should be obtained while naked, and an older child should be dressed in underwear or a lightweight hospital gown.
- Weights and lengths of premature infants should be corrected for gestational age until 24 months of age.
- Special growth charts should be used for infants and children with the following conditions: Down syndrome, Turner syndrome, achondroplasia, and Noonan syndrome.
- A child's weight alone may be insufficient to determine whether he/she is normal weight, overweight or underweight; therefore, a measure of weight-for-height should also be evaluated. For infants (birth to 36 months), weight-for-length may be plotted. For older children (2–20 years), body mass index (BMI)-for-age charts are found on the reverse side of the height and weight charts. The formula for calculating BMI is shown below:

$$BMI = \frac{Weight\ (kg)}{Height\ (m)^2}$$

- A BMI greater than the 95th percentile for age represents overweight status, and a BMI between the 85th and 95th percentiles indicates that a child is at risk for becoming overweight. A BMI less than the 5th percentile for age represents underweight status.
- BMI typically changes with age, decreasing after the first year of life. After it reaches its nadir, typically between 4 and 6 years of life, BMI gradually increases through childhood and adolescence to reach adult levels. This phenomenon is known as adiposity rebound. Having an early adiposity rebound (i.e., before the age of 3 years) places a child at higher risk for being overweight as an adult, regardless of parental BMI or child's BMI at adiposity rebound. It is crucial to monitor BMI-for-age closely. The American Academy of Pediatrics (AAP) recommends that health care providers calculate and plot BMI yearly for all children and adolescents.
- Head circumference should be obtained for all children through the age of 2 years. Children with head circumferences less than the 5th percentile, greater than the 95th percentile, or a rapidly increasing head circumference may require further medical evaluation or imaging studies.

RED FLAG

- Infants whose height or weight decreases more than two percentile tracks merit detailed histories and physicals to detect nutritional or medical problems.

INFANTS (BIRTH TO 1 YEAR)

GROWTH

- Infants usually regain their birth weight within the first 2 weeks of life. During early infancy, they typically gain 5–7 oz/week and double their birth weight by 4–6 months of age. Later in infancy, weight gain velocity slows to about 3–5 oz/week.
- Infants typically grow approximately 1 in./month from birth to 6 months of age and approximately ½ in./month from 6 months to a year of age. During the first year of life, infants gain about 50% of their length.
- During the first 6 months of life, infants require 110–120 kcal/kg/day for growth. By 1 year of age, daily caloric needs decrease to ~100 kcal/kg.

BREAST MILK

- Breast milk is the optimal food for infants. Even if breastfeeding lasts only a few weeks, the benefits are numerous and include improved maternal-infant bonding, decreased gastroesophageal reflux, and decreased frequency of a variety of infections (including otitis media) because of the transfer of maternal immunoglobulins.
- Breast milk contains, on average, 20 kcal/oz. Colostrum, which is produced during the first 1–4 days of life, is extremely protein-rich and has a high concentration of immunoglobulins. Hindmilk has a higher fat content than foremilk, and is about 24 kcal/oz.
- Breast milk provides all of an infant's caloric needs until about 6 months of age. Solid foods should be introduced at that time.
- Infants who are exclusively breastfed should receive a daily vitamin supplement. Maternal vitamin D levels may be inadequate to provide sufficient levels to the infant. Vitamin B_{12} levels may be insufficient in infants whose mothers are strict vegetarians and take no vitamin B_{12} supplements. Fluoride supplementation is usually unnecessary, unless the local water supply contains less than 0.3 ppm of fluoride.
- Contraindications to breastfeeding include
  1. Certain inborn errors of metabolism, such as galactosemia
  2. Maternal infections (such as human immunodeficiency virus [HIV]) that can be transmitted through human milk
  3. Mothers who are undergoing chemotherapy or receiving other drugs that are excreted through human milk
- Breastfeeding should be interrupted under the following circumstances:
  1. Active tuberculosis
  2. Herpes lesions on the breast
  3. Untreated syphilis
- Expressed breast milk should be refrigerated for no more than 48 hours. It may also be stored in the freezer for up to 3–6 months. Thawed breast milk may not be refrozen.

INFANT FORMULAS

- Infant formulas are suitable alternatives for those families who cannot, or choose not to, breastfeed. A variety of formulas are available, including cow's milk based (e.g., Similac or Enfamil), soy based (e.g., Isomil or Prosobee), whey hydrolysate based (e.g., Good Start), or casein hydrolysate based (e.g., Alimentum or Pregestimil). Table 1-1 lists the composition of common infant formulas.
- The long-chain fatty acids docosahexaenoic acid (DHA) and arachadonic acid (AA) are found in breast milk and were recently added to several formulas. DHA is the major omega-3 fatty acid of retinal tissue, and AA is the major omega-6 fatty acid of other

TABLE 1-1   Composition of Common Infant Formulas

FORMULA	PROTEIN	CARBOHYDRATE	LIPID
Cow's milk (Similac, Enfamil)	Whey and casein	Lactose	Soy, coconut and safflower oil
Soy (Isomil, Prosobee)	Soy	Sucrose or corn syrup	Safflower, coconut, soy, palm olein, and sunflower oil
Whey hydrolysate (Good Start)	Whey hydrolysate	Lactose	Palm olein, soy, coconut, and safflower oil
Casein hydrolysate (Alimentum, Pregestimil, Nutramigen)	Casein hydrolysate	Sucrose or corn syrup	Variable—includes safflower, soy, MCT, oil
Elemental (Neocate)	Free amino acids	Corn syrup	Safflower, coconut, and soy oil

TABLE 1-2   Higher Calorie Formula

	CONCENTRATE			POWDER		
CALORIES/OZ	CONCENTRATE (OZ)	WATER (OZ)	TOTAL FORMULA (OZ)	POWDER (SCOOP)	WATER	TOTAL FORMULA (OZ)
20	1	1	2	1	2 oz	2
	13 (1 can)	13	26			
24	3	2	5	3	To the 5 oz line	5
	13 (1 can)	9	22			
27*	2	1	3	3	To the $4\frac{1}{2}$ oz line	$4\frac{1}{2}$
	13 (1 can)	6	19			

* Increasing caloric density above 24 kcal/oz may lead to intolerance because of the increased osmolality and renal solute load.

neural tissue. There is some evidence that infants fed formula with added DHA and AA have improved developmental outcomes compared to infants fed formula without the added long-chain fatty acids.

- Infant formulas are available in three preparations.
  1. *Ready to feed*: No additional water needed
  2. *Concentrate*: Mix 1 oz of formula with 1 oz of water
  3. *Powder*: Mix 1 scoop of formula with 2 oz of water
- Breast milk and all standard infant formulas contain 20 kcal/oz. Higher calorie formula (24 or 27 kcal/oz) can be made by adjusting the amount of water mixed with concentrate or powder (Table 1-2).
- Infant formulas may be prepared in advance and refrigerated. Bottles of formula may be warmed, but avoid warming in a microwave in order to prevent uneven heating. Formula should not remain at room temperature for more than 2 hours. Open containers of ready-to-feed or concentrated formula should be refrigerated and used within 48 hours. Refrigerated bottles of formula prepared from powder should be consumed within 24 hours. Opened cans of formula powder must be kept in cool, dry places (not refrigerators).
- Generic or store brand versions of cow's milk and soy formulas are also available and are suitable options for families that cannot or do not wish to spend as much money on formula. The quality of all commercially prepared infant formulas is regulated by the United States Food and Drug Administration; quality is not sacrificed because of lower price.

CHANGING FORMULAS

- Some infants may have IgE-mediated or non-immune-mediated reactions to the proteins in cow's milk formulas. Symptoms of IgE-mediated reactions have a rapid onset and include wheezing, hives, angioedema, and anaphylaxis. Non-immune-mediated

reactions are more common and have a more gradual onset. Non-immune-mediated symptoms include loose stools (which may or may not be bloody), vomiting, and failure to gain weight.

1. Most infants demonstrate some degree of spitting up. Health care providers should avoid switching formulas for emesis unless weight gain is affected.
2. Thirty to 40% of infants with cow's milk protein allergies will also have reactions to soy formulas. If a cow's milk protein allergy is suspected, then health care provider should recommend a switch to a casein or whey hydrolysate formula. If the infant cannot tolerate a hydrolysate formula, then a free amino acid formula is recommended.

- Other types of infant formula are available, but they may not be medically indicated.
  1. Primary lactose intolerance is exceedingly rare among infants, and secondary lactose intolerance usually occurs later in childhood. Lactose-free cow's milk formulas are also advertised to consumers as beneficial during bouts of diarrhea and the subsequent recovery; however, it is rarely necessary to switch to a lactose-free formula until the infant is severely dehydrated. The AAP's Committee on Nutrition has stated, "Most previously well infants with acute gastroenteritis can be managed after rehydration with continued use of human breast milk or standard dilution of cow milk-based formulas."
  2. Low iron formulas are given to some infants to prevent constipation. This is a myth, and the iron content of these formulas (0.7 mg Fe/5 oz of formula vs. 1.8 mg Fe/5 oz of regular formula) is insufficient for infants.
- Infants should not be switched to whole cow's milk before 1 year of age because of an increased likelihood of developing a cow's milk protein allergy as well as the chance of developing iron-deficiency anemia because of microscopic blood loss in stool.

SOLID FOOD

- Solid foods may be introduced at ~4 months of age. To succeed at eating off a spoon, an infant must be able to sit with support, have sufficient head and neck control, and demonstrate coordinated sucking and swallowing.
- Iron-fortified, single grain cereal (such as rice cereal) is a good first solid food because it is less likely to cause allergic reactions.
  1. Caregivers should avoid adding rice cereal directly to bottles of breast milk or formula as this may lead to excess weight gain. The addition of rice cereal to the bottle (1–2 tsp of rice cereal/oz of formula) is appropriate for infants with significant gastro-esophageal reflux.
  2. Start by mixing a small amount of cereal with breast milk or formula in a bowl to keep the consistency thin, and then offer the mixture to the infant with a baby spoon. When tolerated, gradually increase the thickness of the cereal.
- Several attempts may be needed before the infant can successfully eat off a spoon. Many infants will thrust their tongues out of their mouths and push solid foods out when first trying to eat off a spoon.
- When fortified cereals are tolerated, caregivers may introduce pureed or soft fruits or vegetables.
  1. Introduce new foods one at a time at least 5 days apart in order to more readily identify foods that cause an allergic reaction.
  2. The order in which new foods are introduced is not significant, but caregivers must pay close attention to make sure that the consistency of foods is appropriate. Infants without molars should not be offered foods that must be ground in the mouth before swallowing.
  3. Foods rich in vitamin C promote the absorption of iron.
  4. Egg whites are more allergenic than egg yolks and should not be introduced before 1 year of age; egg yolks may be introduced a few months earlier. If a child has a strong family history of atopy or food allergies, families should opt to further delay the introduction of eggs.
- Infants should not be forced to eat foods that they do not immediately like. Up to 20 exposures to a food may be necessary before an infant accepts a new food because of its taste or texture.
- Honey should not be used to sweeten infant foods because of the risk of botulism. Honey is not pasteurized, and only a few spores are needed to affect infants.
- Infants should be offered developmentally appropriate foods. Finger foods such as crackers or small pieces of soft food should be given when infants can pick up and hold food. Parents should avoid giving foods that are hard, smooth, or difficult to chew because of the risk of choking or aspiration.

RED FLAG

- Infants who have difficulty transitioning to foods with more complex textures may require referral to a speech therapist for a more thorough feeding evaluation.

FEEDING ROUTINES

- Young infants may require feedings every $1\frac{1}{2}$ to 2 hours. After birth, they should be allowed to feed on demand, but they should not be allowed to go more than 4 hours without feeding during the first month of life.
- The volume of breast milk or formula needed each day to ensure growth varies from infant to infant. Infants should be fed when they are hungry, and they should be fed until they are full.
  1. Hunger cues include rooting, crying, grimacing, and placing hands in the mouth.
  2. Satiety cues include closing the mouth, turning away from the breast or bottle, and falling asleep.
  3. Breastfeeding infants should nurse at least 10–20 minutes per breast per feed and demonstrate audible swallowing. Mothers should feel milk letdown but not painful engorgement.
  4. Other evidence that infants are consuming sufficient amounts include >5 wet diapers each day and adequate weight gain.
- Infants should be burped at least once after each feed, and some also need to be burped during feeds. Burping can be facilitated by gently rubbing or patting the infant's back while the infant is seated on the caregiver's lap or resting over the caregiver's shoulder or chest.
- It is not necessary to give young infants water or juice to quench their thirst. Breast milk or formula will provide necessary fluid. Infants' kidneys may not be able to adequately regulate sodium if excessive water is given. Many infants each year suffer hyponatremic seizures because of inappropriate formula dilution or water intake.
- Small amounts of prune or pear juice (1–2 oz/day) may be given to infants with constipation (i.e., small, hard, pebble-like stools, *not* soft, infrequent stools).
- Infants should never be put to bed while drinking bottles. The high sugar content of juice, formula, and milk promotes early dental caries, even in infants whose teeth have yet to break through the gum.

- Bottles should not be automatically offered to crying infants. Infants have a need for nonnutritive sucking and may be consoled by sucking on pacifiers, fingers, or other objects.
- When an infant begins to eat solid foods, he/she should be placed in a high chair during the family meal. This provides the infant with models to demonstrate utensil use and consumption of a variety of foods. Distractions such as television or videotapes should be minimized.
- Parents should be reminded that appropriate portion sizes for infants can vary widely. Many infants eat only a few teaspoons of solid foods per meal at first. It may be months before an infant finishes an entire jar of baby food. Other infants readily enjoy baby food and do not necessarily need to be limited to one jar per meal.
- Older infants should receive two to three snacks each day and should be allowed to drink out of a cup with assistance. When a child can hold a cup, he/she should be weaned from bottles.
- Most infants spit up during or after some feedings. For those infants whose weight gain velocity is suboptimal or who demonstrate signs of oral aversion (e.g., arching the back, turning away from the spoon or bottle), gastrointestinal reflux precautions should be implemented.
  1. Thicken breast milk or formula with rice cereal (1–2 tsp cereal/oz).
  2. Burp infants frequently during and after feeds.
  3. Keep the infant in a seated position for at least 30 minutes after feeding.
  4. Elevate the head of the infant's bed to a 30° angle.

TODDLERS AND YOUNG CHILDREN (1–5 YEARS)

GROWTH

- A child's growth velocity slows significantly around the first birthday.
- Children usually triple their birth weight by their first birthday and quadruple their birth weight by about 2 years of life. Children gain about $4\frac{1}{2}$ to $6\frac{1}{2}$ lb each year between ages 2 and 5.
- Children grow about $2\frac{1}{2}$ to $3\frac{1}{2}$ in. each year between ages 2 and 5.
- Small growth spurts are common.
- It is crucial to start calculating and plotting BMI at this time to look for early adiposity rebound.

RED FLAG

- Children whose BMI nadir occurs before the age of 3 are at higher risk of becoming overweight adults.

EATING PATTERNS

- A child's desire to become more independent during early toddlerhood frequently leads to struggles with parents at mealtime. Many children are more interested in playing and exploring their environment than with eating, which may lead to parental concern that their child's consumption is insufficient.
- Many parents complain that their children are "picky eaters." For most children, this is normal. Few toddlers eat well at all meals, yet most will consume an appropriate variety of foods over time.
- Young children frequently cycle through favorite foods, eating them almost exclusively before tiring of them. Parents should be counseled that most children will again accept these foods if reintroduced at a later time.
- Parents should offer three meals and two to three snacks each day, making sure to offer a variety of developmentally appropriate foods.
- At least 2 hours should pass between feedings. If children are allowed to "graze," or snack more frequently, they often are not hungry at meal time.

RED FLAGS

- Toddlers who are not eating foods with complex textures, such as meats or stews, should be referred to a speech therapist for an oromotor assessment. Some children with very specific food preferences may also exhibit other behaviors suggesting a pervasive developmental disorder; thus, a complete developmental screening is indicated.
- Children with pica are at high risk of iron-deficiency anemia and lead toxicity.
- Although young children typically prefer a more limited variety of foods than adults, health care providers must ensure that a child's food choice is not excessively limited.

FOOD SELECTION

- At 1 year of age, children may be given whole milk. Low fat (2%, 1%, or skim) milk should not be introduced until 2 years of age in order to optimize neuronal development.
- Daily milk intake should be limited to 16–24 oz/day to decrease the risk of iron-deficiency anemia.
- Intake of sugary drinks, including juice, should be limited. A small cup of juice (4–6 oz) at breakfast is sufficient. Drinking large quantities of juice, soda, or fruit punch places children at high risk for becoming overweight. Encourage children to drink water instead.

- Young children remain at high risk for choking and should only eat foods such as hot dogs, popcorn, nuts, and grapes while supervised closely.
- A multivitamin supplement may be given to ensure adequate intake of vitamins. Many parents incorrectly believe that vitamin supplements will increase appetite.

MEAL STRUCTURE

- Children should sit at the table in a high chair or a chair with a booster seat.
- Parents should eat at the table with their children to provide models for good eating behavior.
- Finger foods and child-sized utensils are ideal.
- Young children are often messy eaters. They enjoy touching and playing with their food. Some families may prefer to place a plastic drop cloth under their children's high chairs to expedite cleaning. Parents should be encouraged to wait until after dinner to bathe their children.
- Parents must avoid nagging their children to eat. If they engage in battles with their children over food, they will lose.
- Do not use desserts or sweets as a reward for eating other foods.
- Televisions and videotapes should be turned off to minimize distractions.

PHYSICAL ACTIVITY

- Parents should encourage their children to be physically active at a very early age to prevent overweight later in life.
- Games requiring active movement, such as tag, skipping, and kicking a ball, are appropriate.
- Television and video game time should be limited to less than 2 hours per day.

SCHOOL-AGED CHILDREN (5–10 YEARS)

GROWTH

- Children gain about 7 lb and grow about 2½ in. each year.
- Small, periodic growth spurts are common.

FOOD SELECTION

- Older children should have three meals and one to two snacks each day. Parents should discourage their children from skipping meals, particularly breakfast.

- Portion sizes should gradually be increased, and children should not be encouraged to eat all the food on their plates if they feel full.
- Involving children in the selection and preparation of meals helps to teach them about healthy choices, which is important since they are spending more time away from home.
- Like toddlers, school-aged children like fewer foods than adults and may require several exposures to new foods before accepting them.
- If possible, send a healthy lunch from home instead of choosing a school lunch.
- Parents should be aware of what snacks are provided at after-school activities. If necessary, send a healthier alternative from home.
- Parents should avoid designating "forbidden" foods. Even high-fat foods may be eaten in moderation. Placing excessive restrictions on foods makes them more tempting, and children will seek them out when away from home.
- Foods rich in iron and calcium are essential.
  1. Iron rich foods include red meat, salmon, legumes, and dried fruits.
  2. Dairy products are excellent sources of calcium. For children who do not like or cannot tolerate milk, many other foods, such as orange juice, are now fortified with calcium. Calcium chews or Tums are other alternatives.

PHYSICAL ACTIVITY

- Since physical education is no longer a daily requirement in many schools, children should be encouraged to find other ways of being active, such as organized sports or dance classes.
- Being involved in many activities does not necessarily ensure that a child is active. Parents should be aware of the amount of time their children spend sitting or standing idly during organized activities.
- Parents should incorporate physical activity for the entire family. This does not have to be time-consuming and can include the following small changes:
  1. Taking a daily evening walk.
  2. Always parking at the far end of parking lots to include a small amount of extra walking.
  3. Taking stairs rather than escalators or elevators, or riding the elevator part of the way and finishing on the stairs.
  4. Getting off the bus two or three stops early and walking the remainder of the way.
  5. Doing jumping jacks, sit-ups or jogging in place during commercials when watching television.
- "Screen time" in front of televisions, computers, and video games should be limited to no more than 2 hours

each day. Children should be encouraged to complete their homework and engage in some sort of physical activity before screen time is granted.

ADOLESCENTS (10 YEARS AND OLDER)

GROWTH

- Adolescence is marked in both boys and girls by a significant linear growth spurt and gain of about 50% of adult weight.
- Girls typically experience their linear growth spurt during early adolescence (11–14 years) and complete linear growth about 1–2 years after menarche.
- Boys undergo their linear growth spurt and gain in muscle mass during middle adolescence (15–17 years).

FOOD CHOICES

- Adolescents have increasing independence related to food choices and may eat the majority of their meals away from home; however, their parents should still be encouraged to provide healthy food choices at home.
- All adolescents should be encouraged to eat three meals and a snack each day. Skipping meals and severe caloric restriction frequently lead to binge overeating. Failure to eat breakfast can hinder school performance.
- Adolescents who select a vegan or vegetarian lifestyle may consume an inadequate variety of nutrients, particularly vitamin B$_{12}$, iron, and calcium.
- Health care providers should enquire about fad diets or nutritional supplements to ensure that nutrient intake is neither insufficient nor excessive.
- Menstruating adolescents are at risk of iron-deficiency anemia and should be encouraged to eat foods high in iron (e.g., red meat, shellfish, leafy greens, legumes, or iron-enriched pasta) or to take an iron supplement.
- Peak bone density is reached during the mid-twenties, so adolescents should be encouraged to take in adequate calcium. Good sources of calcium include milk, cheese, yogurt, and calcium-enriched orange juice and bread. If dietary calcium intake is insufficient, adolescents may take a daily calcium supplement.
- The intake of carbonated beverages by adolescent girls should be limited because increased consumption is associated with a higher risk of bone fractures.
- Excessive caffeine intake may cause palpitations, polyuria, and withdrawal headaches.

PHYSICAL ACTIVITY

- Many adolescents do not have daily physical education class. They should be encouraged to engage in at least 30 minutes of vigorous physical activity each day.

- "Screen time" in front of televisions, computers, and video games should be limited to no more than 2 hours each day.

BIBLIOGRAPHY

American Academy of Pediatrics, Committee on Nutrition. Prevention of pediatric overweight and obesity. *Pediatrics* 2003;112(2):424–430.
Conklin CA, Gilger MA, Jennings HC, et al. *The Baylor Pediatric Nutrition Handbook for Residents.* 2001.
Slusser W, Powers NG. Breastfeeding update 1: Immunology, nutrition, and advocacy. *Pediatr Rev* 1997;18(4):111–119.
Story M, Holt D, Clark EM, eds. *Bright Futures in Practice: Nutrition-Pocket Guide.* Arlington, VA: National Center for Education in Maternal and Child Health, 2002.

2 PEDIATRIC HISTORY AND PHYSICAL
Kimberley Dilley and Sandra Sanguino

GENERAL PRINCIPLES

- The pediatric history and physical examination is unique since the majority of information is not obtained directly from the patient.
- It is important to include the patient during the history, addressing conversation and questions even to very young children.
- As with any specialty, it is also important to ensure adequate communication with the patient and family in whatever language is most comfortable for them. This includes the use of trained interpreters. Use of family members to interpret should be avoided if at all possible. Also, the use of written communication for those who sign should be avoided as American Sign Language has a much different vocabulary and syntax from spoken English.
- The pediatric history is similar to the adult history in that you need to elicit the history of present illness, past medical history, and social history. There are, however, many unique aspects of the pediatric history such as birth history and developmental history.
- Performing the physical on a young patient can often be a challenge. It may be necessary to conduct portions of the physical examination on the parents' lap if the child is easily upset.

- If a young child is calm or easily distracted early in the encounter, it is usually prudent to elicit the current complaint, then to start with the cardiac and lung examination, finishing the complete history during the remainder of the examination or after the examination is complete.

HEALTH SUPERVISION RECOMMENDATIONS

- The American Academy of Pediatrics (AAP) has specific guidelines for assessments, anticipatory guidance, and screening evaluations to be performed during well child care at different ages. Please see the AAP policy statement on health supervision for full recommendations (Committee on Practice and Ambulatory Medicine, 2000) and the AAP visit-by-visit description of appropriate well child care published in the AAP Guidelines for Health Supervision III (copyright 1998).
- An integral portion of the health supervision visit is to provide anticipatory guidance, which refers to providing counseling about what can be expected before the next visit.
- Anticipatory guidance regarding issues including but not limited to sleep, introduction of new foods, behavior and discipline, illness management, and safety are an important part of pediatric care.
- Anticipatory guidance is typically provided as specific topics are covered during the history.
- Issues including developmental delays, psychosocial problems, and chronic disease management will generally require additional visits separate from general health supervision visits.

HISTORY OF PRESENT ILLNESS

- The HPI should be a chronologic story of the events leading to the visit seeking care.
- Number of days prior to visit or actual dates should be used because those reading the note later will not get a clear picture of the time course if only days of the week are used to express chronology.
- Any relevant past medical history should be included, but a comprehensive list of all prior medical conditions should be reserved for the past medical history.

PAST MEDICAL HISTORY

- Birth history is important, especially for children younger than 1 year of age. Details of pregnancy include any prenatal illnesses or treatments. Mother's group B beta *Streptococcus* status should always be included, if known. Details of delivery include mode of delivery, gestational age of the infant at delivery, any complications, and the neonatal course for the infant.
- Any hospitalizations or surgeries as well as any major or chronic illnesses in the child's history should be elicited.

FEEDING HISTORY

- At prenatal visits, breastfeeding should be encouraged.
- Infant feeding history includes breast or bottle, type of formula, duration and/or amounts of feedings, and any problems such as emesis or choking.
- Anticipatory guidance around feeding includes waiting to start solids until at least 4 months of age. New foods should be introduced one at a time with a few days of observation for any adverse reactions. Also important is the avoidance of foods with high allergenicity such as berries, eggs, and nuts.
- For toddlers, avoiding struggle over meals and avoiding foods with choking hazard (peanuts, whole grapes, and so on) are important.
- For older children, physicians should stress the importance of five fruits and vegetables per day as well as reasonable portion sizes.

SLEEP HISTORY

- Infants should always be placed on their back (or side) to sleep, never on their stomach. This practice has greatly reduced the incidence of sudden infant death syndrome.
- Important issues for infants include how long they sleep at night and how often they are awakening for feeds. Newborns will not generally sleep more than about 4 hours without waking to eat, but this length of time increases as they grow.
- Families who cosleep with their infants should be counseled on the risk of suffocation. They should also not use alcohol or other drugs that may impair their ability to wake easily to the infant's distress. Further, it may be difficult to transition an infant who has been cosleeping into their own bed after 3–4 months of age, so parents should also be counseled to start early if they intend to have their child cease cosleeping.
- As children grow, issues to be addressed include how to transition a cosleeping child to his/her own bed, dealing with nightmares or night terrors, and nighttime enuresis.

DEVELOPMENTAL HISTORY

- Assessment of a child's development includes both parental report of milestones met at home and physician observation of developmental progress on physical examination. Because early intervention is key to overcoming developmental delays, formal developmental testing should be performed early if there is any suspicion for abnormal progression of development.

- Domains of development to be assessed include gross motor development, fine motor control, cognitive functioning, social interaction, and speech development.

BEHAVIORAL HISTORY

- Discipline methods used by caretakers as well as parental perceptions of the child's behavior are important topics to cover.
- Toddlers should generally be distracted from dangerous or undesirable behaviors, with formal discipline measures being implemented as children grow older.
- Spanking should be avoided, as should trying to reason with a young child about why their behavior is wrong. Firm and consistent application of household rules should be encouraged.

MEDICATION HISTORY

- Always include any medications, including over-the-counter drugs or alternative remedies, which the patient has taken for this illness and on a regular basis.
- Medication history will also include any known allergies to medications and the type of reaction experienced.

IMMUNIZATION HISTORY

- Immunization status should be assessed for children of all ages.
- Documentation, such as a parent's shot records or vaccination records from the primary care provider, should be sought to verify compliance with the recommended immunization schedule.

SAFETY HISTORY

- Guidance regarding safety and prevention of injuries is a very important part of the pediatric encounter. Age-appropriate safety screening should be done at all well child care visits and as relevant at acute care visits.
- Major safety issues for infants include safe bedding and emphasizing supine positioning to prevent sudden infant death syndromes, proper use of car seats, home safety such as water temperature below 120°F and working smoke detectors, prevention of falls, safe toys, and supervision around older children and pets.

- For toddlers, safe storage of weapons, installation of safety devices such as drapery cord holders, avoidance of walkers, avoidance of scald and burn risks, safe foods to eat, and need for constant supervision should be emphasized.
- School age children should have stranger awareness reinforced, use protective gear for biking or skating, continue to use a booster seat until 8 years of age and 80 lb and always have supervision near water.
- For adolescents, issues such as vehicle safety including not to drink and drive also become important.
- For complete recommendations of injury prevention topics to address at specific ages, please see the AAP Guidelines for Health Supervision III (copyright 1998) and the AAP Injury Prevention Program (TIPP) (copyright 1994).

REVIEW OF SYSTEMS

- For young children, the review of systems primarily will be able to assess any outward signs of illness including fever, crying, changes in activity, changes in elimination patterns, and any other indications of pain or discomfort observed by the family.
- For older children, a complete review of systems should attempt to elicit any symptoms in any organ system from head to toe. Pertinent negatives should be included in the written history.
- In general, a focused review of systems with limited organ system involvement is indicative of organic disease while a broadly positive review of systems could indicate either a systemic illness or a psychosomatic condition.

FAMILY HISTORY

- A family history should generally concentrate on first degree relatives.
- Major illnesses in childhood should be sought as should any chronic disease states in adults such as diabetes, hypertension, or hypercholesterolemia. Also of interest would be any early deaths.
- Pertinent negatives should also be included in the written family history.
- A pedigree diagram showing the relationship of affected family members to the patient can be useful when an inherited condition is suspected.

SOCIAL HISTORY

- A good opening question for social history is, "Tell me who lives at home."

- Ages and occupations of parents, the involvement of extended family in care of the patient, and attendance at daycare or school are all important.
- Health habits of the family including smoking should be addressed, and the dangers of secondhand smoke exposure should be emphasized when relevant. Pediatricians can offer smoking cessation assistance to parents who desire to quit.
- Other relevant family health habits include diet and exercise patterns as the family will influence these learned behaviors as children grow.
- Exposure to pets and travel history should also be taken as relevant to the current illness, as should any exposure to others with similar symptoms.
- Adolescents over the age of 12 and perhaps even younger should always have some time alone with the physician. Parents and siblings should step out of the room, allowing time for the teen to discuss issues such as sexual activity and drug use confidentially with the doctor. Sensitive parts of the examination can be performed with the parent present or absent, depending on the adolescent's wishes.

PHYSICAL EXAMINATION

- An important aspect of the pediatric examination is the overall appearance of the child. A toddler who is smiling and playful is not likely to be critically ill. Conversely, if a normally happy and outgoing child is withdrawn and quiet, something could be quite wrong.
- Age-appropriate interpretation of vital signs will often require consultation of a table listing normal values by age. Infants tend to have higher heart rates and respiratory rates which approach adult normal values in preschool age children. Blood pressure values are lower in children and increase with age. Blood pressure measurements are compared to normals based on the child's height and also based on measurements taken in the upper extremities only.
- Growth parameters such as height and weight should always be plotted on growth curves, the latest of which are based on Centers for Disease Control and Prevention (CDC) national reference data released in 2000. Interpretation of some weight-for-height measure such as body mass index (BMI = weight in kg/height in m^2) should be performed routinely so that children can be identified as underweight or at risk for overweight in order to target nutrition and physical activity counseling. Age-appropriate BMI charts (for children ≥2 years of age) can be found on the reverse side of the current CDC growth charts.
- Infants less than 3 years of age should also have head circumference plotted regularly.

- In general, after the first year of life children should not cross more than one growth channel on the growth chart for any of the parameters. Some variation may occur over the first year as infants transition from prenatal growth parameters to their own potential, but dramatic changes should also raise a red flag for infants.
- Included in this chapter are a few key points to the pediatric examination by system, but more complete details of relevant findings can be found in chapters targeting the specific organ systems.

GENERAL APPEARANCE

- It is generally not wise to begin the examination of a young child from the top down as is often done for older children and adults. Many infants will become irate with the examination of the oropharynx and ears, so these should be reserved for the end.
- Overall appearance of the child as mentioned previously is one important aspect of the neurologic examination, particularly for young children.

HEAD AND NECK

- The fontanelle is open in most children under about 18 months of age and should be felt for either bulging indicating possibly elevated intracranial pressure or for a sunken aspect indicating possible dehydration.
- Ophthalmologic examination in young infants includes the presence or absence of a red reflex and the symmetry of the light reflex. Dilation is required for direct observation of the retina and optic nerve. In older children, cooperation may be attained in order to perform fundoscopic examination without pupillary dilation.
- Assessment for lymphadenopathy is routine in children, and parents should be reassured that small and mobile nodes are common. Any erythema, induration, or tenderness should be addressed.
- Inspection of the teeth should not be forgotten, and referral to a dentist for any observable caries is indicated.

CHEST

- As mentioned previously, it is generally prudent to perform this part of the examination first in young children.
- Examination findings of consolidation are often absent in children, so an index of suspicion for pneumonia must be maintained with fever and tachypnea alone.
- Cardiac examination should note any murmurs or extra heart sounds and should include changes with differing positions for cooperative patients.

ABDOMEN

- This is also difficult in upset children and should be performed early and with distraction when possible.
- Notation should be made of the quality of bowel sounds, any palpable masses, whether the liver and spleen are palpable, and any pain that is elicited. Voluntary or involuntary guarding are often elicited without the ability of a child to localize pain.

GENITOURINARY

- If any ambiguity in genitals is noted on newborn examination, the pediatrician should avoid calling the infant by either gender and should consult an endocrinologist for assistance with determination of genotype.
- For males, it is important to note whether the patient is circumcised and whether both testes are palpable.
- Sexual maturity rating (also known as Tanner staging) should be performed at all well child care visits in order to catch any potential disruptions in normal pubertal development.

EXTREMITIES

- Perfusion of extremities is generally commented on with mention of pulses and capillary refill time. Keep in mind that extremities may be poorly perfused in a well child in a cold room, so these findings should be interpreted in light of the overall examination.

SKIN

- Whenever possible, children should be completely undressed and examined in a hospital gown, primarily to allow for an adequate skin examination.
- In the face of neurologic or developmental abnormalities, skin should be examined with a Wood's lamp for neurocutaneous findings which may not be apparent in natural light.
- Rashes should be described by appearance as well as distribution, and history from the caregiver about progression of the rash can also be helpful.

NEUROLOGIC EXAMINATION

- Assessment of primitive reflexes in infants helps to assess development.

- Mental status, quality of speech, motor strength, deep tendon reflexes, and gait analysis can all be helpful in localizing any neurologic findings.

ASSESSMENT AND PLAN

- Any written note of a history and physical concludes with an assessment of the patient's diagnoses and the plans for dealing with those diagnoses.
- The assessment should briefly include supportive evidence including history, physical findings and diagnostic workup such as laboratory values, which are supportive of the diagnosis. Discussion of possible alternate diagnoses that are entertained is also appropriate.
- The plan should include mention of any treatments to be provided as well as plans for follow-up.

REFERENCE

Committee on Practice and Ambulatory Medicine. Recommendations for Preventive Pediatric Health Care (RE9939). *Pediatrics* 2000;105:645.

BIBLIOGRAPHY

Behrman RE, Kliegman RM, Jenson HB (eds.). *Nelson Textbook of Pediatrics*, 16th ed. Philadelphia, PA: W.B. Saunders, 2000, Chaps. 1–6, pp. 1–22.

Hoekelman RA (Ed in Chief). *Primary Pediatric Care*, 4th ed. St. Louis, MO: Mosby, 2001, Chaps. 7–13,16–23, pp. 57–152, 165–324.

McMillan JA (Ed in Chief). *Oski's Pediatrics: Principles and Practice*, 3rd ed. Philadelphia, PA: Lippincott Williams & Wilkins, 1999, Chaps. 7–10, pp. 39–61.

3 HEALTH SUPERVISION: NEWBORN (LESS THAN 1 MONTH)

Barbara Bayldon

- Optimally the first physician visit for an infant will follow a prenatal visit, but the first contact for the family with the pediatrician may be in the hospital after delivery or following discharge. In any case the goals of this visit should be to assess the patient, the patient's family environment, and support the family in adjusting to the addition of a new member by giving anticipatory guidance, explaining the practice's structure and rules. This is a chance to either continue or begin to foster a partnership between the doctor and family toward optimizing the health and development of the child. It is a good idea on entering the room, to introduce oneself, acknowledge all those in the room, and say congratulations prior to the initiation of any interviewing.

THE HISTORY

- The physician may have information from a prior visit, or in the hospital will have the chance to look through a chart for background information; but often during a first office visit one may be relying entirely on the parent for history.

EITHER REVIEW OR ELICIT
- Maternal obstetric history: Maternal age, part obstetric history including prior gestations, outcomes, current obstetrical history, i.e., maternal weight gain, prenatal care, illness/infection, medication, alcohol smoking and substance abuse, prenatal laboratories, and complications.
- Family medical history and risk factors.
- Intrapartum history: Type of delivery, complications such as failure to progress, decelerations, meconium, maternal fever, antibiotics given, Apgar score.
- Hospital and posthospital discharge course if the latter is applicable: It is always a good idea to let the parents know that there are several things you need to know but that you are interested in anything they have noticed or any concerns they have. Topics that need to be covered are
  1. *Hospital course*: (if applicable) any complications while in the hospital and whether the infant was discharged with the mother.
  2. *Behavior and development*: This is a good topic to start with since a concept of what is unique about a child frequently relates to this sphere. At this young age it is often important to highlight the significant although subtle developmental abilities. At this stage parents can note (a) different levels of alertness, (b) symmetric limb movement, (c) response to sound, (d) fixing on faces, (e) even smiling in sleep near age 1 month, (f) primitive reflexes, i.e., Moro, asymmetrical tonic neck reflex (ATNR), rooting reflex.
  3. *Feeding*: Breast vs. Formula: (a) If formula, what type, frequency, and number of ounces can be

elicited, (b) for breastfed infants, the frequency, time sucking at each breast, maternal breast fullness, let down, (c) any complications (too little milk, too much milk, ineffective latching, sore nipples, mastitis, and so forth).
  4. *Elimination*: (a) Urinary frequency and color and stream, (b) stool frequency, color, consistency, and straining are important.
  5. *Sleep*: Newborn infants spend the majority of their time sleeping (up to about 20 hours a day) and have irregular schedules. Major points: (a) total amount of sleep in 24 hours, (b) the sleep-wake cycle, (c) the location of sleep (preferably in a crib) and the importance of being put to sleep on their backs.
  6. *Family/social environment*: It is extremely important to assess the child's environment. This includes (a) people living in the house, (b) parental/caretaker characteristics, (c) maternal (and other) emotional state specifically screening for postpartum depression, (d) SES and work situations.
  7. *Ethnicity and cultural and religious beliefs*: i.e., Are there any cultural or religious beliefs you have that you feel I should know to help care for your child's health? Are there alternative therapies that your family uses?
  8. *Safety*: The major questions at this age are (a) car seats, (b) smoke/CO alarms, (c) sleep situation, as above.
  9. Family medical history.

THE PHYSICAL EXAMINATION

- Even in the hospital, as much as possible the examination should be done in the parent's presence so the doctor can point out physical findings to the parents and reassure them about normal variations which typically may cause concern. As one has been speaking to the parents, one should already have had an opportunity to assess the parent-child interaction, the general appearance of the infant and his/her level of activity. To perform the examination the infant should be completely undressed except for the diaper which will be removed at the appropriate point in the examination. Specific aspects of the examination are
  1. General appearance: General level of alertness, size, responses to stimuli.
  2. Gestational age assessment (at birth).
  3. Weight, length, and head circumference: These should be plotted on a growth chart.
  4. Skin: Mongolian spots, Nevus flammeus, mottling, acrocyanosis, jaundice, other nevi and

neonatal rashes such as erythema toxicum, pustular melanosis, neonatal acne should be noted.

5. Cardiac: Listen carefully for the heart tones and murmur.
6. Lungs/chest: Observe chest movement, respiration rate, and listen for altered breath sounds. Breast engorgement is frequent, normal, and may increase before it resolves.
7. HEENT: Anterior fontanelle, red reflex, conjunctival hemorrhage, fixed vs. intermittent disconjugate gaze, shape of pinna and setting of ears, palate and oral lesions.
8. Neck: Palpate clavicles, check for branchial cleft cyst.
9. Abdomen: Check for bowel sounds, liver and spleen size, abdominal masses; kidneys can often be palpated.
10. Spine: Check for anomalies including sacral dimples, hair tufts.
11. GU: Check for appearance of genitalia, ambiguous genitalia; for girls a mucous discharge with or without blood is a normal finding; for boys check penis and testes. Check patency of anus.
12. Musculoskeletal: Check for developmental dysplasia of the hip with the Ortolani and Barlow techniques.
13. Neuro: Check tone, symmetry of movements (lack of movement in an arm may indicate brachial plexus injury), reflexes such as Moro, ATNR, stepping reflex.

SCREENING

- A metabolic screen is done on each infant prior to hospital discharge. After discharge it is imperative that the doctor checks to make sure that the screening results were normal and do appropriate follow-up on any abnormal results.
- A neonatal hearing screen (most commonly used is otoacoustic emissions, OAE) is also mandated and the results of that should be verified.
- If the hospital test fails then a second should be performed; a second failed test necessitates referral to audiology for further testing.
- In some institutions, bilirubin levels are being done on all newborns to screen for hyperbilirubinemia.

VACCINES

- The hepatitis B vaccine may be given at birth and receipt prior to discharge from the hospital has been

associated with later improved compliance with vaccination schedules.

MEDICATIONS

- A vitamin preparation including vitamin D should be given to all infants consuming less than 16 oz of formula a day by 2 months of age. Fluoride should be provided for infants in areas where fluoride is not added to the water.

ANTICIPATORY GUIDANCE

- It is crucial not to make anticipatory guidance sound like a lecture. One can mention the positives already noted in the parent's care of the infant and one can ask questions regarding feasibility of different recommendations. In reality, much of anticipatory guidance will be done as one takes the history or performs the physical examination but points that should be covered if not already mentioned are the following:

1. *Feeding*: Advantages of breastfeeding if parent is wavering over the decision, support and discussion about breastfeeding techniques and complications, availability of support resources, pumping breasts and growth spurts resulting in increased breastfeeding. For formula discuss type, preparation including not microwaving, not overfeeding. Discuss not giving H_2O and solids at this time. Inform parents of risk of infant botulism after ingestion of honey or corn syrup at less than 12 months.
2. *Development*: A brief review of what can be expected in the next month or two, especially the emergence of social smiling, cooing, increased neck control, and tracking.
3. *Sleep*: Discuss changes in sleep patterns, guiding toward increased night sleeping, risks of co-sleeping, safety of cribs including slats no greater than $2^3/_8$ in. apart, and back to sleep positioning and changing direction of baby in crib so head is not always turned in one direction creating an asymmetry of the skull.
4. *Temperament*: Mention infants have specific temperaments and that they cannot be spoiled at this age.
5. *Safety*: This includes car seat safety, smoke/CO detectors, setting H_2O no higher than 120°F, no walkers in future, issue of parental smoking and secondhand smoke, supervision when patient is around siblings and pets, and not putting in direct sunlight.
6. *Care of the child*: This includes topics of cuddling, bathing (sponge bathing at least until the umbilical

cord falls off), care of the umbilical cord, and care of a circumcision or uncircumcised penis in a male.

7. *Family interactions and friends*: Discuss holding and cuddling infant, how to involve father or other adults, how to involve siblings, and how to create individual times for siblings. The doctor should try to get a feeling of what the childcare plans are in the next months, certainly by the time of the second visit.

REFERENCES

Behrman RE, Kliegman RM, Jensen HB (eds.). *Nelson Textbook of Pediatrics*, 16th ed. Philadelphia, PA, W.B. Saunders, 2000, pp. 30–32.

Committee on Psychosocial Aspects of Child and Family Health 1995–1996. *Guildelines for Health Supervision III*, 3rd ed. Elk Grove Village, IL, American Academy of Pediatrics, 2002, pp. 17–31.

4 HEALTH SUPERVISION: 1–6 MONTHS

Barbara Bayldon

• At the 2-, 4-, and 6-month visits the physician needs to continue to carefully screen for congenital and developmental issues, assess the infant and its environment, and further develop an understanding of the parents while cementing the cooperative relationship toward optimizing the patient's health. Before entering the room it is important to review the patient name, parent names, and any unique aspects of the patient's situation so that each health maintenance visit will be a continuation of the last and an appropriate follow-up of any prior concerns.

THE HISTORY

• An interval history should cover all the major topics relating to health maintenance, particularly emphasizing development, feeding, and issues which frequently give parents problems. While going from open-ended to more specific questions one needs to obtain objective facts rather than vague descriptions of situations which may indicate totally different meanings to the physician and the family (i.e., a lot, only when he needs it, and so on).

BEHAVIOR AND DEVELOPMENT

• One should screen for developmental progress in each domain (i.e., language, cognitive, fine motor, gross motor, and social).

1. At 2 months
   a. Cooing
   b. Responsive smiling
   c. Tracking people's movements by turning the head to the side
   d. Steady head control at least temporarily
   e. Holding a rattle momentarily
2. By 4 months
   a. The infant should be cooing reciprocally
   b. Laughing
   c. Tracking visually through 180°
   d. Have differential response to the mother
   e. No head lag when raised up from lying to sitting
   f. Be reaching and grasping and pulling objects
   g. When prone, raising head and chest off the surface by the hands and may be rolling over
3. By 6 months
   a. Babbling should begin
   b. Making sounds in play
   c. Initiates social interaction by sounds or smiling
   d. Has definite preference for parents/guardians or known caregiver
   e. Holds small bottle with two hands
   f. Transfers objects between hands
   g. Rolls over
   h. May sit or just tripod sit
   i. During this stage the infant is becoming responsive and gaining an ever greater interest in the environment. At each visit encourage the parent to notice specific aspects of the infant's temperament and characteristics or activities that they especially like about the baby.

FEEDING

• It is important to assess the quantity of breast milk/formula the infant is taking (for formula ounce and for breast milk length of feeding time, satiation), the schedule of feeds and any complications of feeds. If the patient is getting less than 16 oz of formula/day, is there supplementation with vitamin D or other vitamins? Assess knowledge of introduction of solids at 4–6 months.

ELIMINATION

• Urine: Frequency, stream, and color
• Stool: Frequency, change in consistency, straining

SLEEP

• By 2 months there should be nighttime sleep pattern and by 4 months most infants can sleep through the night without waking for feeds if managed properly.

There will still usually be between two and three naps a day. Inquire about putting to sleep routine, sleeping situation, and position for sleeping.

FAMILY/SOCIAL ENVIRONMENT

- Each visit is important to assess for changes in the home environment and the impact of the patient on the family.
  1. Maternal emotional state and support. Specifically screen for postpartum depression.
  2. How is the infant affecting the family life? How is any sibling reacting to the baby?
  3. Have they been able to obtain everything for the child?
  4. What are the mother's plans for work/daycare?
  5. What advice has the mother been getting?
  6. Assess for secondhand smoke.

SAFETY

- Major issues are
  1. Check that deficiencies from prior visits have been corrected
  2. Reiterate importance of car seats
  3. Ask about any injuries

THE PHYSICAL EXAMINATION

- A thorough physical examination is a must. It is best to listen to the heart and lungs first and then proceed sequentially from head to toe but leave the most invasive things for last, i.e., the otoscope and oral examination. Again, a major portion of the physical can be accomplished by observation during the interview part of the examination. Important areas include
  1. Head: The status of the fontanelle
  2. Eyes: The red reflex and assessment of conjugate gaze
  3. Cardiac: For each visit it is important to assess for heart tones and murmurs since they may develop at this time
  4. Abdomen: Assess for abdominal masses
  5. Hips: Assess for developmental dysplasia of the hip
  6. Assess for tone, head control, social response, and so on

IMMUNIZATIONS

- Depending on the maker of the vaccine, some of these may be combined together. A vaccine information sheet should be given for each vaccine at each visit and discussed with the parents.
  1. At 2 months
     DTaP #1
     PCV7 #1
     IPV #1
     Hib #1
     Hep B #1 or #2 if previously given
  2. At 4 months
     DTaP #2
     PCV7 #2
     IPV #2
     Hib #2
     Hep B #2 if not given previously
  3. At 6 months
     DTaP #3
     PCV7 #3
     IPV #3
     Hib #3 (unless first two were Pedvax Hib)
     Hep B #3 can be given

LABORATORIES

- Generally no labs are necessary during this time unless there is a specific reason to be concerned about anemia in which case a Hgb and, when appropriate, a hemoglobin electrophoresis can be done.

ANTICIPATORY GUIDANCE

- It is important to give advice and information in a supportive manner. Optimally this is a discussion rather than a lecture. Points to be covered are
  1. Nutrition
     a. Breast milk or formula will be the major nutritional source during this time period. It is important to give reminders of the addition of vitamin D if the baby continues/starts to take less than 16 oz of formula a day. Breastfeeding support without engendering guilt if mother decides against is beneficial. Issues include pumping if going back to work, breastfeeding in public. For both breast- and formula-fed infants, the gradual decreased frequency of feeds should be addressed and not propping bottles in infants' mouths.
     b. A breastfed baby should be having either iron fortified solids or iron supplementation by 6 months. Solid intake may begin between 4 and 6 months and the patient should be assessed for interest and tolerance of solids as well as any allergic reactions.
     c. Introduction of solid foods should be delayed until 4–6 months of age and, if started by 4 months, each new food should be added only every 4–5 days. The first solids should be iron-fortified cereals and then single vegetables and single fruit.
     d. Honey and corn syrup should be avoided in this 1st year.

2. Elimination
   a. Frequent urine changes continue.
   b. Bowel movements are variable and babies can have two or more a day or as infrequently as one every 2–3 days. Babies frequently continue to have some straining but bowel movements should be soft and not hurt.
3. Development
• At each visit incorporate what can be expected to emerge developmentally within the next 2 months or more. In general, infant schedules remain unpredictable at this point but there may be emerging schedule patterns although the pattern may change just as the parent is becoming accustomed to it.
   a. At 2-month visit: Emergence of increased responses to stimuli, particularly social ones, increased cooing, smiling and some laughing, increased head control and movement, reaching, grabbing at small objects and possibly turning over.
   b. At 4-month visit: Continued increased responsiveness and initiation of social interaction, emergence of babbling, increased laughing can all be expected. Differential reaction to the mother/father emerges but the infant will generally be content with all caregivers. Improved reaching, grabbing, holding, turning over from side to side are seen and by 6 months the infant may be able to sit and transfer an object between two hands.
4. Sleep
• Points to discuss are
   a. Changing sleep patterns; there should be more predictable naps.
   b. By 3–4 months if properly managed, babies are physiologically able to sleep through the night.
   c. Back to sleep positioning continues to be important and other safety issues of crib slat separation width and cosleeping may need to be reiterated.
5. Temperament
• It is important to remind parents that infants will have different temperaments, even at this young age.
6. Safety
• Points to discuss are
   a. Car seats/safest in middle back seat
   b. Issue of increasing need of supervision through first year because of first hand-to-mouth activity, turning over, and then ability to crawl and explore
   c. Danger of falls off high surfaces/not placing infants in carriers or car seats off the floor
   d. Danger of carrying hot liquids and infant at same time
   e. Walker use should be discouraged and regarded as developmental down time
   f. Safeguarding of the environment as the infant reaches 6 months, i.e., outlet plugs, removal of poisons, medicines from infant's reach, preferably locked but at least high up, unplugging of electrical appliances after use, a thorough search for small choking hazards on the floor
   g. Emphasize the importance of supervision when in the presence of other small children and pets who may harm infant
   h. Reduction of exposure to direct sunlight and use of sunscreen
   i. Smoke- and gun-free environment
   j. The importance of smoke and carbon monoxide detectors in the home
7. Family interactions and friends
   a. Discuss impact on family of infant and natural jealousy of older siblings
   b. Discuss possibilities for support from father and other adults
   c. Discuss guardian work and daycare plans when applicable
8. Illness detection and emergencies
   a. Review subtle signs and symptoms of illness
   b. Reiterate need for thermometer in the home
   c. Review the practice 24-hour access and make sure parents have the Poison Hotline Telephone number for the area
• At the end of each visit it is important to ask if parents have any other concerns or questions that have not been addressed. Always specify the time of the next appointment and the reason for it while reminding them you are available for problems that crop up before the next health supervision appointment.

REFERENCES

Behrman RE, Kliegman, RM, Jensen HB (eds.). *Nelson Textbook of Pediatrics*, 16th ed. Philadelphia, PA, W.B. Saunders, 2000, pp. 32–36.

Committee on Psychosocial Aspects of Child and Family Health 1995–1996. *Guildelines for Health Supervision III*, 3rd ed. Elk Grove Village, IL, American Academy of Pediatrics, 2002, pp. 25–55.

5 HEALTH SUPERVISION: 6–12 MONTHS

Gwendolyn Wright

• This is an exciting time in infancy. The baby begins to actively explore his/her environment. She/he learns that she/he can manipulate things and people.

Meanwhile, he/she is continuing to grow at a rapid rate and trying new foods.

THE 6-MONTH VISIT

DEVELOPMENTAL MILESTONES

- It is best to elicit a developmental history by asking some broad questions. Examples might include what new things has your baby learned to do? What does he/she understand? How does he/she tell you what he/she wants? How does she/he move?

SPEECH
- Responds to own name
- Understands names, bye-bye, no
- Babbles, imitates

GROSS MOTOR
- No head lag when pulled to sit
- Sits with support
- Rolls over
- Creeps, scoots
- Bears weight when placed

FINE MOTOR
- Transfers objects from hand to hand
- Rakes in small objects
- Interested in toys

SOCIAL
- Smiles, laughs, squeals
- May be outgoing or shy with strangers

NUTRITION

- At this point the baby should be trying a variety of soft foods, including iron-fortified cereal. Emphasize to the parent to give only soft foods and to avoid anything hard and round such as peanuts or popcorn. Some physicians feel that highly allergenic foods such as nuts, citrus, and strawberries should be avoided during this stage; however, this recommendation is not well-supported and should be reserved for markedly allergic families.
- The parents may introduce a cup for water or juice. Juice should be limited to a maximum of 4 oz a day.
- The process of trying new foods can be both fun and also frustrating. Remind parents that a baby may need to try a new food 10–20 times before he/she accepts it!
- Six to 12 months is a critical nutritional phase. The baby must be assessed for risk of iron, vitamin D, and fluoride deficiencies. If the baby is still relying mainly on breast milk, he/she should be given iron, vitamin D, and fluoride supplements. Formula-fed babies should be kept on formula until 12 months of age. If the parent insists on switching to whole cow's milk, consider a multivitamin with iron to prevent anemia. Encourage the parents to give the baby fluorinated tap water (if available in the community). Infants who receive only bottled or well water need fluoride supplementation at this age. Some "nursery water" is sold as fluorinated; however, this is not regulated or tested for content and should not be relied on. Continue to avoid honey until 12 months of age.

ORAL HEALTH

- Do not put the baby to bed with a bottle. Begin to clean the baby's teeth with a soft brush or cloth daily. A fluoride source is needed, as disscussed previously.

BEHAVIOR/SOCIAL ISSUES

SLEEP
- The infant should be sleeping through the night at this point. If the infant is still requiring attention and feedings throughout the night, the family may be exhausted. This and other sleep issues should be addressed. Encourage the baby to console herself/himself and fall asleep on her/his own by putting her/him to bed awake.

DISCIPLINE
- At this age, discipline should consist mainly of distracting the child from dangers or off-limit situations. Structure and routine is useful.

PARENT-CHILD RELATIONSHIP
- Encourage parents to talk to baby, play with infant (peek-a-boo, pat-a-cake, and so on).

LITERACY

- The parents should be encouraged to read to the baby. He/she will mouth the book and bang it—this is normal behavior!

SAFEGUARDING THE ENVIRONMENT

REMINDERS
- Use a rear-facing infant car seat, and place it in the back seat.
- Smoke and carbon monoxide detectors should be installed and checked regularly.
- Check hot water temperature.

- Never leave infant alone, especially in tub or on a high surface.
- Eliminate water hazards: buckets, pools, tubs.
- Keep a smoke-free environment.
- Avoid hot liquids or cooking while holding baby.
- Use sunscreen, hats, and avoid prolonged sun exposure.
- Do not use a baby walker.

NEW ISSUES
- Get down on the floor and check for hazards at the baby's level.
- Make sure small objects are out of the infant's reach.
- Lock up all poisonous substances, including cleaning agents, medications, paint, and so on. Place poison control number somewhere everyone can locate it easily.
- Never give the infant plastic bags or latex balloons.
- Install safety locks on cabinets.
- Install gates on stairs and guards on windows.

PHYSICAL EXAMINATION

- Measure and plot growth parameters.
- In addition to the basic physical exam, pay careful attention to the eyes. Check for a symmetrical red reflex, symmetric light reflex, and perform a cover/uncover test. Teeth may be erupting. Check for developmental dysplasia of the hip.

SCREENING

- Hemoglobin and lead, as appropriate.

IMMUNIZATIONS

- Hib #3 (can be skipped when using certain brands)
- DTP #3
- IPV #3
- HBV #3 (6–18 months)
- PCV7 #3

AT THE END OF THE VISIT

- Ask if the parents' questions and concerns have been answered. Complement the parent and infant on their strengths.

NINE-MONTH VISIT

- A 9-month-old infant will be developing new independence. She/he has strong opinions about food, wants to get down and explore, and may scream when her/his parents leave.
- This is an exciting but challenging time for parents as their cuddly baby begins to makes forays into toddlerhood.

DEVELOPMENTAL MILESTONES

LANGUAGE
- Responds to own name
- Understands no, bye, and so on
- Babbles, imitates, and may say mama/dada non-specifically

GROSS MOTOR
- Sits well
- May pull to stand
- Shakes, bangs, throws, and drops objects

FINE MOTOR
- Inferior pincer grasp
- Pokes with index finger
- Feeds self with fingers
- Tries to use cup

SOCIAL
- Possible stranger anxiety
- Likes games such as peek-a-boo

LITERACY
- Reaches for books
- Looks at pictures and pats them
- Prefers pictures of faces

NUTRITION

- The parents may start giving the infant soft table foods. Encourage finger foods and self-feeding. Continue to avoid choking hazards (as in 6-month visit). The provider should reassess the need for vitamins, iron or fluoride supplementation. Continue to avoid honey.
- It is important to establish structured, family meal times at this age.

ORAL HEALTH

- Continue to avoid bedtime bottles, clean teeth daily, and supplement with fluoride as in 6-month visit. This is a good time to initiate weaning from bottle to cup.

BEHAVIOR/SOCIAL ISSUES

SLEEP

- The infant should be sleeping through the night at this point. If the infant is still requiring attention and feedings throughout the night, the family may be exhausted. This and other sleep issues should be addressed. Encourage the baby to console herself/himself and fall asleep on her/his own by putting her/him in her/his bed when she/he is sleepy but awake.

DISCIPLINE

- At this age, discipline should consist mainly of distracting the child from dangers or off-limit situations. Structure and routine is useful.

PARENT-CHILD RELATIONSHIP

- Encourage parents to talk to baby, play with infant (peek-a-boo, pat-a-cake, and so on).

LITERACY

- Encourage the parent to read daily to their children.

SAFEGUARDING THE ENVIRONMENT

- Baby-proofing the home becomes ever more essential as the infant becomes more mobile!

REMINDERS

- Use a rear-facing infant car seat, and place it in the back seat.
- Smoke and carbon monoxide detectors should be installed and checked regularly.
- Check hot water temperature.
- Never leave infant alone, especially in tub or on a high surface.
- Eliminate water hazards: buckets, pools, tubs.
- Keep a smoke free environment.
- Avoid hot liquids or cooking while holding baby.
- Use sunscreen, hats, and avoid sun exposure.
- Do not use a baby walker.
- Get down on the floor and check for hazards at the baby's level.
- Make sure small objects are out of the infant's reach.
- Lock up all poisonous substances, including cleaning agents, medications, paint, and so on. Place poison control number somewhere everyone can locate it easily.
- Never give the infant plastic bags or latex balloons.
- Install safety locks on cabinets.
- Install gates on stairs and guards on windows.
- Avoid TV.

NEW ISSUES

- Lower the height of the crib mattress.
- Child should eat while seated and observed, never on her/his own and never while running around.
- Provide guidelines for when a new toddler car seat is required (1 year old and 20 lbs.).

PHYSICAL EXAMINATION

- Obtain and plot growth parameters.

SCREENING

- Hemoglobin and lead between 6 and 12 months
- Purified protein derivative of tuberculin (PPD) skin text, now or at 12 months

IMMUNIZATIONS

- Catch-up vaccines as necessary.

AT THE END OF THE VISIT

- Ask if the parent's questions and concerns have been answered. Complement the parent and infant on their strengths.

TWELVE-MONTH VISIT

- The 1-year-old is a handful. He/she may be walking or crawling everywhere. Her/his desire to explore the world will outstrip her/his coordination and she/he will be vulnerable to injuries of all sorts. The parents will be delighted as he/she learns his/her first words. The willful toddler demands things and throws temper tantrums. Sleep and eating issues are the norm.

DEVELOPMENTAL MILESTONES

GROSS MOTOR
- Pulls to stand, cruises, and may take some steps alone

FINE MOTOR
- Precise pincer grasp
- Points with index finger
- Bangs two blocks together
- Drinks from a cup

LANGUAGE

- Has vocabulary of one to three words in addition to "mama" and "dada"
- Imitates vocalizations

SOCIAL/COGNITIVE

- Waves "bye-bye"
- Plays social games (peek-a-boo)
- Looks for dropped or hidden object

NUTRITION

- The growth (and hence the appetite) of infants slows significantly around a year of age. Together with their new-found independence, this decrease in appetite can make meal times a battle. A feeding schedule that includes family meals is very helpful. Parents should avoid force-feeding their children, but may insist they sit through the meal. They should be presented with a healthy variety of foods. The child may prefer to self-feed.
- A 1-year-old should be eating a variety of baby and table foods. Care must be taken to include fruits, vegetables, and protein as toddlers tend to prefer carbohydrates. Most children are switching from formula or breast milk to cow's milk around this age. Parents should be specifically asked about the toddler's milk and juice consumption. Excess of both is common and can cause anemia, obesity, or paradoxically failure to thrive! Milk should be limited to 16–24 oz a day and juice should be limited to 4 ounces a day. Again, all sugar drinks should be avoided and "junk food" should be minimized.

ORAL HEALTH

- If possible, the toddler should see a dentist. Regular brushing and fluoride (usually via tap water) should be continued.

BEHAVIOR/SOCIAL ISSUES

DISCIPLINE

- Continue to use distraction as a major form of control. Parents may begin to use "no" and time-outs. The number of rules should be limited, but enforced consistently.
- Also see "Nutrition" for discussion of feeding issues.

SLEEP

- Maintain a bedtime ritual. Discourage night feedings and arousals using the parent/physician's preferred technique.

SAFEGUARDING THE ENVIRONMENT

REVIEW

- A new car seat may be in order. All the baby-proofing done during 6–12 months needs to be reassessed. The newly walking child may have access to things they couldn't reach before.
- Smoke and carbon monoxide detectors should be installed and checked regularly.
- Check hot water temperature.
- Never leave the toddler alone, especially in tub or on a high surface.
- Eliminate water hazards: buckets, pools, tubs.
- Keep a smoke-free environment.
- Use sunscreen, hats, and such.
- Make sure small objects are out of the toddler's reach.
- Lock up all poisonous substances, including cleaning agents, medications, paint, and so on. Place poison control number somewhere everyone can locate it easily.
- Never give the toddler plastic bags or latex balloons.
- Check safety locks on cabinets.
- Check gates on stairs and guards on windows.
- Avoid TV.

NEW

- Do not leave heavy objects on tablecloths that the toddler may pull down.
- Turn pan handles toward the back of the stove.
- Use gates to keep the toddler away from hot irons, stoves, curling irons, and space heaters.
- There should be no guns in the house at all. If there are, they need to be locked up and the ammunition should be locked up elsewhere.
- Never leave the child to play outside alone.
- Keep cigarettes, lighters, matches, and alcohol out of the child's sight and reach.
- Limit TV to less than an hour a day, or avoid altogether.

PHYSICAL EXAMINATION

- Obtain and plot weight, length, and head circumference.
- In addition to the usual physical exam, extra attention should be paid to the feet and lower extremities. Observe gait. Most parents are concerned about normal variants at this age, including flat feet, intoeing, and varus lower extremities.

SCREENING

- Complete blood count (CBC), lead level, and PPD if not done at 9 months.

IMMUNIZATIONS

- *Measles, mumps, and rubella* (MMR) #1
- VZV #1
- May be given Hib/HBV #3 if appropriate

AT THE END OF THE VISIT

- Ask if the parents' questions and concerns have been answered. Compliment the parent and infant on their strengths.

REFERENCES

Committee on Psychosocial Aspects of Child Family Health 1995–1996. *Guidelines for Health Supervision III*, 3rd ed. Elk Grove Village, IL, American Academy of Pediatrics, 2002.

Committee on Infectious Diseases. *Red Book: 2003 Report of the Committee on Infectious Diseases.* 26th ed. Elk Grove Village, IL, American Academy of Pediatrics, 2003, p. 26.

6 HEALTH SUPERVISION: 13–24 MONTHS

Lisa M. Sullivan

BEFORE THE VISIT

- Note vital signs, plot growth, check immunization status and labs due, note last visit goals, gather handouts for safety/development/nutrition, and select an age appropriate book (e.g., Reach Out and Read Program).

INTRODUCTION

- Take a seat for the interview. Allow the toddler to remain with the parent to acclimate to your presence. Offer the book to the child. Allow the child to roam the room.

INTERVIEW FOR THE PARENT

- How are you and your family? How has your toddler been since last visit? Any illness, ER visits, hospitalizations, or reactions to immunizations? Any questions/concerns? Any WIC or daycare forms needed?

- Review the goals from last visit. Were they met and were follow-up appointments made?

UPDATE THE HISTORY

NUTRITION
- Ask about appetite, milk type, and amount and bottle use or cup. How many cups of juice/soda/sugar drinks a day? How many meals and what types of food/food groups. Is there vitamin use or pica behavior?

ELIMINATION
- Ask about urinary frequency, problems with urination, BM frequency, and character. Is there an interest in toilet training?

SLEEP
- Ask about hours of sleep at night. Where does the toddler sleep and are the parents happy with this arrangement? Is it a crib or bed with safety rails? Is there a bedtime routine, difficulty falling asleep, bedtime resistance or night awakenings? How many naps? Is there a bottle in bed or pacifier use?

BEHAVIOR
- What makes you proud? What new thing does he/she do? How does he/she communicate affection, wants, and dislikes? Are there tantrums? How do you discipline?

DEVELOPMENT
- Observe and inquire about age-specific skills.
  1. *Fine motor*: (a) (15–18 months) pincer grasp, scribbles, stacks two blocks, feeds self with spoon. (b) (18–24 months) buttons, scoops, pours, brushes teeth with help.
  2. *Gross motor*: (a) (15–18 months) walks well, toddle run, climbs. (b) (18–24 months) jumps, kicks and throws ball, navigates stairs, dresses with help.
  3. *Cognitive*: (a) (15–18 months) pretend play (uses toy phone), explores environment, imitates adults. (b) (18–24 months) imitates peers, dramatic play (cooks a meal, cares for a doll), shows self-awareness, seeks "own" things, remembers stories/songs/hidden objects.
  4. *Receptive speech/communication*: (a) (15–18 months) will point to one to two body parts, follows simple commands, points to pictures when asked, listens to stories, repeats words on command. (b) (18–24 months) follows two-step instructions, repeats words heard in conversation.
  5. *Expressive speech/communication*: (a) (15–18 months) 5–15-word vocabulary with additional use of jargon (unintelligible words). (b) (18–24 months)

30–50-word vocabulary, two-word phrases, "conversation."
6. *Social*: (15–24 months) stranger distrust, gives and takes objects, plays games with parents, parallel play with peers, indicates wants/pleasure/displeasure, tests limits of authority and environment, asserts independence.

ENVIRONMENT

- Who cares for at home or at daycare? Is each locale a safe environment and "toddler proofed"? Is the poison control number available at each place? Ask about smokers, pets, water source, sick contacts, travel and car seat use. Does the smoke/carbon monoxide alarm work?
- Review and update past medical history, family history, social history, and review of systems as appropriate.

PHYSICAL EXAMINATION

- Wash your hands and stethoscope.
- Share growth percentiles with parent.
- Position toddler in the parent's lap or upright on the table with a book or toy.
- Perform less threatening exams first (e.g., chest, heart, eyes), saving ears, abdomen, and genitourinary systems for last. Speak softly throughout the exam, using familiar terms like "look at my ear flashlight" (otoscope) and "Popsicle stick" (tongue depressor). Demonstrate that the ear speculum is not sharp. Offer generous praise throughout. Allow toddler to touch and manipulate the stethoscope, noting dexterity and pretend play. Pay close attention to speech and interactions with parent. On exam, watch for bottle caries/malocclusion, strabismus, abdominal masses, hernias, hip dysplasia, gait disturbances (at least 10 strides), and evidence of abuse.

SCREENING

- Screen hearing if toddler has a speech delay or a history of frequent otitis.
- Review screening questions with parent for lead, tuberculosis (TB), and anemia. Test as appropriate.
- Avoid using the words "shot" and "blood" (spell them or use the words *immunization* and *test*).

IMMUNIZATIONS

- Provide vaccine information sheets to parents. Give measles, mumps, and rubella (MMR) and/or varicella if not already given. Give booster diphtheria, tetanus, and pertussis (DTaP #4) between 15 and 18 months.

Refer to American Academy of Pediatrics (AAP)-Red Book for delayed/interrupted immunization schedules.

ANTICIPATORY GUIDANCE

NUTRITION

- Recommend three to five meals a day supervised at the table as a family (approximately 20 minutes). Discuss a well-balanced diet. Give "fist"-sized portions and allow toddler to eat with his/her hands, while encouraging utensil use. It is okay if toddler is a "picky eater" and appetite changes on a daily basis. Toddlers will eat when hungry. Because of choking hazard, no nuts, hard candy, gum, popcorn, hot dogs, grapes or raisins. Discontinue the bottle and encourage a spill-proof cup. Give 16–20 oz whole milk + 4 oz juice a day, no more. No sodas or other sugar drinks, only water. Prescribe fluoride if using well water.

ELIMINATION

- Expect to toilet train at 18 months to 2½ years. Girls usually train early, boys late. Allow toddler to observe parents in the washroom. Once they show interest, parents may get a potty and allow the toddler to sit on it with diapers in place. Toddler is ready when they are dry after naps, complain of soiled diapers, or hide when defecating. Discourage punishment or negative reinforcement. Offer praise for success.

SLEEP

- Stress the importance of a regular bedtime routine. Read a bedtime story. Have child sleep in own toddler bed (close to the floor or with safety rails) and allow child to put self to sleep. Recommend 10–12 hours of sleep + 1–2 naps a day. Discourage bottles or pacifiers in bed.

BEHAVIOR AND DEVELOPMENT

- Encourage independence in eating and play. Offer choices regularly, especially if the toddler is refusing or saying no. Try to deliver more "yes" than "no" messages, praising good behavior. Introduce the family "rules" while setting firm and sensible limits. Enforce with "no," then redirect. If this fails, begin "time-out" (1 minute per year of age). If instead, a tantrum ensues, remove from harm and place in "time-out" without distraction (may need to gently but firmly restrain). Help the child label/name their feelings of frustration (angry, silly, sad). Be a model for good behavior. Be consistent with limits and discipline while providing a safe environment for play and exploration. Allow access to household items of different materials and textures for pretend play (e.g., plastic ware or pans). Encourage imitative behavior. Stimulate language by engaging in conversation. Listen to your toddler and answer questions. Read age-appropriate books (they enjoy the same ones over and over) and allow child to repeat the words. Have toddler point out familiar objects/animals in the story. Encourage them to make up their own stories. Sing songs and teach games of sharing.

INJURY PREVENTION
- Discuss appropriate size and installation of car safety seat. For weights 20–40 lb, use a convertible seat with an internal harness, positioned forward in the rear center seat. At 40 lb, may convert to a booster seat. Never leave a child unattended in the car. Continue to childproof house with stairwell gates, window guards, plastic guards for electric outlets, and cabinet locks. Arrange chairs to discourage climbing to dangerous heights or into forbidden cabinets. Put poison control number in an obvious location (e.g., on phone or fridge). Separate and secure gun and ammunition. Smoke outside and test smoke alarm monthly. No plastic bags/balloons for play. Supervise closely near water, pets, and younger siblings. Keep away from heat sources. Turn pot handles to the back of stove. Set hot water heater to 120°F. Use sunscreen.

CONCLUSION OF VISIT

- Offer handouts reinforcing safety, nutrition, and development goals. Complete and sign any necessary forms.
- Are there any other questions/concerns?
- Conclude with a reminder for the next well-child visit (e.g., 18 months, 24 months, or 3 years) or follow-up as indicated.

BIBLIOGRAPHY

Green M, Palfrey JS (eds.). *Bright Futures: Guidelines for Health Supervision of Infants, Children, and Adolescents* (2nd ed., rev.). Arlington, VA: National Center for Education in Maternal and Child Health, 2002.

Committee on Psychosocial Aspects of Child and Family Health 1995–1996. *Guidelines for Health Supervision III*, 3rd ed. Elk Grove Village, IL, American Academy of Pediatrics, 2002.

ZERO TO THREE: National Center for Infants, Toddlers and Families, 2002. Available at http://www.zerotothree.org.

Committee on Infectious Diseases. *Red Book: 2003 Report of the Committee on Infectious Diseases.* 26th ed. Elk Grove Village, IL, American Academy of Pediatrics, 2003, p. 26.

7 HEALTH SUPERVISION: 2–4 YEARS
Lisa M. Sullivan

BEFORE THE VISIT

- Note vital signs, plot growth, check immunization status and labs due, note last visit goals, gather handouts for safety/development/nutrition, and select an age-appropriate book (e.g., Reach Out and Read Program). Bring an extra pen for the child to use.

INTRODUCTION

- Take a seat for the interview. Introduce yourself to the child and ask simple questions including name, age, sex, favorite toy, and if they would like to sing the ABCs. Allow child to climb onto the examining table and ask him/her to draw (on the table paper) a circle, cross, person, and a scene of their choosing. Have them write their name if able. If unable, then demonstrate and have them copy. Have them point out and name parts of their drawing, prompting as necessary. During this introduction, pay attention to the child's expressive and receptive speech, social skills (eye contact, anxiety level, interactions with parent and examiner), gross motor skills (climbing), fine motor skills (drawing), attention span, ability to follow directions and quality of drawing (cognitive). Obtain the history from the parent while the child is drawing. When the child completes the task, offer praise and a book, further occupying the child and generating trust. Note the child's interest in books.

INTERVIEW FOR THE PARENT

- How are you and your family? How has your child been since last visit? Any illnesses, ER visits, hospitalizations, or reactions to immunizations? Any questions/concerns? Any WIC/daycare/preschool forms needed?
- Review the goals from last visit. Were they met and were follow-up appointments made?

UPDATE THE HISTORY

NUTRITION
- Ask about appetite, milk type, and amount and bottle use or cup. How many cups of juice/soda/sugar drinks

a day? How many meals and what types of food/food groups. Is there vitamin use or pica behavior?

ELIMINATION

- Ask about urinary frequency, problems with urination, BM frequency, and character. Is the child toilet trained?

SLEEP
- Ask about hours of sleep at night. Where does the child sleep and are the parents happy with this arrangement? Is it a bed with safety rails? Is there a bedtime routine, difficulty falling asleep, bedtime resistance or night awakenings? How many naps? Is there a bottle in bed or pacifier use?

BEHAVIOR
- What makes you proud? What new thing does he/she do? How does he/she communicate with parents, siblings, peers, and adults? Are there fewer tantrums? How do you discipline?

DEVELOPMENT
- Observe and inquire about age-specific skills.
  1. *Fine motor*: (a) (3 years) Copies circle and cross, proper pen grasp, draws three-part person, uses utensils, brushes teeth. (b) (4 years) Draws circle and cross, draws six-part person and possibly name, uses utensils well, cuts with scissors, dresses self, buttons, zips.
  2. *Gross motor*: (a) (3 years) Runs well, climbs onto exam table with help, jumps, kicks, navigates stairs well, learning tricycle. (b) (4 years) Climbs onto table by self, hops on each foot, pedals tricycle.
  3. *Cognitive*: (a) (3 years) Inquisitive about everything (mostly why and what), pretend play (emulates adults), knows name and sex, names six or more body parts. (b) (4 years) Asks more questions (how, where, and when), magical thinking, language exceeds understanding of the world, knows colors, learning rules, may sing ABCs.
  4. *Receptive speech/communication*: (3–4 years) Listens attentively to stories, repeats simple phrases, rhymes and songs, and follows directions.
  5. *Expressive speech/communication*: (a) (3 years) Seventy-five percent understandable, short sentences, learning plurals and articles. (b) (4 years) Hundred percent understandable and fluent, longer sentences, adjusts speech to level of listener's understanding.
  6. *Social*: (a) (3 years) Interactive play, learning manners, asserts independence, learning to share. (b) (4 years) Interactive complex play, toilet trained, shares, less tantrums, waits turn, learning board games, helps with chores.

ENVIRONMENT
- Who cares for the child at home, daycare, or preschool? Is each locale a safe environment and "childproof"? Is the poison control number available at each place? Ask about smokers, pets, water source, sick contacts, travel and car seat use. Do the smoke and carbon monoxide alarms work?
- Review and update past medical history, family history, social history and review of systems as appropriate.

PHYSICAL EXAM

- Wash your hands and stethoscope.
- Share growth percentiles with parent.
- Position the child upright on the table.
- Perform less threatening exams first (e.g., chest, heart, eyes), saving ears, abdomen, and genitourinary systems for last. Speak softly throughout the exam, using familiar terms like "look at my ear flashlight" (otoscope) and "Popsicle stick" (tongue depressor). Demonstrate that the ear speculum is not sharp. Offer generous praise throughout. Allow preschooler to manipulate the instruments, noting dexterity and pretend play. End the exam with "exercises" including jumping, hopping, running and skipping down the hallway. On exam, watch for dental caries/malocclusion, strabismus, abdominal masses, hernias, hip dysplasia, gait disturbances (at least 10 strides of each), and evidence of abuse.

SCREENING

- Screen hearing if child has a speech delay or a history of frequent otitis.
- Review screening questions with parent for lead, tuberculosis (TB), and anemia. Test as appropriate.
- Avoid using the words "shot and blood" (spell them or use the words *immunization* and *test*).

IMMUNIZATIONS

- Provide vaccine information sheets to parents. Give booster diphtheria, tetanus, and pertussis (DTaP #5), injectable polio vaccine (IPV #4), and measles, mumps, and rubella (MMR #2) at or after fourth birthday. Refer to American Academy of Pediatrics (AAP)-Red Book for delayed/interrupted immunization schedules.

ANTICIPATORY GUIDANCE

NUTRITION
- Allow child to help plan and prepare the meal, providing choices. Recommend 3 meals a day supervised at

the table as a family (approximately 20 minutes) + 2 snacks. Discuss a well-balanced diet. Give "fist"-sized portions and encourage utensil use. It is okay if child is a "picky eater" and is growing well. Preschoolers will eat when hungry. If child completely avoids one food group (e.g., vegetables) may recommend half a chewable multivitamin a day. Discontinue the bottle and encourage a regular cup. Give 16–20 oz of 0–2% milk + 4 oz juice a day, no more. No sodas or other sugar drinks, only water. Prescribe fluoride if using well water.

ELIMINATION

- Eighty to ninety percent are toilet trained in the day, 60–75% at night. Reassure parent that nighttime wetting is common at this age. Suggest nighttime protection with a diaper or "pull-up." Discourage punishment or negative reinforcement. Offer praise for success.

SLEEP

- Stress the importance of a regular bedtime routine. Read a bedtime story. Have child sleep in own bed (close to the floor or with safety rails) and allow child to put self to sleep. Recommend 10–12 hours of sleep + 1 nap a day. Discourage bottles or pacifiers in bed.

BEHAVIOR AND DEVELOPMENT

- Encourage independence in eating and play. Offer choices regularly and allow child to help with planning and decision making. Try to deliver more "yes" than "no" messages, praising good behavior. Introduce, model, and reinforce social and family "rules" while setting firm and sensible limits. Enforce with "no," and state what the appropriate behavior should be. If behavior persists, punish with an immediate logical consequence (e.g., throws food—must clean up mess and apologize). If this fails, begin "time-out" (1 minute per year of age). If tantrum ensues, remove from situation and place in "time-out" without distraction (may need to gently but firmly restrain). Help the child label/name their feelings of frustration (angry, silly, sad). Be a model for good behavior. Be consistent with limits and discipline while providing a safe environment for play and exploration. Stimulate the imagination with interactive and pretend play. Provide toys and games that require both manual dexterity and simple strategy. Allow access to household items of different types for pretend play (e.g., adult clothing and shoes, broom, plastic ware, pans, tea set). Discourage passive activities (i.e., television). Schedule time alone with child every day. Offer generous praise and affection. Stimulate language by engaging in conversation. Listen to your child and answer questions (including those about gender/sex/birth) simply and accurately. Reassure that masturbation is okay if not disruptive and in private. Read age-appropriate books (they enjoy the same ones over and over) and allow child to repeat the words or make up stories of their own. Sing songs together. Encourage playgroup or preschool experiences. Exercise as a family.

INJURY PREVENTION

- Discuss appropriate size and installation of car safety seat. For weights 20–40 lb, use a convertible seat with an internal harness, positioned forward in the rear center seat. May convert to a booster seat at 40–80 lb. Never leave a child unattended in the car. Continue to childproof house with stairwell gates, window guards, plastic guards for electric outlets, and cabinet locks. Arrange chairs to discourage climbing to dangerous heights or into forbidden cabinets. Keep away from heat sources. Turn pot handles to the back of stove. Set hot water heater to 120°F. Put poison control number in an obvious location (e.g., on phone or fridge). Separate and secure gun and ammunition. Smoke outside and test smoke alarm monthly. Develop a fire escape plan and practice it as a family. No plastic bags/balloons for play. Supervise closely near water and neighborhood animals. Use sunscreen. Wear bicycle helmet. Teach street safety while supervising closely, realizing that preschoolers often forget. Teach that "strangers" are not necessarily "strange." Children should not follow or talk to people they do not know. Instruct children to report inappropriate touching. Teach preschoolers to dial 911 in an emergency.

CONCLUSION OF VISIT

- Offer handouts reinforcing safety, nutrition, and development goals. Complete and sign any necessary forms.
- Are there any other questions/concerns?
- Conclude with a reminder for the next well-child visit (e.g., 4, 5 years) or follow-up as indicated.

BIBLIOGRAPHY

Green M, Palfrey JS (eds.). *Bright Futures: Guidelines for Health Supervision of Infants, Children, and Adolescents* (2nd ed., rev.). Arlington, VA: National Center for Education in Maternal and Child Health, 2002.

Committee on Psychosocial Aspects of Child and Family Health 1995–1996. *Guidelines for Health Supervision III*, 3rd ed. Elk Grove Village, IL, American Academy of Pediatrics, 2002.

Guidelines to Health Supervision III. Elk Grove Village, IL: American Academy of Pediatrics, 1997.

Committee on Infectious Diseases. *Red Book: 2003 Report of the Committee on Infectious Diseases*. 26th ed. Elk Grove Village, IL, American Academy of Pediatrics, 2003, p. 26.

ZERO TO THREE: National Center for Infants, Toddlers and Families, 2002. Available at: http://www.zerotothree.org.

8 HEALTH SUPERVISION: 4 YEARS

Mariana Glusman and Susan Berger

GROWTH AND DEVELOPMENT

- Children's rate of physical growth continues to be steady (approximately 6–8 cm/year and 2 kg/year). In contrast, their developmental maturation continues at an exponential pace.

MOTOR
- Four-year-olds can run fast, go up stairs alternating feet, climb on the jungle gym, and ride a bike with training wheels. They can hold a crayon correctly, draw a person with two to five parts, copy a cross, use scissors, and may be able to write their own name. Handedness is established.

LANGUAGE
- Children this age should be able to say hundreds to thousands of words (more words than can be counted). Their speech should be 100% clear to a stranger, although they may still have some problems with certain sounds (e.g., *r, l, th*). Transient stuttering is normal as long as it is not severe enough that it causes the child frustration (facial grimacing, refusal to speak). Speech dysfluency usually resolves by age 5.

COGNITIVE
- They tend to have magical thinking (*the car is sad*). They should know four colors, ask "w" questions, and be able to identify the function and composition of objects (*What is a spoon for? What is a house made of?*). If taught, they know their phone number and name. If exposed to books, they realize that writing on a page has meaning. They also may be able to recognize their own written name.

PERSONAL
- Can use a fork and spoon, and dress and undress themselves (if no time constraints). Most children are toilet trained during the day by this age.

SOCIAL/EMOTIONAL
- At 4 years children start to play in small groups, learning to play games with simple rules and to take turns. They can identify and be sensitive to other people's feelings, but are still largely egocentric. Their gender identity is well-established. They tend to play gender-stereotyped games. Sexual exploration is common. Pretend play is the most common type of play.

MORAL/ETHICAL
- They are beginning to differentiate truth from fantasy but may bend or not tell the whole truth to avoid punishment. They understand rules but bend them to their benefit.

BEHAVIOR

- As they learn about themselves and others, 4-year-olds try to push the limits of their own abilities and other people's patience. Many children start going to preschool at this age (if not younger) and so may have issues of separation anxiety and learning to interact with groups of other children.

NUTRITION

- Parents often express concerns that their 4-year-olds don't eat enough, or are picky. This is normal and appropriate given their slower growth rate at this age.

SLEEP

- Children this age should sleep 10–12 hours per night. Nightmares are common.

PHYSICAL EXAM

- In previously healthy children, the PE will usually yield little new information. The exam should focus on growth (weight, height, weight/height, body mass index [BMI]), caries and dental problems.

SAFETY

- Children should always be supervised, especially around pools or near the street. They should be taught basic safety rules (pedestrian, playground, water, and bicycle safety). Poisons/medicines/matches should be kept out of reach. They should always use a booster seat if under 60 lb or 59 in. They must be taught safety rules regarding strangers, and "good-touch/bad-touch." They need to know about "private parts," including the correct terms for genitalia. Guns and ammunition should be locked away in separate cabinets. At all visits, parents should be reminded about smoke and carbon monoxide detectors (and batteries).

DISCIPLINE

- Expectations need to be clearly stated, and consistently enforced. Punishment should be fair and logical, e.g., "you can't play in the sandbox if you throw sand." For the most part, children this age respond well to positive attention and individual time with their parents.

HEALTHY HABITS

- Promotion of healthy habits should include using sunscreen, brushing teeth twice a day, seeing a dentist every 6 months, encouraging physical activity, eating healthy meals, avoiding "junk food," and living in a smoke-free environment.

PRESCHOOL

- At this age children go to school to learn to socialize, interact with other children, and begin to separate from their parents. In school, children begin to learn conflict resolution, turn taking, and making friends. They also are exposed to an enriched environment and caring adults beyond their immediate family. Children who do not attend preschool are often inadequately prepared for the kindergarten tasks of separation and socialization.
- Parents also should be encouraged to read interactively with their children at home. This promotes development of language and emergent literacy skills, and provides a link between books/reading and fun. This link can be an important motivating factor as they learn how to read on their own.

ACTIVITIES

- At this age children do not need extensive organized activities, but they do need to play and stay active. TV/video games should be limited to a maximum of 2 hours per day. Parents must also monitor the program content to limit children's exposure to violence.

IMMUNIZATIONS

- After they turn four, children can receive their second measles, mumps, and rubella (MMR), fifth DTaP, and fourth injectable polio vaccine (IPV). Catch-up immunizations may be required for some.

OTHER SCREENING

- Screening should include checking blood pressure and vision/hearing. Lipid profiles and purified protein derivative of tuberculin (PPD) should be done based on risk factors.

REFERENCES

Committee on Infectious Diseases. *Red Book: 2003 Report of the Committee on Infectious Diseases.* 26th ed. Elk Grove Village, IL, 2003.

Dixon SD., Stein MT. *Encounters with Children—Pediatric Behaviour and Development.* Chicago: Year Book Medical Publishers, 1987.

Green, M. *Bright futures: Guidelines for health supervision of infants, children and adolescents—Pocket guide: 2001 update.* Arlington, VA: National Center for Education in Maternal and Child Health, 2001.

Schor EL. Guiding the family of the school-age child. *Contemp Pediatr.* 1998;75–94.

9 HEALTH SUPERVISION: 5–8 YEARS

Mariana Glusman and Susan Berger

- Middle childhood is a time of increasing independence and self-control. Although children this age still require parental supervision and encouragement, as they get older they can take on more responsibility and can make more choices on their own (e.g., clothes, TV shows, snacks). School becomes a very important part of their life, bringing out issues of separation, mastery, and social skills. Children this age have the cognitive and language abilities to understand and respond appropriately to direct questions and should be encouraged to be active participants in the health supervision visit (this can include demonstrating reading ability and making a drawing of themselves with their family).

GROWTH AND DEVELOPMENT

- The changes that take place between kindergarten and third grade are at once gradual and spectacular.
- Children's rate of physical growth slows down (approximately 6 cm/year and 3 kg/year). Their development, however, continues at a rapid pace.

MOTOR
- Strength, speed, and coordination rapidly improve. By 5 years they may start to ride a bicycle, skip, and climb on the monkey bars. By 7 or 8 some begin to participate in dance and sports. *Fine motor* coordination also improves. Tasks that they learn range from drawing a square and tying shoe laces to writing and becoming involved in art or in playing a musical instrument.

LANGUAGE
- By 5 years of age children's speech should be 100% clear and fluent. They can tell coherent stories from start to finish. They follow three-part commands, use at least five-word sentences, use the future tense, and count 10 or more objects. Sentence structure, vocabulary, and language complexity will continue to progressively increase with age. Studies show that language delay is the single best predictor of later learning problems. Therefore it is crucial to identify and address language delays as early as possible.

COGNITIVE
- In this period children go from magical and egocentric thinking (e.g., *the moon is following me*) to more concrete thinking. They are progressively able to think about more than one variable at a time (e.g., length and width of an object) and so can begin to understand concepts such as conservation of length, mass, and volume. Their drawings become more complex (able to draw a person with 8 parts at 5, 12 at 6, and 16 at 7). In school, learning to read, write, and do basic arithmetic are the major cognitive milestones achieved during this period. In kindergarten, children start with grouping and recognizing symbols. By first and second grades children can read simple sentences and do math operations (e.g., addition, subtraction). Children who are unable to grasp these basic skills by the end of second grade will have a much greater risk of school failure as they get into the higher grades.

PERSONAL
- At this stage children are able to take care of their basic personal needs (bathing, brushing teeth, dressing) though they may still require adult supervision.

SOCIAL/EMOTIONAL
- At 5 and 6 years, many children, especially those who did not attend preschool, can have issues with separation from their parents, which can make the transition into school more difficult. As they get older, children become progressively more independent and begin to look more outside the family. Peers become more influential, friendships more important. Gender identity is well-established and boys and girls usually play in separate groups. School plays a crucial role in social development. Children need to learn how to fit in, make friends, control their impulses, deal with teasing and peer pressure, interact with teachers and other adults, sit still, and pay sustained attention (25 minutes to 1 hour in first grade). Children's ability to master these tasks can have a huge and lasting impact on their self-esteem.

MORAL/ETHICAL
- At this age children understand the difference between right and wrong, fair and unfair (the latter being quite devastating!); however, they tend to have rigid beliefs about rules (they have difficulty with gray areas—e.g., when is it okay to *tell on* someone?) When they follow rules they take them to heart. Thus, this is an excellent time to teach and enforce family and safety rules.

BEHAVIOR

- Because of their improved understanding of rules, and their general desire to please the adults in their life, children this age tend to be "good citizens"; however, this can be a difficult time for children as they are faced with increased expectations: to succeed in school academically and socially, to fulfill responsibilities at home (chores, homework, other activities, interacting with siblings), and to take care of their personal needs. Failure to successfully handle these increased expectations can sometimes lead to a sense of inferiority, with long-term consequences.
- Learning delays often emerge as the complexity of the required tasks increases (usually first and second grades), and often manifest themselves as behavior

problems. Conversely, with increasing demands, behavior problems such as attention deficit and impulsivity, which may have been noted before, become more acute and distressing for children and their families.

NUTRITION

- Children this age typically don't eat very much, because they are not growing as fast as before; however, given the increased sedentary lifestyle of many children and the intense marketing of "junk food" to this age group, it is not surprising that 13% of school age children are overweight (weight for age >95%). Therefore nutritional counseling is very important (e.g., serve three meals and two healthy snacks per day, limit *junk food*, limit portion size to the size of the child's fist, model and encourage eating a healthy and balanced diet).

SLEEP

- Children this age should sleep 10–12 hours per night.

ILLNESS

- Recurrent idiopathic pain (e.g., headaches, abdominal pain, limb pain), and habit problems (e.g., nail biting, hair pulling, thumb-sucking) are common in school, aged children and are often associated with stress. Identifying and addressing the sources of stress is often more helpful than embarking on an extensive medical workup.

PAST MEDICAL HISTORY

- It is important to review the PMH because many factors, such as recurrent or chronic otitis media, multiple hospitalizations, in utero exposure to drugs, lead poisoning, and prematurity, may have an impact on school performance.

PHYSICAL EXAM

- The PE will usually provide little new information in children with previously normal physicals. The exam should focus on growth (weight, height, weight/height, BMI), caries and dental problems, and signs of abuse/neglect. As children get older the exam should also include screening for scoliosis and looking for signs of early puberty in girls.

SAFETY

- Forty percent of deaths in this age group are the result of unintentional injury. Children should be closely monitored especially around pools or near the street. Guns should be locked separately from ammunition, and poisons/medicines/matches should be kept out of reach. They should always use seat belts (booster if under 60 lb or 59 in.) in the car/school bus, and helmets/protective gear when riding their bike/scooter/rollerblades. Because they will be exposed to more adults outside the home, they must be taught about "private parts," "good-touch/bad-touch," and "telling mom/dad if anyone makes them feel uncomfortable."

DISCIPLINE

- Expectations and responsibilities (e.g., chores, homework) should be clear, and consistently enforced. Punishment should be fair and logical, e.g., "you can't go out to play because you didn't pick up your toys." For the most part, children this age are eager to please, so it is important to attend to this positive behavior and spend individual time with them. Because their concept of rules is concrete (they should apply equally to everybody), parents also have to model good behavior (e.g., teaching how to resolve conflict without violence) if they expect their child to do so as well. Finally, because peer groups become increasingly more influential in children's choices and behaviors, parents need to know their child's friends and their families.

HEALTHY HABITS

- Promotion of healthy habits should include using sunscreen, brushing teeth twice a day, seeing a dentist every 6 months, encouraging physical activity, having a smoke-free environment, and beginning to discuss avoiding alcohol/tobacco/drugs.

SCHOOL

- Parental involvement is very important for children's success in school. Even before their child starts kindergarten, parents should be encouraged to read to their children. When parents read to their children starting at an early age, they develop improved language and literacy skills. When these children get to school they are more prepared, they love books, want to learn, and are eager to learn to read on their own. Children who are not prepared face the task of learning without context or background. They lack the enthusiasm and even the understanding of why they are learning, so learning to read becomes a boring memorization task. By the end of second grade, children are expected to be able to discuss and write about the meaning of what they read, so those that get stuck, that take so much time figuring out each word that they can't get at the meaning, fall farther and farther behind. For those children who have difficulties learning how to read, intervention (e.g., tutoring, pullout classes) needs to take place as soon as possible, preferably before third grade. Even for children who are not having difficulties, parents should be encouraged to continue reading at home, to meet regularly with the teacher, and be involved in school as much as possible. Parents should have high (though achievable) expectations for their children's academic performance and help them achieve these goals.

AFTER-SCHOOL ACTIVITIES

• Many children start extracurricular activities at this age (team sports, art, music, and so on). Parents need to keep a healthy perspective on these activities, not getting caught up in competition, pressuring kids early on, or overscheduling them so they have no time for independent play, family, or rest. On the other hand, a great number of children spend large amounts of time sitting in front of the TV or playing video games. It is recommended that TV/video games be limited to a maximum of 2 hours per day, and that parents monitor the content of what their children see and play to limit their exposure to violence.

IMMUNIZATIONS

• By this age children should have two measles, mumps, and rubella (MMRs), five DTaPs, four injectable polio vaccine (IPVs), Varivax, four PCV7, and three Hep Bs.

OTHER SCREENING

• Screening should include checking blood pressure and vision/hearing, as well as assessing risk for

hyperlipidemia and tuberculosis (lipid profiles and purified protein derivative of tuberculin [PPD] should be done based on risk factors).

10 HEALTH SUPERVISION: PRE-ADOLESCENCE AND ADOLESCENCE
Robert Garofalo

INTRODUCTION

• Representing the stage of human development between childhood and adulthood, adolescence is a time of tremendous physical, cognitive, social, psychologic, and sexual change. From a traditional medical perspective, adolescence is considered one of the healthiest periods of life, but it also is generally amongst the most problematic. The leading causes of morbidity and mortality among adolescents—including pregnancy, sexually transmitted diseases, unintentional injuries, substance use, and depression and other mental health disorders—are largely preventable. They often arise from health-risk behaviors as adolescents have difficulty coping with the many changes they are faced with. Adolescent medicine therefore focuses on more than narrowly defined medical issues, but takes a holistic approach considering the variety of psychosocial issues that affect daily well-being. Pediatric clinicians caring for adolescents should:

Address acute health care problems.
Provide comprehensive general health care, including clinical preventive services.
Promote health education encouraging teenagers to make appropriate decisions and lead healthy lifestyles.
Support and assist parents in providing supervision and guidance to their adolescents.

LEGAL ISSUES

• For many adolescents, the interface between the health care system and the law revolves around the issues of *consent* and *confidentiality*.

CONSENT

- In the United States, the right of a minor (any individual under age 18) to consent to treatment without parental knowledge is governed entirely by state laws that vary considerably. Adolescents and pediatric health care providers should be keenly aware of state laws surrounding consent and confidentiality, as well as how their individual health care agencies (i.e., hospitals, community health centers, public clinics) interpret them. Most state laws governing adolescents' rights have age limitations generally around age 12–16 years. In particular, exceptions are frequently made empowering adolescents to consent to medical care for public health services such as sexually transmitted disease (STD) treatment, substance abuse or mental health problems, and family planning (i.e., contraceptive) services. The right of an adolescent to get an abortion varies greatly by state. Adolescents may also be exempt from the requirements of parental consent if they meet one of the following requirements:

MATURE MINOR

- Generally individuals 14 years of age or older who understand the risks and benefits of the services being provided and are therefore able to give informed consent. This principle is increasingly invoked to provide to an adolescent health care services that are considered low risk, will benefit the minor, and are well within established medical practice standards. Clinicians caring for adolescents under this provision typically document that the adolescent has acted responsibly.

EMANCIPATED MINORS

- Generally individuals 16 years or older who live away from home, manage their own financial affairs, are married, or are members of the armed services. Emancipation is a legal designation and must be obtained in a court of law. Emancipated minors can receive any form of health care services without parental consent. Pregnant and parenting females are often given the rights associated with emancipation.

MEDICAL EMERGENCIES

- An adolescent may be treated without parental consent if, in a clinician's judgment, delay resulting from attempts to contact a parent might jeopardize the well-being of the minor.

CONFIDENTIALITY

- Legal statutes governing confidentiality of adolescent health care services are far more inconsistent than

policies governing consent. As a general principle, most adolescent medicine providers feel the right to self-consent for health care services carries with it the right to confidentiality about that information. Widely held exceptions to the accepted principles of confidentiality include conditions requiring mandatory reporting such as cases of abuse or when there is the possibility of self-imposed harm to the minor.

FEDERAL LAW

- The *Health Insurance Portability and Accountability Act* (HIPAA) originally passed by President Clinton in 1996 allowed minors to maintain the confidentiality of medical records related to all care that they lawfully consented to under state or federal law (i.e., thus linking the concept of consent and confidentiality). However, the final HIPAA regulations published in 2002 under President Bush severed the link between minors' right to consent and their ability to keep their medical records private. Under HIPAA, minors now only control their medical records when states explicitly authorize them to do so. When state laws either require or permit disclosure to parents, the HIPAA regulation allows the health care provider to comply with that law.

STATE LAW

- Most state laws are *silent* on the subject of confidentiality of adolescents' medical records. Colorado and New York are notable exceptions. It is often left up to the medical provider or health care institution to decide whether to maintain the confidentiality of an adolescent's medical records.

STAGES OF ADOLESCENT DEVELOPMENT

- Because adolescents vary over a wide range of chronological ages, it is useful to characterize an individual within the context of early, middle, or late stages of adolescent development. Each stage is marked by a set of biologic, psychologic, emotional, and sociocultural issues (Table 10-1). These changes do not occur in an all-or-none manner, and individual variation exists in terms of timing and quality.

BIOLOGIC

- Puberty and pubertal changes are the hallmark of the biologic changes associated with adolescence. The somatic and physiologic changes give rise to the sexual maturity rating (SMR) or Tanner stages (Figs. 10-1 and 10-2). Adolescents gain up to 25% of their adult height

TABLE 10-1   Stages of Adolescent Development

VARIABLE	EARLY ADOLESCENCE (AGE 10–13)	MIDDLE ADOLESCENCE (AGE 14–16)	LATE ADOLESCENCE (AGE 17 AND ABOVE)
Biologic	Onset of puberty and secondary sex characteristics (SMR 1-2); beginning of rapid growth	Peak height growth and body composition changes (SMR 3-5); acceptance of body changes	Slower growth; acquisition of adult body composition
Psychologic/Emotional	Concrete thinking; preoccupation with changing body appearance; egocentrism; wide mood swings; reassurance of normalcy ("Am I normal?")	Emergence of abstract thought; sense of invincibility; begin to develop future time perspective	Formal operational thinking; focus on identity in relation to society; increasing sense of vulnerability
Sociocultural	Independence from parents; peer group identification (same sex); sexual interest exceeds activity; idealistic vocational goals	Peak parental conflict and peer conformity; autonomy is chief concern; sexual experimentation and increased risk-taking	Reacceptance of parental values, peers less important than supportive intimate relationships; risk-taking behavior decreases; career planning

and 50% of their adult weight during this period. Individuals vary greatly with regard to onset and rate of pubertal development.

FEMALE PUBERTAL CHANGES

• Typically start between 8 and 13 years of age, and proceed for 3–4 years. Breast development (*thelarche*) generally precedes pubic hair development (*pubarche*). Peak height spurt occurs midway through puberty (SMR 3) and is associated with fat deposition. Average age of menarche approximately 12.5 years (SMR 3-4).

MALE PUBERTAL CHANGES

• Typically start between 9 and 14 years of age, and proceed for 3–3.5 years. Testicular enlargement is the first sign of male pubertal development. Peak height velocity occurs in the latter half of puberty (SMR 4) and is associated with muscle mass development.

PSYCHOLOGIC

• Piaget characterized adolescent thought processes as becoming increasingly sophisticated, from concrete to

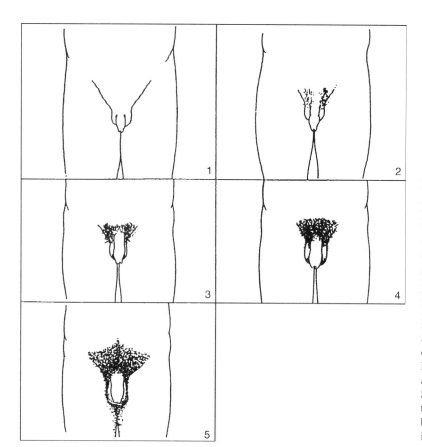

FIG. 10-1 Sex maturity rating (SMR) for male genitalia and pubic hair development. Ratings for pubic hair and genital development can differ in a typical boy at any given time because pubic hair and genitalia do not necessarily develop at the same rate. SMR 1: Prepubertal—no pubic hair; genitalia unchanged from early childhood. SMR 2: Light downy hair develops laterally and later becomes dark. Penis and testes may be slightly larger. Scrotum becomes more textured. SMR 3: Pubic hair has extended across the pubis. Testes and scrotum are further enlarged. Penis is larger, especially in length. SMR 4: More abundant pubic hair with curling. Genitalia resemble those of an adult. Glans penis has become larger and broader. Scrotum is darker. SMR 5: Adult quantity and pattern of pubic hair, with hair present along the inner border of the thighs. Testes and scrotum are adult in size (Daniel and Paulshock, 1979).

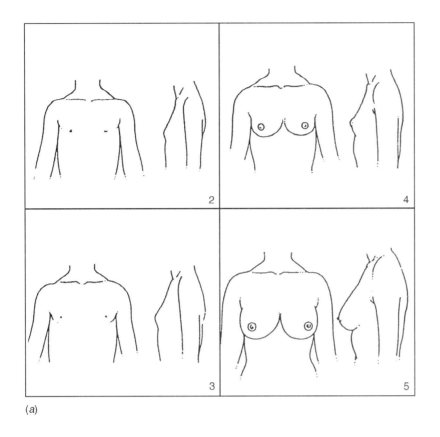

(a)

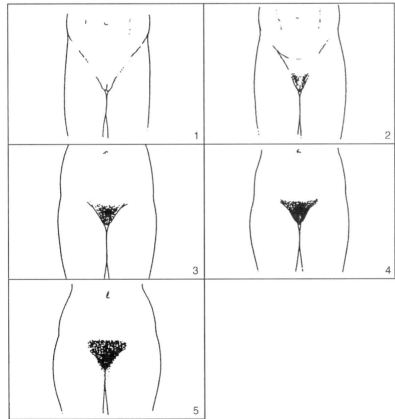

(b)

FIG. 10-2 Sex maturity rating (SMR) for female breast development and pubic hair development. (*a*) SMR 1 (not shown): Prepubertal — elevations of papilla only. SMR 2: Breast buds appear; areola is slightly widened and projects as small mound. SMR 3: Enlargement of the entire breast, with no protrusion of the papilla or nipple. SMR 4: Enlargement of the breast and projection of areola and papilla as a secondary mound. SMR 5: Adult configuration of the breast, with protrusion of the nipple. Areola no longer projects separately from the remainder of the breast. (*b*) SMR 1: Prepubertal — no pubic hair. SMR 2: Straight hair extends along the labia and between ratings 2 and 3, begins on the pubis. SMR 3: Pubic hair has increased in quantity, is darker, and is present in the typical female triangle but in smaller quantity. SMR 4: Pubic hair is more dense, curled, and adult in distribution but is less abundant. SMR 5: Abundant, adult-type pattern; hair may extend onto the medial aspect of the thighs (Daniel and Paulshock, 1979).

formal operational abstract thinking. This cognitive transition is evident in a variety of ways:

SENSE OF INVINCIBILITY

• Early and middle adolescents participate in health-risk behaviors in part because they believe that negative outcomes such as pregnancy, STDs, and serious injury happen to others but not them. As they mature into adulthood they begin to see these activities as increasingly risky.

SENSE OF SELF

• Early adolescents are often preoccupied with bodily changes and are relatively self-centered and egocentric. With the development of formal operational thought, adolescents become more capable of considering perspectives other than their own and develop an adult sense of time and the future.

SOCIOCULTURAL

• The struggle for independence from parents, the emergence of important peer groups and romantic relationships, and the evolution of a sexual identity mark the sociocultural transitions associated with adolescence.

HEALTH ASSESSMENT OF ADOLESCENTS

• The complexities of the physical, psychosocial, and developmental processes that occur during adolescence make routine health maintenance visits critical. The American Medical Association's *Guidelines for Adolescent Preventive Services* (GAPS) is a commonly used set of criteria designed to assist the health care provider with comprehensive adolescent-specific services (Table 10-2). Other commonly used guidelines for the health assessment of adolescent patients include guidelines published by the American Academy of Pediatrics Committee on Practice and Ambulatory Medicine and the Maternal Child Health Bureau's *Bright Futures*. There is much overlap and agreement between these documents and the implementation or utilization of either can be of tremendous assistance to the provision of comprehensive care. It is generally accepted that adolescents *have a scheduled clinical visit at least once per year* whether for anticipatory guidance, health care screening, or physical assessment.

INTERVIEWING THE ADOLESCENT

• Although some time should be spent with the parent(s) to identify their health-related concerns, most of the

visits and patient interviews occur alone with the adolescent, unless he/she specifically requests parental presence. This may be a disconcerting transition for parents and younger adolescents used to a traditional pediatric practice. The health care provider should assist the parent and the adolescent in understanding the importance of privacy and setting an expectation for increasing autonomy in the health care process. Issues of confidentiality and privacy should be addressed with new and established patients along with conditions under which confidentiality might need to be altered (i.e., life or safety threatening situations). In addition to the standard medical history, the goal of the clinical interview is to establish rapport between patient and provider and to identify problems or issues of concern. Since many of the leading causes of adolescent morbidity and mortality are preventable and result from risk-taking behaviors, the hallmark of the adolescent interview is the psychosocial history. The mnemonic HEADDSS is often used to guide the clinicians' systematic review of various systems:

H-HOME

• "With whom do you live?"
• "How are things at home?"
• "How do you get along with your parents and siblings?"
• "What would change in your home or family to make them better?"

E-EDUCATION

• "How is school going?"
• "In what subjects do you do well?"
• "What classes do you find interesting/boring?"
• "Have you ever been suspended from school?"
• "How are your grades in comparison to last year?"
• "How many days this year have you missed school?"

A-ACTIVITIES

• "When you are not in school, what do you do with your free time?"
• "How much television do you watch each day?"
• "What do you do for exercise?" "How often?"
• "Do you have a best friend that you can rely on?"
• "Do you or your friends ever get into fights?"
• "Do you or your friends ever carry weapons?"

D-DRUGS

• "Have you ever tried cigarettes, alcohol, or other drugs?" "Which ones?"
• "With whom do you use drugs or alcohol?" "Alone or with friends?"
• "Do you ever drink alcohol or use drugs at home?" "At school?"
• "Do any of your friends use alcohol or drugs?"

TABLE 10-2   Guidelines for Health Services of Adolescent Patients

| | AGE OF ADOLESCENT | | | | | | | | | | |
| | EARLY | | | | MIDDLE | | | LATE | | | |
PROCEDURE	11	12	13	14	15	16	17	18	19	20	21
Health Guidance											
Parenting[a]	—•—				—•—						
Development	•	•	•	•	•	•	•	•	•	•	•
Diet and Fitness	•	•	•	•	•	•	•	•	•	•	•
Lifestyle[b]	•	•	•	•	•	•	•	•	•	•	•
Injury Prevention	•	•	•	•	•	•	•	•	•	•	•
Screening History											
Eating Disorders	•	•	•	•	•	•	•	•	•	•	•
Sexual Activity[c]	•	•	•	•	•	•	•	•	•	•	•
Alcohol and Other Drug Use	•	•	•	•	•	•	•	•	•	•	•
Tobacco Use	•	•	•	•	•	•	•	•	•	•	•
Abuse	•	•	•	•	•	•	•	•	•	•	•
School Performance	•	•	•	•	•	•	•	•	•	•	•
Depression	•	•	•	•	•	•	•	•	•	•	•
Risk for Suicide	•	•	•	•	•	•	•	•	•	•	•
Physical Assessment											
Blood Pressure	•	•	•	•	•	•	•	•	•	•	•
BMI	•	•	•	•	•	•	•	•	•	•	•
Comprehensive Examination	—•—				—•—			—•—			
Tests											
Cholesterol	–1–	–1–	–1–	–1–	–1–	–1–	–1–	–1–	–1–	–1–	–1–
TB	–2–	–2–	–2–	–2–	–2–	–2–	–2–	–2–	–2–	–2–	–2–
GC, Chlamydia, and HPV	–3–	–3–	–3–	–3–	–3–	–3–	–3–	–3–	–3–	–3–	–3–
HIV and Syphilis	–4–	–4–	–4–	–4–	–4–	–4–	–4–	–4–	–4–	–4–	–4–
PAP Smear	–5–	–5–	–5–	–5–	–5–	–5–	–5–	–5–	–5–	–5–	–5–
Immunizations											
MMR	—•—										
TD					—•—						
HBV[a]	–6–				–6–			–6–			

1. Screening test performed once if family history is positive for early cardiovascular disease or hyperlipidemia.
2. Screen if positive for exposure to active TB or lives/works in high-risk situation (e.g., homeless shelter, jail, and health care facility).
3. Screen at least annually if sexually active.
4. Screen if high-risk for infection.
5. Screen annually if sexually active or if 18 years or older.
6. Vaccinate if high-risk for hapatitis B infection.

[a] A parent health-guidance visit is recommended during early and middle adolescence.
[b] Includes counseling regarding sexual behavior and avoidance of tobacco, alcohol, and other drug use.
[c] Includes history of unintended pregnancy and STD.

- "What do you do if your friends encourage you to use drugs or alcohol?"
- "Have you ever driven a car while drinking or using drugs?"
- "Have you gotten into a car with someone drinking alcohol or using drugs?"

D-Diet

- "How do you feel about your weight?" "What would be your ideal weight?"
- "Do you think you are too heavy, too thin, or just about right?"
- "Have you ever tried to change your diet to either lose or gain weight?"
- "Have you ever used vomiting to keep your weight stable?"
- "Do you eat meat?"
- "How much milk or milk products such as cheese do you eat each day?"

S-Sexuality

- "Have you ever been attracted to boys, girls, or both?"
- "Are you dating or going out with someone?"
- "Do you consider yourself gay/lesbian, bisexual, heterosexual, or not sure?"
- "Have you ever had vaginal or anal sexual intercourse?"
- "Have you had intercourse with men, women, or both sexes?"
- "What do you use for protection against pregnancy or STDs?"
- "What percentage of the time do you use condoms?" "10, 25, 50, 100%?"
- "Have you had any sexual experiences/contact that you did not want to?"
- "Have you ever had an STD?"

S-Suicide/Depression

- "Do you see yourself as generally happy or sad?"
- "Do you ever get down or depressed?"
- "Whom can you talk with when things are difficult or you are feeling sad?"
- "What do you see yourself doing 5 years from now?"
- "Have you ever thought of dying or hurting yourself?"
- "Tell me about the last time you really enjoyed yourself."

PHYSICAL EXAMINATION

- Similar to the patient interview it is generally preferred to perform the physical examination in private without parents present. However, adolescents may be more comfortable with one or both parents present during the examination and should be offered the option if they prefer. From a health maintenance perspective, the physical examination is particularly important for early adolescents who may be concerned about the normalcy of bodily shape, size, and function. Although a comprehensive physical examination should be performed on all adolescents as per recommended guidelines (Table 10-2), special attention should be paid to the following:

Vital Signs

- Height, weight, and body mass index (BMI) are important measures to evaluate in every adolescent patient and should be plotted in the appropriate charts. Hypertension screening through routine blood pressure determination should be performed. Measurement should be evaluated in comparison to established age-specific norms that increase with pubertal maturation.

Skin

- Acne is one of the most common disorders of adolescence. Although it is rarely a serious medical problem, in moderate to severe cases it may be emotionally devastating to an adolescent because of its impact on personal appearance.

Dentition

- Dental hygiene including the frequency of dental care should be evaluated with every adolescent. Encourage daily brushing with fluoridated toothpaste to help prevent dental caries, and regular visits to an oral health care provider.

Breasts

- Examination of the female adolescents' breasts is done not only to detect masses, to evaluate the progression of sexual maturation, but also to educate about what is normal and to teach the technique of self-examination with the hope that this practice will continue into adulthood.

Musculoskeletal

- Progressive idiopathic scoliosis occurs primarily in growing adolescents. Scoliosis is typically manifested during the peak of the height velocity curve (i.e., approximately 12 years in females and 14 years in males). The routine examination should include an assessment of any asymmetries of the neck, shoulders, scapulae, spine, waist, and hips. A scoliometer can be a useful tool in the office setting to determine the angle of trunk rotation (ATR) on the area of greatest asymmetry. If the ATR is <5° this can likely be observed. If the ATR is >5° then a radiograph should be obtained so that a Cobb angle (i.e., degree of curvature of the spine) can be measured. Patients with Cobb angles of >20° on radiograph should be referred to an orthopedic specialist for evaluation.

NECK

- The routine examination of all adolescents should include an evaluation of the size of the thyroid gland.

MALE GENITALIA

- Examination of the male genitalia is done to evaluate for progression of sexual maturity as well as to detect the presence of urethral discharge, inguinal hernias, scrotal masses, or penile lesions. Similar to the breast examination in adolescent females, this represents an opportunity to educate adolescent males on the value and proper technique of the testicular self-examination.

FEMALE GENITALIA

- Although many authorities recommend a pelvic examination in all adolescent females by age 18, there is no absolute consensus. A pelvic examination should be performed at least annually in sexually active adolescents or as symptoms dictate (i.e., unusual vaginal discharge, menstrual dysfunction, or lower abdominal pain). Examination of the external genitalia should be part of all adolescent female routine examinations to evaluate progression of sexual maturity as well as to identify vulvar rash or anatomic abnormality.

LABORATORY TESTING, PROCEDURES, AND IMMUNIZATION

ROUTINE SCREENING LABS

- *Complete blood count (CBC) or hemoglobin*: Although the various adolescent guidelines are not in complete agreement, routine screening among otherwise healthy adolescents is not generally recommended except in adolescent females at increased risk of iron-deficiency anemia because of moderate to heavy menses. Populations at nutritional risk of iron-deficiency anemia should also be monitored.
- *Cholesterol*: Screening tests (i.e., nonfasting cholesterol) are generally performed in individuals with a positive family history of hyperlipidemia or early cardiovascular disease. If levels are >200 mg/dL, then fasting cholesterol, triglyceride, and HDL levels should be measured.
- *STD screening*: All sexually active adolescents should receive annual screening for chlamydia and gonorrhea regardless of symptoms. Although some guidelines recommend human immunodeficiency virus (HIV) and syphilis screening only among high-risk adolescents (young men having sex with other men, persons with multiple sex partners, and persons who exchange sex for money, drugs, or shelter), annual screening remains the standard of care in many communities.
- *Cervical cytology*: Sexually active female adolescents should get annual cervical cytology screening either from a traditional Papanicolaou (PAP) test or using liquid-based medium for sampling (ThinPrep).
- *Urinalysis*: Although not generally recommended, some health care providers may obtain a urinalysis as part of the adolescent health maintenance screening for the possibility of cervicitis, vaginitis, or an asymptomatic urinary tract infection.

PROCEDURES

- Vision screening should be checked as part of routine primary care so that problems may be detected before they affect school performance. Audiometry, although not universally recommended, should be considered in adolescents exposed repeatedly to loud noises (i.e., music), have a history of recurrent ear infections, or report difficulty hearing.

IMMUNIZATIONS

- *Tetanus-diphtheria*: All adolescents who have completed their primary immunization series should receive a tetanus-diphtheria toxoid vaccination booster (Td) during their adolescent years (11–16).
- *Measles, mumps, and rubella (MMR)*: Those who have not previously received their second MMR vaccine should be administered the vaccine during adolescence.
- *Hepatitis B*: All adolescents who have not previously completed the three-injection immunization series should do so during this period.
- *Varicella*: Health care providers should ask all adolescents about a history of chicken pox disease. If negative, they may check serum for varicella antibody before administering the vaccine. In adolescents >12 years of age, the varicella vaccine is administered in two doses. Since this is a live virus vaccine, it is generally contraindicated in individuals with cell-mediated immune deficiencies.
- *Tuberculosis (TB)*: A Mantoux tuberculin skin test (purified protein derivative of tuberculin [PPD]) is recommended only in adolescents at increased risk of acquiring tuberculosis. This includes immediate skin testing for anyone having contact with persons confirmed or suspected of having infectious TB and immigrants from endemic countries or adolescents who have a travel history to endemic countries. Periodic screening is recommended in HIV-infected, homeless, incarcerated, and other high-risk adolescents.
- *Others*: Additional vaccinations such as the influenza, hepatitis A, and pneumococcal vaccines should be administered only in specific subpopulations of adolescents.

MENSTRUAL DISORDERS

NORMAL MENSTRUATION

- Onset of menarche typically between 10 and 16 years of age, with average being approximately 12.5 years.
- Menarche occurs during SMR 3-4, typically 1–3 years after initiation of puberty.
- Age of menarche influenced by family history, stress, exercise, substance use, height/weight, chronic disease, race/ethnicity, and percent body fat (i.e., 17% necessary for onset of menstrual cycles and 22% necessary to maintain regular ovulatory cycles).
- Normal adult ovulatory cycle ranges 21–35 days with average being 28 days and menstrual flow lasts for 3–7 days.
- Normal blood loss: 40–80 cc/cycle.
- Adolescents more likely to have anovulatory cycles particularly in first 2 years after menarche.
- Anovulation, which can be associated with low weight, exercise, and eating disorders, may result in dysfunctional uterine bleeding (DUB), irregular menstrual periods (oligomenorrhea), or amenorrhea.

AMENORRHEA

DEFINITIONS

- Primary amenorrhea: No menses by age 16 despite pubertal development, or no menses and no pubertal development by age 14.
- Secondary amenorrhea: Absence of menses for at least 6 months, or 3 cycle lengths after the establishment of regular cycles. The definition is variable in the adolescent population secondary to concerns about pregnancy.

DIFFERENTIAL DIAGNOSIS

- Primary amenorrhea: Anatomic, chromosomal, or congenital abnormalities such as an imperforate hymen, mullerian agenesis, Turner syndromes (gonadal dysgenesis), and testicular feminization should be considered in addition to the conditions that cause secondary amenorrhea.
- Secondary amenorrhea:
  1. Pregnancy should always be ruled out as a possible etiology of secondary amenorrhea.
  2. Additional considerations include chronic illness, central nervous system causes (i.e., tumor), thyroid disease, hyperprolactinemia, substance use, medications (i.e., phenothiazines), depression, eating disorders, stress, athletic competition, and hyperandrogenism (polycystic ovarian syndromes or PCOS).

EVALUATION

- The laboratory evaluation of amenorrhea requires a stepwise approach driven by the history and physical examination. External or internal genital anomalies suspected as etiologies of primary amenorrhea should be identified by physical examination or radiologic evaluation when necessary. The remaining clinical and laboratory evaluation can proceed as follows:
  1. *Step #1*: A pregnancy test (urine or serum) is a key laboratory test in evaluation of amenorrhea regardless of history of sexual activity.
  2. *Step #2*: A vaginal smear or progestin challenge (10 mg of medroxyprogesterone for 5–10 days) for assessment of estrogen status.
  3. *Step #3*: Labs include FSH (Follicle stimulating hormone), LH (Luteinizing hormone), TSH (Thyroid stimulating hormone), and prolactin. Concern about androgen excess warrants the consideration of DHEAS (Dehydroepiandrostrone sulfate) as well as free and total testosterone.
  4. *Step #4*: (a) An individual with a high FSH (hypergonadotropic hypogonadism) suggests gonadal dysgenesis resulting from chromosomal abnormalities or other causes of ovarian failure. In these individuals a karyotype should be obtained. (b) An individual with a low to normal FSH (hypogonadotropic hypogonadism) suggests either a hypothalamic cause (stress, eating disorder, athletics, substance use, and so on), central nervous system tumor, chronic disease, or other endocrinopathy (i.e., thyroid disease or PCOS).

TREATMENT

- Depends entirely on the diagnosis.
  1. Euestrogenic patients: Regular cycling with either medroxyprogesterone 10 mg orally for 10–12 days at least every 1–2 months or daily administration of the oral contraceptive pill.
  2. Hypoestrogenic patient: Consider decreasing physical activity in athletes or weight gain in patients with eating disorders. In a patient with gonadal dysgenesis conjugated estrogens should be administered first for feminization to progress. This is then followed by medroxyprogesterone, 5–10 mg orally for 12–14 days/month.

DYSFUNCTIONAL UTERINE BLEEDING (DUB)

DEFINITION

- Excessive, prolonged vaginal bleeding in adolescents typically resulting from anovulatory menstrual cycles and unrelated to structural or systemic disease.

DIFFERENTIAL DIAGNOSIS

- Include physiologic anovulation that is often typical of the first 1–2 years postmenarche, foreign bodies (i.e., tampons), trauma, disorders of pregnancy (i.e., ectopic or miscarriage), endometriosis, PCOS, bleeding disorder, endocrinopathy, masses (i.e., polyps or tumors), medications, pelvic inflammatory disease (PID) or other STDs.

EVALUATION

- Patient history: Should focus on possible causes including age of menarche, sexual activity, bleeding problems, history of abuse, and medication use. The level of DUB or estimation of blood loss should be determined (although adolescents are classically poor historians for this estimation).
- Physical examination: A comprehensive examination including vital signs (i.e., blood pressure and evaluation for orthostatic changes) and dermatologic evaluation looking for signs of bruising, bleeding, or androgen excess (i.e., acne, hirsutism, acanthosis nigricans). A pelvic examination should be done in all sexually active adolescents or if there is concern about foreign body. A rectoabdominal examination may also be helpful.
- Laboratory studies:
  1. Should include a CBC and pregnancy test in *all patients*. A sensitive urine pregnancy test or serum human chorionic gonadotropin (hCG) should be used to rule out the possibility of ectopic pregnancy.
  2. An STD screen, clotting studies including liver function tests, pelvic ultrasound, and endocrine evaluation should be considered when clinically appropriate.

TREATMENT

- Depends on extent of anemia and etiology.
  1. Mild DUB (normal hemoglobin and hematocrit): Observation with menstrual calendar to follow subsequent flow patterns; may consider oral iron supplementation or administration of nonsteroidal anti-inflammatory drug (NSAID).
  2. Moderate DUB (hemoglobin 9–11 g/dL): Cycling with monophasic oral contraceptives, barring any contraindications, along with iron supplementation. May also consider oral medroxyprogesterone 10 mg daily for 10–14 days.
  3. Severe DUB (hemoglobin <9 g/dL):
     a. May consider hospitalization, but usually can be stopped with hormonal therapy. Use monophasic oral contraceptive pills, two to four times per day until the bleeding stops, then one pill per day for the remainder of the cycle.
     b. In cases of hemodynamic instability or hemoglobin <7 g/dL, hospitalization pending the cessation of bleeding is recommended. In patients unable to tolerate multiple doses of the oral contraceptive pill, intravenous Premarin 20–40 mg every 4 hours up to 24 hours may be used.
     c. In cases where the bleeding cannot be controlled by these methods, a gynecologic evaluation for possible endometrial curettage may be indicated. This procedure is rarely indicated in the adolescent age group.

DYSMENORRHEA

DEFINITION

- Menstrual pain usually in the lower abdomen. The symptoms may include nausea, vomiting, headaches, or back pain. Menstrual cramps are quite common among adolescent females and are one of the leading causes of school absenteeism in this demographic group.
  1. Primary dysmenorrhea: Painful menstrual cramps characterized by the absence of specific pelvic pathology.
  2. Secondary dysmenorrhea: Results from underlying pelvic pathology such as endometriosis.

EVALUATION

- In patients who do not respond to treatment for primary dysmenorrhea, a pelvic examination should be performed to rule out the possibility of secondary causes.
- Pelvic ultrasound or laparoscopy should be reserved for severe and unresolved cases.

TREATMENT

- Mild-moderate pain: Often responds well to NSAID administration because of the inhibition of prostaglandin activity. These medications should be initiated around or shortly after the onset of symptoms.
- Severe pain: A trial of the oral contraceptive pill is often helpful. In cases associated with endometriosis, an antigonadotropin or gonadotropin-releasing hormone agonist may be warranted.

PREGNANCY AND CONTRACEPTION

PREGNANCY

- The United States has the highest rate of teenage pregnancy in the industrialized world with approximately one million adolescent pregnancies each year, the majority of which are unintended. Adolescent parenting has implications for the mother, father, and child. In comparison to their peers, adolescent mothers are more likely to abandon vocational and educational goals and to live in poverty. They are more likely to delay seeking prenatal care and have higher rates of unfavorable birth outcomes such as prematurity and infant mortality.

DIAGNOSIS AND CLINICAL MANIFESTATIONS
- Pregnancy is the most common diagnosis when an adolescent presents with secondary amenorrhea or a history of "missed periods."
- Additional presenting complaints may be traditional symptoms associated with pregnancy such as morning sickness, swollen tender breasts, or weight gain.
- Adolescents who are pregnant may also present with vague symptoms such as headaches, fatigue, abdominal pain, or urinary frequency.
- On physical examination, an enlarged uterus, cervical cyanosis (Chadwick sign), a soft uterus (Hegar sign), or a soft cervix (Goodell sign) are highly suggestive of an intrauterine pregnancy.

LABORATORY CONFIRMATION
- Urine evaluation for hCG can determine the presence of a pregnancy within 10–14 days of conception.
- Serum hCG evaluations are seldom necessary in the evaluation of a routine pregnancy.
- Serum hCGs are more valuable to either quantifying the duration of the pregnancy or in the presence of troubling signs such as bleeding or pain.

COUNSELING AND DECISION MAKING
- Privacy and confidentiality are critical components to counseling a pregnant adolescent.
- Pregnancy, particularly in younger teenagers, should raise the concern that the sexual activity may have been coercive.
- A negative pregnancy test represents an opportunity for teaching and counseling about reproductive health and family planning options.
- In a pregnant adolescent, options available to manage the pregnancy including adoption/foster care, continuation, and termination. These options should be presented in a nonjudgmental manner.
- Pregnant adolescents should be encouraged to include parents, partners, or other family members in discussions about options. Parents, most often mothers, have a large influence on what a pregnant adolescent decides to do.
- Follow-up is critical as denial or indecisiveness may delay seeking either adult support or appropriate medical care.

MEDICAL MANAGEMENT
- Pregnant adolescents may need assistance with financial or social support, continuation of school or education for successful parenting.

- Adolescents should receive prenatal care as soon as possible since toxemia and anemia of pregnancy are more common in this age group.

CONTRACEPTION

- Approximately one-half of all adolescents are sexually active by about 16 years of age. Adolescents suffer a disproportionate amount of adverse consequences related to their sexual activity including STDs and unintended pregnancy. In general, as few as one-third consistently use effective forms of birth control. Adolescent males should be encouraged to use condoms at all times, and adolescent females should be counseled about the variety of barrier and hormonal contraceptive options available to them. Parental support for contraceptive use typically improves compliance, especially with the oral contraceptive pill.

CONTRACEPTIVE COUNSELING/EVALUATION
- The patient interview should support the adolescent that is abstinent to continue to be so and identify the sexually active adolescent that requires contractive counseling.
- Adolescents with chronic diseases should not be excluded from discussions of sexuality and contraception.
- Goals of contraceptive counseling: (1) to explore patient perceptions and misperceptions of various contraceptive methods and (2) to educate the patient about the risks and benefits of each option vs. the risk of acquiring an STD or becoming pregnant.
- Adolescents should be aware of the differences between contraceptive failure rates with "perfect" vs. "typical" use.
- The use of the withdrawal method as an ineffective method of contraception should be addressed with all adolescents.
- Before starting any form of hormonal contraception, all adolescents should have a complete physical examination including blood pressure measurement. Sexually active youth should receive a pregnancy test, PAP smear, and comprehensive STD screen.

BARRIER METHODS
- Prevent sperm from entering the uterus or vagina.
  1. *Condoms:*
     a. In part related to the fears of acquiring HIV, condom use among adolescents has increased over the past decade.
     b. Most effective barrier method with a 3% failure rate with perfect use and a 12% failure rate typical use.

c. Main advantages: low cost, no major side effects, available without prescription, little need for advanced planning, and are effective against HIV and other STDs.

d. Often used in combination with a spermicide but this may increase the risk for acquiring HIV or another STD.

e. Available in male and female versions. Female condoms somewhat more difficult to use.

2. *Diaphragm and cervical cap:*

a. Diaphragm: Circular dome that when properly placed represents a barrier between the vagina and cervix, thereby blocking sperm from entering the uterus.

b. Cervical cap: A firm plastic structure that fits snugly over the cervical opening.

c. When used with spermicides have 6% failure rates with perfect use and 16–18% failure rates with typical use.

d. Less likely to be used because
   i. Adolescents may have discomfort about touching their genital area.
   ii. They require advanced planning for proper use.
   iii. Disrupt the spontaneity of the sexual act.

Hormonal Methods

• Currently use either estrogen in combination with a progestin or a progestin alone. The estrogen-progestin combination prevents ovulation and thickens cervical mucus. The progestin-only methods may prevent ovulation, but also act to impair fallopian tube transport and thicken cervical mucus making fertilization and/or implantation less likely.

1. Combination Oral Contraceptive Pills (OCP)
   a. Form of contraception most commonly used by adolescent females.
   b. Must be taken daily.
   c. Typically contain 20–35 mg of estrogenic component (i.e., ethinyl estradiol) along with a progestin.
   d. Failure rates <1% with perfect use, but as high as 6% with typical use (i.e., poor adherence).
   e. Additional benefits:
      i. Short term: May include improved acne, reduced dysmenorrheal and shorter menses.
      ii. Long term: Potential help in decreasing risk of benign breast disease, ovarian cysts, and certain gynecologic neoplasm.
   f. Side effects:
      i. Short term/mild: (a) Nausea, weight gain, breast tenderness, acne, mood changes, and headaches. (b) Usually transient. (c) Often interfere with adherence.
      ii. Long term/serious: (a) Thrombophlebitis, hypertension, and myocardial infarction. These are quite rare in adolescents. (b) Amenorrhea occurring after cessation of the OCP lasting up to 18 months.
   g. Contraindications:
      i. Absolute contraindications: Pregnancy, history of breast cancer, estrogen-sensitive neoplasm, thromboembolic disease, hypercoagulability, cerebrovascular accident, malignant hypertension, or hepatocellular disease.
      ii. Relative contraindications: (a) Migraine headaches, borderline hypertension, diabetes, seizure disorder, sickle cell disease. (b) Cigarette smoking warrants special consideration and is a relative contraindication in women aged >35 because of the risk of thromboembolism. This *is not* a contraindication in adolescents. Nonetheless, adolescents on OCPs should be encouraged to quit smoking.

2. Other combination methods: These are recently developed methods that have similar benefits, side effect profiles, and contraindications as the OCP.
   a. Monthly injectable (Lunelle):
      i. As efficacious as the OCP but provides the convenience of a monthly injection.
      ii. Administered by health care provider during first 5 days of menstrual cycle.
      iii. Follow-up doses are given every 28 days (23–33 days).
   b. Transdermal patch (OrthoEvra):
      i. Patch applied to lower abdomen, upper body, or buttocks.
      ii. Applied weekly for 3 weeks and then removed to allow for menstrual bleeding.
      iii. Weekly administration may improve adherence in comparison to the OCP.
      iv. Less effective in obese women weighing over 200 lb.
      v. Additional common side effects include skin irritation and detachment.
   c. Vaginal contraceptive ring (NuvaRing):
      i. Flexible vaginal ring inserted into vagina by the patient.
      ii. Remains in place for 3 weeks.
      iii. Rings accidentally expelled from vagina can be reinserted as long as they have not been out of place for more than 3 hours.
      iv. Not a popular contraceptive option for adolescents squeamish about touching their own genitals.

3. Progestin-only methods:
   a. Progestin-only (mini) pill:
      i. Generally reserved for adolescents in whom estrogen is contraindicated.

ii. Less reliable in preventing ovulation and therefore has a higher rate of contraceptive failure.

iii. Because of the pharmacokinetics, must be taken at the same time each day in order to be maximally effective.

iv. Higher incidence of amenorrhea and irregular menstrual bleeding than with OCPs.

b. Injectable progestin (Depo-Provera):

i. Popular method particularly with younger teens unable to adhere to taking the daily OCP.

ii. Highly effective with failure rates of <1% with perfect or typical use.

iii. Administered intramuscularly by a health care provider every 12 weeks.

iv. Common side effects include (a) weight gain and irregular menstrual bleeding that are frequently problematic for adolescents; (b) amenorrhea with a potential delay of fertility for 6–24 months after discontinuation; and (c) the potential for lowered bone density. Since adolescence is the developmental period in which the accumulation of bone density is maximal, Depo-Provera is generally not recommended in adolescents at risk of osteoporosis.

OTHER

- Intrauterine devices (IUD):
  1. Flexible, plastic objects placed into uterus through the cervix.
  2. May contain pharmacologically active substances such as copper or progesterone.
  3. Mechanism of action unclear, but blocks implantation of the fertilized egg.
  4. Side effects include pelvic infections, uterine perforation, and higher rates of ectopic pregnancy.
  5. Not generally used in adolescents, especially those with multiple sexual partners because of increased risk of sexually transmitted infections.
- Spermicides (Nonoxynol-9):
  1. Refers to a variety of agents available as creams, vaginal suppositories, foams, films, and sponges.
  2. Placed in vaginal cavity shortly before intercourse.
  3. Used in combination with other contraceptives, as failure rates are quite high when used alone.
  4. Side effects may include vaginitis or local irritation, leading to concerns about the mucosal damage and increased risk for acquiring STDs.

EMERGENCY CONTRACEPTION (THE *MORNING AFTER PILL*)

- Oral high-dose estrogen or progestin-only preparations used within 72 hours after intercourse to prevent pregnancy.

- Yuzpe method:
  1. Commonly used in the United States.
  2. Consisting of using *two doses*, *12 hours apart*, of combination OCPs totally 100 µg of ethinyl estradiol in each dose. Common choices for each dose include (a) Ovral two pills. (b) Lo-Ovral four pills. (c) Nordette four pills.
  3. Disrupts hormone pattern to create an unstable uterine lining for implantation.
  4. May come in prepackaged emergency contraceptive kit (Preven).
  5. Effective at reducing risk of pregnancy by 75%.
  6. Common side effects include nausea and emesis, prompting some clinicians to recommend over-the-counter antiemetics (i.e., meclizine hydrochloride or Dramamine) along with each dose.
- Plan B:
  1. Progestin emergency contraceptive kit containing two pills each with 0.75 mg of levonorgestrol.
  2. Nausea and vomiting much less common than with Yuzpe method.
  3. Similar efficacy rate to Yuzpe method.
  4. Recommended in adolescents for whom estrogen use is contraindicated.
- Management and follow-up:
  1. In most health facilities a pregnancy test is administered prior to prescribing emergency contraception. This is somewhat controversial since there is no evidence to suggest that use of emergency contraception would affect early fetal development or adversely affect a previously undetected pregnancy.
  2. All adolescents should receive counseling about the efficacy, mechanism of action, and side effects of the different methods.
  3. A 2-week follow-up visit is recommended to determine the effectiveness of treatment, diagnose a possible early pregnancy, and provide appropriate contraceptive counseling for the future.

SEXUALLY TRANSMITTED AND GENITOURINARY INFECTIONS

STI (Sexually Transmitted Infections)

GENERAL CONSIDERATIONS

- The United States has highest STI rate of any industrialized nation with approximately four million adolescents acquiring an STI annually.
- Adolescent STI risk factors:
  1. Biologic: *Cervical ectopy* (i.e., this maturational process occurs normally in adolescents and is marked by the involution of the cellular lining of the ectocervix changing it from a single layer of

columnar cells to a thicker squamous cell layer) imposes a unique vulnerability to infection to adolescent females.
2. Behavioral: Multiple sexual partners, inconsistent condom use, and sexual activity while using alcohol or other drugs.
3. Social: Lack of access to care, poverty, concerns about confidentiality, unequal power dynamics in sexual relations.
• Almost all adolescent STIs can exist without clinical symptoms making education, screening, early detection, and treatment critically important.
• Annual comprehensive screening for STIs should be done in sexually active adolescents.

VAGINITIS

• Superficial infection of the vaginal mucosa that frequently involves the vulva and typically presents with discharge.
• Differential diagnosis includes bacterial vaginosis, trichomoniasis, and yeast vaginitis (Fig. 10-3).
• Bacterial vaginosis:
1. Sexually- "associated" infection, not STI.
2. Pathogen: *Gardnerella vaginalis*.

3. Classic presentation:
   a. Fishy, malodorous, gray, homogenous discharge.
   b. May also present with irregular menses.
4. Diagnosis: Based on identification of clue cells (i.e., vaginal epithelial cells covered with fragments of gram-negative rods) on wet prep of vaginal discharge.
5. Treatment:
   a. Oral metronidazole 500 mg bid for 7 days or metronidazole intravaginal cream.
   b. Alternative treatment: Single oral dose of metronidazole (2 gm) or oral Clindamycin 300 mg bid for 7 days.
   c. Avoid metronidazole in pregnant adolescents as may be harmful to fetus.
   d. No recommendation to treat partners.
• Yeast vaginitis:
1. Most common form of vaginitis.
2. Pathogen: *Candida albicans*, but other fungal species as well.
3. Classic presentation:
   a. Cheesy, white discharge associated with vulvar pruritus.
   b. Occurs more frequently after systemic antibiotic use and in diabetics, pregnancy, and HIV-infected individuals.

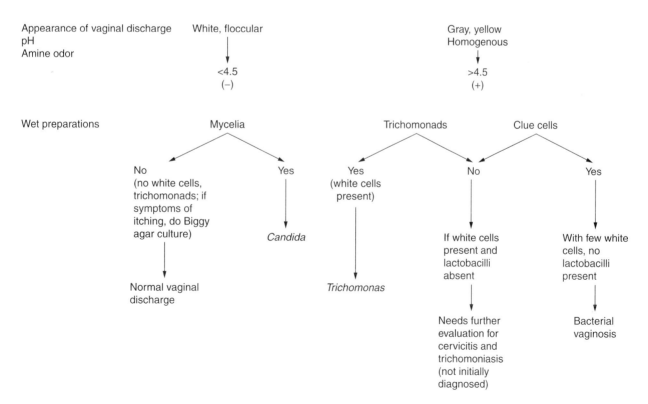

(If purulent endocervical discharge, diagnosis is cervicitis; culture for *N. Gonorrhoeae, C. trachomatis*)

FIG. 10-3 Differential diagnosis of vaginitis.

3. Diagnosis: Based on the presence of hyphae and yeast in vaginal discharge mixed with potassium hydroxide (KOH).
4. Treatment:
   a. Single oral dose of fluconazole (150 mg).
   b. Topical intravaginal antifungal preparation (i.e., suppository, cream, tablet) for 3–7 days.
   c. Topical agents to be used in pregnancy.
   d. Recurrent infections (>4 per year) treated more aggressively.
- Trichomonas:
1. Sexually transmitted infection
2. Pathogen: *Trichomonas vaginalis* (flagellated protozoan)
3. Classic presentation:
   a. Frothy, greenish-yellow, malodorous discharge.
   b. Postcoital bleeding and/or dyspareunia.
   c. Approximately 50% of cases are asymptomatic.
4. Diagnosis:
   a. Based on presence of flagellated organisms and white blood cells seen on wet prep (normal saline).
   b. False-positives seen with some frequency on PAP smear.
5. Treatment:
   a. Single oral dose of metronidazole (2 gm) or oral metronidazole 500 mg bid for 7 days.
   b. All sexual partners should be treated.

URETHRITIS

PRESENTATION
- Inflammation of the urethra presenting most typically as discharge or dysuria.
- Urinary frequency, urgency, pruritus, and erythema of the urethral meatus are less common presentations.
- Asymptomatic or minimally symptomatic presentations are common especially in males.

COMMON PATHOGENS
- *Neisseria gonorrhea* (GC)—most likely to be symptomatic.
- Nongonococcal species (NGU): *Chlamydia trachomatis* (most common), *Ureaplasma* urealyticum, *Trichomonas vaginalis*, and *E. coli*.

DIAGNOSIS
- Typically requires at least one of the following:
1. Mucopurulent discharge from the urethral meatus.
2. Positive leukocyte esterase test on first voided urine specimen (10–15 cc).
3. Gram stain of urethral secretions with >5 WBCs per high-powered field.

4. Other diagnostic tests:
   a. Nucleic acid amplification tests (NAATs) such as polymerase chain reaction for chlamydia.
   b. Culture or DNA probes for gonorrhea.

TREATMENT
- General recommendations:
1. In symptomatic patients, treat presumptively for GC and NGU.
2. Await results of diagnostic testing in asymptomatic screeners.
3. Always treat for both GC and NGU if culture is positive for GC.
4. Treat all sexual partners within 60 days of exposure.
5. Single dose treatments preferable in adolescents because of concerns of poor adherence.
- GC:
1. Singular dose of intramuscular ceftriaxone (125 mg).
2. Single dose of oral cefixime (400 mg).
3. Single dose of oral ciprofloxacin (500 mg) — dependent on geographic area because of the emergence of resistance.
- NGU:
1. Single dose of oral azithromycin (1 g).
2. Oral doxycycline 100 mg bid for 7 days.

CERVICITIS

PRESENTATION
- Inflammation of the cervix resulting in a friable cervix or discharge.
- Irregular menstrual bleeding.
- Asymptomatic presentation.

COMMON PATHOGENS
- Similar to urethritis.
- Most common are gonorrhea and chlamydia.

DIAGNOSIS AND TREATMENT
- See above treatment recommendations for urethritis.

GENITAL ULCER SYNDROMES

- Ulcerative lesions are commonly seen on the vulva and penis, but may also occur on the oral, rectal, and cervical mucosa depending on the sexual behavior of the adolescent.

PATHOGENS
- Most common: *Treponema pallidum* (syphilis) and herpes simplex virus (HSV) (Table 10-3).

TABLE 10-3 Common Pathogens and Presentations for Genital Ulcer Syndromes

DISEASE	ORGANISM	ULCER	LYMPHADENOPATHY
Genital herpes	HSV-2, HSV-1	Small, painful when palpated, vesicles, multiple	Typically associated with primary infection, firm, tender
Syphilis	*Treponema pallidum*	Painless, indurated, well-demarcated, singular	Firm, nontender or minimally tender, rubbery
Chancroid	*Hemophilus ducreyi*	Painful, soft or indurated, purulent, often multiple	Fluctuant, tender, erythema, "bubo" formation, may rupture
Lymphogranuloma venereum	*Chlamydia trachomatis*	Usually absent, singular	Fluctuant, tender
Donovanosis (granuloma inguinale)	*Calymmatobacterium granulomatis*	Painless, chronic, spreading	None

- Others: (a) *Hemophilus ducreyi* (chancroid). (b) *Chlamydia trachomatis* (lymphogranuloma venereum). (c) *Calymmatobacterium granulomatis* (granuloma inguinale).

SYPHILIS (SPIROCHETE)
- Clinical presentation: Three stages of disease
  1. Primary (10–21 days following exposure):
     a. Painless ulcer (chancre) with or without regional adenopathy.
     b. Usually singular, but may be multiple.
     c. Chancre absent in 15–30% of cases.
  2. Secondary (2–6 months after chancre):
     a. Caused by hematogenous spread of spirochete.
     b. Generalized malaise.
     c. Lymphadenopathy, headache, fever, arthralgias.
     d. Rash: Generalized or palms and soles distribution.
  3. Tertiary (years following initial infection):
     a. Unusual presentation in adolescents.
     b. Cardiovascular changes, central nervous system changes, and musculoskeletal involvement.
- Diagnosis:
  1. Dark-field or direct fluorescent antibody testing of lesion.
  2. Screening: Serologic tests for presumptive diagnosis
     a. Nontreponemal tests (Venereal Disease Research Laboratory [VDRL] or rapid plasma reagin [RPR]): (a) Titers correlate with disease activity. (b) False positives: hepatitis, lupus, and so on.
     b. Treponemal tests: (fluorescent treponemal antibody absorption [FTA-ABS]): (a) Used to confirm diagnosis. (b) Remain positive for life.
- Treatment:
  1. Parenterally administered penicillin G is the preferred treatment.
  2. Extent of treatment (i.e., dose and number of doses of penicillin) determined by length or stage of disease.

3. Alternative treatment: Oral doxycycline 100 mg bid for 14 days.
4. Follow nontreponemal titers at regular intervals. Treat all sexual partners within 90 days of exposure.

HERPES SIMPLEX VIRUS (HSV)
- Clinical presentation:
  1. Multiple vesicles on an erythematous base on penile shaft or oral, anal, vaginal, or cervical mucosa.
  2. Associated symptoms may include pain, pruritus, dysuria, and adenopathy.
  3. Two types of virus:
     a. HSV-1:
        i. Typically causes oral lesions.
        ii. Ten to fifteen percent of genital lesions are caused by HSV-1.
     b. HSV-2:
        i. Typically causes genital lesions, although oral disease is possible.
        ii. More likely to cause recurrent disease.
  4. Primary disease associated with more constitutional symptoms.
  5. Recurrent disease associated with prodromal symptoms in 50% of cases.
- Diagnosis:
  1. Largely based on presenting symptoms, clinical inspection and physical examination findings.
  2. Virologic tests (i.e., from scraping of lesion):
     a. PCR HSV DNA—highly sensitive
     b. Tzanck prep (multinucleated giant cells)—insensitive
  3. New serologic tests (type-specific antibodies) are not generally helpful for diagnostic purposes and are not indicated in general screening.
- Treatment:
  1. Generally consists of oral acyclovir or similar medication.

2. Topical therapy offers little clinical benefit.
3. Initiate treatment shortly after onset of symptoms.
4. Duration of treatment varies dependent on primary vs. recurrent disease.
   a. Primary HSV—treat 7–10 days.
   b. Recurrent HSV—treat for 5 days.
5. Can use suppressive therapy for adolescents with >6 recurrences per year.
6. Management should also include counseling.
   a. Natural history: Treatment is not curative.
   b. Transmission: May shed virus asymptomatically particularly during first year after infection.

PELVIC INFLAMMATORY DISEASE (PID)

- Spectrum of inflammatory disorders of the upper genital tract in females—including salpingitis, endometritis, and tubo-ovarian abscess (TOA).
- Disproportionately a disease of adolescents.

COMMON PATHOGENS
- *N. gonorrhea* and *C. trachomatis* are most common (at least 50% of cases).
- May also be a polymicrobial infection with other anaerobic and aerobic bacteria (*Mycoplasma hominis*, *Bacteroides fragilis*, *E. coli*, and so on).

DIAGNOSIS
- Clinical diagnosis is based on the presence of the following *minimum* criteria in the absence of other symptoms:
  1. Lower abdominal pain
  2. Adnexal tenderness
  3. Cervical motion tenderness
- Additional criteria (at least one is recommended to enhance diagnostic specificity) include the following:
  1. Oral temperature >38.3°C
  2. Abnormal cervical discharge
  3. Elevated ESR or CRP
  4. Documented cervical infection with gonorrhea or chlamydia

TREATMENT
- May be treated as inpatient or outpatient.
- Criteria for hospitalization:
  1. If surgical emergencies such as appendicitis cannot be excluded.
  2. If patient fails an outpatient regimen.
  3. If patient is pregnant.
  4. In cases of severe illness (i.e., toxic appearance, vomiting, and so on).
  5. If patient has underlying immune deficiency.

6. Although little data support the hospitalization of all adolescents with PID, this practice should be strongly considered for education and improved compliance with medical therapy.
- Inpatient regimens:
  1. Regimen A: Cefoxitin 2 gm IV q 6 hours plus doxycycline 100 mg orally or IV q 12 hours (if suspect TOA consider adding clindamycin or metronidazole).
  2. Regimen B: Clindamycin 900 mg IV q 8 hrs plus gentamycin 1.5 mg/kg q 8 hours (if suspect TOA consider adding ampicillin).
  3. May consider switching to oral antibiotics following 24–48 hours after clinical improvement to complete a 14-day course.
- Outpatient regimens:
  1. Regimen A: Ofloxicin 400 mg (or levofloxicin 500 mg) plus metronidazole 500 mg bid for 14 days.
  2. Regimen B: Ceftriaxone 250 mg IM as single dose plus oral doxycycline 100 mg bid for 14 days.
- Follow-up: Follow-up in 48–72 hours after outpatient treatment or 1 week after hospitalization.

COMPLICATIONS
- Increased likelihood of future ectopic pregnancy.
- Increased likelihood of tubal infertility.
- Increased likelihood of chronic abdominal pain.

HUMAN PAPILLOMA VIRUS (HPV)

CLINICAL PRESENTATION
- Papular lesions (i.e., warts) on the vaginal, anal, rectal, or cervical mucosa.
- May be asymptomatic or may present with itching, bleeding, or pain).

DIAGNOSIS
- Typically by inspection alone for papular lesions.
- Evidence of HPV may be noted on cytologic sampling of cervix or anal mucosa.

TREATMENT
- Goal is removal of external or visible warts.
- May use one of the following modalities depending on location of lesions and extent of disease:
  1. Patient-applied topicals:
     a. Podofilox 0.5% solution or gel
     b. Imiquimod (Aldara) 5% cream
  2. Provider administered methods:
     a. Cryotherapy with liquid nitrogen
     b. Trichloroacetic acid (TCA)
     c. Surgical or laser excision
- Treatment does not eradicate the HPV.

- Treatment may or may not decrease infectivity.
- Cervical changes noted on PAP smear should be followed at routine intervals.

COMPLICATIONS
- Increased risk of cervical cancer, particularly with HPV serotypes 16 and 18.
- Increased risk of anal cancer has been noted in HIV+ individuals.

HUMAN IMMUNODEFICIENCY VIRUS (HIV)

- See separate chapter on HIV.

DISORDERS OF EATING

OBESITY

GENERAL CONSIDERATIONS
- Obesity and its complications are reaching epidemic proportions in the U.S.
- Multifactorial disease with lifestyle factors (i.e., sedentary lifestyle) thought to be major contributors to increased prevalence of disease.

DIAGNOSIS
- Use body mass index (BMI=kg/m^2) for clinical screening.
- Growth curves from the National Center for Health Statistics now include BMI percentiles (Fig. 10-4).
- BMI >95% for age indicates obesity; between 85th and 95th percentiles indicates at-risk of obesity.

CLINICAL MANIFESTATIONS AND COMPLICATIONS
- Medical:
  1. Can cause complications involving many organ systems including the following:
     a. Endocrine disorders
     b. Hypertension
     c. Dyslipidmias
     d. Sleep apnea
     e. Gall bladder disease
     f. Orthopedic problems
  2. Associated with two endocrine disorders seen with some frequency in adolescents:
     a. PCOS
     b. Diabetes Mellitus Type 2 (DM-2)
  3. PCOS:
     a. Affects 5–10% of women of reproductive age
     b. Although clinical presentation is variable, it is diagnosed by presence of the following:
        i. Menstrual irregularities
        ii. Androgen excess

c. Other common clinical features are the following:
   i. Hirsutism
   ii. Acne
   iii. Obesity (>50% of patients)
   iv. Hyperlipidemia
   v. Acanthosis nigricans
   vi. Anovulatory infertility
4. DM-2:
   a. Affects over 15 million adults and is considered an emerging problem in adolescents
   b. Diagnosis:
      i. Fasting blood glucose greater than or equal to 126 mg/dL.
      ii. Symptoms of diabetes and a random blood glucose greater or equal to 200 mg/dL.
      iii. May use an oral glucose tolerance test for patients at high-risk but who do not meet the above diagnostic criteria.
      iv. Psychosocial: Negative self-image and/or decreased self-esteem may result from societal value placed on being thin. Particularly problematic for female adolescents.

TREATMENT STRATEGIES
- Success traditionally defined as reduction of body weight by 5–10% with prevention of further weight gain.
- Many interventions may achieve the initial weight loss, but treatment failures more common with the maintenance aspects of therapy.
- Primary strategies combine: Nutritional Interventions, and Physical Activity.
- Additional therapies:
  1. Antiobesity medications:
     a. Not generally recommended for adolescents
     b. Include a variety of different classes of medications:
        i. Appetite suppressants
        ii. Fat-absorption inhibitors
        iii. Energy expenditure enhancers
        iv. Insulin sensitizers (i.e., Metformin)
  2. Surgery:
     a. Currently not recommended for adolescents

ANOREXIA NERVOSA (AN) AND BULIMIA NERVOSA (BN)

EPIDEMIOLOGY
- Incidence of AN and BN have increased steadily in past 30 years.
- Females outnumber males 10:1.
- More common in upper and middle socioeconomic groups.
- Runs in families (i.e., familial basis).

2 to 20 years: Girls
Body mass index-for-age percentiles

NAME _____

RECORD # _____

Date	Age	Weight	Stature	BMI*	Comments

*To Calculate BMI: Weight (kg) ÷ Stature (cm) ÷ Stature (cm) x 10,000
or Weight (lb) ÷ Stature (in) ÷ Stature (in) x 703

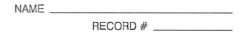

Published May 30, 2000 (modified 10/16/00).
SOURCE: Developed by the National Center for Health Statistics in collaboration with
the National Center for Chronic Disease Prevention and Health Promotion (2000).
http://www.cdc.gov/growthcharts

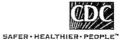

SAFER · HEALTHIER · PEOPLE™

FIG. 10-4 National Center for Health Statistics BMI percentiles.

2 to 20 years: Boys
Body mass index-for-age percentiles

NAME _____

RECORD # _____

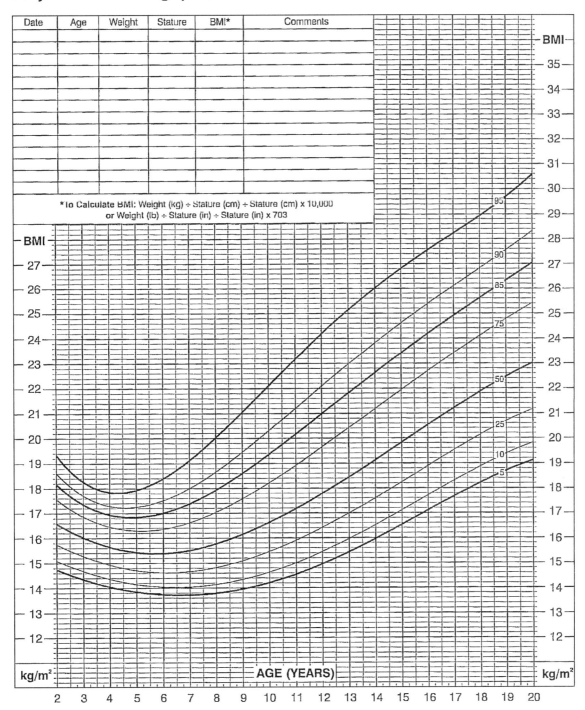

*To Calculate BMI: Weight (kg) ÷ Stature (cm) ÷ Stature (cm) x 10,000
or Weight (lb) ÷ Stature (in) ÷ Stature (in) x 703

Published May 30, 2000 (modified 10/16/00).
SOURCE: Developed by the National Center for Health Statistics in collaboration with
the National Center for Chronic Disease Prevention and Health Promotion (2000).
http://www.cdc.gov/growthcharts

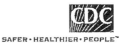

SAFER·HEALTHIER·PEOPLE™

FIG. 10-4   *(Continued)*

DIAGNOSIS (DSM-IV CRITERIA)
- AN:
  1. Two physiologic criteria:
     a. 15% below minimally normal body weight-for-height and age.
     b. Primary or secondary amenorrhea >3 cycles.
  2. Two psychologic criteria:
     a. Intense fear of gaining weight or becoming fat.
     b. Distorted body image.
  3. Two subtypes:
     a. Restricting.
     b. Binge/purge.
- BN:
  1. Two eating binges (i.e., rapid consumption of large amounts of food in a short period of time) per week for at least 3 months.
  2. During food binges, a fear of not being able to stop eating.
  3. Regularly engaging in self-induced vomiting, use of laxatives, diuretics, or rigorous dieting or fasting to prevent weight gain.
  4. Overconcern with body image and weight.

CLINICAL MANIFESTATIONS
- History:
  1. See diet questions in HEADDSS assessment (page 34).
- Review of systems/physical examination:
  1. Weight loss
  2. Abdominal pain
  3. Constipation
  4. Cold intolerance
  5. Hair loss or thinning (lanugo)
  6. Fatigue, weakness
  7. Delayed puberty or short stature
  8. Stress fractures
  9. Dental caries
  10. Calluses on hands/fingers
  11. Vital sign abnormalities (i.e., hypothermia, bradycardia, hypotension)

TREATMENT
- Outpatient treatment requires a multidisciplinary approach:
  1. Nutritional support
  2. Psychologic intervention for patient and family
  3. Medical management
- Consider hospitalization for the following:
  1. Unstable vital signs:
     a. Orthostasis
     b. Severe bradycardia (heart rate <50 bpm)
     c. Severe hypotension (<80/50)
     d. Severe hypothermia
  2. Severe malnutrition (i.e., loss >25% of ideal body weight)

3. Electrolyte abnormalities
   a. Low potassium
   b. Low phosphorous
4. Acute food refusal
5. Suicidality
6. Failure of outpatient therapy

COMPLICATIONS
- Affects multiple organ systems including the following:
  1. Cardiovascular:
     a. Dysrhythmias
     b. Electrocardiographic abnormalities
     c. Cardiac failure
  2. Fluid and electrolyte:
     a. Hypochloremic metabolic alkalosis
     b. Hypokalemia
     c. Elevated blood urea nitrogen
     d. Abnormalities of calcium and magnesium
  3. Gastrointestinal:
     a. Constipation
     b. Delayed gastric motility
     c. Esophagitis
     d. Mallory-Weiss tear
     e. Parotid hypertrophy
  4. Dermatologic:
     a. Acrocyanosis
     b. Brittle hair and nails
  c. Lanugo
     d. Russell sign (calluses over knuckles)
     e. Peripheral edema
  5. Endocrine:
     a. Growth retardation and short stature
     b. Delayed puberty
     c. Amenorrhea
     d. Low thyroid hormone (T3)
     e. Hypercortisolism
  6. Skeletal:
     a. Osteopenia
     b. Stress fractures
  7. Hematologic:
     a. Bone marrow suppression
     b. Low sedimentation rate
  8. Psychologic:
     a. Depression
     b. Increased risk of suicidality

SUBSTANCE USE/ABUSE

DEFINITIONS

- The occasional use of certain substances such as cigarettes, alcohol, or marijuana may be viewed as "normative" given the large proportion of youth who report

having used them. In otherwise normal and healthy adolescents, this may be viewed as *experimentation*.
- *Abuse:* The consumption of cigarettes, alcohol, or other drugs leading to destructive risk-taking behavior negatively affects school, family, or developmental functioning.
- *Dependence:* A psychologic and/or physiologic craving for a drug or other substance.

EPIDEMIOLOGY

- Alcohol and cigarettes are the most commonly reported drugs of use in adolescents.
- Marijuana is the most commonly reported illicit drug used.
- The prevalence of substance use varies by gender, age, geographic region, race/ethnicity, and other demographic factors.
- In general, males are more likely than females to use illicit drugs.
- In general, adolescent substance use has steadily increased over the past 50 years.
- Since the mid-1990s there has been a slight decrease in the prevalence of adolescents' cigarette, alcohol, and marijuana use and an increase in the prevalence of club drugs (i.e., ecstasy) and anabolic steroid use.

DIAGNOSIS

- Ask all adolescents screening questions (see HEADSS assessment) during the annual health maintenance examination.
- The clinician needs to determine:
  1. Patterns of use (i.e., at school, with peers, used alone, by family members).
  2. Level of dysfunction (i.e., school absenteeism, relationship difficulties, problems with the legal system).
  3. Degree of psychiatric or behavioral problems (i.e., anxiety, depression).
- Physical examination findings may include the following:
  1. Weight loss
  2. Skin changes (i.e., track marks)
  3. Mucosal injury (i.e., nose bleeds)
  4. Cough or compromise in pulmonary function
  5. Seizures
  6. Changes in behavior or mood
- Although alcohol detection/levels are determined by blood, the use of most illicit substances is determined by urine screen (i.e., marijuana, amphetamine, and so on).
- Use urine or blood screens only in select circumstances and almost always with the informed consent of the adolescent.

- Stages of adolescent substance use:
  1. Stage 1: Experimentation
  2. Stage 2: To relieve stress
  3. Stage 3: Regular use
  4. Stage 4: Dependence

TREATMENT

- Adolescents in stages 1 and 2 can typically be managed in outpatient settings.
- Adolescents in stages 3 and 4 may require more intensive treatment including hospitalization or placement in a rehabilitation program.
- In the United States, there is a general paucity of adolescent-specific substance abuse treatment programs or facilities.

SPECIFIC AGENTS

TOBACCO
- Most commonly used drug.
- Use among adolescents correlates with use by parents and peers.
- Average adolescent smoker starts by age 12 or 13; regular use usually occurs within 2 years.
- Physically addictive (i.e., nicotine), with greater than 90% of adolescent smokers continuing into adulthood.
- Long-term complications of use kill more people in the United States each year than all other substances/drugs combined.
- Rates of smoking in female adolescents are equal to, if not more than male adolescents.
- Smokeless tobacco (i.e., snuff) is predominantly a male activity.
- Treatment: Smoking cessation programs may include the following:
  1. Nicotine replacement systems (i.e., patch, gum, spray)
  2. Medications (i.e., buproprion)
  3. Community-based counseling

ALCOHOL

- >50% of high school students report a lifetime use alcohol.
- Central nervous system depressant that produces euphoria, disorientation, grogginess, and impaired short-term memory.
- Abuse among adolescents correlates with abuse by parents and peers.
- Male adolescents tend to use and abuse alcohol more than females.
- May see an escalating pattern of use from beer to wine to hard liquor.

- Alcohol consumption contributes to thousands of adolescent deaths and injuries each year, in large part because of drinking and driving and other nonautomotive accidental deaths.

MARIJUANA

- Most prevalent illicit drug, in some communities used more frequently than alcohol.
- Smoked in cigarettes, pipes, or cooked in food.
- Active ingredient is tetrahydrocannabinol (THC).
- Psychopharmacologically similar to alcohol in that it impairs short-term memory, motor coordination, and produces mental cloudiness.
- Metabolized in liver and stored in body fat that results in a long half-life making urine screening for recent use (i.e., last 7–14 days) possible.
- Therapeutic effects include reduced nausea in patients undergoing chemotherapy and reduction of intraocular pressure in patients with glaucoma.

STIMULANTS

- Most frequently used stimulants are amphetamine and cocaine.
- In recent years there has also been an increase in the use of methamphetamine (i.e., crystal meth, ice) especially in the western and southwestern U.S.
- Typically used by snorting, smoking, oral ingestion, or absorption across other mucous membranes (i.e., rectal, vaginal).
- Very physically addictive.
- Multiple central nervous system and cardiovascular effects.
- Clinical effects are dose related and include tachycardia, agitation, insomnia, anorexia, hypertension, and seizures.
- Chronic use can lead to cerebral vascular accidents and psychosis.

ECSTASY (METHYLENEDIOXYMETHAMPHETAMINE)
- Hallucinogen similar to mescaline.
- Classic "club" or "designer" drug.
- Being used with increasing frequency among adolescents.
- Predominantly situational or episodic use (i.e., dances or raves).
- Clinical effects include euphoria, a heightened sensual awareness, and decreased social inhibition.
- Adverse effects: nausea, jaw clenching, anxiety, tachycardia, psychosis, depression, and menstrual irregularities.

GHB (GAMMA HYDROXY BUTYRATE)
- Central nervous system depressant.

ANABOLIC STEROIDS
- Used by adolescents to enhance physical appearance or athletic performance.
- Taken orally, transdermally, or through intramuscular injection.
- Effects include acne, gynecomastia, increased muscle mass, breast pain, testicular atrophy, and menstrual irregularities.
- Psychologic effects include rage/aggression, depression, mood swings, and alterations in libido.
- Oral ingestion associated with hepatic dysfunction.
- Use in early adolescents may result in growth failure because of premature epiphyseal closure.

REFERENCE

Daniel WA, Paulshock BZ. A physician's guide to sexual maturity rating. *Patient Care* 1979;13:129.

11 DRUG THERAPEUTICS IN INFANTS AND CHILDREN
Thomas P. Green

PEDIATRIC CLINICAL PHARMACOLOGY

- The understanding of a few pharmacologic principles will improve a pediatric practitioner's ability to write rational drug prescriptions that are likely to produce the desired effects and avoid toxicity. This chapter outlines the most basic of these principles. The same knowledge is also used to analyze the reasons for an unintended lack of efficacy or untoward drug effect.

DRUG RECEPTOR-EFFECT COUPLING

- A rational framework for understanding the relationship between drug dosing and effect is based on the concept of drug receptor-effect coupling. This principle states that drug effect will occur when drug molecules interact with specific drug receptors at a specific site of action. An important corollary to this idea is that drug disposition is governed by processes that are separate from those that relate to drug effect, and it is ultimately only the drug concentration at the site of action that influences drug effect. Understanding drug disposition involves separate considerations of absorption, distribution, and clearance of a drug, all of which, in turn, determine the concentration of drug at its receptor and site of action at any point in time. The interaction of the drug with its receptor produces the drug effects, both therapeutic and toxic.

DRUG DISPOSITION (PHARMACOKINETICS)

ABSORPTION
- Drugs are given by any of several routes of administration with corresponding effects on the amount and time course of drug that eventually reaches its site of action.
- Intravenous administration is generally regarded as complete, instantaneous absorption, although even homogeneous distribution within blood volume only occurs over several circulation times through the body.
- Other parenteral forms of drug administration may produce nearly complete absorption of the administered dose, but the appearance of drug in plasma will occur more slowly. Drugs administered by subcutaneous and intramuscular routes are examples. Peak drug concentrations are determined by the relative rates of drug absorption on one hand and drug elimination on the other. In the case of intramuscular administration, absorption is determined by factors such as blood flow to the site, the vehicle in which the drug is administered, and the solubility of the drug and vehicle.
- Oral administration and gastrointestinal absorption is the most common method of systemic administration of drug. The fraction of drug administered that reaches the central circulation is usually less than 100% and, in some circumstances, may be only a small and variable fraction of the dose given. Factors that favor absorption in the gastrointestinal track include molecular weight, ionization, and lipid solubility. Factors in various locations within the stomach and small intestine may favor or inhibit absorption. These include the local pH (which may in turn determine the ionization state of the drug) and the presence of active transport mechanisms.
- Drugs pass through the intestinal epithelium and reach the portal circulation, moving toward the liver. For a few drugs, metabolism may occur immediately before reaching the central circulation (first pass effect), thereby adding to the appearance of low absorption.
- Some routes of drug administration are intended to produce high local concentrations of drug, but minimal or no systemic absorption. Examples include inhalational, intrathecal, and topical routes. Each

route is characterized by unique considerations that are beyond the scope of this text.

DISTRIBUTION
- Even while absorption is occurring, drug is beginning to equilibrate with other tissues. The movement of drug between plasma space and other tissue spaces (interstitial space, intracellular space of various tissues) is influenced by many drug factors such as molecular size, ionization, and avidity for protein binding. Other tissue factors are also important, including pH, presence of binding molecules, active and passive transport mechanisms, and bulk fluid movement.
- Distribution volume (V_d) is a theoretical space, the volume of which is calculated based on the ratio of the dose administered (D) and the maximum concentration achieved, C.

$$V_d = \frac{D}{C}$$

- The distribution volume does not correspond to any anatomic compartment, but the relative constancy of this relationship is useful in predicting drug concentrations achieved after doses are administered.
- Complex pharmacokinetic modeling often will identify more than one distribution volume (compartment). Consideration of these additional compartments is necessary for precise research studies, but is not particularly practical for simple clinical predictions.
- Protein binding is an important factor in drug distribution, in that drug bound to protein is generally not available for distribution to other tissues. Factors that decrease protein binding (acidosis, competing drugs or other molecules, hypoproteinemia) may increase free drug and thereby increase the concentration of free drug at the site of action.

METABOLISM
- Most commonly, metabolism is considered in the context of deactivating a drug and facilitating drug elimination. Drug metabolites are excreted because they are generally large ionized molecules that are poorly reabsorbed from bile or urine.
- Metabolism occurs prominently in the liver, where the cytochrome P450 system is particularly important; however, drug metabolism for some compounds occurs in other organs as well, notably the kidney and lungs.
- In some circumstances, the metabolites of active drugs may themselves have activity. In particular, patients with liver or hepatic insufficiency may accumulate higher levels of partially active metabolites, which may account for exaggerated effects in this setting.
- Uncommonly, activation of a drug by metabolism may be required to generate the active form of the drug.

ELIMINATION

- The kidney and the hepatobiliary system are responsible for eliminating many drugs and their metabolites.
- The kidney may clear a drug by glomerular filtration, especially if the drug is small and nonprotein bound. Ionization will decrease the likelihood of reabsorption in the renal tubule. Other drugs may be cleared in the kidney by active tubular secretion, particularly if they are weak acids or bases.
- Clearance is a pharmacologic concept that describes the efficiency of the processes that eliminate the active forms of a drug from the body. Although the concept is analogous to the familiar concept of creatinine clearance that is used to measure renal function, the term applies to all forms of elimination. Clearance is expressed as the ration of the rate of elimination to the simultaneous serum or plasma concentration.

$$Cl = \frac{\text{elimination rate}}{C}$$

- Clearance is most conveniently measured at steady state.
- Half-life can be thought of as the time required, after drug administration has ceased and all distribution has equilibrated, for the concentration of drug in plasma (or the total amount of drug in the body) to fall from one level to half that level. While the half-life is often considered a measure of elimination, both clearance (Cl) and V_d effect half-life in a similar way:

$$t_{1/2} = \frac{0.693V_d}{Cl}$$

- For reasons beyond the scope of this chapter, the half-life is also important in determining the rate at which a drug administered at regular intervals reaches steady state. A drug administered at a dose (D) given at regular intervals (t) will have a dose rate of D/t. It will reach a steady state concentration related to its clearance as given in the following relationship

$$C_{ss} = \frac{D/t}{Cl}$$

- Following the initiation of regular dosing, the drug will reach 50% of this steady state concentration in one half-life, 75% of this concentration in two half-lives (half-way between 50 and 100%), 87.5% of this concentration in three half-lives (half-way between 75 and 100%), and so on. In fact, when a drug concentration is at steady state with one dosing regimen, a subsequent dosage rate change will result in a movement toward the new steady state by the same rule—one-half of the way there in one half-life, and so on.

THE INFLUENCE OF BIOLOGIC MATURATION

- Normal biologic development and maturation influences every aspect of drug disposition. Continuous changes in the functional status of every organ system and in body composition correspondingly alter how drugs are handled by the body.

GASTROINTESTINAL FUNCTION

- Hydrochloric acid secretion is very low at birth and increases slowly in the first year of life. Consequently, there may be little degradation of acid sensitive agents (e.g., penicillin), but a lack of ionization effects that normally favor the absorption of weak acids (e.g., phenobarbital).
- Bile acid secretion is also decreased in the first year of life compared with adult values.

DISTRIBUTION VOLUME

- The ratio of surface area to body weight decreases continuously throughout childhood from very high values at birth to adult values in adolescence. This may be particularly important for topical agents. In addition, the large surface area leads to larger insensible losses and fluid balance that changes more rapidly.
- The fraction of body weight represented by water decreases continuously throughout childhood, beginning with about 80% body weight at birth. This leads to a larger distribution volume for water soluble drugs. As total body water volume decreases with age, there is a marked decrease in the proportion of what is in the extracellular space (equal to intracellular fluid volume at birth).
- The avidity of protein binding also changes for many drugs, usually increasing with age. This may be because of changes in blood proteins or to the presence of endogenous compounds that compete for binding sites.

ELIMINATION

- Hepatic metabolic capacity increases with age, whether normalized for body weight or body surface area; however, studies that have normalized metabolic capacity for estimated hepatic weight have shown similar values in children and adults.
- Renal function increases sharply in the first year of life, both with respect to glomerular filtration and tubular function. Peak glomerular filtration (and corresponding renal clearance of many drugs) is highest

in early childhood and declines slightly in adolescence toward adult values.

DETERMINING APPROPRIATE DOSING REGIMENS

- Based on the foregoing, dosage regimens for drug administration in children must take patient age, size, and coexisting pathophysiologic state into account. In the future, knowledge of genetic factors, for example, those producing variations in rate of hepatic drug metabolism, may be considered. Widely available references exist with drug specific information on these and other factors. A few general principles are noteworthy to assist in this process.
- Extrapolation of adult dosing regimens to pediatric patients based on body size is fraught with pitfalls, based on the considerations above; however, some general guidelines can be offered when recommendations from pediatric trials are not available (Ritschel and Kearns, 1999)

$$\text{if } V_d < 0.3 \text{L/kg} = \frac{\text{Infants surface area (m}^2)}{1.73 \times \text{adult dose}}$$

or

$$\text{if } V_d > 0.3 \text{L/kg} = \frac{\text{Infants body weight (kg)}}{70 \text{kg} \times \text{adult dose}}$$

- These guidelines have been proposed to guide the selection of the drug dose for infants. Determining the dosage interval is a separate process that requires an estimation of the drug clearance relative to the adult value. The dosage interval should be increased proportionately to the decrease in clearance relative to the adult value

$$\text{dosage interval} = \text{adult dosage interval}$$
$$\times \frac{\text{infant drug clearance}}{\text{adult drug clearance}}$$

- Therapeutic drug monitoring can provide supportive information to design appropriate drug regimens or test whether desired blood levels are being achieved. In some circumstances, defining a pharmacokinetic profile can be performed by administering a drug dose and sampling serum drug concentrations. Precise timing of the samples is required and the data are analyzed using principles outlined above. The assistance of a clinical pharmacologist or pharmacist is wise for designing the drug regimen.
- Alternatively, the periodic sampling of serum drug concentrations can be a useful adjunct to improve efficacy

and avoid toxicity. There must be a strong basis for anticipating the likely drug levels as well as a clear understanding of the relationship between drug levels and effect or toxicity in order to choose appropriate sampling times. For example, for some drugs, efficacy is related to middose levels at steady state (anticonvulsants) whereas for other drugs, toxicity may be related to predose levels after several doses have been administered (aminoglycosides). Therapeutic drug monitoring is not useful for all drugs, even those with significant interindividual kinetic variability and toxicity. For example, monitoring of drug effect with coumadin is more useful clinically than the measurements of the drug levels themselves.

DEVELOPMENT OF DRUGS FOR USE IN CHILDREN

- Prior to 1994, there was very little effort to specifically develop information for the rational use of drugs in children. Ethical considerations prevented drug testing in children prior to full testing in adults. Once drugs were approved for use in adults, there was no financial or other incentives for pharmaceutical companies to proceed with drug testing in children. Most drugs were not labeled for, or Food and Drug Administration (FDA) approved for, use in children, and usually carried a disclaimer to this effect. As a result, children were Therapeutic Orphans. While drugs could be used in children by physician order, in most cases there was insufficient research to identify safety, efficacy, toxicity, and appropriate dosing.
- In 1994, the FDA Pediatric Rule went into effect. This allows labeling of drugs for pediatric use based on adult data, provided additional data are developed to demonstrate similar metabolism, safety, and efficacy in children and adults. At the same time the National Institutes of Health established the Pediatric Pharmacology Research Unit Network to promote study of drugs in children. This network of pediatric pharmacologists at medical schools and academic health centers began coordinating research that has improved understanding of pediatric clinical pharmacology and improved rationale drug use in children.
- Further incentives for pediatric drug development occurred in 1997. The FDA Modernization Act provided for 6-month extension of patent exclusivity if drugs are tested in children. This proved to be a substantial financial incentive for pharmaceutical companies to develop drug data in children for commonly used drugs.
- To provide data to guide and support the use of less commonly used drugs which were off patent, the Best

Pharmaceuticals for Children Act took effect in 2002. This empowered the NIH to support pediatric research on FDA-selected drugs where such data did not exist (Pediatric Off-Patent Drug Study).

REFERENCE

Ritschel WA, Kearns GL (eds.). *Handbook of Basic Pharmacokinetics*, 5th ed. Washington, DC: American Pharmaceutical, 1999, pp. 318–319.

BIBLIOGRAPHY

Chiampus EK, Franzenburg A, Sovcik J. *Children's Memorial Hospital Formulary Handbook*, 5th ed. Hudson, OH: Lexi-Comp, 2001.

Kearns GL, Abdel-Rahman SM, Alander SW, Blowey DL, Leeder JS, Kauffman RE. Developmental pharmacology—drug disposition, action, and therapy in infants and children. *N Engl J Med*

EMERGENCY PEDIATRICS

Elizabeth C. Powell, Section Editor

12 RESUSCITATION

Sally L. Reynolds

- The child in arrest is one of the most challenging situations a physician can face. Causes of arrest in the prehospital setting include sudden infant death syndrome, submersion or other trauma, and respiratory illness. As most arrests in children result from respiratory conditions and shock, evaluation and support of the airway is a priority. Intact survival of an out of hospital cardiac arrest is less than 2%.
- The American Heart Association Guidelines (2000) for Pediatric Advanced Life Support of a child in cardiopulmonary arrest are the following:
  1. Begin cardiopulmonary resuscitation (CPR)
  2. Call for help
  3. Call 911 if out of the hospital
  4. Call "code" if in the hospital

CARDIOPULMONARY RESUSCITATION

- Open the airway using the jaw thrust technique. Place your fingers under the lower jaw at the angle of the mandible and move the jaw up and out. Avoid moving the cervical spine in trauma patients.
- Give two breaths—1–1½ seconds per breath. Use a bag-valve-mask (BVM) if it is available. Make sure the chest wall rises with each breath. If the chest wall does not rise, ventilation is probably not effective.
- When using the BVM, use the thumb and index finger to hold the mask on the face and place the third, fourth, and fifth fingers on the lower jaw to help keep the airway open. The bag volume should be at least

450–500 mL. BVM ventilation is much easier with two people: one holds the mask on the face and opens the airway while the other squeezes the bag. If an oxygen source is available, the bag should be attached to it so as to provide oxygen to the patient.

- Check for a pulse (carotid pulse in a child and brachial pulse in an infant). If there is no pulse, or heart rate <60 with poor perfusion, begin chest compressions. The compression rate is 100/minute and the depth one-third to half of the estimated anterior-posterior diameter of the chest. For infants (<1-year-old) compressions can be delivered using two fingers from one hand, or with the thumbs from both hands circling the chest. For children 1–8 years old, use the heel of one hand over the lower half of the sternum, between the nipple line.
- For children older than 8 years old, use the heel of one hand, with the other hand on top of it.
- Check the femoral pulse during compressions to evaluate their effectiveness. Rescue breaths at a frequency of 10–12 breaths/minute should accompany compressions. Place the child on a cardiac monitor to check for ventricular arrhythmias (ventricular fibrillation/ventricular tachycardia).
- In the prehospital setting, if the child is ≥8 years old attach an automatic external defibrillator (AED). An estimated 5–15% of children will be in ventricular fibrillation or ventricular tachycardia and should be defibrillated. In all other children, continue CPR. Observe for chest wall rise with BVM ventilation and check for the presence of a femoral pulse with chest compressions.
- Vascular access options in the child in cardiopulmonary arrest include intraosseous (IO) as well as venous access. Because peripheral or central venous access may be difficult to obtain in pediatric patients, IO line placement is the most efficient method of

vascular access for most care providers. Use an intraosseous needle or a bone marrow needle. The preferred site is the proximal anterior tibia. Alternate sites include the distal femur in infants, the distal tibia in older children, or above the medial malleolus in the adolescent.

- Insert the needle at a 90° angle with a twisting motion as it is difficult to push the needle through the bone cortex. A sudden decrease in resistance suggests the bone cortex has been penetrated and placement is proper. The needle should appear to stand upright. Try to aspirate bone marrow; in some properly placed lines this is not successful. Flush with 10–20 mL of fluid, watching for infiltration around the needle or into the soft tissue. Give fluids, drugs, and blood products through the IO.

- Epinephrine is the drug therapy for asystole. The dose is 0.01 mg/kg (0.1 mL/kg of 1:10,000 concentration) by IV or IO. If access cannot be obtained quickly and an endotracheal tube is in place, use it to administer the epinephrine. The endotracheal dose is 0.1 mg/kg (0.1 mL/kg of the 1:1000 solution), diluted in 3–5 mL of normal saline. In clinical trials, high dose epinephrine (0.1 mg/kg), recommend in the past by the American Heart Association, failed to show a benefit when compared with standard dose epinephrine. It is no longer recommended, but it is an acceptable alternative if there is no response to standard dose epinephrine.

- While establishing vascular access, plan for intubation. Most children can be ventilated and oxygenated effectively with a BVM, thus the intubation can be planned. Assemble equipment including laryngoscope and blade, endotracheal tubes (the estimated correct size, and a half size larger and smaller), stylet, suction (for the mouth and the endotracheal tube), tape, and a CO_2 detection device. Endotracheal tube size can be determined using a length based resuscitation tape, or estimated using the formula [(16+ age years) ÷4].

- The vocal cords of a child are anterior and superior, thus different from an adult. Intubation drugs are not needed in asystolic children. Bag ventilation should be performed until the endotracheal tube is placed, and between placement attempts as needed.

- There is potentially great harm from a misplaced endotracheal tube. Methods to confirm endotracheal tube placement include visualization of the tube going through the vocal cords, listening for equal breath sounds, observing for chest wall rise, and use of a CO_2 detector. Six ventilations should be given before the CO_2 detector is read. If the tube has been misplaced in the esophagus, the six ventilations wash out the residual CO_2 remaining there so that the reading is valid. A change in color from purple to tan confirms the endotracheal tube is in the trachea. In cases of severe circulatory collapse, CO_2 is not delivered to the alveolar space; therefore, a CO_2 detector on a correctly placed endotracheal tube may not change color.

- The endotracheal tube may be used to administer drugs during resuscitation including *l*idocaine, *e*pinephrine, *a*tropine, and *n*arcan (mnemonic LEAN).

- If initial efforts to restore a perfusing rhythm fail, consider *h*ypoxemia, *h*ypovolemia, *h*ypothermia, and *h*yperkalemia, *h*ypokalemia, or other metabolic problems (the four Hs) as well as *t*amponade, *t*ension pneumothorax, *t*oxins/drugs, and *t*hromboembolism (the four Ts).

- Most victims of cardiopulmonary arrest will not be successfully resuscitated. Unless it is a hypothermic arrest (submersion in icy water) the child is unlikely to survive if there is no response with bag ventilation and two doses of epinephrine. For any patient in whom reversible causes of arrest have been addressed, if after 30 minutes of resuscitation a perfusing rhythm has not returned, the resuscitation may be stopped. The clinician should then direct their attention to the family.

- Clinical care of children who are successfully resuscitated includes management of ventilation, perfusion, and temperature. Although resuscitation is performed using 100% oxygen, the concentration of oxygen should be adjusted so as to maintain normal O_2 (as monitored by pulse-oximetry or blood gas analysis). Patients should not be routinely hyperventilated. While this had been recommended in the past, recent data suggest it should be limited to patients with signs of cerebral herniation or suspected pulmonary hypertension. Maintain perfusion with fluids or pressors as needed. Treat hyperthermia, allow mild hypothermia (≥34°C).

- Sudden deterioration of an intubated patient suggests that one of the following may have occurred: *d*isplacement of the endotracheal tube, *o*bstruction of the endotracheal tube, *p*neumothorax, or *e*quipment failure (mnemonic *dope*). If the child is on a ventilator, hand bag and confirm that the oxygen source is functioning property.

SHOCK

- Shock is defined as inadequate perfusion of the vital organs. In compensated shock signs of poor perfusion are present but the blood pressure is in the normal range; in decompensated shock the patient is also hypotensive. An assessment for shock includes heart rate, which may be either fast or slow, blood pressure, and systemic perfusion, which includes mental status, skin color, and temperature, urine output, and pulses. Pulses that are palpable centrally but not peripherally, pulses that are thready or bounding, and capillary refill greater than 2 seconds all suggest shock. The respiratory rate is usually increased.

- Hypovolemic shock is most common. It results from volume loss (vomiting, diarrhea, hemorrhage, fluid redistribution to the extravascular space) or poor intake. Children in hypovolemic shock are usually lethargic, cool, and have poor pulses, a narrow pulse pressure, and capillary refill >2 seconds.
- Distributive shock, caused by sepsis or anaphylaxis, is the inappropriate distribution of blood volume resulting from systemic vasodilation. The pulse pressure is wide and the extremities are cool.
- Cardiogenic shock results from inadequate myocardial function, which limits stroke volume and cardiac output. There is a narrow pulse pressure, an increased work of breathing, and other signs of heart failure including pulmonary edema, peripheral edema, and an enlarged liver.
- Shock is treated initially by managing the airway and breathing (100% oxygen), establishing vascular access (IV or IO), and administering an IV fluid bolus (20 mL/kg 0.9 NS over 5–10 minutes). After the fluid bolus, reassess. If perfusion is improved and the shock is thought to be hypovolumic in origin, give an additional 20 mL/kg 0.9 NS over 20–30 minutes. In trauma patients, if compensated shock is present after 40 mL/kg of 0.9 NS, consider transfusing blood.
- If cardiogenic shock is suspected, fluid volume should be decreased, pressors should be considered, and the child may require intubation earlier in the treatment course. If septic shock is the provisional diagnosis, pressors should also be considered early in the resuscitation. Children in anaphylactic shock should be given epinephrine (IM), corticosteroids and an H_1 or H_2 receptor blocker.
- In children with compensated shock (poor perfusion, normal blood pressure) after IV fluids, consider therapy with one of the following: dobutamine or dopamine (2–20 µg/kg/minute), epinephrine (0.05–3 µg/kg/minute), inarinone (load, 0.75–1 mg/kg over 5 minutes, may repeat up to 3 mg/kg; infusion, 5–10 µg/kg/minute) or milrinone (load, 50–75 µg/kg; infusion, 0.5–0.75 µg/kg/minute). Inarinone or milrinone are particularly well-suited for children in cardiogenic shock.
- In children with decompensated shock (hypotensive), consider dopamine (up to 20 µg /kg/minute), followed by epinephrine (0.1–1 µg /kg/minute), or norepinephrine (0.1–2 µg /kg/minute).
- If a ventilated patient suddenly develops signs of shock, consider tension pneumothorax.

BIBLIOGRAPHY

American Heart Association. Available at http://www.american-heart.org

American Heart Association Guidelines 2000 for Cardiopulmonary Resuscitation and Emergency Cardiovascular Care, 2000.

Hickey RW, Cohen DM, Strausbaugh S, et al. Pediatric patients requiring CPR in the pre-hospital setting. *Ann Emerg Med* 1999;33:174–184.

Mogayzel C, Quan L, Graves JR, et al. Out of hospital ventricular fibrillation in children and adolescents: causes and outcomes. *Ann Emerg Med* 1995;25:492–494.

Ronco R, King W, Donley DK, et al. Outcome and cost at a children's hospital following resuscitation for out-of-hospital cardiopulmonary arrest. *Arch Pediatr Adolesc Med* 1995; 149:210.

Schindler MD, Bohn D, Cox PN, et al. Outcome of out-of-hospital cardiac and respiratory arrest in children. *N Engl J Med* 1996; 335:1473–1479.

Sirbaugh PE, Pepe PE, Shook JE, Kimball KT, Goldman MJ, et al. A prospective, population-based study of the demographics, epidemiology, management, and outcome of out-of-hospital pediatric cardiopulmonary arrest. *Ann Emerg Med* 1999; 33:174–184.

Teach SJ, Moore PE, Fleischer GR. Death and resuscitation in the pediatric emergency department. *Ann Emerg Med* 1995; 25:799–803.

13 INJURY EPIDEMIOLOGY AND PREVENTION
Elizabeth C. Powell

BACKGROUND

- Unintentional injuries are the most frequent cause of death among United States children 1-year-old or older. In 2000, more than 12,441 children and adolescents younger than 20 years old died. The number of unintentional injury deaths is greater than the sum of the next nine causes of death. Causes include motor vehicle collisions, falls, and burns; unintentional injury deaths do not include suicide, homicide, and deaths resulting from child abuse. The magnitude of this problem explains why the prevention of unintentional injuries among youth is a public health priority.
- Nonfatal injuries outnumber injury fatalities for most categories. There are estimated to be 188 emergency department visits for injury and 10 hospital admissions

for each injury death. Unintentional injuries are second to pneumonia as the most frequent cause for hospital admission among youth younger than 15 years old. Injuries account for an estimated 13,562,000 emergency department visits each year. The most common reasons for an injury-related emergency department visit include falls, being struck against a person or an object, and lacerations.

- Rates of unintentional injury deaths have fallen in the past 20–30 years for almost every cause of injury. Injury prevention research and advocacy efforts have contributed to this decline.

- Injury is defined as the transfer of energy (kinetic, thermal, radiation, or chemical) to the human body, resulting in tissue damage. Drowning and choking/asphyxiation are also classified as injuries, although energy transfer causes neither of these mechanisms.

- Injuries are not accidents, which are perceived as "chance" events that are unexpected or random. Rather, many factors that elevate or reduce the likelihood of sustaining a particular injury have been identified. Injury prevention involves identifying and changing the factors related to injury including the agent (i.e., motor vehicle) and the environment (i.e., highway design), as well as modifying individual behaviors (i.e., child safety seat use).

- The causes of childhood injuries are diverse, and the relative importance of different injury mechanisms varies among children and adolescents, depending on their age, gender, and other sociodemographic characteristics. Males, and children living in poverty, appear to be at greater risk for injury-related mortality.

INJURY MECHANISMS AND PREVENTION STRATEGIES

- Motor vehicle trauma is the most common cause of serious and fatal injury. It is the most frequent cause of injury death for most ages, and it accounted for 7842 deaths among children and adolescents in 2000. Common subcategories of motor vehicle injuries include occupant (drivers and passengers) and pedestrian injuries. While teens ages 15–19 years old have the highest death rates from motor vehicle occupant injuries, this mechanism also accounts for the majority of injury deaths among younger children (5–14 years old).

- Motor vehicle crashes result in a significant number of nonfatal injuries, an estimated 730,697 in 2001. Most (69%) were treated in the emergency department only and did not require hospital admission. Adolescents are disproportionately represented in motor vehicle fatalities. The most important risk factors associated with an increased likelihood of a crash involving teenage drivers include driver inexperience in challenging conditions (night, inclement weather, high-volume traffic) and alcohol use. Male teens are more likely to be involved in alcohol-related fatalities than are females.

- Factors associated with the incidence of injury when a crash occurs are often associated with structural features of the car and the availability and use of safety equipment by the occupant. Safety improvements to cars (safety glass, collapsible steering columns, padded interiors, and frame design) have helped to reduce death from frontal impact collisions. A current concern is risk associated with height and weight mismatch between vehicles, such as in collisions involving sport utility vehicles. Limited data suggest that passengers in the smaller vehicle are at a greater risk of injury, particularly from side impact collisions.

- Frontal air bags, a means of automatic occupant protection, are now present in the majority of U.S. automobiles. They reduce the risk of death or serious injury in frontal collisions among adolescents and adults. For infants and children, passenger air bags appear to pose harm, particularly when they are unrestrained and in low-speed crashes. Placing infants and children under the age of 12 in the rear seat is the best protective action against air bag injury.

- The other main protective factor against occupant injury is the use of a child restraint device or seat belt. Car seats are very effective in decreasing the risk of both serious and fatal injury for young children. It is estimated that restraints are used for 85% of infants and 60% of toddlers. A greater challenge is the proper restraint of children who are 4 years old and 40 lb who have outgrown their toddler seats. Children 4–8 years old and between 40 and 80 lb should use a belt positioning booster seat. This maximizes the effectiveness of the restraint and prevents injuries related to improper restraint fit. Belt use by teens is lower than in other age groups. In addition to legislation, education programs to increase seat belt use by preteens and teens are needed.

- Pedestrian injuries, motor vehicle collisions with a person, accounted for more than 1000 deaths among children in 2001. Mortality rates are similar across age groups. There have been steady declines in pedestrian injury deaths in the past 20–30 years, attributed by many to decreasing exposure. Nonfatal injuries, an estimated 66,418 in 2001, far exceed fatal injuries, and include brain injuries, abdominal trauma, and fractures.

- Risk factors for pedestrian injuries include male gender, age 5–9 years old with its developmental limitations, traffic volume and speed, poverty, and the absence of play space. Preschool and school age children are struck when they dart out into the street, mid-block, between parked cars. Toddlers between the ages of 1 and 2 years old are more likely to be injured in nontraffic conditions, in places such as driveways.

- Bicycle-related deaths are usually associated with collisions with motor vehicles. Most are the result of head trauma. There are modest age-specific differences; death rates are highest among those 10–14 years old. Bicycle crashes result in many nonfatal injuries; more than 340,000 injured youth were treated in the emergency department in 2001. Injuries include head trauma, fractures, and skin and soft tissue injuries.
- Use of a protective helmet is effective in reducing head injury, even in collisions with motor vehicles. Helmet use may also help to prevent face injury. Although bicycle helmets have been proven effective in reducing risk for head injuries, the rate of helmet use is low among many youth.
- Drowning is the most common type of injury death among children younger than 5 years old, and the second most common cause for adolescents, accounting for an estimated 1314 child and adolescent deaths each year. Children younger than 5 years old have the highest drowning rate of any age group, including adults. Drowning has a high case fatality rate, as approximately half of children and adolescents treated for a submersion injury will die.
- Drowning is unique in that survival can largely be predicted by the clinical appearance of the child at the time of arrival to the emergency department. The child who is spontaneously breathing will likely survive, whereas the child who requires resuscitation in the emergency department will either die, or survive with extreme disability from brain damage because of prolonged lack of oxygen.
- The circumstances of drowning are age-specific and usually involve poor supervision: infants often drown in bathtubs, while toddlers and young children frequently fall into a body of water such as a pool, a lake, or a river. Adolescent drowning commonly involves males in open water; alcohol is implicated in some cases. As treatment outcomes of drowning victims are poor, prevention strategies are critical. Additional work is needed to better understand risk and protective factors for drowning.
- Fires and burns are implicated in 600–700 deaths among children each year. Young children are at particular risk in residential fires, as they are less able to escape. Most house fire deaths are from smoke inhalation; when burns do occur, the injuries can be quite severe, resulting in prolonged hospitalization and lifelong scars.

- Poverty is strongly associated with risk of death in a house fire. Most occur during the winter months. Faulty heating systems and cigarette smokers in the household are major risk factors for igniting a house fire. A functioning smoke detector reduces the risk of death in a residential fire by 50–70%.
- Most nonfatal burn injuries resulting in admission to the hospital (an estimated 176,492 in 2001) were from scalds from water or hot liquids (coffee, tea, soup). Tap water scalds have become less common since the late 1970s, when this burn injury mechanism was first recognized. Public education and legislation to lower the preset temperatures of hot water heaters contributed to this decline. Other approaches to scald burn injury prevention are limited.
- Falls account for almost 3 million emergency department visits and an estimated 180 deaths each year. Most fatal falls among younger children result from a fall from two or more stories, often from upper-level windows. Falls are the most frequent cause of injury hospitalization among children. Most infant falls are from furniture or infant equipment. Falls among older children usually involve physical activities, play equipment, or sports.
- The severity of a fall-related injury is a function of the height, the characteristics of the impact surface, and the weight of the victim. Injuries from falls range from minor to severe, and include soft tissue injuries, fractures, abdominal injuries, and head trauma.
- Firearm injuries are the second most common cause of death among teens, and accounted for more than 3000 deaths in 2000. Although most firearm deaths are homicides or suicides, among young children a significant number are unintentional. Not all unintentional firearm injuries are fatal: there are estimated to be up to five nonfatal unintentional injuries for every unintentional injury fatality.
- Access to firearms in the home appears to be a risk factor for unintentional firearm injuries. The circumstances often involve playing with loaded guns, resulting in a child shooting himself or another person. Almost one-third of families with children store their guns loaded. In these homes, an estimated 10–20% of guns are stored both unlocked and loaded.
- Child access prevention laws hold the owner of an unsecured gun responsible for injuries inflicted with that gun as a result of a person younger than 18 years of age gaining access to it. States with such laws have been observed to have lower rates of intentional firearm injuries among children. The American Academy of Pediatrics (AAP) currently recommends the best way to prevent firearm injuries is to remove guns from environments in which children live and

play. If that is not possible, guns should be stored unloaded, with the ammunition stored separately, and locked.

- Suffocations are the most common cause of injury death in the first year of life, and account for an estimated 500 deaths among children each year. Like drowning, the mechanism is oxygen starvation, resulting in organ injury and death. Although details of the suffocation events are often lacking, circumstances of suffocation include entrapment of the head and neck in cribs, and choking on food or other objects. It is possible that the actual number of infant suffocations is lower than reported, as some cases of sudden infant death may be mislabeled as suffocation.

- Although a more significant issue in the past, poisonings have become a relatively infrequent cause of injury death among children, and are a fraction of the rates observed among adults. The circumstances of unintentional poisoning deaths include the ingestion of a medication, or the ingestion or inhalation of a commercial product. Poisonings and their management are discussed more comprehensively in Section IV.

- For each poisoning death, approximately 50 per year, an estimated 40,000 ingestions are reported to poison control centers. The substances most commonly ingested among children younger than 6 years old are cosmetics, cleaning substances, analgesics, plants, and cold/cough preparations. An estimated 2–5% of ingestions result in moderate or severe effects. An important protective factor for medication related poisonings is the storage of medication in a childproof container.

- Despite impressive reductions in unintentional childhood injury deaths in the past 25 years, injury remains the most important cause of death and disability for children and adolescents today. Widespread adoption of existing technologies (restraints in motor vehicles, bicycle helmets) could prevent many more injury deaths. Further work is needed to define important risk and protective factors for specific injuries, as well as to determine the characteristics of populations at highest risk.

BIBLIOGRAPHY

Centers for Disease Control and Prevention, National Center for Injury Prevention and Control, National Electronic Injury Surveillance System All Injury Program. Available at http://wonder.cdc.gov.

Centers for Disease Control and Prevention, National Center for Injury Prevention and Control, US injury mortality statistics. Available at http://wonder.cdc.gov.

Centers for Disease Control and Prevention. Update: fatal air bag-related injuries to children-United States, 1993–1996. *MMWR*, 1996;45:1073–1076.

Erdmann TC, Feldman KW, Rivara FP, et al. Tap water burn prevention: the effect of legislation. *Pediatrics* 1991;88:572–577.

Mallonee S, Istre GR, Rosenberg M, et al. Surveillance and prevention of residential fire injuries. *N Engl J Med* 1996; 335:27–31.

Powell EC, Jovtis E, Tanz RR. Incidence and circumstances of non-fatal firearm-related injuries among children and adolescents. *Arch Pediatr Adolesc Med* 2001;155:1364–1368.

Rivara FP. Pediatric injury control in 1999: where do we go from here? *Pediatrics* 1999;103:883–888.

The Future of Children, Unintentional Injuries in Childhood, vol. 10, no. 1. The David and Lucile Packard Foundation, 2000, pp. 23–52.

Thompson RS, Rivara FP, Thompson DC. A case-control study of the effectiveness of bicycle safety helmets. *N Engl J Med* 1989;320:1361–1367.

U.S. Department of Transportation, National Highway Traffic Safety Administration. Children-Traffic safety facts 1996. Washington, DC: U.S. Department of Transportation, NHTSA. Available at http://www.nhtsa.dot.gov.

Weil DS, Hemenway D. Loaded guns in the home: analysis of a national random survey of gun owners. *JAMA* 1992; 267:3033–3037.

Weiss HB, Mathers LJ, Foruoh SN, Kinnane JM. *Child and Adolescent Emergency Department Visit Databook.* Pittsburgh, PA: Center for Violence and Injury Control, Allegheny University of the Health Sciences, 1997.

14 TRAUMA SYSTEMS AND TRAUMA CARE

Elizabeth C. Powell

TRAUMA SYSTEMS

BACKGROUND

- Emergency medicine services systems were derived from military experiences, which demonstrated that appropriate triage, timely transport, and prehospital care improved patient survival. Community-level research suggested outcomes for cardiac patients were improved through better systems for emergency response. Federal legislation, the Emergency Medical Services Systems Act of 1973, provided resources to state and local governments for the implementation of comprehensive emergency medical services systems. Efforts to insure that the specific needs of children were integrated into the system resulted in legislation establishing the Emergency Medical Services for Children program in 1984.

- Emergency medicine services systems vary from community to community and state to state; however, most emergency medicine services programs have similar structures: medical direction, prehospital transport agencies, dispatch, communications, protocols (prehospital triage, prehospital treatment, transport, and transfer), receiving facilities, specialty care units, quality assurance, and public education. It is important that pediatric primary care providers become familiar with the resources in the communities where they practice so as to provide the best care for their patients.

TRAUMA CARE

BACKGROUND

- In caring for a child with traumatic injury, the highest priority is in recognizing and treating life-threatening injuries.

CLINICAL EVALUATION

- The *primary survey* and initial resuscitation, occurring simultaneously, take place in the first 5–10 minutes after the child has arrived to the emergency department. The aim of the primary survey is to identify and treat life-threatening disorders. The *secondary survey*, a repeat assessment that follows, includes a more comprehensive physical examination and diagnostic testing. Children with serious injuries require continual monitoring and ongoing reassessment.
- The primary survey and resuscitation includes the following:
  1. Airway with cervical spine protection: Ascertain airway patency. If the airway is obstructed, perform a chin lift or jaw thrust maneuver, and clear the airway of foreign bodies. Maintain the cervical spine in neutral position (manual immobilization when establishing the airway, use of appropriate devices after the airway is established.)
  2. Breathing and ventilation: Determine the rate and depth of respirations and assess oxygenation (pulse oximeter). Administer high concentrations of oxygen, and ventilate with a bag-valve-mask device if the child is not breathing or if respiratory efforts are inadequate. If there is clinical evidence of a tension pneumothorax (unilateral absence of breath sounds, respiratory distress, tachycardia), perform needle thoracostomy. Place an occlusive dressing on sucking chest wounds.

  3. Indications for endotracheal intubation in the trauma patient are the following:
     a. Inability to ventilate by bag-valve-mask methods.
     b. The need for prolonged control of the airway.
     c. Prevention of aspiration in a comatose child.
     d. The need for controlled hyperventilation in patients with serious head injuries.
     e. Flail chest with pulmonary contusion.
     f. Shock unresponsive to fluid administration.
  4. Circulation and hemorrhage control: Attach a cardiac monitor. Apply direct pressure to sites of external hemorrhage and identify potential sources of internal hemorrhage. Assess perfusion (skin color, quality and rate of pulse, and blood pressure). Place an IV catheter and initiate volume resuscitation with 20 mL/kg of crystalloid. Obtain blood for type and crossmatch, hematologic analysis, and other laboratory tests as indicated. Insert a nasogastric tube and place a Foley catheter.
  5. Disability (brief neurologic examination): Assess the pupils and determine the level of consciousness.
  6. Exposure: Completely undress the patient; prevent hypothermia.
  7. Adjuncts to the primary survey and resuscitation include radiologic studies (AP chest, AP pelvis, lateral cervical spine x-rays), and monitoring of exhaled CO_2 with an appropriate device (intubated patients).
- The secondary survey and management includes the following:
  1. A brief history of the mechanism of injury and patient information (allergies, current medications, past illness, time of last meal, injury event).
  2. Complete head to toe physical examination.
  3. Consider the need for, and obtain diagnostic tests as the patient's condition warrants. These include additional spinal x-rays, extremity x-rays, computed tomography (CT) of the head, chest, abdomen, and/or spine, and others (i.e., contrast urography, angiography).
- Perform continuous monitoring of vital sign and intermittent reassessment of the patient. Provide information to the family about their child's condition. After the child is stabilized, the parents should be permitted at the bedside.

BIBLIOGRAPHY

Advance Trauma Life Support Student Course Manual, 6th ed. Chicago, IL: American College of Surgeons, 1997.

U.S. Department of Health and Human Services, Health Resources and Services Administration, Maternal and Child

Health Bureau. *Five-year Plan: Emergency Medical Services for Children, 2001–2005.* Washington, DC: Emergency Medical Services for Children National Resource Center, 2000.

15 BURNS
Elizabeth C. Powell

BACKGROUND

- Burns are a common cause of death among U.S. children. Burn injuries can be associated with respiratory compromise, sepsis and renal failure; long-term scarring may contribute to functional impairment and psychosocial distress.
- Scald burns, frequent among toddlers and preschoolers, are usually partial thickness burns resulting from a hot liquid spill. House fires are the most lethal burn injury circumstances: injury from inhalation of smoke and other toxic gasses contributes to the injury from the burn.

PATHOPHYSIOLOGY

- Burns cause local inflammatory changes, increased vascular permeability with fluid and protein shifts, tissue edema, and in severe cases, hypoperfusion and shock.

CLINICAL FEATURES

- Burns are described in terms of location, depth, and body surface area involved. The body surface area that is burned is expressed as a percent of the total body surface area.
  1. First-degree burns involve only the epidermis. The skin is red, but there are no blisters and sensation is preserved.
  2. Second-degree burns are partial thickness burns of the dermis, in which the dermal appendages are preserved. The skin has blistering and edema and it is painful, tender, and sensitive to air. The most frequent causes are scalds and flame burns.
  3. Third-degree burns are full-thickness injuries. There is damage to the dermis and dermal appendages, and in some cases to the subcutaneous tissues. The skin appears white or leathery or charred, and the skin surface is dry and nontender. The burn circumstances include prolonged exposure to fire or hot liquids.
  4. The body surface area involved in a burn is important in considering treatment and disposition. In children, there is much age-specific variation in the proportion of body surface area made up by anatomic parts (head, trunk, arms, and legs). Use of a child-specific burn chart is helpful to estimate the percent of the body surface area involved.

MANAGEMENT

- Victims of house fires should be managed in the same manner as a child with traumatic injury, with attention to the airway, and a primary and secondary survey to identify and treat all injuries. Specific attention should be directed to the burn, with an estimation of the extent and depth. Laboratory analysis should include serum electrolytes, renal function tests, urinalysis, and carboxyhemoglobin levels.
- For patients with localized burns from scalds, the size and depth of the burn is estimated. The child should be assessed for pain, and analgesic medications given as needed.
- Restoration or maintenance of tissue perfusion is a priority. The Parkland formula, which has widespread use, is isotonic crystalloid, 4 mL/kg/%BSA over the first 24 hours after the injury. Half of the fluid is given in the first 8 hours, and the remainder is given over 16 hours. Maintenance fluids are added to this. As any fluid resuscitation formula provides only an estimate of fluid need, monitoring hourly urine output is helpful to confirm that fluid resuscitation is adequate.
- Inpatient management. Children with partial thickness burns involving more than 10% of the body surface area or full-thickness burns involving more than 2% of the body surface area or partial thickness burns of the face, hands, feet, or perineum should be admitted.
- Outpatient management. Children with partial thickness burns involving less than 10% of the body surface area or full-thickness burns involving less than 2% of the body surface can be considered for outpatient management if family support appears adequate and there are no other significant injuries or underlying illness. Minor burns are soaked in sterile saline and gently cleaned. The treatment of blisters is controversial—some advocate debridement while others recommend all blisters be left intact. Topical antibiotics and a sterile dressing should be applied. Close follow-up is recommended to insure the wound is healing.

Bibliography

Advance Trauma Life Support Student Course Manual, 6th ed. Chicago, IL: American College of Surgeons, 1997.
Strange G (ed.). *Advanced Pediatric Life Support,* 3rd ed. Dallas, TX: American College of Emergency Physicians, 1998.

16 SHAKEN INFANT
Danny E. Leonhardt

EPIDEMIOLOGY

- Head injury is the most common cause of death from child physical abuse and is the leading cause of trauma-related death in children. Infants and young children comprise the most vulnerable population, with head trauma accounting for an estimated 45–58% of infant homicides. Most victims are younger than 9 months old.
- While social stressors such as poverty, domestic violence, and substance abuse are identified as risk factors for injury, abusive head trauma occurs among all racial and socioeconomic groups. Crying, which increases between 6 weeks and 4 months of age, is often cited as a precipitating factor in abusive head injury; this age range coincides with the peak incidence of abusive head trauma. Male caretakers are the most common perpetrators, followed by babysitters of both sexes, and biologic mothers.
- Mortality from abusive head trauma is estimated to be 13–30%. Survivors often suffer devastating long-term effects including cortical blindness, seizure disorder, profound mental retardation, and quadriplegia.

CLINICAL FEATURES

- In 1972 Caffey described a constellation of findings in infants: subdural and retinal hemorrhages without any indication of external head trauma. He proposed that the injuries were the result of violent shaking, and described the findings as the whiplash-shaken infant syndrome, later referred to as the shaken baby syndrome (SBS).
- The mechanism of injury in SBS is recurring cycles of acceleration-deceleration of the head, creating shearing forces that result in intracranial and retinal hemorrhages. The infant is usually held by the thorax, facing the perpetrator, and is shaken back and forth with its arms, legs, and head moving in a whiplash action.
- The act of shaking which leads to abusive head injuries is so violent that individuals observing the incident would recognize it as dangerous to the child. Anyone with adult strength or size can be a perpetrator. Although most victims are less than 1 year of age, abusive shaking has been reported to occur in children as old as 5.
- While shaking itself is known to cause serious or fatal injuries, shaking is often accompanied by the impact of the child's head against an object or hard surface. Therefore, it has been suggested that terms such as shaken impact syndrome or abusive head trauma may more accurately describe the full range of injuries.
- The clinical signs of severe abusive head injury often occur immediately after the injury event. These signs vary from nonspecific symptoms such as vomiting, decreased feeding, and fussiness, to lethargy, seizures, apnea, and death. Signs of external injuries are often subtle or absent: a bulging fontanel, localized swelling, or minor bruising may be the only appreciable signs of trauma.
- When skull fractures are present, there is frequently swelling over the fracture site; however, the absence of swelling does not exclude a skull fracture, particularly if the fracture was sustained shortly before the infant was brought to medical attention.
- The characteristic features of abusive head trauma are intracranial injury, retinal hemorrhages, and skeletal injuries. While any of these clinical diagnoses may be present in a case of abusive head trauma, it is not necessary for all to be present to confirm the diagnosis of abuse.
- Intracranial injuries include subdural hemorrhage, subarachnoid hemorrhage, cerebral edema/infarction, parenchymal laceration/contusion, diffuse axonal injury, and parenchymal hemorrhage. Subdural hemorrhage results from the tearing of bridging veins in the subdural space because of the shearing forces caused by shaking. Although subdural hemorrhage may be unilateral, it is more commonly bilateral, occurring along the convexity or within the interhemispheric fissure.
- Retinal hemorrhages are found in approximately 80% of shaken infants. The mechanism of retinal hemorrhages is thought to be similar to that of intracranial injuries, a consequence of abnormal shearing forces inside the eye and orbit. They may be unilateral; their presence in the absence of intracranial hemorrhage is rare. The description of the retinal hemorrhages in terms of number, type, location, and distribution is essential for the diagnosis of abusive head injury. A pattern of multiple hemorrhages, distributed

throughout the retina, is virtually diagnostic for abusive head injury. Retinal hemorrhages cannot be used to determine the age of the injury.

- Although any skeletal fracture can be the result of child abuse, the three types of fractures most commonly associated with abusive head trauma are skull, rib, and long bone metaphyseal fractures.
- While a relatively small proportion of skull fractures are a result of child abuse, the incidence of skull fracture in victims of abusive head trauma ranges from 9 to 30%. No type of skull fracture is diagnostic for abusive head injury; however, abuse should be strongly suspected when a child with a story of minor head trauma presents with complex, multiple, diastatic, or occipital skull fractures.
- Rib fractures are the most common fractures present in children with abusive head injury, accounting for up to 50% of all fractures. Rib fractures can be single, multiple, unilateral, or bilateral. Most rib fractures are located posteriorly; however, fractures can occur on any point along the rib arc. Most rib fractures in abusive head trauma are a consequence of direct compression from the perpetrator's hands grasping the child face-to-face by the thorax during a violent shaking event.
- Long bone metaphyseal fractures or classic metaphyseal lesions (CML) are highly specific for child abuse. Metaphyseal fractures most commonly affect the tibia, femur, and proximal humerus and often have a "corner" or "bucket-handle" appearance in radiographic studies. CMLs can occur from acceleration/deceleration forces during shaking or through forceful twisting or pulling of an infant's limb.

DIAGNOSIS/DIFFERENTIAL

- Intracranial hemorrhage in children from causes other than trauma is rare. It is best to assume that all unexplained intracranial hemorrhage in children is because of trauma. Many children with intracranial injury present with a history of a short fall. Although falls are the most frequent cause of injury in children, they are an infrequent cause of death or severe head injury.
- When abusive head trauma is suspected, it is important to obtain a history from each of the child's caretakers. It is often necessary to interview each caretaker separately, focusing on specific questions regarding feeding difficulties, vomiting, irritability, or other subtle neurologic signs.
- It is important to construct a time line of when the child's symptoms began, and when the caretakers last saw the child behaving normally. The history may be inaccurate, as caretakers sometimes misrepresent or

claim to have no knowledge of the cause of the child's symptoms.

- A thorough physical examination should be conducted by a physician familiar with the signs of injuries associated with abusive head trauma. The examination should focus on cutaneous signs of physical abuse, such as bruises, localized scalp swelling, burns, or marks suggestive of trauma. Cutaneous injuries should be documented in the medical record, and when possible, photographed for later reference.
- A head computed tomography (CT) should be obtained in any child in whom abusive head trauma is suspected. The head CT should be performed without IV contrast and should be assessed using bone and soft tissue windows. The head CT allows the clinician to identify injuries that may require urgent intervention, including subarachnoid hemorrhage, mass effect, and large extraaxial hemorrhage.
- An MRI of the head should also be obtained whenever abusive head trauma is diagnosed or suspected. The MRI is more sensitive than head CT for the definition and evaluation of subdural hemorrhage, shear injuries, contusions, and secondary hypoxic-ischemic injury.
- A skeletal survey (skeletal films of the hands, feet, long bones, skull, spine, and ribs) should also be obtained in any infant in whom abusive head trauma is suspected. Acute fractures may be missed on the initial survey, and visualized only on healing (1–2 weeks after the injury event). A skeletal survey should be repeated 2 weeks after the initial evaluation in selected cases in which abuse has been verified or remains a possibility.
- Bone scintigraphy (bone scan) is complementary to the skeletal survey in the evaluation of children in whom abuse is suspected. It is more sensitive than plain films in the assessment of rib fractures, acute nondisplaced long bone fractures, and subperiosteal hemorrhage, as it identifies early periosteal reaction not apparent on plain films.
- An ophthalmology consult should be obtained in all children in whom abusive head trauma is suspected. The pupils should be pharmacologically dilated and the eyes examined by a physician with experience in ophthalmologic signs of child abuse.
- Children suspected of being victims of abusive head injury should undergo laboratory evaluation for abdominal trauma, including liver and pancreatic enzymes and urinalysis. Laboratory findings in abusive head trauma may include abnormal clotting studies (PT and PTT) and anemia. The slight elevation in these clotting studies is an effect of brain injury and should not be confused with a clotting disorder. If abnormal, these studies can be repeated in 2–3 weeks to confirm or refute suspicion of a clotting disorder.

EMERGENCY DEPARTMENT CARE AND DISPOSITION

- The evaluation for possible abusive head trauma needs to be undertaken in any infant or young child where the nature or extent of the injuries is inconsistent with the history given by the caretaker.
- Health care workers are mandatory reporters for child abuse and neglect. A report to child protective services and police should occur when suspicion arises that an injury has been inflicted.
- After a report is made to child protective services, the child needs to remain in a safe environment until the medical evaluation and investigation is completed. This may require admitting the child to the hospital until an alternative safe place can be arranged.

BIBLIOGRAPHY

Alexander RC, Levitt CJ, Smith WL. Abusive head trauma. In: Reece RM, Ludwig S (eds.). *Child Abuse: Medical Diagnosis and Management*. Philadelphia, PA: Lippincott Williams & Wilkins, 2001, pp. 47–80.

American Academy of Pediatrics, Section on Radiology. Diagnostic imaging of child abuse. *Pediatrics* 2000; 105:1345–1348.

American Academy of Pediatrics, Committee on Child Abuse and Neglect. Shaken Baby Syndrome: Rotational Cranial Injuries—Technical Report. *Pediatrics* 2001;108:206–210.

Caffey J. The whiplash-shaken infant syndrome: manual shaking by the extremities with whiplash-induced intracranial and intraocular bleedings, linked with residual permanent brain damage and mental retardation. *Pediatrics* 1974;54:396.

Kleinman PK. Head trauma. In: Kleinman PK (ed.). *Diagnostic Imaging of Child Abuse*. St. Louis, MO: Mosby, 1998, pp. 285–342.

Levin A. Retinal haemorrhage and child abuse. In: David T (ed.). *Recent Advances in Paediatrics*. London: Churchill Livingstone, 2000, pp. 151–219.

17 TOXICOLOGY

Suzan S. Mazor

INTRODUCTION

- The ingestion of a potentially poisonous agent is a common reason for a child to be seen in an emergency department. Young children (ages 1–5 years) have usually inadvertently ingested a small amount of a single toxic substance while adolescents have purposefully ingested larger amounts of one or more substances.
- The management is dictated by the clinical presentation: in the acutely ill patient first the airway, breathing, and circulation are stabilized by intubation, ventilation, venous access, and pharmacologic support. In the stable child the history and physical examination are completed, with emphasis on what and when and how much was ingested, and the management of the poisoning is directed to preventing absorption, enhancing excretion, and providing an appropriate antidote.
- Activated charcoal should be given to all patients with ingestions that are potentially toxic who present to the ED within 4 hours of the event unless the ingested substance is not absorbed by activated charcoal.
- Psychiatric assessment should be obtained for all patients with purposeful ingestions; education and poison prevention information should be provided to those with unintentional ingestions.

SUBSTANCE ABUSE

ETHANOL

EPIDEMIOLOGY
- Ethanol is found in beer, wine, and liquor. In addition, many household products, such as cologne, perfume, and mouthwash contain high concentrations (up to 70%) of ethanol.

PATHOPHYSIOLOGY
- Ethanol is a central nervous system (CNS) depressant and impairs gluconeogenesis. Children with ethanol poisoning are at risk for hypoglycemia because of limited glycogen stores that are rapidly depleted.

CLINICAL FEATURES
- Mild to moderate intoxication presents with nystagmus, ataxia, hypoglycemia, and CNS sedation. At higher levels, hypothermia, coma, and respiratory depression are seen.

DIAGNOSIS AND DIFFERENTIAL
- Serum ethanol levels are available in most hospital laboratories. The differential diagnosis includes head injury, hypoxia, hypoglycemia, sepsis and encephalopathy, as well as sedative-hypnotic drugs,

drugs of abuse and other alcohols (methanol, ethylene glycol and isopropyl alcohol).

EMERGENCY DEPARTMENT CARE AND DISPOSITION
• The care of patients with ethanol intoxication is supportive. Particular attention should be directed to serum glucose replacement and correction of hypothermia. Activated charcoal is not useful in managing an ethanol ingestion, and gastric lavage is helpful only in a recent ingestion (<30 minutes) of a large amount of ethanol.

VOLATILE SUBSTANCES (INHALANTS)

EPIDEMIOLOGY
• Volatile substances of abuse or inhalants include hydrocarbons, nitrites, anesthetic agents, and ketones. Solvent abusers use various techniques in order to induce a "high." "Sniffing" involves inhaling directly from an open container, "huffing" refers to inhaling through cloth soaked in solvent, and "bagging" is breathing the solvent's vapor from a plastic bag.

PATHOPHYSIOLOGY
• Inhalants are toxic to the central nervous system, either directly or because of hypoxia. Some inhalants sensitize the myocardium to catecholamines, resulting in an increased incidence of arrhythmia. Chronic toluene abuse impairs the ability of the distal renal tubule to excrete hydrogen ions, resulting in a distal renal tubular acidosis. Heavy, long-term inhalant abusers may have persistent neurologic deficits.

CLINICAL FEATURES
• A high level of suspicion is required to diagnose inhalant abuse. Residue or odor of the abused substance, such as paint residue, may remain on the victim or his clothing. Early intoxication produces euphoria, ataxia, and slurred speech; lethargy and confusion may follow. In severe cases, seizures or coma develops. Sudden death from dysrhythmia, caused by myocardial sensitization to catecholamines, has also been observed.
• Chronic inhalant abuse may present with muscle weakness, weight loss, hypokalemia, metabolic acidosis, and cognitive dysfunction. Nitrite abuse may oxidize the ferrous ion in hemoglobin, causing methemoglobinemia. Methylene chloride, found in paint stripper, is metabolized to carbon monoxide (CO) by the liver.

DIAGNOSIS AND DIFFERENTIAL
• The diagnosis of inhalant abuse should be suspected in adolescents who present with unexplained mental status changes, dysrhythmias, syncope, hypokalemia, or cardiac arrest. Nitrite abuse should be suspected in unexplained methemoglobinemia, and methylene chloride in unexpected carbon monoxide poisoning.

EMERGENCY DEPARTMENT CARE AND DISPOSITION
• The patient should be removed from the source of exposure and given supplemental oxygen. The skin is decontaminated with copious irrigation. If intubation is indicated, hyperventilation may speed elimination of the inhalant. Pressors and epinephrine should be used with extreme caution because of the possibility of a sensitized myocardium. Seizures and agitation should be treated with benzodiazepines.
• For patients with symptomatic methemoglobinemia, or levels >30%, methylene blue should be administered. Patients with elevated carboxyhemoglobin (COHb) levels should be treated with 100% oxygen.

COCAINE

EPIDEMIOLOGY
• Cocaine is one of the most commonly used drugs of abuse. It is well-absorbed following contact with mucous membranes and can be snorted, smoked, or injected intravenously.

PATHOPHYSIOLOGY
• The effects of cocaine are central nervous system stimulation, vasoconstriction, and local anesthesia. Cocaine has quinidine-like effects on conduction, causing QRS widening and QTc prolongation.

CLINICAL FEATURES
• Cocaine toxicity presents with a sympathomimetic toxidrome: signs and symptoms include hyperthermia, hypertension, tachycardia, tachypnea, altered mental status, seizures, mydriasis, diaphoresis, and hyperactive bowel sounds (Table 17-1). Ischemia of any vascular bed is possible. Arterial vasoconstriction may lead to myocardial ischemia and dysrhythmias. Cerebral infarcts and seizures can occur, as can skeletal muscle injury resulting in rhabdomyolysis.

DIAGNOSIS AND DIFFERENTIAL
• Urine toxicology screens generally measure benzoylecgonine, a cocaine metabolite. Cocaine abuse should be considered in the differential diagnosis of a

TABLE 17-1   Toxic Syndromes

Tricyclic antidepressants/anticholinergics

Hot as a hare—hyperthermic
Dry as a bone—dry mouth
Red as a beet—flushed skin
Blind as a bat—dilated pupils
Mad as a hatter—confused delirium

Sympathomimetics (cocaine, amphetamines)

Mydriasis
Tachycardia
Hypertension
Hyperthermia
Seizures

Narcotics

Miosis
Bradycardia
Hypotension
Hypoventilation
Coma

Cholinergics (organophosphates)

Diarrhea, diaphoresis
Urination
Miosis, muscle fasciculations
Bradycardia
Emesis
Lacrimation
Salivation

patient with the signs and symptoms of a sympathomimetic toxidrome.

EMERGENCY DEPARTMENT CARE AND DISPOSITION

- Benzodiazepines are used to control agitation and to treat hypertension. In addition, nitroprusside or phentolamine can be used to control blood pressure. Beta-blockers may exacerbate hypertension because of unopposed alpha-adrenergic stimulation, and should be avoided. Hyperthermia is treated with active cooling. Sodium bicarbonate may be useful in the management of ventricular arrhythmias. Intravenous hydration and urine alkalinization is recommended if rhabdomyolysis is present.

OPIOIDS

EPIDEMIOLOGY

- Opioids are used clinically for analgesia and anesthesia, and illicitly as drugs of abuse.

PATHOPHYSIOLOGY

- Opioids produce their effects by interacting with mu, kappa, and delta receptors in the central and peripheral nervous systems and in the gastrointestinal tract.

CLINICAL FEATURES

- The classic triad of opioid toxicity is central nervous system depression, respiratory depression, and miosis; however, multiple organ systems can be affected. Cardiovascular effects include hypotension as a result of histamine release and dysrhythmias, seen most often with propoxyphene toxicity. Flushing and pruritus are also caused by histamine release. Bronchospasm and noncardiogenic pulmonary edema have been observed.
- Mydriasis is caused by meperidine, dextromethorphan, or propoxyphene. Seizures may occur following ingestion of meperidine, propoxyphene, tramadol or because of coingestants.

DIAGNOSIS AND DIFFERENTIAL

- Although urine toxicology screens detect opioids, several of the synthetic opioids, methadone, hydrocodone, oxycodone, propoxyphene and fentanyl, are not detected routinely.
- The diagnosis of opioid overdose should be considered in any patient who presents with CNS depression, respiratory depression, and miosis (Table 17-1). The differential diagnosis is broad and includes sedative-hypnotic agents, ethanol, phenothiazines, central alpha$_2$ agonists, such as clonidine, organophosphates and carbamates, as well as nonmedication causes such as trauma, encephalopathy, hypoglycemia, hypoxia, and pontine hemorrhage.

EMERGENCY DEPARTMENT CARE AND DISPOSITION

- Supportive care, with attention to airway, breathing, and circulation, should be initiated. Activated charcoal is useful in managing oral ingestions. Naloxone, a synthetic opioid antagonist, should be administered in patients with poor respiratory effort or depressed mental status; the dose is 0.1 mg/kg with a maximum of 2 mg. Repeat doses can be administered if needed every 3 minutes to a total of 10 mg. Because the half-life of most opioids exceeds that of naloxone, the dose may need to be repeated, or a continuous infusion started.

AMPHETAMINES

EPIDEMIOLOGY

- Prescription amphetamines such as methylphenidate are commonly used in children. The synthetic amphetamines, ecstasy (methylenedioxymethamphetamine [MDMA]) and speed (methamphetamine) are illicit stimulants.

PATHOPHYSIOLOGY

- Amphetamines activate the sympathetic nervous system and stimulate adrenergic receptors, resulting in central nervous system stimulation.

CLINICAL FEATURES

- Mild amphetamine toxicity presents with dilated pupils, tremor, hyperreflexia, tachycardia, and tachypnea (Table 17-1). With more severe toxicity, hyperthermia, cardiac dysrhythmias, seizures, and rhabdomyolysis may occur. Hyponatremia is a rare but serious complication of ecstasy abuse, and is commonly seen after a large amount of water is ingested.

DIAGNOSIS AND DIFFERENTIAL

- A blood or urine toxicology screen is used to confirm amphetamine use. The screen may fail to detect the synthetic amphetamine analogs.
- Amphetamine abuse should be considered in patients with CNS stimulation, psychotic behavior, or hyperpyrexia.

EMERGENCY DEPARTMENT CARE AND DISPOSITION

- Management of amphetamine toxicity is supportive. Gastric lavage should be considered only in recent ingestions. Activated charcoal is useful in adsorbing ingested amphetamines.
- If hyperthermia is present, active cooling and IV fluids are recommended. Urinary alkalinization may be useful for rhabdomyolysis. Benzodiazepines should be administered to patients with seizures, agitation, or muscular rigidity.

IRON

EPIDEMIOLOGY

- Iron is widely used as a vitamin supplement, for prenatal supplementation, and for treatment of anemia. Although it is presumed by many to be harmless, iron is one of the most frequent causes of fatal poisonings in children.

PATHOPHYSIOLOGY

- Iron catalyzes free radical formation and oxidizes a wide range of substances, causing tissue damage and dysfunction, especially in tissues with high metabolic activity.

CLINICAL FEATURES

- The amount of iron ingested is calculated based on the concentration of elemental iron in the compound: ferrous fumarate contains 33% elemental iron, ferrous sulfate contains 20% elemental iron, and ferrous gluconate contains 12% elemental iron.
- There are five phases of iron toxicity:
  1. Phase one lasts 0–12 hours. Iron-induced gastrointestinal mucosal injury results in vomiting, diarrhea, abdominal pain, and gastrointestinal bleeding.
  2. Phase two, 6–24 hours, is known as a "quiescent" phase, although metabolic abnormalities and hypovolemia are often present. The clinician should not be reassured by the patient's benign clinical appearance in this stage.
  3. Phase three, the next 6–48 hours, is characterized by profound shock and metabolic acidosis. Coma, seizures, and renal and hepatic failure can occur. Aggressive intervention to support vital function is essential.
  4. In phase four, the following 2–4 days, iron's direct toxic effects on mitochondria cause fulminant hepatic failure.
  5. Phase five, which may last several weeks, is rare. It is gastrointestinal obstruction resulting from intestinal scarring.

DIAGNOSIS AND DIFFERENTIAL

- The serum iron concentration should be measured 2–6 hours postingestion, when it is expected to peak. Other useful laboratory tests include an arterial blood gas, electrolytes, and liver, renal, and coagulation profiles. Serum iron concentrations over 500 μg/dL indicate significant toxicity. Elevations of the white blood cell count and blood glucose are also suggestive of significant ingestion. An abdominal radiograph may show iron in the gastrointestinal tract, but a negative radiograph does not rule out iron ingestion.
- Iron overdose should be considered in any child who presents with shock, gastrointestinal hemorrhage, or an elevated anion gap metabolic acidosis.

EMERGENCY DEPARTMENT CARE AND DISPOSITION

- Support the airway and ventilate as necessary. Treat hypovolemic shock with IV fluids and blood products. Ipecac induced vomiting may be considered if it is initiated within a few minutes of the exposure. Consider gastric lavage if liquid or chewed tablets were ingested. Activated charcoal, which does not bind iron, is not recommended. Whole bowel irrigation with polyethylene glycol solution via nasogastric tube at a rate of 250–500 cc/hour is very effective in removing ingested tablets.
- Patients with serum iron >500 μg/dL, as well as those with lower serum iron levels associated with shock, gastrointestinal (GI) bleeding, or severe acidosis should be treated with IV deferoxamine

(10–15 mg/kg/hour infusion). Urine color change to "vin-rose" indicates formation of the chelated iron-deferoxamine complex.

• Deferoxamine can be discontinued after the serum iron level has decreased to normal. Prolonged (>24–48 hours) use of deferoxamine is associated with acute respiratory distress syndrome and *Yersinia enterocolitica* sepsis.

LEAD

EPIDEMIOLOGY

• Lead intoxication is the most common metal poisoning encountered today. Lead was used in residential house paint until 1977 and is still present in many older urban homes. Chronic ingestion of lead paint chips and dust are the primary routes of lead exposure in children.

PATHOPHYSIOLOGY

• Lead interferes with hemoglobin synthesis and cellular and mitochondrial function, resulting in multiorgan system effects.

CLINICAL FEATURES

• Central nervous system symptoms of lead toxicity include fatigue, malaise, headache, motor weakness, and encephalopathy. Gastrointestinal effects include constipation and crampy abdominal pain, known as lead colic. A hypochromic, microcytic anemia is commonly seen, and basophilic stippling is characteristic. Renal insufficiency or a Fanconi-like syndrome (aminoaciduria, glucosuria, hypophosphatemia, hyperphosphaturia) may also occur.

DIAGNOSIS AND DIFFERENTIAL

• A whole blood lead level is the most useful laboratory test. Ancillary tests include erythrocyte or zinc protoporphyrin, which is elevated in chronic lead poisoning. Radiographs of the wrists and knees may show "lead lines," dense bands visible in the distal metaphyseal ends of long bones, which are supportive of the diagnosis.

• The diagnosis of lead encephalopathy should be considered in any child with seizures or delirium. The abdominal pain of "lead colic" may be mistaken for appendicitis, renal colic, or peptic ulcer disease.

EMERGENCY DEPARTMENT CARE AND DISPOSITION

• Whole bowel irrigation with a polyethylene glycol solution, 35 mL/kg/hour by nasogastric tube may be helpful in removing lead in patients with lead visible in abdominal radiographs.

• Chelation should be instituted in patients with high lead levels. Options for chelation include IV calcium sodium edetate (ethylene diamine tetra acetate [EDTA]), IM dimercaprol (British-anti-Lewisite [BAL]), and oral succimer. EDTA and BAL are generally used for cases of severe poisoning, lead levels exceeding 70 µg/dL and/or encephalopathy, whereas succimer is used for milder cases. A specialist should be contacted regarding treatment options in lead-poisoned patients.

• The child's home environment should be evaluated and the lead removed. It may be necessary to hospitalize the child to provide a lead-free environment while this occurs.

SEDATIVE/ANALGESICS

ACETAMINOPHEN

EPIDEMIOLOGY

• Acetaminophen, a widely used drug found in many over-the-counter and prescription products, is the most common pharmaceutical agent involved in overdose.

PATHOPHYSIOLOGY

• In therapeutic doses, most acetaminophen is conjugated in the liver by glucuronidation and sulfation. A small percentage is metabolized by hepatic cytochrome P450 to *N*-acetyl-*para*-benzoquinoneimine (NAPQI). NAPQI is bound to glutathione and detoxified. In overdose, glucuronidation and sulfation mechanisms are saturated, and more acetaminophen is metabolized to NAPQI. Hepatic glutathione is rapidly depleted, and NAPQI begins to exert its hepatotoxic effects.

CLINICAL FEATURES

• An acute ingestion of 150–200 mg/kg in a child or 6–7 g in an adult is potentially hepatotoxic. Early after acute overdose of acetaminophen, symptoms are relatively minor or absent. Nausea, vomiting, and anorexia may be seen. Approximately 36 hours after ingestion, transaminase levels rise. Encephalopathy, metabolic acidosis, and an increasing prothrombin time suggest a poor prognosis.

DIAGNOSIS AND DIFFERENTIAL

• After an acute overdose, a 4-hour acetaminophen level should be obtained and plotted on the Rumack-Matthew nomogram (Fig. 17-1). The nomogram is not helpful in assessing the potential toxicity of chronic ingestions or ingestions of extended release products.

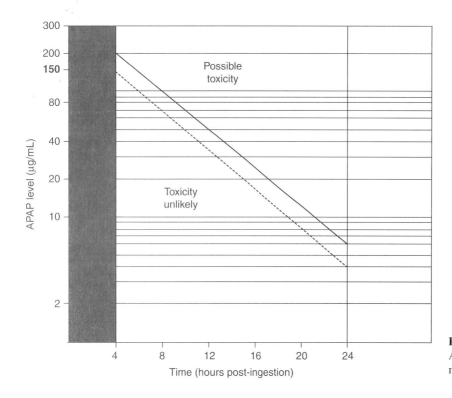

FIG. 17-1 Rumack-Matthew nomogram. APAP: *N*-acetyl-*para*-aminophenol (acetaminophen) (Rumack and Matthew, 1975).

- The differential diagnosis of acetaminophen toxicity includes viral hepatitis, other toxic hepatitides, and hepatobiliary disease.

EMERGENCY DEPARTMENT CARE AND DISPOSITION
- Activated charcoal is useful after acute overdose. It is recommended if the ingestion has occurred within 1–2 hours of presentation or if coingestants are suspected.
- In patients with an acetaminophen level above the "possible toxicity" nomogram line, *N*-acetylcysteine (NAC) oral or via nasogastric tube, is indicated. NAC prevents hepatic toxicity if administered within 8 hours of ingestion. The standard NAC dose is a 140 mg/kg loading dose, then 70 mg/kg every 4 hours for 17 doses. Antiemetics may be necessary. IV NAC, which is not approved for use in the United States, is useful in patients with intractable vomiting, fulminant hepatic failure, and pregnancy.

SALICYLATES

EPIDEMIOLOGY
- Salicylates are widely used for their analgesic and anti-inflammatory properties. Although there has been a dramatic decline since the 1960s in childhood mortality related to aspirin ingestions, toxic exposures continue because salicylates are found in many pre-scription and over-the-counter products, including analgesics, cold medicines, Pepto-Bismol, and oil of wintergreen.

PATHOPHYSIOLOGY
- Salicylate absorption may be erratic. At physiologic pH, salicylate molecules are ionized, but with acidemia, more become nonionized. Nonionized salicylates cross cell membranes and the blood-brain barrier easily, causing toxic effects.
- Initially, salicylates stimulate the respiratory center, resulting in hyperventilation and respiratory alkalosis. Intracellular effects include uncoupling of oxidative phosphorylation and disruption of glucose and fatty acid metabolism, causing metabolic acidosis.

CLINICAL FEATURES
- Acute ingestion produces vomiting, tinnitus, and lethargy. Respiratory alkalosis caused by hyperpnea may be seen early following ingestion, later, metabolic acidosis predominates. Severe poisoning results in hyperthermia, pulmonary edema, hyper- or hypo-glycemia, seizures, and coma.

DIAGNOSIS AND DIFFERENTIAL
- Peak salicylate levels are usually reached within 6 hours after the ingestion; however, with sustained release products, peak levels can occur later (10–60

hours postingestion). Aspirin can also form a gastric bezoar, further delaying absorption. After the level peaks, serial levels should be obtained every 2–4 hours until the level is less than 30 mg/dL. Most toxicologists no longer use the Done nomogram to estimate toxicity.

• Salicylate toxicity should be considered in patients with overdose of any analgesic, and in patients presenting with increased anion gap metabolic acidosis.

EMERGENCY DEPARTMENT CARE AND DISPOSITION

• Attention to airway, breathing and circulation, and ensuring adequate ventilation to prevent respiratory acidosis is important. Consider gastric lavage for alert patients with massive ingestions who present within 1 hour of ingestion.

• Activated charcoal (1 g/kg) should be administered and repeat doses (0.25–0.5 g/kg every 2–4 hours) considered for large ingestions or sustained release preparations. The goal is a ratio of 10 g of charcoal for every 1 g of salicylate ingested.

• Intravenous fluids are crucial to management; urinary alkalinization forces salicylate into ionized form, enhancing its elimination through the kidney. Sodium bicarbonate (3 ampules, 150 meq of 8.4% $NaHCO_3$) is added to 1 L of D5W and given at a rate of 1.5–2 times maintenance. Serum pH should be monitored and maintained between 7.45 and 7.55. Potassium supplementation should be modified to achieve a urine pH of 7.5.

• Hemodialysis is indicated for patients with serum salicylate levels of 100 mg/dL following acute ingestion, or with severe acidosis, electrolyte abnormalities, coma or seizures, regardless of salicylate level.

BENZODIAZEPINES

EPIDEMIOLOGY

• Since their introduction in the 1960s, benzodiazepines have become the most widely prescribed group of psychoactive drugs; they have multiple therapeutic uses. When ingested alone, they are unlikely to result in significant toxicity.

PATHOPHYSIOLOGY

• Benzodiazepines potentiate gamma-aminobutyric acid (GABA), a CNS inhibitory neurotransmitter, causing sedation and anxiolysis.

CLINICAL FEATURES

• Benzodiazepine intoxication causes sedation and CNS depression. Compared to other sedative-hypnotic agents, benzodiazepines are less likely to induce severe

cardiovascular instability or respiratory depression unless combined with other agents.

DIAGNOSIS AND DIFFERENTIAL

• Urine toxicologic screens that determine the presence of benzodiazepines are available at most hospitals. The diagnosis of benzodiazepine overdose should be considered in any patient presenting with CNS depression.

EMERGENCY DEPARTMENT CARE AND DISPOSITION

• Initiate supportive care with attention to airway, breathing, and circulation. Gastric lavage may be considered if the patient presents within 1 hour of a life-threatening ingestion. Administer a dose of activated charcoal.

• Flumazenil is a specific benzodiazepine antagonist that can be used to reverse the effects of benzodiazepine overdose (hypoventilation, coma). Seizures have been reported to result from flumazenil in patients chronically taking benzodiazepines or who have taken coingestants (i.e., tricyclic antidepressants). Therefore, flumazenil should only be used to reverse CNS depression in patients who are not chronically using benzodiazepines who present with a known pure benzodiazepine overdose.

BARBITURATES

EPIDEMIOLOGY

• Barbiturates are widely available and used for seizure control and sedative-hypnotic effects.

PATHOPHYSIOLOGY

• Barbiturates vary in their durations of action based on their lipid solubility. The shortest acting agents have the greatest lipid solubility and thus the greatest CNS penetration. All barbiturates cause CNS sedation, respiratory depression, and hypotension. Their mechanism of action is thought to be through potentiation of GABA, the major inhibitor of CNS activity.

CLINICAL FEATURES

• Typical features of barbiturate toxicity include slurred speech, ataxia, nystagmus, and lethargy, in addition to respiratory depression, hypotension, and hypothermia. Bullous skin lesions on dependent portions of the body (*barb bullae*) have been reported in up to 6% of cases of barbiturate overdose; however, these lesions are nonspecific.

DIAGNOSIS AND DIFFERENTIAL

• Urine toxicology screens commonly detect qualitative presence of barbiturates. Specific serum phenobarbital levels are available in most hospital laboratories. The diagnosis of barbiturate overdose should be considered in any patient with a depressed level of consciousness.

EMERGENCY DEPARTMENT CARE AND DISPOSITION
• Initiate supportive care with attention to airway, breathing and circulation. Gastric lavage may be considered if the patient presents within 1 hour of a life-threatening ingestion. A dose of activated charcoal (1 g/kg) is recommended. Multiple dose activated charcoal (0.25 g/kg every 4–6 hours) has been shown to decrease the half-life of phenobarbital.
• Urinary alkalinization increases the elimination of phenobarbital; it is not effective for short acting barbiturates. Hemodialysis or hemoperfusion may be necessary for patients with severe symptoms, such as hypotension refractory to supportive care.

HYDROCARBONS

EPIDEMIOLOGY
• Hydrocarbon ingestion is one of the most common childhood toxic exposures, usually occurring in children younger than 5 years old. Some children are attracted to the pleasant scents or colorful packaging of these substances; others are exposed because of improper storage in open, or easily opened containers (soda bottles, jelly glasses).
• Aliphatic hydrocarbons are straight-chained carbon molecules saturated with hydrogen atoms. They are commonly used as fuels, polishes, and solvents. Ingested aliphatic hydrocarbons generally produce little systemic toxicity, but during ingestion they pose a serious risk of pulmonary aspiration.
• Hydrocarbons are rarely pure: many contain camphorated, halogenated, or aromatic hydrocarbons, and others are mixed with metals or pesticides. These coingestants are also possibly toxic. Therefore, knowing the exact chemical content of the ingested hydrocarbon is important.

PATHOPHYSIOLOGY
• The aspiration potential of a hydrocarbon depends on its viscosity, volatility, and surface tension. Aspiration potential increases with low viscosity, low surface tension, and high volatility. Hydrocarbons destroy pulmonary surfactant, leading to ventilation-perfusion mismatch, hypoxia, and chemical pneumonitis.

CLINICAL FEATURES
• Prolonged cough, gasping, or choking following ingestion often indicates aspiration. When aspiration

occurs, respiratory distress will usually be evident within 2–6 hours. Fever, caused by direct tissue toxicity, is commonly present early in the clinical course.

DIAGNOSIS AND DIFFERENTIAL
• All symptomatic patients with hydrocarbon ingestion should have a chest radiograph, pulse oximetry, and cardiac monitoring. While the differential diagnosis for hydrocarbon aspiration includes acute respiratory distress because of asthma, foreign body aspiration, or pulmonary infection, most children with a hydrocarbon ingestion have a clear history.

EMERGENCY DEPARTMENT CARE AND DISPOSITION
• Treatment is primarily supportive. For patients who present soon after ingestion of agents with known systemic toxicity (camphorated, halogenated, aromatic, metal containing, pesticides), careful gastric lavage with a small caliber nasogastric tube may be of benefit.
• Patients who remain asymptomatic after 4–6 hours of observation may be discharged. Steroids and antibiotics have not been shown to be effective in treatment of hydrocarbon aspiration, and are not recommended.

CAUSTIC AGENTS

EPIDEMIOLOGY
• Caustic agents, which cause direct tissue injury, are present in many household products as well as in "industrial strength" cleaning products. Fatality is rare but morbidity is significant.
• Household bleach, an alkali, is the most common caustic exposure among children. Other alkalis include sodium hydroxide (lye), drain, oven, and toilet bowl cleaners, and dishwasher detergent. Ingested acids include metal cleaners, rust removers, battery acid, and swimming pool and toilet bowel cleaners.

PATHOPHYSIOLOGY
• Acids cause a coagulative necrosis, which tends to limit further tissue damage. In contrast, alkalines cause a liquefactive necrosis with saponification and continued penetration into deeper tissues, resulting in extensive tissue damage.

CLINICAL FEATURES
• Inhalation of corrosive gases may cause upper airway injury, with stridor, hoarseness, or wheezing. Skin or eye exposure (gases or liquids) often results in immediate pain and redness; burns and blindness can also occur. Oral ingestion usually causes severe pain, followed by spontaneous vomiting.

- Injury to the esophagus from alkaline ingestion has been graded. Grade I injury, mucosal hyperemia without ulceration, carries no long-term risk of stricture formation. Grade II burns, with submucosal lesions and ulcerations, carry a 75% risk of stricture formation, and grade III burns, with deep ulcers and tissue necrosis, invariably lead to strictures and carry a high risk of perforation. Long-term risk of esophageal carcinoma is also markedly increased with grades II and III burns.
- Household liquid bleach is not concentrated enough to cause esophageal injury, but ingestion may cause GI irritation.

DIAGNOSIS AND DIFFERENTIAL
- After oral ingestion of a caustic, oropharyngeal burns may be present; however, their absence does not exclude injury to the more distal GI tract. Chest and abdominal radiographs may show esophageal or gastric perforation.

EMERGENCY DEPARTMENT CARE AND DISPOSITION
- Activated charcoal will interfere with endoscopy and usually does not adsorb caustics, so its use is contraindicated. Syrup of ipecac is also contraindicated. Dilution with milk or water may be helpful if initiated within the first few minutes after exposure in those who have no airway complaints, vomiting, or abdominal pain, and are able to speak.
- Endoscopy should be considered in children with vomiting or drooling. The procedure is ideally performed within 12–24 hours of injury. Patients with grade I injury can resume their diet as tolerated and can be discharged from the hospital when they are able to eat and drink.
- Administration of corticosteroids and antibiotics is controversial but may be beneficial in patients with circumferential grade II esophageal burns. Grade III burns are likely to progress to stricture despite therapy, thus steroids are not recommended.

CARBON MONOXIDE

EPIDEMIOLOGY
- Carbon monoxide (CO) exposure is the most common cause of poisoning death in the United States; children and adolescents account for some of the victims. Exposure to CO results from inhalation of smoke in fires, from motor vehicle exhaust, or from combustion of charcoal, wood, or natural gas for heating or cooking. CO is insidious because it is odorless, colorless, and nonirritating. Many exposures are unrecognized because symptoms are nonspecific.

PATHOPHYSIOLOGY
- CO is absorbed via inhalation and binds to hemoglobin with an affinity 200–250 times that of oxygen. COHb shifts the hemoglobin dissociation curve to the left, making oxygen less available to cells.

CLINICAL FEATURES
- Mild CO exposure presents as a "flu-like" illness with headache, nausea, malaise, and weakness. Moderate exposure results in confusion, lethargy, syncope, and ataxia. In severe exposures coma, seizures, myocardial infarction, and dysrhythmias are seen.
- A delayed neuropsychiatric syndrome after CO exposure has been described. Clinical signs and symptoms include decreased cognition, Parkinsonism and personality changes. This syndrome typically resolves within 1 year.

DIAGNOSIS AND DIFFERENTIAL
- There are no reliable clinical findings for carbon monoxide poisoning; cherry-red skin color and bright-red venous blood are suggestive but infrequently observed. Venous or arterial blood COHb levels should be measured by cooximetry. As pulse-oximetry measures saturated hemoglobin, this value is often normal and this is not a reliable screening test. Arterial blood gas results show metabolic acidosis.
- Children may have symptoms (headache or lethargy) with COHb levels <10%; this low level is associated with no symptoms in most adults.
- The diagnosis of CO poisoning should be considered in patients with "flu-like" illness including influenza, gastroenteritis, alcohol intoxication, and sedative-hypnotic intoxication.

EMERGENCY DEPARTMENT CARE AND DISPOSITION
- The half-life for dissociation of CO from hemoglobin in room air is 6 hours. Administration of 100% oxygen will shorten the half-life to 1 hour. Hyperbaric oxygen at 2–3 atmospheres of pressure reduces the half-life further to 20–30 minutes, and should be considered for cases with severe toxicity (coma or other neurologic symptoms). A poison control center should be contacted for advice when managing severe CO poisoning.

BIBLIOGRAPHY

Cline D, Ma O (eds.). *Just the Facts in Emergency Medicine.* New York, NY: McGraw Hill, 2000.

Ford MD (ed.). *Clinical Toxicology.* Philadelphia, PA: W.B. Saunders, 2001.

Goldfrank LR (ed.). *Goldfrank's Toxicologic Emergencies*, 7th ed. New York, NY: McGraw Hill, 2002.

Leikin JB, Paloucek FP (eds.). *Poisoning and Toxicology Handbook*, 3rd ed. Hudson, OH: Lexi-Comp, 2002.

Ling LJ (ed.). *Toxicology Secrets*. Philadelphia, PA: Hanley & Belfus, 2001.

Olson KR (ed.). *Poisoning and Drug Overdose*, 3rd ed. Stamford, CT: Appleton & Lange, 1999.

Rumack BH, Matthew H. Acetaminophen poisoning and toxicity. *Pediatrics* 1975;55:871.

Tenenbein M. Recent advances in pediatric toxicology. *Pediatr Clin North Am* 1999;46:1179–1188.

18 BIOTERRORISM

Elizabeth C. Powell

INTRODUCTION

- Bioterrorism is the intentional use of biologic agents to produce disease or intoxication in a susceptible population. Biologic agents have been used throughout history; the most recent experience was the anthrax outbreak in 2001 in the United States.
- There are specific disease patterns that are consistent with possible bioterrorism. Most bioterrorist agents initially induce an influenza-like prodrome including fever, chills, myalgias, or malaise. One or more syndromic patterns follow: rapidly progressive pneumonia, fever with rash, fever with altered mental status, or bloody diarrhea. Epidemiologic evidence includes (a) the sudden presentation of a large number of victims with a similar disease or syndrome (cluster), (b) many cases in a similar stage of disease (resulting from a common source of exposure), (c) disease that is more severe or more rapidly progressive than is commonly encountered, and (d) presentation in an unusual geographic area or transmission season.
- When bioterrorism is suspected, physicians must work closely with the public health department so as to effectively diagnose and treat patients.
- The U.S. Centers for Disease Control and Prevention (CDC) has named six pathogenic microbes that pose the greatest risk as bioweapons: anthrax, smallpox, plague, tularemia, botulism, and viral hemorrhagic fever (Ebola, Marburg, Lassa, and others). These agents are the easiest to transmit and they are the most deadly.

ANTHRAX

EPIDEMIOLOGY

- Anthrax spores are common in the soil. The organism infects sheep and cattle and occasionally people, usually through direct skin contact (cutaneous anthrax). Inhalational anthrax, the most lethal form, occurs after the inhalation of anthrax spores. Gastrointestinal anthrax is acquired by the ingestion of poorly cooked contaminated meat.
- There is a vaccine for anthrax; its use has been limited to military and some emergency personnel.

CLINICAL FEATURES

- Onset of illness usually occurs 1–5 days after exposure, but symptoms can take as long as 6 weeks to develop. Symptoms include fever, headache, malaise, and myalgia. In cutaneous exposure, the skin lesion, initially a papule, ulcerates, enlarges, and develops a characteristic black eschar. Inhalational anthrax has an estimated 90% mortality if not treated quickly.
- There appears to be no person-to-person transmission.

DIAGNOSIS AND DIFFERENTIAL

- The symptoms of anthrax are similar to influenza and other acute viral illnesses. Most patients have mediastinitis, suggested by a wide mediastinum (chest computed tomography [CT] or chest radiograph). Many have pleural effusions; some develop pulmonary infiltrates.
- Blood cultures usually grow the organism in 24–36 hours. Specific tests for anthrax (polymerase chain reaction [PCR], immunohistochemistry) can be performed through state health departments.

EMERGENCY DEPARTMENT CARE AND DISPOSITION

- If inhalational anthrax is suspected, treatment with intravenous antibiotics (ciprofloxacin or high dose penicillin with streptomycin) should be initiated.
- Possible prophylaxis regimens for those with a high exposure risk include doxycycline and ciprofloxacin.

SMALLPOX

EPIDEMIOLOGY

- There are two forms of disease: variola major, the more severe form (30% mortality in unvaccinated) and variola minor, the milder form (1% mortality in unvaccinated).
- Transmission is person-to-person via aerosol or droplets. Routine vaccination in the United States stopped in 1972 and global eradication was achieved in 1980. Currently, the world's population is relatively unprotected from this virus.

- The only remaining authorized virus is in two designated labs in the United States and Russia. There is concern that the virus may exist outside the two reference laboratories.

CLINICAL FEATURES

- The incubation period is 7–17 days and the clinical symptoms are similar to those of influenza: fever, headache, and myalgias. The rash develops initially on the face, but spreads to the extremities and the trunk over several days.
- In contrast to varicella (chicken pox), the pustules are deeply embedded in the skin, more concentrated on the face and the extremities, and are in "phase" (i.e., all vesicular) in a specific body area.

DIAGNOSIS AND DIFFERENTIAL

- The early differential includes influenza and other viral diseases. After the rash appears, it must be distinguished from varicella.
- All suspected cases should be reported to the state health department. A confirmed case constitutes a probable bioterrorist event.
- Vesicle fluid can be used for viral culture, examination by electron microscopy, or PCR. This should be done in a designated laboratory. The state health department and the Centers for Disease Control should be contacted concerning specimen transport.

EMERGENCY DEPARTMENT CARE AND DISPOSITION

- There is no known effective therapy. Patients who do not need hospital admission for supportive care should be isolated and cared for at home so as to minimize spread of the disease. Admitted patients should be isolated in negative pressure rooms with aerosol precautions.
- All close contacts should be identified, and vaccinated if it is within 4–5 days of the exposure. Vaccination within 2–3 days of exposure will prevent the disease in most people.

PLAGUE

EPIDEMIOLOGY

- Caused by *Yersinia pestis*, a bioterrorist attack would likely use an aerosolized form than can be inhaled, resulting in pneumonic plague. Secondary transmission would be person-to-person by inhalation of respiratory droplets. The disease has a rapid progression.

CLINICAL FEATURES

- The incubation period for primary pneumonic plague is 1–6 days. Symptoms include fever, malaise, shortness of breath, cough, and sometimes, bloody sputum. Nausea, vomiting, and abdominal pain are also common. There are usually no buboes (painful, swollen regional lymph nodes), the characteristic sign of bubonic plague.
- The chest radiograph typically shows a bilateral, lobar pneumonia.

DIAGNOSIS AND DIFFERENTIAL

- There are no widely accessible, rapid diagnostic tests for plague. Culture of *Y. pestis* from the blood, CSF, or other clinical specimen confirms the diagnosis. Gram-negative bacilli or coccobacilli, sometimes with "safety pin" bipolar staining, are characteristic.
- A positive fluorescent antibody test for *Y. pestis* in direct smears or cultures of sputum, CSF, or blood is presumptive evidence; this is available through some state health departments and the Centers for Disease Control.

EMERGENCY DEPARTMENT CARE AND DISPOSITION

- As disease progression is rapid, antibiotic treatment should be initiated early if the disease is suspected. Streptomycin or gentamicin are the antibiotics used. Among hospitalized patients, isolation procedures to prevent disease spread via respiratory droplets or aerosols are used.
- Among asymptomatic household or hospital contacts, those who were within 6 ft of an infected person, prophylaxis with doxycycline (7-day course) is recommended. Contacts who develop fever or other symptoms should be evaluated, isolated, and treated with intravenous antibiotics until the diagnosis is confirmed or refuted.

TULAREMIA

EPIDEMIOLOGY

- Sources of the organism include small mammals (wild and domestic), blood sucking arthropods that bite these animals (ticks, deerflies, mosquitoes), and water and soil contaminated by infected animals. Research on this organism as a potential bioweapon has occurred in the past in the United States, the Soviet Union, Japan, and other countries.
- Person-to-person transmission has not been observed.

CLINICAL FEATURES

- The incubation period is usually 3–5 days, with a range of 1–21 days. Symptoms include chills, nausea, headache, and fever. There are several tularemic syndromes: the most common is the ulceroglandular syndrome, which is characterized by a painful

macular lesion at the site of organism entry, and inflamed regional lymph nodes. If infection is acquired through inhalation of contaminated particles, pneumonic disease may develop.
• Symptoms may persist for weeks to months.

DIAGNOSIS AND DIFFERENTIAL
• Serologic testing is the most common method to establish the diagnosis. A fourfold or greater change in *F. tularensis* agglutinin titer frequently is evident after the second week of illness; this is considered diagnostic. A single convalescent titer of 1:160 or greater is consistent with prior infection. The indirect fluorescent antibody test of ulcer exudates or aspirate material is also a rapid and specific screening test. Slide agglutination tests are less reliable and PCR assays have limited availability.

EMERGENCY DEPARTMENT CARE AND DISPOSITION
• Although tularemia progresses slowly, it can be fatal without treatment. The antibiotics streptomycin or gentamicin are used.

BOTULISM

EPIDEMIOLOGY
• *Clostridium botulinum* is a spore-forming anaerobic bacterium that makes botulinum toxin; the spores are present in the soil worldwide. Botulism is classically a food-borne disease seen when humans ingest pre-formed toxin present in improperly canned foods.
• A bioterrorist release of botulinum toxin would likely be aerosolized. The clinical syndrome resulting from toxin inhalation is similar to food-borne botulism.
• Botulism is not transmitted person-to-person.

CLINICAL FEATURES
• The incubation period is estimated to be 12–96 hours. Symptoms include diplopia, ptosis, difficulty swallowing, and speech abnormalities. There may be loss of head control, symmetric weakness, and respiratory difficulties as the descending paralysis progresses. Mechanical ventilation may be needed. Disease progression is rapid.

DIAGNOSIS AND DIFFERENTIAL
• A toxin neutralization bioassay in mice, available through state health departments, is used to identify botulinum toxin in serum and stool. Enriched and selective media are used to culture *C. botulinum* from stool.
• Other causes of weakness in the differential include myasthenia gravis, transverse myelitis, poliomyelitis, tick paralysis, and Guillan-Barré syndrome.

EMERGENCY DEPARTMENT CARE AND DISPOSITION
• Supportive care, both respiratory and nutritional, is essential for good outcomes. Botulinum antitoxin has been demonstrated to be effective in infants. It should be started as early in the illness as possible.

VIRAL HEMORRHAGIC FEVER

EPIDEMIOLOGY
• The best known, severe forms in this class of diseases are Ebola and Marburg viruses, but it also occurs in forms that are less severe, such as yellow fever and dengue fever. These diseases are readily transmitted through blood and body secretions. Airborne transmission has been shown only in primates; these agents are included as potential bioterrorist agents because of their virulence.

CLINICAL FEATURES
• The usual incubation period is 5–10 days, but it can range from 2–19 days. Muscle pain, headache, and abrupt onset of fever is followed by nausea, abdominal pain, chest pain, sore throat, cough, and rash. There is bleeding from the skin, the nose, the mouth, or the gastrointestinal tract. The case fatality rate is high, an estimated 30–90%, depending on the viral strain.

DIAGNOSIS AND DIFFERENTIAL
• Hemorrhagic fevers caused by arboviruses may be clinically similar. Both Marburg and Ebola viruses are classified as filoviruses. All specimens from patients with suspected infections must be handled with extreme caution to prevent accidental infection. Identification of the virus is done only in designated laboratories: viral antigens in tissues can be detected by direct immunofluorescence analysis.

EMERGENCY DEPARTMENT CARE AND DISPOSITION
• Patients should be isolated with both contact and droplet precautions. Treatment is supportive: fluids and blood for shock and respiratory support as needed. Antibody-containing serum and interferon therapies have been tried in patients with these infections. There is no vaccine.

BIBLIOGRAPHY

American Academy of Pediatrics. In: Pickering LK (ed.). *2000 Red Book: Report of the Committee on Infectious Diseases*, 25th ed. Elk Grove Village, IL: American Academy of

Pediatrics, 2000, pp. 2t, 85t, 86t, 168–170, 172t, 212–214, 450–452, 618–620.

Khan AS, Levitt AM, Sage MJ, et al. *The CDC Strategic Planning Workgroup. Biological and chemical terrorism: strategic plan for preparedness and response. Recommendations of the CDC Strategic Planning Workgroup*, 2000.

Murray PR, Rosenthal KS, Kobayashi GS, Pfaller MA. *Medical Microbiology,* 3rd ed. St. Louis, MO: Mosby, 1998, pp. 543–544.

Ropeik D, Gray G. *Risk: A Practical Guide for Deciding What's Really Safe and What's Really Dangerous in the World Around You.* Boston, MA: Houghton Mifflin, 2002, pp. 186–194.

Section 3
NEONATAL CRITICAL CARE

Robin Steinhorn, Section Editor

19 NEONATAL RESUSCITATION

Marissa deUngria

SCOPE OF THE PROBLEM

- Five to ten percent of newborn infants will require some degree of delivery room resuscitation to achieve normal transition. One percent require intensive resuscitation measures to survive. Birth asphyxia accounts for ~19% of the 5 million neonatal deaths/year worldwide; therefore >1 million neonatal deaths/year are potentially preventable by adequate resuscitation.
- A delay in establishing effective cardiorespiratory function may increase the risk of hypoxic-ischemic cerebral injury, pulmonary hypertension, and systemic organ dysfunction.

BASIC PRINCIPLES

FETAL LIFE

- Fetal lungs are fluid filled with volumes that are at functional residual capacity (FRC) or 20–25 cc/kg. Fetal lung fluid is expelled by fetal breathing and contributes to amniotic fluid. The placenta is the organ of gas exchange, nutrition, metabolism, and excretion.
- Fetoplacental circulation is characterized by a high-resistance pulmonary circuit and low-resistance systemic circuit. Fetal blood is relatively hypoxemic, with an arterial PaO_2 of 20–30 mmHg and oxyhemoglobin saturations of 75–85%.
- The fetus has compensatory mechanisms for adequate tissue oxygenation and growth that include decreased oxygen consumption, increased red cell mass, and increased affinity of fetal hemoglobin for oxygen.

NORMAL TRANSITION: ADAPTATION FROM INTRAUTERINE TO EXTRAUTERINE LIFE

- The fetus experiences increased oxygen consumption during labor as well as brief periods of asphyxia with contractions because of interruption of umbilical venous blood flow. Compensatory mechanisms to compensate for asphyxia include those described above, as well as greater tissue resistance to acidosis compared to an adult, bradycardia and a "diving reflex" that allows blood to flow preferentially to brain, heart and adrenal glands, and the capability of switching to anaerobic glycolysis (if liver glycogen stores adequate).
- Catecholamine surges during delivery, with levels higher when mothers have labored and in girls compared to boys. Catecholamine levels are lower in preterm infants compared to term infants. Effects include an increase in lung fluid resorption, surfactant release, stimulation of gluconeogenesis, and direction of blood flow to vital organs such as the heart and brain.
- Clamping of the umbilical cord removes the low-resistance placental circuit and increases systemic blood pressure. Postnatal circulation is characterized by a low-resistance pulmonary circuit, and high-resistance systemic circuit, as well as a transition from placental gas exchange to pulmonary gas exchange.
- An increase in negative intrathoracic pressure produces lung expansion; air replaces fetal lung fluid and increases alveolar oxygenation. Because of the viscosity and surface tension forces of lung fluid, large transpulmonary pressures are needed for the first few breaths.

- Pulmonary blood increases because of lung expansion and oxygen-mediated relaxation of pulmonary arterioles. The patent foramen ovale (PFO) and patent ductus arteriosus (PDA) functionally close, and blood previously diverted through ductus arteriosus now flows through the lungs.

DISRUPTED TRANSITION

- Babies may encounter difficulties before, during, or after labor that compromise the transition.
  1. Compromised blood flow in the placenta or umbilical cord may cause decelerations of the fetal heart rate, and may produce hypoxia and ischemia in the fetus.
  2. Insufficient respiratory effort or abnormal lung ion transport because of prematurity, maternal drugs, or anesthesia may lead to incomplete reabsorption of fetal lung fluid, thereby preventing adequate alveolar oxygenation.
  3. Foreign material such as meconium or blood may obstruct the airway thereby preventing adequate lung inflation.
  4. Excessive blood loss or hypoxia-induced cardiac dysfunction or bradycardia may produce systemic hypotension.
  5. Lack of adequate lung inflation and/or oxygenation may lead to sustained constriction of pulmonary arterioles, which may result in persistent pulmonary hypertension (PPHN).
- Clinical signs of disrupted transition include cyanosis, bradycardia, hypotension, and decreased peripheral perfusion, depressed respiratory drive, and poor muscle tone.
- Asphyxia is defined as a failure of gas exchange leading to a combination of hypoxemia, hypercapnia, and metabolic acidemia. Causes include interruption of umbilical blood flow (cord compression), failure of gas exchange across placenta (placental abruption), inadequate perfusion of maternal side of placenta (maternal hypotension), a compromised fetus intolerant to transient, intermittent hypoxia of normal labor (IUGR), or a failure to inflate lungs (RDS).
- A progressive cycle of worsening hypoxemia, hypercapnia, and metabolic acidemia results if adequate ventilation and pulmonary perfusion are not rapidly established. Initially blood flow is preserved to the brain and heart, and blood flow to the intestines, kidneys, muscles, and skin is sacrificed. Ultimately ongoing ischemia, hypoxia, and acidosis lead to myocardial dysfunction and impaired cardiac output. Inadequate blood flow, perfusion, and tissue oxygenation result in brain injury, multiorgan injury, and even death.

OPTIMIZING DELIVERY ROOM (DR) RESUSCITATION

- High-risk infants should be identified early. The resuscitation team should be rapidly activated, and each team member should understand the physiologic mechanisms of adaptation. Data collection and frequent review of resuscitative events are essential.
- Resuscitation equipment should be readily available in the delivery room for every birth, and should be checked at regular intervals and immediately prior to delivery. Expiration dates of medications should be monitored periodically.
- Well-trained personnel must be immediately available in any setting where an infant is likely to be delivered. Every birth should be attended by at least one person whose primary responsibility is the infant and therefore can initiate resuscitation if unanticipated problems can occur. A multiple gestation delivery requires separate personnel for each infant. Personnel must maintain their resuscitative skills and familiarize themselves with new guidelines as outlined by American Academy of Pediatrics (AAP)/American Heart Association (AHA).
- Communication between obstetricians and pediatricians helps identify high-risk deliveries. If a high-risk delivery is expected, prenatal consultation is ideal. Significant maternal medical history, gestational age, prenatal complications, medications, illicit drug use, and prenatal labs should be recorded. Sepsis risk factors including Group B streptococcus (GBBS) carrier status, rupture of membranes, maternal fever, evidence of chorioamnionitis, and use of intrapartum antibiotics should be assessed.

APGAR SCORE

- The Apgar score signifies the overall status of the neonate at birth and response to resuscitation. It does not determine the need for resuscitation or long-term outcome. Scores are assigned at 1 and 5 minutes after birth. If the score remains <7, additional scores are recorded every 5 minutes up to 20 minutes (Table 19-1).

STEPS OF RESUSCITATION

- *Prevent cold stress* and minimize heat loss through use of a preheated radiant warmer, prewarmed blankets, and hat. The newborn head is proportionately larger than the body and therefore can be a major source of heat loss. The goal is a neutral thermal environment with maintenance of normal core temperature with minimal oxygen consumption. The infant should be dried and wet blankets removed to reduce evaporative heat loss (Fig. 19-1).

TABLE 19-1   Apgar Scoring

SIGN	SCORE		
	0	1	2
Heart rate	Absent	Slow (<100 bpm)*	≥100 bpm
Respirations	Absent	Slow, irregular	Good, crying
Muscle tone	Limp	Some flexion	Active motion
Reflex irritability (catheter in nares, tactile stimulation)	No response	Grimace	Cough, sneeze, cry
Color	Blue or pale	Pink body, blue extremities	Completely pink

* bpm indicates beats per minute.

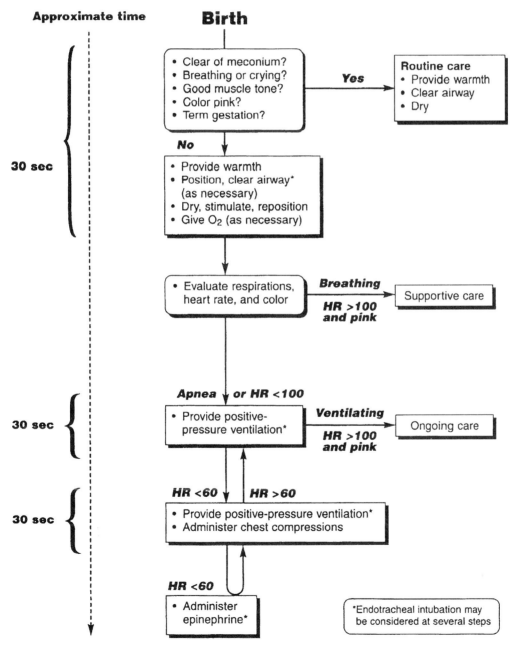

FIG. 19-1   Algorithm for resuscitation of the newly born infant.

- *Position head and suction* to clear the airway with bulb syringe or suction catheter. Suction the mouth first as suctioning nose may lead to gagging and aspiration of oral secretions. Vigorous suctioning of posterior pharynx may produce laryngeal spasm and a vagal response with apnea and/or bradycardia, thereby delaying the onset of spontaneous breathing.
- *Tactile stimulation* can be accomplished through gentle rubbing of back or flicking of heels.
- Evaluate respirations, heart rate, and color. The above steps should take <30 seconds, and if there is no improvement after 30 seconds, move on to next step. Reassess parameters after every intervention.
- *Provide oxygen* as needed via facemask and flow-inflating bag, oxygen mask, or hand cupped around tubing at flow of 5 L/minute. Initially hold as close to face as possible and slowly withdraw as infant responds.
- *Positive-pressure ventilation* (PPV).
- *Chest compressions* with continued assisted ventilation.
- *Medications* are used in the care of only 0.12% of live-born babies as adequate ventilation and lung expansion are the mainstay of resuscitation.

PPV/INTUBATION

- Four percent of newborns require bag-mask ventilation with supplemental oxygen. Indications include insufficient respiratory pattern manifested by gasping and/or apnea, HR <60 bpm for 30 seconds, or persistent central cyanosis despite administration of 100% oxygen.
- Immediate intubation is generally not necessary as bag-mask provides effective ventilation. Important exceptions are in infants with perinatal depression and meconium-stained amniotic fluid, and congenital diaphragmatic hernia (CDH).
- Clear the airway before starting PPV. Place the head in the neutral or "sniffing" position as this aligns the posterior pharynx, larynx, and the trachea, and ensures that the airway is maximally patent. The airway is smaller and located more anteriorly compared to older children and adults. The newborn head is proportionately larger than the body, therefore neck has tendency to be flexed. Both underextension (flexion) and hyperextension can obstruct flow through the airway as well as obstruct visualization of vocal cords. A blanket roll beneath shoulders may be helpful.
- Two types of bags are typically used—should not be >750 mL.
  1. A self-inflating bag (Ambu) may be easier for novice or less experienced resuscitators to use. Significant mixing with room air occurs if an oxygen reservoir is not in place, thereby limiting maximal oxygen delivery to 40%. The valve assembly allows free flow of oxygen only when the bag is compressed or squeezed and therefore cannot be used for blow-by oxygen delivery.
  2. A flow-inflating or "anesthesia" bag requires more experienced resuscitators as it requires continual flow for inflation. It is susceptible to mechanical failure as multiple adjustments need to be considered, including flow of gas into gas inlet, flow of gas out through the flow-control valve, and the seal between mask and infant's face. This bag can deliver higher pressures, which may lead to air leak syndromes (pneumomediastinum, pneumothorax, pneumopericardium); however, in experienced hands they provide a greater range of peak inspiratory pressures and more reliable control of oxygen concentration (of particular concern in preterm infants).
- A tight seal between mask and face is crucial. The mask should be of appropriate size to cover the nose and mouth but not the eyes. Masks with air-filled cushions help maintain a tight seal without inflicting facial or ocular injury. Hold the infant's chin to the mask with the middle finger; do not have fingers on soft tissues of the neck. Supporting the chin also elevates the angle of the jaw, bringing the tongue forward, and opening the airway.
- The first breath must be large enough to ensure alveolar expansion and establishment of functional residual capacity, therefore initial breaths may require higher pressures (25–40 cm H_2O) and longer inflation times. The need for higher initial pressures may be accentuated in preterm infants with noncompliant lungs because of surfactant deficiency. The effectiveness is judged by chest movement, which should approximate .25 to .5 cm. Succeeding breaths need not be as large as FRC is already present. Overdistension and hyperventilation should be avoided: overdistension may impair venous return to heart or lead to pneumothorax and hypocarbia decreases cerebral and myocardial blood flow.
- Continue with a ventilation rate of 30–60 bpm. Often this is the only resuscitation maneuver that will be required, as apnea and bradycardia improve with correction of inadequate lung inflation and hypoxia.
- Evaluate adequacy of bag-mask ventilation by chest rise, audible equal breath sounds, and improvement in HR and color. If response is not adequate, *endotracheal intubation* is required.
- Use appropriate sized laryngoscope blade—size 0 for preterms, size 1 for term infants. If a stylette is used, ensure the tip is at least 0.5 cm from the end of the endotracheal tube (ETT) to avoid trauma. Appropriate

ETT sizes and lengths are based on gestational age and weight.

- Intubation procedure: Place laryngoscope blade into vallecula or onto epiglottis and elevate blade superiorly until the vocal cords come into view. Cricoid pressure may be helpful as the airway is anteriorly located in an infant.
- Proper placement of ETT: In general ETT insertion distance in cm = 6 + infant's weight in kg. Note there is a black line on distal tip of ETT. Insertion of ETT until the black line just passes through vocal cords should position ETT above the carina.
- Placement is initially judged clinically by assessment of adequacy of ventilation. Breath sounds should not be audible over the stomach and stomach should not inflate; however, this can be difficult to assess in preterm infants and if the infant has previously received bag-mask ventilation. Condensation within ETT should be noted on exhalation. A CO_2 detector may be helpful; while false-negative results may occur, false-positive results are very unlikely. If there is any question about whether an ETT is placed appropriately, direct laryngoscopic visualization should be performed. Final confirmation of tube position is via chest radiograph with ETT located between the clavicles and carina.

CHEST COMPRESSIONS/EXTERNAL CARDIAC MASSAGE

- Bradycardia and decreasing blood pressure ensue after a few minutes of hypoxia. The indication for beginning chest compressions is if heart rate is absent or remains ≤60 bpm after 30 seconds of effective ventilation. Heart rate is assessed by auscultation with stethoscope over precordium or by feeling pulsations at base of umbilical cord.
- Two thumb-encircling hands technique is preferred to the two-finger method. This results in better systolic and coronary perfusion pressure, although care must be taken to avoid limiting thoracic expansion during ventilation (Fig. 19-2).
- Compressions are performed on the lower one-third of sternum immediately above xiphoid process. Depth is one-third of the chest anteroposterior diameter or deep enough to generate a palpable pulse. The rate should be 90 compressions and 30 ventilations per minute (ratio of 3 compressions: 1 ventilation).

VASCULAR ACCESS

- Peripheral access can be time-consuming and difficult, especially if hypoxia or acidosis is present.

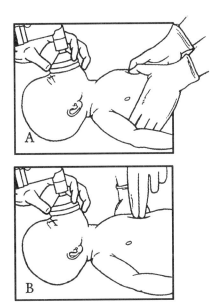

FIG. 19-2 Two techniques for giving chest compressions: thumb (A) and two-finger (B).

Emergency access is via the umbilical vein as it is rapidly accessible. The depth of insertion is ~4–6 cm; blood should flow freely on aspiration assuring that position of catheter is below the liver thereby avoiding potential hepatic injury.

MEDICATIONS

- *Epinephrine*: Alpha vasoconstrictive activity is responsible for returning spontaneous circulation. It is indicated when heart rate remains ≤60 bpm after 30 seconds of effective ventilation and external cardiac massage. Dose is 0.1–0.3 mL/kg of 1:10,000 dilution solution IV (preferred) or intratracheal; can be repeated every 3–5 minutes.
- *Sodium bicarbonate*: Should only be given after adequate ventilation and circulation are established. In the absence of adequate ventilation, blood pH does not significantly improve and respiratory acidosis compounds the metabolic acidosis as bicarbonate is converted to CO_2; however, if ventilation is established, correction of acidosis may increase pulmonary blood flow and may enhance the effect of epinephrine. The dose is 1–2 meq/kg IV, and should always be diluted 1:1 with sterile water and given slowly over at least 2 minutes. Rapid infusions may be associated with intracranial hemorrhage especially in preterm infants. Administration can unmask hypovolemia which may be inapparent because of peripheral vasoconstriction.

- *Narcan* is a narcotic antagonist that should be considered only after ventilation and circulation are established. Significant respiratory depression as a consequence of peripartum administration of narcotics is rare. Narcan is not effective in reversing the effects of other drugs administered to mothers that may depress respiratory function, such as magnesium sulfate, nonnarcotic analgesics. Indications are severe respiratory depression that persists despite normal HR and color following PPV and a history of maternal narcotic administration within the past 4 hours. Narcan is contraindicated in the narcotic-addicted mother or one on methadone maintenance; as it may precipitate acute withdrawal including severe seizures and long-term sequelae. Narcan has a rapid onset of action within 1–2 minutes. The duration of action of narcotics used for labor analgesia is greater than that of narcan; therefore repeated doses of narcan may be necessary. The dose is 0.1 mg/kg IT, SQ, IM, IV.
- *Volume expansion* is considered in conditions associated with hypovolemia or shock clinically manifested by weak pulses, poor capillary filling, and low blood pressure. Clinical reasons that would produce hypovolemia include significant hemorrhage because of placenta previa, placental abruption, or fetomaternal bleed. In addition, cord accidents, tight nuchal cord, or compression by the after-coming head in a breech delivery may impede umbilical venous flow while arterial flow continues, thereby decreasing circulating volume by as much as 20%. Other etiologies for hypovolemia include twin-twin transfusion syndrome and internal hemorrhage. Small aliquots of 10 cc/kg are given with reassessment of BP, perfusion, and oxygenation prior to the next dose. Typical choices are normal saline, Ringer's lactate, 5% albumin, or type O-negative packed red blood cells (PRBCs). Volume should be administered slowly as some vascular beds (especially brain) may be maximally dilated in response to hypotension. Intracranial hemorrhage is a possible consequence of rapid volume expansion, especially in preterm infants.

PITFALLS OF RESUSCITATION—CAN OCCUR AT EACH STEP OR AT MULTIPLE STEPS

- Failure to distinguish secondary apnea from primary apnea: The initial response to hypoxia is increased respiratory effort (primary hyperpnea) followed by primary apnea, which lasts ~1 minute and can be relieved by tactile stimulation. Rhythmic gasping ensues and may last several minutes. This is followed by secondary or terminal apnea, which can *only* be reversed by assisted ventilation. Continued stimulation does not help. Since primary and secondary apnea look the same, consider any apnea as secondary until proven otherwise.
- Vigorous suctioning of posterior pharynx may delay onset of spontaneous breaths.
- Malpositioning of head so that it is not in neutral position.
- Mechanical failures, e.g., oxygen reservoir not in place if Ambu bag used or insufficient oxygen flow. Others include incomplete seal with mask.
- Obstruction of airway.
- Ineffective ventilation pressures will lead to failure to inflate lungs and establish FRC.
- Malposition of ETT in esophagus or in right mainstem bronchus is common. Remember to visualize directly with laryngoscope if ventilation is not effective.
- Pneumothorax can be identified through asymmetric breath sounds and/or asymmetry of chest wall and movement. If under tension, venous return and cardiac output are compromised, and a cardiac arrest may occur. Transillumination is helpful (especially in preterm infants). Chest x-ray is diagnostic; in life-threatening cases, diagnostic thoracentesis should be considered.

SPECIAL CONSIDERATIONS

- *Meconium-stained amniotic fluid* (MSAF) occurs in 10–15% of all pregnancies, and occurs as a reaction to fetal hypoxemia, acidemia, or stress. Approximately; 20–30% of infants will require tracheal suctioning. MSAF is rare before 34 weeks gestation and more common in postterm gestations. Two percent of infants manifest some degree of aspiration, ranging from mild tachypnea to severe pneumonitis and pulmonary hypertension. Pulmonary disease is more likely if MSAF occurs before second stage of labor, if the meconium is thick with particulate material, and/or if meconium is present below the vocal cords. Management includes the following:
  1. Obstetrical suctioning of oropharynx after delivery of head but before delivery of shoulders.
  2. If infant is vigorous and meconium is thin, tracheal suctioning is not necessary. In this setting, suctioning does not reduce incidence of meconium aspiration syndrome or improve outcome, and may instead result in esophageal or tracheal injury.
  3. If meconium is thick or particulate or if infant is depressed, intubation should occur prior to any stimulation or PPV. The ETT should be large enough to remove thick copious meconium, yet fit

easily into infant's trachea. A meconium aspirator should be placed directly onto the ETT, and connected to suction at 80–100 cm water pressure and the ETT should be withdrawn slowly. Repeat intubation and tracheal suctioning with a clean ETT is performed until the return is clear (have several ETTs prepared) unless other resuscitation priorities take precedence.

4. Suction stomach to prevent aspiration of swallowed meconium.

5. Have high index of suspicion for development of pneumothorax.

• *Multiple gestation* is associated with an increased incidence of preterm labor and delivery and separate teams of skilled personnel are needed for each infant. There is a risk of intrauterine growth restriction in one fetus with possible complications in both, including higher sensitivity to asphyxia, hypoglycemia, and polycythemia. There is a risk of twin-to-twin-transfusion syndrome in monozygotic twins with the potential for hydrops in either twin. There is also an increased incidence of congenital anomalies in monozygotic multiple births.

• Infants with *extreme prematurity* (<1000 g) should be delivered in a perinatal center with skilled personnel in obstetrics, anesthesia, and neonatology. A conference with the parents should occur prior to delivery whenever possible. The incidence of perinatal depression is markedly increased in this population because of physiologic immaturity and lability.

1. Multiple factors dramatically increase insensible water loss; therefore drying and providing warmth are very important. In the smallest infants, use of polyethylene wrap, warming mattresses, and warm humidified oxygen and air is helpful.

2. Small infants have weaker muscles of respiration, and are less likely to establish and sustain FRC. This may be further complicated by decreased lung compliance because of surfactant deficiency. Endotracheal intubation is often required, and substantial inspiratory pressure may be needed initially. Surfactant administration in the delivery room is often required. Pitfalls include overventilation, which may impair cardiac output, result in interstitial emphysema or air leak syndromes, and produce hypocarbia and alter cerebral blood flow.

3. There is a high risk of intracranial hemorrhage in this population that may be exacerbated by increased transmitted pressure via PPV, large tidal volumes, and/or chest compressions. Rapid changes in cardiac output also contribute, and may be aggravated by rapid volume administration, hypertension associated with epinephrine, or rapid infusion of $NaHCO_3$.

4. Avoid excessive oxygen concentrations given the possible association of reactive oxygen species with ROP and chronic lung disease.

• *Congenital diaphragmatic hernia* (CDH) occurs in 1 in 2000–5000 live births (see Respiratory Disease section). Prenatal diagnosis is possible, although not all infants are detected on antenatal ultrasound screening. Signs in the delivery room include a flat or scaphoid abdomen and displaced heart sounds to the right (most defects are on the left). Some infants have poor myocardial function requiring inotropic support. Infants with respiratory distress caused by CDH require immediate intubation; bag-mask ventilation is contraindicated as air will expand the herniated bowel and exacerbate lung compression. A gastric tube should be immediately placed to low continuous suction to maintain decompression of herniated bowel and maximize lung inflation. A high index of suspicion should be maintained for the development of a pneumothorax.

• *Hydrops fetalis* may also be detected on prenatal ultrasound; if possible establish the presence and size of pleural effusions and peritoneal fluid. These fluid collections may hinder ventilation, therefore additional skilled personnel are needed to perform thoracentesis and/or paracentesis. High initial inflating pressures and positive end expiratory pressure (PEEP) are usually required because of noncompliant lungs, and pulmonary hypertension is common.

• *Abdominal wall defects* (gastroschisis and omphalocoele) are associated with increased insensible water and heat loss because of the absence of skin covering the intestines. In gastroschisis, the freely mobile intestines may cause traction on, or kink, mesenteric vessels and lead to infarction. Delivery room management includes immediate decompression of the gastrointestinal (GI) tract. Loosely wrap warm salinesoaked gauze around the defect or free intestines, and cover the gauze with plastic wrap or place infant in sterile plastic bag to a level above defect.

• Infants with *spina bifida* should be positioned carefully so the infant is prone or side-lying. There is increased insensible water and heat loss because of skin defects; therefore wrap warm saline-soaked gauze around defect and place the infant in a sterile plastic bag to a level above the defect.

• Infants with *severe malformations* should receive normal resuscitation measures unless certainty exists that the malformations are associated with conditions incompatible with life. This will typically only occur when the malformations are known prenatally and the family requests no resuscitation be performed. Otherwise, resuscitation and stabilization of infant allows time for accurate diagnosis.

OUTCOMES

- Indicators of poor outcome both in terms of survival and subsequent neurodevelopment include the following:
  1. Apgar scores at 5 and 10 minutes of ≤3.
  2. pH <7.0 in the first 2 hours of life.
  3. Absence of heart beat at 5 minutes of life.
  4. Seizures in the first 24 hours of life; presence of seizures in the first 12 hours is particularly ominous.
- Resuscitation should rarely be continued longer than 15–20 minutes in an infant with initial Apgar of 0 and who does not respond rapidly to resuscitation. The incidence of death or severe, irreversible neurologic damage in these infants is very high.

CONTROVERSIAL ISSUES

- A *laryngeal mask airway* (LMA) may be an effective alternative for establishing an airway, especially if bag-mask ventilation is ineffective and attempts at tracheal intubation are unsuccessful. This mask fits over laryngeal inlet, and further training is needed to learn proper insertion technique and use. The LMA cannot be used for tracheal suctioning of meconium or administration of resuscitative medications.
- *Room air resuscitation*: New data indicate that 100% oxygen is associated with a delay in spontaneous ventilation, generation of oxygen free radicals, potential exacerbation of neurologic injury, and the efficacy of resuscitation with room air is being studied. The current standard remains 100% oxygen. As the goal is normoxia and not hyperoxia, monitor oxygen use by pulse oximetry and blood gases and adjust accordingly after completing initial resuscitation measures.
- *High dose epinephrine via ETT*: In general, intratracheal epinephrine is less effective than IV administration. Compensating by using higher ETT doses may exaggerate the hypertensive effect, lower cardiac output, and increase risk of intracranial hemorrhage.
- *Resuscitation at the threshold of viability*: Antenatal counseling is very important as well as maintaining an ongoing dialogue with the family. Assessment of gestational age before and after delivery is accurate within 1–2 weeks. If there is any question of gestational age or prognosis, it is reasonable to provide aggressive resuscitative support as this allows for further assessment of the infant. The infant's response to therapy is an important factor, and if response to resuscitation is poor or if significant complications develop, withdrawal of support may be offered.

BIBLIOGRAPHY

Ballard RA. Resuscitation in the delivery room. In: Taesch HW and Ballard RA, eds. *Avery's Diseases of the Newborn*, 7th ed. Philadelphia, PA, W.B. Saunders Company: 319–333,1998.

Bloom R. Delivery room resuscitation of the newborn. In: Fanaroff A and Martin R, eds. *Neonatal-Perinatal Medicine, Diseases of the Fetus and Infant*, 6th ed. St. Louis, MO, Mosby, 376–402,1997.

Niermeyer S, Kattwinkel J, Van Reempts P, et al. International guidelines for neonatal resuscitation: an excerpt from the guidelines 2000 for cardiopulmonary resuscitation and emergency cardiovascular care: international consensus on science *Pediatrics* 2000:106–29.

Kattwinkel J, ed. *Textbook of Neonatal Resuscitation*, 4th ed. American Heart Association and American Academy of Pediatrics, 2000.

20 BIRTH INJURY

Marissa deUngria

SKULL INJURIES

- *Linear skull fractures* are relatively common and occur most commonly in the parietal bone. The pathogenesis is direct compression during delivery. These may be associated with extracranial or intracranial complications, although serious intracranial complications are not common. They are rarely associated with a dural tear and subsequent development of leptomeningeal cyst, which may be detected by increased transillumination. No therapy is indicated. Skull x-rays several months later may be helpful to document healing and to ensure a leptomeningeal cyst is not developing or enlarging.
- *Depressed skull fractures* are defined as inward buckling of resilient neonatal bone usually without loss of bony continuity. These are usually a result of localized compression of the skull either by pressure against maternal pelvic structures or by forceps, but may rarely occur spontaneously in utero. The most common site is the parietal bone. They can be rarely associated with epidural or subdural hemorrhage (SDH) or cerebral contusion. Management includes computed tomography (CT) scan to exclude intracranial complications and careful neurologic surveillance. Neurosurgical evaluation is indicated.
- *Occipital osteodiastasis* is a form of birth injury characterized by separation of squamous and lateral parts of occipital bone. Seen most commonly after breech

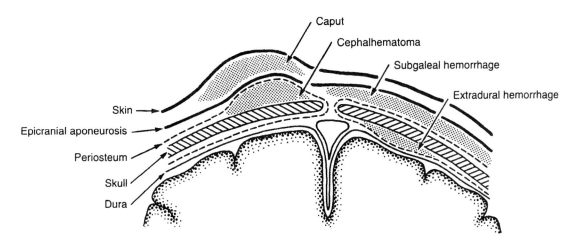

FIG. 20-1 Sites of extracranial (and extradural) hemorrhages in the newborn. Schematic diagram of important tissue planes from skin to dura. (Adapted from Pape KE, Wigglesworth JS. *Haemorrhage, Ischaemia and the Perinatal Brain.* Philadelphia, PA: JB Lippincott.)

delivery, it has become rare because of improved obstetrical techniques. Complications include subdural hemorrhage in the posterior fossa, cerebellar contusion, and cerebellar-medullary compression without gross hemorrhage.

EXTRACRANIAL HEMORRHAGE

- *Caput succedaneum* is subcutaneous hemorrhagic edema commonly seen after vaginal delivery. The most common pathogenesis is compression by the uterus or cervix on the presenting part. It occurs in 20–40% of vacuum-assisted deliveries. It is characterized by soft, superficial, pitting edema that crosses suture lines, and is usually accompanied by marked molding of the head. It spontaneously resolves over weeks to months (Fig. 20-1).
- *Subgaleal hemorrhage* is rare, with an estimated occurrence of 1 in 2500 deliveries. Predisposing factors include vacuum-assisted deliveries, coagulopathies (e.g., factor IX deficiency), prematurity, rapid delivery, and macrosomia. The pathogenesis is external compressive and dragging forces. This hemorrhage can produce massive blood loss because of the large potential space. In severe cases, blood may collect beneath entire scalp, and dissect into subcutaneous tissues of neck. It may be associated with suture diastasis or a linear skull fracture. On examination, there is fluctuant mass that increases in size after birth with a corresponding increase in head circumference. This hemorrhage may be complicated by significant early

hypovolemia, followed by anemia and hyperbilirubinemia. It subsequently resolves over 2–3 weeks.
- A *cephalohematoma* is a hemorrhage between the cranial bones and their surrounding periosteum, and is thereby limited by suture lines. It occurs in 1–2% of live births, and its incidence is more common in males, primiparous mothers, and forceps or vacuum-assisted delivery. It is most commonly seen unilaterally over the parietal bone, although an occipital location is possible. It presents as a firm, tense mass that does not transilluminate, and often increases in size after birth. An underlying linear skull fracture is detected in 10–25% of infants. A cephalohematoma is rarely clinically significant unless accompanied by an intracranial hemorrhage, and it resolves over weeks to months. Rare infectious complications are osteomyelitis and meningitis. A few calcify with initial bony protuberances, but remodel with skull growth over months. No specific therapy is indicated; evacuation of lesion is contraindicated.

INTRACRANIAL HEMORRHAGE

- Clinical signs and symptoms include a bulging anterior fontanelle and circulatory instability because of effects on autonomic nervous system.
- *Epidural hemorrhage* is rare, representing only 2% of all neonatal intracranial hemorrhages seen at autopsy. It is often associated with a cephalohematoma, and almost always associated with linear skull fractures. Clinically the infant displays signs of increased

intracranial pressure, with a bulging anterior fontanelle, seizures, and in severe cases signs of herniation may occur with a fixed, dilated, ipsilateral pupil. An emergent head CT will reveal a convex, lentiform lesion. Death can occur within 24–48 hours, therefore neurosurgical evacuation is imperative.

- *Subdural hemorrhage* (SDH) is an uncommon but serious delivery complication, and is caused by tears of major cerebral veins or dural sinuses. A tentorial laceration with massive infratentorial hemorrhage may occur in the straight sinus, transverse sinus, vein of Galen, or smaller infratentorial veins. In this setting, the hemorrhage may rapidly enlarge and produce lethal compression of the brainstem. A subdural hemorrhage may also occur over the cerebral convexities as a result of rupture of bridging, superficial cerebral veins.
- Predisposing factors include a relatively large infant and relatively small birth canal, unusual deforming stresses such as face or brow presentation, or a history of a difficult forceps or vacuum-assisted delivery.
- While infants may be asymptomatic, recognition of the clinical syndrome is important. There may be an initial period (hours to days) with no neurologic signs, followed by signs of increased intracranial pressure (full fontanelle, irritability, lethargy), followed by symptoms of brainstem compression (apnea, bradycardia, unequal pupils, and oculomotor abnormalities).
- An emergent CT scan is usually diagnostic, and an LP should be avoided because of the possibility of herniation.
- The prognosis depends on the severity of hemorrhage; nearly all infants with lacerations of falx and tentorium present immediately after birth and die.
- Management includes rapid detection and prompt neurosurgical evacuation for tentorial and falx lacerations, occipital osteodiastasis, and posterior fossa subdural hematomas. For convexity SDH, careful and serial examinations are required. Surgical intervention is only indicated if increased intracranial pressure or neurologic deficits occur.
- *Subarachnoid hemorrhage* (SAH) is a relatively common lesion, especially in preterm infants. It refers to blood in the subarachnoid space, usually over the posterior aspect of the cerebral convexities. Predisposing factors are similar to those described above for SDH. Three clinical syndromes may be recognized:
  1. Minimal or no symptoms associated with minor degrees of hemorrhage—most common.
  2. Seizures in an otherwise well infant, typically on the second day of life in term infants.
  3. Massive hemorrhage with catastrophic deterioration and rapidly fatal course—very rare.
- If suspected, a CT scan should be performed as ultrasound is relatively insensitive. The prognosis correlates

with the clinical syndrome, and at least 90% of infants presenting with seizures are normal on follow-up. Complications are rare, and most commonly are hydrocephalus. No specific management is required, unless hydrocephalus develops.

- *Intraventricular hemorrhage* (IVH) is a lesion seen almost exclusively in premature infants (see Prematurity section), but can occur in term infants. Minor degrees of IVH may be an incidental finding in asymptomatic term infants. In symptomatic infants, a history of difficult delivery with forceps or vacuum assistance is found in approximately one-third of cases; however, ~25% have no definable risk factors. Similar to preterm infants, the hemorrhage usually originates in the choroid plexus or subependymal germinal matrix. Clinical features include irritability, stupor, apnea, seizures, fever, jitteriness, and signs of increased intracranial pressure. Seizures occur in 65% of infants and are focal or multifocal. Head ultrasound or CT scan confirms the diagnosis. Initial management is focused on avoiding cerebral hemodynamic disturbances by maintaining adequate arterial blood pressure, avoiding rapid volume expansion and hyperosmolar solutions, and maintaining stable gas exchange without large fluctuations in pH, $PaCO_2$, or PaO_2. Approximately 50% of infants will develop hydrocephalus requiring placement of a ventriculoperitoneal shunt; and an additional 20% will develop ventricular dilatation. Therefore serial head ultrasounds should be performed, and neurosurgical consultation is needed. Complete recovery occurs in ~50% of infants within 2–3 weeks; the remainder improve but may have neurologic abnormalities and subsequent deficits, particularly if there is a history of birth trauma or asphyxia.
- *Intracerebellar hemorrhage* is relatively common, and observed in ~5–10% of autopsy cases. It is more common in preterm infants with a pathogenesis similar to IVH; in term infants it is often related to trauma during birth. The cerebellar vermis is the usual origin of the hemorrhage. The onset of symptoms is variable, and may occur within 24 hours (most common) or as late as 2–3 weeks of age. Infants typically present with signs of brainstem compression (apnea, respiration irregularities, and bradycardia), and obstruction to CSF flow (full fontanelle). More subtle signs such as skew deviation of eyes, facial paresis, and intermittent tonic extension of limbs are possible. An ultrasound or CT scan will confirm the diagnosis. Management is primarily supportive, and surgical intervention is rarely performed. The prognosis for preterm infants is uniformly poor. The outcome in term infants is more favorable but still guarded. All have neurologic deficits, ~50% develop hydrocephalus

requiring shunt placement, and almost all have ongoing cerebellar disturbances including intention tremor, truncal ataxia, and hypotonia. Cognitive deficits are common: consistent but variable.

BIRTH ASPHYXIA

- See neonatal neurology section
- Use of terminology should be limited to describe neonate with all of the following:
  1. Profound metabolic or mixed acidemia (pH <7) on umbilical cord artery blood sample.
  2. Neonatal neurologic manifestations (e.g., seizures, coma, hypotonia).
  3. Multisystem organ dysfunction (e.g., CV, GI, hematologic, pulmonary, renal).

SPINAL CORD INJURY

- These injuries may be responsible for a significant percentage of neonatal deaths; the true incidence is unknown, since the spinal cord is not usually examined at autopsy. Two primary sites of injury occur: lower cervical and upper thoracic sites in breech deliveries, and upper- to midcervical regions after cephalic deliveries. The acute lesions are epidural and intraspinal hemorrhages and edema. The pathogenesis is excessive longitudinal or lateral traction of spine (breech deliveries), or excessive torsion (vertex) deliveries.
- Clinical features are characterized by three syndromes:
  1. Stillbirth or rapid neonatal death with failure to establish adequate respiratory function, especially with lesions involving upper cervical cord or lower brainstem or both.
  2. Severe respiratory failure in first days of life leading to death.
  3. Neurologic instability (*spinal shock*) including weakness and hypotonia in the neonatal period. Survivors develop hyperactive reflexes and spasticity over time that is often confused with cerebral palsy.
- Differential diagnosis includes occult spinal dysraphism, an intravertebral, extramedullary mass (abscess or neuroblastoma), intramedullary lesion (syringomyelia or hemangioblastoma), or a neuromuscular disorder (Werdnig-Hoffman disease).
- Useful studies include spine radiographs to rule out other anomalies. A spinal ultrasound is the most useful test in the acute period, and will help demonstrate cord size and configuration, and can identify blood either within the cord (hematomyelia) or in extramedullary

space. Other helpful studies may include magnetic resonance imaging (MRI) or CT myelography.
- Prevention when there is a known factor such as breech presentation is necessary as there is little specific therapy available once the injury has occurred. Postnatal management is supportive, including ventilation, maintenance of body temperature, prevention of UTIs, and physical therapy to prevent contractures. Exclusion of surgically remediable lesions is necessary. Methylprednisolone is a promising development for acute management of spinal injury in adults, but its role in newborn disease is not clear.

BRACHIAL PLEXUS INJURY

- Brachial plexus injury is weakness or total paralysis of muscles supplied by the nerves of the brachial plexus. The incidence is between 0.5 and 2 per 1000 live births, and is higher in deliveries that require assistance with forceps.
- Predisposing factors include macrosomia, shoulder dystocia, multiparity, prolonged second stage of labor or augmented labor, breech or abnormal vertex presentation (occiput posterior or occiput transverse), and fetal distress or depression.
- The pathogenesis is stretching of the brachial plexus via exertion of extreme lateral traction during delivery. This may produce hemorrhage and edema in the nerve sheath or axon, or in the most severe form, avulsion of nerve root from cord.
- Other traumatic lesions are frequently observed, including fractured clavicle (10%), fractured humerus (10%), facial palsy (10–20%), and laryngeal nerve involvement (2%).
- Two major types of injury are observed; both may occur in the same patient.
  1. *Erb palsy* involves the proximal upper extremity, and makes up 90–95% of brachial plexus injuries as the upper roots are most vulnerable. This injury is usually unilateral, and most commonly on the right; ~50% involve only C5 and C6; C7 is affected in the other 50%. The ipsilateral diaphragm is affected in 5–10% of infants, indicating involvement of C4 and perhaps C3. Clinical features include absent or decreased spontaneous movement of the extremity; and the "waiter's tip" position in which the shoulder is adducted and internally rotated, elbow extended, forearm prone, and wrist and fingers flexed. The palmar grasp reflex is preserved. Deep tendon reflexes (DTRs), particularly the biceps reflex, are decreased or absent.
  2. *Klumpke palsy* involves the distal upper extremity including the hand muscles, and occurs because of

injury to the lower nerve roots or C8 and T1. A true Klumpke palsy is rare; instead infants almost always exhibit proximal extremity involvement also. Clinical features include a flaccid hand, lack of wrist movement or grasp reflex. Sympathetic outflow from T1 is affected in one-third of infants, producing Horner syndrome (ptosis, miosis, and anhidrosis).

- The diagnosis is made clinically by a thorough neurologic examination. Subsequent electromyography (EMG) testing may help delineate injury and monitor recovery. Diaphragmatic involvement may be determined by fluoroscopy or ultrasound. An MRI may be helpful in determining whether there has been partial or complete avulsion of nerve roots.

- Treatment includes immobilization of the arm close to body for 7–10 days to limit further injury. This is followed by gentle passive range of motion exercises to the shoulder, elbow, wrist, and small joints of hand. Supportive wrist splints may help prevent flexion contractures and stabilize fingers. Microsurgical nerve repair is sometimes attempted if there is no appreciable functional recovery by 3 months.

- Prognosis relates to the severity of the lesion, but in general 75–90% resolve without sequelae. Recovery is more likely with Erb compared to Klumpke paralysis, especially if Horner syndrome is present. Onset of recovery within 2–4 weeks of injury is a favorable prognostic sign, and impairment remaining after 15 months of age is likely to be permanent.

DIAPHRAGMATIC PARALYSIS

- Diaphragmatic paralysis is secondary to trauma to cervical roots supplying the phrenic nerve, with a pathogenesis similar to that for brachial plexus injuries. While it may occur as an isolated finding, 80–90% are associated with brachial plexus injury. Approximately 80% involve the right side and less than 10% are bilateral. Phrenic nerve injury is more common after breech than cephalic deliveries.

- The clinical course is variable. Initially, tachypnea and cyanosis may be noted, with blood gases revealing hypercarbia, hypoxemia, and acidosis. This period is often followed by stabilization or improvement as supplemental oxygen and ventilatory support are provided. An elevated hemidiaphragm may not be seen on x-ray during this period, especially if positive pressure ventilation is used. In severe cases, over the subsequent days to weeks, there is respiratory deterioration often associated with atelectasis or infection.

- The diagnosis should be suspected when an elevated hemidiaphragm is noted on chest x-ray. Confirmation is by ultrasound or fluoroscopy, which will show paradoxical movement with spontaneous respiration.

- Initial management is expectant, with a goal to stabilize the infant and provide adequate support of ventilation until natural improvement of the neural injury occurs. Surgical plication of diaphragm is generally performed if no recovery is observed after 2 months of expectant therapy. If there is bilateral paralysis, surgery is recommended only for the more severely involved hemidiaphragm if possible.

- The prognosis for unilateral paralysis is generally good. The majority recover in the first 6–12 months of life, although mortality rates as high as 10–15% have been reported. Mortality is as high as 50% with bilateral paralysis; long-term ventilatory support is typically required.

FACIAL PARALYSIS

- Facial weakness caused by injury to the facial nerve is the most common neurologic manifestation of perinatal trauma, with incidence ranging from 1–6% of live births. Seventy-five percent involve the left side. Pathogenesis is compression of the facial nerve; this is most commonly by the bony sacral promontory, although forceps may be a source of pressure as well. The site of lesion is at or near exit of facial nerve from stylomastoid foramen where it divides into the two major branches (temporofacial and cervicofacial).

- Clinical signs include unilateral weakness of both the upper and lower facial muscles. Weakness is noted at rest; when crying the infant is unable to wrinkle brow, close eye firmly, or move corner of mouth or lower face into effective grimace on the affected side. Dribbling from the corner of mouth during feeding is common.

- Management includes artificial tears and occasionally taping of the eyelid to prevent corneal injury.

- Prognosis is excellent with complete recovery within 1–3 weeks in the great majority of infants.

LARYNGEAL NERVE PALSY

- Laryngeal nerve palsy is important to recognize because it leads to disorders in breathing and swallowing. It may be associated with brachial plexus or diaphragmatic injuries, but may also be related to in utero position before or during delivery where the head is rotated slightly and flexed laterally. The nearby hypoglossal nerve may be affected, resulting in paralysis of the tongue.

- Diagnosis is via direct laryngoscopic examination, which will reveal a paralyzed vocal cord.

- Treatment is symptomatic. Severe lesions may require prolonged gavage feeding or tracheostomy, and noisy breathing and increased risk for aspiration may last >1 year.
- The prognosis is good, and affected infants usually recover completely by 6–12 months of life.

RADIAL NERVE INJURY

- This injury is caused by compression of the nerve in utero by a restricted fetal position, or during difficult labor and delivery by forceps. The site of compression can sometimes be identified by induration with underlying fat necrosis above the radial epicondyle of the humerus. Less common causes include a humeral fracture or septic arthritis at the shoulder.
- Clinical signs include weakness of extensors of wrist, fingers and thumb, producing a characteristic "wrist drop." There is preservation of the grasp reflex and function of intrinsic hand muscles, which differentiates this from a lower brachial plexus lesion.
- The prognosis is good, and recovery occurs in weeks to months.

MISCELLANEOUS INJURIES

- *Retinal hemorrhages* are common, and occur in 19–50% of deliveries. They are more common after vacuum-assisted deliveries. These resolve within several weeks with little long-term morbidity.
- *Intraabdominal hemorrhages* may rarely occur because of a ruptured spleen or hepatic subcapsular hematoma. These hemorrhages should be suspected when there are unexplained symptoms of blood loss or hypovolemia, particularly if there is abdominal distension or discoloration. Emergent surgical evaluation may be needed.

BIBLIOGRAPHY

Mangurten HH. Birth injuries. In: Fanaroff A and Martin R, eds. *Neonatal-Perinatal Medicine, Diseases of the Fetus and Infant*, 6th ed. Mosby, 1997:425–454.

Medlock MD, Hanigan WC. Neurologic birth trauma. Intracranial, spinal cord, and brachial plexus injury. *Clin Perinatol* 1997;24:845–857.

Taeusch HW and Snideman S. History and physical examination of the newborn. In: Taesch HW and Ballard RA, eds. *Avery's Diseases of the Newborn*, 7th ed. W.B. Saunders; 1998: 334–353.

Volpe JJ. *Neurology of the Newborn*, 4th ed. W.B. Saunders; 2001.

21 PREMATURITY

Karen K.L. Mestan and Ruth B. Deddish

HISTORICAL CONSIDERATIONS

- Management of the premature infant has improved dramatically over the past several years because of advances in perinatal care. A greater understanding of fetal and infant nutrition, pharmacology, and pathophysiology combined with the development of improved antenatal care, surfactant therapy, and modern incubator and ventilator technologies have resulted in significant decreases in premature infant morbidity and mortality.
- From 1965 to 1980, the infant mortality rate decreased 47% in the United States, primarily because of the increased survival of high-risk infants with low birthweight (LBW).
- Despite their increased survival rates, low birthweight and very low birthweight (VLBW) infants still account for the majority of neonatal deaths. The contradictory decline in infant mortality without parallel decline in low birthweight infants is because of the increased survival (rather than prevention) of low birthweight and premature infants.
- With the above changes there has been a gradual decrease in the accepted gestational age at which the fetus can survive outside of the womb. Although the exact "limits of viability" remain unclear and vary among institutions, most fetuses born at 23 weeks or less are typically considered nonviable because of the severe immaturity of multiple organ systems.

DEFINITIONS

- According to the World Health Organization (WHO) classification established in 1974, live-born infants delivered before 37 weeks gestation from the first day of the last menstrual period are termed *premature*. This definition is based on the greater likelihood of conditions associated with immaturity, such as hyaline membrane disease (HMD) and intraventricular hemorrhage (IVH), in this group of infants. Although not a formal classification, the term *extreme prematurity* is often used to describe infants born at less than 27 weeks.

- LBW infants are defined by a birthweight of less than or equal to 2500 g. VLBW infants weigh less than 1500 g at birth, and infants of *extremely low birthweight* (ELBW) are less than 1000 g at birth.

- The terms *intrauterine growth retardation* (IUGR) and *small-for-gestational age* (SGA), although related and often used interchangeably, are not synonymous. IUGR is a pathologic deviation from an expected fetal growth pattern. SGA describes an infant whose weight is lower than population norms or lower than a predetermined cutoff weight (<2 SD). The cause may be pathologic, as in infants with IUGR, or nonpathologic, as in infants who are small but otherwise healthy.

- It is important to note that the health of a baby is not only related to its birthweight classification but also to its gestational age. The LBW classification includes infants who are premature, preterm, and SGA or IUGR, and term infants who are SGA or IUGR. For example, an 1800 g infant born at term is very different from an 1800 g infant born at 32 weeks.

INCIDENCE

- The majority of LBW infants are premature; however, because of the significant overlap between preterm infants and term infants who are SGA or IUGR, it is often difficult to separate these two terms when discussing incidences of birth, disease, and mortality.

- During 1997, 7.5% of live-born infants in the United States were LBW. Since the early 1980s, the LBW rate has increased primarily because of an increased number of preterm births. Approximately 9% of all U.S. births are premature, and almost 2% of U.S. infants are born at less than 32 weeks.

- Interestingly, the VLBW rate has remained unchanged for Black Americans but has increased in Whites. The reason for this disparity is not completely clear but at least in part is related to the increase in multiple births in the White population.

RISK FACTORS ASSOCIATED WITH PREMATURITY

- Although most premature births occur for unknown reasons, the most common risk factors associated with preterm delivery are outlined below.

DEMOGRAPHIC FACTORS

- Race has been a well-known and extensively studied risk factor for many years. Black women experience more than twice the rate of premature delivery than White women and account for almost one-third of all premature infants. Lower socioeconomic status (SES) is also associated with higher rates of premature delivery. In addition, women under age 16 and over age 35 are more likely to deliver LBW infants. Age is a more significant factor in White births than in Black births.

BEHAVIORAL FACTORS

- Poor maternal nutrition appears to increase the risk of low birthweight and preterm delivery. Cigarette smoking and substance abuse (in particular, cocaine) play a significant role and are likely to result in the uteroplacental vasoconstriction that leads to an increased rate of abruption. Lastly, inadequate prenatal care often accompanies many of the above risk factors and is commonly associated with preterm delivery.

MATERNAL MEDICAL CONDITIONS

- A previous obstetric history of premature birth or perinatal complications (fetal distress, sepsis) places a woman at higher risk for preterm delivery. In fact, prior poor birth outcome is the single strongest predictor of poor birth outcome, and a premature first birth is the best predictor of a premature subsequent birth.

- Other maternal complications include uterine and cervical abnormalities (bicornuate uterus, incompetent cervix), trauma, vaginal bleeding (placenta previa, abruptio placentae), polyhydramnios, premature rupture of membranes, and chorioamnionitis. Acute or chronic maternal illness such as urinary tract infection, hypertension, preeclampsia, and diabetes are also common risk factors. Delivery may occur either by induced labor to remove the infant from an unfavorable in utero environment or secondary to spontaneous onset of labor.

FETAL FACTORS

- Multiple gestation, chronic fetal infections (e.g., TORCH infections, including *t*oxoplasmosis, *r*ubella, and *c*ytomegalovirus), chromosomal and congenital anomalies, immune and nonimmune hydrops are among the many fetal conditions associated with premature delivery. It is important to note that factors commonly associated with IUGR are frequently seen with prematurity. Again, this relationship is likely because of the fact that preterm births often signify a need for early delivery from a potentially disadvantageous intrauterine environment.

PHYSICAL EXAMINATION: ASSESSMENT OF GESTATIONAL AGE IN THE PREMATURE INFANT

- Accurate assessment of gestational age at birth is particularly important when standard obstetric milestones such as last menstrual period or early fetal ultrasonography are unknown or the infant is IUGR. The Ballard scoring system is commonly used to estimate gestational age at birth (see Newborn section). Some of the neuromuscular and physical findings used in this scoring system may be less reliable because of many conditions that accompany premature birth (e.g., sepsis, edema, respiratory distress, and perinatal depression).
- *Morphologic findings* of the premature infant are helpful in determining gestational age. A paper-thin, *translucent skin* and prominent venous pattern are often characteristic in infants less than 28 weeks. Fine, thin hair on both the scalp and body (*lanugo*) is also present and begins to thin at about 30–32 weeks gestation. A *lack of prominent plantar creases* is characteristic prior to 32 weeks. There is a *lack of prominent breast tissue*, which is a result of maternal hormonal influences. *Underdeveloped cartilage* is evident by the lack of recoil of the folded ear prior to 32 weeks. Lastly, the *distinct appearance of the genitalia* is often a reliable marker of prematurity. In the female, the clitoris and labia minora are prominent until 34–36 weeks. The preterm male lacks prominent rugae on the scrotum, and the testes are often not palpable in the inguinal canal until 28–30 weeks.
- *Neuromuscular findings* in the premature infant are also very distinct. There is a marked *extensor posture* (upper and lower extremities and hips) in the resting supine position as compared to the flexor posture of the term infant. Active tone and reflex responsiveness are markedly decreased in the premature infant, as evidenced by the *lack of arm recoil* when the upper extremities are fully extended and then released. Flexion angles, which measure ligament and tendon laxity, are typically more pronounced in the lower extremities (*popliteal angle test)* and more limited in the upper extremities (*square window test*) in the preterm infant. This pattern of flexion-extension development reverses with increasing gestational age. Lastly, resting tone of both upper and lower extremities is

decreased in the preterm infant as compared to term infants (*scarf sign and heel-to-ear test*).

PROBLEMS ASSOCIATED WITH PREMATURITY

- Immature organ function, complications of therapy, and the specific disorders that may have caused premature onset of labor often increase the severity and obscure the clinical manifestations of many neonatal diseases. Specific problems that are most commonly associated with prematurity are outlined below.

RESPIRATORY

- *Respiratory distress syndrome* (RDS), also called hyaline membrane disease (HMD) is the most common respiratory disease related to prematurity. The incidence is inversely related to birthweight, as RDS occurs in 80% of infants less than 1000 g and in 40% of infants between 1250 and 1500 g. The underlying cause is the physiologic lack of surfactant production in the premature lung which typically begins at 24–28 weeks' gestation. At the time of birth, surfactant deficiency causes collapse of small airways and progressive atelectasis. Clinical manifestations include tachypnea, retractions, and cyanosis that persists or progresses over the first 48–96 hours of life. Chest radiographic findings of a homogeneous reticulogranular pattern and air bronchgrams are characteristic.
- Surfactant replacement therapy has been the mainstay of treatment for over a decade and has accounted for the dramatic decrease in RDS deaths since 1991. It is administered endotracheally as either a prophylactic dose (given within the first hour of life) or as a rescue therapy for infants who acutely develop symptoms. Repeat doses may be indicated depending on the severity and duration of symptoms.
- *Neonatal apnea* defined as the absence of respiratory air flow for a period of greater than or equal to 20 seconds, is another common problem associated with prematurity. The term *apnea of prematurity* (AOP) is a diagnosis of exclusion when all other pathologic causes of apnea (i.e., sepsis, anemia, seizures, necrotizing enterocolitis [NEC], GE reflux) have been ruled out. AOP is thought to be caused by an immaturity of respiratory control mechanisms and may be either central, obstructive, or mixed. If frequent apneic episodes occur that require stimulation or intermittent bag-and-mask ventilation to reinitiate ventilation, treatment with methylxanthine drugs (theophylline and caffeine citrate) should be considered. Positive pressure ventilation via nasal continuous positive airway pressure

(CPAP) or intubation may be required when medical therapy is not effective.

- *Other respiratory problems* associated with prematurity include *congenitally acquired pneumonia, air leak syndromes* (pneumothorax, pneumomediastinum), pulmonary hemorrhage, and *pulmonary interstitial emphysema* (PIE). Chronic lung disease, also known as *bronchopulmonary dysplasia* (BPD), is a late manifestation commonly seen in premature infants who have had severe lung disease in the neonatal period. The incidence of BPD among VLBW infants is about 18% and increases with decreasing gestational age (see Neonatology-Pulmonary section).

CARDIAC

- Congestive heart failure secondary to *patent ductus arteriosus* (PDA) occurs when the large vessel connecting the main pulmonary trunk with the descending aorta fails to close or reopens after functional closure. Normal closure occurs in healthy term newborns by 96 hours of life. The incidence of PDA is inversely related to gestational age, occurring in about 45% of infants under 1750 g and 80% of infants under 1000 g. Typical presentation is in the first 1–2 weeks of life and may include a holosystolic heart murmur, hyperactive precordium, bounding peripheral pulses, and widened pulse pressure. Hypotension and respiratory distress often present without a heart murmur, and echocardiography is almost always necessary to confirm the diagnosis.
- Treatment of PDA includes appropriate ventilatory support and fluid restriction. Indomethacin is a prostaglandin synthetase inhibitor that has proven to be effective in promoting ductal closure, particularly in very premature infants when given within the first 1–2 weeks of life. Surgical ligation of the vessel is indicated in infants who have either failed medical treatment or for whom indomethacin is contraindicated because of its side effects (i.e., renal toxicity, GI bleeding, platelet dysfunction).
- *Other cardiac problems* are nonspecific to the premature infant but occur with increased frequency as compared with term newborn infants. *Hypotension* caused by hypovolemia, cardiac dysfunction, and/or vasodilation secondary to sepsis occurs frequently. The severity of illness is often increased because of the immaturity of the cardiovascular system.

GASTROINTESTINAL

- Necrotizing enterocolitis (NEC) is a disease of serious intestinal injury caused by a combination of vascular and mucosal damage to an immature gut. Although the pathophysiology remains unclear, the most common associated risk factors include prematurity (60–80% of cases occur in high-risk premature infants) and introduction of enteral feedings. NEC should be suspected in any preterm infant presenting with feeding intolerance, abdominal distension, and hematochezia. Early signs are often nonspecific and may mimic neonatal sepsis (i.e., apnea, bradycardia, abnormal white blood cell count, thrombocytopenia). Radiographic findings include the presence of intramural bowel gas (pneumatosis intestinalis) and/or intrahepatic portal venous gas. Acute medical management includes cessation of enteral feedings, gastric compression, sepsis workup, and IV antibiotics. Serial abdominal examinations and x-ray studies are needed to rule out intestinal perforation. Surgical consultation and possible intervention is often required (see Neonatology-Disease of the Digestive Tract section).

NEUROLOGIC

- Intraventricular hemorrhage (IVH) is the most common neurologic complication of premature infants. Although the incidence has decreased significantly in recent years (less than 20% in VLBW infants), IVH remains a major problem because the survival rate of infants <1000 g continues to increase. Bleeding originates in the highly vascularized germinal matrix (GM) which is most prominent and prone to rupture in infants less than 32–34 weeks' gestation. Although several risk factors have been associated with IVH (i.e., fetal distress, disturbances in blood pressure, thermoregulation, acid-base balance, and hemostasis) the exact etiology is unclear, and prevention of severe IVH remains a challenge in caring for the premature infant. Diagnosis is confirmed by ultrasonography and severity is often classified by the Papile system:
1. *Grade I*:   GM hemorrhage
2. *Grade II*:   IVH without ventricular dilatation
3. *Grade III*: IVH with ventricular dilatation
4. *Grade IV*:   GM hemorrhage or IVH with parenchymal involvement
- *Other neurologic complications* include *posthemorrhagic hydrocephalus* (PHH) and *periventricular leukomalacia* (PVL). Approximately 35% of infants with IVH develop PHH. About 30% of these cases eventually require some level of neurosurgic intervention (serial lumbar punctures and/or ventriculoperitoneal shunt placement), while the majority of cases of ventriculomegaly either cease to progress or resolve spontaneously. PVL may or may not accompany IVH,

as the disease is caused by ischemia of the periventricular white matter as a result of decreased cerebral blood flow either in utero or in the early neonatal period. Premature infants exposed to prolonged rupture of membranes, chorioamnionitis, or events thought to cause early IVH (i.e., birth asphyxia or need for vigorous resuscitation) appear to be at increased risk. The diagnosis of PVL may greatly impact prognosis as infants with PVL have a higher incidence of cerebral palsy.

OPHTHALMOLOGIC

- *Retinopathy of prematurity* (ROP) is a disease of the immature retina caused by interruption of the normal development of newly forming retinal vessels. Vasoconstriction and obliteration and subsequent neovascularization of the capillary beds may lead to retinal edema, hemorrhage, and fibrosis. If not reversed in the early stages, retinal detachment and eventual blindness can occur. Although the pathophysiology and etiology of ROP remains unclear, extreme prematurity is known to be the most significant risk factor.
- Serial eye examinations beginning at 4–6 weeks of age are recommended for all infants ≤1500 g or ≤28 weeks and for infants between 1500 and 2000 g with an unstable neonatal course (i.e., requiring significant or prolonged ventilatory support). An International Classification of ROP has been useful in staging the severity of active disease and provides guidelines for when ablative therapy is indicated:

  Stage I: Thin demarcation line between the vascularized and avascular zone of the retina.

  Stage II: Developing ridge extends into the vitreous.

  Stage III: Extraretinal fibrovascular proliferation, neovascular tufts form posterior to the ridge. Plus disease occurs when these vessels become dilated and tortuous.

  Stage IV: Neovascularization extends into the vitreous with fibrosis and scarring, traction, and retinal detachment can occur.

NUTRITIONAL AND METABOLIC DISORDERS

- Careful monitoring of nutrient intake is essential to minimize the risks of malnutrition and failure to thrive. While disorders of glucose metabolism (hypoglycemia and hyperglycemia) are common in the early neonatal period, problems of calcium metabolism (*osteopenia of prematurity*) can occur in chronically ill, poorly supplemented low birthweight infants.

HEMATOLOGIC

- The etiology of *anemia* is often multifactorial (i.e., iatrogenic because of frequent blood sampling, chronic illness, physiologic nadir). *Hyperbilirubinemia* may be caused by many factors as well, and may be either conjugated (often a late finding because of total parenteral nutrition (TPN) cholestasis) or unconjugated (see Hematology section).

IMMUNOLOGIC

- Bacterial, viral, and fungal infections all occur more frequently in premature infants than in full-term infants. Because of immaturity of the immune system, infection can rapidly lead to overwhelming sepsis, with significant morbidity and mortality. Although congenitally acquired bacterial infections caused by *group B beta-hemolytic streptococcus (GBS)* and *E. coli* are most common overall, nosocomial infections secondary to *Staphylococcus, Pseudomonas,* and *Candida* spp. typically occur in the smaller and more chronically ill infants.

MANAGEMENT OF THE PREMATURE INFANT

- Management of the premature infant requires a multisystem, interdisciplinary approach from birth to the time of hospital discharge. Since low birthweight infants are often born acutely ill, delivery in an appropriately equipped and staffed hospital facility can reduce the risk of complications. Poor outcome is associated with a lack of early intensive care and the need to transfer to an outlying hospital.

IMMEDIATE POSTNATAL MANAGEMENT

- The routine measures for resuscitation and stabilization (see Delivery Room Resuscitation section), umbilical cord and eye care, and vitamin K administration in the term newborn infant are essentially the same for premature infants. The American Academy of Pediatrics (AAP) considers delivery of infants at less than 32 weeks or birthweight <1500 g to be high risk and recommends that a pediatric team be readily available for immediate resuscitation and stabilization. Infants older and larger than this may require special care; however, the attendance by a pediatric team at those deliveries should be determined by the individual perinatal history and events (i.e., evidence of sepsis, fetal distress, unsure dates).

NEONATAL INTENSIVE CARE MANAGEMENT

* Following stabilization of the preterm infant, decisions regarding admission for continued intensive care must be carefully considered. The most common indications for specialized care are outlined below.
* *Continuous monitoring* of heart rate, respiratory rate, pulse-oximetry and blood pressure are indicated if the infant exhibits any signs of cardiorespiratory instability. Apnea, increased work of breathing, tachypnea, hypoxia, bradycardia, and hypotension are common indications for admission.
* *The need for thermoregulatory support* is common among low birthweight infants who are otherwise well. Most premature infants are able to maintain their own body temperature at >1800 g. The goal should be to provide an environmental temperature at which oxygen consumption and metabolic stress are minimized but sufficient to maintain body temperature (ideally between 36.4 and 37.1°C). For the very small preterm infant, thermoregulation often requires either an overhead radiant warmer or a closed incubator. Maintenance of environmental humidity between 40 and 60% via a humidified tent or incubator helps to minimize evaporative heat loss.
* *Ventilator management and/or oxygen therapy* is often required in infants presenting with RDS and/or apnea. It is most common in infants who are significantly premature (<32 weeks). The decision to initiate mechanical ventilation is complex. Since premature infants are at high risk of pulmonary injury secondary to barotrauma and hyperoxia that may be induced by positive pressure ventilation, the decision to intubate should not be taken lightly. In addition, every effort should be made to wean the support and supplemental oxygen as rapidly as tolerated to minimize lung injury.
* *Intravenous fluid and electrolyte management* also require close monitoring, particularly in the very low birthweight infant. The immature skin and renal system predispose these infants to significant insensible water losses and electrolyte imbalances that must be replaced based on careful calculation of input vs. output. Overhydration must be avoided as well to minimize complications of pulmonary edema and PDA.
* *Nutritional support* should be initiated as early as possible, ideally within the first 24–48 hours of life. Premature infants typically regain their birthweight more slowly and have higher caloric requirements (110–140 kcal/kg/day for an adequate weight gain of 15 g/kg/day) than term infants. Most infants <1600 g and <34 weeks are unable to bottle-feed because of immaturity of suck/swallow reflexes, and nasogastric tube feedings are a common indication for specialized nursery care. In the extremely premature infant, early parenteral nutrition with intravenous lipids and amino acids is essential to support the exaggerated catabolic state.
* *Enteral feedings* are preferred over the parenteral route because of the complications associated with intravenous parenteral nutrition (i.e., IV site infiltration and burns, long-term central venous access and line infections, TPN cholestasis); however, the decision to advance feeds should take into account the patient's clinical status because of the high incidence of NEC in ELBW and sicker infants. There is recent evidence that early introduction of small-volume enteric feedings of no more than 20 cc/kg/day via continuous or bolus nasogastric tube (minimal enteric feedings) may promote gut development and minimize problems of "feeding intolerance."
* *Suspected neonatal sepsis* is another common indication for specialized care. As compared to their full-term counterparts, premature infants are at much higher risk for congenitally acquired bacterial infections. They often present atypically, with mild or no apparent symptoms, yet their clinical course may deteriorate rapidly and become much more severe if early treatment is not initiated. Therefore, a high index of suspicion should be given to any infant who delivers prematurely. A "rule-out sepsis" workup including a complete blood count, blood culture, and other appropriate studies (i.e., lumbar puncture, urine culture) should be obtained. When sepsis is strongly suspected, broad-spectrum antibiotics should be initiated empirically while awaiting culture results. *GBS, E. coli,* and *Listeria monocytogenes* are the most common pathogens and appropriate coverage includes IV ampicillin and gentamicin.

HOSPITAL DISCHARGE

* For the VLBW infant, hospital discharge requires a multidisciplinary approach. Most infants meet criteria around 36 weeks postconceptional age; however, discharge often occurs much later for infants with multiple medical problems. In addition to routine well-infant health maintenance (i.e., hearing screening, neonatal screening, immunizations), the following specific goals should be met to ensure a safe and successful discharge:
  1. Infant is exhibiting consistent weight gain on current feeding regimen.
  2. Infant is competent in oral feeding either by the bottle or at the breast without cardiorespiratory compromise.
  3. Body temperature is maintained in an open crib with normal ambient temperature.

4. Infant is physiologically mature and has stable cardiorespiratory function of a sufficient duration.
5. Appropriate immunizations have been given.
6. Appropriate metabolic screening has been done.
7. Hematologic status has been assessed and, if indicated, appropriate therapy instituted.
8. Nutritional risks have been assessed and, if indicated, appropriate modifications and therapy instituted.
9. Sensorineural assessments have been completed and follow-up arranged.
10. The primary caregiver has been trained in infant care, including safety issues, car seat use, and sleep position.
11. For patients requiring specialized infant care or monitoring (i.e., nasogastric tube feedings, supplemental oxygen, home medications, apnea monitoring), at least two primary caregivers should demonstrate comprehensive understanding of the supplies and techniques prior to discharge.
12. A primary care physician has been identified and appropriate outpatient follow-up has been arranged, including subspecialty services.

OUTCOMES FOR PREMATURE INFANTS

SURVIVAL OF PREMATURE INFANTS
- In 1997, the VLBW rate was approximately 1.4% and is a reliable predictor of infant morbidity and mortality. Infants born at less than 1500 g continue to account for over 50% of neonatal deaths. Although the exact survival rates may vary from year to year, the trend remains the same: for any given gestational age, the lower the infant birthweight, the higher the neonatal mortality, and for any given birthweight, the younger the gestational age, the higher the neonatal mortality.

LONG-TERM PROBLEMS
- A significant percentage of low birthweight infants will have some degree of long-term morbidity as outlined below. LBW and VLBW infants account for approximately 50% of all disabled infants. Overall, severe impairment occurs in a small percentage of survivors (roughly 10% of VLBW infants) and accounts for the relatively high rate of rehospitalization among former premature infants.
1. Chronic lung disease ranging from mild (minimal oxygen requirement at 1–2 months of age) to severe (tracheostomy and/or ventilator-dependent).
2. Language disorders, learning disabilities, attention deficit and behavior disorders.
3. Major motor and/or cognitive delays (cerebral palsy, mental retardation).
4. Sensory impairments (hearing loss, visual deficits).
5. Poor growth/FTT.
6. Increased risk of child abuse and neglect.

ETHICAL CONSIDERATIONS
- Although the majority of premature infants born today are successfully discharged home with minimal complications, ethical issues continue to arise, particularly in the care of extremely premature and/or severely ill patients. For infants in whom long-term survival and disability is uncertain, it is the obligation of the neonatologist and health care team to routinely discuss the range of treatment options with parents and to work toward agreement of a plan that is in the best interest of the child.

BIBLIOGRAPHY

Behrman RE, Kliegman R, Jenson HB, eds. *Nelson Textbook of Pediatrics*, 16th ed. W.B. Saunders Company; 1999.

Cloherty J and Stark AR, eds. *Manual of Neonatal Care*, 3rd ed. Little, Brown and Company; 1991.

Fanaroff AA and Martin RJ, eds. *Neonatal-Perinatal Medicine: Diseases of the Fetus and Infant*, 7th ed. Mosby; 2001.

Gomella TL, ed. *Neonatology*. 4th ed. McGraw Hill; 1999.

Lucas A, Fewtrell MS, Morley R, Singhal A, Abbott RA, Isaacs E, Stephenson T, MacFadyen UM, and Clements H. Randomized trial of nutrient-enriched formula versus standard formula for post-discharge preterm infants. *Pediatrics* 2001;108:703–711.

Whitaker AH, Feldman JF, Van Rossem R, Schonfeld IS, Pinto-Martin JA, Torre C, Blumenthal SR, and Paneth NS. Neonatal cranial ultrasound abnormalities in low birth weight infants: relation to cognitive outcomes at six years of age. *Pediatrics* 1996;98:719–729.

22 RESPIRATORY DISORDERS OF THE NEWBORN
Nicolas F.M. Porta

DEVELOPMENT OF THE RESPIRATORY SYSTEM

EMBRYOLOGY—STAGES OF LUNG DEVELOPMENT

- **Embryonic** (3–7 weeks): The lung bud originates from the ventral aspect of esophagus, and initial branching and bronchopulmonary segments are defined.

- **Pseudoglandular** (7–16 weeks): Branching of the conducting system occurs, and future airways have a narrow lumen with pseudostratified squamous epithelium. There is a glandular appearance of lung tissue by histology.
- **Canalicular** (16–24 weeks): Diameter of future airways increases, and there is narrowing of epithelial cells lining future airways. Smooth muscle and cartilage appear, respiratory bronchioles appear, and there is increased vascular proliferation within mesenchyme surrounding lung tissue.
- **Saccular** (24–36 weeks): Terminal bronchioles and alveolar sacs appear, with capillaries in closer apposition. There is further thinning of distal airspace epithelium, appearance of type II pneumocytes with early secretion of surfactant, emergence of type I pneumocytes, and closer approximation of capillaries to distal airspaces.
- **Alveolar** (36 weeks—early- to midchildhood): Alveoli appear, and continue to form for several years postnatally. For at least the first 2 years of life there is an increased proportion of lung parenchyma to total lung, subsequently continued growth of lungs is proportional to body growth.

FETAL LUNG GROWTH

- Fetal lung liquid is actively secreted by epithelium into future air spaces and ultimately into amniotic space. Catecholamines and other hormones that increase during labor cause a rapid switch from net secretion to net absorption of liquid in alveolar spaces.
- Mechanical forces producing lung growth include constant distension of lungs caused by relative obstruction of egress of fetal lung liquid at the glottis. These forces maintain positive intrapulmonary pressure relative to amniotic space which is necessary for normal lung growth and maturation.
- Fetal breathing movements (episodic and low volume) are necessary for adequate fetal lung growth to occur.

SURFACTANT

- Surfactant is secreted from and recycled by type II pneumocytes into alveolar spaces. Surfactant decreases surface tension at air-liquid interface within alveoli, thus improving lung compliance and preventing alveolar collapse.
- Surfactant is composed of phospholipids (dipalmitoylphosphatidylcholine [DPPC] ~80%, phosphatidylglycerol (PG), phosphatidylinositol, and phospha-

tidylethanolamine), neutral lipids (cholesterol), and apoproteins (surfactant proteins A, B, C, and D). Surfactant proteins B and C are responsible for organization of surfactant into tubular myelin (the surfactant structure that functions to decrease surface tension at air-liquid interface).
- Surfactant is inactivated by serum proteins, meconium, and oxygen free radicals.

PERINATAL CIRCULATION

- In fetal circulation, respiratory function is maintained by the placenta in fetuses, and pulmonary blood flow is ~10% of biventricular (total cardiac) output. The small cross-sectional area of vessels in early to mid pregnancy, as well as active vasoconstriction at the end of gestation lead to high pulmonary vascular resistance, high pulmonary arterial pressure, and low pulmonary blood flow in the near-term fetus.
- Shortly after birth, pulmonary blood flow increases to half of total cardiac output because of decreased pulmonary vascular resistance in response to an increase in oxygen tension, increase in pH, and cyclic distension of lungs by respiration.
- Pulmonary vascular resistance and blood pressure continue to decrease over the first days to weeks after birth to adult levels.

EVALUATION OF THE NEONATE WITH RESPIRATORY DISEASE

- Respiratory disorders in neonates can be apparent immediately at birth, or after an apparently successful transition from fetus to newborn has occurred.

HISTORY

- Determining gestational age is important. In preterm infants respiratory distress syndrome (RDS) is most common, but it should be remembered that other problems are possible, and there is an increased risk of bacterial sepsis. In term infants, other diagnoses are more likely, although RDS may occur (especially following gestations complicated by diabetes).
- Determine whether there has been fetal evaluation of pulmonary surfactant. The secretion of lethicin (L = phosphatidylcholine) relative to sphyngomyelin (S) by type II pneumocytes increases as the surfactant system matures. A higher L/S ratio in amniotic fluid predicts lower risk of RDS. Secretion of phosphatidylglycerol (PG) occurs late in the maturation of

the surfactant system; the presence of PG in amniotic fluid predicts lower risk of RDS.

- Maternal diabetes increases the risk of RDS at any gestation because of delayed maturation of surfactant. In addition, infants of diabetic mothers have an increased incidence of polycythemia/hyperviscosity, which can lead to poor pulmonary perfusion (pulmonary hypertension) and hypoxemia. Hypoglycemia in the infant may result in agitation or lethargy, which can lead to respiratory insufficiency.
- Chorioamnionitis is associated with an increased risk of pneumonia/sepsis.
- A family history of neonatal death in siblings may have been because of an inherited abnormality, which could be present in the current patient. Examples include congenital heart disease, alveolar capillary dysplasia and congenital deficiency of surfactant protein B or C.
- Many fetal abnormalities associated with neonatal respiratory distress can be identified before delivery by fetal ultrasonography or amniocentesis. Examples include hydrops fetalis, oligohydramnios (associated with pulmonary hypoplasia), trisomy 21 (associated with persistent pulmonary hypertension of the newborn [PPHN]).

EXAMINATION

- Dysmorphic features (craniofacial/thorax)—may suggest underlying neurologic, airway, or lung abnormalities.
- Nasal flaring suggests increased respiratory effort or an airway abnormality. The patency of nasal passages should be determined to rule out choanal atresia or stenosis.
- Examination of the lungs should be assessed for retractions, grunting, quality and symmetry of air movement/symmetry.
- The heart should be examined for a murmur, heart sounds, and the perfusion should be assessed.
- A distended abdomen suggests abdominal pathology; a scaphoid abdomen suggests Potter syndrome or congenital diaphragmatic hernia (CDH).

OTHER TESTS

- A chest x-ray should be performed to evaluate the lungs for infiltrates, perfusion, symmetry, abnormal contents in thorax, pleural effusions, and pneumothorax. In addition, the heart should be evaluated for size and shape, and the vertebrae and ribs should be examined for abnormalities.

- An abdominal x-ray helps evaluate for gastrointestinal distension and for signs of ascites.
- Laboratory studies should include a blood glucose, blood gas analysis to evaluate gas exchange and pH, and hematocrit to evaluate for polycythemia/hyperviscosity or anemia. A white blood cell count with differential and blood culture should be performed to evaluate for infection.
- Direct laryngoscopy may be performed at the bedside to assess for high upper-airway abnormalities and to secure the airway with an endotracheal tube. In some infants, indirect laryngotracheobronchoscopy may be helpful to evaluate for upper and lower airway abnormalities.

CAUSES OF RESPIRATORY INSUFFICIENCY OR FAILURE

AIRWAY

- *Choanal atresia* occurs with a ~1:5000 incidence (90% bony, 10% membranous). Unilateral disease is more common. Choanal atresia should be suspected when a catheter cannot be passed through the nares into oropharynx, and the diagnosis confirmed by computed tomography (CT) evaluation. Approximately half of infants with choanal atresia have other anomalies; in particular CHARGE sequence (*c*oloboma, *h*eart disease, *a*tresia of choana, *r*etarded growth and development, *g*enitourinary anomalies, *e*ar/hearing anomalies) should be considered. Primary repair is frequently successful; in rare cases a tracheostomy is required.
- Micrognathia/retrognathia/*Pierre Robin sequence* should be obvious on physical examination. The airway obstruction from the posterior tongue is more pronounced in supine position. When present, a cleft palate does not cause respiratory distress unless feeding difficulties are severe. These infants may require tracheostomy for several years until the mandible grows enough to maintain the tongue in a more anterior position.
- *Laryngomalacia* is the most common cause of stridor in infants, and may be noted immediately after birth. While symptoms usually resolve spontaneously, a tracheostomy may be needed in severe cases. Laryngomalacia may be associated with subglottic stenosis.
- Laryngeal atresia is rare and requires tracheostomy immediately after birth for survival. Laryngeal webs usually occur at the level of the glottis, and present with symptoms varying from an abnormal cry to severe respiratory distress. Webs may require laser/surgical treatment or tracheostomy. Tracheal atresia

or agenesis is extremely rare, and incompatible with survival.
- Subglottic stenosis presents with stridor and respiratory distress; in severe cases a tracheostomy may be required. Tracheal stenosis is often associated with complete tracheal rings, and may require extensive surgical repair in case of multiple rings or long segment stenosis.
- Excessive oral secretions may obstruct the airway and cause respiratory distress. This may occur in infants with abnormal neurologic function (inadequate swallowing), or in infants with anatomic disease such as esophageal atresia.
- A number of conditions may produce extrinsic airway compression. Vascular rings and slings caused by abnormal development of mediastinal vessels can compress or deviate the trachea causing airway obstruction (most commonly seen with a double aortic arch or aberrant right subclavian artery). Neck or mediastinal masses such as teratomas and cystic hygromas represent large lesions and can cause compression. Some may be amenable to surgical resection. Hemangiomas may be responsive to systemic steroids, but may necessitate tracheostomy for short-term management; 50% of these infants also have skin hemangiomas.
- Vocal cord paralysis is commonly caused by birth or surgical trauma, and is a common cause of stridor in newborn. It is most commonly unilateral, causing hoarse cry and minimal respiratory symptoms. Bilateral paralysis can cause severe respiratory distress, and may necessitate tracheostomy.

CHEST WALL

- Asphyxiating thoracic dystrophy is a rare, autosomal recessive condition that is associated with other skeletal abnormalities. It is fatal without aggressive interventions.
- Anasarca may be caused by fetal hydrops or severe capillary leak from sepsis. It produces decreased compliance of chest wall and therefore decreased compliance of total respiratory system. Treatment is supportive, and diuretic therapy may accelerate resolution.

LUNGS

- Retained fetal lung fluid or *transient tachypnea of the newborn* (TTN) is more common following cesarean deliveries without prior labor. Symptoms usually improve over hours to days. Mechanical ventilation may be necessary in some cases.

- Surfactant deficiency or RDS occurs with an incidence inversely related to gestational age. RDS occurs because of immaturity of the surfactant system in premature lungs. Its incidence is increased in IDM at any gestational age. RDS is frequently further complicated by pulmonary edema.
- Inadequate surfactant function leads to alveolar collapse and decreased lung compliance. Decreased strength of respiratory muscles (diaphragm, intercostals), increased chest wall compliance, and poor nutritional reserve limit the ability of very premature and small infants to compensate for decreased lung compliance.
- Untreated, respiratory insufficiency worsens over several days before spontaneous improvement since surfactant secretion occurs within 2–3 days after birth at any gestation.
- Surfactant deficiency/insufficiency can also occur because of surfactant inactivation by serum proteins (e.g., following pulmonary hemorrhages) and meconium.
- Therapy is aimed at maintaining adequate functional residual capacity (FRC = volume of air in lungs at end of normal expiration, optimizes lung compliance to allow for subsequent inspiration) using continuous positive airway pressure (CPAP), mechanical ventilation with appropriate positive end expiratory pressure (PEEP), and exogenous surfactant.
- *Meconium aspiration syndrome* (MAS):
  1. Meconium stained amniotic fluid (MSAF) complicates 10–20% of deliveries and is more common in the postterm gestation. MAS occurs in ~4% of infants with MSAF, and half of infants with MAS require mechanical ventilation. Although suctioning of the trachea after delivery may prevent aspiration of meconium, infants may still develop MAS when no meconium was suctioned from below the vocal cords.
  2. MAS is characterized by airway obstruction and heterogeneous lung disease manifesting as hyperinflated areas interspersed with atelectatic areas. This results in mismatching of ventilation and perfusion (V/Q mismatching) leading to hypoxemia. In some cases in which meconium (or amniotic fluid) was aspirated deeply into the air spaces, a more homogeneous "parenchymal" lung disease pattern can occur.
  3. Many cases of MAS are further complicated by PPHN.
- *Congenital pneumonia* usually causes diffuse rather than lobar infiltrates in newborn infants. The initial radiograph is frequently indistinguishable from RDS.
  1. Bacterial pneumonia is most common. Pathogens that cause early congenital pneumonia include *group B beta-hemolytic streptococci* (GBS), *Escherichia coli*

(E. coli), and *Listeria monocytogenes*. Congenital chlamydia infection can cause pneumonia that presents between 1 and 3 months of age.

2. Common bacterial pathogens that can cause nosocomial pneumonia include *Pseudomonas* species (esp. *aeruginosa*), *Klebsiella, Serratia, Staphylococcus aureus*, and coagulase negative *Staphylococcus* species.

3. Fungal pneumonias are usually nosocomial, and are most commonly caused by *Candida albicans* and other *Candida* species.

4. Viruses may rarely cause congenital pneumonia (e.g., varicella, cytomegalovirus) or nosocomial/community acquired pneumonia (respiratory syncytial virus, influenza).

• *Pulmonary hypoplasia* may be primary (because of idiopathic pulmonary hypoplasia or pulmonary agenesis) but usually is secondary to external compression and interference with normal growth and development of the fetal lungs.

1. Early and prolonged (second trimester) oligohydramnios can cause pulmonary hypoplasia. Causes include inadequate fetal urine production from renal agenesis/dysplasia or severe urinary obstruction, or chronic amniotic fluid leak caused by preterm premature rupture of membranes.

2. Other less common causes of pulmonary hypoplasia include skeletal abnormalities (e.g., asphyxiating thoracic dystrophy). Because fetal breathing movements are necessary for normal lung development, neuromuscular disease may be associated with pulmonary hypoplasia.

3. Alveolar capillary dysplasia is a rare condition in which there is a deficient pulmonary capillary bed that does not allow for adequate diffusion of gases to and from alveoli. This condition is universally fatal and may involve a genetic predisposition.

• Atelectasis can be diffuse or focal, caused by secretions, branch airway obstruction, or compression from adjacent masses.

• *Air leak syndrome* refers to the group of disorders in which air escapes through ruptured alveoli into any of several potential spaces. Air leak can occur spontaneously, secondary to pulmonary disease, or as a complication of mechanical ventilation. Extraalveolar air may compress air spaces, resulting in decreased lung compliance and respiratory insufficiency. Prompt recognition and evacuation can be lifesaving.

1. Pneumothorax occurs spontaneously in as many as 1% of live births, and complicates 5–10% cases of RDS and 20% cases of MAS.

2. Other locations of air leak are pneumomediastinum, pneumopericardium, pneumoperitoneum, and pulmonary interstitial emphysema (PIE). PIE

is a unique form of air leak in which air from ruptured alveoli dissects into perivascular spaces, causing hyperinflation of nongas exchanging areas of the lungs.

• *Pleural effusions* can compress the ipsilateral (and even contralateral lung in the case of large collections) and cause respiratory insufficiency.

1. Pleural effusions can be the result of hydrops fetalis, congestive heart failure, cardiomyopathy, and some forms of bacterial pneumonia (particularly group B streptococcal pneumonia). Treatment of the underlying cause is essential, and thoracentesis or thoracostomy tubes may be necessary for diagnosis and to relieve symptoms.

2. Chylothoraces are pleural effusions in which chyle from pulmonary lymphatics collects in the pleural space. These may be congenital because of lymphatic abnormalities, birth trauma, or thoracic surgery. Chylothoraces are characterized by high lymphocyte count and high protein and triglyceride content in effusion fluid. Fluid can be milky white in infants who are receiving enteral feedings. Low fat diets may accelerate the resolution of chylothoraces.

• CDH can lead to severe respiratory failure immediately after birth. CDH occurs in ~1:3000 of live births and ~80% are on the left side. CDH occurs because of failure of the complete closure of pleuroperitoneal processes early in gestation. This allows abdominal viscera (intestines, liver, stomach, spleen, and so on) to displace into the thoracic space, which compresses the developing lung, and impedes normal growth and development.

1. In CDH there is ipsilateral and contralateral hypoplasia of the lung parenchyma and vasculature, and the clinical manifestations are consistent with pulmonary hypoplasia and PPHN.

2. CDH presents with cyanosis, heart sounds displaced to the contralateral side, and a scaphoid abdomen. When infants with CDH are symptomatic at birth, mortality is as high as 40%. Ideally, these infants should be delivered in centers that are equipped to provide advanced respiratory techniques such as high frequency ventilation (HFV) and inhaled nitric oxide (NO).

3. Postnatal management includes endotracheal intubation and mechanical ventilation, close cardiopulmonary monitoring with arterial vascular access, echocardiography to rule out anatomic heart disease, and assess for PPHN, gastric decompression, sedation (to minimize swallowing of air into gastrointestinal tract which could further compress the lungs), paralysis for selected cases, and close communication with surgery and extracorporeal membrane oxygenation (ECMO) teams.

4. The use of NO in infants with CDH is controversial. Randomized trials have shown that NO does not improve outcome when used prior to surgical repair; NO may be useful as a bridge to ECMO or when pulmonary hypertension worsens after surgical repair.
- Congenital lung abnormalities are rare but important causes of respiratory distress in the newborn. In most cases infants are asymptomatic, with symptoms developing over time.
  1. *Congenital cystic adenomatoid malformation* (CCAM) is abnormal lung tissue with communication to the bronchial tree. CCAMs are rare, occurring in ~1:30,000 infants, and most commonly occur in the lower lobes. CCAM can be detected in a fetus by ultrasonography, and is very rarely associated with hydrops fetalis. Computed tomography of the chest after birth is diagnostic and helpful to determine surgical approach. Resection shortly after diagnosis is justified by the risk of recurrent infections and theoretical risk of malignant degeneration.
  2. *Pulmonary sequestration* is a rare condition in which abnormal lung tissue receives vascular supply from the systemic circulation (thoracic or abdominal aorta). Intralobar lesions may have communication to bronchial tree and are most commonly found in the lower lobes. Extralobar lesions do not have communication to bronchial tree (but may have communication to adjacent lung tissue) and may be subdiaphragmatic. Sequestrations rarely present in the neonatal period with signs of congestive heart failure because of "run-off" circulation, but usually present later in life with recurrent infections.
  3. *Congenital lobar emphysema* (CLE) is an overinflated, hyperplastic area of the lung surrounded by otherwise normal lung tissue. These are most common in the upper lobes. Symptoms are progressive, but rarely present at birth. Surgical excision is usually curative, although overinflation of remaining lung areas can occur.
- *Secondary causes* of respiratory insufficiency/failure
  1. Birth asphyxia can lead to respiratory insufficiency due to apnea/hypopnea caused by hypoxic-ischemic encephalopathy (HIE), and may be complicated by poor pulmonary perfusion due to associated PPHN.
  2. Although usually due to accompanying pneumonia, sepsis can lead to respiratory insufficiency and may occasionally cause PPHN.
  3. Congenital heart disease (see discussion in Cardiology section) may cause respiratory distress due to congestive heart failure, circulatory failure, pulmonary hypertension, or respiratory insufficiency. Congestive heart failure is more common in lesions categorized by mixing of the systemic and pulmonary circulations (e.g., atrioventricular [AV] canal, ventricular septal defect [VSD], truncus arteriosus) or by systemic outflow obstruction (hypoplastic left heart syndrome [HLHS], coarctation of aorta, interrupted aortic arch, aortic stenosis).
  4. Apnea/hypopnea due to inadequate central nervous system (CNS) regulation of respiration can lead to respiratory insufficiency. This can be seen in premature infants (particularly if the mother has received magnesium), or as a consequence of CNS dysfunction due to malformations/dysgenesis, intracranial hemorrhage, or ischemic brain injury.
  5. Abdominal distension may compress the thorax and interfere with normal respiration. This may be seen as a result of gastrointestinal pathology (obstruction) or large intraabdominal mass effect (renal/genitourinary masses, severe ascites).
  6. Polycythemia can cause PPHN due to increased viscosity of the blood interfering with pulmonary perfusion. This can be seen in IDM, delayed clamping of the umbilical cord, chronic fetal hypoxia (preeclampsia), in the recipient twin of a twin-to-twin transfusion syndrome, and in other fetal conditions (trisomy 21).
  7. Severe anemia can cause respiratory distress because inadequate oxygen delivery to tissues can lead to cellular hypoxia. Anemia may be due to hemolytic disease of the newborn, fetal blood loss due to external hemorrhage (placental abruption, umbilical cord rupture) or fetal-maternal hemorrhage, or the donor twin in twin-to-twin transfusion syndrome.
  8. Hypoglycemia may cause respiratory insufficiency caused by CNS depression and can be seen in small-for-gestational age (SGA) infants, large-for-gestational age (LGA) infants, IDM, birth asphyxia or because of primary hyperinsulinism (e.g., nesidioblastosis or Beckwith-Wiedemann syndrome.)
  9. Metabolic acidosis due to metabolic/genetic causes (inborn errors of metabolism) can present with tachypnea in order to produce compensatory respiratory alkalosis.

THERAPEUTIC MEASURES FOR RESPIRATORY DISORDERS IN NEONATES

ANTENATAL INTERVENTIONS

- Glucocorticosteroids (betamethasone or dexamethasone) are used to induce maturation of the fetal lungs when premature delivery is likely prior to 34 weeks gestation. Use of antenatal glucocorticosteroids leads to decreased morbidity and mortality of premature infants. Efficacy of antenatal steroids is greatest when the first dose is at least 48 hours prior to delivery. Multiple courses of antenatal steroids may not be advantageous compared to a single course and may lead to detrimental effects in the fetal central nervous system.

- Tocolysis is used to postpone threatened premature delivery. Magnesium, calcium channel blockers, terbutaline, and indomethacin are the most commonly used agents. Tocolysis is usually not successful in prolonging pregnancy beyond ~2 days, though this may allow sufficient time for maximal effectiveness of glucocorticosteroid therapy. Tocolysis is contraindicated in pregnancies complicated by chorioamnionitis because of increased risk of neonatal sepsis.
- Antibiotics are indicated in the case of threatened delivery or in cases of chorioamnionitis. Neonatal GBS infections can be decreased by chemoprophylaxis with penicillin during labor when GBS is a known isolate from cervical or urine cultures during the current pregnancy or when there is a prior history of a sibling with invasive neonatal GBS infection.

POSTNATAL INTERVENTIONS

- Oxygen (by free flow, nasal cannula, or hood/tent) can be used to provide adequate tissue oxygenation in cases of decreased pulmonary oxygen diffusion or to facilitate pulmonary vasodilation in transitional circulation.
- Artificial airways may be necessary in cases of airway obstructions. Oral airways are used to provide oropharyngeal patency in such cases as infants with Pierre Robin or choanal atresia. Nasopharyngeal airways are used to provide CPAP without an endotracheal tube or to allow an adequate airway for infants with choanal stenosis.
- Endotracheal tubes (ETT) are used to provide mechanical ventilation when CPAP is not sufficient or when instillation of air into the gastrointestinal tract is contraindicated, such as in infants with CDH, gastroschisis, or omphalocele. Infants with respiratory distress because of CDH should have an ETT placed rapidly in order to provide respiratory support without increasing luminal gas in the intestines, which might further compress the lungs. Infants with respiratory insufficiency and gastroschisis or omphalocele should have an ETT placed in order to avoid gastrointestinal distension, which could be injurious to potentially fragile intestines.
- Mechanical ventilation may be necessary to aid or completely support respiratory function.

1. CPAP is used to maintain FRC and optimize respiratory mechanics. CPAP may be provided by nose/face mask, nasal prongs, nasopharyngeal prongs, or via an endotracheal tube.
2. Intermittent positive pressure ventilation (IPPV) is used to deliver air with variable amounts of oxygen to the airways in order to facilitate alveolar gas exchange. IPPV necessitates an ETT, and its biggest risk is lung injury because of excessive stretching of pulmonary epithelial cells, especially when high concentrations of oxygen are also given. With tidal (conventional) ventilation, physiologic amounts (approximating tidal volume) of air are delivered at physiologic rates. This mode provides bulk flow of air into airways allowing for gas exchange in distal air spaces. With HFV subphysiologic amounts of air are delivered at supraphysiologic rates. This mode facilitates diffusion of gasses to and from distal air spaces.
3. Hyperventilation (not to be confused with overdistention) to cause respiratory alkalosis is sometimes used as a pulmonary vasodilator in cases of PPHN. It should be remembered that this is not a proven therapy, and may decrease cerebral perfusion.
4. Permissive hypercapnia is commonly used, especially in preterm infants, in order to minimize ventilator-associated lung injury when chronic lung disease (CLD) is anticipated or established.
5. Hyperoxia should always be avoided in order to minimize oxygen toxicity to the lungs and other tissues.
6. Appropriate levels of PEEP are essential to optimize respiratory mechanics. Excessive PEEP may interfere with circulatory function, while insufficient PEEP will not adequately maintain FRC and leads to atelectotrauma. Starting levels should be 5–6 cm H_2O in early stages of lung disease; up to 8–10 cm H_2O may be needed in larger infants, or with severe lung/airway disease.

- *Surfactant replacement* is used to maintain alveolar stability in cases of surfactant insufficiency or inactivation. The most efficacious preparations are natural or semisynthetic surfactants extracted from animal airways or lungs (Survanta, Infasurf, and Curosurf). These preparations contain surfactant phospholipids and proteins. Surfactant replacement should be used to complement mechanical ventilation, not as a substitute for it. Maintenance of FRC depends on both mechanical distension of air spaces and alveolar stability.
1. Prophylactic therapy of premature infants at risk for the development of RDS may result in improved outcome (death, interstitial emphysema, pneumothorax, bronchopulmonary dysplasia [BPD]) compared to treatment of infants with established RDS.

Assessment of ETT position is important before giving surfactant, to avoid delivering the dose preferentially to the right side.

2. Treatment of infants with established RDS improves mortality, but does not improve incidence of chronic lung disease.

3. Treatment of term and near-term infants with parenchymal lung disease such as pneumonia or MAS decreases the need for (ECMO). This strategy works best when implemented early in the course of respiratory failure.

4. Surfactant treatment of infants with pulmonary hemorrhage may improve respiratory mechanics by supplementing endogenous surfactant inactivated by blood proteins.

• Circulatory support may be needed in severely ill neonates.

1. Volume infusions may be necessary in cases of circulatory insufficiency that complicates or contributes to respiratory insufficiency. Crystalloid is usually immediately accessible, but should be used judiciously because pulmonary edema frequently complicates respiratory failure. The use of albumin for volume resuscitation of acutely ill patients is associated with increased morbidity and mortality, and is not recommended. Blood products may be particularly useful in the case of hematologic abnormalities. Red blood cell (RBC) transfusions are indicated in cases of severe or symptomatic anemia or acute blood loss. Platelet transfusions are indicated in cases of severe or symptomatic thrombocytopenia or DIC. Fresh frozen plasma (FFP) is indicated in cases of DIC or massive transfusions. Cryoprecipitate is indicated in cases of DIC with decreased blood fibrinogen levels.

2. Cardiovascular-active medications can be useful to improve cardiac output in extremely ill neonates when poor circulatory function aggravates respiratory insufficiency. Ideal dosages of most cardiovascular-active drugs are not clearly defined in neonates, especially premature ones, and caution must be exercised.

   a. Dopamine increases blood pressure in a dose-responsive way. Increasing doses beyond 20–30 μg/kg/minute may not lead to significant clinical improvement and may be associated with decreased tissue perfusion by causing excessive vasoconstriction.

   b. Dobutamine improves myocardial contractility through β-1 effects, but may cause decreased cardiac output if tachycardia develops.

   c. Epinephrine improves contractility and cardiac output. High doses may lead to decreased tissue perfusion by causing excessive vasoconstriction.

   d. Milrinone improves myocardial contractility and causes pulmonary vasodilation, which may be particularly helpful in cases of PPHN. Its use may be limited by systemic vasodilation.

   e. Hydrocortisone may be useful in cases of circulatory failure and shock by improving systemic vascular tone. In addition, steroids may decrease the inflammatory component of many forms of pulmonary diseases such as MAS, pneumonia, and evolving CLD/BPD. The possibility of deleterious side effects such as neurodevelopmental morbidity and intestinal perforation should be considered prior to use in neonates.

• Fluid management should be optimized to help decrease morbidity in infants with severe respiratory failure. Fluid restriction is used to decrease pulmonary edema and progression of CLD/BPD, especially in early or acute settings if tolerated; however, circulatory support with volume may be necessary as previously described.

• Alkalinization is sometimes used to produce pulmonary vasodilation in cases of PPHN. Correction of acidosis that can mediate pulmonary vasoconstriction is essential, but the value of an alkaline pH is less clear. Sodium bicarbonate ($NaHCO_3$) is widely used, but is hypertonic, can lead to respiratory acidosis if ventilation is inadequate, and can lead to hypernatremia if large doses are given. Tris-hydroxymethyl aminomethane (THAM) can also be used to treat acidemia, but is also hypertonic. THAM can correct both respiratory and metabolic acidosis, but can lead to hyponatremia. Rapid or excessive alkali infusions increase the risk of intracranial hemorrhage, especially in premature infants.

• Sedation/analgesia/paralysis

1. Sedation is used to decrease oxygen consumption and to decrease ineffectual respiratory activity when significant respiratory support is necessary. Benzodiazepines with short half-lives such as midazolam can be useful when agitation complicates respiratory function. Symptoms of withdrawal must be carefully monitored when discontinuing benzodiazepines; long-term therapy with longer acting lorazepam may be necessary if tolerance develops.

2. Analgesia is necessary for painful procedures. Oxygen consumption may also be decreased by opioid analgesics. In addition, fentanyl may improve pulmonary vasoconstriction in some infants with PPHN. Symptoms of withdrawal must be carefully monitored when discontinuing narcotic analgesics. When possible, use of infusions should be titrated to effect, and weaned as soon as feasible. Long-term therapy with fentanyl infusions predictably produces

physiologic addition, and methadone may be necessary to accomplish weaning.

3. Paralysis/neuromuscular blockade may improve respiratory mechanics in acute settings if severe asynchrony exists between the patient and the respiratory support; however, long-term pharmacologic paralysis can lead to muscle atrophy and fluid retention, complicating chronic respiratory insufficiency. Paralytic agents can and should be stopped as soon as possible. It is essential to remember that paralytic agents do not provide any sedation or analgesia.

• Pharmacologic pulmonary vasodilation may be necessary in severe cases of PPHN.

1. NO is a natural endothelial derived gas that causes vasodilation by increasing cyclic guanosine monophosphate (cGMP) in vascular smooth muscle cells. Because it has a very short half-life in vivo, NO requires continuous delivery. When given by inhalation, NO is specific to pulmonary vessels because once it reaches the circulation, it becomes inactivated by rapidly binding with hemoglobin to produce methemoglobin.

   a. The most appropriate starting dose is 20 ppm. Higher doses are associated with higher toxicity and no improvement in efficacy. In most infants improvement in oxygenation and pulmonary artery pressures occurs rapidly, and NO can be decreased to 5 ppm within 24 hours. NO can usually be weaned and stopped over 5–7 days.

   b. NO has been shown to decrease use of ECMO in infants with severe hypoxemic respiratory failure and PPHN, and is approved for use in infants >34 weeks gestation. Its role in the treatment of preterm infants is under investigation.

   c. Acute discontinuation of NO may lead to rebound pulmonary hypertension with severe cardiopulmonary decompensation, even in patients without prior evident improvement after initiation of NO.

   d. Use of NO in a center without immediate ECMO availability should be done with caution and only if it can be continued throughout transport of the patient to a center with ECMO availability. Ideally, patients should be transported to an ECMO-capable center prior to use of NO in combination with high frequency ventilation since this therapeutic combination cannot be provided during patient transport.

2. Sildenafil is a Food and Drug Administration (FDA)-approved inhibitor of phosphodiesterase type 5 (PDE5). PDE5 inhibition leads to increased availability of cGMP in vascular smooth muscle cells, thus potentiating the effect of NO. Its use in infants is currently limited to experimental protocols.

• ECMO is used to bypass the lungs using an external circuit to oxygenate the patient's blood through an artificial gas permeable membrane prior to returning it to the body. In order to minimize clotting in the ECMO circuit, anticoagulation or the patient with heparin is necessary.

1. In veno-arterial (VA) ECMO, venous blood is removed through a cannula inserted into the right atrium via the jugular vein. Venous blood is then pumped through the membrane to become oxygenated, then warmed to near body temperature, and returned through a cannula inserted into the aortic arch via the carotid artery. With this circuit, both the patient and the ECMO pump contribute to the cardiac output. The carotid artery is damaged and frequently must be ligated following the ECMO course, potentially increasing the risk of stroke.

2. In veno-venous (VV) ECMO, venous blood is removed through one lumen of a double lumen cannula inserted into the right atrium through a jugular vein. Venous blood is then pumped through the membrane to become oxygenated, warmed to near body temperature, and returned through the other lumen of the double lumen cannula into the right atrium. With this circuit, the ECMO pump does not contribute to cardiac output.

3. ECMO is the only therapy that has been shown to decrease mortality in infants with severe hypoxemic respiratory failure. ECMO use is associated with ~20% risk of neurodevelopmental disability; however, this risk appears to be comparable to outcomes in similar patients with respiratory illness who avoid ECMO.

• Nutritional support is essential in the care of infants with respiratory insufficiency. Parenteral nutrition should be initiated as soon after birth as possible to prevent catabolism and to promote postnatal growth and healing. Enteral nutrition should be initiated as soon as the patient is likely to tolerate it in order to further optimize nutrient uptake and to decrease the risk of infection from long-standing indwelling intravenous catheters.

• Surveillance for infection, and prophylactic initiation of antibiotics in high-risk cases can decrease morbidity and mortality associated with significant bacterial infections in infants with respiratory insufficiency. Prolonged empirical exposure to antibiotics is discouraged because of the increased risk of infection with resistant bacteria and fungi.

• Closure of patent ductus arteriosus (PDA) in premature infants decreases the incidence of chronic lung disease (BPD).

1. Prophylactic therapy with indomethacin (0.1 mg/kg every 24 hours × 3 doses) started within 12 hours after birth to prevent PDA is frequently used in extremely premature infants (<28 weeks gestation).
2. Therapeutic closure of PDA with indomethacin (0.1–0.2 mg/kg every 12–24 hours × 3 doses) is indicated in cases of a symptomatic PDA in any premature infant, or may be considered for an asymptomatic but persistent PDA by Doppler evaluation in an extremely premature infant.
3. Surgical ligation of a PDA should be considered in cases of symptomatic PDA in an extremely premature infant despite appropriate indomethacin prophylaxis/treatment, an asymptomatic PDA by Doppler evaluation in an extremely premature infant despite repeated appropriate indomethacin prophylaxis/treatment, or any PDA in an infant with significant renal dysfunction.

- Diuretics may help weaning ventilator settings in infants with generalized or pulmonary edema, or with CLD/BPD. Loop diuretics are most efficacious, with direct pulmonary effects, but have more severe side effects. Thiazide diuretics may improve respiratory function in infants with CLD/BPD following chronic therapy. They are typically used in combination with spironolactone to protect against potassium wasting, but often lead to electrolyte disturbances.
- Corticosteroids may help in weaning ventilator settings. Long or multiple courses are associated with worse neurodevelopmental outcome (especially cerebral palsy) in premature infants and should be avoided. Systemic vs. inhaled dosing is under investigation.
- Bronchodilators such as albuteral may improve respiratory mechanics in infants with established chronic lung disease; however, excessive dosing can lead to tachyarrhythmias. Bronchodilators are contraindicated in cases of laryngo/bronchomalacia because they may aggravate the hypercompliance of airways.

BIBLIOGRAPHY

Bancalari E. The lung. In: Polin RA, Fox WW, eds. *Fetal and Neonatal Physiology*, 2nd ed. W.B. Saunders; 1998.

Dukarm RC, Steinhorn RH, Morin FC. The normal pulmonary vascular transition at birth. *Clin Perinatol* 1996;23:711–726.

Jobe AH. Lung development. In: Fanaroff AA, Martin RJ, eds. *Neonatal-Perinatal Medicine–Diseases of the Fetus and Infant*, 7th ed. Mosby; 2002:973–990.

Kinsella JP, and Abman SH. Clinical approach to inhaled nitric oxide therapy in the newborn with hypoxemia. *J Pediatr* 2000; 136:717–726.

Kitterman JA. The effects of mechanical forces on fetal lung growth. *Clin Perinatol* 1996 Dec;23(4):727–40.

Sadler TW. *Langman's Medical Embryology*, 8th ed. New York: Lippincott Williams & Wilkins; 2000.

Walsh-Sukys MC, Tyson JE, Wright LL, et al. Persistent pulmonary hypertension of the newborn in the era before nitric oxide: practice variation and outcomes. *Pediatrics* 2000;105:14–20.

Whitsett JA. Pulmonary Surfactant. Polin RA, Fox WW, eds. *Fetal and Neonatal Physiology*, 2nd ed. W.B. Saunders; 1998.

Zwischenberger JB, Steinhorn RH, and Bartlett RH, eds. *ECMO: Extracorporeal Cardiopulmonary Support in Critical Care*. 2nd ed. Extracorporeal Life Support Organization; 2000.

23 HEMATOLOGIC DISORDERS OF THE NEWBORN

Praveen Kumar

ANEMIA IN THE NEWBORN

- The normal hemoglobin value at birth in a term infant ranges from 13.7 to 20.1 g/dL, with a mean of 16.8 g/dL. These values are lower in preterm infants. For example, the normal hemoglobin value at 24–26 weeks of gestation is 12.2 ± 1.6 g/dL.
- *Physiologic anemia* occurs because improved oxygenation after birth leads to suppression of erythropoiesis. This process, combined with shortened survival of fetal red blood cells (RBC) and expansion of blood volume in a growing infant, can lead to a progressive and sometimes rapid decline in the hemoglobin concentration. As a result, hemoglobin concentration gradually falls from 9.0–11.0 g/dL in a normal full-term infant by 8–12 weeks of age.
- The pattern of physiologic anemia differs in preterm infants, and is termed *anemia of prematurity*. The hemoglobin falls to 7.0–9.0 g/dL in a preterm infant by 3–6 weeks of age. The severity of anemia in a sick preterm infant is further exaggerated by iatrogenic blood loss for laboratory samplings. With the resumption of erythropoiesis after the "physiologic nadir" has been reached, the hemoglobin concentration gradually increases to reach a mean level of 11–12 g/dL by late infancy. These changes do not represent any nutritional deficiency and can not be corrected by administration of hematinic agents such as iron and folic acid.
- *Pathologic anemia* in the newborn infant can result from one of the following three processes: (1) blood loss which could either be external or internal and can

occur in antepartum, intrapartum and/or in postnatal period, (2) increased destruction, and/or (3) inadequate production of RBC.

- Some of the common *causes of blood loss* are twin-to-twin-transfusion, feto-maternal hemorrhage, placental abruption, anomalies and traumatic rupture of umbilical cord, obstetric trauma leading to subgaleal, intracranial, and visceral hemorrhage. Many of these infants present with anemia at birth.
- *Anemia caused by hemolysis* is common in the newborn period and can result from intrinsic or extrinsic abnormalities of red blood cells. Some of the common causes of hemolytic anemia are (a) isoimmune hemolytic anemia caused by ABO, Rh, and other minor blood group incompatibility between mother and fetus; (b) erythrocyte enzyme defects such as G6PD and pyruvate kinase deficiency; (c) erythrocyte membrane disorders such as spherocytosis; (d) hemoglobin disorders such as alpha-thalassemia syndromes; (e) infections with or without disseminated intravascular coagulation (DIC).
- Anemia caused by *erythrocyte underproduction* is very uncommon in neonates.
- *Symptoms and signs* of anemia are a result of a decrease in the oxygen-carrying capacity of blood with resultant tissue hypoxia, and depend on the severity of anemia and rapidity of its onset.
  1. *Infants with acute hemorrhagic anemia* present with pallor unassociated with jaundice and vascular instability, which can range from poor capillary refill in mild cases to hypovolemic shock. Initial hemoglobin may be normal with a gradual fall over next 24 hours and reticulocytosis developing 2–3 days after a hemorrhagic event.
  2. *Infants with chronic hemorrhagic anemia* usually present with pallor unassociated with jaundice and stable cardiorespiratory status unless an infant is in congestive heart failure secondary to severe anemia. Hepatosplenomegaly and signs of hydrops fetalis may or may not be present. The hemoglobin concentration is low at presentation with compensatory reticulocytosis.
  3. *Infants with hemolytic anemia* usually present with pallor associated with jaundice, reticulocytosis, and stable cardiorespiratory status. These infants usually present after 48 hours of age, although infants with severe isoimmune disease often present at birth with hepatosplenomegaly with or without hydrops fetalis.
- Treatment of a neonate with anemia depends on the extent of symptoms and signs as well as the underlying etiology of anemia.
  1. Rapid resuscitative measures can be lifesaving for infants with a significant acute hemorrhage.

2. Packed red blood cell (PRBC) transfusions are given to help maintain effective oxygen-carrying capacity. There is no consensus on guidelines for transfusion, but suggested indications are as follows: (a) hematocrit <35% and severe cardiopulmonary disease; (b) hematocrit <30%, moderate cardiopulmonary disease, and before major surgery; (c) hematocrit <25% and mild cardiopulmonary disease; and (d) hematocrit <20% with low reticulocyte count in an asymptomatic infant.
3. Partial exchange transfusion with PRBC is indicated if rapid correction of severe anemia is needed in infants with congestive cardiac failure.
4. Nutritional replacement with iron therapy is particularly important in infants with anemia secondary to blood loss. Other hematinics such as folic acid, vitamin E may also be necessary.
5. Recombinant human erythropoietin (rHuEPO) can increase neonatal erythropoiesis with no significant adverse effects. The effective dose ranges from 600 to 1200 unit/kg/week given subcutaneously in 2–3 divided doses/week. At present, it is considered most beneficial in very low birth weight infants with anemia of prematurity.

POLYCYTHEMIA

- Polycythemia is an increase in the total red blood cell mass and in the newborn is defined as a central venous hematocrit ≥65%. Because of transudation of fluid out of intravascular space after birth, the hematocrit in the newborn peaks at about 2–4 hours of age and then progressively decreases.
- Polycythemia occurs in 2–6% of all newborn infants and the incidence is highest among small-for-gestational age, large-for-gestational age infants and infants of diabetic mothers. Other common risk factors are high altitude, maternal smoking, twin-to-twin-transfusion, delayed cord clamping, placental insufficiency, and intrauterine hypoxia.
- The symptoms observed in a polycythemic infant result from the effects of hyperviscosity which depends on hematocrit, plasma viscosity, RBC aggregation, and deformability of RBC membrane. Increased hematocrit is the most important single factor contributing to hyperviscosity in neonates.
- The clinical signs in infants with neonatal polycythemia-hyperviscosity syndrome are nonspecific and seen in about half of the infants. Signs and symptoms include lethargy, poor feeding, tachypnea, hypoglycemia, hypocalcemia, thrombocytopenia, and plethora. Uncommon symptoms include convulsions,

venous thrombosis, congestive heart failure, and priapism. Short-term and long-term follow-up has shown a higher incidence of neurologic abnormalities in these infants.

• The goal of therapy is to reduce the viscosity by lowering the hematocrit to <60% and to correct associated metabolic abnormalities if present. Partial exchange transfusion is an effective method to achieve this goal. Normal saline is most commonly used as the replacement fluid, although some advocate for use of plasma protein fraction (Plasmanate) or 5% albumin. The volume exchanged is calculated from the following formula:

Exchange Volume

$$= \frac{\text{Blood Volume} \times \text{Observed Hematocrit} - \text{Desired Hematocrit}}{\text{Observed Hematocrit}}$$

• The long-term benefits of partial exchange transfusion in these infants are controversial. There is general agreement that a partial exchange transfusion should be done if the central venous hematocrit is ≥65% in a symptomatic infant and more than 70–75% in an asymptomatic infant.

THROMBOCYTOPENIA IN THE NEWBORN

• The normal platelet counts in both preterm and term newborns are 150,000–450,000/μL. The significance of platelet counts between 100,000 and 150,000/μL, particularly in the preterm neonate, is unclear as it is frequently observed in the absence of an underlying pathology. Thrombocytopenia (platelet count <150,000/μL) is observed in 20–30% of all newborns admitted to NICU.

• Thrombocytopenia in neonates may result from decreased production (less common) or increased destruction (more common) of platelets. In two large studies, no identifiable cause was found in up to 60% of all cases of neonatal thrombocytopenia.

• Congenital disorders associated with *decreased platelet production* include thrombocytopenia with absent radii syndrome (TAR), isolated megakaryocytic hypoplasia, Wiskott-Aldrich syndrome, congenital leukemias, chromosomal abnormalities such as trisomies 13 and 18, and metabolic disorders such as isovaleric acidemia. There is some evidence to suggest that thrombocytopenia observed in SGA infants and infants born to mothers with severe pregnancy induced hypertension is also related to decreased production.

• Causes of *increased platelet destruction* include neonatal alloimmune thrombocytopenia (NAIT),

neonatal autoimmune thrombocytopenia, drug-induced thrombocytopenia, infections, DIC, platelet consumption secondary to indwelling catheters, intravascular thrombosis, and necrotizing enterocolitis. Congenital infections (e.g., TORCH) may cause thrombocytopenia by both decreased production and increased destruction.

• Workup should include evaluation of mother, placenta and the infant.

1. In mothers with a normal platelet count, a history of PIH, hemolysis-elevated liver enzymes-low platelet count (HELLP) syndrome, TORCH infections, or use of agents such as thiazides, hydralazine, and tolbutamide can give a clue to the etiology of thrombocytopenia in the infant. A low maternal platelet count suggests autoimmune or inherited thrombocytopenia. A history of thrombocytopenia in previous child at birth may suggest NAIT.

2. The placenta should be evaluated for the presence of abruption and hemangiomas.

3. In a well-appearing infant with normal physical examination, likely causes of thrombocytopenia are NAIT, neonatal autoimmune thrombocytopenia secondary to maternal immune thrombocytopenia purpura (ITP) or systemic lupus erythematosus (SLE), and drug-induced thrombocytopenia. In a well-appearing infant with an abnormal examination, congenital syndromes such as TAR, giant hemangioma syndromes, and chromosomal anomalies are likely. In a sick infant, usual causes of thrombocytopenia are infections, disseminated intravascular coagulation, and platelet consumption.

• In addition to treating the underlying cause, the treatment options include platelet transfusion, intravenous immunoglobulin, and corticosteroids for immune mediated thrombocytopenia and recombinant thrombopoietin administration.

• The goal of platelet transfusions is to raise platelet count above 100,000/μL and can be achieved by the infusion of approximately 10 cc/kg of platelet concentrate. Washed maternal platelets should be used for infants with alloimmune thrombocytopenia. Platelet transfusions are indicated in any infant with thrombocytopenia with active bleeding. In absence of active bleeding, prophylactic platelet transfusion is recommended at a platelet count of <30,000/μL in stable term infant and <50,000/μL in stable preterm infant. According to the American Association of Blood Banks Pediatric Hemotherapy Committee, platelet transfusions are recommended for counts below 100,000/μL in an unstable infant.

COAGULATION DISORDERS IN THE NEWBORN

- The hemostatic system is not completely developed at birth, and this is even more true in a preterm infant. The prothrombin time (PT) is slightly prolonged, and partial thromboplastin time (PTT) is significantly prolonged compared to the adults. Factors V, VIII, and fibrinogen are present at adult levels by birth but levels of many other coagulation factors such as factors XI, XII are lower. The levels of several anticoagulant proteins such as Antithrombin III, Proteins S and C are low and predispose newborn infants to thrombosis.
- Congenital coagulation disorders are characterized by defects in factor synthesis.
  1. Hemophilia A (factor VIII deficiency) and Hemophilia B (factor IX deficiency) may present with bleeding symptoms in newborn period. Both these disorders are X-linked and occur almost exclusively in males. Factor estimation can establish diagnosis in all infants except those with mild forms of Hemophilia B. Treatment consists of use of fresh frozen plasma (FFP), cryoprecipitate, or lyophilized factor concentrate VIII or IX. Factor IX concentrate should be avoided in newborns because of risk of inducing thrombosis.
  2. Bleeding manifestations are extremely rare in infants with Von Willebrand disease and its diagnosis cannot be made with confidence in the newborn period. Infants with the severe form may behave as hemophilia. Treatment consists of use of cryoprecipitate or desmopressin acetate (DDAVP).
  3. Homozygous forms of factors II, V, VII, X, and XIII can present with bleeding in the newborn period. Delayed bleeding from the umbilical stump is characteristic of factor XIII deficiency and diagnosis requires factor assay as routine clotting studies are normal. The treatment includes infusion of fresh frozen plasma or specific factor concentrate.
- *Acquired coagulation disorders* include hemorrhagic disorders secondary to vitamin K deficiency or liver disease and DIC.
  1. Vitamin K, a fat-soluble vitamin, is essential for normal function of vitamin K dependent factors, factors II, VII, IX and X. Vitamin K is not transported well across the placenta and some infants are vitamin K deficient at birth and at risk of bleeding. Based on its onset, hemorrhagic disease of newborn can be (i) *early*, during or soon after delivery, (ii) *classic*, between 1 and 7 days of life, and (iii) *late*, between 4 and 12 weeks of life. The administration of vitamin K at birth can prevent classic and late disease but has no effect on early-onset hemorrhagic disease of the newborn.
  2. Severe liver disease can produce a hemorrhagic diathesis as a result of vitamin K deficiency or by primary failure of production of coagulation factors.
  3. DIC in the newborn is usually secondary to perinatal asphyxia, sepsis, shock, severe hypothermia, or necrotizing enterocolitis. These infants are usually critically ill and may exhibit widespread bleeding from multiple sites. The diagnosis of DIC is based on laboratory findings of low platelet counts with prolonged PT, activated partial thromboplastin time (aPTT), and decreased fibrinogen. Fibrin degradation products may be elevated. The primary goal of management is treatment of the underlying disorder and control of bleeding by replacement therapy with fresh frozen plasma and platelet concentrate as necessary. Despite aggressive management, DIC has high mortality.

NEONATAL JAUNDICE

- The yellow discoloration of the skin caused by accumulation of bilirubin is called jaundice or icterus. Nearly all newborns develop transient hyperbilirubinemia (serum bilirubin >2 mg/dL) and nearly 65% are clinically jaundiced (serum bilirubin >5 mg/dL).
- Bilirubin is derived primarily from the breakdown of heme in the reticuloendothelial system. Unconjugated bilirubin is released into the circulation and is rapidly bound reversibly to albumin and transported to the liver. Bilirubin enters the liver cell by a process of carrier-mediated diffusion by binding to ligandin (Y protein) and Z protein. Nonpolar and water-insoluble unconjugated bilirubin is conjugated inside liver cells by bilirubin uridine 5′-diphosphate (UDP)-glucuronyl transferase enzyme. Water-soluble conjugated bilirubin is then actively excreted into the bile canaliculi by the liver cells. Conjugated bilirubin cannot be reabsorbed from the intestine and most of it is converted to urobilinoids which are excreted in stool and urine. A small amount of conjugated bilirubin is converted back to unconjugated form by enteric mucosal enzyme, β-glucuronidase, and reabsorbed by way of enterohepatic circulation.
- *Unconjugated hyperbilirubinemia*, also known as indirect hyperbilirubinemia, can be either physiologic or pathologic. In absence of neurologic injury, unconjugated hyperbilirubinemia is not associated with any specific symptoms except those related to the underlying etiology.

- Jaundice is typically apparent first in the face and then follows a cephalocaudal progression as the degree of jaundice increases. Palms and soles are the last to be jaundiced and suggest severe jaundice and an infant at risk for bilirubin encephalopathy. In absence of neurologic injury, unconjugated hyperbilirubinemia is not associated with any specific symptoms except symptoms related to underlying etiology.

- *Physiologic jaundice* in term infants is characterized by a progressive rise in serum bilirubin to a mean peak of 5–6 mg/dL by the third day of life in both White and Black infants and to a peak of 10–14 mg/dL by the fifth day in oriental infants. This peak is followed by a gradual decline to baseline by the fifth day of life in White and Black infants and by the seventh to the tenth day in oriental infants. Physiologic jaundice in a preterm infant appears earlier, can reach a higher peak, and declines more gradually.

The underlying mechanisms for physiologic jaundice in newborn are related to (a) increased bilirubin production because of larger RBC mass and shorter life span; (b) hepatic immaturity resulting in defective uptake, diminished conjugating capacity, and impaired excretion; and (c) increased enterohepatic circulation in newborn.

- *Pathologic jaundice* is diagnosed when there is clinical jaundice in the first 24 hours of life or serum bilirubin level increasing at a rate of >5 mg/dL/day. A peak serum bilirubin level higher than that mentioned above in a term infant and >15 mg/dL in a preterm infant should always be considered pathologic until proven otherwise.
  1. Most disorders causing unconjugated hyperbilirubinemia do so via one or more of the same mechanisms that produce physiologic jaundice described above.
  2. The most common pathologic cause of increased bilirubin production in the newborn is isoimmune hemolytic disease, because of blood group incompatibility between mother and fetus. Other causes of hemolysis as mentioned under causes of hemolytic anemia can also result in pathologic jaundice.
  3. Sepsis, polycythemia, and extravasated blood can lead to increased bilirubin production.
  4. Defects in hepatic uptake of bilirubin such as Gilbert syndrome and defects in hepatic conjugation such as Type I and Type II glucuronyl transferase deficiency are uncommon causes of pathologic jaundice. Other rare causes of glucuronyl transferase inhibition are Lucey-Discroll syndrome and pyloric stenosis.

- *Breast milk jaundice*: Nearly 30–60% of all breast-fed infants develop exaggerated unconjugated hyperbilirubinemia toward the end of the first week of life when physiologic jaundice would normally be decreasing.

1. Breast-fed infants are three times more likely to develop serum bilirubin levels of >12 mg/dL and six times more likely to develop levels of >15 mg/dL than formula-fed infants. Jaundice can persist beyond 2–3 weeks in about 25% of all breast-fed infants and can rarely persist for up to 3 months. It can recur in 70% of future pregnancies.

2. The great majority of infants with breast milk jaundice have serum bilirubin concentrations around 10 mg/dL. Less than 1% have level >20 mg/dL but rarely levels as high as 30 mg/dL have been reported.

3. The etiology of breast milk jaundice is not well-established. Increased enterohepatic circulation appears to be the most important mechanism. Increased concentration of fatty acids and presence of a progesterone metabolite, pregnane-3α-20β diol in breast milk have been suggested to play a role by inhibiting hepatic glucuronyl transferase.

4. Interruption of nursing and use of formula feeding for 1–3 days causes a prompt decline in bilirubin but is only recommended for infants with serum bilirubin concentrations that put them at risk for kernicterus.

- The initial evaluation of a jaundiced infant should include determination of total and direct serum bilirubin in addition to a detailed family, maternal, and infant's history. Evaluation of an infant with pathologic jaundice should include blood group and Rh type determination for mother and infant, direct Coomb's test, hemoglobin or hematocrit, peripheral blood smear and reticulocyte count.

- Treatment options for an infant with unconjugated hyperbilirubinemia include phototherapy, exchange transfusion, and rarely pharmacologic therapy.
  1. Phototherapy is the most common treatment in use for neonatal jaundice. Phototherapy converts bilirubin by isomerization and photooxidation into more water-soluble photoproducts that can bypass the liver's conjugating system and be excreted without further metabolism. Factors that determine the efficacy of phototherapy include spectrum of light, irradiance of light source, distance of infant from light source, and surface area of infant exposed to light. Side effects of phototherapy are minimal and include concerns about light toxicity to the retina, increased insensible fluid loss, bronze baby syndrome, and risk of overheating.
  2. Exchange transfusion is indicated for immediate treatment of severely jaundiced infants at risk of developing kernicterus. A double volume blood exchange transfusion replaces nearly 85% of the circulating red blood cells and lowers serum bilirubin by 50%. The overall mortality is reported to be about 0.3% and significant morbidity occurs in 1–5% of

the patients. In addition, exchange transfusion carries the usual risks of any blood product transfusion.

3. Pharmacologic treatment is not used commonly. Tin and zinc metalloporphyrins have been shown to inhibit enzymes necessary for heme breakdown and can reduce bilirubin production; however, further clinical trials on efficacy and safety are required. Intravenous immunoglobin (IVIG) administration soon after birth can also reduce hemolysis and bilirubin production in patients with isoimmune hemolytic jaundice. Phenobarbital can increase bilirubin elimination by induction of microsomal enzymes in liver. Because it takes 3–7 days to be effective, it is not helpful in the management of majority of infants with unconjugated hyperbilirubinemia.

BIBLIOGRAPHY

Doyle JJ, Schmidt B, Blanchette V, Zipursky A. Hematology. In Avery GB, Fletcher MA, MacDonald MG, eds. *Neonatology: Pathophysiology and Management of the Newborn.* New York: Lippincott Williams & Wilkins; 1999:1045.

Luchtman-Jones L, Schwartz AL, Wilson DB. Blood component therapy for the neonate. In Fanaroff AA, Martin RJ, eds. *Neonatal-Perinatal Medicine.* Philadelphia: Mosby; 2002:1239.

Lindermann R, Haga P. Evaluation and treatment of polycythemia in the neonate. In Christensen RD, ed. *Hematological Problems of the Neonate.* Philadelphia: W.B. Saunders; 2000:171.

Maisels MJ. Jaundice. In Avery GB, Fletcher MA, MacDonald MG, eds. *Neonatology: Pathophysiology and Management of the Newborn.* New York: Lippincott Williams & Wilkins; 1999:765.

24 NEONATAL DISEASES OF THE DIGESTIVE TRACT

Isabelle G. DePlaen and Nicolas F.M. Porta

CONSIDERATIONS IN THE FIRST HOURS OF LIFE

• A term fetus swallows approximately 750 mL of amniotic fluid per day.
• Congenital abnormalities of the gastrointestinal (GI) tract should be suspected when polyhydramnios or bile-stained amniotic fluid exists.

• Shortly after birth, patency of the esophagus is confirmed during delivery room suctioning or during the first feeding. If a baby has difficulties handling oral secretions, feedings, or has significant emesis, an orogastric tube should be placed and x-ray taken to rule out esophageal atresia.
• With the occurrence of intestinal transit, air distributes throughout the GI tract unless a congenital obstruction is present. Concurrently, bacterial colonization occurs.

FEEDING THE PREMATURE INFANT

• The premature infant (especially when extremely premature) is born during the gestational period when body growth rate is at its highest. Nutrients are adequately provided in utero. Therefore, the preterm infant has a higher requirement of many nutrients, and these need to be provided as soon as possible after birth.
• If the infant is too small or too ill to tolerate enteric feeds, early parenteral nutrition with adequate calories, protein, and lipids should be provided.
• Prolonged fasting causes intestinal atrophy and intestinal dysmotility, and should be avoided when possible. There is evidence that early introduction of "minimal enteral feedings" (20 mL/kg/day) is well tolerated even in very preterm infants, and may provide a strategy to maintain intestinal integrity until feedings can be advanced as the primary source of nutrition.
• As soon as the infant is stable, enteral feeds are typically initiated at 10–20 mL/kg/day divided into 8–12 feeds. Breast milk is generally preferred over proprietary formulas. Enteral feeds are slowly advanced as tolerated by 10–20 mL/kg increments up to 140–160 mL/kg/day.
• Once full volumes of feeds are tolerated, "human milk fortifier" is added to the breast milk or the infant is given a 24 cal/oz premature formula. Fortifiers and premature formulas provide the growing premature infant with additional calories, proteins, calcium, and phosphorus to fulfill their higher needs compared to the full-term infant.
• There is conflicting evidence whether faster increases in volume augment the risk for necrotizing enterocolitis (NEC). In most infants, continuous feedings do not have advantages over bolus feeds. Transpyloric feeds are usually avoided, since they bypass the duodenum where up to 20–25% of sugars and fats are reabsorbed.
• Until coordination of suck and swallow occurs (generally between 32 and 34 weeks gestational age), preterm infants will be mostly gavage-fed through an

orogastric tube. When the infant is adequately rooting, bottle-feeding or breastfeeding may be cautiously attempted and advanced as tolerated.

GASTROESOPHAGEAL (GE) REFLUX

- GE reflux is usually a self-limited condition characterized by effortless postprandial regurgitations, which usually resolve spontaneously over time. Treatment is indicated when respiratory problems, such as apnea, persistent oxygen requirement, recurrent infections, airway inflammation, laryngomalacia, or esophagitis are present.
- Treatment includes prone positioning with the head elevated, small frequent feedings, thickening of the feeds with rice cereal or use of antireflux formulas with rice starch (Enfamil AR), metoclopramide (0.1–0.2 mg/kg/dose q 6 hours) and zantac (1 mg/kg/dose q 12 hours).
- Regurgitations should be differentiated from vomiting: An infant who vomits should be investigated urgently to rule out a small bowel obstruction.

INTESTINAL OBSTRUCTION

- Symptoms include vomiting soon after feedings are initiated. A nondistended abdomen and normal passage of meconium is commonly seen in higher GI tract obstructions. Delayed vomiting with a progressively distended abdomen, and delay in passing meconium is more suggestive of a lower GI tract obstruction.
- Nongastrointestinal disorders, such as infections or metabolic disorders can cause vomiting.
- When evaluating infants for possible intestinal obstruction, it should be remembered that intestinal ileus may be seen in other disorders, such as sepsis. Further, maternal treatment with magnesium sulfate prior to delivery is a frequent cause of feeding intolerance in the first week of life, especially in preterm infants.
- *Delayed meconium passage* may also indicate intestinal obstruction.
  1. Meconium, the first infant's stool, is of sticky black-greenish consistency and is an accumulation of intestinal cells, bile, and proteinaceous material formed during intestinal development.
  2. Failure to pass meconium in the first 2 days of life is typically seen in hypothyroidism, preterm infants (50%), and lower intestinal obstruction, such as Hirschsprung disease, anorectal malformations, meconium plug syndrome, small left colon syndrome, hypoganglionosis, and neuronal intestinal dysplasia.

- When intestinal obstruction is suspected, feedings should be stopped, and gastric decompression performed. IV hydration and electrolyte replacement should be provided and broad-spectrum antibiotic therapy initiated while ordering further investigations.

DIAGNOSTIC STUDIES

1. An *abdominal x-ray* might show an absence of air distal to the level of obstruction. A double bubble sign is seen in duodenal atresia, duodenal obstruction by an annular pancreas, a preduodenal portal vein or a mesenteric band. Absence of air in the rectum is seen in Hirschsprung disease. Calcified extraluminal meconium is pathognomonic for meconium ileus.
2. In cases of malrotation with midgut volvulus, *an upper GI* will show an obstructed distal duodenum, an abnormally positioned ligament of Treitz and sometimes the classic "corkscrew" entry into the volvulus complex.
3. *Barium enema* will identify a functional microcolon in intestinal atresia, meconium ileus, and total colonic aganglionosis. In meconium ileus, it might identify characteristic pellets of meconium.

- Specific Etiologies of Intestinal Obstruction:
  1. *Malrotation of the midgut with volvulus* is a surgical emergency. If not treated promptly, ischemic gangrene of the small intestine develops rapidly. In 80% of malrotations, symptoms will develop within the first month of life. The typical presentation is with sudden onset of bilious vomiting with or without bloody stools in a previously well neonate with only minimal other physical findings. Sometimes, pain or a shock-like syndrome is present. The diagnosis is made by an upper GI series. Barium enema has a 10–20% rate of false-negative results because of normally positioned cecum. When suspected, the infant should undergo prompt surgical exploration and treatment.
  2. *Hirschsprung disease or congenital aganglionic megacolon* is the congenital absence of ganglion cells in the Meissner and Auerbach plexus with absence of parasympathetic innervation to the distal intestine. In most cases, it is limited to the rectum and the recto-sigmoid. In 10% of the cases, it extends to the whole colon, or more rarely, to the entire GI tract. Its incidence is 1 in 5000 births, and it is more common in males. It is almost never seen in preterm infants. The most frequent mode of presentation is the failure to pass meconium within 24–48 hours. Other symptoms include abdominal distension, diarrhea, foul smelling stools, and failure to thrive. The

most severe complication of Hirschsprung disease is acute bacterial enterocolitis, characterized by severe abdominal distension, vomiting, bloody stools, and sepsis-like symptoms. Its mortality rate varies between 20 and 25%. The diagnosis of Hirschsprung disease is suggested by barium enema and confirmed by rectal biopsy. Rectal irrigations and anal dilation help maintain gastrointestinal transit until surgical treatment can be performed.

3. *Duodenal, jejunal, or ileal atresia*: Symptoms will vary depending on the level of the obstruction. Duodenal obstruction (atresia/stenosis/web/annular pancreas) presents with bilious emesis within the first day of life. The diagnosis is suspected on the basis of abdominal x-rays; a postnatal abdominal radiograph shows dilated stomach and duodenum (*double bubble* sign). Duodenal atresia is frequently associated with trisomy 21. The diagnosis can be confirmed by an upper GI contrast study showing complete vs. partial obstruction because of stenosis. Gastroesophageal reflux is common after repair because of abnormal peristalsis of the duodenum because of prolonged distension in utero.

4. *Imperforate anus* occurs in 1:5000 births, and is usually noted on the initial newborn examination of the perineum, although low lesions with a perineal fistula or anterior ectopic anus may be more difficult to discern. An abdominal radiograph is usually the only radiologic test that is needed. Placing the patient in a knee-chest position for ~30 minutes before taking a cross-table radiograph may help determine the severity of the malformation and aids in surgical planning. Cardiovascular malformations occur in up to 25% of patients. Low lesions in males may be repaired primarily. In males with high lesions and females, a diverting colostomy is usually performed with a pull-through operation at a later date.

5. *Meconium ileus* is usually because of midileal obstruction by thick hyperviscous meconium, and occurs in 10–15% of patients with cystic fibrosis. It might be simple or complicated by volvulus, intestinal necrosis, perforation, meconium peritonitis, or meconium pseudocyst. *Meconium plug syndrome* is an obstruction of the distal colon by a large white meconium plug. It is most commonly seen with prematurity, magnesium intoxication (maternal treatment), and in infants of diabetic mothers; hypothyroidism and Hirschsprung disease should also be considered. In both conditions, an enema with water-soluble contrast (gastrograffin) is diagnostic, and therapeutic in helping to initiate the passage of meconium. Repeated enemas are sometimes required. When this fails or when complicated

meconium ileus exists, surgical intervention is required. As meconium ileus has nearly 99% association with cystic fibrosis, a sweat test and or genetic testing should be performed to rule out cystic fibrosis.

ESOPHAGEAL ABNORMALITIES

- Esophageal atresia occurs in 1:2500 infants. Approximately 30% have associated cardiac disease, and 20% have associated VACTERL Syndrome (*V*ertebral anomalies, *A*nal atresia, *C*ardiac anomalies, *T*racheo*E*sophageal anomalies, *R*enal anomalies, *L*imb anomalies). Fetal ultrasonography showing polyhydramnios and dilated proximal esophagus can suggest esophageal atresia.
- Esophageal atresia should be suspected in newborn infants with excessive salivation, or who have choking or emesis with first feeding. The diagnosis is confirmed by the inability to pass an orogastric tube beyond several centimeters as confirmed by a chest x-ray.
  1. Esophageal atresia is most commonly associated with associated distal tracheoesophageal fistula (type C), which allows air to enter the rest of the gastrointestinal tract.
  2. Isolated esophageal atresia is more commonly associated with syndromic anomalies.
  3. Short segment atresia is usually repaired in the neonatal period.

ABDOMINAL WALL AND UMBILICAL DEFECTS

- *Omphalocele* is a herniation of abdominal contents (including intestines, stomach, liver, and spleen) into the umbilical cord, covered by parietal peritoneum. Omphalocele occurs in ~1:4000 infants and ~50% of cases have associated anomalies/chromosomal abnormalities (especially with large defects).
  1. Omphaloceles result from incomplete return of abdominal contents into the abdominal cavity during first trimester. Antenatally, they may be suspected by elevated maternal serum alpha fetal protein (AFP) and can be diagnosed by fetal ultrasonography.
  2. Omphalocele is always associated with intestinal malrotation and may be associated with epigastric (Pentalogy of Cantrell) or hypogastric (cloacal exstrophy) defects.
  3. Large omphaloceles that cannot be closed primarily may require staged closure within 1 week to prevent compression of abdominal contents resulting

in ischemia. Alternatively, the covering sac can be covered by a desiccating agent allowing the ventral hernia to mature, and surgical repair delayed until the abdomen is large enough to accommodate the herniated structures.

- *Gastroschisis* is a herniation of abdominal contents through an umbilical defect; 99% occur to the right of the umbilicus. Gastroschisis occurs in 2–5 per 10,000 infants, and is only rarely associated with chromosomal abnormalities. Its rate of occurrence may be increasing.
  1. Gastroschisis is thought to be because of a vascular accident leading to incomplete closure of abdominal wall, and is associated with ~10% incidence of intestinal atresias. Gastroschisis may be suspected by elevated maternal AFP during pregnancy and can be diagnosed by fetal ultrasonography.
  2. Delivery room management includes immediate decompression of the GI tract, prevention of fluid loss by wrapping saline-soaked gauze around the defect, and avoiding compromise of the mesenteric circulation.
  3. Gastroschisis may often not be closed primarily, necessitating staged reduction using a silo. Closure within a 1-week period will decrease the risk of bacterial sepsis.

NECROTIZING ENTEROCOLITIS (NEC)

- NEC is a disease that occurs primarily in premature infants, and affects between 4 and 22% of infants with birth weights less than 1500 g. Its etiology is multifactorial, and risk factors include infectious agents/toxins, enteral alimentation, bowel ischemia or hypoxia, and prematurity.
  1. Although more common in premature infants, NEC can also be observed in term babies. In the term infant, NEC has been associated with polycythemia, gastroschisis, and congenital heart disease.
  2. Initial symptoms vary and may include feeding intolerance, increased gastric residuals, abdominal distension, bloody stools, apnea, lethargy, temperature instability, or hypoperfusion.
  3. Early on, the physical examination may reveal localized abdominal tenderness and decreased reactivity to stimulation. Poor color with decreased perfusion might be noted.
  4. Abdominal x-rays are the radiographic study of choice. Serial studies help assess disease progression. *Pneumatosis intestinalis* is a linear bubbly pattern observed within the bowel wall and is diagnostic of NEC. *Portal venous air* might be seen in the most severe cases. In many cases, the x-ray remains nondiagnostic, but may be notable for a persistent abnormal gas pattern, a localized dilated loop of bowel, or thickened bowel loops.
  5. When intestinal perforation is present, a pneumoperitoneum may be seen on x-ray; however, on supine films, findings may limited to a "football sign," which is a subtle lucency over the liver shadow. Decubitus films are preferred for the detection of free air and are recommended at every evaluation.
  6. NEC is a systemic illness, and should be evaluated with this in mind. Thrombocytopenia, anemia, neutropenia, electrolyte imbalance, metabolic acidosis, hypoxia, or hypercapnia often develop and the complete blood count (CBC), electrolytes, and blood gases need to be monitored closely. As NEC is associated with bacteremia in 11–37% of infants, blood cultures need to be obtained.
  7. Treatment should be undertaken without delay as soon as NEC is suspected. Treatment includes early bowel decompression by effective nasogastric tube suction, prompt broad-spectrum antibiotic coverage (ampicillin, an aminoglycoside, and anaerobic coverage), correction of thrombocytopenia and coagulation defects, pain control, and early parenteral nutrition. Endotracheal intubation and mechanical ventilation are frequently necessary because of apnea and to allow proper bowel decompression. Repeated isotonic fluid boluses (normal saline or fresh frozen plasma [FFP]) are often necessary in the first 48–72 hours to compensate for the tremendous amount of third spacing associated with NEC, and to maintain intravascular volume and adequate mesenteric perfusion. Low dose dopamine (2–3 μg/kg/minute) is sometimes used in an attempt to improve mesenteric perfusion.
  8. Pain control is important, and a fentanyl drip of 2–4 μg/kg/hour is often used. Limiting infant handling and administering additional bolus doses of fentanyl prior to necessary handling will keep the infant as comfortable as possible. Maintaining the infant on a radiant warmer allows close observation of the infant while avoiding hypothermia. Central venous line access and parenteral nutrition with adequate protein and calories is essential to provide substrate for bowel healing.
  9. Surgical intervention is indicated if bowel perforation is suspected (pneumoperitoneum on x-ray) or if there is clinical deterioration despite medical management. While this intervention usually entails exploration, resection of necrotic bowel, and bowel diversion, some surgeons advocate for the use of peritoneal drainage in infants <1000 g.

10. NEC complications include short bowel syndrome, intestinal strictures, and central line and total parenteral nutrition (TPN)-related complications, such as cholestasis and nosocomial infections.
11. NEC mortality ranges from 10–30% and is the result of refractory shock, disseminated intravascular coagulation, multiple organ failure, intestinal perforation, sepsis, or extensive bowel necrosis. Some infants have late mortality because of complications of short bowel syndrome.

DIARRHEA

- Loose stools are common in breast-fed infants, and are not necessarily a sign of disease. Conditions associated with neonatal diarrhea are detailed in Table 24-1. It should be remembered that rotaviral illness is uncommon during the neonatal period, although asymptomatic shedding of the virus is possible.
- The initial evaluation includes stool examination and culture for viral, parasitic, and bacterial agents, stool reducing sugar content, osmolarity measurement, and a CBC.
- When cow's milk protein allergy is suspected, changing to a hydrolyzed formula (e.g., Pregestimil, Nutramigen, or Alimentum) will result in improvement of the symptoms. It should be remembered that soy protein is also highly sensitizing.
- Diarrhea is commonly seen after surgical resection of the intestine in the neonatal intestine. Many factors may lead to diarrhea in this setting, and the length of intestine resected is not always predictive. In general, infants with an intact ileocecal valve and an intact colon do best. In protracted diarrhea, elemental infant formula given continuously by nasogatric feeding may be tolerated, with the nutritional complement given by parenteral nutrition. The rate of enteral feeds is slowly increased over weeks and parenteral nutrition slowly tapered.

HEMATEMESIS

- Hematemesis is most commonly due to swallowed maternal blood. In these cases, an Apt test (alkaline denaturation) of the bloody fluid might confirm the presence of adult hemoglobin. The bloody fluid is mixed with H_2O in approximately a 1:5 ratio and then centrifuged. One milliliter of 1% sodium hydroxide is added to 4 mL of the pink supernatant. If the color changes to yellow-brown, it is maternal blood (HbA). If the color stays pink, it is fetal blood (HbF).

Table 24-1 Conditions Associated With Neonatal Diarrhea

Infectious gastroenteritis

Physical or chemical agents
Antibiotics
Dietary errors: overfeeding, inappropriate dilution of formula
Phototherapy related

Specific enzymatic or biochemical deficiency
Lactase deficiency
Monosaccharide malabsorption (glucose and galactose)
Fatty acid malabsorption
Abeta-lipoproteinemia
Chylomicron retention disease
Wolman disease
Intestinal lymphangiectasia
Congenital chloride diarrhea

Generalized, congenital enterocyte disorders
Microvillus inclusion disease
Intestinal epithelial dysplasia (Tufting disease)

Congenital abnormalities of the intestine
Hirschsprung disease
Neuronal intestinal dysplasia
Malrotation, intestinal stenosis, duplication

Acquired defects of the intestine
Short gut syndrome
NEC

Abnormalities of pancreatic secretion
Cystic fibrosis
Schwachman disease

Abnormalities of liver function
Neonatal hepatitis
Biliary atresia
Congenital cholestatic syndromes

Immunologic disorders

Hormonal disorders
Neural crest tumors
Congenital adrenal hyperplasia
Hyperthyroidism

Inflammatory and allergic disorders
Milk protein allergy

- Gastric bleeding can be caused by stress ulceration, hemorrhagic gastritis because of anti-inflammatory agents (e.g., steroids), gastric volvulus, duplications, and hiatal hernia. Congenital clotting disorders, such as DIC, liver disease, and vitamin K deficiency, may present with gastric bleeding and may be identified by coagulation studies.
- Treatment includes the administration of vitamin K, FFP, placement of a nasogastric tube, and pharmacologic treatment with H_2 blocking agents.

RECTAL BLEEDING

- Isolated rectal bleeding is most commonly seen in infants with anal or rectal fissures or swallowed maternal blood. In more than 50% of infants, no cause can be identified and the bleeding resolves spontaneously.

- Bloody stools, feeding intolerance, and abdominal distension are seen with NEC, malrotation with midgut volvulus, Hirschsprung disease, and intestinal duplication.
- Bloody diarrhea might be seen with infectious diarrhea, or by colitis induced by milk protein allergy (cow's milk or soy protein).

NEONATAL CHOLESTATIC JAUNDICE

- Neonatal cholestasis is defined as a pathologic state of reduced bile formation or flow. It is never normal and should always be investigated. Symptoms are jaundice, hepatomegaly, pale (acholic) stools, and dark urine. Direct hyperbilirubinemia is defined by a conjugated bilirubin level over 2 mg/dL, or a value greater than 15% of the total bilirubin level.
- Parenteral nutrition is the most common cause of cholestasis in the newborn requiring NICU care. It is also seen following intrauterine infections, such as CMV, rubella, toxoplasmosis, excessive bilirubin load from hemolytic disease (*inspissated bile syndrome*), and anatomic disease caused by biliary atresia, choledochal cyst, and biliary hypoplasia. It is more rarely because of metabolic disorders, such as galactosemia, alpha-1 antitrypsin deficiency, cystic fibrosis, tyrosinemia, or neonatal hemachromatosis. Other rare causes include inborn errors of bile acid metabolism, hereditary fructose intolerance, and storage diseases (Niemann-Pick and Gauchers disease).
- Diagnostic tests include alanine aminotransferase (ALT), aspartate aminotransferase (AST), alkaline phosphatase, bilirubin (total and direct), PT, PTT, and albumin. An abdominal ultrasound is useful to rule out gallstones or a choledochal cyst.
- When cholestasis occurs, the diagnosis of extrahepatic biliary atresia needs to be excluded as soon as possible, as early surgical intervention (6–10 weeks of age) is more likely to be successful. Biliary nuclear medicine imaging with hepatoiminodiacetic acid (HIDA scan) is used to differentiate between obstructive causes, such as biliary atresia and hepatocellular cholestasis. When the diagnosis of biliary atresia cannot be excluded before 60 days of life, surgical exploration is necessary, with perioperative cholangiogram and liver biopsy.
- Therapy depends on the underlying cause. The use of choleretic agents, such as phenobarbital or cholestyramine and ursodeoxycholic acid (20–30 mg/kg/day) may increase biliary flow and improve cholestasis. Supplementation of the fat-soluble vitamins A, D, E, and K is necessary.

FULMINANT HEPATIC NECROSIS

- Causes of acute liver failure in the neonate include viral infections (echovirus, herpes, enterovirus), metabolic diseases (galactosemia, tyrosinemia, Niemann-Pick type A, respiratory chain defects, neonatal hemochromatosis, peroxisomal diseases), and asphyxia.
- Manifestations include jaundice, encephalopathy, hypoglycemia, coagulopathy, and hyperammonemia. Although liver enzymes are usually elevated during the acute phases of illness, normalization may occur due to hepatocyte necrosis rather than true improvement.
- Infants with acute liver failure should be immediately admitted to an intensive care facility. Treatment includes support of circulation and respiration, correction of hypoglycemia, replacement of coagulation factors, blood product transfusions, management of associated hyperammonemia and renal failure, and correction of electrolyte disturbances.
- Early involvement of a gastroenterologist is important in determining whether liver transplantation should be considered.

BIBLIOGRAPHY

Altschuler SM. Physiology of the gastrointestinal tract in the fetus and neonate. IN: Polin RA, Fox WW, eds. *Fetal and Neonatal Physiology*, 2nd ed. Philadelphia: W.B. Saunders, 1998.

Cass DL, Wesson DE. Advances in fetal and neonatal surgery for gastrointestinal anomalies and disease. *Clin Perinatol* 2002;29:1–21.

Crissinger KD. Necrotizing enterocolitis. In: Fanaroff AA, Martin RJ, eds. *Neonatal-Perinatal Medicine–Diseases of the Fetus and Infant*, 6th ed. Mosby, 1997.

Flake AW, Ryckman FC. Selected anomalies and intestinal obstruction. In: Fanaroff AA, Martin RJ, eds. *Neonatal-Perinatal Medicine–Diseases of the Fetus and Infant*, 6th ed. Mosby, 1997.

Hsueh W, Caplan MS, Qu XW, Tan DX, De Plaen IG, Gonzalez-Crussi F. Neonatal necrotizing enterocolitis: clinical considerations and pathogenetic concepts. *Pediatr Dev Pathol* 2003;6:6–23.

Kays DW. Surgical conditions of the neonatal intestinal tract. *Clin Perinatol* 1996;23:353–375.

Lee JS, Polin RA. Treatment and prevention of necrotizing enterocolitis. *Semin Neonatol* 2003; 8:449–59.

Stoll BJ. Epidemiology of necrotizing enterocolitis. *Clin Perinatol* 1994;21:205–218.

25 NEUROLOGIC CONDITIONS IN THE NEWBORN

Maria L.V. Dizon, Janine Y. Khan, and Joshua Goldstein

EMBRYOLOGY AND MALFORMATIONS

- Brain development commences very early in gestation. Myelination begins around birth and continues for many years postnatally. Disruption at any point in antenatal or early postnatal development potentially disrupts subsequent neural development.

NEURAL TUBE DEFECTS

- Prenatal diagnosis is made through prenatal ultrasound, and by elevated maternal serum alpha fetal protein (AFP) and elevated amniotic fluid AFP. At birth, if the defect is open, blood cultures should be sent and antibiotics started.
- Head imaging should be obtained to define intracranial anatomy (and extracranial anatomy in the case of encephalocoele) and ventricle size.
- Etiology is multifactorial as suggested by increased incidence amongst the Irish, with extremes of maternal age, with low socioeconomic status (SES), with affected siblings, and with folic acid deficiency.
- Myelomeningocoele is associated with retinoic acid and vitamin A excess.
- It is controversial whether the prenatal diagnosis of a neural tube defect is an indication for Caesarian section.
- Outcome: Seizures and/or epilepsy are expected if there is also cortical dysplasia. Motor deficits are expected especially with myelomeningocoele. Some degree of mental retardation is common.

ANENCEPHALY
- This malformation results from failure of anterior neural tube closure during primary neurulation. Incidence is 0.3 per 1000 live births. The skull is incompletely closed with an exposed, severely malformed forebrain and upper brainstem. The defect may extend from lamina terminalis to foramen magnum with supraciliary frontal, parietal, squamous, and occipital bones missing. Brain tissue is hemorrhagic, fibrotic, degenerated, with ill-defined structure. Facies are frog-like.
- Most anencephalics are stillborn or die in the neonatal period. They can survive longer with supportive care; however, they remain in a permanent vegetative state. As there is no specific treatment, the goal is comfort. Comfort care may or may not include feeding depending on parents, the neonatologist, and local ethics. Debate continues whether organ donation by these neonates is appropriate.

ENCEPHALOCOELE
- This is a less severe failure of anterior neural tube closure. A mass of neural tissue that may or may not be skin-covered extrudes through a skull defect that is usually occipital and midline, but it can also be temporal, parietal, or from the nasal cavity. The protruding tissue may include normal or dysplastic meninges, cerebral cortex, subcortical white matter, parts of the ventricular system, and bone.
- Malformations may also occur in the intracranial brain; this is more likely with giant encephalocoeles.
- Associated malformations include Arnold-Chiari malformation, aqueductal stenosis, and hydrocephalus.
- Encephelocoeles may occur as part of *Meckel syndrome* (occipital encephalocoele, microcephaly, micropthalmia, cleft lip and palate, polydactyly, polycystic kidneys, and ambiguous genitalia). Incidence is 0.15 per 1000 live births.
- Half of infants with encephalocoeles have mental retardation, although outcome is more favorable for anterior encephalocoeles. If protruding tissue includes occipital lobes then cortical blindness is likely.
- Treatment is surgical and is urgent if there is cerebrospinal fluid (CSF) leakage or inadequate skin coverage. Excision/closure may be adequate or ventriculoperitoneal shunting may be necessary. Antibiotics are given until the defect is closed.

MYELOMENINGOCOELE
- Myelomeningocoele results from later failure of posterior neural tube closure. It is controversial whether it is a primary defect or secondary to reopening of an already closed neural tube because of increased hydrostatic pressure. Incidence is 0.41–1.43 per 1000 live births.
- The defect is on the back, and usually caudal, although thoracolumbar, lumbar, or lumbosacral defects exist. The defect includes meninges and dysplastic spinal cord; the vertebral arches are not fused or absent. These elements may or may not be contained in a sac. All lumbar myelomeningocoeles are associated with Arnold-Chiari malformation and aqueduct stenosis.
- Initial treatment includes prone positioning, so that no pressure is applied to lesion. If hip contractures are significant, a platform of blankets may be created to accommodate hip flexion/knee extension. The lesion should be covered with sterile saline-moistened Kerlex or Telfa followed by plastic wrap.

- Up to 50% of children with myelomeningocele may be latex sensitive. Avoid exposing the baby to any latex.
- At birth, the baby may demonstrate apnea caused by brainstem compression; intubation may be necessary.
- Initial physical examination should focus on the head circumference, anterior fontanelle, sutures, reactivity of pupils, level of lesion, spontaneous movement of extremities, withdrawal to soft touch and deep pressure, Babinski sign, cremasteric reflex, anal wink, anal tone, and strength of urinary stream. A normal head circumference does not predict absence of hydrocephalus, and the risk for hydrocephalus increases with higher lesions.
- Treatment is surgical closure with or without placement of a ventriculoperitoneal shunt within 24–48 hours. Most infants develop hydrocephalus by 6 weeks if a shunt is not placed at the time of repair. Follow head circumference closely after surgery and use neuroimaging postoperatively to reassess ventricular size.
- Children with neural tube defects experience a high rate of urinary tract infections, vesicoureteral reflux, kidney failure, hydronephrosis, and obstruction. Most are not continent of urine. Once stable postoperatively, obtain urodynamic studies.
- In general, children with lesions above L2 usually require wheelchairs and have significant scoliosis, while children with lesions at or below L4-5-ambulation will usually ambulate. Early physical therapy should be provided.
- Cognitive outcome is, in part, influenced by hydrocephalus, central nervous system (CNS) infections, and degree of impairment. In most series, 30–40% of the children with myelomeningocele had intelligence quotients less than 80.

DISORDERS OF PROSENCEPHALIC CLEAVAGE

- These disorders are listed below in the order of failure of prosencephalic cleavage, and should be suspected if other midline defects are seen. Apnea may be seen at presentation. As the pituitary may be absent, urine output and electrolytes should be followed.
- Prenatal diagnosis is possible by sonography, but less severe defects can be missed.
- There is no specific treatment for the most severe cases other than antiseizure medications, physical therapy, and special education.

HOLOPROSENCEPHALY
- This is extreme failure of prosencephalic cleavage at fifth to sixth week with an incidence of 1 per 15,000 live

births. There is a single-sphered brain structure with a common ventricle, absent olfactory bulbs, hypoplastic optic nerves, and cerebral cortical dysplasia. The third ventricle is distended into a large posterior cyst.
- Facial deformities are common, and include microcephaly, midface hypoplasia, and hypotelorism. In severe cases, there may be a single eye (cyclopia), severe nasal deformities, cleft lip and palate, or single maxillary central incisor. The face may appear normal, and this finding does not rule out holoprosencephaly.
- Abnormalities of other organ systems (cardiac, genitourinary) occur in ~75% of cases. Etiology is genetic. As many as 50% of cases have chromosomal abnormalities, and holoprosencephaly should prompt evaluation for trisomy 13. An autosomal dominant variety exists, and careful examination of the parents may be helpful. Holoprosencephaly occur in up to 2% of infants of diabetic mothers.
- Outcome is extremely poor with mental retardation, seizures, spasticity, and anosmia. A large posterior cyst requires shunting.

AGENESIS OF THE CORPUS CALLOSUM
- This is a less severe disorder of prosencephalic development between 9 and 20 weeks. The incidence is 4 per 1000 live births.
- Agenesis may be complete or partial; in partial defects, the posterior aspect is deficient. It may be isolated or associated with encephalocoele, holoprosencephaly, pachygyria, and lissencephaly.
- It is associated with *Aicardi syndrome*, which includes agenesis of corpus callosum, chorioretinal lacunae, infantile spasms, and mental retardation. This syndrome is X-linked dominant, so it is seen in females and is lethal in males.

ABSENCE OF THE SEPTUM PELLUCIDUM
- This is a primary disorder of prosencephalic development or can occur as a secondary disorder because of destruction by hydrocephalus or ischemia. It rarely occurs as an isolated anomaly, and is associated with schizencephaly, basilar encephalocoele, and hydrocephalus because of Arnold-Chiari/aqueductal stenosis.
- Septo-optic dysplasia is the most important association. This syndrome includes absence of the septum pellucidum, optic nerve hypoplasia, absent or hypoplastic pituitary, neuronal migration disorders, and cerebellar anomalies.
- Spastic diplegia, seizures, endocrine deficiencies (including panhypopituitarism), visual defects, ataxia, and cognitive defects may be seen.
- Treatment includes hormone replacement for endocrine deficiencies.

DISORDERS OF NEURONAL MIGRATION

- These disorders result from abnormal neuroblast migration and are listed in order of earliest onset to latest although there is overlap of these diseases. Clinically, spastic diplegia, seizures, visual problems, epilepsy, and mental retardation are frequent.
- Prenatal diagnosis by ultrasound cannot be made until the latter half of gestation when gyri become visible. Postnatally, magnetic resonance imaging (MRI) best defines anatomy. Electroencephalogram (EEG) and evoked potential testing may be helpful.
- *Schizencephaly*: This is the most severe defect, and is characterized by a deep cleft in the brain at the position of the Sylvian fissure that extends from pial surface to ventricle. It is believed to be the result of a primary problem in neuroblast migration between 8 and 16 weeks, although it has been associated with infarction of the middle cerebral artery during the second to third trimester. Cocaine exposure may contribute.
- *Lissencephaly*: This disease is characterized by a smooth appearance of the brain because of abnormal neuroblast migration and subsequent abnormal cortical gyration. Two anatomic types exist. Many cases are associated with chromosomal abnormalities (chromosome 17 and X chromosome).
- Treatment includes antiseizure medication, physical therapy, and special education.

HYDROCEPHALUS

- This is the progressive enlargement of ventricles caused by disruption of the CSF circulatory system (development starts at 6 weeks). Prenatal diagnosis may be made by ultrasound. Fetal onset of hydrocephalus is more commonly associated with worse severity and with other brain abnormalities.
- Hydrocephalus differs from *hydranencephaly*, which is an almost entirely fluid-filled brain with very little parenchyma because of necrosis early in gestation. Synonyms for hydranencephaly are porencephaly and multicystic encephalomalacia.
- Etiologies are heterogeneous.
  1. *Aqueductal stenosis* accounts for one-third of cases of congenital hydrocephalus. While most cases are not familial, an X-linked variety exists that is associated with flexion deformity of the thumbs and mental retardation.
  2. *Chiari malformation* is a condition in which the cerebellum portion of the brain protrudes into the spinal canal. The type II Chiari malformation is associated with myelomeningocele, and nearly 90%

of these infants will require a ventriculoperitoneal shunt.
  3. *Communicating or nonobstructive hydrocephalus* occurs when no obstruction to the CSF pathways can be identified. It may result in malfunction of arachnoid villi, and is most commonly seen following intraventricular hemorrhage. Congenital infections may produce hydrocephalus through inflammation of the arachnoid villi. This type may be associated with a higher IQ than other causes of hydrocephalus.
  4. *Dandy-Walker malformation* accounts for 5–10% of congenital hydrocephalus, and is characterized by cystic dilatation of the fourth ventricle and agenesis of the cerebellar vermis. Other CNS abnormalities (e.g., migrational disorders) are seen in 68% of patients.

DISORDERS OF HEAD SIZE AND SHAPE

- Head circumference is a good proxy for brain volume and growth. It should increase by 1 cm/week in term and 0.5 cm/week in preterm neonates. Excessive increases or decreases in head circumference should prompt investigation.
- Macrocephaly is usually isolated and the most common type is autosomal dominant. Measuring parental head circumference is helpful. Consider head imaging to rule out other etiologies.
- Microcephaly also may be familial but is more worrisome than macrocephaly. It is a common feature of intrauterine infections and/or syndromes associated with mental retardation. Evaluation should include evaluation for infectious etiologies, karyotype, head imaging, and eye examination.
- Craniosynostosis is the premature fusion of one or more cranial sutures. It causes abnormal head shape before or after birth. Some cases occur with complex syndromes.

PERINATAL HYPOXIC-ISCHEMIC ENCEPHALOPATHY (HIE)

- HIE should be considered a syndrome, with a number of features that evolve over time. Common events preceding or associated with HIE are depressed Apgar scores, cord blood acidosis, and seizures. The principal underlying mechanism is impairment in cerebral blood flow because of interruption of placental blood flow and gas exchange, resulting in diminished delivery of oxygen and energy substrates to neuronal cells.

- Asphyxia combines a deficit in energy supply (hypoxemia and ischemia) with tissue accumulation of by-products of metabolism (hypercapnea and lactic acidosis). Reduction in cerebral blood flow and oxygen delivery initiates a cascade of adverse biochemical events resulting in a change from aerobic to anaerobic metabolism. These events represent a primary phase of energy failure. Following intrapartum asphyxia, resuscitation results in reperfusion with restoration of cerebral blood flow, oxygenation, and metabolism. HIE is an evolving process in which irreversible neuronal injury may occur over a period of 6–48 hours. Cerebral metabolism deteriorates in a secondary phase of energy failure and brain injury.
- Energy failure results in impaired uptake of glutamate, the major excitatory neurotransmitter in the brain, causing excitatory amino acid (EAA) receptor overactivation. Extracellular accumulation of glutamate causes activation of *N*-methyl-D-aspartate (NMDA) and AMPA receptors expressed on neurons, increasing the permeability of the neuronal cell to sodium and calcium influx. These events produce cellular edema.
- Severity of the secondary energy failure correlates with adverse neurodevelopmental outcome at 1 and 4 years of age. These events may be measured by magnetic resonance spectroscopy: findings include a decrease in the ratio of phosphocreatine/inorganic phosphate, depletion of high-energy phosphates, and accumulation of lactate.
- Five major neuropathologic patterns have been described:
  1. Parasagittal cerebral injury is the major ischemic lesion in term infants. It results from a disturbance in cerebral blood flow, and affects the watershed areas corresponding to the border zones between the anterior and middle cerebral arteries and the middle and posterior cerebral arteries. Pathologic findings are characterized by necrosis of the cortex and subjacent white matter, especially the parietal-occipital region and subcortical white matter. The injury is typically bilateral and symmetrical. The outcome is poor with spastic quadriplegia.
  2. Focal and multifocal ischemic brain necrosis is more common in term infants. The middle cerebral artery is most commonly affected. Necrosis is followed by cyst formation (porencephaly, multicystic encephalomalacia). Outcome may include hemiplegia or quadriplegia.
  3. Selective neuronal necrosis is a common injury pattern in infants who sustain a hypoxic-ischemic injury in the postnatal period, and is secondary to oxygen and glucose deprivation followed by

reperfusion. Neuronal injury is most prominent in the watershed areas of the cerebral cortex and sulci. Long-term sequelae include mental retardation, spasticity, ataxia, and seizures.
  4. Periventricular leukomalacia is a major ischemic lesion in preterm infants, consisting of white matter necrosis involving the frontal horn of the lateral ventricles, optic and acoustic radiations. The long-term sequelae include spastic diplegia and quadriplegia.
  5. Status marmoratus is the least common type of injury. It is predominantly found in term infants, and involves the basal ganglia and thalamus. Survivors may exhibit chorea, athetosis, and cognitive deficits.

CLINICAL FEATURES

- It has been traditionally difficult to define perinatal asphyxia. Findings of infants at risk for HIE include an umbilical arterial blood gas pH <7.0, 5-minute Apgar of ≤3, or continued need for delivery room resuscitation for ≥10 minutes.
- A determination of prognosis is difficult, although this is the most eagerly sought information by the family and care providers for the infant with HIE. The markers for perinatal depression mentioned above may also be indicators of prognosis, to the extent that they indicate severity of injury. For instance, CNS sequelae are more likely when there is severe cord blood acidosis, or a poor response to resuscitation.
- The sequence of clinical features of HIE develops and becomes maximal over the first 72 hours of life. In the first 12 hours, the level of responsiveness of the infant may be depressed. Breathing is often depressed and mechanical ventilation may be required; tone and spontaneous movement may be low.
- Severity of encephalopathy and correlation with outcome are classically described according to Sarnat Staging:
  1. *Sarnat Stage 1*: Irritability, jitteriness, hyperalertness, or mild depression in level of consciousness, normal tone, increased reflexes, and no seizures. Symptoms last for <24 hours and are associated with a good outcome.
  2. *Sarnat Stage 2*: Lethargy, decreased spontaneous activity, hypotonia, increased reflexes, seizures, interictal EEG abnormalities. Approximately 20–40% have neurologic sequelae, although prognosis is good if recovery occurs within 5 days.
  3. *Sarnat Stage 3*: Coma, flaccidity, impaired brain stem function (impaired sucking, swallowing, and gagging reflex), decreased or absent reflexes, seizures uncommon, and abnormalities of interictal

EEG (e.g., burst suppression). Almost all infants have major neurologic sequelae.

- HIE is commonly associated with multiorgan dysfunction, and may affect the kidneys, heart, and liver. Electrolyte abnormalities (particularly hyponatremia and hypocalcemia) are common. Liver function should be assessed with liver enzymes and coagulation testing. The kidneys are commonly affected, and acute tubular necrosis (ATN) or acute renal failure may occur.
- Management is primarily supportive as there are no proven therapies for HIE. Fluid restriction may be needed and hypoglycemia should be avoided. Approximately 50% of affected infants will have clinical seizures requiring anticonvulsant therapy. Phenobarbital is the most common agent used. The typical loading dose for seizures is 20 mg/kg, and additional doses of 10 mg/kg may be provided for breakthrough seizures, to a total of 40–50 mg/kg. Maintenance is 3–5 mg/kg/day and serum levels should be followed. There are experimental interventions being studied to provide neuroprotection before the onset of secondary energy failure, including prophylactic high dose Phenobarbital (40 mg/kg) and hypothermia.

NEONATAL SEIZURES

- Neonatal seizures are one of the few neurologic emergencies encountered in the newborn and require prompt diagnosis and treatment. The precise frequency is unknown, but estimated to occur in 1–2% of neonatal intensive care unit (ICU) admissions.
- Seizures represent the most frequent manifestation of neurologic disease in the newborn and are usually related to significant illness.
- Seizures result from excessive repetitive depolarization of neurons because of an increased influx of Na^+ into neuronal cells and may be caused by disturbance in energy production and failure of Na-K pump (hypoxia, ischemia, hypoglycemia), alteration in the neuronal membrane affecting Na^+ permeability (hypocalcemia and hypomagnesemia), or an excess of excitatory vs. inhibitory neurotransmitters leading to increased depolarization.
- Causes of neonatal seizures
  1. Hypoxic-ischemic encephalopathy is most common cause; onset is usually within 24 hours of birth.
  2. Intracranial hemorrhage (ICH)—subarachnoid, intraventricular, and subdural hemorrhages.
  3. Metabolic—hypoglycemia, hypocalcemia, hypomagnesemia, hyponatremia, hypernatremia, hyperammonemia, pyridoxine deficiency, and amino-acidopathy. Most inborn errors of metabolism do not present until the infant initiates feeding.
  4. Intracranial infections—group B *streptococcus* (GBS), *E. coli*, herpes simplex (HSV), cytomegalovirus (CMV), and coxsackie virus.
  5. Drug withdrawal.
  6. Developmental migrational disorders (see above).
  7. Fifth day seizures occur toward the end of the first week and resolve by the end of the second week. This is a benign condition with an excellent prognosis.

- Clinical manifestations of seizures in the neonate differ from those in the older child. Jitteriness should be differentiated from seizures, and is characterized by the absence of abnormal ocular movements and cessation of abnormal movements with passive movement of the limb.
  1. Subtle seizures: Examples include swimming or bicycling movements, lip-smacking, or ocular movements.
  2. Tonic seizures are usually generalized, characterized by tonic extension of all extremities. They are usually associated with ocular signs or apnea, and seen especially in preterm infants.
  3. Multifocal clonic seizures are characterized by clonic movements originating in one extremity, and then spreading to involve other areas. These are seen especially in term infants.
  4. Focal clonic seizures are characterized by localized rhythmic jerking movements, and are usually associated with focal traumatic or ischemic injury. These may be seen in generalized cerebral insults including metabolic encephalopathies.
  5. Myoclonic seizures are single or multiple jerks of flexion involving the upper or lower extremities. These can be confused with benign sleep myoclonus in the newborn, a condition that occurs during sleep, and is associated with a normal neurologic examination and EEG.

- Recognition of seizure activity may be difficult in the neonate because of the different clinical and EEG findings compared to older child.
- Laboratory evaluation includes glucose, sodium, potassium, calcium, magnesium, and phosphorus. A complete blood count and blood culture should be performed, as well as a lumbar puncture to exclude meningitis. A head-computed tomography (CT) scan should be performed to exclude intracranial hemorrhage/infarction, and a cranial ultrasound should be done in the preterm infant to exclude intraventricular hemorrhage. Other tests depend on suspected etiology.
- An EEG is the preferred investigation to confirm seizure activity and may be a helpful guide to determining prognosis.

- *Management*: Anticonvulsant therapy is not always necessary. Etiology-specific therapy such as glucose infusion, calcium or magnesium, or pyridoxine may be indicated. All anticonvulsants may produce significant respiratory depression, therefore close cardiorespiratory monitoring is necessary and respiratory support is sometimes needed.
- Phenobarbital is the drug of choice and is effective in 85% of newborns with seizures. The loading dose is 20 mg/kg IV, and should be delivered at a rate of ≤1 mg/kg/minute. If seizures persist, additional phenobarbital may be given in 10 mg/kg increments for a total of 40 mg/kg. If seizures are controlled, maintenance of phenobarbital is commenced at 3–5 mg/kg/day.
- Phenytoin is usually given when there is inadequate control of seizures with phenobarbital. *Fos*-phenytoin solution is less irritating to veins and should always be used. The loading dose is 20 mg/kg IV, and is usually given in 10 mg/kg increments. Maintenance dose is 5–8 mg/kg/day, delivered in two divided doses.
- Lorazepam is usually given when there is inadequate response to phenobarbital and phenytoin. Dose of 0.05–0.10 mg/kg—titrate dose as indicated.

INTRACRANIAL HEMORRHAGE

- ICH has multiple causes, including prematurity, trauma, hypoxia-ischemia-reperfusion, coagulation defects, and vascular defects.
- Predisposing factors during pregnancy, labor, delivery, and resuscitation should be identified. Neurologic signs should be recorded and a lumber puncture is usually performed. A head CT or MRI should be performed if an intracranial hemorrhage is suspected in a term infant, but a head ultrasound may be the only feasible test in a preterm infant.
- Etiologies related to birth trauma (*subarachnoid hemorrhage, subdural hemorrhage*) are described in the Birth Injury section.
- *Intraventricular hemorrhage* is almost exclusively seen in the premature neonate (see Prematurity section).
- *Hemorrhagic infarction* occurs when bleeding from capillaries after reperfusion following ischemia; the ischemic may be the result of an initial embolism or vasospasm. Suspect hemorrhagic infarction if hemiparesis, seizures, stupor, or coma are seen in a term neonate.
- Hypercoagulability caused by disseminated intravascular coagulation (DIC), polycythemia, or a coagulation factor deficiency may contribute to intracranial hemorrhage. Evaluation includes prothrombin time (PT), partial thromboplastin time (PTT), fibrinogen, D-dimers, protein C, protein S, antithrombin, factor XI, MTHFR mutation, and gene mutation 20210A.
- Vascular defects such as aneurysms and arteriovenous malformations (usually of the vein of Galen) are rare causes of hemorrhage.

INTRACRANIAL INFECTIONS

- GBS and *E. coli* account for ~70% of all cases of neonatal meningitis (see Neonatal Infectious Disease section). Virtually all organisms that cause neonatal sepsis may produce neonatal meningitis.
- GBS meningitis occurs in 5–15% of early-onset (<7 days) GBS infections and 30–40% of late-onset infections (≥7 days to 3 months).
- *E. coli* expressing the K1 capsular polysaccharide antigen is found in ~75% of cases of *E. coli* meningitis. There is an association between CSF K1 Ag levels and prognosis. As there has been significant emergence of ampicillin-resistant *E. coli* secondary to intrapartum ampicillin therapy, addition of cefotaxime should be considered for suspected gram-negative meningitis. Duration of therapy for gram-negative meningitis is a minimum of 21 days. Acute complications of *E. coli* meningitis include hydrocephalus and subdural effusions. Long-term complications of neurologic impairment are seen in 30–50% of survivors.
- *Candida meningitis* is usually caused by *Candida albicans*, although *Candida parapsilosis* is also seen. Predisposing factors include low birth weight (<1500 g), prolonged total parenteral nutrition, indwelling central venous catheters, and broad-spectrum antibiotic therapy. Diagnosis may be difficult, and repeated peripheral blood cultures may be necessary as cultures may only be intermittently positive. Meningitis and cerebral abscess may be present despite negative CSF cultures. Treatment with combination therapy (amphotericin B and flucytosine [5-FC]) is preferred for neonatal candidal meningitis, as these agents act synergistically. Approximately 50% of premature infants with candida meningitis survived without sequelae; even better outcomes are seen in term infants.
- *CMV* is the most common congenital viral infection. Approximately 40,000 infants are born with a congenital infection each year, although 90% are asymptomatic at birth. CMV specific IgM and urine viral culture readily establishes the diagnosis. Periventricular calcifications, microcephaly, and migrational abnormalities may also be observed. There is a 90% risk of neurologic sequelae, including hearing and

vision impairment in the 10% of infants born with symptomatic, congenital CMV infections.

- *Herpes simplex*: Most HSV infections in the neonate are acquired during delivery because of viral shedding in the female genital tract. Fetal scalp monitoring is a risk factor for neonatal infection. Infants may present with CNS manifestations as part of disseminated disease, or with disease localized to the CNS. Infants with CNS disease usually present during the second to third weeks of life. The characteristic presentation is persistent seizures that are difficult to control. The diagnosis may be made using antigen detection methods on vesicular fluid; CSF may show lymphocytosis and elevated protein, and polymerase chain reaction (PCR) may be performed to detect HSV deoxyribonucleic acid (DNA). The EEG is diffusely abnormal and does not demonstrate focal changes seen in older children. Treatment is acyclovir at 10 mg/kg IV for 10 days. Approximately 50% of infants surviving HSV encephalitis after acyclovir therapy have normal development.

HYPOTONIA AND NEUROMUSCULAR DISEASE

- Hypotonia and weakness can result from lesions anywhere along pathway from cortex to muscle. Lesions above the lower motor neuron produce hypotonia > weakness; in lower motor neuron diseases weakness > hypotonia is observed. A decrease or absence of movement in utero results in contractures rather than hypotonia.
- Presentation and initial management is similar for many of the diseases in this category despite heterogeneous etiologies. There may be a history of decreased movement in utero. Respiratory muscles are weak, and intercostal muscles are usually affected more than diaphragm, leading to paradoxical abdominal movement and pectus excavatum. Handling of respiratory secretions is poor because of weak masticatory and pharyngeal muscles. The cry is often weak. There may be poor central respiratory drive particularly in congenital myotonic dystrophy.
- Treatment is similar and is mostly supportive for these conditions, and includes mechanical ventilation, airway suctioning, aminophylline for poor central drive, chest physiotherapy, tube feedings (small and frequent), metaclopropamide for poor gastric motility, surveillance for pneumonia, antiseizure medications, physical therapy to preserve range of motion, surgical and nonsurgical interventions for joint deformities, and monitoring for scoliosis.
- A chest x-ray (CXR) should be obtained if an infant presents with respiratory distress, and may show a bell-shaped chest or thin ribs. If there are signs of poor cardiac output, an echocardiogram may show signs of cardiomyopathy. Head imaging is needed to rule out a central etiology; other useful tests include liver function tests (LFTs), CPK, electromyelogram, nerve conduction velocity studies, muscle biopsy, and specific genetic testing.
- *Arthrogryposis multiplex congenita* is not a specific etiology, but rather a syndrome of multiple joint contractures and webbing because of decreased movement in utero that can be a manifestation of a problem anywhere along the motor pathway. Upper and lower extremities are affected, and distal joints are more commonly affected. Etiologies other than neuromuscular disease should be considered, including amniotic bands, small/malformed maternal pelvis or uterus, and severe oligohydramnios.
- *Central causes of hypotonia*: Potential causes include maternal anesthetics, hypoxic-ischemic encephalopathy, metabolic disorders, hyperammonemia, organic acidopathies, hypothyroidism, intracranial hemorrhage, and trauma.
- *Prader-Willi syndrome* should be suspected with truncal hypotonia. Many of its classic features are not manifest at birth. This syndrome is caused by a deletion in the paternally derived chromosome 15q11-13. All neuromuscular studies are normal. The etiology for the hypotonia is unknown but is thought to be central.
- *Werdnig-Hoffman disease* or type I spinal muscular atrophy is a disease of anterior horn cell degeneration resulting in very severe hypotonia, weakness, and even flaccid paralysis. The incidence is 0.4 per 1000 births. The onset is early, with half of infants presenting in the first month of life. Severe weakness in a proximal > distal distribution is seen, with minimal movement of hips and shoulders but active movements of hands and feet. Deep tendon reflexes (DTRs) are difficult to elicit. Fasciculations are seen, especially of tongue and fingers. The facial muscles are not weak; the face is active and without ptosis or ophthalmoplegia. The alert state is not affected and intelligence is normal. Laboratory evaluations will show a CPK that is normal. Electromyography (EMG) testing will show fasciculations and fibrillations; nerve conduction velocity is usually normal. Muscle biopsy shows changes of denervation, but this test has been largely replaced by genetic evaluation for the deletion in the q13 region of chromosome 5. Prenatal diagnosis by chorionic villus sampling (CVS) is available.
- *Infant botulism* is a disease of descending hypotonia and weakness caused by presynaptic blockade of cholinergic transmission by toxin from *Clostridium botulinum*; these bacteria have accessed the system via gut colonization. The affected neonate presents as

early as 2 weeks of life with poor feeding, hypotonia, constipation, then progressing to loss of DTRs, cranial nerve dysfunction, papillary paralysis, ptosis, and even sudden death. The diagnosis is confirmed through EMG testing which has a highly specific pattern; a stool culture that is positive for *C. botulinum* is also helpful. Supportive treatment must be provided until spontaneous resolution in 1–2 months.

- *Myasthenia gravis* is a disease of extreme muscle weakness and generalized hypotonia, due to interference with acetylcholine receptors. CPK, CSF, EMG, and nerve conduction velocity testing is normal. Anticholinesterase challenge (neostigmine or edrophonium) gives the definitive diagnosis.

  1. *Transient neonatal myasthenia gravis* is produced by antibodies passively received from the mother. It occurs in 10–20% of infants born with a maternal history of myasthenia gravis. More than 75% of infants present within the first 24 hours of life. Cranial nerve dysfunction is prominent, and while most infants present with feeding difficulties, respiratory compromise is also common. Most infants will require anticholinesterase therapy. This disease is transient and outcome is good.

  2. *Congenital myasthenia gravis* has later onset, and ptosis and ophthalmoplegia are typical presenting symptoms. Anticholinesterase therapy is an essential aspect of management.

- *Congenital myotonic dystrophy* is an inherited disorder, although newborns present with a pattern of disease that is different from adult myotonic dystrophy. The incidence is 1 in 3500 births. During pregnancy polyhydramnios develops because of swallowing disturbances. Infants present with facial diplegia, a tented upper lip, respiratory and feeding difficulties, and hypotonia. This disease should be suspected if there is a maternal history or if myotonia is found in the mother. If affected, the mother will be unable to open her eyes for several seconds after closing them tightly. CPK and CSF are normal; ventricular dilatation is common on head imaging. An EMG will show myotonic discharges. The etiology is a trinucleotide (CTG) repeat on chromosome 19q13.3, with maternal autosomal dominant inheritance. Symptoms are proportional to the number of CTG repeats. Most infants that require mechanical ventilation for >1 month do not survive. Survivors walk by 3 years and have mental retardation or significant learning disabilities.

- *Congenital muscular dystrophy* is a heterogeneous group of disorders sharing clinical and myopathologic features, especially connective tissue proliferation, replacement of muscle by fat, and variation in muscle fiber size. There are many specific varieties that are characterized by myopathy alone (*pure* or *merosin-positive*) or myopathy with central nervous system involvement (*merosin-deficient*). Severe arthrygryposis is often seen early; if not present at birth, contractures develop rapidly. Ventilatory and swallowing disturbances are less commonly associated. The intellect is not necessarily impaired. In most patients, the CPK is elevated early in life. The etiology is genetic and of autosomal recessive inheritance. While some infants may slowly gain milestones during infancy, long-term outcome is poor with progression to severe kyphoscolisis and death.

- *Congenital myopathies* are an incompletely understood group of primary muscle disorders that are present at birth and are not manifest until later. They include nemaline myopathy, central core disease, multicore-minicore myopathy, myotubular myopathy, congenital fiber type disproportion, and minimal change myopathies.

- *Mitochondrial myopathies* result from defects in the electron transport chain. *Cytochrome c oxidase deficiency* is the subtype that most commonly leads to prominent neonatal muscle disease. Suspect these diseases if there is multisystem involvement. Unique features include cardiomyopathy, macroglossia, lactic acidosis, hepatomegaly, and renal tubular defects. Outcome is poor with death in a few months.

- *Pompe's disease* is a rare disease because of a deficiency of acid-maltase activity resulting in glycogen deposits in the anterior horn cells, skeletal and cardiac muscles, liver and brain; it is also known as *type II glycogen storage disease*. This disease may be apparent from the first days of life but usually does not manifest for several weeks. Cardiomyopathy because of glycogen accumulation is a characteristic feature. The tongue is often enlarged. The liver is enlarged and usually firm, and skeletal muscles appear prominent and hypertrophied. A muscle biopsy will reveal large amounts of periodic acid-Schiff (PAS) material with vacuoles. The outcome is dismal with death from cardiac or respiratory causes typical in the first year of life. The etiology is genetic with autosomal recessive inheritance, and prenatal diagnosis is available by fibroblast culture.

BIBLIOGRAPHY

Behrman RE, Kliegman R, Jenson HB, eds. *Nelson Textbook of Pediatrics*, 16th ed. Philadelphia: W.B. Saunders; 1999.

Bianchi DW, Crombleholme TM, D'Alton ME, eds. *Fetology; Diagnosis and Management of the Fetal Patient*. New York: McGraw-Hill; 2000.

Fanaroff AA and Martin RJ, eds. *Neonatal-Perinatal Medicine: Diseases of the Fetus and Infant.* 7th ed., Mosby; 2001.

Fenichel, GM, Neurological examination of the newborn. *International Pediatrics* 1994; 9:77–81.

Gabbe. Obstetrics–Normal and Problem Pregnancies, 4th ed. London: Churchill Livingstone; 2002.

Huppi PS. Advances in postnatal neuroimaging: relevance to pathogenesis and treatment of brain injury. *Clin Perinatol* 2002;29:827–856.

McLone DG, editor. *Pediatric Neurosurgery: Surgery of the Developing Nervous System,* 4th ed. Philadelphia: W.B. Saunders Company, 2001.

Menkes JH, Sarnat HB. *Child Neurology,* 6th ed. New York: Lippincott Williams & Wilkins; 2000.

Scher MS. Seizures in the newborn infant. Diagnosis, treatment, and outcome. *Clin Perinatol* 1997;24:735–772.

Shankaran S. The postnatal management of the asphyxiated term infant. *Clin Perinatol* 2002;29:675–692.

Volpe JJ. *Neurology of the Newborn,* 4th ed. Philadelphia: W.B. Saunders; 2001.

26 GENITOURINARY CONDITIONS

Nicolas F.M. Porta and
Robin H. Steinhorn, MD

- Renal masses are the most common cause of an abdominal mass in the newborn period.

  1. *Hydronephrosis* is the most common congenital condition detected by antenatal ultrasound and occurs in approximately 1 in 700 births. More than 85% of cases of hydronephrosis are due to obstruction at the ureteropelvic, ureterovesical, or bladder neck (posterior urethral valves). After birth, the degree of hydronephrosis may be underestimated in the first few days of life because of the low glomerular filtration rate of the newborn, therefore repeat ultrasonography is mandatory. Consultation with a pediatric urologist or nephrologist is necessary to determine testing for the cause of hydronephrosis. Prophylactic antibiotics are frequently administered to prevent urinary tract infections (UTI).

  2. The most common cystic renal disease in the newborn is *multicystic dysplastic kidney.* It is usually unilateral, although up to 50% of infants will have abnormalities of the contralateral urinary tract. Because the disease is unilateral, prognosis tends to be good. Surgical removal of the affected kidney is controversial, and is often only done when hypertension cannot be controlled. *Polycystic*

kidney disease is less common in the newborn. Newborns presenting with this condition typically have disease inherited in an autosomal recessive fashion, and prognosis is very poor. While autosomal dominant polycystic kidney disease is more common, it usually does not present in the newborn period.

  3. *Renal vein thrombosis* may present in the newborn period with a firm flank mass, hematuria, and thrombocytopenia. Risk factors include dehydration, hypercoagulability, and maternal diabetes. This condition can typically be medically managed; consultation with a hematologist may be helpful in determining whether anticoagulant therapy or thrombolytic is beneficial. Prognosis for survival is good.

- *Vesicoureteral reflux* (VUR) can predispose to upper urinary tract infections and renal damage. VUR can be familial or the result of ureteral or bladder anomalies. Evaluation for VUR should be undertaken for infants with hydronephrosis or a history of urinary tract infection (approximately 30% of infants are found to have reflux after their first UTI). This evaluation typically includes ultrasonography and a voiding cystourethrogram. Management includes prophylactic low dose antibiotics to suppress UTI, urologic consultation, and long-term monitoring.

- *Posterior urethra valves* (PUV) are abnormal values in the urethra that occur only in males, and represent the most common cause of congenital obstruction of the urinary tract in males. PUV are composed of membrane that obstructs the posterior urethra, and can produce a high degree of bladder outlet obstruction, leading to dilation of the urinary bladder, ureters, and renal collecting systems. If severe, it can lead to progressive renal failure and even oligohydramnios associated with pulmonary hypoplasia. PUV can be identified antenatally by fetal ultrasonography. Postnatally, infants may present with a distended bladder, bilateral flank masses, and a history of infrequent voiding or a poor urinary stream. Urgent urologic consultation to immediately decompress the bladder is required. Long-term monitoring of renal function is essential, as there is a 30% risk for the development of progressive renal insufficiency later in childhood.

- *Hypospadius* is the most common penile abnormality noted in the newborn, affecting more than 1 in 300 males. It is a developmental anomaly in which the external meatus is present proximal to, and on the ventral side of the penis, rather than in its normal position on the end of the penile shaft. The degree of hypospadius can be classified according to the location of the meatal opening. Chordee (curvature of the penis) is frequently associated with hypospadius; cryptorchism and inguinal hernias are also commonly observed. While minimal evaluation is required for mild hypospadius, severely affected infants should be evaluated with a karyotype, and conditions such as congenital adrenal hypoplasia should be considered. Surgical correction is usually not attempted in the newborn, but is done later in the first year of life. Circumcision should be avoided in the newborn period, as foreskin may be needed for later surgical correction.

- *Inguinal hernia* is the herniation of intestines through a patent processus vaginalis into scrotum (or labia majora in females).
  1. Inguinal hernias most commonly present as a lump at the pubic tubercle, although the hernia may descend into the scrotum. They occur in ~10% of premature males.
  2. Inguinal hernias may come and go; if a hernia is recognized once it must be surgically repaired even if it is not always apparent. The major risks include incarceration (not able to be reduced) or strangulation (compromise of vascular supply). The risk of incarceration in the first year of life is 5–15%, therefore surgical repair is done early. In premature infants, repair is typically performed prior to hospital discharge.
  3. Postoperative apnea may occur in premature infants, and these patients should be monitored for 24 hours after repair.
- *Cryptorchidism* or undescended testicles occurs in approximately 3% of full-term infants, and is more common in premature infants. The majority of apparent cryptorchid testes are palpable in the inguinal canal at birth. In most infants, full descent of the testicles will occur by 9 months of age without intervention. If not descended by 18 months, orchiopexy is indicated to prevent atrophy and malignant degeneration.
- *Bladder exstrophy* is a very rare congenital malformation of the lower anterior abdominal wall. The anterior wall of the bladder is missing and the bladder mucosa herniates through the lower abdomen. The diagnosis is commonly made antenatally, and is obvious after delivery. The exposed bladder mucosa is typically friable and will not tolerate air exposure; it should be protected after delivery. Staged surgical repair usually begins within the first 72 hours of life with primary closure of the bladder and approximation of the pubic rami.
- Severe cases with more extensive cloacal anomalies and omphalocele are called *cloacal exstrophy*. This condition is frequently associated with imperforate anus, and a vesicointestinal fistula and prolapse of the

bowel into the bladder mucosa. Staged repair begins shortly after birth with separation of the intestinal and genitourinary systems.

BIBLIOGRAPHY

Gonzalez R, Schimke CM. Ureteropelvic junction obstruction in infants and children. *Pediatr Clin North America* 2001;48: 1505–1518.

Kaplan BS. Development abnormalities of the kidneys. In Taesch HW and Ballard RA, eds. *Avery's Diseases of the Newborn*. 7th ed. 1998. Philadelphia: W.B. Saunders: 1136–1143.

McKenna PH, Ferrer FA. Prenatal and postnatal urologic emergencies. In Belman AB, King LR, Kramer SA, eds. *Clinical Pediatric Urology*, 4th ed. Martin Dunitz, 2002.

Vogt BA, Avner ED. The kidney and urinary tract. In: Fanaroff AA, Martin RJ, eds. *Neonatal-Perinatal Medicine–Diseases of the Fetus and Infant*, 7th ed. Mosby; 2002:1517–1536.

Zderic SA. Developmental abnormalities of the genituourinary system. In Taesch HW and Ballard RA, eds. *Avery's Diseases of the Newborn*, 7th ed. Philadelphia: W.B. Saunders Company; 1998:1144–1157.

27 NEONATAL INFECTIONS

Malika D. Shah and Catherine M. Bendel

INTRODUCTION

- Infectious diseases are an important cause of morbidity and mortality in the neonate. A relatively immature defense system renders the neonate particularly susceptible to disseminated systemic infection, rather than localized infections. Neonates may develop bacterial, viral, or fungal infections, depending on their exposure.
- Evaluation and treatment of suspected sepsis is a complex process with many variables. The following guidelines should be individualized to each patient.

RISK FACTORS FOR NEONATAL SEPSIS

- Antenatal risk factors include maternal infection during pregnancy, multiple gestation, young maternal age <20 years old, no prenatal care, and low socioeconomic status. Maternal urinary tract infections, or heavy maternal genital tract colonization, particularly with group B streptococci (GBS) and *Candida* are risk factors. In viral infections, the risk to the neonate is greater with a primary than a recurrent maternal infection.

- Peripartum risk factors include prematurity, very low birth weight (<1500 g), premature rupture of membranes, and prolonged rupture of membranes (>18 hours, with a significant increase in the incidence of infection if >24 hours). Chorioamnionitis is associated with a 5–15% risk of neonatal sepsis; signs of chorioamnionitis include maternal fever (>38°C) and fetal tachycardia. Vaginal births have higher risk than cesarean deliveries. Additional risk factors include a 5-minute Apgar score of <6 and male gender.

- Postpartum risk factors include exposure to a specific pathogen, indwelling devices including intravascular catheters, endotracheal tubes, urinary catheters, and prolonged or frequent courses of broad-spectrum antibiotics. Other factors include hyperglycemia, steroid therapy, and prolonged hospitalization.

CLINICAL MANIFESTATIONS OF NEONATAL SEPSIS

- Early signs may be subtle or nonspecific in the neonate, including poor feeding or decreased responsiveness.
- More specific clinical findings may include the following:
  1. Respiratory distress, apnea, tachypnea, or increasing supplemental oxygen requirement.
  2. Tachycardia, hypotension, poor perfusion, shock.
  3. Temperature instability.
  4. Vomiting, diarrhea, abdominal distention, bloody aspirates, or stools.
  5. Lethargy, seizures, bulging fontanelle, focal neurologic abnormalities.
  6. Hematuria, oliguria.
  7. Jaundice, bruising, petechiae.
  8. Pustules, vesicles, cellulites, omphalitis.
  9. Metabolic acidosis.
  10. Hypoglycemia or hyperglycemia (particularly if previously glucose tolerant).

LABORATORY DIAGNOSIS OF NEONATAL SEPSIS

- Positive cultures of normally sterile body fluids confirm the diagnosis of infection, including the following:
  1. Blood: Must be obtained as a part of every evaluation for sepsis.

2. Cerebrospinal fluid (CSF): Although desirable, especially in symptomatic patients, a lumbar puncture may not be mandatory on all patients. This procedure may be delayed if the infant is unstable and presumed unlikely to tolerate the procedure, or if the reasons for initiating a septic evaluation are weak in an asymptomatic infant. Since meningitis is frequently associated with sepsis, CSF analysis is indicated for all infants with a positive blood culture. Evaluation of the Gram stain and chemical findings (glucose and protein levels) may be helpful in the early diagnostic phase, or if antibiotics have been administered prior to obtaining CSF. A positive Gram stain will confirm suspicions of meningitis, while the chemical studies have limitations based on the wide range of values in normal infants and limited data on normal values in preterm infants.

3. Urine: Sample should be obtained by suprapubic aspiration; sterile catheterization is the alternative method. Urine culture for bacteria may not be mandatory in the first 1–2 days of life, as the yield is extremely low; however, beyond 3 days of age, urine cultures are indicated, as urinary tract infections are a frequent source of infection. Evaluation of the urine for cytomegalovirus (CMV) is often the easiest way to make the diagnosis of congenital CMV.

4. Surface cultures: While once a common practice, the yield of actual infection-causing organisms is low. Results are usually polymicrobial and reflect the entire maternal gastrointestinal (GI)/ genitourinary (GU) normal flora; however, when herpes simplex virus (HSV) is suspected, cultures of the eye and nasopharynx, obtained at 24–48 hours, are indicated and may provide the best diagnostic evidence.

5. Other fluids/sites: Additional cultures should be obtained as indicated by the clinical symptoms and history.

- Hematologic studies, including a complete blood count (CBC) with differential and platelet count are indicated in every sepsis evaluation; however, interpretation is limited because of the wide variations seen among normal infants, especially in the first day of life.
  1. The total white blood cell (WBC) may be difficult to interpret as it rises dramatically over the first 24 hours of life. An extremely elevated (>20,000/mm³) or very depressed (<5000/mm³) count is more suggestive of infection, especially a persistent low WBC (>24 hours).
  2. Persistent neutropenia is a strong indicator of sepsis.
  3. Thrombocytopenia is also associated with sepsis, especially fungal.

- A chest radiograph is indicated in all infants with respiratory symptoms. Focal findings are often absent in neonates and findings of pneumonia may overlap with or be obscured by those of prematurity.
- Serum glucose is indicated in all septic evaluations. Hypoglycemia is frequently associated with early-onset infections, while hyperglycemia in the previously glucose tolerant infant may indicate a late infection.
- C-reactive protein: Interpretation may be limited because of the lack of normative values in the infant; however, a rise in paired samples over a 24-hour period may be helpful in diagnosis. Conversely, values decrease rapidly with adequate therapy. Therefore, persistent elevations may indicate inadequate therapy and may assist in determining length of treatment.
- Coagulation studies are indicated in the unstable symptomatic infant and are frequently prolonged and may indicate disseminated intravascular coagulation (DIC).

BACTERIAL SEPSIS

GENERAL FEATURES OF BACTERIAL SEPSIS
- Bacterial sepsis is generally divided into two patterns of disease presentation in the first month of life, early-onset and late-onset.
- Early-onset bacterial sepsis:
  1. Incidence ranges from 1 to 5 per 1000 live births in the United States.
  2. Onset ≤4 days of age.
  3. The predominant organisms are GBS and *Escherichia coli*, with the maternal genital tract as the source. Other gram-negative enterics, *Staphylococcus aureus*, enterococci, and *Listeria monocytogenes* each account for a few percent of cases per year.
  4. Risk factors are antenatal and perinatal as outlined above.
  5. Complications of pregnancy or delivery are common.
  6. Presentation may be either asymptomatic or symptomatic; but is usually fulminant, rapidly progressive, with multiorgan system involvement and many of the clinical manifestations listed above. Pneumonia is a common presenting sign.
  7. Mortality is high.
- Late-onset bacterial sepsis:
  1. Incidence varies depending on whether community or nosocomially acquired. The incidence of late-onset GBS disease is approximately 0.35–0.5 per 1000 live births in the United States. The incidence of nosocomially acquired infections on the NICU

ranges from 5 to 20%, with the majority of infections occurring among the very low birth weight infants.
  2. Onset ≥5 days of age.
  3. The source of the infection may still be the maternal genital tract, but also includes the postnatal environment (community vs. NICU).
  4. Risk factors include the postpartum category listed above.
  5. Complications of pregnancy or delivery may or may not have been present.
  6. Presentation is more often focal and slowly progressive. Meningitis is frequently present.
  7. Mortality is lower than early-onset, ranging from 2 to 6%.

INDICATIONS FOR A SEPTIC EVALUATION

Bacterial Sepsis: Early-Onset, Suspected
- In ALL symptomatic infants a blood culture, CBC with differential and platelet count, serum glucose, and CSF studies should be obtained as soon as possible and the infant should be started on empiric antibiotics regardless of risk factors. Additional studies are warranted as the specific symptoms and exposure history indicate.
- If truly infected, asymptomatic infants can decompensate rapidly, becoming symptomatic and may benefit from empiric therapy. Therefore, evaluation and treatment of the asymptomatic infant is indicated according to the presence or absence of risk factors which include the following:
  1. Prematurity
  2. Prolonged rupture of membranes
  3. Maternal fever
  4. Maternal chorioamnionitis
  5. Maternal GBS status
- In an asymptomatic infant, risk factors will influence the extent of the evaluation and therapy, as outlined below.

Bacterial Sepsis: Early-Onset, Suspected Asymptomatic With Prematurity as Sole Risk Factor
- Premature infants are at higher risk of infection because of multiple factors including an immature immune status, immature epithelial/mucosal barriers, and the frequent presence of indwelling catheters.
- In evaluating a preterm infant, one should consider the cause of the prematurity.
  1. If the cause of preterm labor is unknown or related to a fetal condition, occult maternal chorioamnionitis should be considered as the etiology. Evaluation of the infant with a blood culture, CBC,

serum glucose is indicated, as well as initiating empiric treatment with antibiotics.

2. If the cause of preterm delivery is solely maternal (such as PIH, bicornate uterus, incompetent cervix), and the child is asymptomatic, and there are no other risk factors, close observation of antibiotics may be justified.

Bacterial Sepsis: Early-Onset, Suspected Asymptomatic With Rupture of Membranes, Maternal Fever, or Chorioamnionitis as Risk Factors

• The presence of either risk factor alone in a term asymptomatic newborn does not routinely warrant cultures and antibiotics; however, PROM is associated with a 1% incidence of neonatal sepsis (increased from a baseline of 0.1–0.5%), therefore close observation is indicated.

• The presence of chorioamnionitis raises the risk of infection in the term infant fourfold. Full diagnostic evaluation with empiric antibiotic therapy for a minimum of 48 hours is indicated.

• In an asymptomatic preterm infant, most centers recommend obtaining blood cultures and a CBC at a minimum and treating with empiric antibiotics if either PROM or maternal fever is present, even in the absence of documented chorioamnionitis.

Bacterial Sepsis: Early-Onset, Suspected Asymptomatic With Maternal GBS Status as a Risk Factor

• GBS is the most common neonatal bacterial infection, characterized by septicemia, pneumonia, and meningitis with a significant degree of mortality and morbidity. As a result, screening in late gestation for carrier status is recommended for all pregnant women.

• Recommendations exist as to whether or not the mother should receive intrapartum antimicrobial prophylaxis. This combined information can then be used to tailor the approach to evaluation and therapy of the asymptomatic infant.

• Current *Centers for Disease Control and Prevention* (CDC) guidelines recommend the following evaluation and treatment. This is not an exclusive course of management and variations that incorporate individual circumstances or institutional preferences may be appropriate.

1. Maternal GBS negative with no other risk factors: no evaluation or treatment required.

2. Maternal GBS positive, gestation less than 35 weeks, no maternal intrapartum antibiotics: full diagnostic evaluation with empiric antibiotic therapy for a minimum of 48 hours is indicated.

3. Maternal GBS positive, gestation greater than 35 weeks, no maternal intrapartum antibiotics: data

are insufficient to recommend a single management strategy.

4. Maternal GBS positive, gestation less than 35 weeks, maternal intrapartum antibiotics (regardless of number of doses): limited evaluation with blood culture and CBC, observation of antibiotics for minimum of 48 hours, if no other risk factors are present and the infant remains asymptomatic.

5. Maternal GBS positive, gestation greater than 35 weeks, less than two doses of antibiotics or antibiotics less than 4 hours prior to delivery: limited evaluation with blood culture and CBC and observation for a minimum of 48 hours.

6. Maternal GBS positive, gestation greater than 35 weeks, two or more doses of antibiotics received by mother with the second dose more than 4 hours prior to delivery: no evaluation, no therapy, observation in-house for at least 48 hours. A healthy appearing infant in this category who is greater than or equal to 38 weeks gestation at delivery may be discharged to home after 24 hours if other discharge criteria are met and a caregiver able to comply with home observation will be present.

Late-Onset Bacterial Sepsis

• Community-acquired late-onset sepsis is usually manifested by meningitis. The differential diagnosis must also include viral infections, as discussed below.

• In the NICU setting, one is more likely to encounter nosocomial infections caused by coagulase-negative staphylococci, gram-negative rods, or other microbes such as *Candida*.

• Most infants will be symptomatic and all should receive blood, urine, and CSF studies with initiation of empiric antibiotic therapy.

• If necrotizing enterocolitis (NEC) or concurrent pneumonia is suspected, radiographs and sputum cultures should be obtained.

• If the child has persistently positive cultures, indwelling catheters should be removed.

CHOICE OF ANTIBIOTICS FOR SUSPECTED BACTERIAL SEPSIS

• Choice of antibiotics is based on knowledge of the most prevalent organisms responsible for neonatal sepsis and the pattern of antimicrobial susceptibility observed for these organisms in the treating institution or community.

• For early-onset sepsis, the combination of penicillin G or ampicillin and an aminoglycoside, most commonly gentamicin, provides adequate coverage for the most prevalent organisms.

1. For suspected late-onset sepsis in nonhospitalized infants greater than 1 month, ampicillin and gentamicin would still provide appropriate coverage; however, to obtain better CSF penetration and to avoid concerns of aminoglycoside toxicity, a third-generation cephalosporin such as cefotaxime may be substituted.

- In hospitalized infants, consideration must be given to other risk factors such as the presence of indwelling catheters (PCVC, ventriculoperitoneal [VP] shunt, urinary catheters, endotracheal tube [ETT]) or abdominal distension (suspected NEC).
  1. MRSA and coagulase-negative staphylococci are likely culprits in the presence of indwelling catheters/shunts and empiric vancomycin frequently needs to be initiated.
  2. In suspected NEC, empiric ampicillin or vancomycin and gentamicin should be initiated. If perforation is suspected, anaerobic coverage with clindamicin may be added.
- Once the causative organism is identified, antimicrobial sensitivities should be determined and empiric antibiotics should be adjusted to provide the most appropriate treatment.
- Length of therapy depends on the specific microbe identified and the severity of symptoms and sites involved. One set of guidelines for length of therapy is as follows:
  1. Mild symptoms with negative cultures: 2–3 days.
  2. Severe symptoms, including pneumonia with negative culture: 5–7 days.
  3. Culture positive: 7–10 days.
  4. Meningitis: 14–21 days (GBS), a minimum of 21 days with *E. coli*, with normal CSF studies at the end of therapy.

OTHER NEONATAL INFECTIONS, NONSEPSIS

CHLAMYDIA TRACHOMATIS

- *Chlamydia trachomatis* is the most common reportable sexually transmitted disease in the United States, with prevalence in pregnant women of 6–12%. There is a significant risk of perinatal transmission from mother to infant. The incubation period varies, but is usually at least 1 week.
- Infants may be asymptomatic or present with either conjunctivitis or pneumonia.
  1. Neonatal conjunctivitis is characterized by ocular congestion, edema, and discharge in the first few weeks of life.
  2. Neonatal pneumonia is usually an afebrile illness with hyperinflation and infiltrates on chest radiograph, with an accompanying repetitive staccato cough, tachypnea, and rales presenting between 2 and 19 weeks after birth.
- *Diagnosis* is based on clinical signs, culture, polymerase chain reaction (PCR), or direct fluorescent antibody staining. *Chlamydia* are obligate intracellular organisms, therefore specimens for diagnostic study must contain actual epithelial cells, not just exudate.
- *Treatment* differs for asymptomatic and symptomatic infants.
  1. The asymptomatic infant born to a mother with untreated chlamydia infection is at high risk for infection and should be observed closely. Currently, there are no recommendations for prophylactic antibiotic therapy, as the efficacy of such treatment has not been shown. Prophylaxis with erythromycin ophthalmic ointment is suggested in the situation when adequate follow-up can be guaranteed.
  2. Infants with chlamydia conjunctivitis or pneumonia should be treated with oral erythromycin (50 mg/kg/day in four divided doses) for 14 days. Topical treatment alone is ineffective. Treatment of the mother and her sexual partner should also be initiated.

GONOCOCCAL INFECTIONS

- *Neiseria gonorrhea* is a gram-negative oxidase-positive diplococcus sexually transmitted organism, with a predilection for mucosal surfaces, which can result in asymptomatic infection of the female genital tract, resulting in transmission from the mother to the infant perinatally. The incubation period is 2–7 days, hence the recommendations for universal prophylaxis of all newborns with erythromycin ophthalmic ointment.
- Infection in the newborn usually involves the eyes— ophthalmia neonatorum—but may present as a scalp abscess (associated with fetal monitoring), vaginitis, or disseminated disease (bacteremia, arthritis, meningitis, or endocarditis).
- Diagnosis can be made based on maternal cultures or cultures from the infant of blood, eye discharge, CSF, or other infected sites such as arthritic joints. Evaluation for other sexually transmitted diseases is also indicated.
- Treatment differs for asymptomatic and symptomatic infants.
  1. The asymptomatic infant born to a mother with untreated gonorrhea should receive a single dose of ceftriaxone (125 mg, IM or IV) in addition to eye prophylaxis with erythromycin eye ointment. An

alternative therapy is cefotaxime (100 mg/kg, IM or IV).

2. Symptomatic infants with ophthalmia neonatorum alone should receive either a single dose of ceftriaxone (125 mg, IM or IV) or cefotaxime (100 mg/kg, IV or IM) in addition to frequent eye irrigations with saline until the eye discharge is eliminated. Topical treatment alone is inadequate.

3. Infants with disseminated disease require 7 days of therapy with ceftriaxone (25–50 mg/kg, IV or IM, once daily) or cefotaxime (50 mg/kg/day, IV or IM, in two divided doses). Cefotaxime is recommended if hyperbilirubinemia present. For documented meningitis, treatment is extended for a total of 10–14 days.

SYPHILIS

- *Treponema pallidum* is a thin motile spirochete responsible for sexually transmitted disease in adults and congenitally acquired syphilis among infants. Infection during pregnancy can result in fetal loss, hydrops fetalis, premature delivery, and congenital syphilis.
- Congenital syphilis can present early or late:
  1. Early congenital syphilis: symptoms occur in the first 2 years of life presenting with snuffles, hemolytic anemia, hepatosplenomegaly, lymphadenopathy, mucocutaneous lesions, periostitis, osteochondritis, thrombocytopenia, and/or meningitis.
  2. Late congenital syphilis: infants may be initially asymptomatic and develop late manifestations after 2 years of age involving the central nervous system (CNS) and musculoskeletal system. These include periostitis of frontal and parietal bones, Hutchinson teeth, mulberry molars, saddle nose, saber shins, eighth nerve deafness (10–14 years), rhagades, and central nervous system abnormalities. Any infant not treated in the newborn period is at risk for late manifestations.
- Definitive diagnosis is made by identifying spirochetes by microscopic darkfield examination, or direct fluorescent antibody testing of infected tissue (such as placenta or umbilical cord) or lesion exudates. Microscopic examination frequently results in false-negative results; therefore presumptive diagnosis is possible using a combination of two types of serologic tests. Nontreponemal tests include the Venereal Disease Research Laboratory (VDRL), rapid plasma reagin (RPR), and the automated reagin test (ART). Treponemal tests include the fluorescent treponemal antibody absorption test (FTA-ABS) and the microhemagglutination test for *T. pallidum* (MHA-TP).

- A complete evaluation for any infant with suspected syphilis includes the following:
  1. Complete physical examination.
  2. Pathologic examination of the placenta or umbilical cord, if possible, using specific fluorescent antitreponemal antibody staining.
  3. Quantitative treponemal and nontreponemal serologic studies (*not* done on cord blood).
  4. CSF sample for VDRL, cell count, and protein.
  5. Long bone radiographs.
  6. CBC with differential and platelet count.
  7. Other tests as clinically indicated.
- Treatment should be initiated for any infant with proven or probable disease as indicated by
  1. Evidence for active disease on examination, laboratory or radiographic studies.
  2. Placenta or umbilical cord positive by darkfield examination or fluorescent antitreponemal antibody staining.
  3. Neurosyphilis: CSF VDRL positive or abnormal CSF cell count or protein measurement.
  4. Serum quantitative nontreponemal titer at least four times greater than the mother's titer.
- Parenteral penicillin G remains the drug of choice for treating syphilis.
  1. Infants with proven or highly probable disease should receive aqueous penicillin G 100,000–150,000 U/kg/day, IV, divided every 12 hours during the first 7 days of life and every 8 hours thereafter, for a total of 10–14 days *or* procaine penicillin G 50,000 U/kg/day, IM, in a single dose for 10–14 days.
  2. For neurosyphilis, aqueous penicillin G 100,000–150,000 U/kg/day, IV, divided every 6–8 hours, for 21 days should be given.
  3. If the patient also is human immunodeficiency virus (HIV)+, treatment with aqueous penicillin should be continued for 21 days.
- Asymptomatic infants born to asymptomatic mothers who have received therapy for syphilis should be managed as follows:
  1. Maternal RPR status at delivery should be checked.
  2. If RPR is positive, an MHA-TP should be done on the infant.
  3. If either the RPR or MHA-TP is positive, the adequacy of the mother's therapy must be determined. Adequate treatment is defined as follows:
     a. Treatment with 2.4 million units once with benzathine penicillin for primary, secondary, or early latent syphilis.
     b. Treatment with 2.4 million units of benzathine penicillin weekly for three consecutive weeks for late latent syphilis.

c. Treatment should be completed at least 30 days before delivery.

d. RPR should be monitored during pregnancy and a greater than or equal to fourfold drop in titer (i.e., from 1:16 to 1:4) should be documented.

e. If any of the above is not present, treatment is considered inadequate. Treatment with erythromycin or any other nonpenicillin regimen during pregnancy is *not* adequate.

4. If the mother is adequately treated, the infant should have a baseline RPR and MHA-TP drawn and should have a follow-up RPR at 1, 2, 4, 6, and 12 months.

5. If the mother has never been treated, is inadequately treated, has undocumented treatment, was treated less than 30 days prior to delivery, received a non-penicillin regimen, has no documentation of declining RPRs or is reinfected: the infant should have a full evaluation (baseline RPR and MHA-TP, LP for CSF VDRL, cell count, and protein).

a. If the evaluation is normal, the infant should be treated with either 10–14 days of therapy or a single dose of benzathine penicillin at the discretion of the neonatology attending.

b. If the evaluation is abnormal, the infant must be treated with a full course of IV penicillin.

TUBERCULOSIS (TB) INFECTION

- *Mycobacterium tuberculosis* is an acid-fast bacillus responsible for tuberculosis infection. The primary indicators for evaluation of the infant are evidence for active disease in the mother or suspicion of latent tuberculosis infection (LTBI) in the mother with a positive tuberculin skin test (TST) and no physical findings of disease.

- Most pregnant women with pulmonary tuberculosis alone are not likely to infect the fetus, but may infect their infant after delivery. Other potential household contacts must also be considered.

- Congenital tuberculosis is rare, but the incidence is increasing with the current increase in overall disease prevalence and in drug resistant organisms.

- Newborns suspected of having tuberculosis should receive the following:

1. A complete evaluation including TST (frequently negative in either congenital or perinatally acquired TB), chest radiograph, lumbar puncture with culture and other appropriate cultures (i.e., gastric aspirate, sputum if possible).

2. Prompt empiric therapy with isonizid, rifampin, pyrazinamide, and streptomycin or kanamycin.

3. Placental histologic examination and culture is indicated.

4. Corticosteroid administration is indicated with confirmation of meningitis.

- Overall assessment, extent of evaluation undertaken, and management of the newborn is based on categorization of the maternal (or household contact) infection. Since most neonatal infections are acquired postnatally, reduction in exposure is key to preventing disease; however separation of the infant from the mother should only be undertaken when absolutely necessary.

1. If the mother (or household contact) has a normal chest radiograph and is asymptomatic: no separation is required and the infant needs no specific evaluation or therapy. Other household contacts should be evaluated.

2. If the mother (or household contact) has an abnormal chest radiograph: the infant must be separated from the mother or household contact until this individual has been evaluated and if tuberculosis disease is found, until the infected individual is receiving appropriate therapy. Other household contacts should be evaluated.

3. If the mother or household contact is found to have possibly contagious TB, the local health department should be notified and the following steps should be taken:

a. The infant should be tested for congenital tuberculosis and HIV and treated as outlined above.

b. All contacts should have a TST, chest radiograph, and physical examination.

c. The placenta should be examined histologically and cultured for tuberculosis.

d. If the maternal physical examination or chest radiograph supports the diagnosis of tuberculosis, the newborn should be treated with regimens recommended for tuberculosis meningitis, excluding corticosteroids. If meningitis is confirmed, corticosteroids should be given.

e. Drug susceptibilities of the organism recovered from the mother and infant should be determined and therapy should be adjusted as necessary.

f. Determination of the length of therapy is dependent on multiple factors and should be done in consultation with a pediatric infectious disease specialist.

NEONATAL VIRAL INFECTIONS

CYTOMEGALOVIRUS (CMV) INFECTION

- Human CMV is a deoxyribonucleic acid (DNA) virus and member of the herpesvirus group. Congenital CMV has a wide spectrum of manifestations, but is usually asymptomatic.

- Five percent of infants with CMV will have profound involvement with intrauterine growth restriction

(IUGR), neonatal jaundice, purpura, hepatosplenomegaly, thrombocytopenia, disseminated intravascular coagulation (DIC), microcephaly, brain damage, intracerebral calcifications (usually, but not exclusively periventricular), and retinitis.

- Approximately 15% of infants born after maternal infection will have one or more sequelae of intrauterine infection; often undiagnosed until later in life, such as hearing loss or developmental delay.
- Transmission occurs transplacentally or perinatally through contact with cervical secretions or through breast milk. Perinatal exposure is not usually associated with disease in term infants, but preterm infants may be infected.
- Transplacental transmission usually occurs during the mother's primary infection with CMV, though it can occur with reactivation. Transmission in the first two trimesters is more likely to cause detriment to the fetus.
- Freezing or pasteurization of breast milk reduces the incidence of transmission.
- Newborns suspected to have congenital CMV should have a urine viral culture sent in the first 3 weeks of life (gold standard), an ophthalmology examination, hearing evaluation, and brain imaging.
- Positive CMV immunoglobulin M (IgM) serology is highly suggestive, but NOT diagnostic.
- No specific treatment other than supportive therapy is currently indicated. Ganciclovir is indicated for the treatment of retinitis and has been used to treat some congenitally infected infants, but insufficient data exist to recommend its routine use.

HERPES SIMPLEX VIRUS (HSV) INFECTIONS

- Neonatal herpes simplex virus infection is uncommon, but can be devastating. The incidence is approximately 1 in every 1500–2000 live births in the United States. Seventy percent of neonatal infections are caused by HSV-2, but the incidence of infections with HSV-1 is rising.
- Most cases occur from a primary maternal genital HSV infection rather than from reactivation of a latent infection. Acquisition of primary HSV infection late in gestation carries a 33–50% chance of neonatal infection vs. a 1–3% chance with latent HSV.
- HSV is most frequently transmitted intrapartum by delivery through an infected maternal birth canal, but ascending infections and intrauterine infections may also occur. Documented in utero and postpartum transmission is rare and accounts for <10% of cases. Prolonged rupture of membranes and scalp electrode monitoring may increase the risk of transmission.

- Neonatal HSV can present as
  1. Disseminated, systemic infection involving predominantly the liver and lung, but also other organs including the CNS (25%)
     a. 35–50% of these infants are born prematurely.
     b. Mean onset of illness is 7 days, with 30–40% presenting in the first week of life.
     c. 30% never have skin vesicles.
  2. Localized CNS disease (35%).
  3. Localized infection involving the skin, eyes, or mouth (40%).
  4. Localized disease (either CNS or mucosal/skin) most often appears in the second to third week of life.
- Early signs of HSV frequently are nonspecific and subtle. The possibility of HSV should be considered in any neonate with vesicular lesions or in any exposed neonate with unexplained illness (including respiratory distress, seizures, or symptoms of sepsis). Since the maternal status is often unknown, and the majority of infected women are asymptomatic, HSV disease should be included in the differential diagnosis of all infants presenting with late-onset sepsis.
- Mortality and morbidity are high, especially with delays in therapy.
  1. Fifty percent of neonates with disseminated disease die despite appropriate therapy.
  2. The majority of infants with HSV encephalitis survive, but most have substantial neurologic sequelae. Early institution of antiviral therapy may decrease morbidity.
- *Diagnostic evaluation* includes obtaining specimens for culture from any skin vesicles present, mouth or nasopharynx, conjunctivae, urine, stool, or rectum. Positive cultures from these sites more than 24–48 hours after birth indicate active viral replication and infection, rather than simple intrapartum exposure. CSF for HSV PCR should be obtained. CBC, LFTs, chest radiographs, and brain imaging studies should be performed if clinically indicated.
- *Treatment* should be initiated with acyclovir (60 mg/kg/day, IV, in three divided doses) for 14 days if disease is limited to the skin, eyes, and mouth, and for 21 days if disease is disseminated or involving the CNS.
- Ocular involvement warrants topical treatment with 1–2% trifluridine, 1% iododeoxyuridine, or 3% vidarabine ophthalmic preparations in addition to parenteral therapy.
- Relapse of CNS, skin, eye, and mouth disease may occur after cessation of antiviral therapy and the optimal approach to preventing such recurrences has not been established. Long-term suppressive therapy may be indicated.

HEPATITIS B (HBV) INFECTION

- Hepatitis B virus may be transmitted vertically from mothers with acute hepatitis during pregnancy or with the hepatitis B surface antigen carrier state. HBV results in a variety of manifestations, ranging from asymptomatic seroconversion to fulminant fatal hepatitis. Chronic HBV infection with persistence of HbsAg occurs in as many as 90% of infants infected by perinatal transmission.
- Most infants are asymptomatic at birth and therapy is based on maternal serologic studies. No specific treatment is available, but both passive (*hepatitis B immune globulin* [HBIG]) and active (hepatitis B vaccine) immunization may prevent development of the disease in infants exposed perinatally.
  1. If the maternal screen is positive, the neonate should receive HBIG (0.5 mL, IM) and the hepatitis B vaccine (at a site different than the HBIG) within 12 hours of birth.
     a. For term infants, this dose of hepatitis B vaccine can be counted toward the three-dose schedule.
     b. For preterm infants who weigh less than 2 kg at birth, this initial vaccine should not be counted toward the three-dose schedule. These preterm infants will receive a total of four doses to complete their series, with the second dose being given once a weight of 2 kg is achieved.
     c. Serologic testing should be performed on all neonates born to HbsAg-positive mothers at 1–3 months of age.
     d. Breastfeeding poses no additional risk of transmission.
  2. If the maternal screen is negative, the infant should receive the vaccine as per the American Academy of Pediatrics (AAP) Recommended Childhood Immunization Schedule (first dose: 0–2 months, second dose: 1–4 months, third dose: 6–18 months).
  3. If the maternal screen is unknown, a postpartum determination should be made and while awaiting results:
     a. Term infants >2 kg should receive the HbsAg vaccine within the first 12 hours of life. Because hepatitis B vaccine is highly effective for preventing perinatal infection when given at birth, the possible added value and the cost of HBIG do not warrant its use when the mother's HbsAg is not known.
     b. If the woman is found to be HbsAg-positive, the infant should receive HBIG as soon as possible, but within 7 days of birth, and be immunized subsequently as per AAP recommendations.
     c. For preterm infants who weigh less than 2 kg at birth, HBIG should be given if the mother's serologic status cannot be determined in the first 12 hours of birth because of the poor immunogenicity of the vaccine in these infants.

HUMAN IMMUNODEFICIENCY VIRUS (HIV) INFECTION/ACQUIRED IMMUNODEFICIENCY SYNDROME (AIDS)

- Perinatal transmission of HIV accounts for >90% of pediatric HIV infection in the USA.
- Zidovudine therapy of selected HIV-infected pregnant women and their newborn infants reduces the risk of perinatal transmission by two-thirds.
- Children born to HIV+ women will typically be asymptomatic. Evaluation of the infant born to an HIV+, or suspected HIV-infected mother includes the following:
  1. Testing by HIV DNA PCR during the first 48 hours of life. Because of possible contamination by maternal blood, this sample should not be obtained as umbilical cord blood.
  2. A second test should be obtained at 14 days to 2 months of age. Obtaining the sample early may enable decisions to be made about retroviral therapy at an earlier age.
  3. A third test is recommended at 3–6 months of age.
  4. Any time the infant tests positive, a second blood sample should be obtained immediately to confirm the diagnosis.
  5. An infant is determined to be infected if two separate samples are positive.
- Infection can be excluded reasonably when two separate HIV DNA PCR assays are negative, at or beyond 1 month of age and one assay must be on a sample obtained at 4 months or older.
- All infants of HIV+ mothers should be treated with zidovudine (2 mg/kg per dose, orally, four times per day), for 6 weeks total, beginning 8–12 hours after birth. If the child is NPO, then zidovudine (1.5 mg/kg per dose, IV, four times per day).
- Breastfeeding should be avoided as 15% of perinatal infection occurs by this route.
- Referral to a pediatric HIV/AIDS clinic is suggested for optimal follow-up and delivery of information to the family.

RESPIRATORY SYNCYTIAL VIRUS (RSV) INFECTIONS

- RSV is an enveloped ribonucleic acid (RNA) paramyxovirus with two major subtypes (A and B), which is responsible for acute respiratory tract illness, particularly bronchiolitis and pneumonia in infants.

- The incubation period ranges from 2 to 8 days.
- Infants at highest risk for developing severe symptoms are those with any form of chronic lung disease (CLD), term infants under 6 weeks of age, infants born prematurely, infants with complicated congenital heart disease, and those with primary immunodeficiency disorders.
- Infants present with lethargy, irritability, poor feeding, and respiratory symptoms manifested primarily by apnea, hypoxia, and radiographic evidence for bronchiolitis/pneumonia.
- Treatment is generally supportive, including hydration and providing supplemental oxygen for hypoxia. Many high-risk infants may need mechanical ventilation.
  1. Ribaviron has antiviral activity against RSV in vitro, but aerosol therapy is controversial and generally no longer advocated.
  2. Respiratory syncytial virus immune globulin intravenous (RSV-IGIV or RespiGam) is approved only for prophylaxis, not treatment of RSV infections; however, some centers have used it to treat extremely ill infants with RSV infection.
- Prevention of disease by passive immunization with palivizumab (Synagis), a humanized mouse monoclonal antibody, is currently recommended for all high-risk infants. Palivizumab is administered IM in a dose of 15 mg/kg once a month during RSV season. In general this would be October–April, but modifications based on regional and seasonal variations may be indicated.
- Palivizumab is not indicated for all infants. The AAP recommends considering the administration of palivizumab to the following:
  1. Infants and children under the age of 2 years with CLD who have received medical treatment for their lung disease in the 6 months preceding the RSV season.
  2. Premature infants according to the following schedule:
     a. <28 weeks gestational age (GA) at birth and <12 months chronologic age at the start of the RSV season.
     b. 29–32 weeks GA at birth and <6 months chronologic age at the start of the RSV season.
     c. 32–35 weeks at birth and <6 months at start of season when other risk factors are present such as
        1. Passive smoke exposure.
        2. Daycare attendance.
        3. Other young or school age siblings (two or more individuals sharing a bedroom, multiple births).

  4. Underlying conditions which would predispose the infant to respiratory complications (i.e., neurologic or airway issues).
  5. Extreme distance to or lack of availability of hospital care for severe respiratory illness
  3. Infants >35 weeks GA with
     a. Complex congenital heart disease or any child with heart disease anticipating surgical correction with weeks.
     b. Underlying conditions which would predispose the infant to respiratory complications (i.e., neurologic or airway issues).
     c. Immunodeficiency disorders or receiving immunosuppressive therapy.
- Palivizumab is not indicated for treatment of RSV infection, nor for inpatient prophylaxis while infants are still on the NICU. Infants hospitalized on the NICU during RSV season should receive their first dose of palivizumab, according to the above criteria, prior to discharge or shortly thereafter.

RUBELLA

- Rubella is an RNA virus classified as a Rubivirus of the Togaviridae family with an incubation period of 14–23 days.
- Postnatal rubella, or infection with the rubella virus after the time of delivery usually results in a mild, self-limited illness characterized by an erythematous maculopapular rash, generalized lymphadenopathy, and low-grade fever. Encephalitis and thrombocytopenia are rare.
- Congenital rubella results from transplacental transmission of the rubella virus to the fetus, occurring with the mother's primary infection. Symptoms range from mild or no clinical manifestations, to severe congenital anomalies including the following:
  1. Ophthalmologic: cataracts, microphthalmia, glaucoma, and chorioretinitis.
  2. Cardiac: patent ductus arteriosis, peripheral pulmonary artery stenosis, atrial or ventricular septal defects.
  3. Sensorineural deafness.
  4. Neurologic: microcephaly, meningoencephalitis, mental retardation, growth retardation, behavioral disorders.
  5. Growth retardation with radiolucent bone lesions.
  6. DIC with hepatosplenomegaly, thrombocytopenia, jaundice, neonatal purpura (resulting in a *blueberry muffin* appearance to the skin).
- The risk of development of congenital anomalies correlates with the gestation at which the mother contracts the disease. The occurrence of congenital defects is at least 50% if infection occurs during the first month of

gestation, 20%–30% if infection occurs during the second month and 5% if infection occurs during the third or fourth month.

- Diagnosis is based on clinical findings, culture of virus (from nasal specimens, throat swabs, blood, urine, and cerebrospinal fluid), and antibody titers.
- Detection of rubella-specific IgM antibody usually indicates recent postnatal or congenital infection in a newborn infant, but false-positive results can occur. A fourfold or greater rise in antibody titer or seroconversion between acute and convalescent serum titers indicates infection.
- Treatment consists of supportive care, neurodevelopmental follow-up, and isolation of infected patients from susceptible persons.

VARICELLA-ZOSTER VIRUS (VZV) INFECTIONS

- Varicella-zoster is a member of the herpesvirus family and primary infection results in chickenpox. Reactivation results in herpes zoster or "shingles."
- Incubation period may be 10–21 days, but averages 14–16 days.
- Primary infection with VZV during pregnancy occurs in 1–5 out of 10,000 pregnancies in the United States; the rate is low as 90–95% of women have antibody to the virus.
- Most neonatal transmission is vertical.
- Intrauterine infection occurs rarely and results in varicella embryopathy, which is characterized by cutaneous scarring of the trunk, limb hypoplasia, encephalitis with cortical atrophy, low birth weight, rudimentary digits, chorioretinitis, optic atrophy, cataracts, microphthalmia, and clubbed feet. This syndrome occurs with first or early second trimester infections; the risk of anomalies in infant born to a mother with a first trimester VZV infection is approximately 2.3%.
- Perinatal exposure to varicella classically occurs when the mother is exposed to VZV in the last 2–3 weeks of pregnancy.
  1. Neonatal disease generally occurs during the first 10 days of life.
  2. Timing of exposure is critical in determining the extent of disease.
     a. If maternal onset of disease is 6 days or more before delivery of a term infant, and the neonate has a clinical infection in the first week of life, the infection will usually be mild because of the transfer of maternal antibodies; however, if the infant is preterm (gestational age <28 weeks), clinical disease in the infant may be severe because of diminished placental transfer of antibodies.
     b. If maternal onset of disease occurs within 5 days before delivery of a term or preterm infant, or within 48 hours after delivery, the neonatal clinical infection will manifest between 5 and 15 days. In these cases, the infection can be fulminant characterized by severe pneumonia, hepatitis, or meningoencephalitis, with a mortality rate of 5–30%.
- Newborn infants whose mothers have had onset of varicella within 5 days before to 2 days after delivery should receive varicella-zoster immune globulin (VZIG) 125 U IM as soon as possible after delivery.
- The mother and baby should be isolated from other patients. If the infant does not have lesions, isolation from the mother is recommended until the child either becomes symptomatic or the mother is beyond the contagious period.
- VZIG should also be given to exposed premature infants. Exposure is defined as contact in the same two- to four-bedroom, adjacent in a ward, or face-to-face contact with an infectious staff member or patient with varicella.

FUNGAL INFECTIONS

- Invasive fungal infection is an increasingly common cause of mortality and morbidity in very low birth weight infants. As the diagnosis is often difficult, and treatment is often delayed, there is significant morbidity and mortality from fungal infections.
- The most common organisms are *Candida* spp. *Malassezia furfur* accounts for a small percentage of catheter infections associated with hyperlipidemia and *Aspergillus* infections are extremely rare.
- The most common *Candida* spp. responsible for infection is *C. albicans*, followed by *C. parapsilosis, C. glabrata, C. krusei, C. stellatoidea*, and *C. lusitaniae*, listed in descending order. This is in marked contradistinction to nonneonatal patients where *C. parapsilosis* rarely causes invasive disease, while *C. glabrata* and *C. tropicalis* rank second and third among invasive strains.
- Risk factors for neonatal candidiasis include both maternal and neonatal factors:
  1. Maternal risk factors include heavy GI/GU colonization with *Candida*, diabetes mellitus, cervical incompetence requiring a cerclage, and prolonged or premature rupture of membranes.
  2. Infant risk factors include heavy colonization with *Candida*, prematurity (especially very low birth weight), broad-spectrum antibiotic exposure, NEC, bowel perforation, mesenteric ischemia, abdominal surgery, presence of indwelling catheters (central

venous, arterial, urinary, peritoneal, ETT), hyperglycemia, administration of intravenous hyperalimentation and intralipid, and corticosteroid administration.

- Common presentations include congenital cutaneous candidiasis, catheter-associated infection, and disseminated infection.
- Congenital cutaneous candidiasis refers to disease present at birth.
  1. Only maternal risk factors are present.
  2. Clinical manifestations are intensely erythematous maculopapular lesions on the trunk and extremities that rapidly become pustular and rupture, leaving denuded skin with well-defined, raised, and scaling borders. Respiratory involvement is rare in the term infant, but may be seen in the preterm infant. Multiorgan involvement is not seen.
  3. Diagnosis is made by clinical examination or by skin fungal culture. Blood cultures are not positive.
  4. Treatment is topical for term infants. If the infant is preterm, parenteral antifungal therapy should be initiated. Breaches of the skin with central catheters should be avoided if at all possible.
  5. The clinical course is a benign, self-limited infection, unless it occurs in an infant weighing less than 1500 g. The prognosis is generally excellent.
- Catheter-associated, nondisseminated candidal infections usually have an age of onset of greater than 7 days, and are directly associated with the duration of catheterization. Many of the risk factors described above are typically present.
  1. Clinical manifestations: Symptoms are subtle, with no respiratory or multiorgan involvement and skin lesions are rarely seen.
  2. Diagnosis: Peripheral and line cultures should be performed. Ultrasound evaluation of the catheter tip for the presence of potentially infected thrombus/endocarditis is indicated.
  3. Treatment includes catheter removal and amphotericin B, with monitoring for toxicity (see below), for 10–14 days following catheter removal and negative culture. Presence of an infected thrombus at the tip of the catheter would require a more prolonged course of treatment. With a right atrial thrombus, treatment for endocarditis is indicated and surgical removal may be necessary for complete resolution.
  4. Clinical course: Most infants respond to a brief course of amphotericin B with a good ultimate prognosis.
- Systemic candidiasis typically has an age of onset of >7 days, with a mean age of onset of 30 days. Multiple risk factors are present, usually for a prolonged period of time.

  1. Clinical manifestations include respiratory deterioration, enteral feeding intolerance, abdominal distension, temperature instability, hypotension, thrombocytopenia, hyperglycemia, and glucosuria. Multiple foci are often involved.
  2. Diagnosis: Complete workup includes blood culture, urine culture, CSF culture, abdominal ultrasound (hepatic, renal, and splenic involvement common), ophthalmologic examination (endophthalmitis with fluffy or hard white infiltrates), and an echocardiogram to evaluate for endocarditis if a central line has been in place.
  3. Treatment is catheter removal and amphotericin B for 3–6 weeks, depending on the extent of dissemination, for an accumulative dose of 30–35 mg/kg.
- Amphotericin B remains the mainstay of therapy.
  1. Initial dose is 0.5 mg/kg, IV over 2–6 hours, then the dose is increased by 0.25 mg/kg/day to a goal of 0.75–1.0 mg/kg/day, adjusting for renal insufficiency.
  2. Monitoring while on amphotericin B includes a daily potassium (K^+), blood urea nitrogen (BUN), creatinine, and platelet count for 1 week. If stable, the K, BUN, creatinine, and platelet count is monitored weekly, and CBC and liver enzymes are also followed weekly. Imaging studies are performed as indicated to follow resolution of intracardiac, renal, or CNS lesions.
  3. Adjunctive therapy with 5-fluorocytosine (50–100 mg/kg/day, orally, divided into two separate doses) is indicated if possible, but has the drawback of oral administration. It is never used as the sole antifungal agent, as rapid development of resistance has been described.
- Alternative therapies include Liposomal amphotericin B and fluconazole but these therapies may have limitations.
  1. Liposomal amphotericin B is used because it has decreased toxicity, but randomized clinical trials are still lacking. Its use is indicated for infants with evidence of toxicity from amphotericin B, or for empiric therapy. Dosing is 3–5 mg/kg/day, IV over 2 hours. As it has decreased renal absorption, it is not indicated for treating renal disease.
  2. Fluconazole is not indicated for empiric therapy. Although most *C. albicans* strains are sensitive, decreased sensitivity is seen with *C. glabrata* and *C. parapsilosis*, with complete resistance found with *C. krusei*. After identification the infecting spp. therapy may be switched to fluconazole if *Candida* strain determined to be sensitive. Dosing is dependent on gestational age and levels must be monitored:
     a. ≤29 weeks: 5–6 mg/kg/72 hours, IV
     b. 30–35 weeks: 3–6 mg/kg/48 hours

c. Term: 6–12 mg/kg/24 hours
   1. Renal, hepatic, and hematologic side effects may occur, but are less pronounced than amphotericin B.

BIBLIOGRAPHY

American Academy of Pediatrics. *Red Book: Report of the Committee on Infectious Diseases*. 25th ed. Elk Grove Village, IL: American Academy of Pediatrics; 2000.

Benjamin DK Jr, Miller W, Garges H, Benjamin DK, et al. Bacteremia, central catheters, and neonates: when to pull the line. *Pediatrics* 2001;107:1272–1276.

Edwards MS, Baker CJ. Bacterial infections in: Long S, Pickering LK, Prober C, eds. *Principles and Practice of Pediatric Infectious Diseases*. New York, Churchill Livingstone; 1997: 606–14.

Fanaroff AA and Martin RJ, eds. *Neonatal-Perinatal Medicine: Diseases of the Fetus and Infant*. 7th ed. Mosby; 2001.

Guidelines for the Acute Care of the Neonate. James M. Adams, Jr., MD, Joseph A. Garcia-Prats, MD, Richard J. Schanler, MD, Michael E. Speer, MD, and Leonard E. Weisman, MD, Editors. Section of Neonatology, Baylor College of Medicine, 2002, 10th edition, 101 pages.

Remington JS and Klein JO, eds. *Infectious Diseases of the Fetus and Newborn Infant*. 5th edition. Philadelphia: WB; 2001.

Denise M. Goodman, Section Editor

28 SEPSIS, SHOCK, AND OXYGEN DELIVERY

Maria Luiza C. Albuquerque

PATHOPHYSIOLOGY/EPIDEMIOLOGY

HOW DO WE THINK ABOUT SEPSIS TODAY?

- Different from several years ago, we view patients with sepsis not as having an immune system that has gone out of control, but rather as having a system that is extremely compromised and unable to clear critical pathogens.
- We still do not understand the mechanisms of organ failure and death in patients with sepsis, and autopsy studies in children and adults do not reveal widespread necrosis of organs.
- Exciting new advances in the treatment of sepsis include therapy with activated protein C, tight control of blood glucose in the 80–110 mg/dL range, and early aggressive therapy to optimize oxygen delivery and minimize cellular oxygen deficit.
- With the advent of critical care medicine, the mortality from sepsis in the pediatric population (9%) is markedly better than in adults (28%).

CLINICAL FEATURES

DIAGNOSIS OF SHOCK

- Shock is a clinical state characterized by inadequate tissue perfusion resulting in delivery of oxygen and metabolic substrates that is insufficient to meet tissue metabolic demands.

- Shock occurs with normal, increased, or decreased blood pressure.
- Hypovolemic shock means there is inadequate intravascular volume relative to the vascular space and is the most common form of shock in children.
- Cardiogenic shock indicates myocardial dysfunction and shock that may be associated with hypovolemia or inappropriate distribution of blood flow in the body. It will be present in all forms of shock after a prolonged time.
- Distributive shock is defined by inappropriate distribution of blood flow to the organs and skin, and is commonly seen in sepsis and anaphylaxis.
- *Compensated* shock is defined as a clinical state of tissue perfusion that is inadequate to meet metabolic demand in the presence of normal blood pressure. In *decompensated* shock, hypotension is present (systolic blood pressure is less than 5th percentile for age). An important example of decompensated shock is patients with septic shock who have a high cardiac output but concomitant hypotension and severe deficits in end organ perfusion. Urgent treatment is required to prevent progression to cardiac arrest.

DIAGNOSIS OF SEPTIC SHOCK

- Fever, tachycardia, and vasodilation are common in children with infections.
- Suspect septic shock when the above signs are accompanied by a change in mental status (inconsolable irritability, lack of interaction with parents, or inability to be aroused).
- A more definitive diagnosis of septic shock may be made in children who have a probable infection, hypo- or hyperthermia, and decreased perfusion.
- Decreased perfusion may be noted by the following signs and symptoms: (1) decreased mental status,

(2) capillary refill of >2 second (cold shock) or flash capillary refill (warm shock), (3) decreased (cold shock) or bounding (warm shock) peripheral pulses, (4) mottled and cool extremities (cold shock), or (5) decreased urine output of less than 1 mL/kg/hour. Note: Hypotension is not necessary for establishing the diagnosis of septic shock (see compensated and decompensated shock above).

THE IMPORTANCE OF OXYGEN DELIVERY

- Since shock is defined by inadequate substrate delivery to meet tissue metabolic demands, and oxygen is the major substrate of aerobic metabolism, it becomes critical to understand the determinants of oxygen delivery.
- Oxygen delivery or systemic oxygen transport is equal to the amount of oxygen delivered to the entire body per minute, and it is the product of arterial oxygen content and cardiac output, CO (or cardiac index, CI, if referenced to the child's surface area).
- Arterial oxygen content = Hgb (g/dL) $\times$ 1.34 (mL O_2/g Hgb) $\times$ SaO_2 + (PaO_2 $\times$ 0.003) and is expressed in mL of oxygen per dL of blood (normal range is approximately 18–20 mL/dL).
- Oxygen delivery (mL/min) = Arterial oxygen content (mL/dL) $\times$ CO (L/minute) $\times$ 10 (dL/L).
- CO (L/minute) = Heart rate $\times$ stroke volume (and stroke volume is determined by preload, afterload, and contractility).
- Oxygen delivery falls if either arterial oxygen content or cardiac output decreases without an increase in the other component. In respiratory failure associated with shock, the increased work of breathing that occurs in children adds to their metabolic demands and increases their likelihood of developing decompensated shock and a critically low oxygen delivery to their tissues.
- To optimize oxygen delivery in septic shock and shock in general, the arterial oxygen content should be kept normal by assuring a normal Hgb level with packed red blood cell transfusions, if necessary. CO should be optimized with volume resuscitation via the use of crystalloids such as lactated ringers or normal saline. In addition, vasopressor, inotropic, or inodilator medications (depending on the type of shock) may need to be initiated to enhance CO.

INITIAL EVALUATION

- Initial labs include the following:
  1. Arterial pH
  2. Glucose
  3. Ionized calcium
  4. WBC (severe infection if >2 standard deviations above normal for age or <4000/mm^3)
  5. Hemoglobin
  6. Platelet count
  7. DIC panel (includes PT, PTT, fibrinogen, FDPs)
  8. Electrolytes
  9. Blood and urine culture

GUIDELINES FOR THE TREATMENT OF PEDIATRIC SHOCK

- Step 1: In the first 0–5 minutes of presentation recognize the child's decreased mental status and perfusion. Remember the ABCs, maintain the airway, and establish access according to Pediatric Advanced Life Support (PALS) guidelines. The preferred access, especially in the case of decompensated shock, is the one most readily available. If need be, establish intraosseous access if peripheral or central venous access is not immediately possible.
- Step 2: Manually, push 20 cc/kg of normal saline or lactated ringers or colloid boluses up to 60 cc/kg. The first 20 cc/kg of fluid should be administered in 15 minutes or less. Placing the first 20 cc/kg fluid bolus on an infusion pump to run over an hour is not appropriate, and may significantly compromise oxygen delivery to the tissues and lead to decompensated shock. Decreased morbidity and mortality have been associated with rapid infusion of the first 40 cc/kg of volume during the first hour of resuscitation.
- Step 3: After 15 minutes have elapsed, and initial fluids have been administered, determine if the patient has fluid responsive or fluid refractory shock. If the patient seems to be responding to fluid, observation in the pediatric intensive care unit (PICU) is the next appropriate step.
- Step 4: If the patient has fluid refractory shock, make every attempt to establish central venous access (often by route of the femoral vein). Ideally, use a central venous catheter with a length appropriate to measure the central venous pressure (CVP) accurately, and the inferior vena cava or superior vena cava oxygen saturation (SVC O_2). It has recently been shown that maintaining a normal perfusion pressure reduces morbidity and mortality from shock. The perfusion pressure is the mean arterial pressure – central venous pressure (MAP – CVP).
- Step 5: Once the second line, the central venous catheter, has been placed and the patient has been deemed to have:
  - Fluid refractory shock—begin a dopamine infusion. At this point arterial monitoring is warranted.
- OR

- Fluid refractory and dopamine resistant shock— begin epinephrine for cold shock or norepinephrine for warm shock. Do not maintain the patient on dopamine for an extended period of time without giving consideration to epinephrine and norepinephrine for maintenance of perfusion pressure.
- Step 6: If after 60 minutes, the patient appears to still be resistant to the above vasopressors, consider that the patient may be at risk for adrenal insufficiency, and administer hydrocortisone. For stress coverage a dose of 1–2 mg/kg as a bolus is usually administered, but in profound shock doses as high as 50 mg/kg have been used.
- Generally, pediatric patients begin to respond to the therapies delineated above; however, there are three subclassifications of shock that require further refinement of fluids, vasopressors, inotropes, inodilators, and vasodilators in addition to continuation of volume resuscitation.
- Step 7:
  1. Subclassification 1: The patient has normal blood pressure, persists with cold shock, and the SVC O$_2$ saturation is <70%. In this case, consider adding a vasodilator (dobutamine) or inodilator such as milrinone (type III phosphodiesterase inhibitor), and continue judicious volume loading.
  2. Subclassification 2: The patient has low blood pressure, persists with cold shock, and the SVC O$_2$ saturation is <70%. In this case, further titration of epinephrine is warranted as well as judicious volume loading. One may want to consider a low dose infusion of vasopressin if this situation persists.
  3. Subclassification 3: The patient has low blood pressure and warm shock (SVC O$_2$ saturation is >70%). The norepinephrine and volume infusions should be further titrated, and if the situation persists, a low dose infusion of vasopressin should be considered.
- In all of the above situations, the perfusion pressure (MAP-CVP) should be normalized as much as possible with the vasoactive and volume infusions used. In addition, the physical examination, blood pressure, temperature, urine output, and glucose and ionized calcium should be carefully monitored.

EMPIRIC ANTIBIOTICS

- In neonates use ampicillin and gentamicin (in doses appropriate for meningitis).
- In children use cefotaxime (200–300 mg/kg/day divided q 6 hours) or ceftriaxone (50–100 mg/kg/day divided q 12 hours) plus vancomycin (40–60 mg/kg/day divided q 6 hours).

BIBLIOGRAPHY

American Heart Association. *PALS Provider Manual*, pp. 24–41.

Bernard GR, Vincent JL, Laterre PF, et al. Efficacy and safety of recombinant human activated protein C for severe sepsis. *N Engl J Med* 2001;344:699–709.

Carcillo JA, Davis AI, Zaritsky A. Role of early fluid resuscitation in pediatric septic shock. *JAMA* 1991;266:1242–1245.

Carcillo JA, Fields AI. Clinical practice parameters for hemodynamic support of pediatric and neonatal patients in septic shock. *Crit Care Med* 2002;30:1365–1378.

Gorelick MH, Shaw KN, Baker MD. Effect of ambient temperature on capillary refill in healthy children. *Pediatrics* 1993; 92:699–702.

Matthay MA. Severe sepsis—a new treatment with both anticoagulant and anti-inflammatory properties. *N Engl J Med* 2001; 344:759–762.

Perkin RM, Levin DL, Webb R, Aquino A, Reedy J. Dobutamine: a hemodynamic evaluation of in children with shock. *J Pediatr* 1982;100:977–983.

Rivers E, Nguyen B, Havstad S, Ressler J, Muzzin A, Knoblich B, Peterson E, Tomlanovich M. Early goal-directed therapy in the treatment of severe sepsis and septic shock. *N Engl J Med* 2001;345:1368–1377.

Van den Berghe G, Wouters P, Weekers F, et al. Intensive insulin therapy in critically ill patients. *N Engl J Med* 2001; 345:1359–1367.

29 ACUTE RESPIRATORY DISTRESS SYNDROME
David M. Steinhorn

DEFINITIONS

- *Acute lung injury (ALI)*: Any acute alteration in lung function resulting from pathologic changes in lung structure.
- *Acute respiratory distress syndrome (ARDS)*: A syndrome of inflammation and increased capillary permeability that is associated with a constellation of clinical, radiologic, and physiologic abnormalities not primarily resulting from heart failure.
- *Ventilator associated lung injury (VALI)*: A syndrome of secondary lung injury seen in patients with ARDS as a result of the effects of mechanical ventilation on the injured lung.

OVERVIEW OF NORMAL PULMONARY GAS EXCHANGE

- Pulmonary gas exchange consists of (1) *oxygenation*, i.e., oxygen (O_2) uptake from the alveoli and (2) *ventilation*, i.e., carbon dioxide (CO_2) elimination from the body.
- Pulmonary alveolar surfactant facilitates effortless inspiration and helps maintain a residual volume within the alveoli between breaths, serving as an oxygen reservoir.
- The thoracic and diaphragm muscles must move respiratory gases in and out of the alveoli repetitively without fatiguing. Significant work of breathing occurs during inspiration to expand the thoracic volume, to overcome resistance during gas flow in airways, and to stretch the elastic tissue of the chest; exhalation tends to be passive unless increased airways resistance or thoracic abnormalities exist.
- Work of breathing in infants is relatively higher than in older individuals, leading more rapidly to respiratory distress when airways resistance or thoracic compliance is abnormal.

DETERMINANTS OF OXYGENATION

- Oxygenation depends on the percentage of O_2 in the alveolar gas and the lungs' ability to direct the pulmonary blood flow to oxygenated alveoli (ventilation-perfusion matching: *V/Q*). The alveolar gas equation (29-1) describes the *maximal* arterial oxygen level (PaO_2) which depends on $PaCO_2$ and FiO_2. The difference between the $P_{Alveolar}O_2$ and the measured PaO_2 (alveolar-arterial oxygen difference: $P_{(A-a)}O_2$) is generally 5–10 torr in healthy individuals and increases with increasing age and supine positioning. It is markedly increased in ARDS.

$$P_{Alveolar}O_2 = P_{insp}O_2 - P_{Alveolar}CO_2$$

$$\cong FiO_2 \times (P_{barometric} - 47) - \frac{PaCO_3}{0.8} \quad (29\text{-}1)$$

where PO_2 and PCO_2 are measured in units of mmHg; FiO_2 is the fraction, i.e., 0.5 = 50%.

DETERMINANTS OF VENTILATION

- Arterial PCO_2 is determined by CO_2 production vs. clearance. Central respiratory drive responds to the $PaCO_2$ or decreased pH (medullary drive), hypoxemia, and mechanical loading of the respiratory muscles. Normal neuromuscular integrity is vital to maintaining the $PaCO_2$ in a physiologic range; end-tidal CO_2 ($PetCO_2$) measured by capnography is within 2–4 mmHg of $PaCO_2$ in healthy individuals—it may be inaccurate in ARDS (Table 29-1).

CAUSES OF ACUTE RESPIRATORY DISTRESS SYNDROME AND ACUTE RESPIRATORY FAILURE

PRIMARY PULMONARY ETIOLOGIES

- Pulmonary infections
  1. Bacterial pneumonia: *S. pneumoniae*, group A streptococcus, *S. aureus*, mycoplasma
  2. Viral pneumonitis: RSV, parainfluenza, influenza, adenovirus
  3. Opportunistic infections, especially in immune-compromised host: PCP, fungi
- Trauma (local and remote), aspiration pneumonia, thromboembolism, thermal or toxic inhalation injury, near drowning, and strangulation/airway obstruction.
- Anatomic/developmental/metabolic: Abnormal surfactant function (immaturity, congenital deficiency), connective tissue disease/vasculitis, and cystic fibrosis.

NONPULMONARY ETIOLOGIES

- Shock of any cause with associated acidemia, altered tissue perfusion, and capillary leak.

TABLE 29-1 Mechanisms of Hypoxemia

FACTORS AFFECTING PaO_2 AND $PaCO_2$	UNDERLYING MECHANISM	CLINICAL EXAMPLES
Inspired oxygen	↓ Alveolar PO_2	Elevated altitude; $FiO_2 < 0.21$
Hypoventilation	↓ CO_2 elimination	Muscle fatigue; obstruction; sedation
Low *V/Q* mismatch	↓ Gas exchange; → blood flow	Pneumonia; atelectasis; ↓ surfactant
Intracardiac shunt	Right → left shunt	Septal defects; patent foramen ovale
Abnormal diffusion	Interstitial/alveolar edema	Congestive heart failure; capillary leak

- Generalized septicemia, generalized inflammatory states (e.g., connective tissue, pancreatitis), multiple transfusions, paraneoplastic syndrome, and asphyxia.
- Toxic ingestions.
- Nonpulmonary organ failure, especially liver and kidney.

PATHOGENESIS OF ARDS

- Typically follows an inciting stimulus:
  1. Exudative phase (days 1–3): Initial injury → oxidants and proteolytic enzyme release → tissue damage → increased capillary permeability, inflammatory response, alveoli flooded by plasma proteins, impaired surfactant function → atelectasis → increased work of breathing and ↓V/Q → hypoxemia, hypercarbia → [death likely *if no intervention*].
  2. Proliferative phase (days 3–7): Proinflammatory mediators amplify inflammation → further tissue damage, altered gas exchange, altered alveolar cell phenotype, capillary microthrombi → stage set for repair or further damage leading to subsequent fibrosis.
  3. Fibrotic phase (>7 days): Alveoli may either restore normal architecture or may progress to fibrosis with decrease in Type II cells and thickened alveolar septae chronically impairing gas exchange. Specific mechanisms leading to these outcomes are unclear.

RECOGNITION OF ARDS AND IMPENDING RESPIRATORY FAILURE

- Increased work of breathing, e.g., tachypnea, hyperpnea, retractions (intercostal, supra- or substernal) suggesting decreased thoracic compliance or airway obstruction, nasal flaring, grunting, use of accessory respiratory muscles, +/– prolonged expiratory phase.
- Cyanosis, altered sensorium (suggests ↓cerebral O_2 delivery) or impending exhaustion.
- Evidence for abnormal pulmonary gas exchange:

  $PaCO_2 > 50$ mmHg; $PaO_2 < 60$ mmHg with $FiO_2 > 0.6$ ($SpO_2 < 90\%$ on 60% FiO_2)

- Bilateral diffuse infiltrates on chest x-ray (CXR) without left-sided heart dysfunction; $PaO_2/FiO_2 \leq 200$.
- Hemodynamic changes with respiratory effort (pulsus paradoxus).

INITIAL MANAGEMENT OF ACUTE RESPIRATORY FAILURE AND ARDS

- Immediately provide *supplemental oxygen* via face mask, nasal cannula, or oxygen hood for all dyspneic, cyanotic, or severely distressed patients. Initially, higher concentrations of oxygen are preferred while assessing the cause of acute respiratory distress. Make *NPO*.
- *Assess adequacy of gas exchange* by auscultation of chest, obtain CXR if condition permits.
- *Assess work of breathing* by observing for retractions, nasal flaring, and use of accessory muscles.
- Attempt to *relieve obvious causes* of respiratory distress, e.g., removal of foreign bodies in the upper airway, bronchodilators for asthma exacerbations, epinephrine for anaphylactic reactions.
- *Assess hemodynamic* status by examining peripheral perfusion, determine blood pressure, mental status (assesses cerebral oxygen delivery); place pulse oximeter if available. Provide fluids for hypotension and consider pressors to support systemic blood flow.
- *Continuous presence of nurse* or physician to intervene in the event of rapid deterioration.
- *Obtain arterial blood gas* and other initial laboratory studies, as needed.

SUBSEQUENT MANAGEMENT OF IMPENDING RESPIRATORY FAILURE AND ARDS

- If patient can *maintain* $PaCO_2 < 50$ *and* $PaO_2 > 60$ mmHg on no more than 60% oxygen, therapy should be continued with noninvasive oxygen support as begun above.
- If the work of breathing or blood gas suggests the presence of respiratory failure or impending failure, *plans for intubation by a skilled practitioner* should be made immediately. Patients with respiratory failure or impending failure should not be observed without airway support unless the cause can be reversed within minutes. It is always safer and more defensible to *place an endotracheal tube in patients with severe respiratory distress before a respiratory arrest ensues*. Intubation under emergency conditions is always more difficult and risky for the patient.
- *Intubated patients should be managed in a facility with 24-hour intensive care nursing* and physician presence. Transfer to such an institution is critical for the timely diagnosis, treatment, and support of patients with ARDS.
- Noninvasive positive pressure ventilation techniques (NIPPV) e.g., face mask bi-level positive airway pressure or nasal CPAP, require careful nursing and

respiratory therapy care, especially in young children. *NIPPV may obscure an evolving pulmonary process* leading to a more risky intubation when no longer supportable by NIPPV techniques. Patients supported with NIPPV must be managed where the support staff is familiar with their use and maintenance in children and where immediate intubation and advanced life support can be provided.

PRINCIPALS OF MECHANICAL VENTILATION SUPPORT FOR ARDS

GOALS DURING MECHANICAL VENTILATION: MINIMIZE SECONDARY DAMAGE TO INJURED LUNG

- Treat underlying causes of ARDS, i.e., infection, shock, infarcted tissue.
- Use effective tidal volume <10 mL/kg (ideal: 5–8: skillful optimization of mechanical ventilation to the *patient's* status is critical. *Avoid* excessive tidal volumes and airway pressures >40 cm H_2O following the initial stabilization. VALI begins in the first hours of supporting the injured lung). Use volume mode and switch to pressure limited mode if peak airway pressure is >30 cm H_2O; rate to keep $PaCO_2$ < 50 mmHg.
- Keep lungs "open" between breaths with PEEP initially 8–12 cm H_2O may need 14–16 cm H_2O of PEEP (the hallmark of acute ARDS is reduced lung volume as atelectasis evolves; thus, the mainstay of the initial management is to *gently* open the lung with moderate inflation pressure [ideally less than 35–40 cm H_2O] and to maintain the lung in an open state between breaths utilizing PEEP settings of 8–12 cm H_2O. PEEP should be adjusted to permit a reduction in the FiO_2 to less than 0.6 while achieving saturations >90%. Paralysis of the patient may be necessary).
- Achieve saturations >90% and pH >7.2 with minimal FiO_2 (*lungprotective strategy*: "Perfect" blood gas values are not the goal during the management of ARDS. Achieve "acceptable" physiologic values, i.e., a $PaCO_2$ which allows an acceptable pH (>7.2) and PaO_2 > 55 mmHg, rather than inflict repeated damage to the injured lung through repetitive positive pressure breaths).

ADVANCED MANAGEMENT OF ARDS AND RESPIRATORY FAILURE

- Provide 24-hour critical care services. The use of advanced techniques, e.g., extracorporeal membrane oxygenation (ECMO) and oscillatory ventilation, requires a full complement of services available only at tertiary care centers. Prone positioning may

improve gas exchange but must be done with care to avoid extubation. Transfer of the patient intubated for respiratory failure before requiring advanced modalities will maximize the potential for recovery.

PROGNOSIS

- With judicious and timely intervention by practitioners skilled in the care of children with ARDS, current survival should be 75–85% depending on the etiology and other associated diseases. Patients with underlying malignancies or immune-compromised states have a worse prognosis but should receive the same aggressive and lung-protective strategy outlined above.

BIBLIOGRAPHY

Matthews BD, Noviski N. Management of oxygenation in pediatric acute hypoxemic respiratory failure. *Pediatr Pulmonol* 2001;32:459–470.

Pinhu L, et al. Ventilator-associated lung injury. *Lancet* 2003; 361:332–340.

Singh JM, Stewart TE. High-frequency mechanical ventilation principles and practices in the era of lung-protective ventilation strategies. *Respir Care Clin N Am* 2002;8:247–260.

30 NEAR-DROWNING
Ranna A. Rozenfeld

DEFINITIONS

SUBMERSION INJURIES

- Drowning—death from asphyxia caused by submersion in water.
- Near-drowning—survival, even if temporary, after asphyxia from submersion.
- Dry-drowning—asphyxia without ever aspirating water into lungs (10–15%).

EPIDEMIOLOGY

- Over 6000 deaths occur each year in the United States.
- Frequency is highest during summer months.
- Accidental drowning is the third most common cause of death in children under the age of 15 years, exceeded only by motor vehicle accident and malignancy.

- Drowning rate is twice as high for Whites as Blacks for children under 5 years, while Blacks are at a higher risk at all other ages.
- Males are four times more likely to drown than females.
- Ninety-eight percent of drownings occur in fresh water, and 50% occur in private swimming pools.
- Bathtub drownings mainly involve infants and those with seizure disorders. This is increasingly recognized as a form of child abuse among infants and toddlers.
- Drowning in buckets is increasing among toddlers. This has to do with the toddler's high center of gravity and poor coordination.

PATHOPHYSIOLOGY

- A specific sequence of events has been described in animal studies. After the initial panic and struggle, breath-holding occurs followed by either aspiration (85–90%) or laryngospasm (10–15%) resulting in hypoxemia.
- The single most important and prognostically significant consequence of submersion is a decreased oxygen delivery to the tissues.

PULMONARY EFFECTS

- Aspiration of fluid results in persistently abnormal gas exchange with resultant hypoxia and hypercarbia.
- With adequate resuscitation, normocapnea or hypocapnea is achieved while hypoxemia persists, indicating a significant ventilation/perfusion mismatch and diffusion defect leading to intrapulmonary shunting and venous admixture.
- Aspiration of stomach contents and other debris such as sand, mud, and algae may also impair gas exchange. Bacterial pneumonia may further cause pulmonary compromise.
- Between 10 and 15% of drowning victims have severe laryngospasm after submersion resulting in dry-drowning from asphyxia without aspiration of water into their lungs.
- Patients without significant fluid aspiration recover from asphyxia rapidly if they are successfully resuscitated before cardiac arrest or irreversible brain damage occurs.

CARDIOVASCULAR EFFECTS

- Profound cardiovascular instability is often seen after an episode of severe near-drowning and it poses an immediate threat to survival after the initial rescue.
- Life-threatening arrhythmias such as ventricular tachycardia or fibrillation and asystole are most often a result of hypoxemia rather than electrolyte abnormalities.
- Cardiogenic shock may result from hypoxic damage to the myocardium.
- Metabolic acidosis may further impair myocardial performance.
- Most patients have low left ventricular filling pressures because of excessive permeability of pulmonary and systemic capillaries resulting in hypovolemia.

CENTRAL NERVOUS SYSTEM EFFECTS

- Hypoxia, sufficiently prolonged, causes profound disturbances of central nervous system (CNS) function.
- The severity of brain injury depends on the magnitude and duration of hypoxia.
- Progressive oxygen depletion and impaired neuronal metabolism result in loss of consciousness.
- Significant neuronal damage may continue to occur even after restoration of circulation and oxygenation.
- Several mechanisms have been proposed to explain postresuscitation cerebral hypoperfusion and progressive CNS injury. These include increased intracranial pressure (ICP), cerebral edema, accumulation of cytosolic calcium, and oxygen-derived free radical damage.
- With improved cardiopulmonary support, the extent of CNS injury has become the major determinant of survival and morbidity in patients after near-drowning.

MANAGEMENT AND TREATMENT

- Since the full extent of CNS damage cannot be determined at the time of rescue, all patients should receive aggressive basic and advanced life support at the scene, in the ED, and the pediatric intensive care unit (PICU).

MANAGEMENT AT THE SCENE

- The success or failure of cardiopulmonary resuscitation (CPR) at the scene often determines the outcome.
- Basic life support should be started immediately.
- The victim should be removed from the water as soon as possible, but mouth-to-mouth resuscitation can begin in the water.
- Chest compressions should not be performed in the water since they are ineffective.
- There is no evidence to suggest that the Heimlich maneuver is effective in removing water from the lungs and may cause aspiration of stomach contents;

however, if there is an obvious foreign body, then it needs to be removed for effective ventilation.

MANAGEMENT IN THE EMERGENCY DEPARTMENT

- Other forms of associated trauma must be considered
  1. Slips and falls into pools may sustain external head injuries such as abrasions, lacerations, and contusions.
  2. With bathtub drownings, if child abuse is suspected, look for fractures and other evidence of previous injury.
  3. In adolescents, submersion is often associated with illicit drug or alcohol use, therefore urine and blood toxicology tests should be considered.
  4. Spinal injuries are not uncommon, especially with diving injuries.
- All patients should be observed in the ED for 4–6 hours, and those with significant submersion and possible aspiration should be observed for 6–12 hours.
- Observation includes clinical examination of respiratory status and cardiovascular status, oxygen saturation, cardiac rhythm, acid-base status, and electrolytes.
- The need for hospitalization should be determined by the severity of the submersion episode and clinical evaluation. Patients with respiratory symptoms, decreased O_2 saturation, and altered sensorium should be hospitalized.

MANAGEMENT IN THE PICU

- Patients often require intubation and ventilation with high FiO_2 and high PEEP.
- Ventricular arrhythmias, asystole, and hypotension are frequently seen early.
- Hypovolemia is commonly encountered, so diuretics should not be given to treat pulmonary edema and patients will often need fluid resuscitation.
- If patients remain hypotensive after appropriate fluid resuscitation, inotropic support may be required.
- Arterial and central venous pressure (CVP) monitoring is required in most patients requiring intensive care unit (ICU).
- Extracorporeal membrane oxygenation (ECMO) may be considered in patients with severe lung injury or severe hypothermia.
- Secondary bacterial infection due to aspiration or from prolonged ventilation has been seen; however, prophylactic antibiotics are not recommended.
- Once the patient is successfully resuscitated, the severity of encephalopathy is the main determinant of mortality and morbidity from near-drowning.

- The occurrence of cerebral edema and intracranial hypertension 2–3 days after a submersion injury is a reflection of the earlier hypoxic injury rather than a manifestation of a reversible process.
- Routine use of ICP monitoring is debatable.

OUTCOME

- The outcome of near-drowning victims depends largely on the success of resuscitative measures at the scene of injury.
- Patients who are successfully resuscitated and who are conscious on arrival at a hospital have an excellent chance of intact survival.
- Pulmonary injury can be managed in most patients.
- For those who require continued resuscitation in the ED, a variety of prognostic factors have been evaluated. Variables such as age, length of submersion, serum pH and body temperature, although previously thought to influence outcome, have not been shown to be reliable prognostic indicators.
- The need for continued CPR at the hospital, fixed and dilated pupils, seizures, flaccidity, and GCS ≤5 are poor prognostic signs in the absence of hypothermia.
- GCS >5 on arrival in the ED or ICU is highly predictive of good outcome.
- Severe hypothermia has been shown to influence the outcome favorably even after prolonged submersion; however, not all hypothermic near-drowning victims are fortunate enough to escape serious neuronal damage.
- Quan et al. (1990) has identified two risk factors for death or severe neurologic impairment: duration of CPR >25 minutes and submersion duration >9 minutes. Predictors of good outcome were submersion duration <5 minutes and CPR <10 minutes.

PREVENTION

- The greatest tragedy in submersion episodes is that a previously healthy child either dies or is left with permanent neurologic deficits the majority of which are preventable.
- Placing proper fencing around pools is the most effective method of prevention.

REFERENCES

Ibsen LM, Koch T. Submersion and asphyxial injury. *Crit Care Med* 2002;30(Suppl.):S402–S408.

Quan L, Wentz KR, Gore EJ, Copass MK. Outcome and predictors of outcome in pediatric submersion victims receiving prehospital care in King County, Washington. *Pediatrics* 1990;86:586–593.

Zuckerman GB, Conway EE. Drowning and near drowning: a pediatric epidemic. *Pediatr Ann* 2000;29:360–366.

31 MECHANICAL VENTILATION

Steven O. Lestrud

INDICATIONS

- The goal of pediatric artificial respiration is to ensure adequate oxygenation and minute ventilation in a variety of clinical situations involving different lung pathophysiology.
- Indications to improve oxygenation include pneumonia, pulmonary edema, and acute respiratory distress syndrome (ARDS).
- Clinical situations requiring maintenance of minute ventilation include postoperative patients, asthma, and bronchiolitis.
- Other common indications include respiratory failure from neuromuscular disease and central nervous system disorders. The variety of indications has resulted in many therapeutic goals and ventilatory techniques to achieve these goals. Several modes of mechanical ventilation are available to optimize patient recovery by normalizing pulmonary gas exchange while minimizing lung disease.

GENERAL PRINCIPLES

- Gas flow generated from the mechanical ventilator has to be signaled from the machine or from the patient. A machine initiates breath by time and this is referred to as a control mode. Patient efforts trigger breaths by pressure or flow changes in the circuit and are referred to as assist modes.
- The signal stopping the breath is called cycling and this signal can be the volume delivered, time, flow, or pressure. The delivered gas is limited by volume or pressure. The terminology of mechanical ventilation revolves around these three signals, initiation, cycling, and limits.

MODES OF ARTIFICIAL VENTILATION

- *Volume ventilation*: Primary input is volume of gas to be delivered from the ventilator. Airway and alveolar pressures generated as a result of the volume delivered will vary depending on the resistance to flow and the compliance of the respiratory system.
    1. *IMV—intermittent mandatory ventilation* (time initiated, volume limited, volume/time cycled): Volume is fixed, as is respiratory rate and inspiratory time (IT). The volume is delivered at the set rate independent of patient efforts. In pediatrics this mode is usually only used when there is no patient effort.
    2. *SIMV—synchronized intermittent mandatory ventilation* (flow/pressure initiated, volume limited, volume/time cycled): The volume set can be delivered in synchrony with patient effort, decreasing work of breathing. With apnea, the set rate and the volume delivered provide the minute ventilation the patient receives.
    3. *Assist-control* (flow/pressure/time initiated, volume limited, volume/time cycled): Volumes delivered are consistent. There is a rate set when there is no patient effort. In contrast to SIMV, patient efforts result in the entire delivered tidal volume with each breath.
- *Pressure ventilation*: Primary input is a pressure limit. Variable tidal volumes will result based on the respiratory system compliance and resistance.
    1. *Pressure control* (time initiated, pressure limited, time cycled): A control mode of ventilation in which gas flow is rapid at initiation of breath but decreases when the pressure limit is reached, resulting in a constant airway or alveolar pressure during the inspiratory cycle. This leads to a higher mean airway pressure (MAP) than would be seen in volume modes achieving similar peak inspiratory pressures.
    2. *Pressure limited* (flow/pressure/time initiated, pressure limited, time cycled): A synchronized mode of ventilation delivering flows as in pressure control but where a breath can be triggered by patient effort.
    3. *Pressure support* (flow/pressure initiated, pressure limited, flow cycled): The patient initiates each breath, and then flow from the ventilator generates the pressure level set. Tidal volume will vary and each respiratory effort will be supported when triggered. The pressure is maintained until the inspiratory flow decreases to preset levels designed by the ventilator software. There is no backup respiratory rate, thus the patient must have an adequate respiratory rate and drive to breathe. This mode is used as a weaning method from support.
    4. *Pressure regulated volume control*: The minute ventilation (tidal volume and respiratory rate) is set as a guarantee; the volumes delivered will be pressure limited.

HIGH FREQUENCY OSCILLATORY VENTILATION (HFOV)

- Generally described as nonconventional ventilation. Parameters set include MAP, frequency measured in hertz (cycles per second), and pressure swing referred to as delta pressure (ΔP).

SETTING UP CONVENTIONAL MECHANICAL VENTILATION

RESPIRATORY RATE (FREQUENCY) AND INSPIRATORY TIME (IT)

- Respiratory rate is set initially for physiologic normative rate for the patient's age; rates generally are higher for younger children.
- Inspiratory time defines the time allowed for gas to flow and is lower for infants and children than for adults. Times vary from 0.4 to 1 second. With higher rates, short IT is necessary to allow for exhalation time, avoiding breath stacking. When exhaled time is prolonged such as in acute asthma, the IT may again be shortened to allow complete exhalation.

VOLUME

- Volumes generally are calculated at 8–12 mL/kg of body weight. Ideal body weight calculations may be necessary in very obese patients as the tidal volumes used based on actual weight will result in overdistention of the lungs and high peak inspiratory pressure. Peak inspiratory pressure and plateau pressure are monitored closely with this mode of ventilation as they may increase greatly with decreased lung compliance. High peak pressure (around 30 cm H_2O) is associated with alveolar overdistention and lung damage. With conditions such as ARDS, poor lung compliance frequently results in high peak pressure. Strategies for volume ventilation in this instance include using small tidal volumes, approximately 6 mL/kg, and increased frequency to achieve the desired level of gas exchange.

PRESSURE LIMIT

- The pressure limit input limits peak pressures. The minute ventilation the patient achieves is the product of the resultant tidal volume and the set frequency. Tidal volumes in this mode are variable based on resistance to flow and compliance of the respiratory system. Pressure limits for neonates are lower than

children. Pressure limits should be set 12–30 cm H_2O above end expiratory pressure.

PRESSURE SUPPORT

- Pressure support generally is set at levels to overcome resistance of flow through the endotracheal tube. The optimal pressures for the various diameters of endotracheal tubes are unknown, but pressures that result in tidal volumes of 6–10 mL/kg are commonly used. This is accomplished with pressure support set between 5 and 15 cm H_2O.

VOLUME SUPPORT

- This mode to enhance weaning from mechanical ventilation requires a stable respiratory system and adequate respiratory drive. Volumes are set and the pressure needed to generate the volume is monitored. Volumes limited to 5–8 mL/kg are set; as pressure decreases to 5–15 cm H_2O, the patient should be evaluated for readiness to extubate.

POSITIVE END EXPIRATORY PRESSURE (PEEP)

- Flow is maintained through the ventilator circuit to keep alveolar pressures at set levels. With minimal lung disease PEEP is set at 3–5 cm H_2O. Increasing PEEP increases alveolar surface area, increasing functional residual capacity, and improving oxygenation. With ARDS, higher PEEP levels have been used and are not uncommonly 15–20 cm H_2O. Higher levels of PEEP may lead to interstitial emphysema, pneumothorax, and pneumomediastinum as well as alveolar over distention and increased perfusion-ventilation mismatch.

FiO_2

- Supplemental oxygen can be supplied from 21 to 100% oxygen. Many newer generation ventilators can substitute gases other than nitrogen such as helium for therapeutic use while maintaining appropriate tidal volumes.

SETTING UP HFOV

- MAP is the main determinant of oxygenation. MAP is set 3–5 cm H_2O above the MAP measured during conventional ventilation. Overdistention with high MAP may result in decreased oxygenation by worsening perfusion to alveolar units.

- Hertz, ΔP, and occasionally IT alter ventilation. Small babies are placed initially on Hz of 12–15; in larger children Hz down to 3 are used based on carbon dioxide (CO_2) removal. Lowering Hz results in increased CO_2 removal. Increased pressure swings (ΔP) also improve CO_2 removal. Adequate pressures are clinically evaluated by assessing chest movement and wiggle of toes. The IT is only rarely changed but may be increased in attempts to improve ventilation.

BIBLIOGRAPHY

Donn SM, Sinha SK. Newer modes of mechanical ventilation for the neonate. *Curr Opin Pediatr* 2001;13:99–103

Hill LL, Pearl RG. Flow triggering, pressure triggering, and autotriggering during mechanical ventilation. *Crit Care Med* 2000;28:579–581.

Tobin MJ. Medical progress: advances in mechanical ventilation. *N Engl J Med* 2001;344:1986–1996.

32 ACID–BASE BALANCE

Ranna A. Rozenfeld

DEFINITIONS

- pH is the Power of Hydrogen defined by the Henderson-Hasselbalch equation:

$$pH = pK + \log ([HCO_3^-]/0.03\ PCO_2)$$

- Acidosis—decrease in arterial pH, or a process that tends to do this.
- Respiratory acidosis—this is caused by CO_2 retention, which increases the denominator in the Henderson-Hasselbalch equation and so depresses the pH. Hypoventilation and ventilatory failure can cause respiratory acidosis.
- Metabolic acidosis—reduced pH not explained by increased PCO_2. This is caused by a primary fall in the numerator $[HCO_3^-]$ of the Henderson-Hasselbalch equation. It is usually associated with an increased anion gap (see below).
- Alkalosis—this means an increase in arterial pH.
- Respiratory alkalosis—this is seen in alveolar hyperventilation. The decreased PCO_2 explains the increased pH.

TABLE 32-1 Normal Values for Infants and Children

MEASUREMENT	NEWBORN INFANT	INFANT AND CHILD
Respiratory rate	40–60	20–30 <6 years 15–20 >6 years
pH	7.3–7.4	7.3–7.4 <2 years 7.35–7.45 >2 years
PCO_2 mmHg	30–35	30–35 <2 years 35–45 >2 years
HCO_3^- (meq/L)	20–22	20–22 <2 years 22–24 >2 years
O_2 saturation (%)	≥ 95	>95
PO_2 mmHg	60–90	95

- Metabolic alkalosis—raised pH out of proportion to changes in PCO_2. It is associated with hypokalemia, exogenous alkali administration, or with volume contraction, as in severe prolonged vomiting, when the plasma bicarbonate concentration rises.
- Anion gap—to differentiate between acid gain and HCO_3^- loss.

$$\text{Anion gap} = [Na^+] - ([Cl^-] + [HCO_3^-])$$
$$\text{Normal gap 8–12 meq/L}$$

- Anion gap acidosis: gap >12 meq/L, caused by decrease in HCO_3^- balanced by an increase in unmeasured acid ions, not by an increase in chloride. Causes include salicylates, methanol, paraldehyde, ethylene glycol, lactic acidosis, ketoacidosis (from diabetes or starvation), and uremia.
- Nonanion gap acidosis: gap 8–12 meq/L, caused by a decrease in HCO_3^- balanced by an increase in chloride. Causes include renal tubular acidosis, carbonic anhydrase inhibitor, and diarrhea.
- Table 32-1 gives normal values for infants and children.

EXPECTED COMPENSATORY CHANGES IN BLOOD GASES AFTER A PRIMARY DERANGEMENT

- Metabolic acidosis: $PCO_2 = 1.5 \times [HCO_3^-] + 8$
- Metabolic alkalosis: $PCO_2 = 40 + 0.7 \times ([HCO_3^-(\text{measured})] - [HCO_3^-(\text{normal})])$
- Acute metabolic changes will have a change in pH by 0.15 for every change in $[HCO_3^-]$ of 10 mmHg.
- Respiratory acidosis:
  1. Acute: $[HCO_3^-]$ increases by 1 meq/L for each 10 mmHg rise in PCO_2.

TABLE 32-2   Compensation after a Primary Derangement

DISORDER	pH	PRIMARY CHANGE	EXPECTED COMPENSATION
Acidosis			
Metabolic	↓	↓ HCO_3^-	↓ PCO_2 by 1–1.5 × fall in HCO_3^-
Acute respiratory	↓	↑ PCO_2	↑ HCO_3^- by 1 meq/L for each 10 mmHg rise in PCO_2
Chronic respiratory	↓	↑ PCO_2	↑ HCO_3^- by 3.5 meq/L for each 10 mmHg rise in PCO_2
Alkalosis			
Metabolic	↑	↑ HCO_3^-	↑ PCO_2 by 0.25–1 × rise in HCO_3^-
Acute respiratory	↑	↓ PCO_2	↓HCO_3^- by 1–3 meq/L for each 10 mmHg fall in PCO_2
Chronic respiratory	↑	↓ PCO_2	↓HCO_3^- by 2–5 meq/L for each 10 mmHg fall in PCO_2

2. Chronic: [HCO_3^-] increases by 3.5 meq/L for each 10 mmHg rise in PCO_2.
- Respiratory alkalosis:
  1. Acute: [HCO_3^-] decreases by 1–3 meq/L for each 10 mmHg fall in PCO_2.
  2. Chronic: [HCO_3^-] decreases by 2–5 meq/L for each 10 mmHg fall in PCO_2, but usually not to <14 meq/L.
- Acute respiratory changes will have a change in pH by 0.08 for every change in PCO_2 of 10 mmHg (Table 32-2).

OXYGEN CARRIAGE

- Oxyhemoglobin dissociation curve: relates O_2 saturation to PO_2.
  1. Curve shifted to the left (increased hemoglobin affinity for oxygen): alkalosis, hypothermia, hypocarbia, decreased 2,3-diphosphoglycerate (2,3-DPG), increased fetal hemoglobin, and anemia.
  2. Curve shifted to the right (decreased hemoglobin affinity for oxygen): acidosis, hyperthermia, hypercarbia, and increased 2,3-DPG.

CLINICAL APPROACH TO BLOOD GAS INTERPRETATION

- Blood gases provide measurements of pH, PCO_2, PO_2, total hemoglobin, and derivation of indices such as oxygen content, HCO_3^-, base deficit/excess, and oxyhemoglobin saturation.
- Blood gases allow for the determination of pathologic states and whether the abnormalities are primarily respiratory or metabolic.
- When evaluating acid-base disorders it is best to take a stepwise approach (see Figure 32-1).

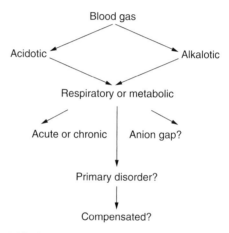

FIG. 32-1 Stepwise approach to blood gas interpretation.

1. Determine whether the patient is acidotic or alkalotic.
2. Determine whether the primary process is respiratory or metabolic.
3. If respiratory, is it acute or chronic?
4. If metabolic, is there an anion gap?
- Determine the primary disturbance and then evaluate for mixed disorder by the degree of compensation (see formulas and Tables 32-1 and 32-2).
- A simple disturbance should have one acid-base disorder.
- A mixed disorder can be detected by calculating the expected compensation and then comparing that to the actual value.

BIBLIOGRAPHY

West JB. *Pulmonary Pathophysiology: The Essentials*, 5th ed. Philadelphia, PA: Williams & Wilkins, 1998.

Williams AJ. Assessing and interpreting arterial blood gases and acid-base balance. *BMJ* 1998;317:1213–1216.

33 TRAUMATIC BRAIN INJURY

Zehava L. Noah

EPIDEMIOLOGY

- Traumatic brain injury (TBI) affects 200–300 children/ 100,000 per year. Motor vehicle accidents, falls, and child abuse are the leading causes.
- TBI is the leading cause of death, approximately 7000 per year, in children over 1 year of age. Eighty percent of the children who die with multiple trauma die of head injury. Overall mortality in children with TBI is 2.5% compared to 10.4% in adults.
- Each year there are 25,000 children with new permanent disabilities as a result of TBI.
- Preventive measures such as appropriate car seats well secured and positioned according to child's size and age, appropriate booster seats for older children, effective restraining devices, seat belts, air bags, helmets, screens, and rails over windows, are the most effective strategies in decreasing the risks of TBI.

MECHANISM OF INJURY

- Children are more vulnerable to TBI than adults because of their size, the larger head to body ratio, the thinner cranial bones, less myelinated tissue, and a greater incidence of diffuse injury and brain edema.
- The primary insult causes a direct injury. Secondary injury results from the brain response to the primary injury and includes inflammatory and biochemical processes; it may be further complicated by secondary insult with events such as hypoxia and hypotension.
- The primary injury may be focal, resulting in skull fracture, brain contusion, or intracranial hemorrhage, or it may be diffuse.
- Spinal cord injury occurs in approximately 1% of all children admitted to the hospital with TBI.
- Nonaccidental trauma: Patients present commonly with altered mental state, seizures, vomiting, and irritability. Injuries include subdural hematoma, subarachnoid hemorrhage, skull fractures, or diffuse axonal injury with or without cerebral edema. History in these patients is often lacking while the findings suggest repeated events.

PATHOPHYSIOLOGY

- In the first year of life a child's brain almost triples in weight. The intracranial contents include 80% brain,

10% blood, and 10% cerebrospinal fluid (CSF). CSF production is 0.35 mL/minute. CSF volume is lower in infancy. Cerebral blood flow (CBF) in children changes with age. Cerebral blood velocity is lower in infancy, increases in childhood, and decreases again during adolescence.

- Cerebral autoregulation in adults is constant between a mean arterial pressure (MAP) of 60–160 mmHg. With the exception of premature and very young infants those numbers seem to hold true for most infants and children.
- Normal intracranial pressure (ICP) in children is 2–4 mmHg compared to adults 5–15 mmHg. Despite open fontanels and sutures infants cannot tolerate even small rapid intracranial volume expansion.
- In the presence of adequate oxygen supply the main substrate for brain metabolism is glucose. In healthy children the metabolic rate for O_2 and glucose is higher than in adults.
- Three phases have been suggested post TBI. *Initially* there may be hypoperfusion. Hyperventilation during this phase may result in secondary ischemia and worse outcome. The *second phase* starts approximately 24 hours after TBI. CBF increases out of phase with oxygen utilization. *Later* in the course there may be vasospasm. The incidence of hyperemia in children post-TBI is not known.

INITIAL EVALUATION AND STABILIZATION

- A *history* is essential in understanding the nature of the injury and assessing its potential severity.
- The *initial* assessment starts with the ABCs (airway, breathing, circulation). Hypoxia and hypotension must be treated aggressively.
- A brief *neurologic* examination includes Glasgow coma score (GCS) (Table 33-1) which assesses the state of wakefulness, motor and verbal function, pupillary function, and presence of signs of transtentorial or brain stem herniation.
- A brief *head to toe examination* follows to evaluate for the presence of additional injuries.
- Initial *monitoring* includes heart rate, blood pressure, and oxygen saturation.
- Initial *actions* include stabilization of the cervical spine with a size and age appropriate hard collar, supplemental oxygen, and intravenous access.
- Patients with GCS ≤8 must be *intubated and ventilated*. Important points in intubating these patients are (1) the intubation must be performed with in-line traction of the cervical spine, (2) cricoid pressure must be applied throughout the process to avoid aspiration,

TABLE 33-1 Glasgow Coma Scale

OLDER CHILDREN		INFANTS AND YOUNGER CHILDREN
RESPONSE	SCORE	RESPONSE
Eye opening		
Open spontaneously	4	Open spontaneously
To verbal command	3	React to speech
To pain	2	To pain
None	1	None
Best verbal response		
Oriented, converses	5	Appropriate words, smiles, fixes, and follows
Confused, disoriented and converses	4	Consolable crying
Inappropriate words	3	Persistently irritable, moaning
Incomprehensible sounds	2	Restless agitated, inconsolable
None	1	None
Best motor response		
Obeys verbal command	6	Spontaneous or obeys verbal command
Localizes pain	5	Localizes pain
Withdraws in response to pain	4	Withdraws in response to pain
Abnormal flexion	3	Abnormal flexion
Extension posturing	2	Extension posturing
None	1	None

SOURCE: Adapted and modified from Teasdale G, Jennett B. Assessment of coma and impaired consciousness: a practical scale. *Lancet* 1974;2:81 and Vavilala. *Int Anesth Clin* 2002;40(3):69–87.

and (3) care must be taken in the choice of medications to protect from surges of increased intracranial pressure. Medications for induction may include thiopental, or alternatively morphine and midazolam, followed by a short-acting muscle relaxant. Lidocaine may be given as an adjunct. The patient's state of volemia must be assessed prior to the administration of medications. If hypovolemia is suspected, volume resuscitation with normal saline or hypertonic saline (3%) is indicated. In patients with suspected increased intracranial pressure it is important to avoid straining or coughing by the judicious administration of sedatives, analgesics, and muscle relaxants.

• *Mannitol* (0.25–1 g/kg) should be given if the patient's examination suggests increased intracranial pressure, or signs of imminent herniation (pupillary inequality, fixed dilated pupils, decerebrate or decorticate posturing).

• If *seizures* are suspected or diagnosed the administration of lorazepam followed by fosphenytoin or phenobarbital may be indicated.

• *Radiologic studies* usually require an intrahospital transport of the patient. Untoward events must be avoided, such as hypoxia, hypotension, or increased intracranial pressure. The patient must be escorted and monitored. Computed tomography (CT) scan of the head is indicated for patients with altered mental state, focal neurologic examination, or physical evidence of head trauma. Potential findings include skull fractures, intracranial bleeds, intraparenchymal contusions, cerebral edema, and obliteration of the basal cisterns. CT angiography and venography, Xenon CT, and magnetic resonance imaging (MRI) may help with the patient's therapy and prognosis, but are not necessarily a part of the initial evaluation.

TREATMENT OF SEVERE TRAUMATIC BRAIN INJURY IN CHILDREN

• Infants and children with head injury are best treated in a pediatric trauma center.

• The goals in the treatment of severe traumatic brain injury are optimal brain perfusion and oxygenation. This is achieved by controlling ICP, maximizing CPP (cerebral perfusion pressure) and by preventing events such as hypoxia or hypotension.

• The application of a protocol for the treatment of traumatic brain injury in the intensive care unit is recommended.

MONITORING

• Intracranial pressure: ICP monitoring is indicated in patients with severe brain injury and requires the insertion of an intraparenchymal monitor, or an intraventricular catheter. The latter allows drainage of CSF in addition to ICP monitoring.

- Arterial pressure requires the insertion of an arterial catheter. This provides constant monitoring of blood pressure and arterial blood gases, and thus continuous monitoring of CPP, calculated as MAP—ICP.
- Central venous pressure requires the insertion of a central venous catheter, providing secure intravascular access, monitoring of central venous pressure in order to optimize volemia, and monitoring of venous blood gases.
- Jugular bulb. A venous catheter is placed at the level of the jugular bulb, monitoring venous blood gases and oxygen saturation of blood draining from the brain. May help in assessing the global perfusion and oxygenation of the brain.
- Continuous monitoring of exhaled (end tidal) CO_2 allows close monitoring of ventilation.
- Continuous monitoring of oxygen saturation is essential.
- Electroencephalogram (EEG): Indicated in the evaluation and treatment of seizures and in the evaluation of the depth of coma resulting from the injury, or induced by drugs.
- Metabolic
  1. Glucose. Rationale: Surveillance for both hyper- and hypoglycemia
  2. Sodium. Rationale: Surveillance for hyponatremia (SIADH, cerebral salt losing), hypernatremia (dehydration as a result of osmotherapy)
  3. Osmolarity
  4. Hemoglobin
  5. Coagulation

TREATMENT OF INCREASED INTRACRANIAL PRESSURE

- Euvolemia must be maintained.
- Monitoring goals:
  1. ICP <15 for infants and young children, ICP <20 for older children.
  2. CPP >40 for infants, CPP >50 for young children, CPP >60 for older children.
- Ventilation goal:
  $PaCO_2$ 38–40 mmHg.

INTERVENTIONS

- These interventions are applied stepwise. If the patient fails to improve or deteriorates, the CT is repeated.
  1. EVD drainage of CSF is indicated if the ICP is consistently above the target value. Concerns:

Excessive drainage may result in ventricular collapse. Invasive device increases the risk of infection, typically with *Staphylococcus aureus*.

  2. Analgesia and sedation. Rationale: To prevent pain and discomfort that may result in increased ICP. Relatively short-acting agents are recommended such as fentanyl or morphine and midazolam. Concerns: May alter mental state and thus inadvertently prolong therapeutic interventions.
  3. Muscle relaxation. Rationale: To prevent cough and gagging with the endotracheal tube, which can increase ICP. Concerns: Neurologic examination impossible except for pupillary reflex.
  4. Hyperventilation. Rationale: To produce mild cerebral vasoconstriction and thus lower ICP. $PaCO_2$ 35–38 mmHg. Concern: Hyperventilation may aggravate cerebral circulatory deficiencies.
  5. Position: Head at midline. Elevation of the head to 30°. Rationale: To promote maximal intracranial venous drainage. Concern: Possible effect on blood pressure.
  6. Osmotic agents. Rationale: To decrease the amount of water in the brain. Mannitol reduces blood viscosity and extravascular volume. Dosage: 0.25–1 g/kg/dose every 2–8 hours. Concerns: Excessive dehydration, hypovolemia, and hyperosmolar state resulting in renal failure or disruption of blood-brain barrier. With prolonged use of mannitol and abrupt discontinuation of therapy, cerebral edema may increase.
  7. Hypertonic saline (3%) may also be used for the same purpose. End points for this therapy include high sodium level and high osmolarity (330–350 mOsm/kg).
  8. Aggressive hyperventilation. $PaCO_2$ 30–35 mmHg. Rationale: Refractory ICP.
  9. Barbiturates. Rationale: Used in the management of refractory ICP. Barbiturates alter vascular tone, decrease metabolic demands of the brain, and may improve tolerance to hypoxia and free radical injury. Both pentobarbital and phenobarbital are used. End points: Desired effect on ICP or burst suppression on EEG. Concerns: May affect cardiac function and cause hypotension; most patients require inotropic support. Alters mental state and neurologic examination. May prolong course.
  10. Temperature control. Rationale: Control metabolic rate, and thus control oxygen demands. Fever must be avoided. Moderate hypothermia (temperature 32–35°C) has been used recently in TBI. Preliminary studies hint at improved outcomes.
  11. Decompressive craniotomy is performed in some centers for refractory increased intracranial pressure.

• As the patient improves, therapies are withdrawn gradually in the order they were added. The intraventricular monitor is withdrawn as soon as possible in order to avoid the risk of infection.

GENERAL CARE

• Fluids. First 24–48 hours normal saline without glucose unless the patient has low glucose (<75). Rationale: Risk of CNS (central nervous system) acidosis through lactate production as a result of anaerobic metabolism of glucose, and possible increased risk of cerebral edema. Total fluids at maintenance. Guide fluid therapy by monitoring CVP and BP.
• Nutrition. Start nutrition within 72 hours. Enteral nutrition preferred, via jejunal feeding tube if necessary. Patients may require intravenous alimentation. Estimation of nutritional requirements in TBI patients is difficult. Trauma increases energy expenditure whereas sedation, paralysis, and high dose barbiturates decrease energy expenditure. In intubated patients metabolic measurements of energy expenditure may be helpful.
• Antibiotics: Antibiotic prophylaxis is not recommended for these patients with the possible exception of intraventricular catheter placement.
• Corticosteroids: Steroids are not recommended for traumatic brain injury.

CONCLUSIONS

• In the last two decades there have been considerable advances in the understanding of the pathophysiology of TBI and secondary injury. The institution of rigid protocols in order to achieve uniform management of these patients has resulted in improved outcomes; however, morbidity and mortality still remain high in children under 4 years of age and in adolescents. Many of the strategies used in the pediatric protocols are based on adult information, and may not apply to some infants or children.

BIBLIOGRAPHY

Mazzola CA, Adelson PD. Critical care management of head trauma in children. *Crit Care Med* 2002;30(Suppl. 11): S393–S401.
Vavilala MS, Lam AM. Perioperative considerations in pediatric traumatic head injury. *Int Anesth Clin* 2002;40(3):69–87.

34 TECHNOLOGY DEPENDENT CHILDREN

Zehava L. Noah and Cynthia Etzler Budek

THE PATIENTS

• Infants and children who have impaired respiratory capacity because of inadequate central control of breathing, significant residual lung disease secondary to a catastrophic illness, severe airway malacia, or those who suffer from a severe neuromuscular condition.
• This is a heterogeneous group of patients whose only common denominator is chronic respiratory failure. Patients with residual lung disease have the best possibility of weaning off ventilatory support. Patients with central hypoventilation or profound neuromuscular weakness have the least.
• Other common problems in this patient population include loss of oromotor skills related to prolonged intubation (requiring alternate feeding route such as gastrostomy), gastroesophageal reflux disease (GERD) (requiring a Nissen operation or jejunal feedings), vision and hearing deficits commonly related to prematurity, and abnormal bone mineralization commonly related to immobility.
• These patients are delayed in their development when compared to age appropriate peers, and need help through therapies to achieve milestones.
• Developmental gains, however, continue throughout infancy and childhood.

RATIONALE FOR HOME CHRONIC VENTILATORY SUPPORT

• The assumption that a child's potential for normal growth and development and integration into family and community are far better at home in the least restrictive environment, as compared to long-term institutionalization, and the realization that home discharge on a ventilator is less costly than hospital stay.

THE GOAL

• Discharge home with the parents assisted by nurses, respiratory care practitioners, and therapists, under the care of the pediatrician. Pulmonary and/or critical care practitioners continue to manage the ventilatory care and assist with coordination of care.

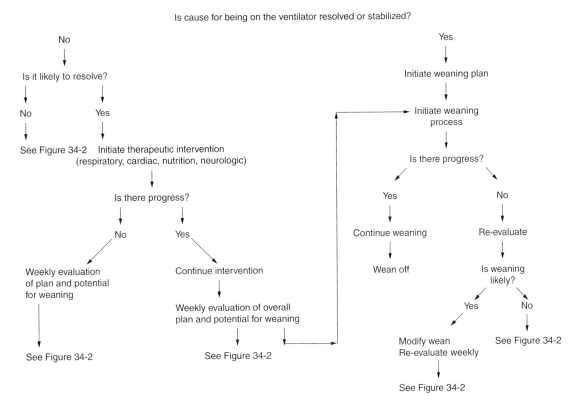

FIG. 34-1 Decision tree for weaning off the ventilator.

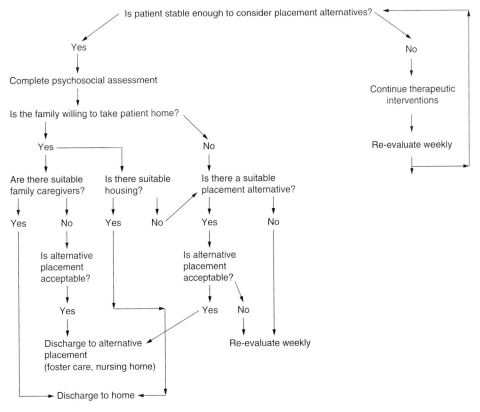

FIG. 34-2 Decision tree for discharge.

TABLE 34-1   Equipment

TYPE	PRINCIPLE	DEVICE	INDICATION	ADVANTAGES	DISADVANTAGES
Noninvasive	Positive pressure	CPAP	OSA	Relatively easy and safe, applied via face mask or nasal pillows, does not require gas source	Midface dysplasia, requires power source
	Positive pressure	Bi-level	OSA	Applied via face mask or nasal pillows, does not require gas source	Midface dysplasia, requires power source
		Rocker bed	Muscular weakness	Does not require face mask	Not very effective, requires power source, moving parts may be hazardous to young children
	Negative pressure	Cuirasse	Muscular weakness	Device applied externally to chest	Not very effective, requires power source
	Negative pressure	Iron lung	Muscular weakness	Does not require tracheostomy	Child confined to iron lung space, ventilation interrupted for care delivery, requires power source
Invasive	Diaphragmatic pacing	Pacing leads activated by radio pacing device	Central hypoventilation, high spinal cord injury	Very light, easy to carry around	Requires surgical placement of pacing wires and receiver, and tracheostomy, less effective with obesity
	Positive pressure ventilation	LP-10	Respiratory failure	Entrains room air, has internal battery, may be attached to wheelchair	Child needs tracheostomy, requires power source, relatively heavy, volume ventilator, may be pressure limited, limited range of settings
	Positive pressure ventilation	LTV	Respiratory failure	Entrains room air, continuous flow, has internal battery, wide range of volume and pressure parameters, easy to transport, resistant to EMI	Child needs tracheostomy, requires power source, sensitive to airway leak

ABBREVIATION: CPAP, continuous positive airway pressure.

THE STEPS

• Perform a thorough *evaluation of the child's condition and weaning potential* by a multidisciplinary team and appropriate specialty consultants as determined by the child's underlying diagnoses.

MULTIDISCIPLINARY TEAM

1. Medicine (neonatology, critical care)
2. Nursing
3. Respiratory care
4. Therapies: OT, PT, speech, developmental
5. Nutrition
6. Child life
7. Family
8. Case management
9. Social work

CONSULTANTS

1. Pulmonary medicine
2. ENT (bronchology)
3. Cardiology
4. Sleep medicine
5. Physiatry
6. Medical psychology
7. Pediatric surgery
8. Mineral/bone metabolism
9. Orthopedics
10. Neurology

TABLE 34-2 Chronic Respiratory Failure

CATEGORY	COMMON CONDITIONS	SYMPTOMS	DIAGNOSTIC WORKUP	MANAGEMENT
Disorders of central control of breathing	Ondine's curse Myelomeningocele Arnold-Chiari malformation Brain-stem tumors	Severe bradypnea or apnea during some or all sleep states Child does not recognize hypercarbia, and at times hypoxia. Does not increase breathing effort	Sleep study: documentation of hypoxia and hypercarbia during sleep coupled with no flow and no respiratory effort Brain CT, MRI, and EEG may be helpful	Noninvasive or invasive ventilation during sleep
Airway disorders	Obstructive sleep apnea: large tonsils, adenoids, redundant pharyngeal tissue	Snoring and irregular breathing during sleep Hypercarbia and hypoxia Somnolence and lack of energy during wake period	Sleep study documenting hypercarbia, hypoxia, and increased effort of breathing with poor or nonexistent flow Airway radiogram may also be helpful	Tonsillectomy, adenoidectomy, surgical removal of redundant pharyngeal tissue Noninvasive end expiratory or bi-level positive pressure
	Extrathoracic airway malacia	Stridor, increased work of breathing, suprasternal retractions	Direct laryngoscopy, bronchoscopy	Surgical supraglottoplasty Noninvasive positive end expiratory pressure Tracheostomy
	Intrathoracic airway malacia: associated with tracheoesophageal fistula, vascular ring, and pulmonary artery sling s/p repair	Prolonged exhalation and wheezing unresponsive to or aggravated by bronchodilators, copious secretions, distinctive cough increased work of breathing	Bronchoscopy, preferably with patient breathing spontaneously	Noninvasive or invasive positive end expiratory pressure
Significant lung disease	Bronchopulmonary dysplasia Children recuperating from ARDS Chronic aspiration	Poor growth and development, evidence of increased work of breathing, intercostal and subcostal retractions, tachypnea, and lower airway obstruction partially responsive to bronchodilators and anti-inflammatory agents	Chest radiogram, CT of chest, infant PFTs, bronchoscopy Sputum cultures	Optimal nutrition, fluid restriction, diuretics, bronchodilators, anti-inflammatory Tracheostomy and positive pressure ventilation
Neuromuscular weakness	Spinal muscular atrophy (type I)	Profound weakness, inability to increase work of breathing	Muscle biopsy, nerve conduction, genetic testing	Negative or positive pressure breathing Tracheostomy
	High quadriplegia	Paralysis below level of cord injury Autonomic dysfunction when hollow viscus distended	Spinal MRI	Tracheostomy Positive pressure ventilation

ABBREVIATIONS: ARDS, acute respiratory distress syndrome; CT, computed tomography; MRI, magnetic resonance imaging; EEG, electroencephalogram; PFTs, pulmonary function tests.

- Determine if the child *fails to wean off* the ventilator despite (Fig. 34-1)
  1. Optimal cardiorespiratory state (may include use of oxygen, bronchodilators, diuretics, steroids)
  2. No intercurrent illness
  3. Optimal nutrition
  4. No medications contributing to weakness (sedatives, analgesics, muscle relaxants)
- Evaluate for *tracheostomy and gastrostomy*
- Transition to *portable ventilatory device*
- Evaluate *potential for home discharge* (Fig. 34-2)

1. Psychosocial evaluation of child and family
2. Availability of two family care-givers
3. Willingness and ability of the family to learn care
4. Suitability of home (size, accessibility, temperature control, safety)
5. Approval of home owner for likely requirement of electrical upgrade
6. Need for access-related modifications
7. Telephone service
- Assess *growth and development* of child on current plan of care including tracheostomy, portable

ventilator, bronchodilators, anti-inflammatory drugs, diuretics as appropriate, and nutrition.

• Provide *parent/caregiver teaching* to include all aspects of child's care
  1. CPR.
  2. Tracheostomy care including hand ventilation, suctioning, tracheostomy tube change, stoma care, and recognition of emergencies such as malposition or obstruction of tracheostomy tube.
  3. Ventilatory management including assembling ventilator circuit, and recognition and troubleshooting of equipment (Table 34-1) malfunction.
  4. Gastrostomy or central line care if applicable.
  5. All aspects of well-child care.
  6. A 24-hour period when parents demonstrate their ability to independently care for the child.

HOME DISCHARGE

• Finalize discharge plans at discharge conference that includes the multidisciplinary care team, consultants, funding agency, case manager, home-care nursing agency, and durable medical equipment provider.

FOLLOW-UP

• Develop plan for outpatient follow-up.
• Common conditions leading to chronic respiratory failure—see Table 34-2.

BIBLIOGRAPHY

Mallory GB, Jr., Stillwell PC. The ventilator-dependent child: Issues in diagnosis and management. *Arch Phys Med Rehabil* 1991;72:43–55.

Nelson VS, Carroll JC, Hurvitz EA, Dean JM. Home mechanical ventilation of children. *Dev Med Child Neurol* 1996; 38:704–715.

O'Donohue WJ, Jr., Giovannoni RM, Goldberg AI, et al. Long-term mechanical ventilation. Guidelines for management in the home and at alternate community sites. Report of the Ad Hoc Committee, Respiratory Care Section, American College of Chest Physicians. *Chest* 1986;90:1S–37S.

Oren J, Kelly DLH, Shannon DC. Long-term follow-up of children with congenital central hypoventilation syndrome. *Pediatrics* 1987;80:375–380.

Panitch HB, Downes JJ, Kennedy JS, et al. Guidelines for home care of children with chronic respiratory insufficiency. *Pediatr Pulmonol* 1996;21:52–56.

35 BRAIN DEATH

Denise M. Goodman

WHAT IS DEATH?

• The traditional definition is cardiorespiratory death, i.e., cessation of breathing and loss of heartbeat.
• Modern cardiorespiratory support permits maintenance of vital signs even after neurologic function is lost.
• The concept of brain death was developed in an effort to detect irreversible absence of brain function before cardiovascular demise.

GOAL OF BRAIN DEATH CRITERIA

• To attempt to identify complete lack of function of the cerebral hemispheres and the brain stem = "whole-brain" brain death.

HISTORY OF DEVELOPMENT OF CRITERIA

• 1959—Mollaret and Goulon introduced the term of coma depasse or irreversible coma.
• 1968—Harvard Criteria were published—first published criteria, did not include children.
• 1987—Task Force on Brain Death in Children published guidelines simultaneously in four journals.

REQUIREMENTS FOR DETERMINING BRAIN DEATH

• The cause of death *must be* known.
• There is irreversible loss of brain and brain-stem function (requires comprehensive examination and persistence over time).
• Confounding factors have been excluded (such as hypothermia, circulatory shock, and drug intoxication).
• Coma and apnea must coexist.

COMPONENTS OF THE BRAIN DEATH EXAMINATION

• Absence of brain-stem function
  1. Midposition or fully dilated pupils unreactive to light.

2. Absence of reflex or spontaneous eye movement, including oculocephalic and oculovestibular tests (doll's eyes, calorics).
3. Absence of corneal, gag, cough, sucking, and rooting reflexes and no spontaneous movement of bulbar musculature.

- Apnea using standardized testing
- Patient is flaccid with no spontaneous or induced movement *excluding* spinal reflexes.
- Examination is consistent, with the observation period differing by age.

OBSERVATION PERIOD

- Ages 7 days to 2 months—two examinations and electroencephalogram (EEGs) 48 hours apart.
- Ages 2 months to 1 year—two examinations and EEGs 24 hours apart, or one examination and EEG plus absent cerebral blood flow.
- Age >1 year—two examinations 12–24 hours apart, corroborative tests are optional.

SPINAL REFLEXES

- Several studies have demonstrated spinal reflexes to be present in patients for whom there is no intracerebral circulation by angiography.
- The current understanding is that spinal stretch and deep tendon reflexes can be preserved in brain death.

CORROBORATIVE TESTING

- May include EEG, angiography, or radionuclide brain flow examination.
- Results can be "consistent with" brain death but not "diagnostic of" brain death.
- Requirements differ by country—the physician should adhere to his or her local published guidelines.

THE EXAMINATION—AN ORDERLY APPROACH

BEFORE BEGINNING THE EXAMINATION

- Ensure that the etiology of coma is known.
- Ensure that the coma is deemed to be irreversible.
- Exclude drug intoxication.
- Correct any confounding metabolic conditions, such as acid-base disorders, electrolyte disorders, and endocrinopathies.

- Make sure the patient is normothermic.
- Make sure the patient is normotensive.
- Ensure that pharmacologic neuromuscular blockade is not present—use a nerve stimulator to demonstrate the absence of neuromuscular blocking drugs.
- The patient should exhibit no cerebral motor response to pain.

EXAMINE THE CRANIAL NERVES

- The pupils should be midposition or fully dilated and unresponsive to light (CN II, III).
- There should be no spontaneous extraocular motion (CN III, IV, and VI).
- Test for the corneal reflex (CN V sensory, CN VII motor). A normal response is eyelid closure and upward deviation of the eye. This is absent in brain death.
- Test for the gag reflex (CN IX sensory, CN X motor).
- Test the oculocephalic reflex (doll's eyes). A normal reflex is for the eyes to deviate to the left as the head turns right, so that the eye looks at the examiner. In brain death this is absent, and the eyes do not change position with head movement (*painted on* appearance).
- Test the oculovestibular reflex (Cold calorics). Instill ~100 mL (less for smaller children) of ice water into the ear canal. A normal response induces nystagmus with the fast component toward the opposite side. In brain death this is absent and there is no eye deviation.

PERFORM AN APNEA TEST

- Preoxygenate with 100% oxygen for at least 10 minutes.
- Place the patient on continuous high flow oxygen throughout the trial (such as by using an anesthesia bag connected to the endotracheal tube).
- Wait for the $PaCO_2$ to exceed 60 torr. The $PaCO_2$ rises approximately 3–4 torr/minute during apnea.
- Observe for any respiratory effort by watching for chest rise, listening to the chest, and gently feeling the anesthesia bag.

DOCUMENTATION OF THE EXAMINATION

- The note should be separate and specifically titled as an examination of brain and brain-stem function.
- The time should be noted.
- Each component of the examination should be listed and the findings described.
- The apnea test should include all blood gases with their times as well as the means by which evidence of respiratory effort was assessed.

FINDINGS WHICH MAY BE ASSOCIATED WITH BRAIN DEATH

- Diabetes insipidus
- Hypothermia
- Hyperglycemia
- Acidosis, electrolyte imbalances
- Cardiopulmonary instability
- No tachycardic response to atropine
- No bradycardic response to vagal stimulation

BIBLIOGRAPHY

Report of Special Task Force. Guidelines for the determination of brain death in children. *Pediatrics* 1987;80:298–300.

Saposnik G, Bueri JA, Maurino J, Saizar R, Garretto NS. Spontaneous and reflex movements in brain death. *Neurology* 2000;54:221–223.

Wijdicks EFM. The diagnosis of brain death. *N Engl J Med* 2001;344:1215–1221.

PEDIATRIC HOSPITAL CARE

Jennifer A. Daru, Section Editor

36 ADMITTING A PATIENT

Jennifer Daru and Robert Listernick

- Once the decision has been made to admit a patient to the hospital, several things must occur. Parental and, occasionally, insurance approval for the admission must be obtained. After a full history and physical examination is performed, the location and type of care a patient needs must be determined. In addition, an attending physician needs to be identified to care for the patient on the inpatient unit.

THE ADMIT HISTORY AND PHYSICAL

- The admitting history and physical examination must be as complete as possible in order to facilitate both problem-focused and future comprehensive care of the patient. A properly obtained history alone can lead to the correct diagnosis in over 80% of cases.
- Elements of a pediatric history include the following:
  1. The *source* of the history should be recorded. Both the patient and family should be interviewed together. If the patient is older than 11 years, he or she also should be interviewed alone and a psychosocial and medical social interview should be performed using the HEADDS outline. HEADDS refers to questions for the adolescent regarding his or her *home, education, activities, drugs, sexuality, and suicide/depression.*
  2. *History of the present illness.*
  3. *Past medical history.*
  4. *Birth history.*

5. *Developmental history*: screen fine and gross motor, cognitive and perceptive language, and personal-social skills.
6. *Immunization history.*
7. *Social history.*
8. *Family history*: ask about a history of consanguinity, when appropriate.
- Special comments on the physical examination:
  1. Remember that *vital signs* change with age.
  2. The patient's *growth parameters* should be plotted on standardized charts.
  3. Be prepared to play with a child or stand away from the child and observe.

MEDICAL INSURANCE CONSIDERATIONS

- *Health Maintenance Organization (HMO)*: In general, the hospital must be part of the patient's HMO network for the insurance to cover the admission. In emergent or unscheduled admissions, the patient's primary care provider (PCP) must be contacted. If the hospital is not a part of the HMO network and the PCP allows the transfer, HMO insurance will cover the visit. If the PCP does not approve transfer, the patient may be responsible for the hospital bill.
- *Preferred Provider Organization (PPO)*: A patient pays a percentage of the hospital bill based on whether or not the hospital is a part of the patient's PPO network. A PCP is not required to approve the admission.
- *Medicaid (non-HMO)*: Visits are not restricted and no approval is required for admission.
- *Self-pay/uninsured patients*: These patients should be referred immediately to a financial services representative. Many of these children may qualify for Medicaid or other state-based plans of which parents may not be aware.

CONSENTING TO ADMISSION OF A PEDIATRIC PATIENT

- In general, a parent or recognized legal guardian of a patient must sign consent to allow a child's admission to the hospital. A few special scenarios include the following:
  1. *Missing parent or guardian*: When the parent/legal guardian is missing, attempts must be made to contact this person via phone for permission to treat and admit the patient. Until this person is found, the physician of record takes responsibility for the patient. While a close relative may be present, they do not have the right to give legal approval for admission.
  2. *Emergency situations*: Consent is not required if it creates a delay in care that would endanger the patient; the physician takes responsibility. In general, the law supports the physician's right to perform life-saving therapy without consent.
  3. *Nonemancipated minors and the Mature Minor Rule*: The right of a minor to give consent without parental knowledge is governed by state law. In many states, this includes the ability to consent for treatment and diagnosis of a sexually transmitted disease, drug abuse, and psychiatric therapy. Abortion rules also vary by state; however, if abuse or neglect is suspected, this must be reported immediately to the appropriate local agency. There is an emerging concept of the "mature minor rule"; this states that low risk care, within standard practices that will benefit the patient, can be given with the minor's consent alone.
  4. *Emancipated minor*: The definition of an emancipated minor varies by state. In general, minors who (1) live separately from their parents, (2) support themselves, (3) are married, (4) have a child or are pregnant, (5) are part of the military, or (6) have been granted emancipation by the court can give consent for their own treatment and admission. Documents proving emancipation are usually not required.
  5. *Patients 18 and older*: These patients may give their own consent to admission; however, parents cannot give legal approval for admission of patients 18 years or older who have mental problems or disabilities leading them to be unable to give their own consent, unless they have petitioned the court for guardianship.
  6. *Refusing care*: A child who is neither emancipated nor a mature minor cannot refuse care when the parent and physician agree that it is in the child's best interest; however, competent parents/guardians have the right to refuse care for their children in situations in which the problem is neither life threatening nor likely to cause serious impairment. A physician must be ready to seek legal custody of a patient if it is deemed that the patient is placed at risk by parental refusal of care. This includes the situation when the child's life or well-being is in danger because of their place of residence or with the person responsible for their well-being. This is usually performed by taking *temporary protective custody* while notifying the local child protective agency. Hospital ethical teams should also assist in the decision-making process. Courts have determined that parents do not have the right to refuse life-saving treatment, even if such treatment is against their religious convictions.

METHODS OF CARE DELIVERY

- *Attending physician*: All patients must be admitted under the care of an attending physician who assumes the responsibility and liability for the admission. The attending may be the patient's PCP, the on-call physician, a hospitalist, or a specialist. If a nonpediatric attending admits a patient (e.g., a family practitioner or a surgeon), guidelines should exist for pediatric attending consultation. Hospitalist physicians, defined as physicians who spend the majority of their time providing inpatient care, act as independent attending physicians; they should communicate regularly with the patient's PCP.
- *Resident physicians*: These doctors play an important role in the care of hospitalized patients, performing daily examinations and writing patient orders; however, liability and final decision-making remain with the attending of record.
- *Nurse practioners (NP) and physician assistants (PA)*: A NP is a registered nurse who has further education and clinical training, usually through a certificate or masters program. A PA has at least 2 years of undergraduate education followed by up to a year of preclinical training and a year of physician supervised clinical education. The role of these physician extenders varies across hospital units and states. The American Academy of Pediatrics (AAP) recommends that a hospital have written protocols outlining their involvement in patient care.

LOCATION

- After deciding that a patient needs inpatient care, the treating physician must determine if a patient should be admitted to the hospital's observation unit, the pediatric inpatient floor, or the intensive care unit. At times, the patient may require transfer to another facility. A secondary consideration is the type of room a patient will need.

1. *Observation unit*: This unit was established to allow for patient care and evaluation beyond the emergency room for patients who do not require a prolonged inpatient stay. Usually, patients may stay in observation units for as long as 24 hours. Potential benefits of an observation unit include improved patient care, increased patient satisfaction, and cost effectiveness. Patients may be monitored for longer periods of time than are possible in the emergency room, potentially decreasing hospital liability. Third party payers recognize *observation status* as a special billing code, and reimburse it differently than the standard admission. Of note, a patient does not need to be in an observation unit to be admitted under observational status. Potential diagnoses that would qualify for admission to an observation unit include (1) mild respiratory distress associated with asthma, pneumonia, bronchiolitis, and croup, (2) mild gastroenteritis and dehydration, (3) children with suspected appendicitis who warrant observation, (4) children with mild head trauma, or (5) minor ingestions. Patients do not qualify for an observation admission if they require (1) intensive care, (2) oxygen, or (3) treatment for a serious bacterial infection.

2. *Pediatric intensive care unit (PICU)*: A level one PICU has higher acuity patients and immediate pediatric subspecialist availability. A level two PICU usually has less medically complex patients who have stable disorders; it has limited subspecialist availability. Considerations for admission to a PICU are based on the type of admitting institution and the spectrum of care delivered.

3. *Transfer to another hospital*: If a patient cannot be appropriately cared for at a hospital, the treating physician must assist in the patient's stabilization and the transfer process. Options for the transport of patients include the use of either a basic or advanced life support team (ALS or BLS), or a critical care team. BLS and ALS teams are staffed by paramedics and emergency medical technicians (EMTs), while critical care teams may involve a combination of EMTs, paramedics, critical care nurses, respiratory therapists, and, when necessary, physicians. The type of care provided by each team varies by state. It is important that the transport team used is qualified to care for all of the patient's needs. The mode of transport required is dependent on the severity of the patient's illness, skills of the initiating hospital team, distance from the receiving facility, and the weather. All teams may travel by ambulance. Critical care teams and some ALS or BLS teams, depending on the region, may also be involved in transports requiring helicopter or fixed wing travel. In general, the tertiary care center's transport team can assist with transport decision making; however, the final decision remains with the treating physician.

4. *Isolation beds*: Most hospitals have an infection control team and established patient isolation policies (Table 36-1).

TABLE 36-1 Types of Isolation

Airborne Precautions	Measles*, varicella*, rubella*, tuberculosis*
Droplet Precautions	Invasive Hib or neisseria meningitidis infection (i.e., meningitis, pna, sepsis), pneumonia (mycoplasma, streptococcal), scarlet fever, pertussis, adenovirus, influenza
Contact Precautions	*Gastrointestinal*: any acute diarrheal illness, enteric infections with clostridium difficile, diapered patients with rotavirus, ecoli 0157, shigella
	Respiratory: any viral infection (pneumonia, bronchiolitis, croup) including rsv, parainfluenza, enteroviral
	Skin: herpes simplex, impetigo, scabies, staphylococcal and group A streptococcal infection, zoster*
	Other: colonization with a multi-drug resistant organism (MRSA, VRE), small pox*
Protective Isolation	Immunocompromised patients

* negative air flow room

SOURCE: *Recommendations for Isolation Precautions in Hospitals*—1996 and the *Children's Memorial Hospital Isolation Policies*—2000.)

ADMISSION ORDERS

- Standardized admission orders prevent physicians from forgetting important details (Table 36-2).
- Special caveats include the following:
  1. Record the weight at the beginning of the admission orders, so that pharmacists and nurses can double-check fluid and medication orders.

TABLE 36-2 Admit Orders

Weight
Full or Observation Admit
Admit to (Attending Physician)
Diagnosis
Condition
Vitals
Allergies
Ambulation
Nursing Orders (monitors, record of in and outs)
Diet
IV Fluid
Medications
Special orders (Radiologic tests, and so on)
Lab Tests
Call House Officer for: Temperature, Heart Rate,
Respiratory Rate Parameters
Other Orders

2. State vital sign parameters for which nurses should call the physician; normal values for vital signs are dependent on age.
3. When dosing medications (1) write out dose in dosage units by weight, such as milligrams or micrograms (i.e., do not write 15 mg/kg/dose of acetaminophen or 5 mL amoxicillin), (2) use a zero to the left of a dose less than one, but (3) avoid use of a terminal zero to the right of a decimal point (i.e., write 0.5 mg or 5 mg but not 5.0 mg).

37 THE INPATIENT UNIT
Jennifer Daru and Robert Listernick

• The pediatric floor and its staff should be child friendly and safe, supporting both the medical and developmental needs of pediatric patients.

PEDIATRIC FLOOR GENERAL SETUP

• The American Academy of Pediatrics (AAP) has recommended that pediatric floors have the following:
  1. Rooms set up for close observation of young patients.
  2. Areas for play and education.
  3. Child-proofed rooms with electrical outlet covers and both window and door locks.
  4. Supplemental oxygen and suction equipment, along with standard electrical outlets by each bed; all should have access to emergency power.
  5. Safe beds for patients, including cribs with hoods, isolettes for young infants when appropriate, and other age-appropriate furniture.
  6. A treatment room to be used for all patient procedures.
  7. Sufficient area in patient rooms so that the parent may sleep in the room with the patient, if desired.

PEDIATRIC FLOOR OR BEDSIDE EQUIPMENT

• Bedside and floor equipment will need to include the following:
  1. Monitors: (1) *Cardiac/apnea monitors* should be available for any patient less than 3 months of age who has either respiratory problems or who is at risk for apnea or bradycardia. (2) *Pulse oximetry* may be used to monitor patients in acute respiratory distress or any patient who receives supplemental oxygen. Care should be taken to discontinue use of monitors when they are no longer needed, so as to avoid overtreatment of minor changes in vital signs. Alarms on monitors must be easily heard by nursing staff.
  2. Humidified oxygen delivery systems with flow meters that have the ability to adjust oxygen concentration from room air to 100%.
  3. Suction equipment.
  4. Thermometers, blood pressure equipment with appropriate cuff sizes for infants and young children, otoscope, and ophthalmoscope.
  5. Scales and stadiometer for weight and height measurements of both infants and children.
  6. Portable lamps.
  7. Resuscitation equipment, including a standardized pediatric resuscitation cart, backboard for resuscitation, and pediatric-sized defibrillator.
  8. Papoose board.
  9. Appropriately sized intravenous, phlebotomy, and lumbar puncture trays.

EMERGENCY PREPAREDNESS

• Staff should be certified in neonatal resuscitation and pediatric advanced life support as appropriate; However, all staff members should know the location of code buttons and oxygen masks on the inpatient floor and in the patient rooms. Mock codes involving all floor staff should be performed on a regular basis.

38 THE MEDICAL RECORD, BILLING, AND MEDICOLEGAL CONSIDERATIONS
Jennifer Daru and Robert Listernick

PHYSICIAN CHARTING AND THE BILL

• The medical record should be a sequential recording of the patient's course, including the emergency room visit, events during the hospitalization, and the discharge summary.

- All information in the record should be signed, dated, timed, and written in legible handwriting. The amount of time spent both with the patient and writing the note is relevant for billing purposes. Insurance companies will deny claims if they cannot read the doctor's note.
- Each visit to the patient should be charted. When more than one visit is made in a day, each charted visit can be billed or can affect billing.
- Daily charting should include a SOAP progress note. (a) *Subjective*: This part of the note should include details of the patient's overnight course and current concerns and complaints. (b) *Objective*: This should include a physical examination, including vitals signs, relevant physical findings, and pertinent laboratory data. (c) *Assessment* of patient. The stated diagnosis will be part of the patient bill and should justify the patient's admission to the hospital. If the diagnosis is unclear, the assessment should include a summary of the patient's symptoms and a discussion of the differential diagnoses. (d) *Plan*: The plan should address problems included in the assessment and any other patient needs.
- When an error is made in charting the medical record, a single line should be placed through the erroneous text, with the change dated and initialed by the physician.
- Daily billing should be done based on the information provided in the physician's note and the time spent by the physician. There are large fines for billing for services without a record of care.
- Bills for prolonged admissions should be submitted at least once a week to ensure faster reimbursement.

THE HEALTH INSURANCE PORTABILITY AND ACCOUNTABILITY ACT OF 1996 (HIPAA)

- HIPAA covers three major areas of health care: insurance portability, fraud enforcement (accountability), and administration simplification (reduction in health-care costs).
- Importantly, it governs the use and disclosure of a patient's protected health information (PHI). The act outlines national standards for protecting an individual's medical records and holds hospitals and physicians accountable with civil and criminal penalties for violating a patient's privacy rights.
- Hospitals are now required by HIPAA to issue new patients a written Notice of Privacy Practices outlining the hospital's privacy practices and the patient's rights. This document explains to patients how their PHI may be used and disclosed, in addition to who has received their information. It limits release of information to the minimum number of people reasonably needed for the purpose of the use and disclosure.

MEDICAL ERRORS

- Because of the complexity of the practice of medicine, medical errors will occur. It is critical to try to reduce these occurrences through strict review and implementation of protective systems throughout the hospital. If an error is made, it needs to be charted as it happened without opinion or emotion, just as any part of the patient course is charted. Risk management teams, where available, should always be contacted.

39 INPATIENT CARE
Jennifer Daru and Robert Listernick

MONITORING INTAKE AND OUTPUT

- A strict record of oral intake and urine and stool output needs to be maintained for almost all patients admitted to a pediatric unit. Both parents and nurses will need to participate in this process.
- Stool output should be charted by nurses; abnormal characteristics (i.e., blood, acholic stools) require further evaluation.
- A minimum urine output of 1 cc/kg/day should be maintained. In situations where accurate measurement of urine output is essential, placement of a urinary catheter may be necessary.
- Daily weights also help monitor a patient's fluid balance.

INTRAVENOUS FLUID THERAPY ON THE PEDIATRIC FLOOR

- A patient should be acutely rehydrated in the emergency room using one or more boluses of 20 cc/kg of isotonic fluid, generally normal saline. In patients with ongoing circulatory issues, other fluids may be considered, such as blood or plasma.
- Once a patient comes to the floor, a number of factors should be considered in providing continuous intravenous fluid (IVF) support, including maintenance needs, ongoing losses, and any other special circumstances. With proper rehydration and reintroduction of oral liquids, most children will wean quickly from intravenous fluid.

STEP 1: CALCULATING MAINTENANCE REQUIREMENTS

- IVF: Multiple methods exist to calculate maintenance IVF requirements, but for the average child, the Holliday-Segar method will suffice. This method estimates that for every 100 cal metabolized, a patient will need 100 cc of free water.
  a. Using this method: For the first 10 kg of body weight a patient requires 100 cc/kg/day, for the second 10 kg a patient needs 50 cc/kg/day, and for each additional kilogram of body weight above 20 kg, a patient needs 20 cc/kg/day. Residents writing fluid orders on a per hour basis often approximate this using the "4-2-1 rule": for the first 10 kg of body weight the patient requires 4 cc/ kg/hour, for the next 10 kg they require 2 cc/kg/ hour, and then for each kilogram above 20 kg they require 1 cc/kg/hour.
  b. Most physicians use a maximum IVF rate of 100–125 cc/hour for larger children or adults.
- Electrolytes: Maintenance sodium needs are 2–4 meq/kg/day. For most children this need is somewhere between 0.2 and 0.45 normal saline. Maintenance potassium needs are 2–3 meq/kg/day. Potassium should be added only if a child is urinating, usually in between a concentration of 10 and 20 meq KCl per liter IVF given.
- Glucose: In a child with normal glucose homeostasis, a 5% dextrose solution is given.

Example

- A 15-kg child comes to the floor after being hydrated in the emergency room for gastroenteritis. He has just urinated 100 cc. Calculate maintenance IVF.
- **Solution:** Child's weight = 15 kg.
- *Fluid*
  For the first 10 kg give 100 cc/kg/day or 1000 cc/day.
  For the next 5 kg give 50 cc/kg/day or 250 cc/day.
  Total fluid (or free water) need equals 1250 cc/day or 52 cc/hour.
- *Sodium*

$$4 \text{ meq Na/kg/day} \times 15 \text{ kg} = 60 \text{ meq Na/day}$$

This 60 meq sodium is given mixed into the fluid the child requires per day (1250 cc/day). To determine a concentration of saline (usually described as a per liter amount):

$$60 \text{ meq Na required/1250 cc IVF required}$$
$$= X \text{ meq Na given/liter IVF given}$$

where $X = 48$ meq Na

- While a pharmacist can make a solution to any concentration of sodium necessary, certain concentrations are readily available:

0.9 NS = 154 meq/L NaCl
0.45 NS = 77 meq/L NaCl
0.2 NS = 34 meq/L NaCl

- For this patient it is appropriate to choose 0.2 NS.
- *Potassium*

$$2 \text{ meq KCl/kg/day} \times 15 \text{ kg} = 30 \text{ meq KCl/day}$$

Again, this amount must be given across the 1250 cc of fluid:

$$30 \text{ meq KCl required/1250 cc IVF required}$$
$$= X \text{ meq KCl given/liter IVF given}$$

$$X = 24 \text{ meq KCl}$$

- *Final order*
  D5 0.2 NS + 20 meq/L KCl at 52 cc/hour

STEP 2: REPLACEMENT OF LOSSES

- Many children who have been rehydrated appropriately in the emergency room and who are then started on maintenance intravenous fluid will begin to recover. No further calculations to replace losses should be needed unless a child does not keep up with ongoing losses.
- If a child does not begin to recover, ongoing losses should be assessed and replaced regularly.

METHODS OF INTRAVENOUS FLUID DELIVERY

- Peripheral intravenous lines (PIVs) usually last between 0 and 4 days. PIVs need to be checked on a regular basis as they carry the risk of subcutaneous infiltration, thrombosis, and infection. If a PIV infiltrates the subcutaneous tissue, it should be removed immediately, and the extremity should be elevated. If necessary, hyaluronidase can be used to prevent scarring. Serious infiltrations with caustic agents (e.g., calcium) should be evaluated by a plastic surgeon. Nursing and physician notes should record the occurrence. The need for intravenous therapy always should be reevaluated prior to the replacement of a PIV.
- Occasionally, intravenous access is necessary, but a PIV cannot be placed. In nonemergent situations, a peripherally inserted central catheter (PICC) or other central venous catheter can be placed. A PICC is inserted into a peripheral vein and threaded such that the distal end lies in a central vein. In emergent situations, it may be necessary to place an intraosseous line.
- PICC lines are used for long-term intravenous needs, lasting as long as 3 months. The risk of infection

increases the longer the catheter is in place, by port number, and each time the catheter is accessed. Nurses must be trained in the proper use and care of PICC lines. If concern arises for infection, removal of the line must be strongly considered. Occasionally, PICC lines may also become occluded.

FEVER

- Parents should be educated that fever, defined as a temperature over 100.4°F (38°C), is a natural response to infection that aids the body in recovery; however, fever can also be uncomfortable for the patient and may contribute to the development of dehydration.
- When a child has been hospitalized, it is most precise to take the child's temperature either rectally, orally (in children older than 4 or 5), or with an infrared otic thermometer. Axillary temperatures should not be used in the hospital.
- It is crucial to support a febrile patient's fluid needs either orally or intravenously.
- In a child with an established reason for fever, it may be appropriate to prescribe acetaminophen (15 mg/kg/dose every 4–6 hours) or ibuprofen (10 mg/kg/dose every 6 hours). There are no data to support the simultaneous use of these two medications.

OXYGEN THERAPY

- Clear parameters for oxygen use in a patient should be written in the admission orders.
- Patients on oxygen for more than a few hours will require a humidified source to decrease insensible water losses and aid in comfort.
- The delivery of supplemental oxygen to young children may be difficult. Delivery modalities include a face mask, nasal cannula, or head hood. The delivery vehicle should be individualized to the patient. In general, use of an oxygen tent is discouraged, as it limits access to the child and may also affect a child's body temperature.

HOSPITAL SERVICES FOR CHILDREN

- Hospital services for children will be dependent on the institution. The physician must understand a hospital's capabilities in order to provide children with the best possible services.
- A *social worker's* job in the hospital is to assist in the further assessment of an at-risk child's life outside the

hospital. This includes, but is not limited to (1) ensuring the patient's safety from neglect and/or physical abuse both in the hospital and on return home, (2) further evaluating a caregiver's ability to provide proper food and housing, and (3) reviewing the home environment. Social workers are often aware of community and state agencies that can assist in patient care. They can make referrals to food, public aid, and support systems, as well as assist with transportation planning on discharge.

- *Child protection agencies* exist in all states. Although workers are not hospital staff, they may work closely with hospital teams to provide for the safety of children. Child protection agencies can be contacted by anyone concerned about a child's well-being. Once a child protection worker is contacted, the claim will be investigated quickly. In some cases, the agency will take custody of the child or give temporary custody to another family member or friend until a child's safety can be ensured. Discharge of a patient may have to be delayed until these arrangements are made.
- *Developmental teams* may exist at higher level facilities to help assess and treat developmental problems.
- *Educational services* during brief admissions may be provided by some hospitals, but state-provided tutors are mandated by a state's board of education once certain criteria are met, such as prolonged admission. If a patient requires prolonged recovery at home after discharge, the social worker may need to obtain state-provided tutors.
- *Respiratory care* should be provided by therapists familiar with the needs of children. Therapists should assist in pediatric nebulizer dosing and administration, as well as with pediatric and neonatal ventilation. Prior to patient discharge, they can also help educate families of children with reactive airway disease on use of home nebulizers or metered dose inhalers.
- *Occupational and physical therapy* services for children may exist at higher level facilities or for specific common problems in community hospitals.
- *Nutrition services* are required by the Joint Commission for Accreditation of Hospitals (JACHO). Nutrition services should closely review patients who are (1) less than the 5th percentile for weight, (2) greater than the 95th percentile in weight or, (3) less than the 5th percentile in weight/height. They should also review patients who are receiving hyperalimentaion or who are not being enterally fed for prolonged periods.
- A *child life representative* can make a large difference in the child's interpretation of disease through play and discussion. This person should address the patient's fear in an open and honest way in order to help facilitate patient care.

• *Financial services* exist in all hospitals. Patients with limited or no insurance should be seen by a financial representative as soon as possible in order to assist in arranging payment plans or determine if a patient is eligible for coverage. It should be made clear to the patient that care will not be withheld for financial reasons.

40 DISCHARGE PLANNING
Jennifer Daru and Robert Listernick

• Many hospitals have *discharge* planners who will assist with providing the patient home services on discharge (such as nebulizers or home nursing) or finding physicians to care for patients following discharge.
• If the patient's primary care provider (PCP) differs from the inpatient attending, outpatient follow-up and continuity of care must be assured through phone calls and faxed copies of the relevant record.
• Plans for follow-up after discharge should be written with clear instructions in laymen's terms. Caregivers must be advised as to what symptoms and signs should prompt return, and whom they should call with concerns. These instructions must be written and discussed in the caregiver's primary language.
• Awareness of the patient's financial situation is crucial for ensuring compliance with outpatient medicines. On occasion, it may be appropriate to have the caregiver purchase medicines prior to patient discharge.

41 DEATH IN THE HOSPITAL
Jennifer Daru and Robert Listernick

THE ANTICIPATED DEATH

• Legal guardians and patients have the right to make an informed decision regarding forgoing further treatment. They may decide to either forgo all further treatment (which may include withdrawal of current treatment), limit further treatment of the patient, or

provide any possible treatment for the child. It is crucial that the family be provided with adequate support both during and after the decision-making process.
• If the decision is made to forgo resuscitation or intubation, a clear order must be written in the chart by the attending physician. An explanatory note must accompany this order.
• It is crucial that when a patient passes away, the family be allowed appropriate time to be with their child. Families who have chosen to continue all possible therapies may benefit from watching practitioners attempt resuscitation.
• After death, an appropriate physician should approach the family about postmortem examination. Benefits of such an examination to the patient's family as well as to future patients should be explained. There is usually no charge for this examination.

THE UNANTICIPATED DEATH

• In the case of an unanticipated death, the family should be contacted as resuscitation efforts are begun. Support teams should assist the family in understanding what may have happened; following the child's death, the family should be allowed time alone with their child. As before, autopsy services should be made available.
• Death of a child in the emergency department or on the inpatient floor from unclear causes deserves investigation; however, only medical examiners have the legal authority to investigate deaths that are unexplained or occur unexpectedly. At the time of death, the physician should take a history and perform a standard physical examination, and help provide support. The American Academy of Pediatrics (AAP) supports the need for autopsies for all infants who die suddenly and unexpectedly; an international standardized autopsy protocol is available. The available history should be given to the medical examiner who will do skeletal x-rays, examine tissue, and perform cultures, metabolic studies, and drug screens on the body. Examination of the death scene will be done by the medical examiner's team.

ORGAN DONATION

• The Omnibus Reconciliation Act of 1986 requires that hospitals discuss organ donation with families of deceased patients, as well as refer all potential organ donors to their local organ procurement organization.

42 CULTURAL, RELIGIOUS, AND OTHER MAJOR CONSIDERATIONS IN PATIENT CARE

Jennifer Daru and Robert Listernick

- When interviewing patients, the physician should consider the impact the following factors have on patient care, as well as on the family-physician relationship:
  1. The religious and cultural background of the patient.
  2. Whether the child or child's parents may be gay.
  3. The role of extended family in the child's life, e.g., half-siblings, step-parents, or noncustodial parents.
  4. The family's use of alternative medications or providers.
- The physician may wish to involve a religious leader or social worker to ensure that parents feel comfortable with and understand the medical process.
- The physician must take care that his/her own religious beliefs and social biases do not negatively affect his/her interaction with patients and their families.
- In cases when a patient is placed at risk by the religious or cultural beliefs of a family, a physician should consider taking temporary custody, involving ethical teams, and child protective services.

OVERCOMING LANGUAGE BARRIERS

- When working with families who do not speak the same language as the physician, it is always better to use a medical translator than a family member or staff person who may have limited language skills and/or medical understanding.
- Whenever possible, a patient's siblings (if less than 18) should not be used for translation.
- Translators should be used to update the family on a daily basis and prior to any patient procedures.
- All patient prescriptions and discharge instructions should be translated and labeled in the patient's native language.

RELIGIOUS AND CULTURAL AWARENESS

- Religious and cultural views or customs vary from region to region, family to family, and person to person. It is best for the physician to ask the patient and family directly if they have a religious or cultural

belief of which the health care team should be aware. Examples of the impact of religious and cultural views on medicine include the following:
1. *Christian scientists* promote the healing of mental and physical illness through prayer. They often will not seek care from a standard medical practitioner. In situations where the health of a child is in danger, it may be necessary to take custody of the child for further treatment.
2. *Jehovah's Witness* practices have changed over time. Previously, the use of any blood products or organ transplantations was forbidden, as this was a sin for which a person would forgo eternal life. The Associated Jehovah's Witness for the Reform on Blood are working to change customs. Jehovah's Witness has reversed its views on the receipt of different blood components such as platelets, bone marrow transplants, and other transplants, now saying that their use is "up to individual conscience." Many will still refuse packed red blood cell transfusions, although some will accept a chemically modified hemoglobin. Taking custody of a child may be necessary in cases where life is placed at risk. Some families may feel that the receipt of a "forced" transfusion is not commission of a sin. While vaccination was prohibited before the 1950s, the church now states that it is up to an individual's conscience whether vaccination is appropriate.
3. *Christian practices* other than those mentioned above vary widely. Both Catholic and Protestant Christian families traditionally baptize infants at birth. Some baptize by full immersion in water while others sprinkle holy water over the face of the person being baptized. In the Catholic faith, the baptism saves the infant from original sin, while in the Protestant faith the process welcomes a newborn to the church. Some families may wish that a sick newborn be baptized by a priest before death, while others will accept baptism with holy water by a well-meaning individual either before or immediately after death.
4. *Muslims* whisper the calls of prayer into a child's ear just after birth. This is often accompanied by placing a drop of honey in the mouth. Male circumcision is usually performed after the seventh day of life. Breastfeeding is addressed in sacred scripture and many women consider it their sacred duty. Modest dress is very important after the onset of maturity (bulugh). After bulugh, girls wear the hejab, or head covering, which only reveals their face. At puberty, it becomes preferable for the child to see a same-sex physician. When a child is critically ill without possibility of cure, the physician is

expected to give a positive message to the family and to speak with the head of the family separately. Of note, while Muslims fast the entire month of Ramadan from sun-up to sun-down, children and those who are ill are not expected to fast. Patients may require a special halal diet and usually do not eat pork.

5. *Jewish* circumcision is performed on the eighth day after the child is born along with a naming ceremony. This marks the child's entrance into the covenant (brit) with God. Patients may require a kosher diet (a diet requiring special preparation that does not combine dairy and meat). Orthodox Jews may require special attention if in the hospital on the Sabbath. Both men and women who are strictly orthodox may refuse to shake hands with physicians of the opposite sex.

6. The *Hindu patient* may use a combination of therapies including reiki (healing touch) and ayurveda (traditional herbal medicine) as well as traditional western medicine. Hindus believe in a continuing cycle of birth, life, death, and rebirth (samsara) until enlightenment (moksa) is achieved. Distribution of wealth, prestige, and suffering are consequences for one's acts in this lifetime and previous ones.

7. *Roma (Gypsy) patients*, who may be of varied religious backgrounds, have intense loyalty to the family. Illness is not individualized, but is shared by the clan. In the health-care setting, elder males expect to lead, even though many older Roma may be illiterate. A woman is not permitted to interrupt a man or be alone with a man who is not her husband. There are strict rules about "pollution"; the upper half of a woman's body is pure (wuzho) and the lower half is polluted (marime). Failure to keep secretions or impurities originating from the lower half of the body from contaminating the upper half is believed to cause illness. Once ill, the Roma may use charms, talismans, amulets, or female faith healers (drabarni). Patients may request a famous physician, prefer older practitioners, or may demand treatment that is inappropriate. Anesthesia is thought to be a "little death" and may be feared.

BIBLIOGRAPHY (SEC. 5)

American Academy of Pediatrics, Committee on Hospital Care and Pediatric Section of the Society of Critical Care Medicine. Guidelines and levels of care for pediatric intensive care units. *Pediatrics* 1993;92:166.

American Academy of Pediatrics, Task Force on Interhospital Transport. *Guidelines for Air and Ground Transport of Neonatal and Pediatric Patients.* Elk Grove Village, IL: American Academy of Pediatrics, 1993.

American Academy of Pediatrics, Committee on Hospital Care. Staffing patterns for patient care and support personnel in a general pediatric unit. *Pediatrics* 1994;93:850.

American Academy of Pediatrics, Committee on Bioethics. Guidelines on forgoing life-sustaining medical treatment. *Pediatrics* 1994;93:532.

American Academy of Pediatrics, Committee on Bioethics. Informed consent, parental permission, and assent in pediatric practice. *Pediatrics* 1995;95:314.

American Academy of Pediatrics, Committee on Bioethics. Religious objections to medical care. *Pediatrics* 1997; 99:279.

American Academy of Pediatrics, Committee on Hospital Care. Facilities and equipment for the care of pediatric patients in a community hospital. *Pediatrics* 1998;101:1089.

American Academy of Pediatrics, Committee on Hospital Care. The role of the nurse practitioner and physician assistant in the care of hospitalized children. *Pediatrics* 1999;103:1050.

American Academy of Pediatrics, Committee on Child Abuse and Neglect. Distinguishing sudden infant death syndrome from child abuse fatalities. *Pediatrics* 2001;107:437.

American Academy of Pediatrics, Committee on Child Abuse and Neglect. Addendum: Distinguishing sudden infant death syndrome from child abuse fatalities. *Pediatrics* 2001; 108:812.

American Academy of Pediatrics and American College of Emergency Physicians, joint statement. Death of a child in the emergency department. *Ann Emerg Med* 2002;40:409.

American Academy of Pediatrics, Committee on Hospital Care. Pediatric organ donation and transplantation. *Pediatrics* 2002;109:982.

Asser SM, Swan R. Child fatalities from religion-motivated medical neglect. *Pediatrics* 1998;101:625.

Barnes LL, et al. Spirituality, religion and pediatrics: Intersecting worlds of healing. *Pediatrics* 2000;106:899.

Barnes LL, et al. Spirituality, religion and pediatrics: Intersecting worlds of healing. *Pediatrics* 2002;106:899.

Hedayat KM, Pirzadeh R. Issues in Islamic biomedical ethics: A primer for the pediatrician. *Pediatrics* 2001;108:965.

James SE (ed.). *Air and Surface Transport Nurses Association: Standards for Critical Care and Specialty Ground Transport.* Lexington, KY: Myers Printing, 2002.

Mace SE. Pediatric observation medicine. *Emerg Clin North Am* 2001;19:239.

McCarthy PL. Fever. *Pediatr Rev* 1998;19:401.

Sheahan E (ed.). *HIPAA Training Handbook for the Medical Staff: An Overview of HIPAA.* Marblehead, MA: HCPro, 2003.

Sullivan DJ. Minors and emergency medicine. *Emerg Med Clin North Am* 1993;11:841.

The Hospital Infection Control Practices Advisory Committee: guideline for isolation precautions in hospitals. *Am J Infect Control* 1996;24:24.

Tsai AK, et al. Evaluation and treatment of minors: reference on consent. *Ann Emerg Med* 1993;22:1211.

Available at *www.religioustolerance.org.*

ALLERGIC AND IMMUNOLOGIC DISORDERS

Jacqueline A. Pongracic, Section Editor

43 ANAPHYLAXIS

Richard Evans III

EPIDEMIOLOGY

- Increased exposure to an allergic trigger (antigen) is the major risk factor for anaphylaxis. Race, sex, age, geographic location, atopy, or season of the year are not considered major risk factors.
- The most common causes of anaphylaxis are antibiotic injections, especially penicillin (fatality rate = 0.002% injection) followed by Hymenoptera stings (fatality rate = 23 deaths per 150 million stings).

PATHOPHYSIOLOGY

- Anaphylaxis is the clinical manifestation of immediate hypersensitivity. This adverse event occurs rapidly, often dramatically, and is unanticipated.
- Anaphylaxis is the most severe form of allergy and must always be considered a medical emergency.
- Death may occur suddenly through airway obstruction or irreversible vascular collapse.
- Tryptase and histamine are considered to be the important mediators of anaphylaxis. Tryptase is found in normal serum at levels of 1 ng/mL. Histamine is not present in normal serum. Serum levels of both are elevated after anaphylaxis. Tryptase and histamine levels correlate with clinical severity of anaphylaxis. Tryptase is a mast cell-derived mediator that diffuses more slowly than histamine. Tryptase levels peak around 60 minutes; after 1–2 hours they begin a decline with a half-life of 1.5–2.5 hours. Histamine levels peak at 5 minutes and decline with a half-life of 1–2 minutes.

- Small amounts of common proteins can trigger anaphylaxis (Table 43-1).

CLINICAL FEATURES

- Anaphylaxis can vary in severity and is potentially fatal. It is a multisystem disease, especially affecting the skin, the respiratory tract, and the cardiovascular system (Table 43-2).

NOTE

- Anaphylaxis can present with symptoms of only one system. For example, urticaria and/or angioedema is not mandatory. Some patients (as many as 11%) do not have dermatologic symptoms at the time of presentation. A rare patient will present with cardiovascular collapse or acute pulmonary obstruction.

TABLE 43-1   Elicitors of Anaphylaxis/Anaphylactoid Reactions

COMMON	UNCOMMON
Food: peanuts, tree nuts, fish, shellfish, cow milk, eggs	Gelatin
Insect stings and bites: yellow jackets, hornets, wasps, fire ants, honeybees	Immunotherapy
Medications: antibiotics, aspirin, nonsteroidal anti-inflammatory drugs, general anesthetic agents, opioids, insulin, protamine, streptokinase, blood products, progesterone, radio contrast media, antithymocyte globulin	Dialysis membranes Seminal fluid Summation-anaphylaxis
Latex	Idiopathic
Exercise	

TABLE 43-2   The Spectrum of Presentation of Anaphylaxis

GRADE	SKIN	ABDOMEN	RESPIRATORY TRACT	CARDIOVASCULAR SYSTEM
I	Pruritus Flush Urticaria Angioedema			
II	Pruritus Flush Urticaria Angioedema	Nausea Cramping	Rhinorrhea Hoarseness Dyspnea	Tachycardia (Δ>20 beats per minute) BP change (20 mmHg systolic) Arrhythmia
III	Pruritus Flush Urticaria Angioedema	Vomiting Defecation Diarrhea	Laryngeal edema Bronchospasm Cyanosis	Shock
IV	Pruritus Flush Urticaria Angioedema	Vomiting Defecation Diarrhea	Respiratory arrest	Cardiac arrest

DIAGNOSIS AND DIFFERENTIAL

- Some reactions mimic anaphylaxis. These are called pseudoallergic (non-IgE mediated) or anaphylactoid reactions. Causes include direct release of mediators (e.g., morphine, vancomycin), direct activation of complement system (bypass), interaction with kallikrein-kinin system, platelet activation, and psychoneurogenic reactions.

THERAPY

- Drugs and other agents used in the treatment of anaphylaxis and anaphylactoid reactions are listed in Table 43-3. Epinephrine administered intramuscularly is the treatment of choice for anaphylaxis. Other general principles of therapy include treatment of hypoxia, hypotension, and hypovolemia. Bronchospasm should be treated with epinephrine and albuterol.

PROGNOSIS

- Prognosis is generally good; however, this depends on accuracy of early diagnosis and prompt treatment.

PREVENTION

- Prevention is dependent on correct diagnosis, identification, and strict avoidance of the offending agent (trigger). A careful allergy history is essential in the identification of the trigger.
- Educating the patient is key to successful prevention of subsequent reactions. Limiting use of new agents for strict indications only is advised. Hyposensitization should be considered when possible (Hymenoptera

TABLE 43-3   Treatment of Anaphylaxis

Immediate Action

Assessment

Check airway and secure if needed
Rapid assessment of level of consciousness
Vital signs

Treatment

Epinephrine
   (Adult) 1:1000 0.3–0.5 mL IM q 15 minute prn
   (Child) 1:1000 0.01 mL/kg IM q 15 minute prn
Supine position, legs elevated
Oxygen
Tourniquet proximal to injection site (for parenteral allergen exposure)

Dependent on Evaluation

Start peripheral intravenous fluids
H_1 and H_2 antagonist
   Diphenhydramine
      (Adult) 25–50 mg po, IM or IV
      (Child) 12.5–25 mg po, IM or IV
   Ranitidine: 1 mg/kg IV
Corticosteroids
   Methylprednisolone (2 mg/kg q 6 hours) IV
   Hydrocortisone
   <10 kg: 15 mg IV
   10–20 mg: 25 kg IV
   20–40 kg: 40 mg IV
   >40 kg: 50 mg IV
Glucagon—(children) 0.025–0.1 mg/kg/dose, not to exceed
   1 mg/dose IV
Atropine—(children) 0.01–0.02 mg/kg/dose up to a maximum of
   0.4 mg/dose; repeat every 4–6 hours as needed; maximum dose:
   1 mg IV
Electrocardiographic monitoring
Transfer to hospital

Hospital Management

Medical antishock trousers
Continued therapy with above noted agents and management
   of complications

sensitivity). Premedication is useful in preventing ana-phylactoid reactions because of radiocontrast media.

BIBLIOGRAPHY

Anonymous. The diagnosis and management of anaphylaxis. Joint Task Force on Practice Parameters. American Academy of Allergy, Asthma and Immunology, American College of Allergy, Asthma and Immunology, and the Joint Council of Allergy, Asthma and Immunology. [Erratum appears in J Allergy Clin Immunol 1998 Aug;102(2):264]. *Journal of Allergy & Clinical Immunology* 1998;101:S465–528.

Morritt J. Aszkenasy M. The anaphylaxis problem in children: community management in a UK National Health Service District. *Pub Health* 2000;114:456–459.

Rusznak C, Peebles RS Jr. Anaphylaxis and anaphylactoid reactions. A guide to prevention, recognition, and emergent treatment. *Postgrad Med* 2002;111:101–104, 107–108, 111–114.

Kemp SF. Current concepts in pathophysiology, diagnosis and management of anaphylaxis. Immunol Allergy. *Clin North Am* 2001 Nov; 21(4):611–634.

44 ALLERGIC RHINITIS

Patricia Keefe and Richard Evans III

EPIDEMIOLOGY

- Allergic rhinitis affects up to 20% of children in the United States. Although the onset may be at any age, it is a disease that first occurs most commonly in childhood and adolescence.
- Allergic rhinitis to perennial allergens such as mold and dust mite has been described in children as young as 6 months of age. In the case of seasonal allergic rhinitis, such as that seen with grass and tree pollen, the individual must have at least two full seasons of exposure before symptoms can develop.
- The incidence of allergic rhinitis has been on the rise since the 1970s. Potential causes include the increasing urban population, increasing concentration of airborne pollution, and increases in the indoor dust mite population.

PATHOPHYSIOLOGY

- Allergic rhinitis results from the inhalation of allergen to which the patient has specific IgE antibody. Allergen binding causes this IgE to cross-link on the surfaces of mast cells in the nasal mucosa and submucosa resulting in the release of histamine and leukotrienes which mediate symptoms and cytokines.
- The allergic response occurs in two phases. The acute phase is an immediate reaction following exposure to allergen and consists of rhinorrhea, sneezing, and nasal pruritus. This phase is mediated mostly by histamine. The late phase occurs 4–6 hours after exposure with persistent symptoms of nasal congestion and rhinorrhea. This phase is mediated by cellular infiltration into the nasal mucosa and submucosa and the resulting inflammatory reaction. The distinguishing cell in allergic rhinitis is the eosinophil, which can be identified by nasal smear.
- The disease may be caused by perennial allergens, such as mold, cockroach, animal dander, and dust mite. Perennial allergic rhinitis results in year round symptoms. More typically, the pattern of allergic rhinitis is seasonal, with a predictable pattern year after year. In the upper Midwest, for example, spring symptoms come from tree pollens, summer symptoms from grass pollens, and autumn symptoms from ragweed pollen or molds. These patterns vary from one part of the country to another and are based on climate and indigenous botanical populations.

CLINICAL FEATURES

- Rhinitis is a term used to describe symptomatic inflammation of the nasal mucosa characterized by rhinorrhea, sneezing, pruritus, and congestion. Allergic rhinitis is rhinitis attributable to a known allergen and is often accompanied by ocular allergy with symptoms of injected sclera, pruritus, and tearing.
- Typical allergic facies are often noted in children with allergic rhinitis. Findings include open mouth breathing, dark coloration under the eyes (allergic shiners), and a crease across the lower eyelid (Dennie's sign) caused by conjunctival edema. There may be a transverse crease across the lower nose caused by chronic upward rubbing on the tip of the nose; a motion called the "allergic salute." Inspection of the nasal cavity reveals pale, boggy, and sometimes bluish mucosa. Polyps may be present and appear as pearly, smooth, and glistening lesions. They may also take the form of grapelike masses.

DIAGNOSIS AND DIFFERENTIAL

- The differential diagnosis includes nonallergic rhinitis (vasomotor rhinitis), rhinitis medicamentosa, recurrent infectious rhinitis, chronic sinusitis, nasal foreign bodies, nasal polyps, tumors, and anatomic abnormalities of the nasal structures, ciliary disorders, hypothyroidism, and cystic fibrosis.

- Diagnosis is based on symptom complex, seasonal or perennial nature of the symptoms, personal and/or family history of other allergic diseases, physical examination, and evidence of allergen sensitization.

- Skin tests provide confirmatory evidence of specific IgE to an allergen after clinical relevance has been established by the history and physical examination. Positive skin tests without a clinical correlation to history and/or physical examination are clinically insignificant. Skin tests are highly sensitive. False negatives and false positives do occur, usually because of poor technique. False negative results may be the result of concomitant use of antihistamine medication.

- Skin testing for perennial allergens is possible in the very young child; however, for seasonal allergens, skin testing is not reliable until the child is 2–3 years of age, after the child has been exposed to at least two seasons of the allergen in question.

- RAST (radioallergosorbent test) is an in vitro technique for the detection of specific IgE antibodies to various allergens. While not as sensitive as skin testing, it may be employed in place of skin testing when antihistamines have been taken by the patient, high-quality skin testing extracts and well-trained personnel to use them are unavailable, or in the case of widespread eczema or other skin disease precluding skin testing.

TREATMENT

- The treatment of allergic rhinitis includes allergen identification and avoidance of exposure, pharmacotherapy, and in some cases, allergen immunotherapy.

- Successful avoidance of an allergen results in complete resolution of symptoms. If the patient has a pet allergy, the family should be advised to remove the pet from the home. Dust mite control measures include avoidance of down bedding, encasing of bedding in dust mite impermeable covers, and washing bedding in hot water at least biweekly. Mold may be minimized by use of an air conditioner/dehumidifier in the humid summer months and routine cleaning of areas in the home that promote mold growth, such as shower stalls and basements. Of course, avoidance of ubiquitous outdoor pollens is much more problematic and medical treatment and/or immunotherapy is often required.

- Preferred pharmacotherapy includes second-generation antihistamines. The second-generation antihistamines are preferred over first-generation antihistamines because in general they are less sedating. Topical nasal corticosteroids are useful for nasal congestion. Topical cromolyn sodium may be useful particularly for very young children or those individuals who cannot toler-

TABLE 44-1   Pharmacotherapy of Allergic Rhinitis

Second-generation H1 antagonists

Cetirizine (Zyrtec)
Desloratine (Clarinex)
Fexofenadine (Allegra)
Loratadine (Claritin)

Nasal corticosteroids

Budesonide (Rhinocort AQ)
Fluticasone (Flonase)
Mometasone (Nasonex)
Triamcinolone (Nasacort AQ)

Nonsteroid anti-inflammatory nasal spray

Cromolyn Sodium (Nasalcrom)

Ocular preparations

Ketotifen (Optivar)
Levacobastine (Livostin)
Olopatadine (Patanol)

ate or wish to avoid corticosteroids. A variety of ocular preparations are also available. See Table 44-1 for specific medications. Prescribe medications in a stepwise approach based on symptom severity:

Mild episodic symptoms	Oral nonsedating antihistamine PRN OR Topical antihistamine, topical cromolyn sodium to nose, eyes or both
Moderate continuous symptoms	Intranasal corticosteroid daily starting before season AND Oral nonsedating antihistamine daily with or without decongestant Topical treatment as needed
Severe refractory symptoms	Consider other diagnoses/coexisting disease Consider oral corticosteroid therapy for a few days to alleviate symptoms Immunotherapy

- Immunotherapy should be considered in patients with disease refractory to the above interventions, intolerance to medications or intolerable side effects to medications, and when the allergen is hard to avoid or symptoms last more than two seasons of the year. It is proven effective to decrease severity of symptoms in most patients. A minimum of 3 years is required for treatment and a frequent cause of treatment failure is premature discontinuation of therapy. The mechanism of action is not fully understood but may be through modification of the late phase response and the formation of blocking antibodies.

PROGNOSIS

- Without treatment, allergic rhinitis tends to persist indefinitely although remissions do occur. Symptoms, however, may vary from season to season based on patient exposure to allergens. With proper treatment, the prognosis is excellent.

PREVENTION

• Prevention of symptoms is accomplished by decreasing exposure to relevant allergens as much as possible. Keeping windows closed and air-conditioning on during seasons of pollen exposure is helpful. Avoiding pets in the home is essential. Maintaining a dry environment through the use of dehumidifiers and cleaning areas of known mold growth with bleach may minimize mold in the home. Dust mite avoidance, particularly in the bedroom, is also essential.

BIBLIOGRAPHY

Grammer L, Greenberger P, et al. (eds.). *Patterson's Allergic Diseases,* 6th ed. Philadelphia, PA: Lippincott Williams & Wilkins, 2002.

Leiberman P, Anderson J. *Current Clinical Practice: Allergic Diseases: Diagnosis and Treatment,* 2nd ed. Totowa, NJ: Humana Press, 2000.

Middleton E, Reed CE, Ellis EF, et al. (eds.). *Allergy Principles and Practice,* 5th ed. St. Louis, MO: CV Mosby, 1998.

45 ASTHMA
Kristen Koridek and Richard Evans III

EPIDEMIOLOGY

• Asthma is the most common chronic disorder in children and adolescents. About 5 million children under 18 years of age have asthma. This includes an estimated 1.3 million children under the age of 5 years.
• Each year, children with asthma miss more than 10 million school days (on average more than three times the school absences of children without asthma).
• Children living in poverty and/or inner cities have higher rates of hospitalizations and mortality from their asthma.
• Children with asthma often limit activities unnecessarily.

PATHOPHYSIOLOGY

• Asthma is a chronic inflammatory disorder of the airways in which many cells play a role, including mast cells and eosinophils. In susceptible individuals this inflammation causes symptoms which are usually associated with widespread but variable airflow obstruction that is often reversible either spontaneously or with treatment, and causes an associated increase in airway responsiveness to a variety of stimuli.

CLINICAL FEATURES

• Symptoms tend to remit and recur and typically include cough and wheeze.
• Physical examination of the upper respiratory tract, chest, and skin should evaluate for the following findings: hyperexpansion of the thorax; sounds of wheezing during normal breathing or a prolonged phase of forced exhalation; increased nasal secretions, mucosal swelling, sinusitis, rhinitis, or nasal polyps; and atopic dermatitis/eczema or other signs of allergic skin problems.

DIAGNOSIS AND DIFFERENTIAL

• The diagnosis of asthma in adults and children over 5 years of age is often established by thorough history. Recurrent episodes of coughing or wheezing are almost always because of asthma in these age groups. Cough can be the sole symptom. Findings that increase the probability of asthma include episodic wheeze, chest tightness, shortness of breath, or cough; symptoms worsen in presence of aeroallergens, irritants, or exercise; symptoms occur or worsen at night, awakening the patient; patient has allergic rhinitis or atopic dermatitis; and close relatives have asthma, allergy, sinusitis, or rhinitis.
• Objective assessment of pulmonary function is also useful in making the diagnosis. Since asthma symptoms are episodic, PEFR or FEV_1 may be normal. Spirometry may show an obstructive pattern with FEV_1 <80% predicted. A beta-agonist, such as albuterol, may be administered to assess for reversibility of airway obstruction. Fifteen percent improvement in FEV_1 is touted to be diagnostic of asthma.
• Chest radiography is rarely used for the diagnosis of asthma. Findings may include hyperexpansion, flattened diaphragms, and atelectasis but imaging is often normal. Chest x-ray is useful in determining the presence of pneumomediastinum or pneumothorax in acute asthma.
• The diagnosis of asthma in infants and children younger than 5 years of age is usually more difficult than in older children. Young children with asthma are often mislabeled as having bronchiolitis, bronchitis, or pneumonia. As a result, many do not receive adequate therapy. The diagnostic steps listed previously are the same for this age group except that spirometry

TABLE 45-1 Features of Asthma Severity and Corresponding Therapy*

	INTERMITTENT STEP 1	MILD PERSISTENT STEP 2	MODERATE PERSISTENT STEP 3	SEVERE PERSISTENT STEP 4
Day Symp	Symptoms ≤2 times a week	Symptoms >2 times a week, < daily	Daily symptoms/uses bronchodilator daily	Continuous symptoms Limited physical activity Frequent attacks
Noc Symp	≤2 times a month	>2 times a month	>1 time weekly	Frequent
PF	Normal	Normal	60–80% predicted	≤60% predicted
Therapy	Short-acting bronchodilator, inhaled beta$_2$-agonist, prn. Alb 2 puffs q 4–6 hours	One daily long-term preventive medication low-dose steroid,** short-acting bronchodilator, inhaled beta$_2$-agonist, prn **Age ≤ 12 years** Bud DPI 200 mcg/dose = 200 mcg qd Pulm resp 0.5 mg qd Flu MDI 44 μg, 88–176 μg/day = 2–4 puffs of 44 μg/day Alb 2 puffs q 4–6 hours, prn **Age > 12 years** Bud DPI 200 μg/dose 200–400 μg = 1–2 inh qd Flu MDI 44 μg, 110 μg, 88–264 μg/day = 2–6 puffs of 44 μg or 2 puffs of 110 μg/day Alb 2 puffs q 4–6 hours, prn	Daily long-term preventive medications. Inhaled steroid, medium dose. Short-acting bronchodilator, inhaled beta$_2$-agonist, prn **Age ≤ 12 years** Bud DPI 200 μg/dose 200–400 μg = (1–2 inh)/day Pulm resp 0.5–1 mg qd Flu 44 or 110 μg, 176–400 μg = 4–10 puffs of 44 μg/day or 2–4 puffs of 110 μg/day Adv 100/50 1 puff bid or 250/50 1 puff bid Alb 2 puffs q 4–6 hours, prn no more than 3 doses **Age > 12 years** Bud DPI 200 μg/dose, 400 μg = (2–3 inh)/day Flu 264–660 μg = 2–6 puffs of 110 μg Adv 100/50 1 puff bid or 250/50 1 puff bid Alb 2 puffs q 4–6 hours, prn	Multiple daily long-term preventive agents. Inhaled steroid, high dose. Corticosteroid tablets or syrup qd Short-acting bronchodilator, inhaled beta$_2$-agonist, prn. **Age ≤ 12 years** Bud DPI 200 μg/dose >400 μg = >2 inh/day Pulm resp 0.5–1 mg qd Flu >440 μg = >4 puffs of 110 μg or >2 puffs of 220 μg/day Adv 250/50 1 puff bid or 500/50 1 puff bid Alb 2 puffs q 4–6 hours, prn no more than 3 doses **Age > 12 years** Bud DPI 200 μg/dose, >600 μg = >3 inh/day Flu >660 μg, =>6 puffs of 110 μg or >3 puffs of 220 μg/day Adv 250/50 1 puff bid or 500/50 1 puff bid Alb 2 puffs q 4–6 hours, prn

*The presence of one of the features of severity is sufficient to place a patient in that severity level.

**If symptoms persist or increase, increase steroid dose.

ABBREVIATIONS: PF = peak flow; Alb = Albuterol; Bud = Budesonide; Pulm resp = Pulmicort Respules; Flu = Fluticasone; Adv = Advair; MDI = Meter Dose Inhaler.

SOURCE: Modified from Tables 3-4a and 3-4b (pp. 45–46) in *Guidelines for the Diagnosis and Management of Asthma*, Expert Panel Report II, 1997.

is not possible. A trial of asthma medications may aid in the eventual diagnosis.

- Diagnosis is not needed to begin to treat wheezing associated with an upper respiratory viral infection, which is the most common precipitant of wheezing in children under age 5. Patients should be monitored carefully.
- There are two general patterns of illness in infants and children who have wheezing with acute viral upper respiratory infections: a remission of symptoms in the preschool years and persistence of asthma throughout childhood. The factors associated with persistence of asthma are allergies, a family history of asthma, and early exposure to aeroallergens and passive smoke.

THERAPY

- Classify asthma severity as intermittent, mild persistent, moderate persistent, or severe persistent based on combined assessments of symptoms and lung function. Therapy of asthma is based on the assessment of severity (see Table 45-1).
- Acute asthma management includes the use of beta-agonists for quick relief. When beta-agonists are ineffective or required more than four times a day, add oral corticosteroids (1–2 mg/kg/day) for 3–5 days.

PROGNOSIS

- There is no cure for asthma. Symptoms sometimes decrease over time. With proper self-management and medication treatment, most people with asthma can lead normal lives.

PREVENTION

- Asthma management and prevention has six interrelated parts:
  1. Educate patients to develop a partnership in asthma management.
  2. Assess and monitor asthma severity with objective measures of lung function.
  3. Avoid or control asthma triggers.
  4. Establish medication plans for chronic management.
  5. Establish plans for managing exacerbations.
  6. Provide regular follow-up care.

REFERENCES

Expert Panel Report 2 Guidelines for the Diagnosis and Management of Asthma. NIH Publication No. 97-4051, 1997.

46 DRUG ALLERGY
Rajesh Kumar

IgE-MEDIATED REACTIONS AND PSEUDO-ALLERGIC REACTIONS

EPIDEMIOLOGY

- Drug allergy is the disease state resulting from an abnormal immune response to a drug. This includes IgE-mediated reactions to drugs reviewed in this section. It should be clear that this is distinct from known side effects, drug interactions, genetically predisposed intolerances (such as G6PD deficiency), or idiosyncratic reactions.
- Fifteen to 30% of adult hospitalized patients experience adverse drug reactions and allergic/immunologic drug reactions accounted for 6–10% of them. Skin reactions are the most frequent manifestation occurring in 80% of cases compared to anaphylaxis (9–15% of cases).
- In a drug surveillance program, 0.04% of people registered had anaphylaxis.
- While these numbers represent adult data for the most part, there are no similar large studies of children.
- Drug allergy is not associated with allergic status in general. The greatest risk factor for drug allergy is repeated exposure. Topical and parenteral routes seem to be more likely to sensitize than oral routes of drug administration. Also while there are some studies suggesting a genetic predisposition in families with multiple drug allergy, this does not correspond to the general population.

PATHOPHYSIOLOGY

- Typically, these reactions include those which are associated with either IgE-mediated reactions to a drug or non-IgE-mediated mast cell activation such as occurs with opioids or radiocontrast media.

CLINICAL FEATURES

- The manifestations of both types of reactions are similar. Symptoms may be limited to the skin (pruritus, urticaria, erythematous flushing, or angioedema) or they may be systemic. Systemic manifestations include bronchospasm, laryngeal oedema, hypotension, hyperperistalsis, and emesis. These events may be present alone or in combination.

- Symptoms typically have rapid onset within an hour of exposure.
- An IgE-mediated reaction does not usually occur on first exposure to a drug; however, pseudo-allergic reactions may occur on first exposure.

DIAGNOSIS AND DIFFERENTIAL

- Most essential for diagnosis is history and good documentation. Standardized testing is available for penicillins and is reliable. Large adult studies show that penicillin skin testing is 98.8% sensitive. Specificity is less clear since intentional challenges are not routinely carried out in patients with clear histories and positive skin tests.
- Testing is available for a number of anesthetic agents with good negative predictive value, but this is not standardized. Testing for IgE-mediated reactions is also suggested for certain protein macromolar drugs such as insulin, streptokinase, chymopapain, and tetanus toxoid.
- Testing with most other drugs is limited by scanty data where optimal concentrations and predictive values are not well-established.
- Skin testing is clearly not appropriate for anaphylactoid reactions since these reactions are not IgE-mediated. Examples include radiocontrast media, opiates, nonsteroidal anti-inflammatory drugs (NSAIDs), and red man syndrome with Vancomycin.

TREATMENT

- STOP THE ADMINISTRATION OF THE OFFEND-ING AGENT!!
- The treatment of purely cutaneous urticarial reactions involves the use of a short-acting, faster onset antihistamine such as diphenhydramine and may include the short-term use of corticosteroids.
- Treatment of anaphylaxis has as its cornerstone epinephrine (1:1000 at a dose of 0.01 mL/kg up to 0.5 mL intramuscularly) and aggressive supportive care. For further treatment on anaphylaxis, refer to the section on Anaphylaxis.
- If the drug is essential and the only option for care, desensitization for IgE-mediated reactions may be considered with the help of an allergist/immunologist. This should not be taken lightly as it is a potentially life-threatening procedure which can only be considered in a monitored setting capable of early response to anaphylaxis.

PROGNOSIS

- While most urticarial reactions are easily controlled, anaphylaxis can be severe and biphasic in 5–20% of cases. There are also cases of protracted anaphylaxis. As such, the physician must act quickly to treat anaphylaxis as soon as it is recognized.

PREVENTION

- *Avoid* agents known to cause these reactions.
- For previous *pseudo-allergic* reactions to radiocontrast media, ensure that low ionic contrast media is used. For essential procedures, use a premedication regimen of prednisone 1 mg/kg/dose (at 13 hours preprocedure/7 hours preprocedure/and 1 hour preprocedure) along with a dose of diphenhydramine 1 mg/kg (1 hour preprocedure). This protocol may decrease the incidence and severity of anaphylactoid reactions. *This protocol should not be used for prevention of anaphylactic reactions.*
- Another key issue in prevention is to minimize the number of courses of medications that a patient receives to decrease chance of sensitization.

OTHER COMMON (NON-IgE-MEDIATED) REACTIONS

DELAYED MACULAR OR PAPULAR CUTANEOUS DRUG ERUPTIONS

EPIDEMIOLOGY
- This is the most common drug-induced eruption.
- Estimates in adult and mixed populations suggest that this occurs in up to 10% of patients on aminopenicillins and 2% of patients on other penicillins.
- These types of eruptions are also common in acquired immunodeficiency syndrome (AIDS) patients receiving sulfonamides (up to 50–60%).
- Other higher risk groups include patients with Epstein-Barr virus (EBV), cytomegalovirus (CMV), and chronic lymphocytic leukemia.

CLINICAL FEATURES
- These eruptions usually develop within a week of initiation of the offending drug.
- Simple eruptions do not typically involve eosinophilia, fevers, arthralgias, hepatitis, or adenopathy. Such features would suggest hypersensitivity syndrome or serum sickness.
- The eruptions have a variable course and may range from erythematous, morbilliform, and macular to

papular rashes. They do not include purpura or blistering lesions, which may indicate vasculitis or target-toid lesions, respectively.
- Pruritus is not uniformly present.

DIAGNOSIS AND DIFFERENTIAL
- No reliable clinically available laboratory tests are available. The diagnosis is established by history and clinical features.

TREATMENT
- The most prudent course of action is discontinuation of the offending agent and avoidance of this agent in the future.
- Pruritus and mild cutaneous reactions may be treated with antihistamines. Desensitization protocols are available for these types of reactions in HIV patients who must have sulfadiazine for prophylaxis and cannot use alternative agents.

PROGNOSIS
- In the absence of features of serum sickness, hypersensitivity syndrome, Stevens-Johnson syndrome (SJS), or toxic epidermal necrolysis (TEN), these reactions remit with withdrawal of the agent. Usually, resolution occurs within a few days.

PREVENTION
- Avoid amino-penicillins in cases where EBV is suspected. As always, minimize drug use (especially antimicrobials) to clearly indicated usage.

SERUM SICKNESS

EPIDEMIOLOGY
- Since heterologous sera are used very infrequently (except for treatment of evenomation, botulism, diphtheria, and rabies), these are now an uncommon cause of serum sickness.
- Serum sickness-like reactions are seen more commonly with beta-lactams or other antimicrobials, anticonvulsants, or Thiouracil. Cefaclor is estimated to cause this syndrome in 1.8/100,000 courses and may be the most common cause of this reaction.

CLINICAL FEATURES
- Symptoms start 6–21 days after the administration of the agent if the person has not been previously exposed. Symptoms include fever, malaise, skin eruptions, adenopathy, and joint symptoms of arthralgias or arthritis.

DIAGNOSIS AND DIFFERENTIAL
- The diagnosis is clinical but laboratory features may be supportive. These features are variably present and transient such as hematologic abnormalities (leukopenia/leukocytosis/plasmacytosis) liver transaminase elevations, creatinine elevations, and complement consumption (decreased $C_3/C_4/CH_{50}$ and presence of positive immunoassays for immune complexes).

TREATMENT
- Stop the offending agent!!
- Severe cases may benefit from a course of systemic corticosteroids with a taper.
- Antihistamines may be used for pruritus.
- Supportive care is important for any end-organ damage.

PROGNOSIS
- Mild disease is usually self-limited, but more severe disease requires hospitalization and several weeks to fully resolve.

PREVENTION
- Limit use of antibiotics. Avoid agents such as Cefaclor if equally effective drugs are available.
- Never readminister the offending agent.
- If foreign serum was the cause, then subsequent skin testing with antisera should be employed to avoid potential anaphylaxis on reexposure.

TWO RARE BUT IMPORTANT SEVERE REACTIONS: STEVENS-JOHNSON SYNDROME (SJS) AND TOXIC EPIDERMAL NECROLYSIS (TEN)

EPIDEMIOLOGY

- TEN has an incidence of 0.4–1.2 cases/million population with a mortality rate of 30%.
- SJS has a prevalence of 1–6 cases/million people years with estimated rates of mortality of 5%.
- Drugs are felt to cause 50% of these reactions. More commonly implicated drugs include sulfonamides, anticonvulsants, barbiturates, piroxicams, allopurinol, and amino-penicillins.

CLINICAL FEATURES

- Usually these diseases begin within 1–3 weeks of initiation of therapy.
- SJS has features which include mucosal lesions at ≥2 sites, target lesions or initially papular lesions with

rare areas of confluence, detachment of ≤10% of body surface area, and lesions of the respiratory or gastrointestinal tracts. Ten to thirty percent of cases may involve fever, and serious ocular complications may occur in 10% of patients.

- TEN has features which are similar to SJS, but more severe. Mucosal lesions at ≥2 sites are present. Individual cutaneous lesions may be similar to those seen in SJS. Lateral pressure results in separation of the upper layer of the epidermis from the basal layer (Nikolsky's sign) with large sheets of necrotic epidermis. As compared to SJS, TEN has >30% detachment of epidermal body surface area. Leukopenia is common. Gastrointestinal and respiratory epithelial involvement is extremely common, and ocular complications may occur in 10%.

DIAGNOSIS

- The pediatrician must evaluate for the clinical features noted above.
- Dermatology should be consulted if the diagnosis is suspected but not fully established yet (immunofluoresence and electron microscopy of skin samples may be helpful).

TREATMENT

- Supportive treatment in high acuity units is essential.
- Intensive care unit (ICU) care is important for all cases of TEN where fluid losses may be great. Allergy and dermatology consultations may be helpful in current and future management. Ophthalmology should be involved in all severe SJS and in all cases of TEN.
- The role of corticosteroids is controversial with some centers reporting improved outcomes in large series. Others suggest that infection and ocular complications may be more common with the use of corticosteroids.
- Most other treatments have not been well studied, including recent experience with IVIG in TEN.

CLINICAL FEATURES OF HYPERSENSITIVITY SYNDROME AND OTHER DISEASES

HYPERSENSITIVITY SYNDROME/VASCULITIS

- This reaction usually starts 7–10 days after the onset of drug therapy. The rash may range from macular to palpable purpura. There may be associated fever, joint disease, nephritis, hepatitis, pleuropulmonary and cardiovascular manifestations (usually milder).

- Peripheral eosinophilia may be marked with associated leukocytosis and elevated erythrocyte sedimentation rate (ESR).
- Small vessel granulocytic/mononuclear infiltration is often present on biopsy. Leukocytoclastic changes do not have to be present.
- Treatment includes withdrawal of the agent and supportive care. Corticosteroids have been used in those severely affected.
- Anticonvulsants are a known cause with significant cross-reactivity between phenytoin, phenobarbital, carbamazapine, and possibly lamotrigine. In these cases, the prognosis is usually worse and may be associated with eosinophilic infiltration and noncaseating granuloma formation.

DRUG-INDUCED SYSTEMIC LUPUS ERYTHEMATOSUS (SLE)

- The most common causes include hydralazine and procainamide. Anticonvulsants are also noted to cause this syndrome.
- The onset is usually more abrupt than idiopathic systemic lupus erythematosus (SLE) and the course usually milder, with less frequent renal and neurologic involvement.
- Other drug-related adverse reactions include some of those listed below. For more extensive discussion of these diseases, refer to the Bibliography section.
- Organ system manifestations of systemic diseases may occur, e.g., pulmonary infiltrates with eosinophilia, eosinophilic nephritis, allergic hepatitis, end-organ damage associated with lupus, like syndrome, and drug-associated vasculitis.
- Other cutaneous reactions to drugs are important to note including fixed drug eruption, contact dermatitis, photoallergic and phototoxic reactions, purpura fulminans, acute generalized exanthematous pustulosis, and erythema multiforme minor.

BIBLIOGRAPHY

Adkinson NF. Drug allergy. In: Middleton E, Reed C, Ellis E, Adkinson NF, Busse W (eds.), *Allergy Principles and Practice*, 5th ed. St. Louis, MO: Mosby, 1998.

DeShazo RD, Kemp S. Allergic reactions to drugs and biologic agents. *JAMA* 1997;278(22):1895–1906.

Ditto AM, et al. Drug allergy. In: Grammer LG, Greenberger PA (eds.), *Patterson's Allergic Diseases*, 6th ed. Philadelphia, PA: Lippincott Williams & Wilkins, 2002.

47 FOOD ALLERGY

Jennifer Kim and Jacqueline Pongracic

EPIDEMIOLOGY

- Six to 8% of children younger than 3 years have food allergy. The overall prevalence of food allergy in children younger than 18 years is only 1–2%. Although parents perceive the prevalence to be higher at 28%, only one-quarter of cases in children are confirmed to be because of food hypersensitivity.
- Food allergy is increasing in prevalence, but the etiology of this trend is unclear. The rise in children may be due to introduction of foods to an immature immune system and/or gastrointestinal tract. The mechanisms have yet to be fully elucidated.
- The incidence is higher in children with a family history of allergic diseases such as asthma, allergic rhinitis, and atopic dermatitis (AD). Up to 40% of children with AD have associated food allergies.
- Food allergy is the most common cause of severe anaphylaxis outside the hospital setting. Actual mortality rates are unknown, but an estimated 100 Americans die of food-induced anaphylaxis each year. There are four major risk factors for fatal food-induced anaphylaxis: concomitant asthma (especially if it is poorly controlled), delay in administration of epinephrine, previous severe allergic reaction to the same food, and denial of symptoms.

PATHOPHYSIOLOGY

- Exposure to a particular food protein may induce two aberrant immune responses: IgE-antibody-mediated food allergy (T cells direct B cells to produce IgE) in which the primary effector cells are basophils and mast cells or non-IgE-mediated food allergy (cell-mediated).
- IgE-mediated (Gell and Coombs Type I) hypersensitivity accounts for most food allergies. Onset of symptoms is usually within minutes but most reactions occur within 2 hours of exposure or ingestion. This acute response may be followed by a late-phase response 4–6 hours later. Approximately one-third of food-induced anaphylactic reactions are biphasic.
- Food allergens are composed of glycoproteins. In general, they are water soluble, heat-stable, and resistant to acid and enzymatic degradation. Food processing can potentially alter antigenicity. For example, fish allergens may be changed with the canning process. In some cases, the allergen is degraded by cooking (such as in fruits and vegetables), but most food allergens are unaltered by heat.
- Any food may cause allergy, but the "big 8" cause 93% of food allergy in young children. In order of frequency, beginning with the most common, these are egg, peanut, cow milk, soy, tree nuts, fish, shellfish or crustacea, and wheat.
- In older children and adults, common allergens include peanut, crustacea, tree nuts, and fish.
- Other foods that are commonly listed as allergens but rarely have true significance include corn, tomato, strawberry, citrus, chocolate, food dyes, and preservatives.

CLINICAL FEATURES

- Cutaneous reactions are the most common reactions but are not required for diagnosis. Acute urticaria, angioedema, flushing, and morbilliform pruritic dermatitis may develop. Exacerbations of AD also occur; food allergies have been confirmed by double-blind placebo-controlled food challenges (DBPCFC) in 15–30% of children with AD. Contact urticaria is defined as hives that develop at sites of direct contact with food; it is difficult to assess the risk of systemic involvement in these situations.
- Gastrointestinal reactions are the second most frequent manifestations of food allergy. Symptoms include nausea, vomiting, diarrhea, and abdominal pain or cramping. Oral symptoms include pruritus, tingling, and edema of the lips, tongue, palate, and throat.
- Respiratory symptoms usually occur as part of a generalized anaphylactic reaction. Symptoms include sneezing, rhinorrhea, congestion, nasal pruritus, dysphonia, bronchospasm, and laryngeal edema. Patients may describe a feeling of tightness or a "lump" in the throat, itchiness in the throat, a dry hacking cough, dysphonia, or pruritus in the ear canals. Six percent of children with asthma have food-induced wheezing.
- Anaphylaxis is defined as an acute severe reaction involving one or more organ systems. Up to 11% of anaphylactic reactions are not accompanied by skin manifestations. Other generalized symptoms include dizziness or a feeling of "impending doom." (Please see anaphylaxis section for further explanation.)
- There is no evidence that food allergy induces otitis media, attention deficit/hyperactivity disorder (ADHD), autism, or seizures.

DIAGNOSIS AND DIFFERENTIAL

- The history is paramount to establishing the diagnosis. Identify the *food* suspected and the quantity ingested. Also identify the *symptoms* of the reaction and when they last occurred. Focus on the *timing* of the ingestion to the onset of symptoms (within 2 hours for an IgE-mediated reaction). Ascertain the *consistency* of reactions that occur with repeated exposure to the particular food. Consider other factors (such as exercise) that may be associated with the reaction. Investigate if occult ingredients may have triggered a reaction; consider foods included in processing or contamination (in preparation or from shared equipment at a factory).
- The diagnosis is confirmed by the determination of the presence of food-specific IgE antibody, results of elimination diets, and responses to oral food challenges. A dietary diary may also be a helpful tool but is limited by recall bias.
- Skin prick tests (SPT) assess for the presence of specific IgE antibody. SPT is a relatively quick and inexpensive procedure that is generally performed in an allergy office setting. If allergen specific IgE antibody is present, mast cells will release mediators that will cause a wheal and flare response. There is no age limit; even infants may undergo SPT. The false positive rate is 50–60%, but SPT have a high negative predictive value (more than 95%).
- Radioallergosorbent test (RAST) is an in vitro test that determines the presence and concentration of food-specific IgE antibody. This test is less sensitive, less specific, more expensive, and more time-consuming than SPT; however, RAST is preferred in patients with dermatographism, skin eruptions, or if antihistamines cannot be withheld. RAST is used to assist in the confirmation of a diagnosis or in monitoring patients with a known food allergy. There is no uniform measure at which results indicate a true or severe food allergy, and the level of the RAST score is not necessarily predictive of severity of reaction. There is a high false positive rate, especially in highly atopic children. Ordering "panels" of food allergy tests can be disastrous. Tests should be performed based only on potential triggers as established by history.
- The CAP System FEIA-RAST (Pharmacia & Upjohn, Bridgewater, NJ) is a particular method of RAST that is useful in the measurement of IgE to specific allergens. The CAP-RAST has increased sensitivity compared to other RASTs; the positive predictive value is similar to SPT for cow milk, fish, egg, and peanut. Studies have determined values for which there are 95% confidence limits that a child

with AD has clinical reactivity or not. Values have been established for cow milk, fish, egg, peanut, soy, and wheat.
- Note that SPT and RAST cannot be used as sole proof of clinical allergy.
- Cross-reactivity can be demonstrated on SPT and RAST, but this often does not correlate clinically. For example, peanuts and other legumes have immunologic cross-reactivity, but allergic reactions to more than one legume are rare in a given individual.
- Oral food challenges are indicated when the history and testing are equivocal or contradictory and when multiple foods are implicated. Challenges may be helpful in the diagnosis but must be performed in an appropriate clinical setting where emergency resuscitation can be easily performed if necessary. DBPCFC are considered the gold standard for the diagnosis of food allergies. One may also proceed with an open or single-blinded oral challenge in the office setting, again with appropriate emergency medical equipment available. Open challenges are also used to determine if the child has developed tolerance to the food after a period of strict avoidance.
- An elimination diet may be necessary to establish the diagnosis of food hypersensitivity. If confounding factors are eliminated and the patient is able to exclude the correct allergen(s) from the diet, a lack of response to the elimination diet excludes the culprit foods as a cause of the disorder; however, if multiple foods are potentially responsible but difficult to ascertain by history and laboratory tests, an elemental diet may be tried to establish a diagnosis. A trial of casein hydrolysate (Alimentum, Nutramigen) or amino acid-derived (Neocate, EleCare) formula may be useful. If symptoms resolve, a food challenge is generally required to confirm the diagnosis and allergen.
- A variety of disorders mimic the presentation of food allergy. Structural gastrointestinal disorders in infants and young children present with abdominal pain, vomiting, and diarrhea following feedings or with chronic cough and wheezing associated with recurrent aspiration. Examples include hiatal hernia, pyloric stenosis, and the H-type tracheoesophageal fistula.
- Deficiencies of enzymes such as disaccharidase, lactase, or sucrase produce abdominal cramps and diarrhea. Pancreatic insufficiency and gallbladder/liver disease should also be considered as potential causes of malabsorption.
- Various bacterial toxins (such as *Staphylococcus* and *E. coli*) cause abdominal pain, vomiting, and diarrhea.
- Many toxins produce symptoms that may appear indistinguishable from immediate hypersensitivity reactions, such as scromboid poisoning. Ingestion from histamine-like spoilage products may result in

sudden angioedema, hives, abdominal pain, or throat tightness. Tuna, mackerel, and skipjack are the most commonly implicated fish.

- Methylxanthines (such as caffeine) cause nervousness, tremor, and tachycardia.
- Ethanol may cause flushing, tachycardia, hypotension, somnolence, nausea, and vomiting in sensitive individuals.
- Vasoactive amines (epinephrine, dopamine) are found in bananas, tomatoes, avocados, cheeses, pineapples, and wines. Chocolate also contains phenylethylamine. Symptoms from these foods, however, are rarely confused with true allergic reactions.
- Bulemia and anorexia should also be considered.

TREATMENT

- For the acute allergic reaction, treatment is dependent upon the severity of symptoms. When symptoms are limited to the skin (urticaria or angioedema, not affecting the airway), diphenhydramine (5 mg/kg/day divided q 6 hours) or other antihistamine therapy may be the only medication required. More significant symptoms, such as respiratory distress or cardiovascular collapse, require rapid administration of epinephrine (1:1000) 0.01 mg/kg/dose IM q 15 minutes as necessary. (Please see Anaphylaxis discussion.)
- All patients with IgE-mediated allergic reactions to foods should be prescribed and trained in the use of injectable epinephrine. It must be carried at all times. All caregivers, including school staff, should be familiar with its administration. Epinephrine administration should immediately trigger a call to emergency medical services or transport to the nearest hospital for further evaluation. Patients should be observed for a minimum of 4 hours in case of a biphasic reaction.
- A written emergency health care plan should also be given to the family, which outlines indications for antihistamines and epinephrine. A medical emergency bracelet or necklace is also highly recommended.
- Avoidance of subsequent reactions is achievable only through strict dietary avoidance of the culprit food. Education regarding food labeling and avoidance, including potential hidden food sources, should be directed to parents and caregivers of young patients.
- Support groups such as the Food Allergy and Anaphylaxis Network (www.foodallcrgy.org, 800-929-4040) are invaluable in assisting families successfully eliminate allergenic foods.
- A dietician may also be helpful in optimizing the nutrition of a child with multiple food allergies.

PROGNOSIS

- Strict avoidance gives the child the best chance possible for outgrowing their food allergy. Of course, the likelihood of the development of tolerance also depends on the particular allergen. Approximately 85% of children will outgrow their allergy to egg, milk, soy, or wheat by the age of 5 years whereas those with peanut, tree nut, fish, or shellfish allergy are less likely to develop tolerance.
- A decline in specific IgE antibody is associated with loss of clinical reactivity. SPT and RAST may remain positive in children who become clinically tolerant.

PREVENTION

- The Committee on Nutrition of the American Academy of Pediatrics has published recommendations for infants at risk to develop atopic disease given a strong family history but these guidelines have not been proved to prevent food allergy consistently. Breastfeeding is recommended for the first year of life. The mother should also avoid peanuts and tree nuts with consideration of elimination of egg, milk, and fish. No specific recommendations are available for diet during pregnancy. Foods commonly associated with allergy should be introduced to the child as follows: solid food (after 6 months), milk (after 12 months), egg (after 24 months), and peanut, tree nuts, and fish (after 36 months).

OTHER RELATED DISEASES

- Oral allergy syndrome (OAS) results in oral pruritus and mucosal edema associated with ingestion of some fresh fruits and vegetables. This reaction occurs mainly in patients with concurrent pollen allergy and is caused by IgE antibodies that cross-react with proteins found in the pollens and fruits/vegetables. OAS rarely progresses to involve other organs except in the case of celery root ingestion in birch pollen-allergic patients. Interestingly, patients often tolerate the cooked form of these same foods because the responsible allergens are typically destroyed in the heating process. OAS may affect up to 40% of adults with pollen allergy.
- Food-dependent exercise-induced anaphylaxis or urticaria typically occurs only when the patient exercises within 2–4 hours of ingestion of the food allergen. In the absence of exercise, the patient ingests the food without any reaction. SPT is usually positive. Avoidance of the food prior to any anticipated exercise is recommended.

• Allergic eosinophilic gastroenteropathy is characterized by eosinophilic infiltration of the gastrointestinal (GI) tract, most commonly the mucosal layer. Approximately 50% of adult cases have evidence of an IgE-mediated process, supported by positive skin tests to multiple foods. Signs and symptoms may include those of reflux, postprandial abdominal pain, vomiting, early satiety, and diarrhea. Weight loss and failure to thrive are hallmarks of this disorder in infants and children. If allergy testing does not easily identify the culprit foods, trial of a strict elimination diet may be necessary.

BIBLIOGRAPHY

Pastorello EA, Ortolani C. Oral allergy syndrome. *Food Allergy: Adverse Reactions to Foods and Food Additives*, 2nd ed., 1997, pp. 221–234.

Sampson HA. Immediate reactions to foods in infants and children. *Food Allergy: Adverse Reactions to Foods and Food Additives*, 2nd ed., 1997, pp. 169–182.

Sampson HA. Food allergy. Part 1: immunopathogenesis and clinical disorders. *J Allergy Clin Immunol* 1999;103(5):717–728.

Sampson HA. Food allergy. Part 2: diagnosis and management. *J Allergy Clin Immunol* 1999;103(6):981–989.

Sicherer S. Food allergy. *Lancet* 2002;360(9334):701–710 .

48   SINUSITIS

Kelly Newhall and Rajesh Kumar

• Sinusitis is inflammation of one or more of the paranasal sinuses. Because bacterial infection of the sinuses usually involves the nasal epithelium as well, one might describe this infection as rhinosinusitis.
• Sinusitis is classified by duration as acute (less than 4 weeks), subacute (1–3 months), chronic (at least 3 months) and recurrent (>3 infections/year).

EPIDEMIOLOGY

• Each year over 20 million cases of acute sinusitis are diagnosed. Sinusitis is the fifth most common reason for which antibiotics are prescribed.
• In normal children, approximately 5–13% of viral infections with sinus involvement will be complicated by acute bacterial sinusitis (Brook et al., 2000). The peak incidence at the ages of 3–6 years correlates with the peak incidence of viral upper respiratory infections (URIs).
• Pathogens most frequently implicated in pediatric cases of acute bacterial sinusitis are *Streptococcus pneumoniae* (30–66%), *Haemophilus influenzae* NT (nontypeable) (35%), and *Moraxella catarrhalis* (4–12%). Little data exist for the pathogens of chronic bacterial sinusitis in children; however, in adults pathogens include those listed above as well as *Staphylococcus aureus*, group A *Streptococcus*, *Pseudomonas aeruginosa*, and anaerobes.
• The prevalence of allergic or nonallergic fungal sinusitis in immunocompetent children is unknown. In adults, however, approximately 7% with chronic sinusitis will have an underlying fungal pathogen. The most common species recovered from children are *Bipolaris* sp., *Curvularia* sp., and *Aspergillus* sp. Aspergillus fumigatus may be the most common cause of fungal sinusitis in immunocompetent adults.
• Risk factors for the development of sinusitis include frequent URIs (i.e., children in daycare), a history of allergic rhinitis, nasal polyposis, and anatomic abnormalities of the ostiomeatal unit (OMU). In addition, other underlying diseases such as cystic fibrosis, ciliary dyskinesia, and other immunodeficiencies place children at risk for the development of chronic or recurrent sinus disease. Conflicting epidemiologic data exist regarding the relationship of environmental tobacco smoke (ETS) and risk of sinusitis. One study found that children exposed to ETS had poorer surgical outcomes after endoscopic sinus surgery.

PATHOPHYSIOLOGY OF SINUSITIS

See Table 48-1 for age of onset of sinusitis.

TABLE 48-1   Age of Onset of Sinusitis

Sinus	Age of development	Age radiographically apparent
Ethmoid and maxillary	4 months gestation	birth
Frontal	6–12 months of age	3–7 years of age
Sphenoid	3 years of age	9 years of age

• Ostial blockage is important in the development of bacterial sinusitis. The ostia most frequently affected are those that drain into the OMU, which are the maxillary and ethmoid sinuses. The OMU is a region within the middle meatus, under the middle turbinate. The ostia which drain into this compact area are easily obstructed.

- Over 80% of episodes of sinusitis are preceded by a viral URI. The remaining 20% of cases arise in children affected by complications of allergic rhinitis.
- The following basic physiologic derangements predispose the patient to an overgrowth of bacteria: inflammation with diminished mucociliary transport and increased mucus production; mucosal edema/mucus impaction with decreased patency of the sinus ostia, and subsequent impaired ventilatory exchange. The combination of stagnant secretions, decreased oxygen tension, and decreased pH create an ideal medium for the overgrowth of bacteria.

CLINICAL FEATURES

- Symptoms of acute bacterial sinusitis may include rhinorrhea, nasal congestion, fever, cough, halitosis, snoring, mouth breathing, feeding problems, and postnasal drip. Chronic sinusitis symptoms may include facial pain, headache, and chronic cough in addition to those symptoms of acute sinusitis. Cough is the most frequent manifestation of chronic sinusitis in children. Older children may complain of facial pain and tooth pain, whereas younger children are less likely to do so.
- Signs (variably present) include the presence of purulent nasal mucus and posterior oropharyngeal drainage, sinus tenderness, and middle ear effusions. The presence of unilateral facial dysmorphism, such as proptosis or telecanthus, should increase suspicion for an underlying fungal sinusitis.
- Younger children do not typically display the localizing clinical signs and symptoms that aid physicians in diagnosing adults.
- Symptoms must be present for a minimum period of time, usually greater than 10 days. Symptoms for less than 7 days are unlikely to indicate bacterial sinusitis. Also, a change in color of nasal secretions from clear to white, yellow, or green is not predictive of acute bacterial sinusitis.

DIAGNOSIS AND DIFFERENTIAL

- The diagnosis of acute bacterial sinusitis is dependent on symptoms lasting for a minimum of 10 days and based on history and physical examination.
- Further diagnostic testing, either imaging or culture, is not necessary for the diagnosis and treatment of acute bacterial sinusitis.
- Imaging should be used for the following situations: evidence of an intracranial or intraorbital complication; failure of a full course of antibiotic therapy; chronic or recurrent sinusitis; and assessment of anatomy in anticipation of sinus surgery. Studies might also be obtained when the physician is faced with a vague history and equivocal physical examination. Computed tomography (CT) scanning is the preferred imaging modality for the assessment of sinusitis; however, plain radiographs might be acquired when a CT scan cannot be obtained.
- Plain radiographs poorly visualize the ethmoid air cells and are generally useful only in children over the age of 2. The three most useful views include a Caldwell (AP) view, Waters (occipitomental) view, and a lateral view. Radiographic findings consistent with sinusitis include opacification of a sinus (85% specific), air fluid levels (80% specific), and mucosal thickening >4 mm. Inflammation from other causes, for example, allergic rhinitis, may cause mucosal thickening, lowering the specificity of this finding. In addition, there is a high false negative rate associated with this imaging modality especially in assessment of the ethmoid sinuses that are prominently affected in children.
- A CT scan for the diagnosis of bacterial sinusitis has the advantage of increased sensitivity, and better anatomic definition compared to plain radiographs. Coronal views are recommended to determine the patency of the OMU; however, if not used judiciously (i.e., in patients with more than 10 days of symptoms), CT may overdiagnose sinusitis. Ninety-seven percent of infants and children with a common cold had significant abnormalities on CT scan, which were transient and self-limited. A CT scan of the sinuses is also useful in the diagnosis of fungal sinusitis. Classic findings of fungal sinusitis include unilateral complete opacification of a sinus with heterogenous attenuation, and possible bony erosion.
- It is not necessary to confirm the diagnosis of bacterial sinusitis through culture for uncomplicated bacterial sinusitis. If culture is necessary, for example, after treatment failure, the "gold standard" is needle puncture and aspiration of sinus contents; however, direct fiber endoscopic culture of discharge from the middle meatus correlates well with aspiration and is less invasive. Tissue specimens should also be sent for fungal staining and culture to assess for a fungal pathogen.
- The differential diagnosis of bacterial sinusitis includes viral URIs and allergic rhinitis in the pediatric patient. Viral URIs should improve within 10 days. Other diagnoses to consider include adenoidal hypertrophy, reflux pharyngitis, rhinitis medicamentosa (if self-medicating with adrenergic topical preparations), foreign body (in a younger child with unilateral symptoms), and allergic fungal sinusitis. If cough is the primary symptom, one must be alert for alternative diagnoses such as asthma and image the sinuses if response to therapy is poor.

TREATMENT

- Sinusitis is treated empirically secondary to the limited number of organisms involved and to the invasive techniques required to obtain a culture.
- First line therapy for children with acute bacterial sinusitis is high-dose amoxicillin (80–90 mg/kg/day). For β-lactam allergic patients consider azithromycin, clarithromycin, or trimethoprim-sulfamethoxazole. Refer to Table 48-2 for doses. Should the patient be acutely ill and fail to respond to treatment within 48–72 hours, consider changing antibiotic therapy. Second line treatment options include amoxicillin/clavulanate, cefprozil, cefdinir, or cefuroxime.
- Duration of treatment for acute sinusitis is 10–14 days. Duration of treatment for chronic sinusitis is 21–28 days. One clinical pearl is treating the patient for 7 days after they have noted substantial improvement in symptoms. Patients may require as much as 6 weeks of treatment before resolution of symptoms.
- Adjunctive treatments are primarily used to improve symptoms, and decrease edema. Refer to Table 48-3 for a list of such treatments. Most treatments lack definitive evidence of benefits.
- Consider referral to an allergist or an otolaryngologist for the following situations: recurrent or chronic sinusitis; a strong personal or family history of allergic disease; nasal polyposis; immunocompromised patients; and failure of aggressive medical treatment.
- If the child is toxic appearing despite antibiotic therapy or if complications of sinusitis are present, the patient should be urgently assessed and hospitalized.

TABLE 48-2 Antimicrobial Therapy for Acute Sinusitis

First-line antibiotics

Amoxicillin	80–90 mg/kg/day ÷ tid × 10 days Max (adult) dose 250–500 mg tid
TMP-SMX (Bactrim/Septra)	8–10 mg trimethoprim/kg/day × 10 days Max (adult) dose 160 mg /800 mg bid

Second line antibiotics

Amoxicillin/Clavulanate (Augmentin)	80–90 mg amoxicillin/kg/day ÷ bid × 10 days; max (adult) dose 500–875 mg bid
Azithromycin (Zithromax)	10 mg/kg/day on day 1 then 5 mg/kg/day for days 2–5; max (adult) dose 500 mg on day 1 then 250 mg/day for days 2–5
Cefprozil (Cefzil)	30 mg/kg/day ÷ bid × 10 days Max (adult) dose 250–500 mg bid
Cefdinir (Omnicef)	14 mg/kg/day ÷ bid × 10 days Max (adult) dose 300 mg bid
Clarithromycin (Biaxin)	15 mg/kg/day ÷ bid × 10 days Max (adult) dose 500 mg bid

TABLE 48-3 Adjunctive Treatments for Sinusitis

TREATMENT	DESIRED EFFECT
Nasal saline spray or lavage	May loosen crusts, and help to thin and clear mucus improving drainage providing symptomatic relief. Studies imply but do not confirm this role.
Topical decongestants	Help to shrink edematous mucosa, and relieve obstruction. It is important to caution patient to limit the use of these medications for 3 days to avoid rhinitis medicamentosa.
Oral decongestants	May help to relieve nasal congestion and improve symptoms. When decongestants were combined with antibiotics for treatment of sinusitis, studies in adults showed total costs and symptoms decreased. This has not yet been shown in children.
Nasal steroids	May assist in decreasing the inflammatory response especially when the patient has a component of allergic rhinitis causing their sinusitis. Studies show a more rapid decrease in edema and improvement in obstruction when used with antibiotics.
Antihistamines	May have a role in decreasing symptoms in patients with an allergic component of their disease, otherwise no evidence to routinely recommend their use.
Oral steroids	These have no proven role in improving outcomes of acute or chronic sinusitis in children.

PROGNOSIS

- Spontaneous resolution of acute bacterial sinus disease occurs in anywhere from 50–67% of cases usually within 4 weeks of the onset of symptoms.
- Serious complications of sinusitis are rare. Such complications include intracranial abscesses, meningitis, and orbital infections.
- Aggressive medical therapy successfully treats approximately 90% of patients with chronic sinusitis.

PREVENTION

- Approximately 55% of patients with chronic sinusitis have a history of allergic rhinitis. Aggressive medical treatment including avoidance of relevant allergens may help prevent recurrence of this disease.
- Anatomic abnormalities should be corrected if felt to be contributing to sinus disease, and nasal polyps should be either treated aggressively with nasal corticosteroid sprays or surgically removed.
- Prophylactic antibiotics may be considered for recurrent infections occurring greater than three times in 6 months, or four times in 1 year. An immunologic evaluation should be initiated in these patients to assess for immunodeficiency.

BIBLIOGRAPHY

Brook I, Gooch WM, Jenkins SJ, Pichichero ME, Reiner SA, Sher L, Yamauchi T. Medical management of acute bacterial sinusitis: Recommendations of a clinical advisory committee on pediatric and adult sinusitis. *Ann Otol Rhino Laryngol* 2000;109:2–20.

Conrad DA, Jenson HB. Management of acute bacterial rhinosi-nusitis. *Curr Opin Pediatr* 2002;14:86–90.

Hamilos DL. Chronic sinusitis. *J Allergy Clin Immunol* 2000; 108(2):213–227.

McClay JE, Marple B, Kapadia L, Biavati MJ, Nussenbaum B, Newcomer M, Manning S, Booth T, Schwade N. Clinical pres-entation of allergic fungal sinusitis in children. *Laryngoscope* 2002;112(3):565–569.

Poole MD, Jacobs MR, Anon JB, Marchant CD, Hoberman A, Harrison CJ. Antimicrobial guidelines for the treatment of acute bacterial rhinosinusitis in immunocompetent children. *Int J Pediatr Otorhinolaryngol* 2002;63:1–13.

Spector SL, Bernstein IL, Li JT, Berger WE, Kaliner MA, Schuller DE, Blessing-Moore J, Dykewixz MS, Fineman S, Lee RE, Nicklas RA. Complete guidelines and references for treatment of sinusitis. *J Allergy Clin Immunol* 1998;102(6): S108–S144.

49 URTICARIA/ANGIOEDEMA

Jacqueline Pongracic

EPIDEMIOLOGY

- Acute urticaria is more common than chronic urticaria. Chronic urticaria is defined as hives lasting longer than 6 weeks.
- Urticaria and angioedema occur in all age groups and coexist in 50% of individuals.
- Ten to twenty percent of the population experiences urticaria at some point in their lives. The prevalence in children is unknown, probably because of the tran-sient nature of this disorder. Estimates suggest that 2–3% of children are affected.
- Certain types of urticaria are more common in allergic children, but most cases occur in nonallergic individuals.
- In children, urticaria is more common than angioedema and the two coexist in approximately 10% of cases.

PATHOPHYSIOLOGY

- Urticaria develops when plasma extravasation occurs within the dermis in association with release of vasoac-tive mediators from mast cells. A role for histamine (a mast cell-derived mediator) has been hypothesized in acute urticaria, since injection of histamine into the skin generates a wheal and flare response. When extravasation occurs in the deep dermis, angioedema ensues.
- Chronic urticaria may be an autoimmune process, since autoantibodies to IgE and the high-affinity IgE receptor have been demonstrated in a subgroup of individuals with this disorder. Although associations with autoimmune diseases have been reported in adults with chronic urticaria, such reports are lacking in children.
- Biopsy of a typical acute urticarial lesion reveals edema and vascular dilatation with little to no inflammatory infiltrate. Immunofluorescence does not demonstrate the deposition of complement or immunoglobulin.
- Biopsy of a lesion of urticarial vasculitis demonstrates leukocytoclastic inflammation (nuclear dust), perivenu-lar infiltrates (polymorphonuclear cells), endothelial cell proliferation, and fibrin deposits. Immunofluore-scence shows deposition of C_3, IgM, and fibrin.
- Complement and kinins contribute to the development of angioedema. Angioedema may be acquired or hereditary. Hereditary angioedema is an autosomal dominant disorder in which there is a deficiency of C_1 esterase inhibitor, causing disregulation of comple-ment cleavage and activation leading to angioedema.

CLINICAL FEATURES

- The typical lesion of urticaria is pruritic, with a raised central wheal and surrounding erythema. It may have a highly variable size and shape. The lesion typically lasts several hours, no longer than 24 hours, leaving no mark or sequelae.
- The characteristic lesion of cholinergic urticaria is that of a small wheal (1–3 mm) with large areas of sur-rounding erythema, the so-called "fried egg appear-ance."
- Dermographic lesions are usually linear.
- In urticarial vasculitis, lesions often affect the lower extremities, persist longer than 24 hours, and leave residual purpura.
- Common in toddlers, papular urticarial lesions are grouped together and possess central punctae. Occasionally, bullous features are seen. Papular urticaria also tend to persist longer than 24 hours.
- While urticaria is pruritic, angioedema is not and is usually associated with a painful or burning sensation. The lesions of angioedema often affect the face, hands, and feet and are not well demarcated. Hereditary angioedema usually presents in adolescence and is characterized by recurrent attacks of swelling of the face, extremities, and throat. Abdominal pain may also

occur. This entity has a significant mortality rate of 30% because of airway involvement. Triggers include trauma and dental procedures, but swelling may also occur spontaneously.

DIAGNOSIS AND DIFFERENTIAL

- The diagnosis is often established by thorough history and physical examination. Particular attention should be given to preceding infectious illnesses, medications (prescription and over the counter), nutritional supplements and alternative medicines (vitamins and herbs), physical factors, and underlying diseases. Careful physical examination should evaluate for the presence of fever, weight loss, evidence of infection, lymphadenopathy, hepatomegaly, arthritis, and muscle weakness.
- The most common causes of acute urticaria include infections (viral, parasitic), food allergens (cow milk, egg, peanut, tree nuts,), drugs (antibiotics, antiseizure agents), and physical causes (cholinergic, cold, dermographism, pressure). The cause of chronic urticaria is identified in only 20% of cases. Chronic urticaria is usually related to physical factors or infections but is not usually related to food or environmental allergens.
- Since the lesions have a characteristic appearance, visualization of the lesion is very helpful in cholinergic urticaria, papular urticaria, and dermographism.
- The location may help to identify the cause. Involvement of exposed areas suggests solar or cold urticaria. Lesions primarily over the lower extremities point to urticarial vasculitis. Waistline distribution is associated with physical causes, such as pressure-induced urticaria.
- Laboratory evaluation usually has a low yield in identifying the cause, but may be considered for the evaluation of chronic urticaria. Complete blood count (CBC) with differential, C_3, C_4, CH_{50}, erythrocyte sedimentation rate (ESR), and urinalysis are sometimes useful. Additional studies may be appropriate as determined by history and physical examination.
- Biopsy is not recommended and is rarely necessary in acute urticaria, but it may be helpful in chronic urticaria, particularly when urticarial vasculitis is suspected.
- Hereditary angioedema should be considered when the typical manifestations are evident. Family history is positive in 25% of cases. The laboratory diagnosis of hereditary angioedema includes a low serum C_4 and demonstration of deficiency or dysfunctional serum C_1 esterase inhibitor.
- The differential diagnosis of papular urticaria includes early varicella, neurotic excoriations, lymphomatoid papulosis, acute parapsoriasis, Gianotti-Crosti syndrome and pityriasis lichenoides.

- The differential diagnosis of angioedema includes cellulitis and erysipelas (usually warm, red, and tender), lymphedema (usually accompanied by thickened skin), acute contact dermatitis (generally associated with overlying vesicles and papules), idiopathic scrotal edema, and Melkersson-Rosenthal syndrome (accompanied by furrowed tongue and cranial nerve palsy).

THERAPY

- Avoidance of the inciting agent or trigger factor (e.g., keep exposed areas covered, use sunscreens containing PABA, avoid excessive cold, and avoid food allergens) is important when a cause has been established.
- Treatment of the underlying disease is important.
- H_1 receptor antagonists are the mainstay of medical management. Suggestions include diphenhydramine 1–2 mg/kg q 6 hours, hydroxyzine 0.5 mg/kg q 6 hours, cetirizine 2.5 mg/day for children younger than age 6 years and 5–10 mg/day for older children. For cases of cold-induced urticaria, cyproheptadine is the drug of choice.
- A trial of H_2 receptor antagonists may be added when H_1 blockers are inadequate although the efficacy of this intervention has not been clearly established in children.
- Systemic corticosteroids should be reserved for severe cases or angioedema. High doses followed by a taper may help to gain control.
- Acute attacks of hereditary angioedema should include emergency airway management when necessary, fresh frozen plasma, or epsilon-aminocaproic acid.
- Preventive therapy of hereditary angioedema using androgenic steroids such as stanazolol should be employed when frequent or life-threatening attacks occur. Management of this disorder should be directed by an experienced specialist.

PROGNOSIS

- Most episodes of acute urticaria resolve in 1 month and more than half of all cases of urticaria resolve in 1 year.

PREVENTION

- Secondary prevention of urticaria/angioedema includes avoiding identified triggers (drugs, foods, environmental allergens—especially animals, contact allergens, cold, sun exposure, tight clothing).

TREATMENT
- Treatment with subcutaneous rG-CSF improves the quality of life in affected patients by increasing the ANC without exhaustion of myelopoiesis.
- The subcutaneous dose of rG-CSF required for the maintenance of an ANC above $1.0 \times 10^3/\mu L$ in cyclic neutropenia is typically less than that for SCN.

PROGNOSIS
- Death from overwhelming infections is uncommon.
- Some patients may experience improvement in clinical symptoms, with the cycles being less noticeable as they grow older.

AUTOIMMUNE NEUTROPENIA

- Autoimmune neutropenia (AIN) is caused by peripheral destruction of neutrophils by granulocyte-specific autoantibodies present in a patient's serum.

PRIMARY AUTOIMMUNE NEUTROPENIA (AIN)

EPIDEMIOLOGY
- This is the most common form of neutropenia seen in young children and equally affects both genders.

PATHOPHYSIOLOGY
- Neutrophil counts usually vary between 0 and $1500/\mu L$ during the neutropenic phase with the majority of patients presenting with a neutrophil count greater than $500/\mu L$ at the time of diagnosis.
- The ANC may transiently increase two- to threefold during a severe infection and return to neutropenic levels following resolution.
- Bone marrow shows normal or increased cellularity. In some cases maturation arrest may occur but myeloid precursors reach at least to the myelocyte/metamyelocyte stage.
- Antibodies are most commonly directed at the isolated glycoproteins of the granulocyte membrane and are designated neutrophil antigens (NA).
- The etiology of this disease remains unknown without clear association with parvovirus infection.

CLINICAL FEATURES
- Predominantly seen in infancy, AIN is not associated with other systemic immune mediated disorders such as systemic lupus erythematosus (SLE).
- Patients usually present with mild skin and upper respiratory tract infections. A small minority may suffer from severe infections such as pneumonia, meningitis, or sepsis.

DIAGNOSIS AND DIFFERENTIAL DIAGNOSIS
- The diagnosis of primary AIN may be coincidental since some patients remain asymptomatic despite low neutrophil counts.
- Detection of granulocyte-specific antibodies is the gold standard for diagnosing primary AIN. In some patients detection of these autoantibodies may require repeated testing.
- Granulocyte immunoflorescence testing (GIFT) is one of the most sensitive methods available for detection of antigranulocyte antibodies.

TREATMENT
- Symptomatic treatment with antibiotics for infections is usually sufficient.
- Prophylactic antibiotic treatment should be reserved for those with recurrent infections. Cotrimoxazole, ampicillin, or first generation oral cephalosporins are the most commonly used prophylactic antibiotics.
- Other treatment options include high-dose IVIG, corticosteroids, and rG-CSF. rG-CSF is clearly most effective in increasing the ANC.

PROGNOSIS
- The prognosis of primary AIN is very good since it is self-limited. Neutropenia usually remits spontaneously within 1–2 years. Disappearance of the autoantibodies from the circulation precedes normalization of neutrophil counts.

SECONDARY AUTOIMMUNE NEUTROPENIA (AIN)

EPIDEMIOLOGY
- Can be seen at any age but is more common in adults and has a more variable clinical course.

PATHOPHYSIOLOGY
- Other systemic or autoimmune diseases such as hepatitis, SLE, or Hodgkin's disease often accompany the neutropenia.
- Large granular lymphocyte (LGL) proliferation or LGL leukemia, Epstein-Barr virus (EBV), cytomegalovirus (CMV), human immunodeficiency virus (HIV), and parvovirus B19 infections may be associated with secondary AIN.
- Even if not evident at the time of diagnosis, patients are at risk for developing other autoimmune problems.
- Antineutrophil antibodies have pan-FcγRIII specificity.

CLINICAL FEATURES
- Patients may present with similar infections as seen with primary AIN.

DIAGNOSIS AND DIFFERENTIAL DIAGNOSIS

- Detection of granulocyte-specific antibodies and identification of the underlying or associated disease is important.
- Differential diagnosis include other forms of neutropenia and hematologic malignancies.

TREATMENT AND PROGNOSIS

- Secondary AIN responds best to therapy directed at the underlying cause.
- Neutropenia poorly responds to high-dose IVIG, corticosteroids, and rG-CSF.

ALLOIMMUNE NEONATAL NEUTROPENIA (ANN)

PATHOPHYSIOLOGY AND EPIDEMIOLOGY

- First described by Lalezari in 1966, ANN is caused by the transplacental transfer of maternal antibodies against the neutrophil antigens NA1, NA2, and NB1 leading to immune destruction of neonatal neutrophils.
- These complement activating antineutrophil IgG antibodies can be detected 1 in 500 live births.
- Antibody coated neutrophils in ANN are phagocytosed in the RES and removed from circulation.

CLINICAL FEATURES

- The neutropenic neonate is therefore predisposed to infections.
- Omphalitis, cellulitis, and pneumonia present within the first 2 weeks of life.

DIAGNOSIS AND DIFFERENTIAL DIAGNOSIS

- Diagnosis can be made by detection of neutrophil-specific alloantibodies in the maternal serum.

TREATMENT AND PROGNOSIS

- ANN responds to G-CSF or high-dose IVIG, but most patients improve without specific treatment in a few weeks to 6 months.

DEFECTS OF LEUKOCYTE ADHESION

LEUKOCYTE ADHESION DEFICIENCY TYPE 1

EPIDEMIOLOGY

- The first reports related to this disorder date back to 1970s.
- This is a rare disease with true incidence not known.

PATHOPHYSIOLOGY

- Integrins are cell surface receptors of noncovalently associated heterodimeric chains, comprised of one α subunit (either $CD11_a$, $CD11_b$, or $CD11_c$) and a common β chain (CD18). These proteins mediate leukocyte adhesion to the endothelium.
- LAD1 results from mutations in the gene encoding the common β chain CD18, located at chromosome 21q22.3 leading to defective chemotaxis, adherence, phagocytosis of complement coated particles, bacterial killing, as well as low natural killer (NK) and cytotoxic T-lymphocyte activity.
- Because of defective chemotaxis and adhesion, leukocytes fail to migrate to sites of infection, accounting for the inability to form pus and erythema at the site of infection.

CLINICAL FEATURES

- It is often manifested by delayed umbilical cord separation, omphalitis, persistent leukocytosis, destructive periodontitis, and recurrent infections with *Staphylococcus aureus, Pseudomonas aeruginosa*, and *Klebsiella*.
- Oral ulcers, severe periodontitis, gingivitis with apical bone loss, and eventual loss of permanent teeth are major problems encountered in LAD1.
- Necrotizing cutaneous ulcers with delayed wound healing and eschar formation are common complaints.
- Ulcerative gastrointestinal (GI) disorders resembling idiopathic inflammatory bowel disease may be seen.

DIAGNOSIS AND DIFFERENTIAL DIAGNOSIS

- Persistent neutrophil leukocytosis in the absence of infection is the hallmark of the disease.
- A history of delayed umbilical cord separation, persistent leukocytosis, recurrent bacterial infections of the skin, lungs, upper airways, perirectal area, bowels, necrotizing skin ulcers with poor healing, severe gingivitis, and periodontal disease suggest the diagnosis of LAD1.
- Definitive diagnosis can be made with flow cytometry analysis of patient's white blood cells showing a decreased or absent CD18 and its associated heterodimers: $CD11_a$, $CD11_b$, and $CD11_c$.

TREATMENT

- Definitive therapy of LAD1 is bone marrow transplantation. Infections must be managed aggressively since the inflammatory responses and clinical signs are unreliable. Surgery is essential for the debridement of nonhealing ulcers, which may be followed by tissue grafts.

PROGNOSIS

- Mostly prognosis is very poor without bone marrow transplantation.
- Rarely, patients live beyond childhood with less frequent or severe infections than the severely affected

and do not typically have delayed umbilical cord separation.

LEUKOCYTE ADHESION DEFICIENCY TYPE 2 (LAD2)

EPIDEMIOLOGY
- LAD2 is a very rare autosomal recessive inherited disease of fucose metabolism.

PATHOPHYSIOLOGY
- First described in 1992 by Etzioni et al., LAD2 is caused by a defect in fucose metabolism.
- Lack of expression of different fucosylated molecules leads to a complex phenotype, including neurologic and immunologic features.
- Impaired expression of sialyl-Lewis X and other fucosylated proteins that function as ligands for the selectins leads to impaired neutrophil adhesion to the endothelium resulting in defective leukocyte migration to sites of infection.

CLINICAL FEATURES
- Infection susceptibility, leukocytosis, and poor pus formation are typical.
- Infections, predominantly of the skin, lung, and gums are not as severe as seen in LAD1.
- Severe mental retardation, hypotonia, seizures, dysmorphic features, short stature, strabismus, persistent periodontitis, and Bombay (hh) blood phenotype are also part of the syndrome.

DIAGNOSIS AND DIFFERENTIAL DIAGNOSIS
- Leukocytosis in the absence of infection is a striking clinical finding. In contrast to LAD1, wound healing is not impaired.
- Absence of CD15s on patient neutrophils shown by flow cytometry analysis in the setting of clinical findings confirms the diagnosis of LAD2.

TREATMENT AND PROGNOSIS
- Effective and prompt treatment of infections is the key in the management of LAD2.
- Oral fucose supplementation has been reported to induce a clinical and laboratory improvement in some patients.

CHRONIC GRANULOMATOUS DISEASE

EPIDEMIOLOGY
- CGD occurs with a frequency of 40.5–1/100,000.

PATHOPHYSIOLOGY
- CGD comprises a group of four inherited disorders with a common phenotype, characterized by recurrent severe bacterial and fungal infections and tissue granuloma formation.
- Today it is known that CGD is the result of deficient superoxide (O_2^-) generation via the nicotinamide adenine dinucleotide phosphate (NADPH) oxidase system by activated phagocytes.
- It is inherited in X-linked and autosomal recessive patterns.
- The most common form of CGD is caused by mutations in the gene encoding the gp91^{phox}.
- Carrier detection revealed a functionally abnormal phagocyte population in 89% of mothers, making for a spontaneous mutation rate of approximately 11%.
- In several patients with large enough deletions, affected adjacent genes lead to McLeod syndrome (compensated hemolysis, acanthosis, progressive neurodegenerative symptoms, absent erythrocyte Kx protein, and diminished levels of Kell-blood group antigens), Duchenne's muscular dystrophy, or X-linked retinitis pigmentosa in addition to CGD.
- Mutations in the genes encoding the NADPH oxidase components p47^{phox}, p67^{phox}, and p22^{phox} cause the autosomal recessive forms of CGD, accounting for approximately 35% of all cases.

CLINICAL FEATURES
- Onset of first severe infection is usually in infancy or childhood although several adults have been diagnosed with CGD following a severe infection.
- Common clinical problems are related to recurrent infections with catalase positive bacteria and fungi.
- Patients with CGD often present with pneumonia, liver abscess skin infections, lymphadenitis, and osteomyelitis.
- Recurrent pyogenic infections with *Staphylococcus aureus, Burkholderia* sp., *Serratia marcescens, Chromobacterium violaceum, Aspergillus* sp., *and Nocardia* sp. are common for CGD.
- Infections may be widely disseminated and fatal but are most commonly skin abscesses, cervical lymphadenitis, pneumonia, osteomyelitis, liver or perianal abscesses, and gingivitis.
- Staphylococcal liver abscesses, are common in CGD and cause significant morbidity. Because of their fibrocaseous consistency, percutaneous drainage is rarely successful and open surgery is required.
- Invasive pulmonary aspergillosis is the primary cause of death in American CGD. *A. fumigatus* and *A. flavus* are commonly isolated, but *A. niger* and *A. nidulans*, species with low pathogenicity in the normal host, have been frequently reported in CGD.
- *Aspergillus* pneumonia is usually detected via computerized tomography as a well circumscribed

consolidation in the peripheral lung parenchyma. Thoracic-wall invasion may occur, leading to osteomyelitis of the ribs, perforation of the diaphragm, or cutaneous abscesses.

- Septicemia is uncommon, but can occur with *B. cepacia, C. violaceum,* or *S. aureus* in the setting of osteomyelitis.
- Exuberant tissue granuloma formation at the sites of infection, at surgical wounds, and hollow viscera is a frequent problem, seen more often in patients with the X-linked form of CGD.
- Granuloma formation, an inflammatory process, is one of the hallmarks of CGD. Pyloric outlet obstruction, bladder outlet obstruction, and ureteral obstruction are commonly encountered problems resulting from granuloma formation.
- A Crohn's disease-like inflammatory bowel disease is part of this inflammatory spectrum and may involve esophagus, jejunum, ileum, cecum, rectum, and perirectal area in about 30% of patients.
- In the setting of GI involvement, manifestations include diarrhea, malabsorption, and lipid-laden pigmented histiocytes are found in biopsies.
- Autoimmune or rheumatologic problems, such as discoid lupus erythematosus, SLE, and polyarthritis resembling juvenile rheumatoid arthritis, have been reported in patients with CGD.

DIAGNOSIS AND DIFFERENTIAL DIAGNOSIS

- In the setting of severe, recurrent infections with catalase positive organisms involving the lung and liver or granuloma formations in the GI or genitourinary tract, CGD should be considered.
- The diagnosis is established by the inability of neutrophils to reduce nitroblue tetrazolium dye, the absence of chemiluminescence, or the failure to oxidize dihydrorhodamine (DHR assay).
- The DHR assay (flow cytometric assay of oxidative burst) is the most sensitive and enables quantitation of the oxidative capacity of neutrophils.
- This can also show the genotype-dependent variability in reduced NADPH oxidase function.

TREATMENT

- Prophylactic trimethoprim-sulfamethoxazole (TMP-SMX) reduces the frequency of major infections especially those caused by *S. aureus.*
- TMP-SMX prophylaxis is ineffective against fungal infections but does not encourage them. Prophylactic itraconazole appears to be effective in preventing fungal infections.
- Leukocyte transfusions are used during severe infections in addition to antibiotics, although the benefits are unproven.

- Conventional bone marrow transplants have been tried in CGD with limited success.
- Interferon (IFN)-γ is crucial in prophylaxis against infections. The exact mechanism of action of IFN-γ is not known.
- Subcutaneous administration of recombinant IFN-γ three times a week at a dose of 50 μg/m^2 (for those with body surface area greater than 0.5 m^2) is recommended in addition to TMP-SMX as prophylaxis in CGD.
- The adverse effects of recombinant IFN-γ in patients with CGD have been limited to fever, chills, headache, erythema, flu-like illness, and diarrhea.
- Granulomas respond very well to low-dose steroids and regress completely with tapering over several weeks. Exuberant formation of granulation tissue and dysregulated cutaneous inflammatory responses lead to wound dehiscence and impaired wound healing in CGD.

PROGNOSIS

- Mortality is about 5% per year for the X-linked form of the disease and 2% per year for the autosomal recessive varieties. The most common causes of mortality are *Aspergillus* pneumonia, followed by *Burkholderia cepacia* pneumonia or sepsis.
- Patients with the p47^{phox}-deficient genotype have better prognosis and less severe clinical phenotype overall (Curnutte, 1993 #166).

HEREDITARY MYELOPEROXIDASE DEFICIENCY (HMD)

EPIDEMIOLOGY

- Has a frequency of 1:4000 (Parry, 1981 #394).

PATHOPHYSIOLOGY

- Characterized by the lack of myeloperoxidase (MPO) activity, a heme containing enzyme necessary for the conversion of H_2O_2 to hypochlorous (HOCl) and the subsequent killing of phagocytosed bacteria, fungi, and viruses.
- Neutrophils of MPO-deficient individuals fail to produce HOCl on stimulation, while the NADPH oxidase system remains unaffected.
- Neutrophils have no apparent defect in phagocytosis of bacteria and fungi; however, microbicidal activity is affected in a time-dependent manner with a prolonged respiratory burst.
- It is caused by germline mutations and inherited as an autosomal recessive trait.
- There is heterogeneity among patients in the degree of MPO deficiency; both total and partial deficiencies have been described.

- Patients with primary MPO deficiency do not usually have an increased incidence of infections, probably because MPO independent mechanisms compensate for the lack of MPO for microbicidal activity.

CLINICAL FEATURES
- Most individuals are diagnosed incidentally when MPO activity is used for specific neutrophil staining such as in some automated differential readers.
- In some patients visceral candidiasis occurs if concurrent diabetes is present.
- Other problems are nonfungal recurrent infections, malignancies (solid or hematologic tumors), and certain skin disorders.

DIAGNOSIS
- The diagnosis of MPO deficiency can be made using anti-MPO monoclonal antibodies for flow cytometric analysis of the neutrophil population.

TREATMENT AND PROGNOSIS
- There is no specific treatment. Treatment of candida infection or nonfungal infections is the key.
- Prognosis is very good.

HYPER IgE RECURRENT INFECTION SYNDROME (HIES) OR JOB SYNDROME

EPIDEMIOLOGY
- HIES occurs in all racial and ethnic groups.

PATHOPHYSIOLOGY
- This is a multisystem autosomal dominant disorder characterized by recurrent infections of the lower respiratory system and skin, chronic eczema, extremely elevated IgE levels, and eosinophilia.
- There is strong evidence for autosomal dominant inheritance.
- There are sporadic cases born to consanguineous parents that may be autosomal recessive.
- HIES syndrome may represent mutation of a single gene, mutations in different genes in different families, or deletion of contiguous genes over a short chromosomal distance.
- Efforts to identify a single gene responsible for this phenotype have not yet been successful.

CLINICAL FEATURES
- Facial abnormalities are protruding, prominent mandible and prominent forehead, hypertelorism, broad nasal bridge and a wide, fleshy nasal tip with increased interalar distance.

- Midline anomalies common in this disorder are high-arched palate and midline sagittal clefts of the tongue. A single patient with HIES was reported to have a cleft lip and a palate.
- Skeletal abnormalities are common in this disorder. A high incidence of fractures and scoliosis has been recognized. Hyperextensibility of joints is also common.
- A unique dental abnormality seen in this syndrome is retained primary teeth causing delayed eruption of the permanent teeth. This may be because of reduced resorption of primary tooth roots.
- Moderate to severe eczema presenting within the first hours to weeks of life is almost universal in HIES.
- Mucocutaneous candidiasis involving finger and toenails, mouth, vagina, and intertriginous areas is seen in approximately half of the patients.
- Lung abscesses requiring surgical drainage are almost always staphylococcal. Primary pulmonary infections are predominantly with *Staphylococcus aureus* and *Hemophilus influenzae*. These pneumonias usually lead to the development of pneumatoceles.
- Lung cavities provide three environments for *Pseudomonas* or *Aspergillus* superinfection.
- Thoracotomy is frequently required for removal of pneumatoceles or drainage of infected cavities.
- Inflammatory bone lesions are relatively common and can be sterile or septic.
- *Pneumocystis carinii* pneumonia, *Cryptococcus neoformans* esophageal infection, and intestinal *Histoplasmosis* have been reported.
- Characteristic of this syndrome is an extremely elevated serum IgE level, usually above 2000 IU/mL.
- Fluctuations in IgE levels have been recorded over time and the IgE levels do not correlate with disease activity.
- Abnormal T-cell activation or defective suppressor T-cell function may underlie the excess production of IgE.
- Total serum IgG levels are usually within the normal range.
- Also, antigen-specific antibody responses are impaired against both polysaccharide and protein antigens, which may contribute to the increased susceptibility to infections.
- Eosinophilia is common. See Table 50-2 for the frequency of clinical features in HIE syndrome.

DIAGNOSIS AND DIFFERENTIAL DIAGNOSIS
- Elevated IgE levels in addition to recurrent pulmonary infections and eczema suggest a diagnosis of HIE syndrome; however, there is no single diagnostic test. Diagnosis is established based on clinical features.
- Severe atopia is a close mimic.

TABLE 50-2 Clinical and Laboratory Findings in Patients with the Hyper-IgE Syndrome

FINDINGS	INCIDENCE (%)
Eczema	100
High IgE levels (above 2000 IU/mL)	97
Eosinophilia (>2 SD above the mean for normals)	93
Boils	87
Pneumonia	87
Candidiasis	83
Characteristic facies (in those ≥16 years)	83
Lung cysts	77
Scoliosis (for those ≥16 years)	76
Hyperextensible joints	68
Delayed dental shedding	72
Bone fractures	57

SOURCE: Adapted from Grimbacher et al. *N Engl J Med* 1999;340(9):692–702.

REFERENCES

Lekstrom-Himes J, Gallin JI. Immunodeficiency Diseases Caused by Defects in Phagocytes. *N Engl J Med* 2001;343:1703–1714.

Grimbacher B, Holland SM, Gallin JI, et al. Hyper-IgE Syndrome with Recurrent Infections-an Autosomal Dominana Multisystem Disorder. *N Engl J Med* 340(9);692–702.

Rosenzweig SD, Holland SM. Phagocyte Immunodeficiencies and their Infections. *J Allergy Clin Immunol* 2004;113(4):620–626.

II. *Antibody Deficiency Syndromes*

AGAMMAGLOBULINEMIA

EPIDEMIOLOGY

- Eighty-five percent of patients with early onset hypogammaglobulinemia are male with X-linked agammaglobulinemia (X-LA).

PATHOPHYSIOLOGY

- Agammaglobulinemia is caused by mutations in genes that are critical for the maturation of B cells and development of antibody mediated immunity. The most common form is X-LA, caused by mutations in the Btk gene, affecting the early stages of B-cell differentiation.

- Autosomal recessive forms of B-cell development disorders are rare forms that can be caused by mutations either in μ-heavy chain gene or B-cell linker protein.
- B cells are very few or absent, but T cells are present with preserved functions. Pro-B cell numbers in the bone marrow are normal or increased.
- All immunoglobulins are significantly decreased or absent. Patients are not able to mount primary antibody responses to antigens.

CLINICAL FEATURES

- Pyogenic bacterial infections of the sinopulmonary tract may present as early as 4–6 months of age when maternal antibodies fall below protective levels. *Streptococcus pneumoniae* and *H. influenza* are commonly encountered pathogens.
- Other infections include pyoderma, chronic conjunctivitis, gastroenteritis, arthritis, meningitis-encephalitis, and osteomyelitis.
- Lymphoid tissues are reduced in size.
- Chronic enteroviral meningoencephalitis and disseminated polio following OPV administration can complicate the clinical course.
- Compared with patients with X-LA, patients with μ-heavy chain defect have an earlier onset of disease and more complications.

DIAGNOSIS AND DIFFERENTIAL DIAGNOSIS

- Early onset infections, profound hypogammaglobulinemia, and very low or absent B cells (<2%) warrant a diagnosis of agammaglobulinemia. Definitive diagnosis is achieved by mutational analysis.

TREATMENT

- Early diagnosis, broad spectrum antibiotics, and IVIG replacement are critical aspects of treatment.
- Trough serum IgG level >500 mg/dL is important in preventing acute severe bacterial infections and bronchiectasis. A level >800 mg/dL is necessary to prevent chronic sinusitis and enteroviral infections.

PROGNOSIS

- Bronchiectasis with chronic lung disease is the major morbidity.
- It is not clear if patients with X-LA are predisposed to malignancies.

HYPER-IGM SYNDROME (HIGM)

EPIDEMIOLOGY

- HIGM mainly affects boys (55–65% of cases).

PATHOPHYSIOLOGY

- The X-linked form is a T-cell deficiency with molecular defects in the gene encoding for CD40L, which is essential for immunoglubulin class-switch recombination.
- Non-X-linked forms of the disease exist, and three other molecular defects (autosomal recessive) have been described.
- Peripheral blood B-cell counts are normal. B cells express surface IgM and IgD, but cannot switch from IgM to IgG production.

CLINICAL FEATURES

- HIGM is characterized by severe recurrent bacterial infections in the sinopulmonary and gastrointestinal tracts with decreased serum levels of IgG, IgA, and IgE but normal or high IgM levels.
- *Pneumocystis carini* pneumonia (PCP), central nervous system histoplasmosis and toxoplasmosis, *Cryptosporodium* diarrhea, sclerosing cholangitis, parvovirus-induced aplastic anemia and neutropenia are among the complications.

DIAGNOSIS AND DIFFERENTIAL DIAGNOSIS

- Severe recurrent bacterial infections in the sinopulmonary tract with decreased serum IgG, IgA and IgE but normal or high IgM levels, and normal B-cell numbers warrant a diagnosis of HIGM.
- For the X-linked form, absence of CD40L expression on activated T cells documented by flow-cytometry establishes the diagnosis.
- Definitive diagnosis is achieved by mutational analysis.

TREATMENT AND PROGNOSIS

- IVIG replacement, PCP prophylaxis, and anti-bacterial antibiotic prophylaxis should be administered when needed. Granulocyte colony stimulating factor (GCSF) may be required to treat neutropenia.
- Bone marrow transplant has been successful in this setting.

COMMON VARIABLE IMMUNODEFICIENCY (CVID)

EPIDEMIOLOGY

- CVID affects ~1 in 10,000–100,000 individuals worldwide.
- CVID occurs in two peaks at ages 1–5 years and 16–20 years. The average age of onset of symptoms is 25 years, and the average age of diagnosis is 28 years.

PATHOPHYSIOLOGY

- CVID is a late onset, highly variable immunodeficiency characterized by hypogammaglobulinemia, mostly normal B-cell numbers, and variable degree of T-cell dysfunction.
- Serum concentrations of IgG are reduced 2 standard deviations below normal for age. Most patients also have reduced IgA levels; 50% of patients have low IgM concentrations.
- Affected individuals have abnormal responses to protein and polysaccharide antigens.

CLINICAL FEATURES

- Recurrent otitis media and pneumonia, and chronic sinusitis are the most frequent presenting infections. Recurrent pulmonary infections lead to bronchiectasis and chronic lung disease.
- Bacterial pathogens are similar to those in X-LA.
- Other infections include *Mycoplasma* and *Ureoplasma* associated with arthritis.
- Malabsorption, chronic diarrhea, and gastroenteritis are usually caused by *Giardia, Campylobacter*, and *Yersinia* species.
- Hypertrophy of lymphoid tissues and autoimmune disorders are common.
- The incidence of malignancy is increased.

DIAGNOSIS AND DIFFERENTIAL DIAGNOSIS

- Recurrent sinopulmonary infections, hypogammaglobulinemia, with detectable circulating B cells suggest a diagnosis of CVID once other causes of hypogammaglobulinemia are ruled out.
- X-linked lymphoproliferative disease (XLP) should be considered if the proband is a male with family history of male deaths due to lymphoproliferative disease or fulminant EBV infection.

TREATMENT AND PROGNOSIS

- Aggressive treatment of infections and IVIG replacement are critical.
- The mortality rate over a 25-year period is 24%, due to lymphoma and chronic lung disease.

SELECTIVE IGA DEFICIENCY

- This is the most common immune deficiency (1/400–1/600).

PATHOPHYSIOLOGY AND CLINICAL FEATURES

- Most patients are asymptomatic and diagnosed incidentally.
- Selective IgA deficiency may co-exist with other selective antibody deficiencies (i.e., polysaccharide unresponsiveness). It may be a variant of CVID and progress to panhypogammaglobulinemia.
- Sinopulmonary infections, conjunctivitis, and gastroenteritis may develop.
- Selective IgA deficiency may be associated with autoimmune disorders.

DIAGNOSIS AND DIFFERENTIAL DIAGNOSIS

- An undetectable level of serum IgA with normal IgG and IgM levels warrants the diagnosis.
- Pneumococcal titers should be checked to rule out associated selective antibody deficiency.

TREATMENT

- IVIG therapy is not indicated in selective IgA deficiency without other immunologic abnormalities.

TRANSIENT HYPOGAMMAGLOBULINAEMIA OF INFANCY

PATHOPHYSIOLOGY

- This disorder is the result of maturational delay and presents when maternal antibody disappears at 4–6 months.

CLINICAL FEATURES

- Sinopulmonary tract infections with encapsulated bacteria present as early as 4–6 months of age as maternal antibodies decrease.
- *S. pneumoniae* and *H. influenza* are commonly encountered pathogens.

DIAGNOSIS AND DIFFERENTIAL DIAGNOSIS

- Immunoglobulin levels are low but not absent.
- Diagnosis can only be confidently established when recovery has occurred.
- The differential diagnosis includes atypical forms of X-LA with few circulating B cells, and XLP disease.

TREATMENT AND PROGNOSIS

- IVIG replacement is not indicated except for rare cases. The prognosis is excellent. It usually resolves by age 18–24 months.

BIBLIOGRAPHY

Ballow M. Primary immunodeficiency disorders: antibody deficiency. *J Allergy Clin Immunol* 2002;109(4):581–591.

Conley ME, Rohrer J, Minegishi Y. X-linked agammaglobulinemia. *Clin Rev Allergy Immunol* 2000;19(2):183–204.

Gaspar HB, Conley ME. Early B cell defects. *Clin Exp Immunol* 2000;119(3):383–389.

Gulino AV, Notarangelo LD. Hyper IgM syndromes. *Curr Opin Rheumatol* 2003;15(4): 422–429.

Minegishi Y, Lavoie A, Cunningham-Rundles C, et al. Mutations in activation-induced cytidine deaminase in patients with hyper IgM syndrome. *Clin Immunol* 2000; 97(3):203–210.

Winkelstein JA, Marino MC, Ochs H, et al. The X-linked hyper-IgM syndrome: clinical and immunologic features of 79 patients. *Medicine (Baltimore)*. 2003; 82(6):373–384.

Yel L, Minegishi Y, Coustan-Smith E, et al. Mutations in the mu heavy-chain gene in patients with agammaglobulinemia. *N Engl J Med* 1996;335(20): 1486–1493.

III. *T-Cell Immunodeficiencies*

SEVERE COMBINED IMMUNODEFICIENCY

EPIDEMIOLOGY

- The frequency of SCID has been estimated to be 1 in 50,000 to 1 in 500,000 births.
- X-linked SCID accounts for 45% of all cases.
- Adenosine deaminase (ADA) deficiency has been observed in approximately 16% of all SCID patients.

PATHOPHYSIOLOGY

- SCID is a rare inherited immune disorder, which is fatal in the absence of immune reconstitution.
- SCID leads to severe bacterial and viral infections within the first 6 months of life. SCID is characterized by profound T-cell lymphopenia, lack of cellular (lymphocyte proliferative responses to mitogens, antigens, and allogeneic cells in vitro) and humoral (B-cell) immunity and, in some cases, decreased NK-cell number and function.
- The genetic and molecular bases of SCID include mutations in genes encoding the interleukin-2-receptor common gamma chain (IL2RG), V(D)J recombination/DNA repair factor (ARTEMIS), recombinase-activating gene-1 and -2, (RAG1, RAG2), (ADA), the common leukocyte surface protein (CD45), Janus kinase 3 (JAK3), and interleukin-7-receptor (IL7R).
- X-linked SCID (few or no T or NK cells but a normal or elevated number of B cells) caused by mutations in the gene encoding the IL2RG accounts for 45% of all cases.
- In the autosomal recessive SCID, caused by absence of enzyme ADA, pronounced accumulations of adenosine and its metabolites lead to apoptosis of thymocytes and circulating lymphocytes, which causes the immunodeficiency.
- Most patients with Omenn syndrome have autosomal recessive SCID caused by mutations in RAG1 or RAG2 genes, resulting in partial and impaired V(D)J recombinational activity. Circulating activated, oligoclonal T lymphocytes that do not function normally, absence of circulating B cells, and abnormal lymph node architecture lacking germinal centers are the pathologic features.
- The bare lymphocyte syndrome (BLS) or major histocompatibility complex deficiency is a rare form of SCID, characterized by the absence of constitutive and inducible expression of MHC determinants on immune cells.
- Mutations in unidentified genes may also cause SCID.

CLINICAL FEATURES

- Affected children present with failure to thrive, frequent episodes of diarrhea, oral candidiasis, pneumonia, otitis, sepsis, and cutaneous infections in the first few months of life. Persistent opportunistic infections, such as those due to *Candida albicans, Pneumocystis carinii*, varicella zoster virus, parainfluenzae virus, respiratory syncytial virus, adenovirus, cytomegalovirus, EBV, and BCG may lead to death.
- A complete physical examination of lymphoid organs reveals absent tonsillar tissue and lymph nodes.
- Since infants with SCID lack the ability to reject foreign tissue, they are at risk for graft-versus-host disease (GVHD) caused by transplacentally transferred maternal T cells or from T lymphocytes in nonirradiated blood products. GVHD occurs in as many as 20% of patients with SCID and may manifest as rash occurring at birth.
- The distinguishing features of ADA deficiency include the presence of multiple skeletal abnormalities of chondro-osseous dysplasia on radiographic examination.
- Generalized erythroderma and desquamation, diarrhea, hepatosplenomegaly, hypereosinophilia, and markedly elevated serum IgE levels are characteristic for Omenn syndrome.

DIAGNOSIS

- Chest radiographs help to assess the thymic shadow, which is absent in SCID.
- Lymphopenia together with very low or undetectable immunoglobulins suggest SCID. Low absolute lymphocyte count when compared with age-matched normal infants, is a very helpful clue in diagnosing SCID. Normal range for the cord blood absolute lymphocyte count is 2000 to 11,000/mm³. In neonates with values less than this range, SCID should be suspected and T-cell phenotypic and functional studies should be performed. The normal absolute lymphocyte count is higher at 6–7 months of age when most SCID patients are diagnosed. Therefore any count less than 4000/mm³ at 6–7 months is considered lymphopenic.
- Flow cytometric evaluation of lymphocyte subsets reveals significantly low numbers of T cells. Assessing the absence or presence of NK cells and B

cells help to determine the SCID phenotype. For example, patients with X-linked SCID usually have few or no T or NK cells but a normal or elevated number of B cells that do not produce immunoglobulin.

Molecular causes of SCID	Lymphocyte phenotype
X-linked SCID	
(γc gene mutations)	T($-$),B($+$),NK($-$)
Autosomal recessive SCID	
ADA gene mutations	T($-$),B($-$),NK($-$)
Jak3 gene mutations	T($-$),B($+$),NK($-$)
IL7Rα-chain gene mutations	T($-$),B($+$),NK($+$)
RAG1 or RAG2 mutations	T($-$),B($-$),NK($+$)
Artemis mutations	T($-$),B($-$),NK($+$)
CD45 gene mutations	T($-$),B($+$)

- ADA-deficient infants usually have a much more profound lymphopenia, with mean lymphocyte counts of less than 500/mm^3.
- If T cells that are highly positive for HLA-DR expression are detected, transplacentally transferred maternal T cells should be suspected (maternal T cell engraftment).
- In vivo screening of T-cell function by delayed hypersensitivity skin test measuring the lymphocyte memory to previously encountered antigens such as *C. albicans*, tetanus toxoid, or mumps is performed by intracutaneous injection of 0.1 mL of these antigens and measuring the induration 48–72 hours later. The detection of induration 2 mm or larger at more than one test site is considered to be evidence of intact cell-mediated immunity.
- Proliferative responses to mitogens and antigens are significantly diminished or absent.

DIFFERENTIAL DIAGNOSIS

- Other primary or secondary immunodeficiencies that may present with similar symptoms as SCID include DiGeorge anomaly, Wiskott-Aldrich syndrome (WAS), ataxia-telangiectasia (A-T), or perinatally transmitted HIV.
- Profound immunodeficiency characterized by low or absent T lymphocytes can occasionally be seen in patients with DiGeorge syndrome (DGS). Most patients with DGS have a deletion in the long arm of chromosome of 22 (del22q11.2), which is detected by fluorescence in situ hybridization (FISH). Affected patients may have cardiac defects, abnormal facies, thymic hypoplasia, cleft lip/palate, and hypocalcemia.
- Infants with HIV usually present with failure to thrive, lymphadenopathy, hepatosplenomegaly, persistent diarrhea, or oral candidiasis. In advanced stages, when T lymphocytes are low, opportunistic infections

such as *P. carinii, C. albicans,* or *Mycobacterium avium* are seen. Diagnosis is determined by HIV-DNA by polymerase chain reaction (PCR) or HIV antibody by enzyme-linked immunosorbent assay.
- *A-T* manifests with progressive cerebellar ataxia and oculocutaneous telangiectasias during infancy. Patients with A-T usually have recurrent sinopulmonary infections and a high incidence of malignancy. The range of immunodeficiencies described in A-T include antibody deficiency and, less commonly, moderate-to-severe lymphopenia.
- Patients with WAS typically present with eczema, recurrent infections, and thrombocytopenia with small platelet size on peripheral smear. Impaired humoral immune responses such as increased serum IgA and IgE levels and decreased level of IgM are prominent immunologic features in WAS. In contrast to profoundly deficient humoral and cell-mediated immunity seen in SCID, patients with WAS may occasionally have moderately decreased T-cell numbers and functions.

TREATMENT AND PROGNOSIS

- Early diagnosis and treatment is vital. Hematopoietic stem-cell transplants are the standard treatment.
- The probability of successful allogeneic bone marrow transplantation is high (95%) when performed before 3–4 months of life. Stem-cell transplantation is most effective in the short asymptomatic period after birth.
- Patients should only receive CMV negative and irradiated packed red blood cells (PRBCs) if transfusion is necessary.
- In anticipation for bone marrow transplant, patients should receive PCP prophylaxis and IVIG if needed.

COMBINED IMMUNODEFICIENCY (CID) SYNDROMES

CID distinguishes patients with low, but not absent, T-cell function from those with SCID.

PURINE NUCLEOSIDE PHOSPHORYLASE (PNP) DEFICIENCY

EPIDEMIOLOGY

- PNP deficiency is a rare autosomal recessive immunodeficiency.
- More than 40 patients with CID have been found to have PNP deficiency.

PATHOPHYSIOLOGY

- Mutations in the gene encoding PNP (14q13.1) are responsible for this immunodeficiency.
- In the absence of PNP, the urate precursors hypoxanthine and xanthine are not formed and guanosine and deoxyguanosine build up, becoming toxic for T cells while decreased GTP causes CNS injury.

CLINICAL FEATURES

- Generalized vaccinia, varicella, lymphosarcoma, and GVHD mediated by T cells from nonirradiated allogeneic blood or bone marrow are fatal in this disorder.
- Neurologic abnormalities range from developmental delay, behavioral problems, and spasticity to mental retardation.
- Autoimmune diseases, such as autoimmune hemolytic anemia, thrombocytopenia, and vasculitis may be seen.

DIAGNOSIS AND DIFFERENTIAL DIAGNOSIS

- SCID with neurologic deficits should be considered PNP deficiency until proven otherwise.
- Most patients have normal or elevated concentrations of immunoglobulins.
- PNP-deficient patients are profoundly lymphopenic with absolute lymphocyte counts usually less than $500/mm^3$.
- T-cell function is low but not absent and varies with time.
- Serum and urinary uric acid are deficient.
- Measurement of erythrocyte PNP activity confirms the diagnosis.

TREATMENT AND PROGNOSIS

- PNP deficiency is fatal in childhood unless immunologic reconstitution is achieved.
- Bone marrow transplantation is the treatment of choice but has limited success.

IMMUNODEFICIENCY WITH THROMBOCYTOPENIA AND ECZEMA-WISKOTT-ALDRICH SYNDROME (WAS)

EPIDEMIOLOGY

- WAS affects 4 males per 1,000,000 male births.

PATHOPHYSIOLOGY

- The mutated gene responsible for this defect is limited in expression to lymphocytic and megakaryocytic lineages.
- The product of WAS gene is designated as WASP (WAS protein) which is an intracellular signaling molecule involved in T-cell receptor signaling and actin polymerization.
- WAS is an X-linked recessive syndrome, but isolated X-linked thrombocytopenia is also caused by mutations in the same gene.

CLINICAL FEATURES

- WAS is characterized by eczema, thrombocytopenia with small platelets and susceptibility to infections with pneumococci and other encapsulated bacteria.
- Patients usually present during infancy with prolonged bleeding and atopic dermatitis.
- Commonly encountered infections are otitis media, pneumonia, meningitis, or sepsis.
- Infections with *Pneumocystis carinii* and the herpes viruses may arise.
- Autoimmune cytopenias and vasculitis occur after infancy.

DIAGNOSIS AND DIFFERENTIAL DIAGNOSIS

- In WAS, impaired humoral immune responses to polysaccharide antigens occur, as evidenced by poor or absent antibody responses to polysaccharide antigens. Low serum IgM, elevated IgA and IgE, and a normal or slightly low IgG concentration may be seen.
- Moderately reduced percentage of T cells may be seen with flow cytometry. Lymphocyte responses to mitogens are moderately depressed.
- The mean platelet volume in WAS is 3.8–5.0 fL (normal: 7.1–10.5 fL)
- Detection of the mutated gene confirms the diagnosis. Prenatal diagnosis of WAS is also available for affected families.

TREATMENT AND PROGNOSIS

- Survival beyond the teenage years is rare.
- The most common cause of death in WAS is EBV-induced lymphoreticular malignancy.
- Complete corrections of platelet and immunologic abnormalities may be achieved with bone marrow transplants from HLA-identical siblings.

- Splenectomy for uncontrollable bleeding may lead to increased platelet counts.
- Administration of prophylactic antibiotics and IVIG are other treatment modalities.

BIBLIOGRAPHY

Becker-Catania SG, Gatti RA. Ataxia-telangiectasia. *Adv Exp Med Biol* 2001;495:191–198.

Buckley RH. Primary cellular immunodeficiencies. *J Allergy Clin Immunol* 2002;109(5):747–757.

Buckley RH. Primary immunodeficiency diseases due to defects in lymphocytes. *N Engl J Med* 2000;343(18):1313–1324.

Imai K, Nonoyama S, Ochs HD. WASP (Wiskott-Aldrich syndrome protein) gene mutations and phenotype. *Curr Opin Allergy Clin Immunol* 2003;3(6):427–436.

Kalman L, Lindegren ML, Kobrynski L, et al. Mutations in genes required for T-cell development: IL7R, CD45, IL2RG, JAK3, RAG1, RAG2, ARTEMIS, and ADA and severe combined immunodeficiency. *Genet Med* 2004;6(1):16–26.

Myers LA, Patel DD, Puck JM, Buckley RH. Hematopoietic stem cell transplantation for severe combined immunodeficiency in the neonatal periods leads to superior thymic output and improved survival. *Blood* 2002;99(3):872–878.

Ochs HD. The Wiskott-Aldrich syndrome. *Semin Hematol* 1998;35(4):332–345.

Perlman S, Becker-Catania S, Gatti RA. Ataxia-telangiectasia: diagnosis and treatment. *Semin Pediatr Neurol* 2003;10(3):173–182.

Section 7
DISEASES OF THE HEART AND GREAT VESSELS

Rae-Ellen W. Kavey, Section Editor

51 CARDIAC EVALUATION: NORMAL AUSCULTATION, MURMURS AND CLICKS

Rae-Ellen W. Kavey

- At least 50% of normal children have an innocent murmur noted at one time or another, so differentiation of functional from organic murmurs is an important role for pediatric care providers.
- The physical examination is the single best means of suspecting the presence of congenital heart disease.
- Cardiac evaluation should begin with a general impression of the child's state of health, charted height and weight compared with norms for age/gender, vital signs especially blood pressure, and visual evaluation for dysmorphic features. This is important since congenital heart disease is associated with a number of different syndromes (see Table 51-1 for known syndromes and associated cardiac pathology).
- The focused cardiovascular examination begins with visual inspection of the thorax for asymmetry due to underlying cardiomegaly and displaced cardiac impulses. This should be followed by palpation of the precordium and the suprasternal notch. In normal children, there is a small impulse along the left sternal border and a localized point of maximal impulse (PMI) in the fifth to sixth intercostal space. Presence of abnormal impulses *always* means there is underlying cardiac pathology.
- Cardiac evaluation includes abdominal examination for hepatosplenomegaly, assessment of perfusion in the extremities, and pulse evaluation in all four extremities.
- Coarctation of the aorta is the most commonly missed congenital cardiac diagnosis: the combination of hypertension (which can be mild in younger patients) and decreased pulses in the lower body should alert the clinician to this important diagnosis.
- On auscultation, the heart sounds are the normal framework for the cardiac cycle. In children, heart sounds are easily heard. The first sound is single and the second has two components related to closure of the aortic and pulmonary valves. On inspiration, there is increased venous return to the right side of the heart which delays pulmonary closure and widens the normal split of the second sound. This is reversed with expiration when the second sound should narrow to a single sound. *Presence of normal respiratory variation in S2 is a strong indicator of a normal cardiovascular examination.*
- Murmurs are classified by their *intensity* and their *timing.*

INTENSITY

- Grade 1: soft, difficult to appreciate.
- Grade 2: readily heard but not loud.
- Grade 3: loud but no thrill.
- Grade 4: with a thrill.
- Grade 5: heard with stethoscope half off the chest.
- Grade 6: audible without stethoscope or with head of the stethoscope lifted off the chest.
- Because the chest wall is thin in children, grades 5 and 6 murmurs are not uncommon.

TIMING

- Systolic ejection murmurs begin after S1, peak in early systole and decrescendo in intensity to end before S2. They are typical of innocent murmurs and of murmurs secondary to narrowing of outflow from the heart.

TABLE 51-1   Syndromes Associated with Congenital Heart Defects

SYNDROME	CHARACTERISTICS	CARDIAC DIAGNOSIS
Down (trisomy 21)	Mental retardation (MR), ⇓ muscle tone, antimongoloid slant to eyes	AV canal, VSD
DiGeorge (del. 22q11)	Variable MR/immune deficiencies/facial anomalies	TOF, truncus arteriosus, right aortic arch
Turner (XO)	Short stature, webbed neck, widely spaced nipples, lymphedema	Coarctation of the aorta, bicuspid aortic valve, aortic stenosis, hypoplastic left heart syndrome
Noonan	Phenotypic Turner but occurs in males and females, normal chromosomes	Dysplastic pulmonary valve, HCM
William	Neonatal hypocalcemia, mild MR, "cocktail" personality	Supravalvar aortic stenosis, pulmonic stenosis
Marfan	Tall lean habitus, arachnodactyly hyperextensibility, dislocated lens	MVP, aortic root dilation, aortic dissection
Alagille	Neonatal jaundice/cholestasis	Pulmonic valve stenosis, pulmonary artery branch stenosis
Holt-Oram	Digitized thumb	ASD, common atrium

ABBREVIATIONS: AV canal, atrioventricular canal; HCM, hypertrophic cardiomyopathy; MVP, mitral valve prolapse; TOF, Tetralogy of fallot.

- Holosystolic/regurgitant murmurs begin with S1 and continue with the same intensity right into S2. A typical holosystolic murmur is that caused by a ventricular septal defect (VSD). Holosystolic murmurs are always organic.
- Diastolic murmurs are never louder than grade 4 and are always abnormal.
- Continuous murmurs are usually abnormal, the one exception being the innocent venous hum. A continuous murmur occurs when there is flow throughout the cardiac cycle with the best example being a patent ductus arteriosus.
- A click is an additional heart sound related to movement of one of the valves and is always an abnormal finding. *Systolic ejection clicks* occur right after S1 and are related to opening of a semilunar valve. If the valve abnormality is very mild, the only positive finding could be an isolated systolic ejection click. If there is stenosis, the click will occur at the beginning of a systolic ejection murmur. A *midsystolic click* is related to retrograde movement of an AV valve toward

the atrium behind it at peak ventricular systole. A classic example is the click of mitral valve prolapse.
- General characteristics of an innocent murmur:
  1. Soft, ≤grade 3.
  2. Vary significantly with change in position.
  3. Systolic in timing (with the exception of the venous hum).
  4. Do not radiate off the precordium.
  5. Occur in a normal child.
  6. Rare in infancy; usually heard in children over the age of 2.
- Specific characteristics of the individual functional murmurs are in Table 51-2.
- Most studies have concluded that skilled auscultation alone is adequate for evaluation of the innocent murmur in the vast majority of cases.
- Referral to a pediatric cardiologist should occur whenever a murmur does not meet the innocent criteria or whenever there is an associated question such as failure to thrive, potential history of cardiac symptoms, or extreme parental anxiety.

TABLE 51-2   Functional Murmurs

TYPE	DESCRIPTION	LOCATION	ETIOLOGY	AGE
Still's	Systolic ejection murmur, twanging, vibratory, musical	Mid-LSB (left stenal border) to apex	?	3–8 years
Pulmonic ejection	Nondescript systolic ejection murmur	Best at base, louder lying down, no radiation	Flow across right ventricular outflow tract	8–14 years
Venous hum	Continuous low-pitched murmur, louder in diastole	Sitting up, leaning head back elicits murmur; lowering chin or lying down eliminates it	Flow in great veins returning to heart	3–6 years
Peripheral pulmonic stenosis	Systolic ejection murmur	Axillae, back, less well at base of the heart	Bifurcation of pulmonary artery	Newborn

- In infancy, any murmur heard has a much greater chance of being organic and deserves further evaluation.
- Cardiac evaluation should be one of the first steps in the workup of failure to thrive.

BIBLIOGRAPHY

Castle RF, Craige E. Auscultation of the heart in infants and children. *Pediatrics* 1960;Suppl.:511–520.

Danford DA, Nasir A, Gumbiner C. Cost assessment of the evaluation of heart murmurs in children. *Pediatrics* 1993;91:365–368.

Fogel DH. The innocent systolic murmur in children: a clinical study of its incidence and characteristics. *Am Heart J* 1959;59:844–855.

Newburger JW, Rosenthal A, Williams RG, Fellows K, Miettiren, A. Noninvasive tests in the evaluation of heart murmurs in children. *N Engl J Med* 1983;308:61–64.

Rosenthal A. How to distinguish between innocent and pathologic murmurs in childhood. *Pediatr Clin North Am* 1984;31:1229–1240.

Van Oort A, Le Blanc-Botden M, De Boo T, Van Der Werf T, Rohmer J, Daniels O. The vibratory innocent heart murmur in schoolchildren: difference in auscultatory findings between school medical officers and a pediatric cardiologist. *Pediatr Cardiol* 1994;15:282–287.

52 CHEST PAIN

Rae-Ellen W. Kavey

- Chest pain in children is a common complaint but is only very rarely associated with any organic disease.
- Almost invariably, pain in the chest—whatever its characteristics—is viewed as coming from the heart by children and their parents.
- Families often have overwhelming concerns that the child has serious heart disease and can be very difficult to reassure.
- In general, chest pain at rest recurring over many months is benign.
- Exertional chest pain deserves cardiac evaluation with electrocardiogram (ECG), echo, and exercise test to exclude important but rare cardiac ischemic causes.
- Characteristics of the pain and physical examination findings help determine subsequent evaluation as outlined in Table 52-1.

TABLE 52-1   Evaluation of Pediatric Chest Pain

DIAGNOSIS	SYMPTOMS/SIGNS
Idiopathic	>6 months history of recurrent pain, usually at rest. No associated symptoms. Normal examination.
Chest wall	
Traumatic	History of trauma. Pain at site.
Musculoskeletal	History of unusual effort, exertion. Pain elicited by movement of neck, shoulders, thorax.
Costochondritis	Inflammation at costochondral junction. Pain at site.
"Catch pain"	Sudden onset of sharp, severe pain, at rest. Lasts seconds to minutes at most. Pain increased with breathing, motion. "Catches" patient in midinspiration. Normal examination.
Bronchopulmonary	History of respiratory symptoms, asthma. Often with fever. <48 hours duration. Cough reproduces pain. Rales, rhonchi, wheezes on examination.
Cardiac	
Coronary ischemia	Exertional onset of substernal pressure/pain, often radiating to back, neck, left arm. Associated with pallor, diaphoresis, and syncope. Associated tachycardia with cocaine.
Left ventricular outflow obstruction Coronary anomaly Cocaine abuse	Must have cardiac evaluation.
Arrhythmias	
Supraventricular tachycardia, Ventricular tachycardia	History of rapid forceful beats rather than pain.
Gastrointestinal	
Gastroesophageal reflux	Postprandial, often begins when patient lies down. Relieved by antacids

BIBLIOGRAPHY

Brown RT. Costochondritis in adolescents. *J Adolesc Health Care* 1981;1:198–201.

Driscoll DJ, Glicklich LB, Gallen WJ. Chest pain in children: A prospective study. *Pediatrics* 1976;57:548–651.

Fyfe DA, Moodie DS. Chest pain in pediatric patients presenting to a cardiac clinic. *Clin Pediatr* 1984;23:321–324.

Kloner RA, Hale S, Alker K, Prezkalla S. The affects of acute and chronic cocaine use on the heart. *Circulation* 1992;85:407–419.

Miller AJ, Texidor TA. Precordial catch, a neglected syndrome of precordial pain. *JAMA* 1955;159:1364–1365.

Pantell RH, Goodman BW. Adolescent chest pain: A prospective study. *Pediatrics* 1983;71:881–887.

Rowe BH, Dulberg CS, Peterson RG, Vlad P, Li MM. Characteristics of children presenting with chest pain to a pediatric emergency department. *Can Med Assoc J* 1990;143:388–394.

Selbst SM, Ruddy RM, Clark BJ, Henretig FM, Santalli T. Pediatric chest pain: A prospective study. *Pediatrics* 1988;82: 319–323.

Selbst SM, Ruddy BR, Clark BJ. Chest pain in children: follow-up of patients previously reported. *Clin Pediatr* 1990;29: 374–377.

Wiens L, Sabath R, Ewing L, Gowdamarajan R, Portnoy J, Scagliotti D. Chest pain in otherwise healthy children and adolescents is frequently caused by exercise induced asthma. *Pediatrics* 1992;90:350–353.

53 SYNCOPE

Jatin N. Patel and Wayne H. Franklin

- Syncope in pediatrics is a common complaint although the true incidence has not been elucidated. The standard definition of syncope is the sudden, transient loss of consciousness, and postural tone that results in impaired cerebral function. When applying the standard definition of syncope in the preambulatory patient, it can be difficult to identify syncopal episodes, as this group does not have upright posture. Syncope has heterogeneous causes, but the majority of syncope is related to problems of the autonomic nervous system. Malignant causes, potentially leading to sudden cardiac death, must be excluded.

EPIDEMIOLOGY

- No good population based studies have identified the true incidence and prevalence of syncope.
- Syncope is not a common diagnosis in infants and newborns because they typically do not fit into the classic definition of syncope. In addition, the most common cause of syncope, vasodepressor syncope, is unlikely to occur unless the patient is in an upright position.
- Reports have shown that between 10 and 50% of adolescents have had at least one syncopal episode.
- In children and adolescents, the cause of syncope in over 90% of the patients is vasodepressor syncope.
- Hypertrophic cardiomyopathy (HCM) is the most common cause of sudden death in young competitive athletes and may present first with an episode of syncope.

PATHOPHYSIOLOGY

- Multiple causes of syncope, both cardiac and noncardiac, have intrinsic differences in their pathophysiology; however, they all lead to the ultimate endpoint of diminished perfusion to the cerebrum and resultant loss of consciousness.
- Vasodepressor syncope results from a complex interplay of the autonomic and cardiovascular systems that cause vasodilation and/or bradycardia, leading to hypotension and syncope. On arising, blood pools in the lower extremities causing decreased right and left ventricular filling. In response to decreased filling, the left ventricle contracts vigorously and stimulates mechanoreceptors (C-fibers) in the posterior ventricular wall. Stimulation of C-fibers causes a reflex increase in vagal tone that results in bradycardia (cardioinhibitory response). In addition, the stimulation of C-fibers causes a reflex vasodilation of the peripheral vasculature that results in hypotension (vasodepressor response). Both the bradycardia and/or the hypotension can cause syncope. Baroreceptors in the carotid arteries and mechanoreceptors in the heart respond to hypovolemia by decreasing their firing rates leading to increased sympathetic tone. Sympathetic activity may then lead to C-fiber stimulation and syncope. Serotonin may be involved with central blood pressure regulation, and a lack of adequate serotonin may lead to syncope.
- Cardiac syncope results from impairment of blood flow, myocardial dysfunction, arrhythmias, or any combination of these. Examples of impaired blood flow include aortic stenosis, pulmonary vascular obstructive disease (pulmonary hypertension), and hypertrophic cardiomyopathy. Myocardial dysfunction leading to inadequate cardiac output may occur in the presence of myocarditis, cardiac ischemia (e.g., an anomalous coronary artery), or dilated cardiomyopathy. Tachyarrhythmias (e.g., ventricular tachycardia and ventricular fibrillation) and bradyarrhythmias (e.g., heart block) are causes of arrhythmia induced syncope. Conditions such as acquired or congenital long QT syndrome or Wolff-Parkinson-White syndrome may predispose to tachyarrhythmias. In a child or adolescent with structural heart disease, supraventricular tachycardia is an unlikely etiology of syncope.
- Noncardiac syncope results from primary central nervous system (CNS) disorders (e.g., seizures), apnea, gastrointestinal disease (e.g., gastroesophageal reflux in the infant), drug exposure, metabolic abnormalities (e.g., hypoglycemia in the infant), psychiatric disorders (e.g., conversion disorder and malingering), dysautonomia (e.g., Riley-Day syndrome), and hypovolemia.
- The various substrates mentioned above for syncope may manifest in any pediatric age group. Certain entities are seen more frequently in some age groups than others. For example, gastroesophageal reflux is a cause of syncope in the infant, but not seen outside of this age group.

CLINICAL FEATURES

- The onset of vasodepressor syncope is usually seen in teenage patients with the average age of presentation being 13 years old. A slight preponderance of females may be present. Episodes usually occur when sitting or standing. Symptoms occur several minutes after a position change. Blood loss, pain, intercurrent illness, dehydration, and heat can exacerbate the potential for syncope. Additionally, coughing, micturition, deglutition, and hair combing cause syncope in a neurally-mediated fashion. Associated symptoms that may occur prior to the actual syncopal event include dizziness, visual and auditory disturbances, weakness, pallor, tachycardia, and diaphoresis.
- Cardiac syncope has multiple causes that may lead to syncope or change in tone.
  1. *Impairment of blood flow lesions*: Patients may be previously asymptomatic, have easy fatigability, a heart murmur and/or chest pain. Syncope during exercise has a higher chance of being cardiac in origin compared to patients who have syncope when upright. These patients may present with sudden cardiac death.
  2. *Myocardial dysfunction*: Shortness of breath, fatigue, or tachycardia prior to syncope.
  3. *Tachyarrhythmias*: Chest discomfort, palpitations, light-headedness, or blurry vision before syncope occurs.
  4. *Bradyarrhythmias*: Dizziness, nausea, decreased energy, or exercise intolerance in addition to syncope.
- Noncardiac syncope has a diverse scope of clinical features that will not be outlined in detail in this section. Both vasodepressor syncope and other cardiac etiologies of syncope can cause a seizure due to lack of cerebral perfusion. They both can be associated with tonic or tonic/clonic movements; however, primary seizures usually have a longer postictal phase.

DIAGNOSIS AND DIFFERENTIAL

- The goal is to identify malignant causes. The key data that differentiate malignant and nonmalignant causes are obtained in a careful, directed, and detailed history and physical examination along with limited studies.
- Malignant causes are considered if the family history is positive for sudden cardiac death (especially one at an early age), heart disease, arrhythmias, or neurologic disease. A past history of cardiac disease, cardiac surgery, palpitations, or drug use may predispose the patient to having a malignant cause of syncope.

- Events surrounding the syncopal event should be explored. If the patient had syncope with standing, pain, or fear then vasodepressor syncope is likely. They may also experience warmth, diaphoresis, headache, or nausea. Syncope during exercise, on awakening to an alarm, or during swimming may indicate a more malignant cause of syncope.
- Patients with a hypertrophic cardiomyopathy or aortic stenosis may have a harsh systolic ejection murmur at the right upper sternal border along with an increased left ventricular impulse. One can decrease the murmur of hypertrophic cardiomyopathy by having the patient do a hand-grip maneuver (increases afterload). The murmur will increase after release of hand-grip. A gallop with tachycardia indicates myocardial dysfunction as seen with myocarditis or cardiomyopathy. Hepatomegaly may also be present.
- Diagnostic testing should include an electrocardiogram (ECG). An ECG may help to identify patients with hypertrophic cardiomyopathy (left ventricular hypertrophy, ST-T-wave changes, and deep Q waves), long QT syndrome, Wolff-Parkinson-White syndrome, Brugada syndrome, or Arrhythmic Right Ventricular Dysplasia. Additional tests are as directed by the history, physical examination, and ECG.
  1. *Tilt test*: The tilt test is one potential tool used in the evaluation of vasodepressor syncope. The patient is kept supine on a table and then the head is elevated to 70°. Blood pressure and ECG is monitored. A test is positive if symptoms are reproducible with an associated drop in blood pressure and/or heart rate. A negative test does not completely exclude vasodepressor syncope, and a positive test does not exclude malignant causes. Isoproterenol may be used to reproduce symptoms if the tilt test is negative at baseline; however, this may further decrease the specificity of the test. Tilt testing should be interpreted with caution so as not to miss a potentially lethal cause of syncope.
  2. *Holter monitor/event recorder*: The 24-hour ambulatory electrogram (Holter monitor) can pick up arrhythmias that a 12-second ECG does not detect. Holter monitors are useful for a syncope evaluation if the symptoms occur daily. Rare episodes of syncope are unlikely to be picked up on a Holter monitor. An event recorder may be more useful because symptom-specific data are obtained. Several types of event monitors are available and can be used depending on the clinical situation. An event monitor that the patient places on himself/herself when the event occurs is not helpful when the symptom is syncope. The alternative is

an event monitor in a "loop mode" that a patient can wear continuously (usually for a month). The monitor is continuously recording and erasing the patient's ECG. When the patient presses a button, the ECG is recorded from a preset time prior to pressing the button and records for a preset time after the button is pressed. This ECG is stored and can be transmitted over the telephone after the event. This type of recording device is helpful in patients who have a premonitory symptom (e.g., dizziness). Event recording is more cost-effective than Holter monitoring. A newer type of event recorder is now available that is used in the loop mode; however, certain parameters such as a high and low heart rate can be programmed in so that if the patient's rate goes out of the specified range, the monitor will record. This is helpful in patients who have no warning about the syncopal episode.

3. *Implantable loop recorder (ILR)*: This device is similar to the event monitor; however, it is implanted subcutaneously in the chest region. It can record an ECG that is either patient activated or when the heart rate goes outside of specified parameters. The ILR can be interrogated, much like a pacemaker, noninvasively after an episode. This type of monitor is rarely indicated in the usual pediatric patient with syncope.

4. *Exercise testing*: Used to provoke ischemia or arrhythmia. A negative test does not exclude cardiovascular disease if indicators are present. This test is potentially useful in patients who have syncope during exercise.

5. *Echocardiogram*: Very low yield for associated cost. Not routinely recommended for evaluation of syncope unless the event occurs *during* exercise. At that point a directed echocardiogram should be considered to evaluate for myocardial function, hypertrophic cardiomyopathy, right ventricular dysplasia, and abnormal coronary artery origins.

• A good history, physical examination, and ECG will help diagnose most cases of syncope. The cost of ancillary tests remains high with very low diagnostic yield. Selective tests should be performed as indicated by the history, physical examination, and ECG.

TREATMENT

• Vasodepressor syncope may not need treatment and is often self-limiting. Whether to treat or not to treat depends on the number and severity of the events.

Identifying predisposing risk factors and avoiding them is potentially effective but not always practical. Additional primary therapy includes an increase in fluid and salt intake. Patients should be encouraged to take in at least their maintenance fluids as calculated by their body weight. Fludrocortisone, alpha-agonists, beta-blockers, and selective serotonin reuptake inhibitors may be helpful.

• Treatment for cardiac syncope involves either removing the obstruction to flow, augmenting cardiac output, or antiarrhythmia therapy, i.e., cardioversion, medication, radiofrequency catheter ablation, pacemaker, or an implantable cardioverter-defibrillator (ICD).

• Treatment for noncardiac syncope is tailored to addressing the specific underlying cause.

PROGNOSIS

• Vasodepressor syncope has a good prognosis. Episodes may be isolated. If there is recurrence, it will likely be self-limiting with improvement over time. Some patients have more difficulty and may require referral to a cardiologist for more specialized management.

• Cardiac causes of syncope have a worse prognosis including the potential for sudden cardiac death.

PREVENTION

• The primary prevention of vasodepressor syncope is recognition of precipitants and avoiding them when possible. Additionally, maintaining adequate hydration offers benefit.

• For cardiac causes exercise limitation (hypertrophic cardiomyopathy, long QT syndrome, Wolff-Parkinson-White syndrome, myocardial dysfunction, and pulmonary vascular obstructive disease), medications (beta-blockers for long QT syndrome), radiofrequency catheter ablation (WPW), pacemakers and ICDs are a few preventive measures that may be employed. Several genes have been identified for long QT syndrome and hypertrophic cardiomyopathy. Although routine gene screening is currently impractical because of the genetic heterogeneity of these diseases, a proband's genes can be investigated to identify an abnormality in a specific family. Once this gene is identified in the proband, other members of that family can be screened for that specific gene defect. Those asymptomatic patients then have the option for preventive strategies.

BIBLIOGRAPHY

Cook S, Franklin WH. Evaluation of the athlete who 'Goes to Ground'. *Prog Pediatr Cardiol* 2001;13:91–100.

Daniels CJ, Franklin WH. Common cardiac diseases in adolescents. *Adolesc Med* 1997;44:1591–1601.

Deal BJ, Wolff GS, Gelband H. Syncope diagnosis and management. *Current Concepts in Diagnosis and Management of Arrhythmias in Infants and Children,* Armonk, NY: Future; 1998;223–240.

Kochilas L, Tanel RE. Evaluation and treatment of syncope in infants. *Prog Pediatr Cardiol* 2001;13:71–82.

Sokoloski MC. Evaluation and treatment of pediatric patients with neurocardiogenic syncope. *Prog Pediatr Cardiol* 2001; 13:127–131.

Steinberg LA, Knilans TK. Costs and utility of tests in the evaluation of the pediatric patients with syncope. *Prog Pediatr Cardiol* 2001;13:139–149.

54 CONGENITAL HEART DISEASE
Rae-Ellen W. Kavey

- Congenital heart disease is common, occurring in just under 1 in 1000 live births.
- Congenital heart defects cover the range from trivial abnormalities of no functional consequence to complex/critical problems presenting catastrophically in the newborn.
- During the first year of life, congenital heart disease is the leading cause of death from birth defects.
- Detecting the presence of congenital heart disease is an important role for the pediatric care provider.

Acyanotic Congenital Heart Disease

VALVE LESIONS

PULMONARY VALVE STENOSIS

- Pulmonary stenosis occurs in 8–12% of all children with congenital heart disease and is more common in females.

PATHOPHYSIOLOGY
- Pulmonary stenosis refers to obstruction of right ventricular outflow which may occur below, at, or above the pulmonary valve.

- In classic *valvular* pulmonic stenosis, valve leaflets are thickened with fusion of the commisures. In *infundibular pulmonic stenosis,* there is thickening of the muscle and narrowing of the path leading from the body of the right ventricle to the pulmonic valve. This type of obstruction tends to increase as cardiac output increases. With *supravalvar pulmonic stenosis* there is a waistline above the pulmonic valve before the bifurcation of the pulmonary artery branches at the level of the valve sinuses.
- In children with Noonan syndrome, pulmonic valve stenosis is the characteristic lesion and the valve leaflets can be thickened and dysplastic.
- Whatever the level of obstruction, the narrower the outflow from the right ventricle, the higher the RV pressure and the greater the compensatory right ventricular hypertrophy of the ventricle.

CLINICAL COURSE/FINDINGS
- In childhood, most patients with pulmonic stenosis are asymptomatic. Examination reveals increased right ventricular impulse along the left sternal border and possibly a thrill across the RV outflow tract if the obstruction is severe. There is a systolic ejection murmur over the RV outflow tract with the loudness of the murmur increasing as narrowing increases. The murmur radiates along the path of outflow, from the base of the heart to the lungs.
- With mild-to-moderate valvular pulmonic stenosis, there is usually a systolic ejection click at the outset of the murmur.
- The maximum intensity of the murmur will occur closest to the site of an actual RV outflow tract narrowing, often allowing discrimination between obstruction below, at, or above the valve.
- Narrowing due to muscle bundles in the body of the right ventricle (called double chamber right ventricle) produces obstruction below the level of the infundibulum. This kind of narrowing can progress rapidly.
- The electrocardiogram (ECG) is normal in children with mild pulmonary stenosis; there is increasing right axis deviation and right ventricular hypertrophy as the severity of narrowing increases, regardless of the level of obstruction. With two-dimensional echo pulse and color Doppler imaging, there is visualization of the site of narrowing and the degree of right ventricular hypertrophy. Doppler allows estimation of severity of the narrowing.

CLINICAL COURSE/NATURAL HISTORY
- Critical pulmonary stenosis in the neonate is a cyanotic lesion and will be reviewed in that section.

- Patients are generally asymptomatic with pulmonic stenosis even when the degree of narrowing is moderate to severe.
- Beyond the first year or two of life, mild pulmonic stenosis is not progressive; this means that if a child has mild pulmonic stenosis at the age of 2, only infrequent pediatric cardiology follow-up is required subsequently.
- Treatment is needed if there is moderate-to-severe narrowing defined as an outflow tract gradient between the RV body and the pulmonary artery of more than 50 mmHg or, a right ventricular pressure greater than one-half to two-thirds of aortic pressure.
- For moderate to severe pulmonary valve stenosis, cardiac catheterization and balloon valvuloplasty are indicated. This technique has been successfully performed for more than 20 years with an excellent safety record; the majority of patients require only one dilation.
- If the site of narrowing is above or below the valve and the narrowing moderate to severe, surgical intervention is needed.
- After successful intervention (catheter based or surgical), children are allowed unlimited activity. There is no cardiac limitation to their life span. They continue to require antibiotic prophylaxis for potentially bacteremic procedures.

AORTIC VALVE STENOSIS

- Left ventricular outflow tract obstruction occurs with a prevalence of 3–6% in children with congenital heart disease. It occurs more often in males than in females.

PATHOPHYSIOLOGY
- Narrowing of the left ventricular outflow tract at valvar, subvalvar, or supravalvar level is associated with increased left ventricular pressure and left ventricular (LV) hypertrophy corresponding to the severity of the obstruction.
- In *valvular aortic stenosis* (AS), the pathology can range from bicuspid aortic valve without measurable stenosis to a critically obstructed valve associated with congestive heart failure in the newborn.
- *Subaortic stenosis* can arise from a discrete membrane across the left ventricular outflow tract below the valve or from a fibromuscular tunnel. In either case, turbulence arising from the subvalvular narrowing can lead to progressive aortic insufficiency.
- *Supravalvular aortic stenosis* is an annular constriction above the aortic valve at the level of the sinuses

of Valsalva. Supravalvar AS is commonly seen in children with Williams syndrome.

CLINICAL COURSE/NATURAL HISTORY
- The vast majority of children with aortic stenosis are asymptomatic.
- With severe untreated obstruction, exertional chest pain, easy fatigability, syncope, or even sudden death can occur.
- Aortic stenosis at any level is progressive over time, both with growth during childhood and with calcification during adult life.
- Because of the risks associated with severe obstruction and the progressive nature of aortic stenosis, children with moderate aortic stenosis are restricted from strenuous sports in a competitive setting. After intervention, exercise recommendations depend on the extent of residual pathology.
- Aortic stenosis is one of the congenital lesions most commonly associated with bacterial endocarditis. For valvular aortic stenosis, intervention is recommended for severe narrowing (defined as a gradient ≥75 mmHg across the left ventricular outflow tract) and for moderate aortic stenosis (gradient 50–75 mmHg) associated with symptoms, or with electrocardiographic evidence of left ventricular strain at rest or induced by exercise. Children with valvular aortic stenosis and a gradient < 50 mmHg are followed prospectively.
- Valvuloplasty can be performed in the cath lab or surgically with very similar long-term results: there are varying degrees of residual aortic stenosis and insufficiency after either procedure.
- At some point in their lives, most individuals with congenital valvular aortic stenosis will require valve replacement with either their own pulmonary valve (Ross procedure) or a mechanical valve.
- For subvalvular aortic stenosis, surgery is usually recommended when the gradient approaches 50 mmHg with any evidence of aortic insufficiency.
- For supravalvar aortic stenosis, surgery is recommended for a gradient ≥50 mmHg, or when there is any evidence of coronary compromise related to the supravalvular narrowing.

FINDINGS
- Aortic stenosis at any level causes a systolic ejection murmur heard best at the base of the heart, particularly the second right intercostal space, with transmission along the outflow tract from the heart to the suprasternal notch, neck, and apex.
- Even with mild stenosis, there is often a faint thrill felt in the suprasternal notch.
- With mild-to-moderate valvular aortic stenosis, a systolic ejection click can be heard at the outset of the

murmur—this often disappears as obstruction progresses.

- With bicuspid aortic valve, an isolated systolic ejection click can be the only finding; bicuspid aortic valve is very commonly associated with coarctation of the aorta.
- The greater the narrowing, the louder the murmur; when a thrill is felt over the precordium the degree of stenosis is usually at least moderate.
- Electrocardiograms are often completely normal in children with aortic stenosis. The extent of left ventricular hypertrophy and the presence of ST segment and T-wave changes in the inferior and left lateral leads (LV strain pattern) can be helpful in decision-making regarding the severity of the obstruction. Development of LV strain is a sign that intervention is indicated.
- Echo/Doppler evaluation allows visualization of the level of obstruction and the degree of severity as well as the extent of left ventricular hypertrophy. The Doppler gradient leads to an estimate of LV outflow tract obstruction, which can be correlated with other findings for decision-making.
- Children with aortic stenosis should undergo complete echo/Doppler evaluation at least every 1–2 years.

COARCTATION OF THE AORTA

- Coarctation of the aorta occurs in 8–10% of all cases of congenital heart disease. As with all LV outflow tract diagnoses, it is more common in males than in females.

PATHOPHYSIOLOGY
- A posterior shelf indents the upper thoracic aorta just opposite the mouth of the ductus arteriosus.
- In the neonatal period, when the ductus is still open, the aortic mouth of the ductus can allow a detour around this narrowing. For this reason, the diagnosis of coarctation is very difficult to make in newborns. When the ductus closes, usually by 2 weeks of age, the obstruction becomes manifest with higher blood pressure in the upper body and lower blood pressure and reduced pulses below the coarctation.
- In 10–20% of patients with coarctation of the aorta, the obstruction is severe enough to induce congestive heart failure at this time.
- Eighty to ninety percent of patients are asymptomatic with classic findings for upper body hypertension and reduced blood pressure and pulses in the lower body.
- At least 60% of patients with coarctation have a bicuspid aortic valve.

- Coarctation of the aorta is the classic cardiac lesion associated with Turner syndrome.

FINDINGS
- Classic findings are elevated blood pressure in the upper body and reduced blood pressure and pulses in the lower body; there is a midsystolic murmur over the left back related to flow past the coarctation site.
- Auscultation of the heart itself is normal in 40% of patients and positive for the click of a bicuspid aortic valve in the other 60%.
- In older patients, continuous murmurs of collaterals bypassing the coarctation site are heard over both sides of the back.
- In neonates, findings of congestive heart failure may predominate with the only feature specifically suggestive of coarctation being the difference in pulses and perfusion between the upper and lower body.
- In newborns, the electrocardiographic pattern is right axis deviation and right ventricular hypertrophy. In older children, a left ventricular hypertrophy pattern develops secondary to LV pressure overwork.
- Echocardiography will demonstrate the posterior shelf protruding into the descending aorta; Doppler evaluation will predict the arm/leg gradient.
- With color Doppler, collateral vessels can be demonstrated as can the presence of associated bicuspid aortic valve and the extent of left ventricular hypertrophy.

CLINICAL COURSE/NATURAL HISTORY/ INTERVENTION
- Newborns who present with coarctation and congestive heart failure can present with shock and profound acidosis. Prompt recognition of the diagnosis and initiation of prostoglandins will lead to reopening of the ductus and restoration of effective flow past the coarctation site to the lower body.
- In these babies, surgical repair of coarctation is required.
- If left untreated, patients with coarctation develop severe cardiovascular problems such as myocardial infarctions, strokes, and aortic rupture related to the upper body hypertension early in adult life.
- Average age at death in untreated coarctation is the fourth decade.
- For the 80–90% of patients who are asymptomatic, coarctation repairs should be accomplished as soon as the diagnosis is made.
- Asymptomatic infants and children should be referred for repair as soon as the diagnosis is made since the older the patient at the time of repair, the more likely they are to develop hypertension postoperatively unrelated to any residual narrowing at the repair site.

- For the neonate with critical coarctation in congestive heart failure, surgical repair is required immediately. Best results are achieved with an extended end-to-end repair, which augments the transverse arch and eliminates the coarctation shelf completely.
- Surgical repair has been successfully accomplished with very low mortality and good long-term results for greater than 50 years.
- Balloon dilation/stenting has been used to effectively treat native coarctation in older children and adults; however, questions about the potential for aortic dissection and aneurysm development await long-term follow-up.
- After successful coarctation repair, patients still need regular follow-up for recurrent coarctation (10% of repairs in infancy), hypertension (at least 30% of patients even when repaired in early childhood), and bacterial endocarditis prophylaxis, as well as the possibility of progressive aortic stenosis and insufficiency related to the bicuspid aortic valve.

AORTIC INSUFFICIENCY

- Isolated congenital aortic insufficiency is extremely rare; however, aortic insufficiency secondary to a bicuspid aortic valve, subaortic stenosis, or prolapse of an aortic valve leaflet into a ventricular septal defect (VSD) increases the prevalence.
- Most cases of aortic insufficiency in children are secondary to intervention for aortic stenosis, either surgical or balloon valvuloplasty.
- As with all regurgitant lesions, aortic insufficiency is progressive over time.

PATHOPHYSIOLOGY
- Aortic insufficiency results in volume overload of the left ventricle and increased stroke volume in systole; diastolic pressure is low because of flow back across the aortic valve. This combination leads to a widened pulse pressure.
- The degree of aortic insufficiency is reflected in the severity of left ventricular volume overload.
- When aortic insufficiency develops as a result of aortic valve leaflet prolapse into a ventricular septal defect, this is an indication for surgical repair of the ventricular septal defect (VSD).

FINDINGS
- Regurgitation across the aortic valve results in a high-pitched decrescendo diastolic murmur heard best at the midleft sternal border but well transmitted to the apex; the murmur is heard best with the patient sitting. Systolic blood pressure may be mildly increased and pulse pressure is wide.

- With moderate-to-severe aortic insufficiency, the regurgitant flow back across the aortic valve intersects the forward flow across the mitral valve to produce a middiastolic flow rumble (an Austin Flint murmur).
- Associated lesions like aortic stenosis and ventricular septal defect will contribute their findings to auscultation.
- *Electrocardiogram*: As would be anticipated, increasing left ventricular overload produces the electrocardiographic picture of left ventricular hypertrophy. With severe aortic insufficiency, relative coronary insufficiency can be reflected in ST/T-wave changes in the inferior and left lateral leads (LV strain).
- *Echocardiographic findings*: The two-dimensional study will identify the etiology of aortic insufficiency whether that is an abnormal aortic valve, a subaortic membrane, or a prolapsing aortic valve leaflet. With color Doppler, the width of the regurgitant jet correlates with the severity of regurgitation as does the left ventricular dimension.
- Serial ECG and echo findings can be used to assess the volume work of the left ventricle and guide the need for valve replacement.

CLINICAL COURSE/NATURAL HISTORY
- Whatever the etiology, aortic insufficiency tends to progress over time.
- Symptomatic patients should be referred for surgery, usually the Ross procedure in which the patient's own pulmonary valve is placed in the aortic position with a homograft in the right ventricular outflow tract.
- When aortic insufficiency develops as a result of prolapse into a ventricular septal defect, surgical closure of the ventricular septal defect ± plasty of the affected aortic valve leaflet is required to prevent progressive aortic insufficiency.
- In asymptomatic patients with AI, there are no definitive guidelines for surgical referral. From adult studies, progressive severe left ventricular dilation and/or reduced LV systolic function are indications for surgery. Left ventricular function returns to normal postoperatively in the vast majority of cases.

NATURAL HISTORY/OUTCOME
- Once a competent valve is in place, findings of LV volume overload resolve.
- Mechanical valves necessitate long-term anticoagulation and this is associated with significant morbidity primarily related to trauma.
- Unfortunately, any valve placed in the aortic position in childhood will require replacement in the future and each successive operation is at higher risk.
- The Ross procedure has the potential to "cure" aortic stenosis, but there are no long-term follow-up studies after the Ross procedure performed in childhood as yet.

- In the short term, additional surgery is often required to replace the bioprosthetic valve in the pulmonary position and eliminate dilation of the aortic root with secondary insufficiency.
- Antibiotic prophylaxis for any potentially bacteremic procedure is required.
- Children with mechanical valves are limited from contact sports because of the risks of anticoagulation.
- Children with mild aortic insufficiency, normal electrocardiogram, and normal treadmill exercise test results are unlimited in their activities.

PULMONIC INSUFFICIENCY

- Isolated pulmonary insufficiency is extremely rare, but pulmonary insufficiency after surgical or interventional procedures for RV outflow tract obstruction is relatively common, occurring most frequently after tetralogy of Fallot repair.

PATHOPHYSIOLOGY
- Pulmonary insufficiency causes a volume overload of the right heart.
- In isolation, pulmonary insufficiency is very well tolerated with patients asymptomatic through childhood and into middle adult life.
- However, after tetralogy of Fallot repair, the valve insufficiency is often associated with residual pulmonary stenosis and RV outflow tract fibrosis and dysfunction because of prior resection at surgery.
- In this context, findings of progressive right ventricular dilation and reduced function are common.

FINDINGS
- The murmur of pulmonary insufficiency is a low-pitched decrescendo diastolic murmur directed down along the left sternal border. The murmur increases significantly when the patient is lying down. In isolation, pulmonary insufficiency will produce a mild right ventricular hypertrophy pattern on the ECG. If it occurs after surgery for tetralogy, the ECG will reflect the usual complete right bundle branch block pattern.
- With echo/Doppler, the width of the regurgitant jet, backflow from the pulmonary branches, and the extent of RV dilation allow estimation of the severity of pulmonary insufficiency.
- Echo also allows serial evaluation of the hemodynamic impact of pulmonary insufficiency on the right ventricular size and function over time.

CLINICAL COURSE/NATURAL HISTORY
- Patients with isolated mild-to-moderate pulmonary insufficiency are asymptomatic and unlimited in their activity.

- With isolated severe pulmonary insufficiency or pulmonary insufficiency with distal stenosis, progressive RV dilation/dysfunction can develop associated with reduced exercise tolerance and atrial and ventricular arrhythmias. Such patients are limited from strenuous sports in a varsity team setting.
- If severe pulmonary insufficiency is left untreated, progressive RV dilation and dysfunction will develop.

INTERVENTION
- When findings of severe RV volume overload develop, pulmonary valve replacement with a bioprosthetic valve is indicated.
- Unfortunately, all current valves become obstructed over 5–15 years; thus pulmonary valve replacement in childhood sets the stage for repeated valve replacements throughout life. Research is ongoing to develop alternatives to preclude this problem.

NATURAL HISTORY/OUTCOME
- Patients with pulmonary insufficiency require long-term follow-up for development of severe RV volume overload.
- After pulmonary valve replacement, patients need serial evaluation for development of progressive stenosis of the bioprosthetic valve.
- Antibiotic prophylaxis to reduce the risk for bacterial endocarditis for any potentially bacteremic procedure is indicated.
- Exercise limitation depends on the degree of right ventricular overwork.

TRICUSPID INSUFFICIENCY

- Tricuspid insufficiency in childhood is usually associated with Ebstein's anomaly of the tricuspid valve. This is a very rare diagnosis, occurring in less than 1% of patients with congenital heart disease.

PATHOPHYSIOLOGY
- Septal leaflet of the tricuspid valve is displaced from its normal position down toward the apex of the right ventricle. This results in incorporation of part of the right ventricle into the right atrium and concomitant decrease in right ventricular size.
- The more the septal leaflet is displaced, the greater the degree of tricuspid insufficiency.
- The most severe cases present as neonates with cyanosis due to right-to-left shunting through a patent foramen ovale—this situation will be discussed in the section on cyanotic congenital heart disease.

FINDINGS
- The greater the degree of tricuspid regurgitation, the more pronounced the findings of right atrial

volume overload. With mild-to-moderate tricuspid insufficiency in childhood there will be a soft holosystolic murmur, heard best at the lower right and lower left sternal border, that increases with inspiration and when lying down.

- In Ebstein's anomaly, the murmur of tricuspid insufficiency is often associated with a triple or quadruple rhythm.
- With greater degrees of tricuspid insufficiency, there will be an associated soft, low-pitched middiastolic murmur of relative tricuspid stenosis related to the increased flow across the tricuspid valve in diastole. Often this murmur is only heard with the patient lying down.
- Right atrial and to a lesser degree right ventricular enlargement are commensurate with the degree of regurgitation.
- With severe regurgitation, pulsation of engorged neck veins and liver can be felt.
- The electrocardiogram will show right atrial enlargement and incomplete right bundle branch block pattern. First degree AV block occurs in 40% of patients. Twenty percent will have ECG evidence of Wolff-Parkinson-White.
- On chest x-ray, increasing right atrial enlargement will be reflected in an increasing cardiothoracic ratio.
- With echo/Doppler evaluation, the diagnosis is easily made with clear demonstration of the downward displacement of the septal leaflet of the tricuspid valve on two-dimensional imaging in the four-chamber view. Right atrial enlargement and relative right ventricular hypoplasia are seen reflecting the degree of anatomic severity. Color Doppler will visualize the extent of tricuspid insufficiency and the possible presence of a patent foramen ovale with potential for right-to-left shunting.

CLINICAL COURSE/INTERVENTION

- The clinical course depends on the degree of anatomic displacement and secondary tricuspid insufficiency. Patients with severe tricuspid insufficiency present as cyanotic newborns.
- Patients with mild-to-moderate tricuspid insufficiency are usually asymptomatic in childhood.
- The degree of tricuspid regurgitation tends to progress over time and most patients begin to develop symptoms of easy fatigability ± recurrent atrial arrhythmias in their late teens or early twenties.
- Surgical repair of the tricuspid valve is technically challenging with variable results.
- Tricuspid valve replacement with a bioprosthetic valve is an alternative, but due to the low pressures in the right heart, valve dysfunction frequently occurs.

- Atrial arrhythmias tend to occur in 10–20% of patients even after successful surgery.
- Antibiotic prophylaxis is indicated for all potentially bacteremic procedures.
- Exercise limitation depends on the degree of insufficiency: Children with mild-to-moderate TR and normal exercise tests are unrestricted. Those with severe TR and/or abnormal response to exercise testing are limited from participation in strenuous sports in a team setting.

MITRAL VALVE INSUFFICIENCY

- The majority of patients with mitral insufficiency have developed the regurgitation secondary to acute rheumatic fever.
- Isolated congenital mitral regurgitation is very rare, but can occur secondary to a cleft in the anterior leaflet of the mitral valve in patients with an endocardial cushion defect and rarely due to shortened tethered cords, the so-called parachute mitral valve.
- Mitral valve prolapse is a common substrate for MR and may occur in as many as 5% of children with a significant female preponderance.

PATHOPHYSIOLOGY

- The physiologic consequence of mitral insufficiency is volume overload of the left atrium and left ventricle.
- The greater the degree of regurgitation, the larger the LA and LV volumes.
- The etiology of the insufficiency (rheumatic, cleft mitral valve, mitral valve prolapse) determines the pathophysiology: *Rheumatic mitral regurgitation* tends to be greatest during acute rheumatic carditis and can be very severe with associated congestive heart failure at that time. Mitral regurgitation due to a *congenital cleft* is usually mild with findings and course dominated by the associate congenital heart lesions. In *isolated mitral valve prolapse*, the degree of mitral regurgitation in childhood is usually very mild.
- Mitral regurgitation tends to progress over time.
- Echocardiography is the diagnostic test of choice allowing visualization of the valve abnormality leading to regurgitation.
- The degree of left atrial and left ventricular enlargement on echo/Doppler evaluation reflects the severity of mitral regurgitation and can be used for serial follow-up.

CLINICAL COURSE

- Most patients with mitral insufficiency of any etiology are asymptomatic in childhood, the exception being the child with acute rheumatic carditis. No exercise limitation is required for mild mitral insufficiency except in the setting of acute rheumatic fever.

- Bacterial endocarditis prophylaxis is indicated for all patients with mitral insufficiency; patients with rheumatic MR also require penicillin prophylaxis against recurrent strep infections.
- With severe mitral insufficiency, symptoms of exertional fatigue develop.
- Severe mitral insufficiency is often associated with atrial arrhythmias.
- Progressive severe left heart dilation, the onset of symptoms and/or the development of atrial arrhythmias are indications for surgical intervention.

INTERVENTION
- Cleft mitral valves are repaired at the time of surgery for the associated endocardial cushion defect.
- In some patients with mitral insufficiency, mitral ring annuloplasty can decrease the degree of mitral insufficiency significantly.
- Usually, mitral valve replacement is required and this mandates chronic anticoagulation.
- If valve replacement is required in childhood, serial replacements will be required through adult life with each surgery at increased risk for morbidity and mortality.

LEFT-TO-RIGHT SHUNTS

VENTRICULAR SEPTAL DEFECT (VSD)

- VSDs are the most common congenital cardiac diagnosis accounting for 15–20% of all cases.
- VSDs can occur anywhere in the ventricular septum, see Table 54-1 for the description of the VSD location.

PATHOPHYSIOLOGY
- The clinical course of a patient with ventricular septal defect depends on the size and location of the defect.
- A *large VSD* is defined as a defect that has essentially the same diameter as the aortic root.
- With large VSDs, LV and RV systolic pressures are equalized with pulmonary artery pressure at systemic levels.
- LV-to-RV shunting occurs because of the lower diastolic pressure (resistance) in the pulmonary vascular bed.

TABLE 54-1 VSD Classification by Location

VSD TYPE	INCIDENCE	LOCATION
Membranous	80%	Beneath septal leaflet of TV from RV, beneath AoV from LV side
Outlet	5–7%	In RV outflow tract, just beneath PV
Inlet	5–8%	Beneath septal leaflet of TV, below membranous defects
Muscular	5–20%	Apical septum, frequently multiple

- With a large defect, shunting will increase progressively as pulmonary vascular resistance undergoes the normal decline beginning at birth and reaching the nadir at approximately 3 months of age. The left-to-right shunt will increase progressively during the first 6 weeks of life.
- The congestive heart failure associated with a VSD is a high output failure reflecting primarily the increased workload of the left ventricle pumping both to the lungs and the body.
- Most ventricular defects can become smaller through a variety of different mechanisms; however, if a large defect is not closed by 1–2 years of age, there will be a progressive increase in pulmonary vascular resistance reflecting trauma to the small arteries in the pulmonary bed. Ultimately, right-to-left shunting and cyanosis will develop. This is now a very rare situation called Eisenmenger syndrome. In this setting, closure of the ventricular septal defect will result in acute right ventricular failure and death.
- A *small ventricular septal defect* is restrictive, preventing any transmission of left ventricular pressure to the right ventricle and pulmonary arteries. The degree of left-to-right shunting is limited by the size of the defect and so will not change as pulmonary vascular resistance declines.
- A *moderate ventricular septal defect* can be associated with a significant left-to-right shunt which becomes manifest as pulmonary vascular resistance declines; however, the size of the defect prevents the development of systemic level pulmonary hypertension.
- While a significant left-to-right shunt can develop, it is not usually large enough to produce congestive heart failure.
- One of the mechanisms for closure of a ventricular septal defect is prolapse of the right coronary cusp into a membranous or outlet defect. This results in secondary aortic insufficiency. If this is not treated, progressive aortic insufficiency can develop.

CLINICAL COURSE/FINDINGS
- On auscultation, the murmur of a ventricular septal defect is holosystolic with the same intensity throughout.
- With a *small defect*, the murmur runs into the second heart sound and can obscure it. Often there are high-pitched components in the murmur of a small VSD.
- The murmur is heard best over the site of shunting, so muscular VSDs can be heard best toward the apex and outlet VSDs at the upper- to midleft sternal border.
- Even small defects can have a localized thrill associated with them.

- With *large ventricular septal defects*, the precordium is diffusely active with a thrill. Although the murmur is holosystolic, the second sound will be readily heard and P2 will be accentuated.
- With a *moderate-to-large VSD*, there will often be an associated low-pitched middiastolic flow rumble at the apex related to increased flow across the mitral valve. When this is present, pulmonary blood flow (PBF) is at least two times the systemic flow.
- *ECG findings* will reflect the size of the defect: Normal with small VSDs; reflecting mild left ventricular hypertrophy with moderate VSDs; and demonstrating significant combined ventricular hypertrophy with large VSDs.
- In Eisenmenger syndrome, there is severe right ventricular hypertrophy.
- *Echocardiography* is an essential part of the evaluation of a ventricular septal defect allowing visualization of the size and location, plus measurement of LV volumes, and estimation of right heart pressures.
- In addition, echo will allow identification of associated prolapse of an aortic cusp and secondary aortic insufficiency before this becomes audible on auscultation.
- Serial echocardiograms support clinical decision-making regarding the need for and timing of surgical intervention.
- Clinically, large ventricular septal defects result in typical VSD findings on auscultation plus tachypnea, tachycardia, and diaphoresis. There may be hepatomegaly but peripheral edema is rare. Growth failure and frequent respiratory infections can be associated with a large ventricular septal defect.
- Since most VSDs can become smaller with time, a period of medical management is traditional; however, if there is growth failure, current management is surgical closure within the first 6 months of life. Morbidity and mortality are very low, ≤ 2% for surgical repair.
- Children with small VSDs are entirely asymptomatic.
- Surgical management is never needed for an intrinsically small VSD.
- Usually patients with moderate VSDs are asymptomatic and grow normally.
- If a moderate VSD does not become small on its own, surgical closure is considered for those defects in which there is evidence of persistent volume overload beyond the first or second year of life.
- If a moderate VSD is associated with prolapse of a coronary cusp and secondary AI, surgical closure is recommended to increase fibrous support for the aortic valve and prevent progressive aortic insufficiency.
- Although currently experimental, catheter closure of ventricular septal defects is under investigation and is likely to become an option in the future.

- On long-term follow-up post-VSD closure, the majority of patients do extremely well with normal growth and activity and normal life span. Rarely, patients can develop surgical heart block late after surgery and this is most common in patients who have required repair in early infancy and experienced transient heart block in the early postoperative period.
- Small VSDs are associated with a significant risk for endocarditis so recommendations for good dental hygiene and antibiotic prophylactics for dental work are indicated.
- Beyond 6 months postsurgical VSD closure with no residual defect, antibiotic prophylaxis is no longer required.

ATRIAL SEPTAL DEFECT (ASD)

- Atrial septal defects are common, representing 5–10% of all congenital heart defects.
- ASDs are more common in females than in males.

PATHOPHYSIOLOGY
- The defect in the atrial septum can occur in three different positions:
  1. *Secundum ASD*: The most common, accounting for 60% of all ASDs. The defect occurs in the midportion of the atrial septum at the site of the fossa ovalis.
  2. *Ostium primum ASD*: Account for 30% of all atrial defects. This is an incomplete endocardial cushion defect with deficiency of the inferior part of the atrial septum just above the AV valves. A primum ASD is associated with clefts in the mitral and tricuspid valves. There is a relative deficiency of the superior portion of the ventricular septum but no VSD.
  3. *Sinus venosus ASD*: Ten percent of atrial septal defects are in this location, superiorly, just below the entrance of the SVC to the right atrium. Sinus venosus ASDs are often associated with anomalous pulmonary venous return of the upper right lung vein to the right atrium.
- Left-to-right shunting through the atrial defect occurs when left atrial pressure exceeds right atrial pressure. Because atrial pressures reflect end diastolic pressures in the ventricles and RV end diastolic pressure is often higher than LV end diastolic in the neonate, shunting is minimal in this time period and increases throughout infancy.
- If untreated, shunting through an atrial septal defect will increase further in adult life as end diastolic pressure rises in the left ventricle with age.

CLINICAL FINDINGS/COURSE

- Children with an atrial septal defect are asymptomatic.
- Because the pressure difference between the atria is low, no murmur is produced by the left-to-right shunt; however, the increased pulmonary blood flow produces a grade 2-3/6 ejection murmur heard best at the upper left sternal border with radiation to both lungs.
- Increased flow across the right ventricular outflow tract delays pulmonary valve closure producing the classic "fixed split" of the second sound.
- With the child lying down, a soft middiastolic flow murmur of increased flow across the tricuspid valve can be heard.
- In patients with primum ASD, mitral insufficiency due to the cleft in the mitral valve can cause a holosystolic murmur heard best at the apex with radiation to the left axilla.
- *Electrocardiographic findings*: In secundum and sinus venosus ASDs, there is right axis deviation and mild right ventricular hypertrophy with an rsR prime pattern in V1. In primum ASDs, the mild RVH pattern is the same but there is left axis deviation.
- *Echocardiography* allows visualization of the defect and of the RV volume load seen as increased RV size and flattened or paradoxical motion of the ventricular septum. With sinus venosus ASD, the drainage of the pulmonary veins can be evaluated. With primum ASD, the inferior defect and the associated cleft mitral valve can be seen and the degree of mitral regurgitation quantified.
- While patients with ASD are asymptomatic in childhood, problems with congestive heart failure, atrial arrhythmias, and pulmonary hypertension can develop in the third decade of life and beyond.
- Spontaneous closure of secundum ASDs diagnosed when an echocardiogram is performed in infancy are relatively common and these likely represent simply persistent patency of the foramen ovale. Spontaneous closure beyond 2 years of age is rare. In addition, if an atrial septal defect in the secundum position is more than 8 mm in diameter, spontaneous closure is unlikely.
- Neither sinus venosus nor primum ASDs can undergo spontaneous closure.
- Intervention for closure of atrial septal defects with significant left-to-right shunts (defined as evidence of RV volume overload) is recommended beyond 2 years of age.
- Secundum ASDs can be closed using a device in the cath lab with proven safety and efficacy.
- Primum atrial septal defects require surgical repair including suture closure of the cleft mitral valve. There is a small risk of heart block associated with primum ASD repairs.
- Sinus venosus atrial septal defects also require surgical repair with routing of the pulmonary veins to the left atrium as needed.
- Postoperatively, the vast majority of patients with effective closure of an atrial level shunt do extremely well.
- After primum ASD repair, follow-up for development of progressive mitral insufficiency is needed.
- After sinus venosus defect repair, follow-up for development of sinus node dysfunction is recommended.

PATENT DUCTUS ARTERIOSUS (PDA)

- Patent ductus arteriosus is a relatively common congenital heart defect, occurring in 5–10% of patients.
- Among premature infants, PDA is almost universally present. This discussion will focus on full-term babies with patent ductus arteriosis.

PATHOPHYSIOLOGY

- Patent ductus represents failure of complete closure of the fetal ductal arch.
- Beyond the immediate neonatal period, systemic vascular resistance exceeds pulmonary vascular resistance. This results in left-to-right shunting throughout the cardiac cycle.
- With a large patent ductus, there can be pulmonary hypertension and rarely, the ductus is so large that progressive changes in pulmonary vascular resistance occur as they can with a large VSD.

CLINICAL COURSE/FINDINGS

- Because there is left-to-right shunting throughout the cardiac cycle, there is a continuous murmur heard best at the base of the heart with transmission to both lungs.
- The precordium is active and there a may be a thrill at the upper left sternal border. Pulses are bounding.
- When the PDA is large, there can be signs of pulmonary overcirculation and congestive heart failure—tachypnea, tachycardia, failure to thrive, and susceptibility to respiratory infections.
- More often, a persistently patent ductus arteriosus is small to moderate and the patient is entirely asymptomatic.
- The *electrocardiogram* will reflect the degree of cardiac overwork. With a large PDA there will be evidence of combined ventricular hypertrophy. With a small PDA, the ECG will be normal.
- *Echocardiography* is diagnostic, demonstrating the width and length of the patent ductus, estimating PA pressure, and revealing the extent of LV volume overload. Echocardiography also excludes associated

lesions. Of particular note is the possibility of coarctation, which can be masked in the presence of a patent ductus arteriosus.

- Beyond the newborn period, persistence of a ductus is abnormal. Spontaneous closure is unlikely in a full-term infant.
- With a large ductus, findings of heart failure and failure to thrive can be present.
- When a large PDA is diagnosed, closure is recommended. This can be achieved in the cath lab using a device or surgically. Cath lab closure is the procedure of choice for infants greater than 6 months of age; however, surgical ligation and division can be preformed at any age with extremely low morbidity and mortality.
- Postoperative course following PDA closure is completely benign with no subsequent need for endocarditis prophylaxis.

PATENT DUCTUS ARTERIOSUS IN PREMATURE INFANTS

- Among premature infants, the patent ductus arteriosus is almost universally present. The greater the degree of prematurity, the more likely it is for a PDA to persist.
- In preterm babies whose course is often complicated by lung disease, clinical findings of the ductus can be atypical with an active precordium, bounding pulses, and a crescendo systolic murmur at the base or no murmur at all.
- The presence of a left-to-right shunt through a PDA definitely worsens premature lung disease.
- Echocardiography can be used to diagnose the PDA, estimate PA pressures, and LV volume overload.
- The electrocardiogram shows nonspecific findings.
- For premature babies, pharmacologic closure of the ductus with indomethacin, a prostaglandin inhibitor, is recommended. If the ductus persists after a total of three courses of indomethacin or if renal or hemorrhagic complications prevent its use, surgical ligation is recommended.
- Post-PDA ligation, there are usually no significant residua.

ATRIOVENTRICULAR CANAL

- Complete AV canal represents 2% of all congenital heart disease. It is the most common heart defect in children with Down syndrome. Half of the children with trisomy 21 have congenital heart disease and in 40% of these, the defect is a complete AV canal.

PATHOPHYSIOLOGY

- Failure of development of the endocardial cushions, the central part of the heart, results in a large confluent atrial/ventricular septal defect and a common atrioventricular valve.
- Partial forms exist with a relatively small ventricular component, large atrial component, and single AV valve, the so-called intermediate AV canal.
- An ostium primum ASD is a partial AV canal—there is no ventricular component, a central low ASD, and cleft mitral and tricuspid valves (see ASD section).

CLINICAL COURSE/FINDINGS

- In each case, the clinical course is governed by the presence and size of the atrioventricular defect.
- For a complete AV canal, findings are those of a large VSD with pulmonary hypertension; an additional murmur of mitral insufficiency can sometimes be appreciated.
- In babies with Down syndrome, pulmonary vascular resistance often does not undergo the normal decline. Findings of a left-to-right shunt can be minimal and congestive heart failure may never develop even with very large defects.
- It can be difficult to suspect congenital heart disease from clinical findings in children with Down. For this reason, *arbitrary cardiac evaluation is recommended for all newborns with this diagnosis.*
- For complete AV canal, the course is that of a large VSD. Since there is no chance for spontaneous closure, surgery is performed when significant congestive heart failure and/or failure to thrive develop, always in the first year of life.
- For babies with Down syndrome and complete AV canal, repair is recommended by 6 months of age to minimize development of pulmonary vascular disease.
- For intermediate AV canal, findings are those of a small-to-moderate VSD with an additional pulmonary flow murmur and fixed split of S2 reflecting the atrial level shunt.
- With an intermediate canal, there is usually no significant heart failure or risk of pulmonary vascular disease; however, there is also no chance for spontaneous closure. Complete repair is recommended at 1–3 years of age, sooner if there are associated symptoms.
- With complete AV canal repair, there is often residual mitral or tricuspid insufficiency, which requires long-term follow-up. Ten percent of patients will require additional surgery for the mitral valve late after AV canal repair. This is somewhat more common after an intermediate canal repair than after a complete AV canal repair.
- On *electrocardiogram*, there is a superior QRS axis with a prolonged PR interval and combined ventricular hypertrophy. With an intermediate canal the axis can be leftward and the degree of hypertrophy will reflect the ventricular overwork.

- *Echocardiography* reveals all elements of the anatomy of an AV canal including the size of the central AV septal defect, the attachments of the common AV valve, and the presence of any associated defects. With pulse and color Doppler, the extent of intracardiac shunting and of AV valve regurgitation can be visualized and RV and PA pressures estimated.
- Postoperative follow-up and activities will be dictated by the extent of the residual mitral valve abnormality.
- Endocarditis prophylaxis is required even after surgery for an endocardial cushion defect.

CYANOTIC

- Cyanotic defects account for less than 5% of patients with congenital heart disease, but are major focus of the pediatric cardiologist's time.
- Most cyanotic lesions present in the neonatal period and that will be the focus of this section.
- At least 5 g/100 mL of unsaturated hemoglobin are required to produce central cyanosis by any mechanism. The higher the total hemoglobin content, the smaller the degree of desaturation necessary to reach this level of reduced hemoglobin. This explains why anemic patients may not appear cyanotic even with severe arterial desaturation.
- Evaluation for cyanotic heart disease requires exclusion of cyanosis from the other major causes:
  1. Pulmonary
  2. Central nervous system (CNS)
  3. Methemoglobinemia
- Newborns with cyanosis on a pulmonary basis have evidence of respiratory distress (retractions, nasal flaring, rales, or abnormal parenchymal sounds on auscultation).
- In babies who are blue because of CNS problems, other findings such as poor tone, weak cry, abnormal posturing, and seizures lead to diagnosing the hypoventilation that underlies the cyanosis.

- In general, babies with methemoglobinemia appear completely well with the exception of their cyanosis.
- Arterial blood gas findings can be used to effectively identify the child with cyanosis on a cardiac basis as shown below:

ABG Findings in Cyanotic Newborns by Etiology

CNS, Pulmonary	vs.	Cardiac
pH		pH Normal to reduced
Normal to reduced		
PCO_2 Increased		PCO_2 Normal/decreased
PO_2 Mildly to		PO_2 Moderately/severely
moderately reduced		reduced

- Pulmonary blood flow on chest x-ray can be used to effectively divide patients with cyanotic heart disease into groups that define the critical cause of their cyanosis. Echo/Doppler evaluation will then almost always allow complete anatomic diagnosis to be made; however, *chest x-ray and ECG findings can be used to triage the cyanotic newborn and develop an initial management plan. See Fig. 54-1.*

DECREASED PULMONARY BLOOD FLOW

- In all patients with decreased pulmonary blood flow on chest x-ray and a small heart, the critical issue is obstruction to outflow of venous blood to the lungs, a problem that becomes manifest as the ductus closes.
- Characteristic ECG findings can distinguish between the diagnoses: Remember that normal newborns have right ventricular dominance as a reflection of prenatal physiology. The normal newborn electrocardiogram, therefore, shows a pattern of right axis deviation and right ventricular hypertrophy.

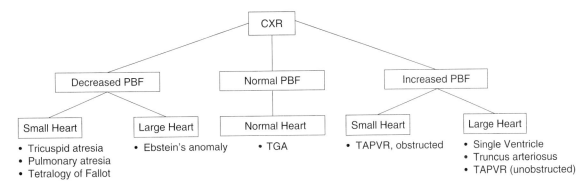

FIG. 54-1 Management Plan

TRICUSPID ATRESIA

- Classic atresia of the tricuspid valve is associated with significantly reduced right ventricular size. For this reason, the dominant cardiac mass is the left ventricle and the electrocardiogram shows left axis deviation and left ventricular hypertrophy.

PULMONARY ATRESIA

- With atresia of the pulmonary valve, the right ventricle is present but relatively hypoplastic. This results in a relatively leftward axis for a newborn (0–90°) and an unusual neonatal pattern of LV dominance.

TETRALOGY OF FALLOT

- This is the most common cyanotic congenital heart defect. The classic components are RV outflow tract obstruction, large ventricular septal defect, overriding aorta, and right ventricular hypertrophy. Time of presentation for tetralogy of Fallot depends on the severity of the RV outflow tract obstruction. When this obstruction is critical, the baby presents as a cyanotic newborn. The electrocardiogram will show right axis deviation and right ventricular hypertrophy, a normal newborn pattern. With less severe RV outflow tract narrowing, patients present with milder degrees of cyanosis later in early infancy.
- In *Ebstein's anomaly*, downward displacement of the septal leaflet of the tricuspid valve results in inclusion of part of the right ventricular inflow in the right atrium and, therefore, hypoplasia of the effective right ventricle plus varying degrees of tricuspid insufficiency. When presentation occurs in the newborn, each of these components is maximized with right to left shunting through a patent foramen. The baby presents with cyanosis shortly after birth and chest x-ray shows extreme cardiomegaly as well as decreased pulmonary vascular markings. This is the classic "wall to wall" heart picture. The electrocardiogram will show right atrial enlargement and an RV conduction delay or even complete right bundle branch block plus right atrial enlargement.
- In all of these lesions, initial therapy is improving pulmonary blood flow by establishing patency of the ductus with institution of prostaglandin therapy.
- For *tricuspid atresia*, the next step is surgical creation of a systemic-to-pulmonary shunt to provide a stable source of pulmonary blood flow and subsequent management is that of a single ventricle.
- For *pulmonary atresia*, shunt creation is combined with opening of the pulmonary outflow. If the right ventricle grows and becomes adequate in size, the shunt can then be subsequently eliminated leaving a four-chambered heart. If right ventricular size is inadequate, the patient is managed as a single ventricle.

- For *tetralogy of Fallot*, both right and left ventricles are well-developed and thus complete repair can be performed in the newborn. Alternatively, a systemic to pulmonary shunt can be placed to stabilize pulmonary blood flow with complete repair occurring later in infancy. When tetralogy presents with less severe RV outflow tract obstruction, beyond the immediate neonatal period, complete repair is performed electively within the first 6 months of life.
- For *Ebstein's anomaly*, the degree of tricuspid regurgitation tends to decrease as pulmonary vascular resistance undergoes the normal neonatal decline and forward flow from the RV increases. Usually, as oxygen saturations improve, the ductus can be allowed to close and the patient will do well as an infant and child, developing problems related to tricuspid insufficiency later in childhood or in adult life (see *Ebstein's anomaly* in the section on valvular lesions). If the right ventricular hypoplasia and tricuspid regurgitation are too severe to allow this, a systemic to pulmonary shunt is placed and subsequent management will depend on the adequacy of the right ventricle to support normal pulmonary blood flow.

NORMAL PULMONARY BLOOD FLOW

TRANSPOSITION OF THE GREAT ARTERIES

- The only cyanotic lesion with normal pulmonary blood flow is *transposition of the great arteries (D-TGA)* in which the aorta arises from the right ventricle and the pulmonary artery from the left.
- This is the most common cyanotic lesion presenting in the newborn and represents approximately 3% of congenital heart defects. It occurs more often in males than in females.
- In more than half of patients with *transposition*, the arterial malposition is the only abnormality. When other diagnoses are present, the course will be altered. This discussion is confined to isolated transposition of the great arteries with intact ventricular septum.
- The electrocardiogram shows the normal newborn pattern of right axis deviation and right ventricular dominance.
- Initial survival is dependent on bidirectional flow through persistent fetal channels, the foramen ovale, and the ductus arteriosus.
- Initiation of prostoglandins will maintain the patency of the ductus arteriosus in the immediate neonatal period; balloon septostomy of the foramen ovale is used to enhance bidirectional flow at atrial level.
- Current management of *transposition of the great arteries* is the arterial switch operation in the newborn. At surgery, the proximal great arteries are reversed and

coronary arteries are transplanted to the neoaortic root. Follow-up for up to 20 years reveals that the majority of patients do extremely well with minimal incidence of aortic insufficiency on follow-up.

- Prior management (Mustard or Senning procedure) used redirection of the systemic and pulmonary venous return at atrial level. These procedures are complicated by major postoperative problems including loss of sinus rhythm, atrial arrhythmias, and progressive systemic right ventricular dysfunction and are no longer used for simple transposition.

INCREASED PULMONARY BLOOD FLOW

SINGLE VENTRICLE
- This category combines all forms of *single ventricle* in which the common denominator is one functioning ventricular pumping chamber; the important diagnosis of *hypoplastic left heart syndrome* (HLHS) will be reviewed separately.
- The clinical picture of single ventricle is of mild cyanosis, often associated with signs of tachypnea and tachycardia.
- The ECG findings reflect ventricular hypertrophy (left, right, or both) and echo/Doppler findings allow visualization of the specific anatomic diagnosis.
- Management entails limitation of pulmonary blood flow and pulmonary artery pressures since low pulmonary vascular resistance is essential for palliation of single ventricle.
- Often, relief of associated obstruction of systemic outflow is necessary.

HYPOPLASTIC LEFT HEART SYNDROME
- HLHS is the most common cause of death from cardiac defects in the first month of life. In this diagnosis, mitral and aortic atresia are associated with virtual absence of the left ventricle. There is hypoplasia of the ascending aorta and aortic arch.
- Systemic blood flow is dependent on right-to-left shunting through the ductus arteriosus and then retrograde flow around the aortic arch to perfuse the head and neck vessels and the coronary arteries plus forward flow from the ductus to the descending aorta to perfuse the lower body.
- Survival is dependent on both continued patency of the ductus and left-to-right shunting at atrial level of pulmonary venous return into the right atrium. Initial management is prostaglandins to maintain ductal patency ± balloon atrial septostomy as needed.
- There are two options for initial palliation of HLHS—cardiac transplantation or the Norwood procedure followed by single ventricle palliation.

- Transplantation is limited by scarcity of donor organs and problems with pulmonary vascular disease developing while waiting for transplant.
- The Norwood procedure involves combining the aortic and pulmonary roots as a single outflow from the right ventricle and widening the aortic arch to provide systemic flow plus a systemic-to-pulmonary shunt to provide flow into the detached pulmonary arteries. Subsequently, patients are managed as a single ventricle. Current best results for the technically demanding Norwood procedure are an approximately 80% survival of the first stage.
- For patients with double inflow forms of *single ventricle*, management entails securing patency of systemic outflow and banding of the pulmonary artery to reduce pulmonary blood flow and pressure and maintain low pulmonary vascular resistance.
- After initial palliation, *single ventricle* patients (including those with Norwood palliation of HLHS) are managed currently with a bidirectional Glenn that connects the superior vena cava directly to the pulmonary arteries, usually by 6 months of age. This is followed by the Fontan procedure in which inferior vena cava (IVC) flow is directed entirely into the pulmonary arteries. There are many variants of the Fontan procedure including the original direct connection between the right atrium and pulmonary arteries and both intra- and extracardiac conduits. Survival for staged palliation of *single ventricle* through the bidirectional Glenn to the Fontan is currently 80%. For HLHS, the most complex and challenging single ventricle, survival through the Fontan is lower, averaging 60%.

TRUNCUS ARTERIOSUS
- *Truncus arteriosus* is a rare form of congenital heart disease, representing less than 1% of all patients. Patients present in early infancy with an enlarged heart, increased pulmonary blood flow, and mild cyanosis.
- In this diagnosis, the pulmonary arteries arise directly from an overriding aorta above a large ventricular septal defect.
- Thirty percent of patients have an associated right aortic arch.
- There is a strong association with 22q11 deletion (DiGeorge syndrome).
- The electrocardiogram usually shows combined ventricular hypertrophy; the specific diagnosis can be made with echo/Doppler evaluation.
- Patients with truncus arteriosus present like patients with single ventricle with mild cyanosis and tachypnea as pulmonary vascular resistance undergoes its normal decline.

- Current management involves early complete repair before 3 months of age. The ventricular septal defect is patched so that the arterial trunk arises exclusively from the left ventricle. Pulmonary arteries are detached from the truncus and flow is established between the right ventricle and pulmonary arteries using either autologous tissue or a conduit.
- After initial surgery, subsequent follow-up for development of RV to PA obstruction ± truncal valve insufficiency is needed.

TOTAL ANOMALOUS PULMONARY VENOUS RETURN

- The final diagnosis in this category is *total anomalous pulmonary venous return* (TAPVR). In TAPVR, the pulmonary veins drain into a confluence behind the heart that does not connect to the left atrium. Drainage occurs to the right atrium through an anomalous pathway, which is a remnant of a fetal venous channel.
- The path of drainage determines the clinical course: *Supracardiac* (50%)—pulmonary venous confluence drains through a left vertical vein into the innominate and thus the right atrium. *Cardiac* (20%)—pulmonary venous confluence drains into the coronary sinus. *Infracardiac* (20%)—pulmonary veins drain below the diaphragm through the portal vein/ductus venosus/hepatic vein or IVC into the right atrium. *Mixed* (10%)—combination of drainage sites.
- For survival, an atrial septal defect is essential.
- Clinical presentation depends on whether there is obstruction along the pathway of pulmonary venous return. This is most common with the infradiaphragmatic type. The patient presents with marked cyanosis and respiratory distress. Chest x ray shows a small heart and an intense pulmonary interstitial edema pattern.
- The *electrocardiogram* shows right axis deviation and severe right ventricular hypertrophy.
- On *echo/Doppler*, the path of pulmonary venous drainage is outlined; marked right atrial and right ventricular enlargement and pulmonary hypertension are shown plus right-to-left shunting at atrial level, a small left atrium, and compressed left ventricle.
- Urgent corrective surgery is needed to anastamose the pulmonary venous confluence to the left atrium. Postoperatively, severe pulmonary hypertension can persist and require aggressive management. In the past, persistent pulmonary hypertension was the cause of significant mortality after successful surgery. Current mortality is less than or equal to 10%.
- Postoperatively, recurrent pulmonary venous obstruction can develop in approximately 10% of patients requiring reoperation.
- Unobstructed total anomalous venous return presents with mild cyanosis and mild congestive heart failure; patients may be only minimally symptomatic.

- Chest x-ray shows an enlarged heart and increased pulmonary blood flow. Electrocardiogram shows right axis deviation and right ventricular hypertrophy.
- With echo/Doppler, the site of anomalous venous return is identified plus the right-to-left shunt at atrial level is visualized. The right heart is enlarged and the left relatively small, but there is no pulmonary hypertension.
- Repair involves anastomosis of the pulmonary venous confluence to the left atrium plus ASD closure. The mortality rate is <3%.
- After repair of unobstructed pulmonary venous return, patients generally do very well.

BIBLIOGRAPHY

Allen HD, Gutgesell HP, Clark EB, Driscoll DJ (eds.). *Moss and Adams' Heart Disease in Infants, Children and Adolescents, Including the Fetus and Young Adult*, 6th ed. Philadelphia, PA: Lipincott Williams & Wilkins, 2001.
Fyler DC (ed.). *Nadas' Pediatric Cardiology*. St. Louis, MO: Mosby, 1992.
Park MK. *Pediatric Cardiology for Practitioners*, 3rd ed. St. Louis, MO: Mosby, 1996.
Smith DW. *Recognizable Patterns of Human Malformation*, 3rd ed. Philadelphia, PA: W.B. Saunders, 1982.
Zuberbuhler JR (ed.). *Clinical Diagnosis in Pediatric Cardiology*. New York, NY: Churchill Livingstone, 1981.

55 ARRHYTHMIAS
Kendra Ward and Barbara J. Deal

- The management of pediatric patients with arrhythmias can be challenging yet rewarding: patients may present with arrhythmias during well child neonatal visits, or with palpitations, chest pain, or hypotensive shock. This chapter is intended to help the clinician recognize and diagnose pathologic arrhythmias, guide initial and emergency management, and understand indications for timely referral to a pediatric cardiologist or pediatric electrophysiologist. The differential diagnosis for pediatric arrhythmias is outlined in Table 55-1. Finally, specific antiarrhythmic medications pediatricians should be familiar with will be covered.

TABLE 55-1   Arrhythmia Classification

IRREGULAR RHYTHM	BRADYCARDIA
Sinus arrhythmia	Sinus bradycardia
Premature beats: atrial or ventricular	Blocked premature atrial contractions
Atrial fibrillation	Atrioventricular conduction disorders
Ventricular fibrillation	Second degree, third degree
Wenckebach conduction	Junctional rhythm
NARROW COMPLEX TACHYCARDIA	**WIDE COMPLEX TACHYCARDIA**
Sinus tachycardia	Supraventricular tachycardia conducted with bundle branch block
Supraventricular tachycardia	
Accessory connection mediated:	Ventricular tachycardia
AV reentrant	Preexcited atrial tachycardia
Orthodromic reciprocating	Junctional tachycardia with bundle branch block
Antidromic reciprocating	
Atrioventricular nodal	SVT with antidromic conduction via an accessory connection
Reentrant	
Automatic	Ventricular fibrillation
Primary atrial tachycardia	
Atrial reentrant/atrial flutter	
Automatic atrial tachycardia	
Multifocal atrial tachycardia	
Atrial fibrillation (usually irregular)	

DEVELOPMENTAL CHANGES IN THE ELECTROCARDIOGRAM

- *Rate*: Recognizing an abnormal rhythm requires familiarity with the normal range of acceptable heart rates as it changes from birth through adolescence (Table 55-2). These values vary slightly when sleep data are evaluated.
- *QRS axis*: The QRS axis is normally rightward in the newborn, reflecting the work of the RV in utero and postnatally against higher pressures in the lungs. The mean QRS axis in a newborn is approximately +137° (range +59 to −163). By approximately 6 months of age the QRS axis approximates the adult axis with a mean of +56 (range +6 to +100). A leftward axis in an infant is always abnormal.
- *QRS duration*: A normal QRS duration in an infant is 80 ms or less and in the child is less than 100 ms.
- *T wave*: The T wave in lead V1 is upright for the first few days of life. By 4–5 days it inverts and remains inverted until adolescence.

TABLE 55-2   Normal Heart Rates for Age by ECG

AGE	HEART RATES
Infant	90–160
3–5 year-old	70–140
5–8 year-old	65–130
8–16 year-old	60–125

- *Intervals*: The PR interval changes with age. On day 1 of life the normal PR interval ranges from 80 to 160 ms. From 1 day to 3 months, the normal PR interval is up to 140 ms; from 6 months through early adolescence normal is up to 160 ms; and then in the teenage years the normal PR interval is up to 180 ms.

IRREGULAR CARDIAC RHYTHMS

SINUS ARRHYTHMIA
- *Electrocardiogram (ECG) appearance*:
  1. Irregular rhythm with phasic variation in PP intervals sinus P wave before each QRS.
  2. Rate varies with respiration.
- *Characteristics*: Normal variant.
- *Ages*: Commonly occurs in early childhood, less prominent with older ages.
- *Treatment*: None.

PREMATURE ATRIAL CONTRACTIONS (PACs)
- *ECG appearance*:
  1. Premature P waves differing in axis and morphology from sinus P waves.
  2. Conduction to the ventricles may be normal, aberrant (conducted with bundle branch block), or blocked (not conducted). Premature P waves may be obscured in the preceding T wave.
- *Characteristics*: Infrequent PACs are common and occur in 13–77% of normal individuals.
- *Ages*: Occurs at any age; commonly detected in utero or first days of postnatal life.
- *Associated conditions*: Isolated, infrequent PACs are rarely associated with underlying conditions. Frequent PACs should prompt an evaluation for predisposing causes. These include structural heart disease, especially atrial defects, or myocardial dysfunction (including myocarditis), intracardiac lines, electrolyte abnormalities (hypokalemia, hypercalcemia), hypoxia, hypoglycemia, thyroid disease, and cardiac stimulant drugs (ephedrine, antihistamines, asthma medications).
- *Special considerations*: Wide complex extra beats in a patient who has PACs likely represent PACs with aberrant conduction.
- *Treatment*: Majority do not require treatment, other than evaluation for predisposing causes as noted above. Frequent PACs require follow-up, as they may be associated with sick sinus syndrome and later development of supraventricular tachycardia (SVT).

PREMATURE VENTRICULAR CONTRACTIONS (PVCs)
- *ECG appearance*:
  1. Premature QRS complex without preceding conducted P wave.

2. QRS morphology differs from sinus conducted QRS complex.
3. QRS duration usually but not always prolonged.
- *Ages*: Rare isolated PVCs are seen in newborns and older adolescents; may be seen in 6–27% of normal infants and children by Holter.
- *Associated conditions*: Usually secondary to another condition, similar to frequent PACs as described above. Careful evaluation of the patient for predisposing causes is needed: medication use, electrolyte abnormality, intracardiac central lines, myocardial disease, hypoxia, and long QT syndrome (LQTS).
- *Special considerations*: Frequent PVCs should prompt referral to a cardiologist for further evaluation. PVCs associated with syncope may be associated with a life-threatening condition.
- *Treatment*: Depends on the underlying condition, as correcting predisposing causes may eliminate the arrhythmia. PVCs in the ostensibly normal heart only require treatment when associated with symptoms or cardiac dysfunction.

ATRIAL FIBRILLATION
- *ECG appearance:*
  1. Absence of discrete organized atrial activity.
  2. Atrial fibrillation waves best seen in leads V1 and V2.
  3. Irregularly irregular ventricular response.
- *Characteristics*: Quite rare in childhood, with a prevalence less than 0.4% in patients under 40 years of age. The presence of atrial fibrillation in childhood is always abnormal, and requires thorough cardiac evaluation by a specialist.
- *Ages*: Bimodal: Rarely seen in infants with SVT associated with Wolff-Parkinson-White (WPW) syndrome, and older patients with significant valvar heart disease.
- *Associated conditions*: Advanced structural heart disease (including valvar disease, hypertrophic cardiomyopathy), thyrotoxicosis, SVT with WPW, highly trained athletes, and rarely in a familial form.
- *Special considerations*: Cerebral embolization of clot. In patients with an accessory connection (AC), atrial fibrillation can conduct rapidly to the ventricles and initiate ventricular fibrillation (VF). Digoxin and calcium-channel blocking medications such as verapamil may enhance accessory connection conduction, increasing the risk of ventricular fibrillation, and should be avoided in the presence of preexcitation.
- *Treatment*: Virtually always requires treatment in children: cardioversion or rate control. Rate control can be achieved with digoxin, beta-blockers, calcium-channel blockers, or atriovertricular node modification. Conversion to sinus rhythm may be achieved with medications including ibutilide, procainamide, amiodarone, or interventions including catheter ablation or surgery.

VENTRICULAR FIBRILLATION
- *ECG appearance*:
  1. Irregular, wide QRS rhythm.
  2. Very rapid ventricular rates greater than 200 bpm.
  3. Polymorphic ventricular complexes.
- *Characteristics*: Terminal lethal arrhythmia; may be a very rare cause of sudden cardiac death as a primary arrhythmia.
- *Ages*: Any, although as a terminal arrhythmia VF is more frequently seen in older patients; younger patients have a higher incidence of asystole as terminal arrhythmia.
- *Associated conditions*: Shock, severe heart failure, cardiomyopathy, ischemic cardiac disease, other structural heart disease, LQTS, WPW, hypoxemia, halothane anesthesia, potassium or other electrolyte abnormalities, and infection.
- *Special considerations*: In healthy individuals, may be produced by sudden blunt chest trauma, such as direct blow from baseball or hockey puck, known as "commotio cordis"; treated successfully by prompt defibrillation.
- *Treatment*: Immediate defibrillation using 2–4 J/kg of energy, Advanced Cardiac Life Support algorithm. After successful resuscitation, treatment depends on underlying cause; automatic implantable defibrillators are implanted in some patients.

WENCKEBACH, MOBITZ TYPE I SECOND-DEGREE AVB
- *ECG appearance*:
  1. Progressive lengthening of the PR interval.
  2. Eventual failure to conduct an atrial impulse to the ventricles.
- *Characteristics*: Seen in normal children during sleep and other times when vagal tone predominates.
- *Ages*: Adolescents, less commonly in younger children.
- *Associated conditions*: High vagal tone, athletes, and myocarditis in the acutely ill patient.
- *Special considerations*: Exclude underlying disease as a cause.
- *Treatment*: Usually asymptomatic and not usually progressive: intervention is rarely necessary. If the patient experiences associated symptoms such as syncope, especially with exertion, further evaluation and referral are indicated.

BRADYCARDIA

SINUS BRADYCARDIA
- *ECG appearance*:
  1. Sinus rhythm with rate less than normal for age.
  2. P waves before every QRS complex with a normal PR interval and normal QRS morphology.

- *Characteristics*: Depends on clinical setting: may range from a coincidental finding to a catastrophic prearrest rhythm.
- *Ages*: Any age, but uncommon in normal infants and young children; incidence increases with age beyond early adolescence.
- *Associated conditions*: Conditioned aerobic athlete, concurrent medication use such as clonidine or toxic ingestion, anorexia or depression, hypothyroidism, sick sinus syndrome, previous congenital heart disease surgery, increased intracranial pressure, obstructive sleep apnea, gastroesophageal reflux, and long QT syndrome.
- *Special considerations*: Stable patients should be evaluated for obvious symptoms such as dizziness, presyncope, or syncope, as well as for subtle symptoms: fatigue and sedentary lifestyle.
- *Treatment*: Emergency management for unstable bradycardic patients includes atropine, isoproterenol, or emergency pacing. Treatment of predisposing causes is usually sufficient to improve the heart rate. Symptomatic bradycardia is unusual in patients with structurally normal hearts and no associated underlying conditions; pacing is rarely required.

SECOND-DEGREE ATRIOVENTRICULAR BLOCK
- Failure to conduct some but not all atrial activity to the ventricles.

MOBITZ TYPE I (WENCKEBACH)
(See also above.)

MOBITZ TYPE II
- *ECG appearance*:
  1. A relatively constant PR interval.
  2. P wave fails to conduct to ventricle, without preceding progressive lengthening of the PR interval.
- *Characteristics*: Usually associated with pathology within the atrioventricular (AV) node or distally in the His-Purkinje system; referral to cardiac specialist indicated.
- *Ages*: All ages; uncommon.
- *Associated conditions*: Congenital AV block associated with maternal antibodies may initially present as first- and second-degree AV block, and progress with time to complete AV block. Other conditions: surgical repair of congenital heart disease; atrial septal defects, myocarditis; familial conduction disorders.
- *Treatment*: Generally not associated with symptoms, but requires monitoring due to risk of progression of AV block or development of symptoms. Symptomatic children (exercise intolerance, dizzy spells, syncope, or ventricular enlargement) require a pacemaker.

COMPLETE ATRIOVENTRICULAR BLOCK (TYPE III AVB, CAVB)
- *ECG appearance*:
  1. Complete dissociation of the P wave and QRS.
  2. Atrial rate greater than the ventricular rate, with failure to conduct P waves that fall outside the T wave of the preceding QRS.
- *Characteristics*: Acquired or congenital. The acquired form occurs with surgical damage to the His bundle or AV node: resolution may occur in the first 2 postoperative weeks. Late onset CAVB in postoperative patients is associated with syncope or death. Congenital CAVB occurs in approximately 1:20,000 births; half of these infants have a congenital heart defect (CHD); others are usually infants of mothers with collagen vascular disease, which may be subclinical. The infants and mothers should be tested for SSA/Ro and SSB/La antibodies.
- *Ages*: Congenital form usually recognized in infancy; caused by progressive form of AV conduction disorder in some, may infrequently be detected in older children.
- *Associated conditions*: Myocarditis, rheumatic fever; surgical repair of congenital heart disease. Infants with long QT syndrome may also have CAVB, a combination associated with significant mortality.
- *Special considerations*: Always requires urgent evaluation by a cardiac specialist.
- *Treatment*: Pacing indicated for significant bradycardia for age, wide QRS escape rhythm, significant ventricular ectopy, symptoms (including syncope or seizures, fatigue, poor growth parameters), ventricular enlargement, or dysfunction.

Blocked Premature Atrial Contractions (PACs)
- *ECG appearance*:
- The ECG criteria are described above.
- *Characteristics*: Nonconducted or *blocked* PACs occur when the PAC occurs quite prematurely, thus exceeding the ability of the AV node to conduct normally; slightly later PACs may be conducted with aberrancy. Blocked PACs are a frequent cause of pauses noted on monitors in neonates, and may be mistaken for sinus bradycardia or AV block. See above section on PACs for additional details.

JUNCTIONAL RHYTHM
- *ECG appearance*:
  1. Regular rhythm with narrow QRS complex, without preceding atrial activity.
  2. Junctional rates typically between 40 and 100 bpm; vary with age.
  3. P waves may be absent or infrequent (sinus bradycardia); dissociated (AV block), or follow each QRS (retrograde conduction).

- *Characteristics*: This is a common arrhythmia in pediatric patients and is seen in 13–45% of children by Holter monitoring. Junctional rhythm often occurs during times of increased vagal tone or sinus arrhythmia as an escape rhythm.
- *Ages*: Can occur at any age, although infrequent in infants; increased incidence with advancing age, most commonly seen in adolescents during sleep.
- *Associated conditions*: Sick sinus syndrome or sinus bradycardia in athletes; prior surgery for congenital heart disease, especially Senning/Mustard procedures for transposition of the great arteries, or Fontan procedures.
- *Treatment*: Rarely requires treatment, as symptoms are uncommon. In patients with repaired congenital heart disease, maintenance of normal atrial rates may decrease the incidence of developing atrial tachycardia.

NARROW COMPLEX TACHYCARDIA

SINUS TACHYCARDIA

1. *ECG appearance*: P waves precede each QRS complex with a regular RR interval.
2. Normal P-wave axis (0–90°), morphology, and PR interval.
3. Sinus rate is faster than upper limit of normal for age.

- *Characteristics*: Occurs in the presence of underlying cause, resolves when underlying cause resolves.
- *Ages*: Can occur at any age.
- *Associated conditions*: Sinus tachycardia is a symptom of a systemic illness. Possible causes include fever, hypovolemia, anxiety, anemia, circulatory shock, thyrotoxicosis, tachycardia causing medications, congestive heart failure, and myocardial disease.
- *Special considerations*: Due to inability to distinguish sinus tachycardia from other arrhythmias, particularly automatic atrial tachycardia (AAT), by rate alone, an ECG should always be obtained in infants with heart rates greater than 180 bpm, or in older children with elevated heart rates for their age.
- *Treatment*: Usually not associated with hemodynamic compromise; identification and treatment of underlying cause usually sufficient. Patients with thyrotoxicosis may require beta-blocking medications.

Supraventricular Tachycardia (SVT)

- The mechanism of SVT can usually be determined by analysis of the electrocardiogram. The incidence of different types of SVT varies with age. Reentrant mechanisms account for most SVT, most commonly using an accessory connection or dual AV nodal pathways. Infants often present with evidence of congestive heart failure including tachycardia, pallor,

irritability, congestion, or poor feeding, although in at least 20% of infants with SVT, the arrhythmia is detected during routine examination. Older children usually complain of palpitations, or chest or abdominal pain.

Atrioventricular (AV) Reentrant Tachycardias

- AV reentrant tachycardia uses an AC as one limb of the tachycardia circuit and the AV node as the other limb. Tachycardia cannot continue if block occurs in any part of this circuit. In general, patients with AC-mediated tachycardia tend to be younger with faster tachycardia rates. Associated structural heart disease is present in approximately 20% of these patients, including Ebstein's anomaly of the tricuspid valve, ventricular and atrial septal defects, and congenitally corrected transposition of the great arteries.

ORTHODROMIC RECIPROCATING TACHYCARDIA (ORT)

- *ECG appearance*:
  1. Typically regular, narrow QRS morphology (Fig. 55-1).
  2. Retrograde P waves follow QRS, by at least 70 ms.
  3. 1:1 VA relationship; SVT terminates in presence of AV block.
- *Characteristics*: Orthodromic reciprocating tachycardia (ORT) can occur using a concealed or a manifest AC, with antegrade conduction via the AV node, and retrograde conduction via an AC. Patients with a concealed AC will have a normal ECG when not in tachycardia. WPW syndrome: the AC is manifest during sinus rhythm producing a slurred upstroke of the QRS (delta wave) and shortened PR interval. The incidence of WPW is approximately 0.3–1.0% in children.
- *Ages*: In childhood, 40% of first episodes of SVT take place during the first 2 months of life, with age-related peaks of occurrence in older children aged 5–8 and 10–13. SVT presenting in infancy may "resolve" after the first year of life, but will recur at an older age in up to 70% of patients.
- *Associated conditions*: Structural heart disease; WPW on resting ECG.
- *Special considerations*: Patients with WPW have a higher incidence of atrial fibrillation than the general population. Digoxin and calcium-channel blocking medications may increase conduction over the AC, and are therefore avoided in the presence of manifest preexcitation.
- *Treatment*: Acute treatment: DC cardioversion in the unstable patient; otherwise vagal maneuvers, adenosine, or atrial pacing will terminate acute episodes. The decision for chronic treatment is based on severity and frequency of episodes. Beta-blocking agents

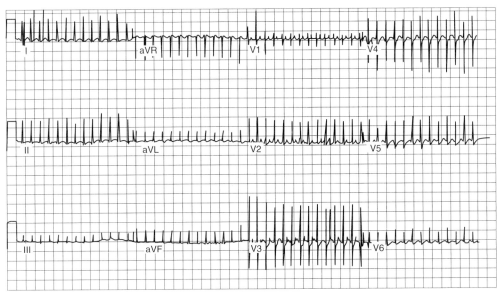

FIG. 55-1 Orthodromic reciprocating tachycardia (ORT).

are used commonly; catheter ablation is often performed in older children, particularly if manifest pre-excitation is present.

Permanent Form of Junctional Reciprocating Tachycardia (PJRT)

- *ECG appearance*:
  1. Regular, narrow QRS morphology tachycardia.
  2. Inverted retrograde P waves in leads II, III, and AVF, with long RP interval.
  3. 1:1 AV relationship: SVT terminates in presence of AV block.
- *Characteristics*: A subset of orthodromic reciprocating tachycardia, with retrograde conduction via a very slowly conducting AC, which is catecholamine sensitive.
- *Ages*: Most commonly seen in infants and toddlers, less frequently in older children.
- *Associated conditions*: Congestive heart failure, fatigue, and wheezing.
- *Special considerations*: Due to its slower rates and incessant nature, PJRT may not produce symptoms of palpitations, but congestive heart failure may be present as a result of long-standing tachycardia. Adenosine may terminate this tachycardia, but due to sinus tachycardia following adenosine, PJRT promptly reinitiates: this is commonly misinterpreted as "failure of adenosine." Recording rhythm strips during administration of adenosine can detect this phenomenon.
- *Treatment*: Usually difficult and multidrug therapy is often needed. Catheter ablation is the treatment of choice in older children.

AV Nodal Reentrant Tachycardia (AVNRT)

- *ECG appearance*:
  1. Regular, narrow QRS morphology (Fig. 55-2).
  2. Rates 150–300 bpm (mean, 170 bpm in older patients).
  3. Retrograde P waves with a short RP interval, less than 70 ms.
  4. Retrograde P waves may simulate an R in lead V1.
- *Characteristics*: A reentrant rhythm in which the AV node has two functional and likely two anatomically distinct pathways. Functional dissociation of conduction over the two pathways allows antegrade conduction over the more slowly conducting pathway, with retrograde conduction over the other pathway. Dual AVN physiology is reported in 35–46% of children and up to 85% of adults. The "typical" form travels antegrade over the slow pathway and retrograde over the fast pathway, resulting in a short RP interval as described above. Symptoms are common, and episodes are frequently terminated with vagal maneuvers. Visible neck pulsations are often described during this form of SVT.
- *Ages*: Rarely presents in infancy, but by 6–10 years of age accounts for 31% of SVT, and >50% of regular SVT in adults.
- *Associated conditions*: Slightly more common in females; not associated with congenital heart defects.
- *Special considerations*: Verapamil, especially when administered intravenously, is usually avoided in infants because of profound hypotension.
- *Treatment*: Acute management can include vagal maneuvers or adenosine. Long-term medical management

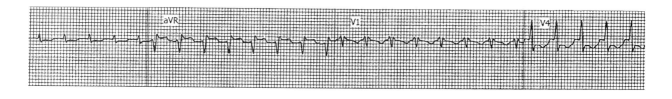

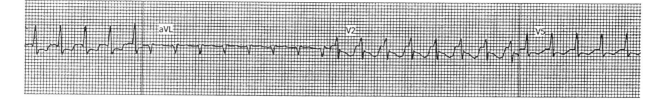

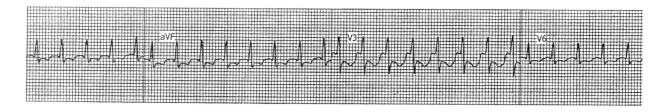

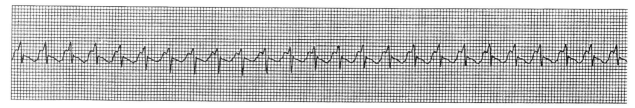

FIG. 55-2   AV nodal reentrant tachycardia (AVNRT).

is directed at blocking the AVN and can include calcium-channel blockers, digoxin, or beta-blockers. AV node slow pathway modification using catheter ablation is highly successful, although associated with a very small risk of creating AV block.

Primary Atrial Tachycardias
• Primary atrial tachycardia includes all forms of SVT where the electrical disturbance takes place within atrial tissue. The AVN and ventricles are not necessary for the arrhythmia to continue, and tachycardia persists in the presence of AVB. These arrhythmias are not common and account for up to 15% of SVT across all age groups.

Atrial Flutter (AF)
• *ECG appearance*:
  1. Rapid, regular sawtooth atrial flutter waves.
  2. Variable AV conduction, usually 2:1.
  3. Atrial rates 250–480 bpm.
  4. Persists in presence of AV block.

• *Characteristics:* A "macroreentrant" rhythm usually occurring in the right atrium. Atrial flutter occurring in the postoperative patient with CHD is often referred to as "atrial reentrant tachycardia" or "incisional atrial tachycardia" due to its association with atrial scars.
• *Ages*: A bimodal distribution in childhood: initially in the fetus or neonate, and later in the older child/adolescent in the setting of structural heart disease.
• *Associated conditions*: In infants, frequently associated with SVT due to accessory connections. In the older patients, atrioventricular valve disorder or prior extensive atrial surgery is usually present.
• *Special considerations*: In older patients, due to slow or variable AV node conduction, the ventricular rate may be only 120–140 bpm: suspect this condition in the older patients with repaired CHD and a heart rate greater than 100 bpm.
• *Treatment*: Acute treatment is always necessary to achieve sinus rhythm or at least rate control: electrical cardioversion, atrial pacing, or medications. In the

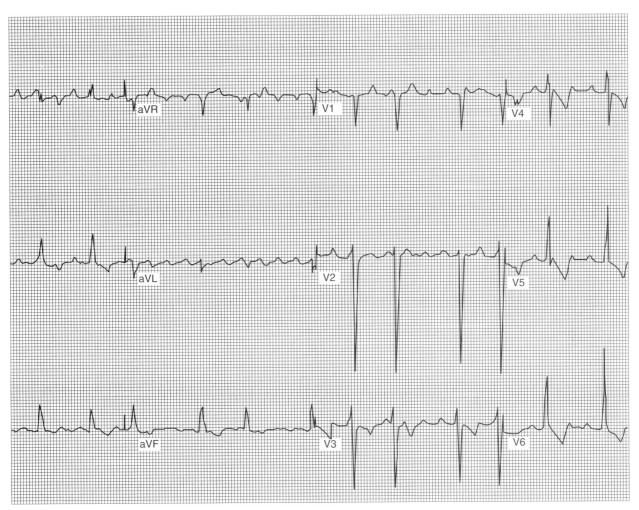

FIG. 55-3 Atrial reentry tachycardia.

presence of atrial tachycardia of uncertain duration, evaluation for the presence of atrial thrombus is necessary, usually involving transesophageal echocardiogram. Definitive treatment with catheter ablation or arrhythmia surgery may be effective.

Atrial Reentry Tachycardia
- *ECG appearance*:
  1. Discrete abnormal appearing P wave precedes QRS (Fig. 55-3).
  2. PR interval usually prolonged.
  3. SVT persists with AV block.
  4. Variable RR intervals may occur due to varying conduction.
  5. Atrial rates usually <250 bpm.
- *Characteristics*: This arrhythmia typically occurs in the setting of CHD, and uncommonly is seen in patients with ostensibly normal hearts. It can be distinguished from atrial flutter by slower atrial rates and discrete

low amplitude P waves. See discussion above regarding atrial flutter.

Automatic Atrial Tachycardia (AAT)
- *ECG appearance*: Distinctly visible P waves with abnormal morphology or axis. Prolonged PR interval, particularly with faster rates. Atrial rates 130–280 bpm; may vary with catecholamines. Warm up and cool down seen in atrial rates at initiation and termination of tachycardia.
- *Characteristics*: A form of incessant tachycardia caused by enhanced automaticity of an ectopic atrial focus. Twenty to thirty percent of patients have more than one ectopic focus. AAT accounts for 4–6% of SVT.
- *Ages*: Occurs at all ages.
- *Associated conditions*: Usually occurs in children with structurally normal hearts; however, due to incessant nature, patients may present with tachycardia induced cardiomyopathy. Heart failure may be reversible with control of the arrhythmia.

• *Special considerations*: Patients with "idiopathic" or unexplained cardiomyopathy should be carefully evaluated for the presence of this tachycardia.
• *Treatment*: Medical control is often difficult; beta-blocking medications may be effective, but often requires multiple antiarrhythmic medications. Catheter ablation is highly effective; very rarely surgery may be required for treatment.

MULTIFOCAL ATRIAL TACHYCARDIA (MAT)
• *ECG appearance*:
  1. Irregular atrial rate >100 bpm.
  2. At least three different, distinct, nonsinus P-wave morphologies present and firing randomly.
  3. Varying PP, PR, and RR intervals.
• *Characteristics*: Extremely rare in children, seen in 0.36% of hospitalized adults, and less commonly in children.
• *Ages*: Seventy-five percent of pediatric patients with MAT present in infancy.
• *Associated conditions*: Noncardiac abnormalities such as pulmonary disease, dysmorphic syndromes, and neurologic abnormalities are frequently present. Structural heart disease is present in about half of infants with MAT; hypertrophic cardiomyopathy may be present.
• *Special considerations*: Pulmonary disease may be present, and improvement in pulmonary status may ameliorate the tachycardia.
• *Treatment*: Antiarrhythmic therapy is not highly effective, and is reserved for incessant and rapid tachycardias. There is a high incidence of spontaneous resolution after infancy.

ATRIAL FIBRILLATION (USUALLY IRREGULAR)
• See description in previous section.

JUNCTIONAL ECTOPIC TACHYCARDIA (JET)
• *ECG appearance*:
  1. Narrow QRS tachycardia, without preceding P waves.
  2. Ventriculoatrial dissociation may be present, or retrograde conduction to the atrium may be present at slower rates.
  3. Warm up and cool down at initiation and termination may be seen.
• *Characteristics*: Originates from the compact AVN or tissue immediately surrounding the node, due to abnormally enhanced automaticity of that tissue. Due to incessant nature of congenital form, may produce significant cardiomyopathy, and requires aggressive treatment.
• *Ages*: Two forms: congenital (rare) and early postoperatively following surgery for congenital heart disease.

The postoperative form is usually seen in infants or toddlers.
• *Associated conditions*: Seen most commonly in first 24–72 hours following surgery for ventricular septal defects, atrioventricular canal defects, and tetralogy of Fallot.
• *Special considerations*: The rate of tachycardia can vary with administration of sympathomimetic agents, autonomic tone, hydration status, and body temperature. Postoperative JET usually resolves after 2–5 days.
• *Treatment*: Congenital JET is difficult to treat and most success has been seen with amiodarone or combination therapy; due to risk of progressive AV node disease (apoptosis), mortality is significant and a pacemaker is frequently implanted. In the postoperative setting, JET may cause significant hemodynamic compromise at higher rates; treatment with hydration, removal of inotropic medications, procainamide, diltiazem, or amiodarone may be effective in slowing the tachycardia rate.

WIDE COMPLEX TACHYCARDIA

VENTRICULAR TACHYCARDIA (VT)
• *ECG appearance*:
  1. Ventricular origin, rate >120 bpm.
  2. QRS duration >15 ms longer than 98th percentile for age.
  3. VA dissociation usually present.
  4. Fusion beats.
• *Characteristics*: Originates at a level below the AVN and has a rate > 120 bpm or 25% faster than the sinus rate; mechanisms include reentry, abnormal automaticity, and triggered activity.
• *Ages*: Any, but overall uncommon in childhood.
• *Associated conditions*: Electrolyte disorders, drug or toxin ingestion, myocarditis, cardiomyopathy, infantile Purkinje cell hamartomas, and postoperative congenital heart disease.
• *Special considerations*: Torsades de pointes (twisting of points) is an undulating rapid polymorphic wide QRS tachycardia associated with LQTS.
• *Treatment*: Appropriate medical therapy depends on the underlying cause of VT and may include cardioversion, amiodarone, lidocaine, or beta-blockers; catheter ablation or implantable cardioverter defibrillator (ICD) therapy; surgery.

Antidromic Tachycardia
• *ECG appearance*:
  1. Wide QRS tachycardia.
  2. Preexcited QRS morphology identical to preexcitation pattern during sinus rhythm.

3. 1:1 AV relationship.
4. Terminates in the presence of AV block.
- *Characteristics*: Although rare, patients with WPW may have SVT which conducts antegrade over the accessory connection and retrograde via the AV node, resulting in a wide complex tachycardia that resembles the preexcited baseline ECG.
- *Ages*: Very uncommon, at any age.
- *Associated conditions*: Wolff-Parkinson-White syndrome.
- *Special considerations*: If atrial fibrillation occurs, a rapid irregular wide QRS rhythm results, usually requiring urgent cardioversion.
- *Treatment*: Cardioversion, adenosine, procainamide, amiodarone; catheter ablation of accessory connection.
- Other wide complex tachycardias from differential (Table 55-1) are described in previous sections.

ARRHYTHMIA MANAGEMENT

- *Assess patient*: If hemodynamically unstable, prompt cardioversion/defibrillation, and advanced cardiopulmonary resuscitation (CPR) algorithms. Energy requirements are higher for ventricular or atrial fibrillation (2 J/kg).
- *Obtain 12-lead ECG*: Attempt to identify mechanism of arrhythmia. Treatment is mechanism-specific.
- *Identify predisposing causes*: Electrolyte disturbance, concurrent medications, hypoxia, heart failure, and so on.
- *Estimate natural history*: Rhythm may be transient due to predisposing causes, and electrolyte correction or removal of central line may treat arrhythmia.
- *Determine therapeutic end-points*: Conversion to sinus rhythm or rate control.

BRADYCARDIA MANAGEMENT OPTIONS

- Initiate Basic Life Support (BLS) if needed
- Epinephrine
- Atropine
- Isoproterenol
- Transthoracic pacing
- Intracardiac pacing

Narrow complex tachycardia management options
- Initiate BLS if indicated
- Vagal maneuvers
- Adenosine
- Other agents sometimes used—calcium-channel blockers, esmolol
- Electrical cardioversion

Wide complex tachycardia management options
- Initiate BLS if indicated.
- VF or VT without pulses → defibrillate.
- VT with pulses but poor perfusion → immediate synchronized cardioversion.
- VT with pulses and good perfusion → evaluate electrocardiogram, establish vascular access for medications (amiodarone or procainamide or lidocaine).
- Wide complex tachycardia of unknown etiology in stable patient → attempt adenosine to help determine etiology, procainamide or amiodarone, and cardioversion.

ANTIARRHYTHMICS

- A review of all the antiarrhythmics used for pediatric arrhythmias is beyond the scope of this text and the reader is referred to the *Physician's Desk Reference*, pediatric formulary, or cardiology texts for comprehensive information. A pediatric cardiologist would prescribe these medications. This section will cover common indications and special considerations for the primary care physician.

ADENOSINE

- *Action*: Blocks conduction through AVN for approximately 10 seconds.
- *Indication*: Drug of choice for acute treatment of SVT in children.
- *Dose*: The initial dose 0.1 mg/kg, with a maximum initial dose of 6 mg.
- *Special considerations*: Because of the extremely short half-life, a two-syringe method for rapid administration should be used. A defibrillator should be on hand during administration of adenosine, due to risk of proarrhythmia. Use with extreme caution in heart transplantation patients, as profound asystole may occur. Although adenosine is not effective for atrial flutter, atrial fibrillation, or VT, it may help diagnostically when the underlying rhythm is not clear from the 12-lead ECG.

AMIODARONE

- *Action*: Wide effects: inhibits alpha- and beta-adrenergic receptors producing vasodilation and AVN suppression; inhibits outward potassium current that prolongs the QT interval.
- *Indication*: Refractory SVT or VT and life-threatening arrhythmias.

- *Dose*: In arrhythmias associated with shock, initial dose of 5 mg/kg over 20–60 minutes; after the initial stabilization up to 15 mg/kg/day as needed.
- *Special considerations*: Other drugs that prolong the QT interval should not be used with amiodarone in most situations. The major side effect is hypotension and the patient must be monitored throughout administration of the bolus dose; worsening of congestive heart failure may also occur. Pediatric Advanced Life Support recommendation of 5 mg/kg bolus dosing may cause the patient to become unstable/hypotensive; in unstable patients should only be administered by the cardiologist/intensivist. In general, avoid settings of prolonged QT intervals, hypokalemia, and severe CHF.
- *Side effects*: Chronic therapy has a high incidence of side effects affecting the thyroid, lungs, skin, liver, and eyes.

ATROPINE

- *Action*: Parasympatholytic drug that accelerates sinus/atrial pacemakers and enhances AV conduction.
- *Indication*: Used in emergency situation for vagally-mediated bradycardia.
- *Dose*: IV/IO 0.02 mg/kg with a minimum dose of 0.1 mg, can repeat 1× in 5 minutes.
- *Special considerations*: The minimum dose is 0.1 mg as lower doses can cause paradoxical bradycardia.
- *Side effects*: Flushing, warm skin, papillary dilatation, tremor, and delirium.

BETA-BLOCKERS

- *Action*: Beta-adrenergic blockade. There are several different preparations available (propranolol, metoprolol, atenolol, pindolol, esmolol) and they differ in their half-lives, beta-selectivity, and intrinsic sympathomimetic activity.
- *Indication*: SVT, other arrhythmias where rate control is desired, and prophylactically in patients with LQTS.
- *Dose*: The dose and dosing schedule vary with preparation; however, a general range is 1–2 mg/kg/day.
- *Special considerations*: Use extreme caution or avoid intravenous administration of long-acting beta-blocking medications such as propranolol; esmolol preferred for intravenous use. Do not administer intravenous beta-blockers with concurrent usage of calcium-channel blocking medications.
- *Side effects*: Sleep or behavioral disturbance, exacerbation of reactive airway disease, cold extremities,

fatigue, and depression. Toddlers may rarely experience profound hypoglycemia with resultant seizures or coma.

Calcium-channel blocking medications

- *Action*: Calcium-channel blockade. Verapamil is the agent used most extensively in pediatrics; it has its greatest effect on the sinus and AV node, producing slowing.
- *Indication*: AV nodal reentrant tachycardia (AVNRT), verapamil sensitive VTs, rate control of atrial flutter/fibrillation.
- *Dose*: 4–8 mg/kg/day divided tid or qid. For intravenous use, diltiazem may be preferred.
- *Special considerations*: Calcium-channel blockers can cause profound bradycardia and hypotension in infants: avoid intravenous use in young patients. Have calcium chloride 10 mg/kg available for treatment of hypotension.
- *Side effects*: Hypotension, bradycardia, headache, dizziness, and constipation.

Digoxin

- *Action:* Binds to the Na-K ATPase transport complex and inhibits outward flux of sodium ions; autonomic effects mediated by the parasympathetic nervous system.
- *Indication*: Digoxin is used as an inotropic agent and a weak AVN blocker. It may also decrease atrial irritability.
- *Dose*: Loading dose is approximately 30 µg/kg with 50% given initially and each successive 25% given at 6-hour intervals. Maintenance doses are 7–10 µg/kg/day.
- *Special considerations*: Generally not used in patients with WPW as can increase conduction over the AC and can lead to ventricular fibrillation.
- *Side effects*: Bradycardia, arrhythmias, fatigue, headache, gastrointestinal distress, and visual changes.

Procainamide

- *Action:* Sodium channel blocking agent, decreases myocardial excitability and conduction velocity, prolongs refractory periods, prolongs PR, QRS, and QT intervals.
- *Indication*: Atrial fibrillation, atrial flutter, and refractory SVT; ventricular tachycardia, postoperative JET.
- *Dose*: IV loading dose 7–10 mg/kg in infants and 15 mg/kg in older patients over 30–50 minutes. Chronic oral therapy 40–100 mg/kg/day, divided q 4–8 hours.
- *Special considerations*: Can increase AVN conduction and increase HR when used for automatic atrial tach of atrial fibrillation. Must give slowly to avoid heart

block and myocardial depression. Avoid other QT prolonging drugs or hypokalemia/hypomagnesemia.

- *Side effects*: Hypotension, AV block, ventricular arrhythmias, central nervous system (CNS), and gastrointestinal (GI) disturbances, and lupus-like syndrome.

Lidocaine

- *Action*: Sodium channel blocker, suppresses automaticity of conduction tissue, homogeneity of repolarization.
- *Indication*: Ventricular irritability associated with ischemia or electrolyte abnormality; digoxin toxicity. Not as effective as either procainamide or amiodarone for acute termination of sustained VT.
- *Dose*: Load 1 mg/kg, follow with infusion 20–50 μg/kg/minute.
- *Special considerations*: Not used for narrow complex tachycardias.
- *Side effects*: Bradycardia, hypotension, CNS, and GI.

Sotalol

- *Action*: Nonselective beta-blocker, prolongs action potential duration of atria and ventricles, slows sinus rate and AV nodal conduction. The beta-blocker effect is dominant at lower doses.
- *Indication*: Refractory SVT, fetal SVT, atrial tachycardia following surgery for congenital heart disease, and VT.
- *Dose*: The starting dose is 90–100 mg/m^2/day (1–4 mg/kg/day) divided bid or tid with a maximum dose of 200 mg/m^2/day.
- *Special considerations*: Can prolong the QT and should not be given concurrently with other QT prolonging agents.
- *Side effects*: Fatigue, dizziness, rash, GI distress, and bleeding.

Flecainide

- *Action:* Blocks slow sodium channels with mild potassium channel blocking effects: decreases automaticity, prolongs action potential duration and refractory periods, QRS prolongation.
- *Indication*: Refractory SVT.
- *Dose*: Infants 80–90 mg/m^2/day (3–6 mg/kg/day) divided bid, older patients 100–110 mg/m^2/day q 8 or q 12.
- *Special considerations*: May result in a slow incessant tachycardia during SVT. A wide QRS may result due to bundle branch block. Negative inotropic effect. Increased risk of cardiac arrest in patients with heart disease.
- *Side effects*: Blurry vision, paresthesia, and proarrhythmia.

BIBLIOGRAPHY

Bink-Boelkens MTE. Pharmacologic management of arrhythmias. *Pediatr Cardiol* 2000;21(6):508–515.

Deal BJ, Wolff GS, Gelband H. *Current Concepts in Diagnosis and Management of Arrhythmias in Infants and Children.* New York, NY: Futura Publishing, 1998.

Ganz LI, Friedman PL. Supraventricular tachycardia. *N Engl J Med* 1995;332(3):162–173.

Tipple MA. Usefulness of the electrocardiogram in diagnosing mechanisms of tachycardia. *Pediatr Cardiol* 2000;21(6):516–521.

56 HEART FAILURE AND CARDIOMYOPATHY

Elfriede Pahl

- Definition: The diagnosis of heart failure is based on the clinical history and the physical examination, and suggests that the child's myocardium is unable to meet the body's demands either at rest or with exertion.
- The etiology depends on age. This section will focus on cardiomyopathy and exclude congenital malformations, which are reviewed in Chapter 54.
- Incidence of cardiomyopathy in children was recently reported as 1.1 new cases annually per 100,000 children living in New England or the South.
- The disease process directly affects cardiac muscle leading to altered myocardial function, with symptoms varying depending on the anatomic/pathologic type.
- Four major categories of cardiomyopathy are recognized:
  1. Dilated cardiomyopathy (DCM): 75–80%
  2. Hypertrophic cardiomyopathy (HCM)
  3. Restrictive cardiomyopathy (RCM)
  4. Right ventricular dysplasia, arrhythmogenic (ARVD)

DILATED CARDIOMYOPATHY (DCM)

- Most cases are idiopathic in etiology; however, specific causes include the following:
  1. *Inflammatory* viral myocarditis or collagen vascular
  2. *Ischemic*—either from a congenital coronary anomalies or Kawasaki disease with coronary aneurysms

3. *Metabolic*—e.g., storage disorders or mitochondrial abnormalities
4. *Primary tachycardia*—incessant
   a. Supraventricular—i.e., atrial, junctional
   b. Ventricular tachycardia—in infants, may be due to a cardiac tumor
5. *Miscellaneous*—e.g., anthracyclines, neuromuscular disorders, other toxins

PATHOPHYSIOLOGY AND SYMPTOMS OF DCM

- The heart becomes dilated and may also develop hypertrophy, with concomitant decreased systolic function. Patients may be asymptomatic or have symptoms of cardiac congestion.
- Infants generally present with tachypnea, diaphoresis, feeding intolerance, and growth failure.
- Symptoms in older children include orthopnea, exercise intolerance, chest pain, and often flu-like symptoms in the case of acute myocarditis; abdominal pain may be the result of hepatic congestion or low output.

DIAGNOSTIC TESTS FOR DCM

- Echocardiography is the standard for diagnosis of DCM, excluding structural abnormalities and specifing chamber size, % contractility, and presence of valvar regurgitation.
- Electrocardiogram (ECG) should be performed to assess rhythm, axis, chamber enlargement, and to look for signs of ischemia or Q waves.
- A chest x-ray (CXR) usually shows cardiomegaly and may show pulmonary vascular congestion (± pleural effusion).

PHYSICAL EXAMINATION FINDINGS OF DCM

- These include abnormal vital signs with tachycardia, tachypnea, and if severe, hypotension. Rales may be heard, and an apical S3 gallop as well as a systolic murmur if tricuspid or mitral insufficiency is present. The liver may be enlarged. The extremities should be examined for pulses, perfusion, and presence of edema.

TREATMENT OF DCM

- Acute treatment may require intravenous inotropes and careful diuresis.
- Digoxin is appropriate as standard therapy of symptomatic heart failure.

- Chronic therapy is aimed at affecting chronic neurohormonal imbalance. Although angiotensin-converting enzyme (ACE)-inhibitors (captopril, enalapril) and now betablockers (metoprolol, carvedilol) are often started with the supervision of a pediatric cardiologist, few pediatric studies exist.
- The use of steroids, intravenous immunoglobulin, or immunosuppressive therapy for myocarditis is controversial.
- Long-term prognosis is quite variable. Some children may make a complete recovery, especially if the etiology is myocarditis. Others require long-term medications and have persistent abnormalities on echocardiography, even though they may be asymptomatic. The most severe cases may progress to death from an arrhythmia or severe heart failure and are listed for heart transplantation.
- DCM is the most common indication for heart transplant in children beyond 1 year of age.

HYPERTROPHIC CARDIOMYOPATHY (HCM)

- HCM is synonymous with idiopathic hypertrophic subortic stenosis and may be obstructive. Although more commonly detected in adults, children are being diagnosed from asymptomatic screening of children of affected parents.
- The pathophysiology involves thickening of the intraventricular system with resultant abnormal compliance of the left ventricle leading to impaired diastolic relaxation and filling.
- Fifty percent of cases are inherited (dominant); the remainder are new mutations.
- HCM is a common cause of sudden death in young athletes.

Clinical Features
- Symptoms in the first decade are uncommon; patients presenting with syncope or chest pain have a more ominous prognosis. Patients may be aware of palpitations and dyspnea on exertion.
- The physical examination may reveal a hyperdynamic apical impulse and an ejection murmur at the apex.

Diagnostic Tests
- The ECG may show left ventricular hypertrophy, deep Q waves, and diffuse ST-T wave changes.
- The chest x-ray may be normal.
- Echocardiogram is diagnostic.
- Genetic testing is being performed on a research basis and may help risk stratify patients in the future.

Prognosis of HCM
- Patients may remain asymptomatic for years.

- Patients should avoid vigorous exercise and competitive sports.
- The risk of sudden death is increased in patients with malignant Holter (ventricular tachycardia, VTACH), family history of sudden death, or syncope.
- Beta-blockers are the mainstay of treatment and surgical subaortic resection is reserved for children with high obstructive gradients and/or symptoms.

RESTRICTIVE CARDIOMYOPATHY (RCM)

- This is a very rare form of cardiomyopathy, but is associated with a poor prognosis since it often presents late.
- Most cases in children are idiopathic; however, adult cases have been associated with sarcoid, amyloid, scleroderma, and hypereosinophilia.
- The hallmarks are small ventricles with normal thickness and very poor compliance, and marked dilation of both atria.
- The clinical symptoms include congestion with dyspnea, orthopnea, and pulmonary hypertension.
- Physical examination may reveal pulmonary rales, an S4 gallop, hepatomegaly, pedal edema, and ascites.

DIAGNOSIS OF RCM

- ECG shows biatrial enlargement, with nonspecific ST changes.
- The CXR shows pulmonary congestion but no cardiomegaly.
- Echocardiography shows severely dilated atrial with preserved systolic function.

PROGNOSIS OF RCM

- The prognosis is poor, especially if diagnosed in young children.
- Cardiac catheterization is indicated, and if there is pulmonary hypertension, the patient should be listed for heart transplantation.
- Medical therapy is limited to diuretics and anticoagulation if thrombus or atrial arrhythmias occur.

ARRYTHMOGENIC RIGHT VENTRICULAR CARDIOMYOPATHY (ARVD)

- This very rare form of cardiomyopathy should be suspected from ECG in a patient with history of unexplained syncope or near sudden death.
- It is very uncommon in children.

Pericarditis, Acute

- Etiology is usually idiopathic, but has been seen in rheumatic heart disease and Kawasaki disease.
- Inflammation of the pericardium can be due to infection (viral, bacterial, fungal), malignancy, uremia, drugs, and collagen vascular.
- The most common symptom is sharp stabbing chest pain, which changes with position.
- A friction rub may be heard on auscultation.
- Rapid pericardial fluid accumulation can lead to cardiac tamponade, manifesting with tachycardia and hypotension.
- Treatment is symptomatic, but may include nonsteroidal anti-inflammatory drugs (NSAIDs), steroids, and pericardial damage for large or persistent effusions.

CONCLUSIONS

- The causes of heart failure in children are multitude and carry variable etiologies.
- Treatment depends on symptoms, age, and type of cardiomyopathy.
- Long-term prognosis is variable.

BIBLIOGRAPHY

Basso C, et al. Arrhythmogenic right ventricular cardiomyopathy. Dysplasia, dystrophy, or myocarditis? *Circulation* 1996;94(5): 983–991.

Boucek MM, Edwards LB, Keck BM, et al. The registry of the international society for heart and lung transplantation: fifth official pediatric report—2001 to 2002. [Journal Article] *J Heart Lung Transplant* 2002;21(8):827–840.

Boucek MM, et al. The registry of the international society of heart and lung transplantation: Fifth official pediatric report—2001 to 2002. *J Heart Lung Transplant* 2002;21(8): 827–840.

Bruns LA, Kichuk M, Lamour J, et al. Carvedilol as therapy in pediatric heart failure: An initial multicenter experience. *J Pediatr* 2001;138(4):505–511.

Drucker NA, Colan SD, Lewis AB, et al. Gamma-globulin treatment of acute myocarditis in the pediatric population. [Journal Article] *Circulation* 1994;89(1): 252–257.

Duncan BW, Haraska V, Jonas RA, et al. Mechanical circulatory support in children with cardiac disease. *J Thorac Cardiovasc Surg* 1999;117:529–542.

Friedman RA, Moak JP, Garson A, Jr. Clinical course of idiopathic dilated cardiomyopathy in children. *J Am Coll Cardiol* 1991;18:152.

Kimberling MT, Balzer DT, Hirsch R, Mendeloff E, Huddleston C, Canter CE. Cardiac transplantation for pediatric restrictive cardiomyopathy: Presentation, evaluation, and short-term outcome. *J Heart Lung Transplant* 2002;21(4):455.

Lewis AB, Chabot M. Outcome of infants and children with dilated cardiomyopathy. *Am J Cardiol* 1991;68:365.

Lipshultz SE, Sleeper LA, Towbin JA, et al. The incidence of pediatric cardiomyopathy in two regions of the United States. *N Engl J Med* 2003;348:17:1647–1655.

Maron BJ, Fananapazir L. Sudden cardiac death in hypertrophic cardiomyopathy. *Circulation* 1992;85(I):57–63.

Maron BJ, Thompson PD, Puffer JC, et al. Cardiovascular preparticipation screening of competitive athletes: Statement for health professionals from the Sudden Death Committee (Clinical Cardiology) and Congenital Cardiac Defects Committee (Cardiovascular Disease in the Young). American Heart Association. *Circulation* 1996;94:850.

Mason JW, O'Connell JB, Herskowitz AL, et al. A clinical trail of immunosuppressive therapy for myocarditis. *N Engl J Med* 1995;333:269.

Montigny M, Davignon A, Fouron JC, et al. Captopril in infants for congestive heart failure secondary to a large ventricular left-to-right shunt. *Am J Cardiol* 1989;63:631–633.

Ostman-Smith I, Wettrel G, Riesenfeld T. A cohort study of childhood hypertrophic cardiomyopathy: Improved survival following high-dose beta-adrenoceptor antagonist treatment. *J Am Coll Cardiol* 1999;34:6.

Pinkney KA, Minich LL, Tani LY, et al. Current results with intraaortic balloon pumping in infants and children. *Ann Thorac Surg* 2002;73:887–891.

Rivenes SM, Kearney DL, Smith EO, Towbin JA, Denfield SW. Sudden death and cardiovascular collapse in children with restrictive cardiomyopathy. *Circulation* 2000;102(8):876–882.

Shaddy RE, Curtin EL, Packer M, Sower B, Tani LY, Burr J, LaSalle B, Boucek MM, Mahony L, Hsu D, Pahl E, Burch GH, Schlencker-Herceg R. The pediatric randomized carvedilol trial in children with heart failure: Rationale and design. [Clinical Trial. Journal Article. Randomized Controlled Trial] *Am Heart J* 2002;144(3):383–389.

Shaddy RE, Tani LY, Gidding SS, Pahl E, Orsmond GS, Gilbert EM, Lemes V. Beta blocker treatment of cardiomyopathy with congestive heart failure in children: a multi-institutional experience. *J Heart Lung Transplant* 1999;18(3):269–274.

Spirito P, Seidman CD, McKenna WJ, et al. The management of hypertrophic cardiomyopathy. *N Engl J Med* 1997;336:775.

Spodick DH. Pathophysiology of cardiac tamponade. *Chest* 1998;113:1372.

Towbin JA. Pediatric myocardial disease. *Pediatr Clin North Am* 1999;46(2):289–312.

Weller RJ, Weintraub R, Addonizio LJ, Chrisant MR, Gersony WM, Hsu DT. Outcome of idiopathic restrictive cardiomyopathy in children. *Am J Cardiol* 2002;90(5):501–506.

Wiles HB, Conner D, Thierfelder LC, et al. Mutations in the cardiac myosin binding protein-C gene on chromosome 11 cause familial hypertrophic cardiomyopathy. *Nat Genet* 1995;11: 434.

Yetman AT, Hamilton RM, Benson LN, McCrindle BW. Long-term outcome and prognostic determinants in children hypertrophic cardiomyopathy. *J Am Coll Cardiol* 1998;32(7): 1943–1950.

57   ACQUIRED HEART DISEASE
Rae-Ellen W. Kavey

INFLAMMATORY

RHEUMATIC FEVER

- Definition: A post-streptococcal autoimmune inflammatory disease of connective tissue.
- Epidemiology: Major cause of heart disease in developing countries; declining incidence in North America but with an upsurge in cases since the mid-1980s.
- Clinical manifestations follow an untreated group A streptococcal infection after a period of latency in children 6–15 years of age. In 60% of patients, the streptococcal infection was subclinical or medical care was not sought.
- There is a genetic susceptibility to acute rheumatic fever with a specific B-cell alloantigen identified on lymphocytes in greater than 90% of rheumatic fever patients, but less than 4% of controls; clinically, this is expressed as a positive family history of rheumatic fever or rheumatic heart disease.
- Streptococcal pharyngitis occurs on an average of 3 weeks before the onset of symptoms. The streptococcal infection may be atypical and therefore undiagnosed.
- Diagnosis is based on the revised Jones criteria (Table 57-1). Acute rheumatic fever is present if there are two major criteria or one major and two minor criteria plus evidence of prior group A streptococcal infection.

TABLE 57-1   Revised Jones Criteria for Diagnosis of Acute Rheumatic Fever

MAJOR	MINOR
Carditis	Fever
Arthritis	Arthralgia
Chorea	Lab findings:
Erythema marginatum	+ Acute phase reactants
Subcutaneous nodules	(ESR, CRP)
PLUS	Prolonged PR on ECG
Evidence of antecedent group A streptococcal infection (+) throat culture or rapid streptococcal Ag test Elevated or rising streptococcal antibody titers	

SOURCE: Dajani AS, Ayoub E, Bierman FZ, et al. Guidelines for the diagnosis of rheumatic fever: Jones criteria, updated 1992. *Circulation* 1993;87:302–307.

- *Arthritis* is the most common manifestation of rheumatic fever, occurring in 70% of patients. There is swelling, erythema, heat, pain, and limitation of motion affecting large joints either simultaneously or successively.
- *Carditis* occurs in 50% of patients with clinical findings of disproportionate tachycardia, murmurs of mitral and/or aortic insufficiency, pericarditis, or congestive heart failure.
- *Erythema marginatum* is a rash occurring in less than 10% of patients. The transient pattern is red, nonraised, and in a lattice pattern, exaggerated by heat and eliminated by cold.
- *Subcutaneous nodules* are a rare manifestation occurring late in the illness in approximately 5% of cases. The nodules are firm, painless, less than 2 cm in diameter, found singly or in clusters on the extensor surfaces of large joints or along the spine.
- *Sydenham's chorea* is a distinct manifestation of rheumatic fever occurring 2–6 months post streptococcal infection and usually in isolation. Patients initially have emotional lability and personality changes progressing to random spontaneous movements. These are exaggerated by any attempt to perform a purposeful action. The movement disorder varies from mild to incapacitating.
- In applying the Jones criteria, acute rheumatic fever can be diagnosed with Sydenham's chorea alone plus evidence of preceding streptococcal infection.
- Echocardiography plays an important role in the diagnosis of rheumatic fever confirming the clinical diagnosis of mitral and/or aortic insufficiency and allowing quantification of cardiac enlargement and ventricular function.
- Controversy exists about whether echo documentation of mitral or aortic insufficiency alone without clinical findings should be considered as evidence of carditis. Till now, echo evidence alone is not considered diagnostic of carditis.
- Treatment is streptococcal eradication (penicillin either orally for 10 days or IM) and anti-inflammatory:
  1. For arthritis alone or mild carditis, acetylsalicylic acid (ASA), 80–100 mg/kg/day; salicylate level of 20–25 mg/dL.
  2. For moderate-to-severe carditis, prednisone is recommended, 2–4 mg/kg/day.
  3. Duration of therapy depends on the severity of presentation and the response to therapy ranging from 2–6 weeks. ASA is started when prednisone taper begins.
- Patients with congestive heart failure are treated as described in the section on heart failure.
- Bed rest followed by activity restriction is a time-honored part of rheumatic fever therapy. The duration of activity limitation increases with the severity of the initial illness and especially the extent of carditis. Children with severe carditis are often limited from normal activity for a period of several months. The sed rate is a very useful way to judge the persistence of rheumatic inflammation—full activity is permitted after the sed rate returns to normal.
- Chorea does not respond to anti-inflammatory agents. Treatment focuses on reducing involuntary movements and agitation and includes haldol, valproic acid, thorazine, and valium.
- Post rheumatic fever, antibiotic prophylaxis to prevent recurrent streptococcal infection is mandatory since the severity of cardiac involvement increases with each recurrence. Prophylaxis can be oral (pen-V, 125–250 mg PO bid), or IM (benzathine penicillin, 1.2 million units q 28 days). For those allergic to penicillin, sulphadiazine, 1 g/day is used.
- Past the acute phase, findings of valve involvement can regress significantly; however, aortic and mitral insufficiency tend to progress over time and dramatic mitral insufficiency in the acute stage can evolve to present in adult life as mitral stenosis. For these reasons, lifelong cardiology follow-up is recommended for all patients postrheumatic fever with cardiac involvement.
- Duration of prophylaxis should extend beyond the circumstances of high risk for streptococcal infection, usually the mid-20s. Patients with long-term exposure to children should continue prophylaxis indefinitely.

KAWASAKI DISEASE

- Kawasaki disease is an acute inflammatory panvasculitis of unknown etiology.

Epidemiology
- This acute illness develops in 4–8 children per 100,000 per year, often on an epidemic basis. There is a seasonal pattern peaking in the late winter and spring. The disease primarily affects young children with the peak incidence between the ages of 1 and 5, but infants and older children are also affected. There is a male to female predominance of 1.5:1. Incidence in Asian children is much higher than in other racial groups.

Pathophysiology
- Although the specific etiology of Kawasaki disease is unknown, pathologic studies have demonstrated that there is likely to be an autoimmune basis as a response to some as yet unidentified trigger. All of the small arteries of the body are affected and it is the inflammatory response at this level that leads to the characteristic clinical picture.

Diagnosis

- This is a clinical diagnosis based on established criteria with five of six needing to be met for the diagnosis of classic Kawasaki disease. In the acute phase, fever is a universal finding, present for at least 5 days and unresponsive to antipyretic therapy.
- An easy way of thinking of Kawasaki disease is to remember the swollen erythematous appearance of these children. This is secondary to the generalized red rash, which involves primarily the trunk and perineum, swollen red chapped lips, strawberry tongue, nonexudative conjunctivitis, and puffy hands and feet. Cervical lymphadonapathy less than 1.5 cm is a less common finding.

Clinical Course

- The acute phase of the illness lasts approximately 10 days. During this time, cardiac findings are those of tachycardia and possibly myocarditis (distant heart sounds, gallop rhythm, decreased perfusion). Children with Kawasaki disease are strikingly irritable with spinal fluid findings of a sterile encephalitis.
- In the subacute phase, 10 days to 3 weeks post onset, the rash, fever, and lymphadenopathy resolve and there is peeling of the tips of the fingers and the toes. It is during this stage that the important cardiac finding of coronary aneurysms can manifest. Approximately 20% of patients will manifest coronary artery aneurysm development on echocardiography if untreated.
- In the first week of the illness, there is marked elevation of the white count, erythrocyte sedimentation rate (ESR), and C-reactive protein. In the second week of the illness, mild anemia develops along with marked thrombocytosis.
- Following the resolution of the clinical findings, there is a convalescent phase during which the ESR and platelet count gradually return to normal. This can last several months.
- Cardiac management is an important part of Kawasaki disease. During the acute phase of the illness (first week to 10 days), an electrocardiogram (ECG) will show sinus tachycardia and often nonspecific ST/T-wave changes. An echocardiogram will usually be normal in this time period or may show a small pericardial effusion. During the second week of the illness, coronary artery aneurysms develop. These can involve the entire coronary system and are usually quite easily seen on echocardiography. In some patients, massive coronary artery aneurysms develop and these can be associated with thrombus visible within the vessels.

Treatment

- Fortunately, there is usually a dramatic response to therapy with intravenous gammaglobulin. A single dose of 2 g/kg is given over 6–10 hours with often prompt resolution of fever, erythema, and edema over the next 24 hours. In children who are treated with gammaglobulin, the incidence of coronary artery aneurysm is 2–4% compared to 20% in those who are not treated.
- In the acute phase, patients are also treated with high dose aspirin, 80–100 mg/kg/day. This is continued until day 14 or when fever lysis occurs. Following this, aspirin is used in antiplatelet doses, 5–10 mg/kg/day, because of hypercoagulability related to the elevated platelet count.
- When giant coronary aneurysms develop, the primary risk is that of thrombosis so anticoagulation with Coumadin and aspirin is recommended.
- Long-term management of children who have had Kawasaki disease depends on the degree of coronary artery involvement. Those who have never shown any evidence for coronary artery involvement on echocardiography require follow-up for the first year to be certain that nothing develops. While there are no protocols for this, many cardiologists feel that a child who has had Kawasaki disease should be seen again at least once in childhood since the long-term natural history of this disease is still evolving.
- Those children in whom coronary aneurysms develop during the acute phase of the illness require coronary angiography 3–12 months after the acute illness to evaluate for the extent of coronary aneurysms and the presence of coronary artery stenosis. Obviously, if stenosis is present, surgical intervention is indicated at any stage.
- Following the initial angiogram, a follow-up angiogram is recommended at 18 months to 2 years post the acute illness since 50% of aneurysms will regress spontaneously within this time period.
- In those children who have residual coronary aneurysms, a yearly stress test with imaging for myocardial ischemia is recommended with angiography to be repeated if any abnormalities of perfusion are identified.
- In the small group of children with persistent giant coronary aneurysms >6–8 mm in diameter, long-term anticoagulation is recommended.
- In the Japanese literature, there are case reports of early myocardial infarction late after Kawasaki disease in childhood. Reports such as these suggest that children with Kawasaki disease who have had evidence for coronary involvement at any stage require long-term follow-up.

INFECTIOUS

MYOCARDITIS

- Myocarditis is an inflammation of the cardiac muscle, usually on an infectious basis but also present as part of inflammatory illness.

Epidemiology

- Subclinical myocarditis is felt to be present in many viral illnesses. Clinical myocarditis is rare: the true prevalence of myocarditis in childhood is unknown because of undetected subclinical cases; however, myocarditis is a known cause of sudden unexpected death in childhood and is the leading cause for acute heart transplantation in young adults.

Pathophysiology

- Most cases of myocarditis have a viral etiology with the most common pathogens being the enterovirus group (coxsackie B, echo, and polio) and the adenovirus group; however, almost every virus has been shown to have the potential to cause myocarditis. Nonviral causes include bacteria, fungus, and autoimmune reactions including rheumatic fever, lupus, Kawasaki disease, and acute drug reactions. The illness is most severe in the acute viral setting. There is an inflammatory infiltrate of the myocardium with necrosis and/or degeneration of myocytes. As the process continues, the degree of active inflammation decreases.
- In most patients, the acute process resolves with complete recovery. In a smaller percentage, there are findings of overt severe congestive heart failure and if they do not respond to conventional measures there may be an associated progressive downhill course.
- A small percentage who present with either subclinical or clinical myocarditis go on to develop a picture of dilated cardiomyopathy.

Clinical Course

- There is often a preceding history of viral illness, but this is less common in infants. Patients then develop findings of congestive heart failure including easy fatigability, dizziness on exertion, lethargy, poor appetite or poor intake, paroxysmal nocturnal dyspnea, and presyncope or syncope.
- On examination, there is tachypnea and tachycardia. Heart tones are decreased with a gallop rhythm. Murmurs of mitral insufficiency can be heard. An electrocardiogram will show decreased QRS voltages, diffuse ST/T changes, and often arrhythmias including atrial premature complexes (APCs), ventricular premature complexes (VPCs), atrial and ventricular tachyarrhythmias, and heart block.
- Chest x-ray will show cardiomegaly with associated pulmonary edema when present.
- Echocardiography demonstrates normal cardiac anatomy but striking chamber enlargement particularly of the left ventricle with reduced LV systolic function. A small pericardial effusion may be seen.
- The vast majority of patients, especially those with subclinical myocarditis will improve spontaneously

and require no long-term therapy. A very small percentage will have a steep downhill course and require aggressive cardiac support including potentially left ventricular assist devices and even acute heart transplantation. Another small group will appear to recover from the acite illness but go on to develop findings of chronic congestive heart failure due to a dilated cardiomyopathy.

Therapy

- Even in mild cases, bed rest is recommended. Depending on the degree of congestive heart failure, anticongestive therapy including inotropes, afterload reduction, diuresis, and oxygen are recommended. For patients in shock, aggressive use of pressors and intubation are indicated and it is in this situation that extracorporeal membrane oxygenation or a left ventricular assist device as a temporary measure to support the circulation can be considered. The echocardiogram can be used to follow the response to therapy.
- At least half of patients with myocarditis will have a complete recovery. An additional smaller group will recover significantly but will be left with depressed ventricular function and require long-term treatment with afterload reduction and digoxin plus diuretics. Finally, a small group will have progressive heart failure and circulatory collapse requiring emergent heart transplantation or ending in a fatal outcome.
- In general, noninfectious myocarditis is much less severe and responds to treatment of the underlying diagnosis.
- Viral cultures and acute and convalescent viral titers are indicated to evaluate for potential etiologies.

PERICARDITIS

- Pericarditis is an inflammation of the pericardium caused by either an infectious or a noninfectious process. As the pericardium is a closed space, collection of fluid in response to pericarditis can result in significant cardiac compromise.

Pathophysiology/Clinical Course

- Inflammation of the pericardium can occur in response to a viral infection, a bacterial infection, or as part of the inflammatory response in a variety of settings.
- In acute viral pericarditis, the patient has fever and often a history of an upper respiratory tract infection. There is complaint of pain over the chest which is exacerbated by breathing and movement and relieved by leaning forward in the upright position. When significant pericardial fluid develops, there is no chest pain and patients are initially asymptomatic. When

there is rapid accumulation of a large amount of peri-cardial fluid, compression of the heart occurs (cardiac tamponade) with symptoms of low cardiac output and venous congestion.

- On physical examination, the classic finding is of a pericardial friction rub. This is a grating sound, to-and-fro, in systole and diastole. A friction rub increases in intensity when the stethoscope is pressed against the chest. When there is significant pericardial fluid, heart tones are distant and there is no friction rub. There will be findings of hepatomegaly and pulsus alternans.

- In the rare case of purulent bacterial endocarditis, patients present with high fever and with chest pain and dyspnea. On examination, heart tones are very distant and there is often impending circulatory collapse.

Diagnosis

- The history and physical examinations strongly suggest the diagnosis. The electrocardiogram will show low voltage QRS complexes and ST segment elevation. Chest x-ray will show varying degrees of cardiomegaly with a water bottle silhouette characteristic of a large effusion. Echocardiography is the diagnostic test for pericarditis demonstrating the effusion even when it is very small. With large effusions, echocardiography will show signs of cardiac tamponade with collapse of the right atrium and the right ventricle.

Therapy

- With purulent pericarditis, urgent surgical drainage is necessary. With viral pericarditis without significant pericardial effusion, no therapy is indicated—as the viral process resolves, so will the pericarditis. With large pericardial effusions that compromise cardiac output, drainage and anti-inflammatory therapy are needed. With pericarditis as part of the picture of collagen vascular disease or rheumatic fever, anti-inflammatory therapy is indicated.

- Occasionally, patients with pericarditis have severe precordial pain and require steroid therapy and aggressive pain medication.

- Rarely viral pericarditis will develop a chronic relapsing picture and ultimately may require removal of the pericardium for relief of pain and recurrent pericardial effusion.

BACTERIAL ENDOCARDITIS

- Bacterial endocarditis is a microbial infection of the endocardial surface of the heart.

- Incidence: This is a rare illness occurring in 1:2000 to 1:4000 admissions to a pediatric hospital. In the general population, there are 5 cases per 100,000 patient years. In a high-risk population (patients with underlying heart disease), the incidence is 1230 cases per 100,000 patient years.

- Pathogenesis: Local turbulence promotes a sterile network of platelets and fibrin on the endocardial surface, which is then colonized by microorganisms entering the blood stream from a distant site.

- The most common predisposing factor to endocarditis is structural heart disease. In recent years, indwelling lines represent an additional significant risk since the line can traumatize the endocardial surface creating the substrate for infection even in structurally normal hearts.

- Bacteremia is secondary to nonsterile invasive procedures (e.g., Oral, GI, GU), extracardiac systemic infection, and usually outside the pediatric population, intravenous drug use.

- Most common underlying cardiac diagnoses are aortic valve disease, mitral valve prolapse, ventricular septal defect, and postoperative tetralogy of Fallot.

Clinical Course

- The presentation may be acute, with fever and shaking chills suggesting an infectious etiology. More commonly, the presentation is indolent with low-grade fever, anorexia, lack of energy, and weight loss.

- Findings at presentation include fever in 90%, splenomegaly in 50–60%, and petechiae in 26%. Twenty percent present with congestive heart failure and/or a new murmur. In 40%, there are finite neurologic findings including focal neurologic deficits or new onset seizures.

- A preceding event explaining bacteremia is identified in roughly 40% of cases, most commonly unprotected dental work, a systemic infection, or preceding cardiac surgery.

- Blood cultures are positive in 90% of patients. There is evidence of an acute inflammatory state with an elevated sed rate or C-reactive protein (CRP) in 90% of cases. Approximately 80% of patients have a normochromic normocytic anemia and 41% have hematuria.

- The most common pathogens are *Staphylococcusaureus* and *Streptococcus viridans* but all microorganisms including fungi have the potential to cause endocarditis. For this reason, the illness is sometimes called infective endocarditis. In patients who acquire their infection in the hospital, either related to an indwelling line or after cardiac surgery, *Staphylococcus epidermidis* and fungus are more common causative organisms. In 10% of patients with proven endocarditis, blood cultures are negative.

- Because the presentation can be relatively indolent and highly variable, and because the diagnosis is rare making recognition difficult, the time to diagnosis is frequently prolonged, averaging 30 days. A definitive diagnosis of endocarditis requires pathologic confirmation. In clinical practice, the diagnosis is based on a combination of findings known as the Duke criteria that include echocardiographic results. The Duke criteria are summarized in Table 57-1.
- *Echocardiographic findings are a critical part of both the diagnosis and management of patients with endocarditis in childhood.* In patients who have not undergone prior cardiac surgery, the initial echocardiogram demonstrates vegetations diagnostic of endocarditis in 80% of cases. In postoperative patients where abnormal densities can be part of the residua of cardiac surgery, echocardiograms are diagnostic of endocarditis in 45% of cases.
- The diagnosis of endocarditis can be confirmed quickly by an echocardiogram but obviously a negative study does not exclude the possibility.
- Demonstration of intracardiac vegetations predicts a more malignant course.
- Serial echocardiograms can be used to inform the clinical management since a progressive increase in the size of the vegetation, findings of a perivalvular abscess, or evidence of valve destruction indicate the need for early surgical intervention.
- *In older children or those in whom a transthoracic echocardiogram is suboptimal, transesophageal echocardiography is strongly recommended.* In adults, a transesophageal echocardiogram is a mandatory part of the investigation for possible endocarditis.
- After cardiac surgery, prosthetic valves are an important underlying substrate for endocarditis, whether the valve is mechanical or bioprosthetic.
- Once the diagnosis is made and appropriate antibiotic therapy is in place, patients remain at significant risk for systemic embolization, extension of infection within the heart, progressive valve destruction, and intractable congestive heart failure particularly in the first 2 weeks of treatment.
- Outcome: After treatment for endocarditis in the current era, there are significant cardiac residua in 59% of patients, central nervous system (CNS) residua in 60%, and chronic renal failure in 2.5%. *Current mortality is 10%.*
- In 65% of patients, therapy is medical only but in 25%, early surgical intervention is necessary.
- In 30–40% of cases, the course is complicated by peripheral emboli including CNS emboli in 10–20%

of cases. One-third of patients develop congestive heart failure and 10% develop renal failure.
- *Endocarditis should always be suspected when a child with known heart disease of any kind develops fever without an identified cause.* This high index of suspicion and rigorous use of blood cultures should optimize the potential for early diagnosis and effective management.

TABLE 57-1 Duke Criteria

Major Criteria
- Positive blood culture (two separate cultures at least 12 hours apart) (Durack et al., 1994).
- Evidence of endocardial involvement.
  1. Positive echocardiogram
  2. New valvular regurgitation

Minor Criteria
- Predisposition: Structural heart condition or intravenous drug use
- Fever
- Vascular phenomena
- Immunologic phenomena
- Microbiologic evidence
- Echocardiographic evidence

DIAGNOSIS OF ENDOCARDITIS

- Definite
  1. Pathologic
  2. Clinical
     a Two major criteria
     b One major, three minor criteria
     c Five minor criteria
- Possible
- Findings consistent with endocarditis that fall short of definite but not rejected.
- Rejected
  1. Firm alternative diagnosis.
  2. Resolution of findings with antibiotic therapy for ≤4 days.
  3. No pathologic findings at autopsy after ≤4 days of treatment.

BIBLIOGRAPHY

Awadallah SA, Kavey REW, Smith FC, et al. The changing face of infective endocarditis in childhood. *Am J Cardiol* 1991;68:90–94.

Carapetis JR, Currie BJ. Rheumatic fever in a high incidence population: The importance of monoarthritis and low grade fever. *Arch Dis Child* 2001;85:223–227.

Dajani AS, Ayoub E, Bierman FZ, et al. Guidelines for the diagnosis of rheumatic fever: Jones criteria, updated 1992. *Circulation* 1993;87:302–307.

Dajani AS, Taubert KA, Takahashi M, et al. Guidelines for long term management of patients with Kawasaki disease. *Circulation* 1994;89:916–922.

Dajani AS, Taubert KA, Wilson W, et al. Prevention of bacterial endocarditis. Recommendations by the American Heart Association. *JAMA* 1997;277:1794–1801.

Durack DT, Lukas AS, Bright DK. New criteria for diagnosis of infective endocarditis. Utilization of specific echocardiographic findings. *Am J Med* 1994;96:200–209.

Ferrieri P. Proceedings of the Jones criteria workshop. *Circulation* 2002;106:2521–2523.

Martin AB, Webber S, Fricker FJ, et al. Acute myocarditis: Rapid diagnosis by PCR in children. *Circulation* 1994;90:330–333.

Minich LL, Tani LY, Dagotto LT, et al. Doppler echocardiography distinguishes between physiologic and pathologic "silent" mitral regurgitation in patients with rheumatic fever. *Clin Cardiol* 1997;20:924–926.

Newburger JW, Takahashi M, Beiser AS, Burns JC, et al. A single intravenous infusion of gamma globulin in the treatment of acute Kawasaki disease. *N Engl J Med* 1991;324:1633–1639.

Pinsky WW, Friedman RA. Pericarditis. In: Garson A, Jr. (ed.), *The Science and Practice of Pediatric Cardiology*. Philadelphia, PA: Lea and Felsinger, 1990, pp. 1590–1604.

Rheuban KS. Pericardial diseases. In: Allen HD, Gutgesell HP, Clark EB, Driscall DJ (eds.), *Moss and Adams Heart Disease in Infants, Children and Adolescents, Including the Fetus and Young Adult*, 6th ed. Philadelphia, PA: Lippincott Williams & Wilkins, 2001, pp. 1287–1296.

Sainer L, Prince A, Gregary WN. Pediatric infective endocarditis in the modern era. *J Pediatr* 1993;122:847–853.

Towbin JA. Myocarditis. In: Allen HD, Gutgesell HP, Clark EB, Driscall DJ (eds.), *Moss and Adams Heart Disease in Infants, Children and Adolescents, Including the Fetus and Young Adult*, 6th ed. Philadelphia, PA: Lippincott Williams & Wilkins, 2001, 1287–1296.

interpretation of BP for age and body size is essential. *At a minimum, blood pressure should be measured at every pediatric visit from 3 years of age and charted against norms for age/gender/height.*

- To be accurate, blood pressure needs to be measured using the correct size cuff for the child's arm so a variety of cuff sizes need to be available. An approximation of the correct size is a cuff whose bladder will cover 80–100% of the circumference of the arm. Blood pressure should be measured with the child at rest after 3–5 minutes with the arm supported at heart level. It should be taken at least twice and the average used.
- Systolic BP is determined by the onset of Korotkoff sounds and diastolic blood pressure is determined by the disappearance of the Korotkoff sounds.
- The National Heart Lung and Blood Institute commissioned a series of Task Forces to define appropriate evaluation and management of high blood pressure in childhood. The most recent update in 1996 confirmed the use of the Second Task Force report of 1987 as the basis for the evaluation of high blood pressure in children.
- From that report, *the younger the child and higher the blood pressure, the more likely it is for hypertension to be secondary*. A summary of the most common etiologies of hypertension at different ages is included in Table 58-1.
- Because blood pressure variation is under multiple physiologic controls including cardiac, vascular, central nervous system (CNS), and endocrine, derangements in any of these systems can cause high blood pressure.
- From the algorithm of the Second Task Force, evaluation for high blood pressure is indicated after a series of systolic and/or diastolic pressures are recorded above the 95th percentile for age/gender/height (Fig. 58-1).

58 HYPERTENSION

Rae-Ellen W. Kavey

- In childhood, high blood pressure (HBP) is defined as systolic and/or diastolic pressure above the 95th percentile for age, gender, and height.
- Over the last decade, normal values for blood pressure in childhood have been defined based on more than 60,000 BPs in children. These standards are available online at http://www.nhldi.nih.gov/health/prof/agart/hbp/hbp ped.htm.
- Primary and secondary hypertension can manifest at any time in childhood so measurement and correct

TABLE 58-1 Etiology of Hypertension: Prevalence by Age Group

AGE GROUP	CAUSE

Newborn	Abnormal renal blood flow
	   Renal artery thrombosis (indwelling umbilical catheter)
	   Renal artery atresia
	Congenital malformation of the kidney
	Coarctation of the aorta

Infancy to 6 years	Renal parenchymal disease Coarctation of the aorta Renal artery stenosis
6–10 years	Renal artery stenosis Renal parenchymal disease Essential hypertension
>10 years	Essential hypertension Renal parenchymal disease

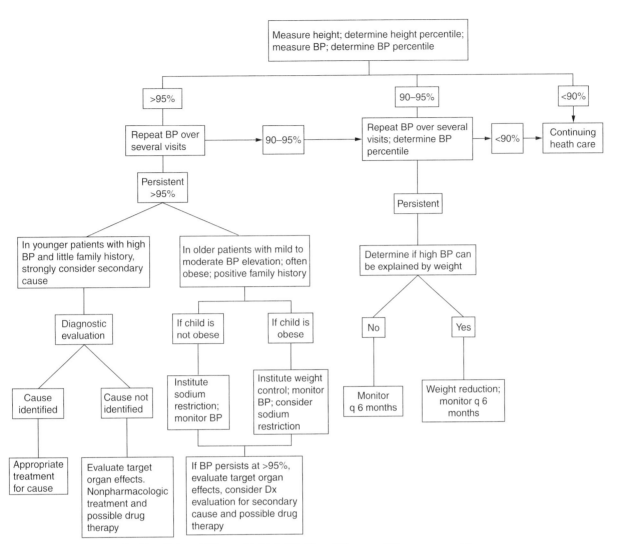

FIG. 58-1 Algorithm for identifying children with high BP. Note: Whenever BP measurement is stipulated, the average of at least two measurements should be used.
Source: Report of the Second Task Force on blood pressure control in children. *Pediatrics* 1987; 79:16–23.

- Body size and blood pressure are very closely linked throughout childhood. If repeated blood pressure measurements are above the 95th percentile in a child who is overweight, few diagnostic tests are needed other than a urinalysis, blood urea nitrogen (BUN), and creatinine (Cr) to exclude renal dysfunction.
- A summary of the important historic information and the relevant necessary testing for the most common diagnoses leading to hypertension in childhood is contained in Table 58-2.
- In adolescents, the phenomenon of *white coat hypertension* is quite common. This is high blood pressure seen in medical care settings but not present at any other time. The best way to evaluate for white coat

hypertension is the use of ambulatory monitoring which measures blood pressure using an automated cuff away from the office. Norms for wake and sleep blood pressure on ambulatory monitoring in childhood are now available. If BPs are normal on ambulatory monitoring, no additional evaluation is needed so this is a good first test for evaluation of potential hypertension in teenagers.
- *Whenever obesity is seen in conjunction with hypertension, weight loss is the primary therapy.* Even small amounts of weight loss often result in complete normalization of the blood pressure in both children and adults.
- Therapy for hypertension in childhood focuses on elimination of the etiology when one is present. Drugs

TABLE 58-2   History, Physical Examination Findings, and Targeted Workup for HBP in Childhood

HISTORY	PHYSICAL EXAMINATION	POTENTIAL DIAGNOSIS	EVALUATION
Indwelling U/A catheter	+/–Abdominal bruit	Renal artery thrombosis/stenosis	Plasma renin level, renal artery doppler flow; renal arteriogram
Family history of HBP	High BP alone	Essential hypertension	Echocardiogram for LV mass, U/A, BUN, Cr to exclude renal disease
Progressive weight gain, muscle cramps, weakness, acne	Truncal obesity, hirsution, striae, buffalo hump	Cushing syndrome	Urinary 17-OHCS excretion, plasma cortisol
Leg cramps post exertion	Upper extremity hypertension. Decreased pulses, BP in lower body. Murmur over left back.	Coarctation of the aorta	Cardiac echo/doppler with evaluation of aortic arch; +/– aortic arch angiogram/CT/MRI
Dysuria, frequency, UTIs	Pallor, edema	Chronic renal disease	U/A; urine culture, BUN, Cr; renal ultrasound, IVP
Episodic flushing, diaphoresis	Tachycardia, diaphoresis	Phaeochromocytoma	Plasma and urine catecholamines and metabolites; abdominal CT
Poor growth, developmental delay	Elfin facies, small size, cardiac murmur, abdominal bruit	Williams syndrome	Cardiac echocardiogram for peripheral pulmonary stenosis, supravalvar aortic stenosis; renal artery doppler flow/arteriogram, serum calcium
Muscle cramps, weakness, constipation, polyuria	Edema	Hyperaldosteronism	Electrolytes, plasma aldosterone
Drug use—prescription steroids, contraceptives; nonprescription stimulants, anabolic steroids	Tachycardia, cushingoid facies	Drug response	Drug withdrawal
Weight loss, family history of autoimmune disease	Tachycardia, decreased weight for height, brisk deep tendon reflexes	Hyperthyroidism	Thyroid function tests
Obesity, decreased linear growth, cold intolerance, constipation	Increased weight for height, decreased linear growth velocity	Hypothyroidism	Thyroid function tests

ABBREVIATIONS: U/A, urinary analysis; UTI, urinary tract infection; OHCS, hydroxycorticosteroids; CT, computed tomography; MRI, magnetic resonance imaging; IVP, intravenous pyelogram.

TABLE 58-3   Antihypertensive Drugs

	INITIAL DOSE	MAXIMUM DOSE (MGM/KG/DAY)
Converting enzyme inhibitors		
Captopril		
Neonates	0.03–0.15	2
Children	1.5	6
Enalapril	0.15	0.6
Calcium channel blockers		
Nifedipine	0.25	3
Diuretics		
Hydrochlorothiazide	1	2–3
Furosemide	1	12
Bumetadine	0.02–0.05	0.3
Metolazone	0.1	3
Spironolactone	1	3
Beta-adrenergic blockers		
Propanalol	1	8
Atenolol	1	8
Metoprolol	1	8
Alpha-adrenergic blockers		
Prazosin	0.05–0.1	0.5
Central alpha-adrenergic agonists		
Methyldopa	5	40
Clonidine	0.005	0.03
Vasodilators		
Hydralazine	0.75	7.5
Minoxidil	0.1–0.2	1

are used on a short-term basis while this is being accomplished or chronically when the diagnosis is essential hypertension and there is significant elevation of BP plus increased left ventricular (LV) mass on echocardiography, indicating end-organ response to sustained BP elevation. In Table 58-3, antihypertensive drug therapy recommendations from the Second Task Force report are summarized.

• There are no long-term clinical trials evaluating the risks of chronic antihypertensive therapy in children. For this reason, a very conservative approach should be taken to the initiation of drug therapy for hypertension in young children.

BIBLIOGRAPHY

Harshfield GA, Alpert BS, Pulliam DA, Somes GW, Wilson DK. Ambulatory blood pressure monitoring in healthy and hypertensive children. *Arch Dis Child* 1994;94:180–184.

Mirkin BL, Newman TJ. Efficacy and safety of captopril in the treatment of severe childhood hypertension: report of the International Collaborative Study Group. *Pediatrics* 1985;75:1091–1100.

Report of the Second Task Force on blood pressure control in children—1987. *Pediatrics* 1987;79:1–25.

Rocchini AP, Katch V, Anderson J. Blood pressure in obese adolescents: effect of weight loss. *Pediatrics* 1988;82:16–23.

Soergel M, Kirschstein M, Busch C, Thomas D, et al. Oscillometric twenty-four-hour ambulatory BP values in healthy children and adolescents: a multicenter trial including 1141 subjects. *J Pediatr* 1997;130:178–184.

Sorof JM, Poffenbarger T, Franok PR. Evaluation of white coat hypertension in children: Importance of the definitions of normal ambulatory blood pressure and the severity of casual hypertension. *Am J Hypertens* 2001;14:855–860.

Update on the 1987 Task Force Report on high blood pressure in children and adolescents: A working group report from the National High Blood Pressure Education Program. *Pediatrics* 1996;98:649–658.

59 HYPERLIPIDEMIA

Rae-Ellen W. Kavey

- Pathologic studies have now shown that both the presence and extent of atherosclerotic lesions at autopsy after unexpected death of children and young adults correlate positively and significantly with known hypercholesterolemia. This information supports recommendations for early identification and management of hyperlipidemia in childhood.
- Cholesterol is one of the body's major lipids and acts as a precursor for steroids, hormones, and bile acids as well as providing an important structural component in all cell membranes.

- For most individuals, control of cholesterol metabolism is polygenic, representing the sum of additive small effects on a number of different genes. In this setting, hypercholesterolemia will often only be expressed in childhood if there is an environmental stimulus like obesity or a high-fat diet.
- A small number of individuals inherit specific single gene disorders of lipid metabolism. A classic example of this is familial hypercholesterolemia (FH) in which reduced low-density lipoprotein (LDL) receptors in the liver result in elevated cholesterol levels dating from birth. Heterozygous FH is inherited in an autosomal recessive pattern and occurs at a frequency of 1 in 500 in the American population. In these individuals, symptomatic coronary heart disease develops in the forties.
- Regardless of the genetic basis, management of hypercholesterolemia is based on serum lipid levels.
- Researchers have shown that cholesterol levels "track" from childhood into adult life, meaning that extremely high levels in childhood will be predictive of similar elevation in adult life; however, *for the majority of children, a single screening cholesterol is a relatively weak predictor of future cholesterol levels.*
- For this reason, the National Cholesterol Education Program (NCEP)-Pediatric Panel, recommends a "selective screening" approach to hyperlipidemia in childhood as outlined in Figs. 59-1 and 59-2. The panel recommends that lipid levels be measured in children with a positive family history of early cardiovascular disease in an expanded first-degree pedigree or with a parental history of hypercholesterolemia.

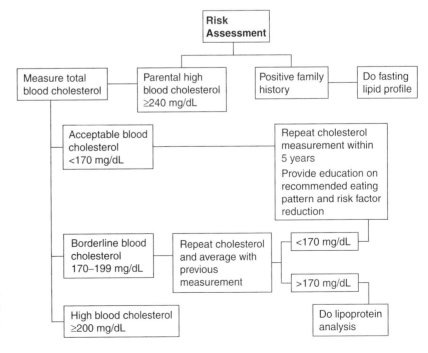

FIG. 59-1 Algorithm for selective screening of lipid levels in children from the National Cholesterol Education Program—Pediatric Panel Guidelines.

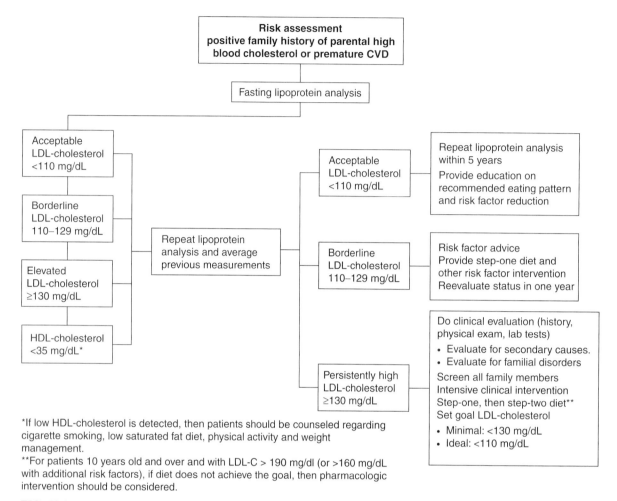

FIG. 59-2 Algorithm for classification and management of children with measured LDL cholesterol from the National Cholesterol Education Program—Pediatric Panel Guidelines.

- A *positive family history* means evidence for cardiovascular disease, treated angina, angioplasty, stenting of the coronary arteries, myocardial infarction, or coronary artery bypass surgery in a male below the age of 55 or a female below the age of 60 in an expanded first-degree pedigree comprised of parents, grandparents, aunts, and uncles.
- To address the second group, those children with *a parental history of hypercholesterolemia,* pediatric care providers should obtain lipid levels in parents where this information is needed to determine the screening status of their patients. In adults, a total cholesterol >240 mg/dL has been designated as abnormal.
- In addition to checking lipids in children with a positive family history of either hypercholesterolemia or premature coronary disease, I would add *obesity,* diabetes mellitus, and chronic renal disease as additional reasons to obtain a lipid profile in childhood.
- The best age to measure lipids in an identified child is approximately 3–5 years when the 12-hour fast necessary is tolerable. Total cholesterol and high-density lipoprotein (HDL) cholesterol levels can be measured accurately from a nonfasting specimen; however, determination of triglycerides requires a fasting specimen and triglyceride level is necessary to calculate LDL cholesterol (Friedewald equation: $LDL\text{-}C = TC\text{-}HDL\text{-}(TG/5)$)
- Normal values for lipids in children are lower than they are in adults and are similar from 1 to 18 years of age with the 75th percentile being roughly 170 mg/dL and the 95th percentile being 200 mg/dL.
- The NCEP-Pediatric Panel recommends use of the 75th percentile of the normal distribution (170 mg/dL) to designate a total cholesterol level as abnormal, similar to the adult guidelines; however, tracking studies indicate that this approach would erroneously identify many children as having elevated cholesterol levels which will not track into adult life. For this reason, most pediatric specialists use the 95th percentile to designate an abnormal level in childhood. Practically

speaking, this means that a *total cholesterol >200 mg/ dL is abnormal.*

- Lipid levels vary from day to day; thus an average of at least two results should be reviewed before labeling a child as hypercholesterolemic.
- Total cholesterol level is often used as a proxy for LDL cholesterol; however, in order to know the LDL cholesterol level, all the elements in the lipid panel need to be measured.
- The two most common patterns of lipid abnormality identified in children are type 2A (FH) where there is marked elevation in total and LDL-C levels with the remainder of the profile usually normal; and type 2B, a pattern associated with obesity where there is mild elevation in cholesterol, moderate-to-severe elevation in triglycerides, and reduced HDL. The type 2B pattern is associated with adult onset diabetes and with premature atherosclerotic disease. This pattern is almost always seen with obesity when it appears in children. Initial management for either of these two forms of hypercholesterolemia is dietary.
- Other very rare forms of hyperlipidemia exist. If a fasting lipid profile reveals an unusual pattern not consistent with 2A or 2B hypercholesterolemia, referral to a lipid specialist is recommended at that time.
- When a child is identified as having true hypercholesterolemia (i.e., an average of at least two cholesterol levels >200 mg/dL), secondary causes which include hypothyroidism, diabetes, nephrotic syndrome, hepatic disease, and exogenous factors like steroid and oral contraceptive use must be excluded.
- Once secondary hypercholesterolemia has been excluded, the first step in management of hypercholesterolemia is institution of the American Heart Association Step One diet. This is actually the diet recommended by the American Academy of Pediatrics for all normal children with <30% of calories from fat and <10% from saturated fat, plus cholesterol intake below 300 mg/day.
- The most effective way to implement this diet is for the hypercholesterolemic child and parent(s) to meet with a nutritionist at least twice for training.
- On average, on a well-maintained low-fat and low-cholesterol diet, total and LDL cholesterol levels decrease by 10–20%. This diet has been shown to be both safe and effective in children.
- For obese children, response to diet change can be very impressive. In obesity, a decrease in calorie intake needs to be associated with the shift toward lower fat and lower saturated fat and with this combination even small amounts of weight loss can be associated with complete normalization of the lipid profile.

- If lipid levels do not decline significantly, the Step Two diet is recommended. This contains <30% of calories from fat and <7% from saturated fat. *The low-fat, low-cholesterol diet should be maintained for at least 1 year before drug therapy is considered.*
- The NCEP-Pediatric Panel recommends drug therapy be considered only for children >10 years of age if LDL cholesterol remains >190 mg/dL (equivalent to a total cholesterol of >300 mg/dL); or if LDL cholesterol is greater than 160 mg/dL (equivalent to a total cholesterol of 250 mg/dL) with a positive family history of premature cardiovascular disease and at least two additional risk factors.
- Drug therapy should be implemented in conjunction with a specialist for lipid disorders in children.
- While other lipid elements have not been addressed by guidelines, low-HDL cholesterol is known to be a strong predictor of early atherosclerotic disease in adults and can be anticipated to track in the same way as the total and LDL cholesterol levels do from childhood. Certainly, HDL levels below 35 mg/dL should be taken into consideration in the decision to initiate drug therapy for hypercholesterolemia in childhood.
- In all children with hypercholesterolemia, attention needs to be paid to optimization of all the risk factors: elimination of cigarette smoking in the home, maintenance of a normal weight for height proportion, normalization of blood pressure, and promotion of a very active lifestyle.

BIBLIOGRAPHY

Kavey REW, Daniels SR, Lauer RM, et al. American Heart Association guidelines for primary prevention of atherosclerotic cardiovascular disease beginning in childhood. *Circulation* 2003;107:1562–1566.

Lauer RM, Lee J, Clarke WR. Factors affecting the relationship between childhood and adult cholesterol levels: The Muscatine study. *Pediatrics* 1988;82:309–318.

National cholesterol education program: Report of the expert panel on blood cholesterol levels in children and adolescents. *Pediatrics* 1992;S9(3 Part 2):525–584.

Obarzanek E, Kimm SY, Barton BA, et al. Long-term safety and efficacy of a cholesterol-lowering diet in children with elevated low-density lipoprotein cholesterol: Seven year results of the DISC study. *Pediatrics* 2001;107:256–264.

Williams CL, Hayman CC, Daniels SR, et al. Cardiovascular health in childhood: a statement for health professionals from the committee on atherosclerosis, hypertension and obesity in the young of the American Heart Association. *Circulation* 2002;106:1178–1185.

Sarah L. Chamlin, Section Editor

60 BIRTHMARKS

Annette M. Wagner

HEMANGIOMAS

EPIDEMIOLOGY AND PATHOPHYSIOLOGY

- One of most common tumors of infancy.
- Present in 2.5% of newborns and 10% of infants at 1 year of age.
- More common in premature infants <30 weeks gestation and in girls.
- Eighty percent of hemangiomas are solitary and 38% occur on the head and neck.
- Comprised of endothelial cell proliferation with dilated vascular channels.
- Resolution occurs by apoptosis of cells.
- Pathophysiology is unknown but hemangioma cells contain similar histochemical markers to maternal placental cells.

DIFFERENTIAL DIAGNOSIS AND CLINICAL FEATURES

- Deep lesions can be mistaken for other rapidly growing infantile tumors including rhabdomyomas, infantile myofibromas, sarcomas, or hemangioendotheliomas.
- Early lesions may be mistaken for port-wine stains.
- Hemangiomas appear in the first month of life and undergo proliferation for 8–12 months followed by involution with 50% gone by age 5, 60% by age 6, and so on.
- Can be superficial, deep, or mixed in type.

- Superficial hemangiomas begin as small telangiectatic papules that are surrounded by a white halo that rapidly enlarge into a raised lobulated tumor with a "strawberry" appearance.
- Deep hemangiomas are large subcutaneous masses often with an overlying blue hue or telangiectasias on the surface.
- Congenital hemangiomas rarely occur and can persist without involution (NICH—*non*involuting *c*ongenital *h*emangioma) or undergo more rapid involution with resolution by age 2 (RICH—*r*apidly *i*nvoluting congenital *h*emangioma).
- Complications of hemangiomas requiring intervention are ulceration, visual obstruction, disfigurement, and airway occlusion.
- Patients studded with multiple hemangiomas may have hemangiomatosis with liver involvement (diffuse hemangiomatosis) and be at risk for high output heart failure.
- Large segmental facial hemangiomas are associated with PHACES syndrome (*p*osterior fossa malformations, *h*emangioma, *a*rterial or *a*ortic defects, *c*ardiac anomalies, *e*ye anomalies, and *s*ternal defects).

TREATMENT AND PROGNOSIS

- Most hemangiomas do not require treatment and have excellent prognosis.
- Large facial hemangiomas or hemangiomas overlying the cervical or lumbosacral spine should be imaged by magnetic resonance imaging (MRI) for evidence of posterior fossa malformations or spinal dysraphism.
- Ulcerated hemangiomas may require treatment with antibiotics, occlusive dressings, analgesics, and occasionally oral steroids or pulsed dye laser.
- Oral steroids are the mainstay of treatment for visual or airway obstruction, disfigurement or diffuse

hemangiomatosis, and are effective during the proliferative phase.
- Other treatments for complicated hemangiomas include interferon-α or vincristine.
- After involution, skin changes of atrophy, redundancy and fibrofatty tissue deposition can be present and may require surgical correction.

PORT-WINE STAINS AND STURGE-WEBER SYNDROME

EPIDEMIOLOGY AND PATHOPHYSIOLOGY

- Port-wine stains are congenital vascular malformations comprised of dilated and ectatic capillary-like vessels.
- Occur in 0.3–0.5% of infants at birth; an occasional acquired form occurs.
- Five to eight percent of facial port-wine stains are associated with Sturge-Weber syndrome.
- Sturge-Weber syndrome is port-wine stain involving the first branch of the trigeminal nerve associated with vascular malformation of the ipsilateral meninges and cerebral cortex.
- Dysmorphogenesis of cephalic neuroectoderm due to a somatic mutation arising during development is proposed pathogenesis of Sturge-Weber.
- No sex or race predilection is seen.

DIFFERENTIAL DIAGNOSIS AND CLINICAL FEATURES

- May be mistaken for early superficial hemangioma.
- Stains are brightly erythematous irregular patches at birth.
- Progressive deepening of color to bluish-purple occurs with time.
- Hypertrophy of underlying tissue and angiomatous papules can develop within the stain.
- Klippel-Trenaunay syndrome is the association of limb overgrowth, a venous or lymphatic malformation with a port-wine stain.
- CMTC (*cutis marmorata telangiectatica congenita*) is a mottled form of vascular malformation with cutaneous atrophy and limb hypotrophy.
- Sturge-Weber syndrome is the association of V1 facial port-wine stain with ipsilateral eye abnormalities (glaucoma, buphthalmos, or choroids vascular anomalies) in 30% of patients, and brain abnormalities (vascular anomalies, cerebral atrophy, and calcifications) manifesting as seizures (80%), developmental delay (60%), or hemiplegia (30%).

- Diagnosis of Sturge-Weber can be aided by MRI with gadolinium but may be nondiagnostic.

TREATMENT AND PROGNOSIS

- Pulsed dye laser can be used to lighten port-wine stains.
- Multiple treatments at 2–3 month intervals are required for maximum improvement.
- Infants affected with Sturge-Weber require regular eye examinations, treatment of glaucoma to prevent vision loss, neurologic follow-up for control of epilepsy, early developmental intervention, treatment for overgrowth of the jaw.
- Cosmetic improvement of the port-wine stain can be obtained with laser treatment but some darkening of the stain with time and sun exposure is anticipated and recurrent treatment may be required.

CONGENITAL AND ACQUIRED MELANOCYTIC NEVI

EPIDEMIOLOGY AND PATHOPHYSIOLOGY

- Small congenital nevi occur in 1–2% of infants.
- Large congenital nevi occur in 0.02% of infants.
- Comprised of proliferations of melanocytes in nests occurring at or shortly after birth that track along hair follicles and extend deeply into the skin.
- Acquired nevi usually appear after 18 months increasing in number until age 30 with two peaks of acquisition in the preschool years and at puberty.
- Acquired nevi are less common in pigmented races.

DIFFERENTIAL DIAGNOSIS AND CLINICAL FEATURES

- Can be mistaken for café au lait macules, urticaria pigmentosa, smooth muscle hamartoma, mosaic hyperpigmentation, or lentigines.
- All congenital nevi have an increased risk of melanoma estimated at 1% for small lesions (<1.5 cm in adult) and as high as 12% for garment-type congenital nevi (>20 cm in adult).
- Congenital nevi are usually larger than acquired nevi and often have a papillated surface; many develop hypertrichosis with time.
- Congenital nevi often have irregular borders and multiple colors.
- Acquired nevi are tan to dark brown macules that may become elevated with time.

- Nevi with features concerning for malignancy are *A*symmetric, have *B*order irregularity, multiple *C*olors, and a *D*iameter >6 mm (ABCDs).
- Changes of rapid growth, color, or shape should be evaluated in all nevi.
- Family history of melanoma in first-degree relatives increased the risk of melanoma in a child.
- Atypical nevus syndrome is a familial condition associated with the development of multiple acquired nevi with atypical features and an increased risk of melanoma.
- Spitz nevi are dome-shaped red-brown to pink or flat jet-black nevi that may appear suddenly and grow rapidly; they often have a concerning histopathologic appearance.

TREATMENT AND PROGNOSIS

- Excision of small congenital nevi without atypical features is not recommended.
- Excision of medium-sized and large congenital nevi with atypical features should be considered due to the increased risk of melanoma in these lesions.
- Excision should be considered for Spitz nevi; histopathologic evaluation by an experienced dermatopathologist is suggested.
- Large congenital nevi associated with neurocutaneous melanosis (a benign or malignant melanocytic infiltration of the meninges) has a poor prognosis; infants with large congenital nevi overlying the spine or with large congenital nevi should be evaluated with an MRI to look for this finding.
- Children with a family history of melanoma or atypical nevus syndrome should be routinely evaluated by a dermatologist.
- Melanoma is rare in children; the prognosis for melanoma in a child, like in an adult, depends on the depth of the lesion.

CAFÉ AU LAIT MACULES AND NEUROFIBROMATOSIS TYPE 1

EPIDEMIOLOGY AND PATHOPHYSIOLOGY

- A café au lait spot occurs in up to 18% of newborns and 36% of older children.
- More common in pigmented races.
- Increased epidermal melanin is present in keratinocytes and melanocytes without melanocyte proliferation.
- Can be markers of genetic disease including neurofibromatosis (NF), McCune-Albright syndrome, or Watson syndrome.

- Neurofibromatosis Type 1 (NF-1) is autosomal dominant, occurs in 1/3000 infants and results from a mutation in the gene for neurofibromin (17q22.2), a tumor suppressor which controls cell proliferation.

DIFFERENTIAL DIAGNOSIS AND CLINICAL FEATURES

- Can be mistaken for nevi, mastocytomas, lentigines.
- Café au lait spots are flat, light to dark brown macules and patches with well-defined borders that occur on any body part except the palms, soles, and scalp.
- New lesions can be acquired with time and lesions grow proportionately.
- NF-1 is diagnosed in prepubertal children by the presence of at least two of the following criteria: ≥6 café au lait macules ≥5 mm, ≥2 neurofibromas of any type or one plexiform neurofibroma, axillary or inguinal freckling, optic glioma, ≥2 Lisch nodules, bony abnormality (pseudoarthrosis or sphenoid dysplasia), or a first-degree relative with NF-1.
- Other manifestations of NF-1 include learning disabilities, scoliosis, leukemia, and other malignancies.

TREATMENT AND PROGNOSIS

- Some successful treatment of café au lait spots with laser have been reported, but repigmentation after treatment occurs.
- Children with neurofibromatosis Type 1 have highly variable disease expression.
- Comprehensive follow-up is indicated; ideally in the context of a multidisciplinary clinic.

BIBLIOGRAPHY

Arbuckle HA, Morelli JG. Pigmentary disorders: Update on neurofibromatosis-1 and tuberous sclerosis. *Curr Opin Pediatr* 2000;12(4):354–358.

Brown TJ, Friedman J, Levy ML. The diagnosis and treatment of common birthmarks. *Clin Plast Surg* 1998;25(4):509–525.

Chamlin SL, Williams ML. Pigmented lesions in adolescents. *Adolesc Med* 2001;12(2):195–212.

Drolet BA, Esterly NB, Frieden IJ. Hemangiomas in children. *N Engl J Med* 1999;341(3):173–181.

Fishman C, Mihm MC, Jr., Sober AJ. Diagnosis and management of nevi and cutaneous melanoma in infants and children. *Clin Dermatol* 2002;20(1):44–50.

Garzon MC, Frieden IJ. Hemangiomas: when to worry. *Pediatr Ann* 2000;29(1):58–67.

Kihiczak NI, Schwartz RA, Jozwiak S, Silver RJ, Janniger CK. Sturge-Weber syndrome. *Cutis* 2000;65(3):133–136.

Lynch TM, Gutmann DH. Neurofibromatosis 1. *Neurol Clin* 2002;20(3):841–865.

Makkar HS, Frieden IJ. Congenital melanocytic nevi: An update for the pediatrician. *Curr Opin Pediatr* 2002;14(4):397–403.

Marghoob AA. Congenital melanocytic nevi. Evaluation and management. *Dermatol Clin* 2002;20(4):607–616.

Metry DW, Dowd CF, Barkovich AJ, Frieden IJ. The many faces of PHACE syndrome. *J Pediatr* 2001;139(1):117–123.

North PE, Waner M, Mizeracki A, Mrak RE, Nicholas R, Kincannon J, Suen JY, Mihm MC. A unique microvascular phenotype shared by juvenile hemangiomas and human placenta. *Arch Dermatol* 2001;137(5):559–570.

Rothfleisch JE, Kosann MK, Levine VJ, Ashinoff R. Laser treatment of congenital and acquired vascular lesions. A review. *Dermatol Clin* 2002;20(1):1–18.

Tekin M, Bodurtha JN, Riccardi VM. Café au lait spots: The pediatrician's perspective. *Pediatr Rev* 2001;22(3):82–90.

Further information: www.sturge-weber.com; www.nf.org

61 INFLAMMATORY SKIN DISEASE

Sarah L. Chamlin

ATOPIC DERMATITIS

EPIDEMIOLOGY AND PATHOPHYSIOLOGY

- Chronic inflammatory skin disorder occurring in 17% of school-aged children in United States.
- Ninety percent of affected children will have onset of disease by 5 years of age.
- Atopic dermatitis often improves or resolves with age with a 10-year clearance rate between 50 and 70%.
- Underlying abnormalities include increase in CD4+ TH2 helper T cells, elevated serum IgE levels, increased mediators such as histamine and prostaglandins, and genetic predisposition.
- Exacerbating factors: weather changes, sweating, environmental allergens (dander, dust mites), cutaneous infection, food allergies, and stress.

CLINICAL FEATURES AND DIFFERENTIAL DIAGNOSIS

- The distribution of atopic dermatitis varies with age. Infants will more commonly have facial and extensor surface involvement and older children and adults have flexural involvement or localized disease (particularly hands). The scalp is also commonly involved in infants and children.
- Lesions are typically erythematous, poorly demarcated papules and plaques with scale. Lichenification as a result of chronic scratching and rubbing commonly occurs. Nummular, "coin-shaped," lesions of atopic dermatitis are often confused with tinea corporis. Common features also seen in patients with atopic dermatitis include xerosis, keratosis pilaris, infraorbital folds, and hyperlinear palms.
- Signs of bacterial superinfection include crusting, oozing, and follicular-based papules and pustules. Bacterial, viral, and fungal infections occur more commonly in individuals with atopic dermatitis.
- Pruritus is common and often disrupts initiation and maintenance of sleep.
- The differential diagnosis includes psoriasis, allergic and irritant contact dermatitis, scabies, seborrheic dermatitis, and immunodeficiency syndromes (Wiskott-Aldrich syndrome, hyper-IgE syndrome).
- Many infants have clinical features of both atopic and seborrheic dermatitis.
- Pityriasis alba, a mild variant of atopic dermatitis, typically presents with hypopigmented patches or plaques on the face, but these lesions can occur elsewhere on the body.

TREATMENT AND PROGNOSIS

- Emollients are a mainstay of therapy. Twice daily application of a thick cream or ointment is recommended.
- Bathing restriction is not necessary unless frequent baths worsen the dermatitis. A short (5–10-minute) daily bath with a mild fragrance-free soap followed by a thick emollient is recommended.
- Use of lightweight, nonocclusive clothing is recommended.
- Topical corticosteroids are a mainstay of treatment. Low-potency (Class VI or VII) steroids are recommended for the face or intertriginous areas. Low- to midpotency steroids are suggested for the trunk, extremities, or scalp. Ointments are more efficacious and typically preferred over creams. A lotion, solution, or foam is preferred for the scalp. Twice daily use of topical corticosteroids is recommended.
- Calcineurin inhibitors (pimecrolimus 1% cream and tacrolimus 0.03 or 0.1% ointment) are effective in treating atopic dermatitis. Both drugs are approved for use in children >2 years of age. Twice daily use is recommended.
- Oral sedating antihistamines (diphenhydramine or hydroxyzine) are effective when given at night for symptoms of pruritus and sleep disruption.

- When signs of bacterial infection (*Staphylococcus aureus*) are present, systemic antibiotics (cephalexin, dicloxicillin, erythromycin) are indicated for a 10–14 day course. Topical antibiotics (e.g., mupirocin) are only indicated for very localized disease. Bacterial colonization without clinical signs of infection may be trigger atopic dermatitis.
- Antiviral agents are indicated for herpes simplex infections, eczema herpeticum. Children with eczema herpeticum, if systemically ill, may require hospitalization for intravenous acyclovir and fluids.
- Systemic therapy is rarely indicated. For severe refractory cases, systemic agents such as corticosteroids (followed by a long taper) or cyclosporin can be helpful.
- Both ultraviolet B (UVB) and psoralen with ultraviolet A (PUVA) may be effective in refractory cases. UVB therapy is preferred in the pediatric population and requires treatment three times per week for several months.
- Food allergy is rarely a contributing factor to atopic dermatitis. Approximately one-third of children with severe atopic dermatitis have food allergy that contributes to the severity of skin disease. If food allergy is suspected a referral to an allergist is indicated.
- Avoidance of environmental allergens (house dust mite and dander) may improve the severity of dermatitis in some sensitized individuals.

PSORIASIS

EPIDEMIOLOGY AND PATHOPHYSIOLOGY

- Chronic inflammatory skin disorder with a prevalence of 1–3% in the general population with one-third of individuals presenting before 20 years of age.
- Genetic, immunologic, environmental, and infectious factors all play a role in the pathogenesis of psoriasis. A family history of psoriasis is present in 35% of affected individuals.

CLINICAL FEATURES AND DIFFERENTIAL DIAGNOSIS

- Plaque type is the most common form of psoriasis seen in children and adults. Lesions are erythematous, well-demarcated asymptomatic plaques with silvery scale and can be localized or generalized on any body site. Scalp is a common site of involvement. Infants presenting with diaper involvement often do not have the typical silvery scale.
- Guttate type psoriasis presents with multiple small "teardrop" lesions usually in a generalized pattern.

Less commonly, psoriasis can be pustular or erythrodermic.
- Nails can be involved with pitting, yellowing, subungual hyperkeratosis, and "oil drops" (proximal onycholysis).
- Arthritis, typically of the distal interphalangeal joints occurs in a small percentage of children with psoriasis. This can precede development of skin lesions.
- Streptococcal infection may be a trigger for appearance of disease.
- The differential diagnosis includes seborrheic dermatitis, atopic dermatitis, and bacterial folliculitis (pustular variant).

TREATMENT AND PROGNOSIS

- Mid- to high-strength topical corticosteroids are used twice daily as monotherapy or once daily when used in combination with daily topical calcipotriene (trunk, extremities, or scalp). One is applied in the morning and the other is applied in the evening. Low-potency corticosteroids are recommended for the face or intertriginous areas.
- Topic refined tar preparations such as liquor carbonis detergens (LCD 5–10%) can be combined with mid-potency corticosteroids and used once or twice daily.
- Topical tazarotene used in combination with a potent topical steroid may be effective for some children. The side effect of irritation often limits the use of tazarotene in the pediatric population.
- Both UVB and PUVA may be effective for widespread cases. UVB therapy is preferred in the pediatric population and treatment three times per week for several months is suggested.
- Severe refractory cases may require systemic therapy with methotrexate, cyclosporin, or other agents.

SEBORRHEIC DERMATITIS

EPIDEMIOLOGY AND PATHOPHYSIOLOGY

- Seborrheic dermatitis often appears in the first month of life and may persist for the first year.
- Although the etiology is unknown, the yeast, *Pityrosporum ovale*, may play a role.

CLINICAL FEATURES AND DIFFERENTIAL DIAGNOSIS

- Eruption occurs in "seborrheic" areas, face (eyebrows), scalp, posterior auricular area, and intertriginous areas including the diaper area. Itch is uncommon and when present suggests the diagnosis of atopic dermatitis.

- Scalp may have greasy yellow plaques with scale. Other areas often have erythematous papules and plaques. Moist areas may not have visible scale.
- The differential diagnosis includes atopic dermatitis, psoriasis, scabies, *Candida* infection, tinea capitis, deficiency dermatoses (acrodermatitis enteropathica, fatty acid deficiency, biotin deficiency), and Langerhans cell histiocytosis.

TREATMENT AND PROGNOSIS

- Antiseborrheic shampoos (selenium sulfide, zinc pyrithrione, tar, salicylic acid) can be used to help loosen scale. These can cause eye irritation and should be left on for 5 minutes.
- Oils can be applied to the scalp and left on several hours. A soft brush may help loosen the adherent scale.
- Low-potency steroid solutions or lotions are effective for scalp disease. Low-potency steroid ointments or creams are suggested for the trunk, face, and extremities.
- Antistaphylococcal antibiotics are suggested when oozing or crusting is present.

CONTACT DERMATITIS (ALLERGIC AND IRRITANT)

EPIDEMIOLOGY AND PATHOPHYSIOLOGY

- Diaper dermatitis is the most common form of irritant contact dermatitis in children. This is caused by contact with urine, feces, detergents, soaps, and antiseptics in diapers.
- Common causes of allergic contact dermatitis include poison ivy, poison oak, poison sumac, nickel, cosmetics, dyes, and rubber products.
- Approximately 85% of the population is susceptible to poison ivy after adequate exposure.

CLINICAL FEATURES AND DIFFERENTIAL DIAGNOSIS

- The eruption site may be a clue to the cause. Lesions occur where the contactant touched the skin (lines, streaks, angles).
- Irritant diaper dermatitis usually spares the creases. Perianal dermatitis is often caused by diarrhea.
- Acute lesions: Erythema, pruritus, vesicles, bullae, and crust and scale.
- Chronic lesions: Hyperpigmentation, fissures, lichenification, xerosis, and scale.

- Nickel allergy often presents with chronic periumbilical lesions due to exposure to metal closures on clothing.
- The differential diagnosis includes psoriasis, atopic dermatitis, fungal infection, and seborrheic dermatitis.

TREATMENT AND PROGNOSIS

- Avoidance of the irritant or allergic trigger is the most successful therapy.
- Patch testing can be performed to identify suspected contact allergens.
- The dermatitis can be treated with topical corticosteroids twice daily for 1–2 weeks until the eruption is resolved (mid- to high-potency for localized disease and midpotency for extensive disease). Systemic corticosteroids (1–2 mg/kg tapered over 10–21 days) are indicated for severe extensive disease.
- Antihistamines are indicated for the associated pruritus. Systemic antibiotics with *Staphylococcus aureus* coverage should be prescribed if infection occurs. A cool compress may provide symptom relief.
- Frequent diaper changes, low-potency corticosteroids, and diaper barrier creams are indicated for irritant diaper dermatitis.

BIBLIOGRAPHY

Barros MA, Baptista A, Correia TM, Azevedo F. Patch testing in children: A study of 562 schoolchildren. *Contact Dermatitis* 1991;25:156–159.

Boguniewicz M, Fiedler VC, Raimer S, Laurence ID, Leung DY, Hanifin JM. A randomized vehicle-controlled trial of tacrolimus ointment for treatment of atopic dermatitis in children. *J Allergy Clin Immunol* 1998;102:637–644.

Burks AW, James JM, Hiegel, et al. Atopic dermatitis and food hypersensitivity reactions. *J Pediatr* 1998;132:132–136.

Hanifin JM, Saurat JH. Understanding atopic dermatitis: Pathophysiology and etiology. *J Am Acad Dermatol* 2001;45:S1–68.

Hoare C, Li Wan Po A, Williams H. Systematic review of treatments for atopic eczema. *Health Technol Assess* 2000;4:1–191.

Laughter D, Istvan JA, Tofte SJ, Hanifin JM. The prevalence of atopic dermatitis in Oregon schoolchildren. *Adv Dermatol* 2000;43:649–655.

McAlvany JP, Sherertz EF. Contact dermatitis in infants, children, and adolescents. *Adv Dermatol* 1994;9:205–223.

Menni S, Piccino R, Baietta S, et al. Infantile seborrheic dermatitis: A 7-year follow-up and some prognostic criteria. *Pediatr Dermatol* 1989;6:13–15.

Williams HC, Strachan DP. The natural history of childhood atopic eczema: Observations from the British 1958 birth cohort study. *Br Med J* 1998;139;834–839.

Further information: www.nationaleczema.org

62 ACNE

Jill Nelson and Amy S. Paller

ACNE VULGARIS

EPIDEMIOLOGY AND PATHOPHYSIOLOGY

- Acne vulgaris is a chronic multifactorial disease of the pilosebaceous unit. Most commonly, acne occurs during teenage years and represents an early manifestation of puberty. Persistence of acne into the third decade and beyond occurs more frequently in young women and may signal an endocrinologic abnormality. Occasionally, acne lesions are seen in infants, most commonly in boys.
- Androgenic stimulation of sebaceous glands, located in the follicular apparatus, leads to sebaceous gland enlargement and increased sebum production.
- Abnormal keratinization of the follicle occurs, at least in part because follicular keratinocytes become lipid-laden.
- The plugging of the follicle with sebum and desquamated keratinocytes manifests as a comedo (blackhead or whitehead).
- *Propionobacterium acnes* is the primary organism found in follicles of patients with acne and is largely responsible for inflammatory lesions.
- *P. acnes* derives nutrients from sebum and produces chemotactic factors, proteases, and lipases, which break down the follicle wall and attract inflammatory cells.
- Although hyperandrogenism is usually associated with severe acne, as in patients with congenital adrenal hyperplasia, ovarian or adrenal tumors, and polycystic ovarian disease, most adolescents with acne have normal endocrine function.

CLINICAL FEATURES AND DIFFERENTIAL DIAGNOSIS

- Acne occurs primarily on the face, upper chest, and back, areas with the greatest density of sebaceous glands.
- Comedones are noninflammatory lesions with either a widely dilated follicular opening, thereby exposing its contents (open comedo, blackhead), or a small follicular opening (closed comedo, whitehead).
- Inflammatory lesions may be inflammatory papules, pustules, or nodules, and represent ruptured microcomedones.

- Sequelae of acne include scars, erythema, and postinflammatory hyperpigmentation.
  1. Scars may be superficial, pitted, hypertrophic, or keloidal.
  2. Erythema may persist for 1–2 years after clearance of active lesions.
  3. Postinflammatory hyperpigmentation is usually seen in patients with darker skin types. In the absence of continuing inflammatory activity, the pigmentation tends to fade over several months to years.
- Diagnosis is usually straightforward. Acne vulgaris may be confused with folliculitis, rosacea, inflamed epidermal cysts, or the multiple facial angiofibromas seen in tuberous sclerosis.
- Acne can be triggered or worsened by administration of medications, particularly corticosteroids, methotrexate, lithium, and phenytoin.

TREATMENT AND PROGNOSIS

- Treatment should be targeted to the type of acne lesions present. Patients should be encouraged to be persistent with therapy, as clinical changes occur over 6–8 weeks or longer.
- Comedonal acne is best treated with topical retinoids, such as adapalene, tretinoin, or tazarotene. In general, micronized forms and creams are less irritating than gels or solution, but may also be less effective.
- Topical retinoids should be applied once daily; a pea-sized amount should be enough to cover the face. Optimal tolerance is achieved by initiating therapy every other day and gradually increasing application frequency to nightly as tolerated.
- Small inflammatory lesions are treated best with topical benzoyl peroxide, available in concentrations of 2.5–10%. Emollient bases are less drying than gels. The higher strengths tend to be more irritating. Benzoyl peroxide is applied one to two times per day and can bleach clothing, towels, or bedding.
- Benzoyl peroxide is available in combination with topical erythromycin or clindamycin; combination therapy may increase compliance and decrease the risk of antibiotic resistance.
- For patients who do not tolerate benzoyl peroxide, topical antibiotics such as topical clindamycin or erythromycin may be effective.
- Most patients have mixed comedonal and inflammatory acne, and thus are treated with both an anticomedonal agent and an anti-inflammatory agent. Benzoyl peroxide may be used with topical retinoids, but the medications should never be applied together; generally one is applied in the morning and the other at night.

- Waiting for 30 minutes or more after cleansing before application of topical medication decreases the tendency for medication-induced irritation or stinging.
- Deeper inflammatory papules, pustules, and cysts or acne resistant to topical therapies require oral agents in addition to the application of topical medications.
- Oral tetracycline is generally the first choice agent in dosages of 500 mg bid. For optimal absorption, tetracycline must be administered in the absence of food to avoid interaction with calcium or iron. Nausea or abdominal discomfort, not uncommonly, occurs with ingestion of tetracycline, but sun sensitivity is unusual. Tetracyclines can stain developing teeth, and should not be used in children under the age of 9 years or in pregnant women. A rare side effect of all tetracyclines is pseudotumor cerebri, which may present with headaches and/or blurred vision.
- When tetracycline cannot be used or is ineffective, doxycycline or minocycline (also in the tetracycline family) should be considered. Both medications are usually initiated at dosages of 100 mg bid. Gastrointestinal upset occurs less commonly, and ingestion concurrent with food causes significantly less interference with absorption than tetracycline. Sun sensitivity is a concern, especially with doxycycline, and patients should be warned that sunburn may occur with relatively little sun exposure. Minocycline has rare but potentially serious side effects, including drug-induced lupus, nephritis, serum sickness, drug hypersensitivity syndrome, and autoimmune hepatitis. Occasionally, minocycline administration leads to vertigo or the development of blue-gray pigmentation of acne scars, the gingivae and roof of the mouth and the shins.
- Erythromycin and azithromycin are less commonly used because of the higher rate of resistance and thus lower efficacy. Erythromycin usage should be reserved for children less than 9 years of age, including patients with infantile acne, and pregnant patients who require oral therapy.
- Other antibiotics, such as cephalexin and amoxicillin, have been reported anecdotally to improve acne; however, they do not tend to concentrate in the follicle as tetracyclines and erythromycins do, and both cephalosporins and penicillins are commonly used for other childhood bacterial infections. Oral administration of clindamycin tends to be quite efficacious, but carries the risk of development of pseudomembranous colitis. The use of trimethoprim-sulfamethoxazole, although effective, should be discouraged because of the potential for life-threatening drug reactions.
- Isotretinoin is reserved for patients with severe inflammatory acne that is recalcitrant to systemic antibiotic therapy. Isotretinoin causes involution of the sebaceous gland, and is the only therapeutic agent that suppresses sebum production. Although it has no direct antibacterial effect, growth of *P. acnes* is inhibited because of the sebum depletion. The typical 5-month course is effective in >90% of patients and may suppress acne for months to years. Many patients will eventually require some form of treatment for acne again, especially if the patient is young. In the United States, isotretinoin can only be prescribed by a physician enrolled in the prescriber program. Isotretinoin administration requires careful clinical and laboratory monitoring, and has been associated with several potential side effects, most of which are reversible when the medication is discontinued. Isotretinoin is a major teratogen; care must be taken to avoid pregnancy while the medication is administered. Virtually all patients develop cheilitis and most note dryness of the skin and mucous membranes. Approximately 25% of patients experience hypertriglyceridemia, emphasizing the need for monthly fasting laboratory testing. Rare but potentially serious adverse effects of isotretinoin include pseudotumor cerebri and possibly psychologic abnormalities. Concurrent administration of a systemic antibiotic should be avoided to minimize the risk of pseudotumor cerebri. Although the link with depression and suicide ideation with isotretinoin has not definitively been established, patients must be warned about this possible problem and monitored carefully.
- Hormonal therapy with estrogen predominant oral contraceptives is an option for girls with inflammatory acne; this therapy tends to be more effective in girls who notice fluctuations in their acne severity with menses. Improvement is usually seen within 3–6 months of initiation.
- Laboratory evaluation is not indicated for acne unless hyperandrogenism is suspected. Excess androgens may be produced by the adrenal gland or ovary.
- Hyperandrogenism should be considered if there is sudden explosive onset of severe acne, precocious puberty, premature adrenarche, menstrual irregularity, hirsutism, or evidence of insulin resistance (obesity, acanthosis nigricans). An evaluation should be performed in collaboration with a pediatric endocrinologist or gynecologist.

NEONATAL AND INFANTILE ACNE

- Acne may occur in neonates or infants. Males are most frequently affected. Usually the face is affected although the chest or trunk can be involved. The sebaceous glands of neonates are actively producing sebum in the first weeks of life secondary to maternal androgens. The glands gradually atrophy over a 2–3-month period until puberty when they become active again.

- Infantile acne begins between ages 3 months and 1 year. In infantile acne the lesions tend to be more pleomorphic and may include comedones, inflammatory papules, and pustules. Occasionally inflammatory cysts or nodules may occur, sometimes without other types of lesions. The cause of infantile acne remains unknown and the role of androgens is less clear. Some have postulated an end organ hypersensitivity to androgens, resulting from increased androgen receptor to ligand affinity, increased 5-alpha-reductase activity, or other variations in androgen metabolism.
- Neonatal cephalic pustulosis is clinically similar to classic neonatal acne, but has been linked to *Malassezia furfur* infection. In contrast to neonatal acne, cephalic pustulosis is a nonfollicular process beginning in neonates less than 1 month. Confirmation of *M. furfur* can be made by direct microscopy of pustular material and response to topical ketoconazole therapy.
- Neonatal acne generally does not require intervention. For infants with acne of mild-to-moderate severity, topical benzoyl peroxide and/or a topical retinoid may be effective depending on the type of lesions. If moderate inflammatory papules or cysts predominate, scarring is a concern and administration of oral erythromycin in addition to topical therapy is appropriate. Oral isotretinoin has been safely administered to infants or young children with cystic acne who are unresponsive to oral antibiotic therapy.

BIBLIOGRAPHY

Bergman JN, Eichenfield LF. Neonatal acne and cephalic pustulosis: Is Malassezia the whole story? *Arch Dermatol* 2002; 138(2):255–257.

Cunliffe NJ. Acne. In: Harper J, Oranje A, Prose N (eds.), *Textbook of Pediatric Dermatology*, Vol. 1. Oxford: Blackwell Science 2000, pp. 639–653.

Leyden JJ. Drug therapy: Therapy for acne vulgaris. *N Engl J Med* 1997;336(16):1156–1162.

Mengesha YM, Hansen RC. Toddler-age nodulocystic acne. *J Pediatr* 1999;134(5):664–648.

Strauss JS, Thiboutot DM. Diseases of the sebaceous glands. In: Freedberg IM, Eisen AZ, Wolff K, Austen KF, Goldsmith LA, Katz SI, Fitzpatrick TB (eds.), *Fitzpatrick's Dermatology in General Medicine*, Vol. 1. New York: McGraw-Hill, 1999, pp. 769–783.

63 VIRAL INFECTIONS, MISCELLANEOUS EXANTHEMS, AND INFESTATIONS

Anthony J. Mancini

VIRAL INFECTIONS

VERRUCA VULGARIS

EPIDEMIOLOGY AND PATHOPHYSIOLOGY
- Synonyms: common wart; plantar wart (verruca plantaris), flat wart (verruca plana).
- Caused by human papillomavirus (HPV), a double-stranded deoxyribonucleic acid (DNA) virus; multiple serotypes.
- Transmission by direct contact, autoinoculation, and fomites (especially plantar warts).

DIFFERENTIAL DIAGNOSIS AND CLINICAL FEATURES
- Differential diagnosis includes skin tag, nevus, molluscum contagiosum, juvenile xanthogranuloma, epidermal nevus.
- Flesh-colored, verrucous (rough-surfaced) papules, often clustered or in a linear configuration (Koebner phenomenon).
- Distribution variable (verruca plana most common on face).
- Occasionally filiform (numerous projections from a slender stalk).
- Tiny black dots (representing thrombosed capillary vessels) may help to differentiate from other entities.

TREATMENT AND PROGNOSIS
- Spontaneous involution common (may take up to several years).
- Effectiveness of therapy must be balanced by discomfort and trauma for the child.
- Salicylic acid liquids useful, especially with occlusion (duct tape, plasters); not appropriate for facial lesions.
- Cryotherapy (liquid nitrogen) effective, of limited use in young children.
- Cimetidine (30–40 mg/kg/day for 8 weeks) may be useful.
- Other therapies include chemovesicants, laser therapy, topical immunotherapy.
- Verruca plana may respond to topical tretinoin cream.

MOLLUSCUM CONTAGIOSUM

EPIDEMIOLOGY AND PATHOPHYSIOLOGY
- Caused by molluscum contagiosum virus (MCV), a double-stranded DNA virus.
- Peak age of 2–12 years.
- Transmission by direct skin contact, fomites, auto-inoculation.
- Although common in acquired immunodeficiency, pediatric disease usually not a marker for human immunodeficiency virus (HIV).

DIFFERENTIAL DIAGNOSIS AND CLINICAL FEATURES
- Differential diagnosis includes verruca vulgaris, nevus, juvenile xanthogranuloma, Spitz nevus, folliculitis.
- Discrete, flesh-colored, pearly or waxy papules, usually 1–5 mm.
- Central depression (*umbilication*) may be present.
- Variable distribution, but most commonly neck, axillae, thighs, face, and abdomen.
- Associated inflammation and scaling (*molluscum dermatitis*) common, especially in atopic patients.

TREATMENT AND PROGNOSIS
- Nearly always resolve spontaneously (months to years).
- Aggressive therapy unwarranted; "watchful waiting" appropriate if desired.
- Cantharidin (blister beetle extract) 0.9% in flexible collodion very effective, safe when used correctly (not recommended for facial, genital, or perianal lesions).
- Cryotherapy and curettage useful but limited by pain, emotional trauma in young children.
- Topical chemovesicants, tretinoin, immunotherapy used with variable success.

MISCELLANEOUS EXANTHEMS

PAPULAR ACRODERMATITIS OF CHILDHOOD

EPIDEMIOLOGY AND PATHOPHYSIOLOGY
- Synonym: Gianotti-Crosti syndrome.
- A distinct exanthematic eruption in response to a variety of viral infections.
- Classically associated with hepatitis B infection and acute anicteric hepatitis (mainly Japan and Europe).
- Most common etiologic agent in United States is Epstein-Barr virus.
- Young children most frequently affected, especially during spring/early summer.

DIFFERENTIAL DIAGNOSIS AND CLINICAL FEATURES
- Upper respiratory prodrome common.
- Abrupt onset of monomorphous, flesh-colored to pink papules on the extensor extremities, face, and buttocks.
- Trunk is usually relatively spared.
- Vesicular or purpuric lesions, lymphadenopathy, fever occasionally present.
- Differential diagnosis includes drug reaction, molluscum contagiosum, erythema multiforme, other viral exanthems.

TREATMENT AND PROGNOSIS
- Evaluate for hepatitis only if clinical suspicion present.
- Symptomatic therapy with antihistamines, emollients.
- Spontaneous involution occurs over 4–10 weeks.

UNILATERAL LATEROTHORACIC EXANTHEM

EPIDEMIOLOGY AND PATHOPHYSIOLOGY
- Synonym: asymmetric periflexural exanthem of childhood.
- A distinct exanthem of probable viral etiology; exact organism(s) not confirmed.
- Average age of onset 24 months.
- No seasonal predilection.

DIFFERENTIAL DIAGNOSIS AND CLINICAL FEATURES
- Upper respiratory or gastrointestinal prodrome may precede cutaneous eruption.
- Initially unilateral and localized, most often in axillary and/or thoracic regions.
- Less common sites of initial involvement include inguinal region, lower extremity.
- May subsequently generalize, but maintains a unilateral predominance.
- Morphology most commonly eczematous or morbilliform, less often scarlatiniform, urticarial or purpuric.
- Variable features include pruritus, fever, lymphadenopathy.
- Differential diagnosis includes contact dermatitis (most common), other viral exanthems, drug eruption, scabies, scarlet fever, miliaria.

TREATMENT AND PROGNOSIS
- Symptomatic therapy with emollients, antihistamines.
- Spontaneous resolution occurs over 2–10 weeks.

PITYRIASIS ROSEA

EPIDEMIOLOGY AND PATHOPHYSIOLOGY
- An acute, self-limited exanthematous skin eruption.
- Viral etiology (including human herpesvirus-7) postulated but unconfirmed.
- Most common in spring and fall.

DIFFERENTIAL DIAGNOSIS AND CLINICAL FEATURES

- May begin with a single, scaly erythematous plaque (*herald patch*).
- Within 1–2 weeks, multiple secondary erythematous papules and plaques develop.
- Lesions are oval, with long axis following lines of skin cleavage (*inverted Christmas tree*).
- Most common areas involved are trunk and proximal extremities, less often neck, face, or distal extremities.
- Surface scale has free edge pointing inward (*trailing scale*).
- "Inverse" pityriasis rosea presents with lesions localized to axillae and groin.
- Differential diagnosis includes tinea (herald patch stage), atopic dermatitis, psoriasis, secondary syphilis, pityriasis lichenoides chronica.

TREATMENT AND PROGNOSIS

- Spontaneous involution occurs over 6–12 weeks.
- Therapy is symptomatic; ultraviolet light may accentuate involution.
- Serologic testing for syphilis indicated in sexually-active patients or those with any signs of sexual abuse.

INFESTATIONS

SCABIES

EPIDEMIOLOGY AND PATHOPHYSIOLOGY

- A common skin infestation caused by *Sarcoptes scabiei*.
- Acquired through direct skin-to-skin contact, less often via fomites.
- Most common symptom is pruritus, caused by the allergic reaction of the host.
- Occurs in all ages, races, and socioeconomic backgrounds.
- Female mite burrows under stratum corneum, lays eggs that give rise to adult mites in 2 weeks.

DIFFERENTIAL DIAGNOSIS AND CLINICAL FEATURES

- Initial symptom is pruritus, especially at night, and occasionally in absence of lesions.
- Skin lesions include erythematous papules, vesicles, crusting, and linear burrows.
- Common sites include wrists, finger webs, palms and soles, belt line, areolae, axillae, and penis.
- Nodules, scalp involvement seen mainly in infants.
- Immunosuppressed individuals may present with crusted, scaling plaques, especially of hands and feet (*crusted* or *Norwegian* scabies).
- Secondary bacterial infection/pyoderma common.
- Differential diagnosis includes atopic dermatitis, seborrheic dermatitis, Langerhans cell histiocytosis, impetigo, arthropod bites, papular urticaria, contact dermatitis.
- Diagnosis confirmed by visualizing mites, eggs or fecal pellets on direct microscopy of mineral oil scrapings (highest yield from burrows).

TREATMENT AND PROGNOSIS

- Treatment of choice is 5% permethrin cream, applied for 8–14 hours then rinsed.
- In infants, scalp and face should also be treated, with care taken to avoid eyes and mouth.
- Family members, close contacts, and housemates should all be treated.
- Some advocate repeat treatment in 1 week, although single treatment is quite effective.
- Clothing and linens should be washed in hot water, dried on high-heat setting.
- Treat itch and secondary infection if necessary.
- Other treatment options include lindane, sulfur, oral ivermectin (off-label).

PEDICULOSIS CAPITIS

EPIDEMIOLOGY AND PATHOPHYSIOLOGY

- Common infestation in children, caused by *Pediculus humanus capitis*.
- Affects all socioeconomic groups; most common in children ages 3–12 years.
- Less common in African-Americans, related to oval-shaped and larger-diameter hair shafts.
- Spread by direct head-to-head contact, less often fomites (hats, combs, brushes).
- Adult female louse lays up to 10 eggs (nits) per day, which attach to hair shaft close to scalp with strong cement.

DIFFERENTIAL DIAGNOSIS AND CLINICAL FEATURES

- Itch is main symptom, less often secondary impetiginization or lymphadenopathy present.
- Differential diagnosis includes hair casts (keratin debris that can easily be slid off the hair), seborrheic dermatitis, tinea capitis.
- Diagnosis confirmed by finding a live louse; nit can be confirmed by hair shaft microscopy.
- Nits located more than 1 cm from scalp unlikely to be viable.

TREATMENT AND PROGNOSIS

- Over-the-counter treatment options include 1% permethrin creme rinse and pyrethrin with piperonyl butoxide (various concentrations).
- Prescription treatment options include 5% permethrin cream, 0.5% malathion lotion, and 1% lindane shampoo.

- Nit combing a useful adjunct, but difficult and tedious.
- Resistance reported to lindane, permethrin, and pyrethrins, but more often treatment failure due to noncompliance or reinfestation.
- Oral ivermectin may be useful as off-label therapy in severe or resistant infections.
- Environmental decontamination important, including grooming items, clothing, linens, and furniture.
- "No-nit" school policies discouraged by American Academy of Pediatrics, American Public Health Association.
- No adverse sequelae; head lice do not transmit other infectious diseases.

BIBLIOGRAPHY

Bodemer C, de Prost Y. Unilateral laterothoracic exanthem in children: A new disease? *J Am Acad Dermatol* 1992; 27:693–696.

Caputo R, Gelmetti C, Ermacora E, et al. Gianotti-Crosti syndrome: A retrospective analysis of 308 cases. *J Am Acad Dermatol* 1992;26:207–210.

DelGiudice P. Ivermectin in scabies. *Curr Opin Infect Dis* 2002; 15:123–126.

Drago F, Ranieri E, Malaguti F, et al. Human herpesvirus 7 in pityriasis rosea. *Lancet* 1997;349:1367–1368.

Frankowski BL, Weiner LB, et al. Clinical report—head lice. *Pediatrics* 2002;110:638–643.

Hofmann B, Schuppe HC, Adams O, et al. Gianotti-Crosti syndrome associated with Epstein-Barr infection. *Pediatr Dermatol* 1997;14:273–277.

McCuaig CC, Russo P, Powell J, et al. Unilateral laterothoracic exanthem. A clinicopathologic study of forty-eight patients. *J Am Acad Dermatol* 1996;34:979–984.

Peterson CM, Eichenfield LF. Scabies. *Pediatr Ann* 1996; 25(2):97–100.

Roberts RJ. Head lice. *N Engl J Med* 2002;21:1645–1650.

Silverberg NB, Sidbury R, Mancini AJ. Childhood molluscum contagiosum: Experience with cantharidin therapy in 300 patients. *J Am Acad Dermatol* 2000;43:503–507.

Spear KL, Winkelmann RK. Gianotti-Crosti syndrome. A review of ten cases not associated with hepatitis B. *Arch Dermatol* 1984;120:891–896.

Williams LK, Reichert A, MacKenszie WR, et al. Lice, nits and school policy. *Pediatrics* 2001;107:1011–1015.

DISORDERS OF THE ENDOCRINE SYSTEM

Donald Zimmerman, Section Editor

64 DIABETES MELLITUS AND HYPOGLYCEMIA

Donald Zimmerman, Reema L. Habiby, and Wendy J. Brickman

Diabetes Mellitus

CLASSIFICATIONS

- Type 1 diabetes mellitus: Autoimmune or idiopathic
- Type 2 diabetes mellitus
- Gestational diabetes mellitus
- Other forms: Maturity onset diabetes of youth (MODY), atypical, cystic fibrosis (CF)-related, medication induced, and neonatal

DIAGNOSIS

Diabetes
- Fasting plasma glucose ≥126 mg/dL (American Diabetes Association, 2003)[*]
- Two-hour stimulated glucose ≥200 mg/dL (repeated)[*]

Impaired Fasting Glucose
- Fasting plasma glucose ≥100 mg/dL (recent change from 100 mg/dL).

Impaired Glucose Tolerance
- Two-hour stimulated glucose ≥140 and <200 mg/dL

---

[*]During oral glucose tolerance test (OGTT), diagnosis of diabetes needs to be confirmed on separate day.

GLUCOSE HOMEOSTASIS

INSULIN PRODUCTION/PROCESSING
- Preproinsulin is processed to form proinsulin which is processed to form insulin (A chain [21 aa] and B chain [30 aa] connected by two disulfide bonds) and c-peptide (C chain).

INSULIN SECRETION
- The GLUT-2 transporter in the beta-cell takes up glucose, which is then metabolized. Glucose metabolism is coupled with insulin secretion. With increasing adenosine triphosphate/adenosine diphosphate (ATP/ADP) ratio, the ATP sensitive K+ channel (KATP) closes, depolarizing the cell, causing an influx of calcium which subsequently leads to insulin secretion.
- Insulin secretion occurs in two phases. The first phase reflects a rapid insulin release over 5–10 minutes after exposure to glucose. This is followed by an increasing second phase of insulin release.

INSULIN ACTION (VIA INSULIN RECEPTOR SUBSTRATE-1 [IRS-1] AND IRS-2 AND SIGNAL TRANSDUCTION PATHWAYS)
- *Liver*: Decreases hepatic glucose production, stimulates lipogenesis, and inhibits ketogenesis.
- *Adipose tissue*: Suppresses lipolysis, inhibits free fatty acid mobilization, and stimulates lipogenesis.
- *Muscle tissue*: Increase in protein accretion, glycogen synthesis, and glucose oxidation.

TYPE 1 DIABETES MELLITUS

EPIDEMIOLOGY

- Individuals with type 1 diabetes account for 5–10% of the estimated 17 million Americans with diabetes.
- Incidence (/100,000/year) ranges from 3.3 to 11 in non-Hispanic Blacks and 13.3 to 20.6 in Caucasians in America (LaPorte et al., 1995). Highest incidence in Finland (35.3) and lowest in Korea (0.7).
- Incidence increases in winter and with increasing distance from equator. Slight preponderance in males.
- Increased prevalence in siblings (2–17%) and offspring (2–5%) of probands with type 1 diabetes.

PATHOPHYSIOLOGY

- HLA susceptibility: Chromosome 6: DR3 (DQA1* 0501, DQB1*0201) and DR4 (DQA1*0301, DQB1* 0302). DR2 and DR7 are protective.
- Other genetic loci may also confer susceptibility and/or protection, i.e., insulin-dependent diabetes mellitus (IDDM2) in which the number of variable number of tandem repeats (VNTRs) to the insulin gene may contribute to susceptibility or protection (Bennett et al., 1995).
- Appears to be an environmental component as well (i.e., viruses, toxins) which triggers T-cell activation (only 50% concordance in identical twins).
- Development of antibodies to cell surface and cytoplasmic antigens, i.e., insulin, protein tyrosine phosphatase-like molecule (ICA512/IA2), glutamic acid decarboxylase (GAD).
- In studies of relatives of those with type 1 diabetes, presence of multiple antibodies and loss of first phase insulin release are predictive of the development of type 1 diabetes (Verge et al., 1996; Chase et al., 2001).
- Silent autoimmune destruction of islet cells.
- With loss of critical mass of beta cells, insulin release is suboptimal, glucose uptake diminishes, and lipolysis, ketogenesis, glycogenolysis, and proteolysis increases. Metabolic decompensation ensues. This may be amplified by other hormones (i.e., epinephrine, cortisol, and glucagons). Glucose toxicity further impairs islet-cell insulin release. As process deteriorates, diabetic ketoacidosis (DKA) develops.

PRESENTATION

- Asymptomatic, noticed on routine examination: Glycosuria ± ketonuria.
- Typical: Polyuria, polydipsia, polyphagia, abdominal pain, weight loss, and emesis.
- Common: DKA.

EVALUATION

- Urine analysis: Glycosuria and ketonuria.
- Serum glucose
- Serum electrolytes: Acidosis, potassium, sodium (correct for glucose: sodium is falsely decreased by 1.6 meq/L for every 100 mg/dL glucose is above the normal range).
- VBG/ABG
- HgbA1c
- Insulin and c-peptide concentration.
- Diabetes autoimmune antibodies: GAD, insulin, IA2.

TREATMENT

- In asymptomatic individuals, the confirmation of a diagnosis of diabetes will need to be made. This can be with preprandial and 1–2-hour postprandial glucose concentrations. Typically, fasting blood glucose is greater than 200 mg/dL. Infrequently, oral glucose tolerance test (1.75 g/kg glucose, up to 75 g) is given orally in 5-minute time frame. Serum glucose and insulin are obtained at time 0 (30 and 60 minutes optional) and 120 minutes from start, with time starting when patient begins to take glucose solution. Once confirmed, insulin therapy and education is started.
- In mildly symptomatic individuals, able to tolerate food intake, insulin therapy is begun as discussed below. Education, nutrition, and diabetes survival skills are taught as well.
- In cases of DKA, initiation of therapy should be as swift as possible. See below.

INSULIN
- New insulin compounds bring increased flexibility and additional options for insulin regimens. See Table 64-1 for a list of the more common insulins available in the United States.
- Choice of regimen will often depend on patient motivation, financial resources, lifestyle, age, and personal choice as well as experience of care team. In general the regimens can be grouped into two types:
1. Split dose (2–3 Injections/day): Rapid and intermediate acting insulin is given in the morning. Rapid is also given at dinner time. Intermediate acting may be given with dinner injection or prior to bedtime. Number of carbohydrates is usually set per meal or snack. Additional rapid insulin is given at breakfast, dinner, and possibly bedtime to correct hyperglycemia.
   a. Two-thirds of daily dose given in morning and one-third in evening (dinner and bedtime combined).
   b. Morning dose consists of one-third rapid acting and two-thirds intermediate acting.

TABLE 64-1 Types of Insulin

NAME OF INSULIN	TYPE OF INSULIN	ONSET OF ACTION	PEAK ACTION	ENDS
Humalog/novolog	Rapid	10 minutes	1–2 hours	3–4 hours
Regular	Fast	20–40 minutes	2–4 hours	6–8 hours
NPH/lente	Intermediate	2–4 hours	6–10 hours	16–20 hours
Ultralente	Long	4–6 hours	10–20 hours	24–36 hours
Glargine	Long	2 hours	No peak	At least 24 hours
Regular 70/30 70% NPH/30% regular	Fast and intermediate	Combined pattern	Combined pattern	Combined pattern
Novolog 70/30 70% NPH/30% novolog	Rapid and intermediate	Combined pattern	Combined pattern	Combined pattern

c. Dinner dose: one-third of evening dose: consists of rapid acting.

d. Bedtime dose: two-thirds of evening dose in intermediate acting insulin (in two-injection regimen, this is given at dinner time).

2. Basal-bolus: Continuous subcutaneous infusion (CSI) with insulin pump or multiple injections of rapid insulin with long-acting, daily. Basal insulin is provided with continuous rapid insulin via pump therapy or with long-acting insulin injection. Rapid insulin is given at meals and snacks based on needed correction for hyperglycemia as well as number of carbohydrates to be eaten. More flexibility in meal timing and composition. More closely reflects normal endogenous insulin secretion.

a. Usually 40–50% of daily insulin is given as long-acting insulin.

b. Insulin to carbohydrate ratio: Range: 1 unit for 30 g carbohydrates to 1 unit for 8 g (varies by age and personal experience).

c. Correction dose: Range: 1 unit insulin to lower glucose 125 mg/dL to 1 unit to lower glucose by 25 mg/dL (varies by age and personal experience).

• Initial insulin therapy is often with split mixed regimen. With experience may go to basal-bolus regimen if appropriate for age and lifestyle. Initial insulin dose for split mixed is 0.5–0.75 u/kg/day for those with mild presentations.

• Dose changes should be based on trends seen in the glucose monitoring. Glucose monitoring is recommended before each meal and at bedtime. At times, additional blood glucose testing before snacks, 2 hours after meals, or in the middle of the night will be necessary to adequately assess the insulin regimen and direct appropriate changes. Changes up or down 10% are reasonable to make as needed, with one change being made no more frequently than every 3–4 days.

• Elevated morning glucose concentrations may be caused by (1) waning insulin coverage, (2) dawn phenomenon: due to increased counterregulatory hormones in early morning hours or to decreased available insulin, or (3) Somogyi phenomenon in which hypoglycemia occurs during sleep, causing an increase in counterregulatory hormones which lead to subsequent hyperglycemia.

• During illness, especially those causing decreased food intake or malabsorption, increased exercise, and times of stress more significant changes in insulin may need to be made and blood glucose should be monitored more frequently. Insulin therapy may need to be lowered (not further than two-thirds to half normal intermediate dose), but never stopped. Development of ketonuria needs to be monitored whenever insulin is markedly decreased.

• While NPO because of illness or in preparation for procedure, insulin drip offers best control. Determine insulin dose by initially providing 1 g of insulin for every 5 g of dextrose provided through intravenous fluids.

• With the onset of therapy in type 1 diabetes, near euglycemia is restored. As a result glucose toxicity resolves and remaining functional islet cells are again able to secrete insulin. Consequently exogenous insulin needs dramatically decrease. Individuals may have small insulin requirements and little deviation in their glucose concentrations during this time period, often referred to as the honeymoon phase. This phase frequently lasts 6 months to 1 year.

TREATMENT GOALS

• Majority of blood glucose concentrations in target zone (see Table 64-2).

• Minimize hypoglycemia (especially in those less than 6 years of age).

• Target HgbA1c as close to normal as possible without frequent hypoglycemia.

DIABETIC KETOACIDOSIS (DKA)

• An outline of treatment is included, but a chapter of this scope is not able to give due justice or the needed details for DKA. Fatalities occur in approximately 1% of cases, mainly from cerebral edema or electrolyte abnormalities. The premise of DKA is insulinopenia and subsequent lack of glucose uptake and uninhibited lipolysis and ketogenesis.

TABLE 64-2   Target Blood Glucose and HgbA1c

AGE (YEARS)	BEFORE MEALS (GLUCOSE, mg/dL)	2 HOURS AFTER MEAL (GLUCOSE, mg/dL)	BEDTIME (GLUCOSE, mg/dL)	HgbA1c (%)
0–3	100–200	150–250	150–200	<9.0
3–5	100–200	150–250	150–200	<8.5
6–8	80–180	80–180	120–180	<8.0
9–11	80–180	80–180	100–180	<7.5
≥12	80–180	80–180	100–180	<7.2

- Definition: Arterial pH <7.30, bicarbonate <15 meq/L, glucose >250 mg/dL.
- Flow sheet to follow: Glucose, Na, K, HCO_3, pH, insulin drip, type of fluids, fluid rate, total fluids in, total fluids out, urine ketones, heart rate, and neuro check.
- Foley, nasogastric suction, electrocardiogram (ECG) as appropriate.

Laboratory Studies
- Initial: Same as above. Consider studies for underlying infection as well, i.e., chest x-ray, urine analysis and culture, blood culture, and throat culture.
- Subsequent: Electrolytes and VBG every 2 hours, phosphorous and calcium every 4 hours, hourly glucose.

Fluids (Usually About 10% Dehydrated): NPO (Even for Ice Chips)
- Initial: Cardiovascular stabilization with 0.9 NS bolus (restrict to 10–20 cc/kg unless otherwise indicated).
- Subsequent: Remainder of fluid deficit should be estimated and replaced over 36 hours. Because of hyperosmolality, continue to use 0.9 NS. Rapid correction of osmolality is thought to contribute to risk of cerebral edema. Fluids should not exceed 4 $L/m^2/day$. Electrolytes—see below.

Electrolytes (Total Body Potassium and Phosphorous Depleted in DKA)
- Hypokalemia can occur despite total body depletion because of intracellular shifts with therapy. Phosphorous infusion can lead to hypocalcemia. Therefore monitor Ca^{++}.
- Once potassium is ≤5 meq/L, potassium should be added to fluids at 40 meq/L composed of half KCl and half KPhos.
- Potassium may need to be increased for hypokalemia and a higher proportion given as KPhos in face of decreasing phosphorous.

Dextrose
- Lower glucose ideally 100 mg/dL every hour.
- Maintain glucose around 200 mg/dL for at least the first 12 hours. Increase dextrose in fluids once glucose is below 250 mg/dL.

- Begin with 2.5% dextrose and increase as needed to 10% dextrose. Rarely 12.5% is required.
- Can use 2-bag system where dextrose is 0 in one and 10% in the other. Titrate ratio of fluid from each bag to create desired dextrose concentration, i.e., fluids in 3:1 ratio will give 2.5%.

Insulin
- Continuous intravenous infusion of regular insulin at 0.1 u/kg/hour.
- May need to increase insulin if glucose is not responding. Rarely need to go above 0.14 u/kg/hour.
- Insulin should be continued at 0.1 u/kg/hour until bicarbonate is greater than 16–18 meq/L. Adjust dextrose as needed if glucose concentrations are lower than target range.

Bicarbonate Therapy
- Recent study suggests administration is associated with cerebral edema. Cannot recommend bicarbonate therapy across the board. In cases of cardiovascular and respiratory compromise, especially at pH <7.0, administration needs to be considered on an individual basis.

Cerebral Edema
- Low pH, low bicarbonate, sodium bicarbonate therapy, and hyponatremia may each be associated with cerebral edema. Although uncommon, cerebral edema can occur at presentation of DKA, but usually evolves 6–12 hours after initiation of insulin therapy.
- Have high suspicion, treat early.
- Symptoms: Decrease in mental status (this may wax and wane), headache (do not give acetaminophen or nonsteroidal anti-inflammatory drugs [NSAIDs] during DKA therapy, so as not to mask the headache). Unequal dilated pupil, delirium, incontinence, vomiting, and bradycardia.
- Diagnosis: Can usually be seen on computed tomography (CT) scan. If suspicious, treat, and then get CT scan.
- Treatment: (a) Mannitol: 1/2–1 g/kg IV. (b) Intensive care unit. (c) May require intubation and mechanical ventilation.

Converting to Subcutaneous Therapy (Most Easily Done at Breakfast or Dinner)

- Once bicarbonate is greater than 18 meq/L and DKA resolved, can switch to subcutaneous therapy.
- Have meal tray at bedside. Give subcutaneous insulin. Wait 30 minutes if regular insulin given and 5 minutes if humalog or novolog given. Turn off insulin drip and have patient start to eat. If patient tolerates meal without difficulty, turn off dextrose containing fluids 45 minutes later. In severe cases of dehydration, may need to continue IV fluids without dextrose at maintenance for an additional 12–24 hours.

HYPOGLYCEMIA

- A common side effect of insulin therapy. With repeated hypoglycemia, individuals may have hypoglycemia unawareness, and subsequently have severe episodes without prior symptoms.
- Symptoms: Pallor, diaphoresis, confusion, jitteriness, weakness, hunger, and seizure.
- Treatment:
  1. If conscious: Simple carbohydrate, i.e., juice, candy, and glucogel. Begin with one carbohydrate serving (15 g). May need more. Recheck glucose in 10–15 minutes.
  2. If unconscious: Glucagon injection subcutaneously (may cause nausea) or IV dextrose (0.5 g/kg slow IV infusion, repeat as necessary).
  3. With severe episodes: Patient may have some nausea. Confirm patient can tolerate PO intake prior to discharge. More frequent blood glucose monitoring will be needed for the next 24 hours. Look for precipitating event. May need to alter insulin therapy or nutritional intake in the next 24 hours.

ASSOCIATED AUTOIMMUNE DISEASE

- Hashimoto thyroiditis
- Celiac disease
- Adrenal insufficiency
- Every 3 years or as indicated check thyroid antibodies, adrenal antibodies, and celiac panel (transglutaminase or endomysial antibodies). If thyroid antibodies are positive, then check thyroid functions at least once a year.

DIABETES LONG-TERM COMPLICATIONS

- Retinopathy: Initial eye examination and then annual, after 5 years of diabetes. Individuals have been known to present with cataracts.
- Nephropathy: Spot microalbuminuria determination at least every year. If positive, then overnight collection for proteinuria. Ace inhibitors are being used to treat microalbuminuria. Hypertension should be assessed and treated if >90th percentile for age, gender, and height norms.
- Cardiovascular disease: Fasting lipids initially (after glucose control is stable) and then periodically as indicated. Diet intervention is mainstay of therapy.
- Neuropathy: Physical examination, delayed gastric emptying.

TYPE 2 DIABETES IN YOUTH

EPIDEMIOLOGY

- Prevalence in Pima Indians: 15–19-year-old males and females: 3.8 and 5.3%, respectively (Dabelea et al., 1998). Prevalence has increased over the past 30 years and is thought to be the result of increase in obesity and in utero diabetes exposure.
- Now type 2 diabetes accounts for 8–45% of new cases presenting to pediatric diabetes clinics (Fagot-Campagna et al., 2000).
- Common in Japan, where all school children are screened, increasing reports in Europe.
- Increased prevalence of type 2 diabetes has been temporally related to increase in overweight in America. Current prevalence of overweight reported at 15% by Third National Health and Nutrition Examination Survey (NHANES III) (Ogden et al., 2002), with higher prevalences (just under 30%) for African-American females and Hispanic males.
- Increased sedentary activity and decreased physical activity of youth also thought to contribute to increased insulin resistance.
- In the adult population, one-third of individuals with type 2 diabetes are undiagnosed. There have been no studies to date that show similar findings in youth.
- The prevalence of impaired glucose tolerance in the overweight pediatric population reported at 25% (Sinha et al., 2002).
- There appears to be a preponderance of adolescent females with type 2 diabetes (3:2).

PATHOPHYSIOLOGY

- Has not been elucidated in children specifically. In adults, type 2 diabetes refers to probably a group of disorders of carbohydrate metabolism that are associated with insulin resistance and impairment of insulin secretion. Either aspect may predominate.
- Because of dramatic increases in reporting of type 2 diabetes in youth over a short time span (15–20 years), factors, other than genetic, have been implicated in the rise in type 2 diabetes in youth. These may include increases in insulin resistance with overweight or lack of physical activity or changes in the intrauterine environment.

- Some evidence suggests that insulin secretion may be decreased in some individuals at high risk of developing type 2 diabetes (i.e., offspring of individuals with diabetes, individuals from specific ethnic groups)(Elbein et al., 2000; Arslanian, 2002; Goran et al., 2002). Whether there are other factors that are also leading to impaired insulin secretion in individuals is not clear.
- Impaired glucose tolerance may precede the development of type 2 diabetes, as it does in type 1 diabetes. But in this case, the fasting and stimulated insulin concentrations are elevated signifying the presence of compensated hyperinsulinism which is seen during insulin resistance. In type 2 diabetes there is a relative impairment of insulin secretion, and increased needs, secondary to insulin resistance cannot be met, resulting in hyperglycemia.

PRESENTATION

- Many youth with type 2 diabetes are asymptomatic. Females often will be diagnosed after presentation with monolial infection. Glycosuria without ketonuria.
- Acanthosis nigricans (AN) is a frequent physical finding in youth with type 2 diabetes, but not all youth with AN have type 2 diabetes.
- Others have mild symptoms including polyuria, polydipsia, unexplained weight loss, blurry vision, glycosuria, ± ketonuria, and hyperglycemia.
- Severe presentation of DKA (see above) or hyperglycemic hyperosmolar syndrome (HHS) (see below).

TREATMENT

- Currently treatment for insulin resistance and impaired glucose tolerance is limited to institution of lifestyle changes. No study has been done in youth to determine if oral medication delays the progression to diabetes. In the presence of impaired glucose tolerance (IGT) a repeat OGTT should be done in 1 year, unless symptoms warrant it being completed earlier.
- Most important, yet most difficult component, of treatment plan is institution of lifestyle changes (see below).
- If HgbA1c is >8%, despite lifestyle changes, then introduction of oral medication is reasonable.
- Treat with insulin initially if (1) any possibility individual has type 1 diabetes (overweight youth can have type 1 diabetes as well) and (2) if fasting glucose is over 250 mg/dL and/or postprandial glucose concentrations are greater than 300 mg/dL (secondary to glucose toxicity).

- Wean insulin once the goal of HgbA1c has been achieved and clinical picture is suggestive of type 2 diabetes.
- Ideal treatment goal is HgbA1c below 7%. Changes are made when HgbA1c is greater than 7–8%.

LIFESTYLE CHANGES
- Probably the most difficult, yet most important aspect of therapy: Nutrition and activity component.
- *Nutrition*: No specific diet given. Healthy food choices emphasized. Close interaction with nutritionist to educate whole family, especially individuals who do the shopping and cooking. Assist individuals with finding options. Works best when child and/or family are ready for change. Need to help family find barriers and prepare to bypass them.
- *Activity*: Two components: Decreasing sedentary activity and increasing physical activity. Again need to find barriers to physical activity and help families find ways to bypass them, i.e., financial resources, supervision after school, and transportation.

ORAL MEDICATION
- Metformin: Only Food and Drug Administration (FDA) approved medication for youth.
- Decreases hepatic gluconeogenesis. Possibly decreases insulin resistance (may be secondary effect).
- Therapeutic dose: 1000–2000 mg/day in two divided doses with meals. Start with 500 mg/day and increase by 500 mg/day.
- Gastrointestinal (GI) side effects (flatus, abdominal discomfort, and anorexia) frequent, improve with slow titration. Major side effect is lactic acidosis and potential for fatality.
- Contraindicated with renal or liver impairment or hypoxia.
- Hold with any vomiting illness or pneumonia till resolved.
- Also hold 72 hours prior to elective surgery or iodine containing dye study.

Sulfonylurea and Metiglinides
- Act on the KATP channel, keeping it closed, and therefore increasing insulin secretion. Metiglinides are glucose stimulated and given with each major meal.
- Side effects include hypoglycemia and hyperinsulinemia. Possibly some weight gain. Hypoglycemia may be less of an issue for metiglinides, given they work only with food intake.

Alpha Glucosidases
- Slow carbohydrate absorption.
- Ideal for youth with primarily postprandial hyperglycemia.

- Side effect of GI system, flatus and abdominal discomfort, may limit its use. Frequent dosing.

Thiozolidinediones (Glitazones)
- Act on peroxisome proliferator-activated receptor gamma (PPAR-gamma) receptor. Decrease insulin resistance.
- Side effects: Hepatic toxicity may be less common in newer glitazones. Previously troglitazone was removed from the market because of hepatic failure. Little experience with youth. Also causes weight gain.
- Insulin (See above)
- DKA (See above)

HYPERGLYCEMIC HYPEROSMOLAR SYNDROME (HHS)
- High morbidity and mortality in adults. Complications of HHS not well studied.
- Malignant hyperthermia-like syndrome with subsequent rhabdomyolysis has been reported with fatality in 4/6 subjects. Fever developed with administration of insulin therapy (Hollander et al., 2003).
- Often a precipitating factor is present, i.e., medication or infection. Consider further testing as appropriate.
- Usually more severe dehydration than in DKA, thought to develop over days to weeks. Most often individual has blunted response to thirst, i.e., emesis or limited access to water.
- Given dehydration, course may be complicated by morbidities associated with dehydration, i.e., thrombosis.

Definition
- Glucose ≥600 mg/dL
- pH ≥7.3, HCO_3^- ≥15 meq/L
- Dehydration in the absence of severe ketosis, serum osmolality ≥320 mOsm/kg

Treatment
- Similar to DKA. See above.

Screening
- Methods of screening and who to screen are not well established.
- The American Diabetes Association (ADA) recommends screening with a fasting blood glucose in all youth with a body mass index (BMI) >85th percentile and at least two risk factors for diabetes: (1) high risk race/ethnicity, (2) family history of type 2 diabetes, or (3) evidence of insulin resistance (i.e., hypertension, acanthosis nigricans, or polycystic ovarian syndrome).
- A normal fasting glucose does not eliminate a possible diagnosis of impaired glucose tolerance or diabetes.

COMPLICATIONS

Metabolic Syndrome
- Syndrome found in youth with insulin resistance, IGT, and diabetes.
- Definition in youth not established.
- In adults, based on presence of low high density lipoprotein (HDL), elevated triglycerides, hypertension, impaired fasting glucose or impaired glucose tolerance, and/or abdominal obesity (elevated waist circumference).
- May confer increased risk for cardiovascular disease and diabetes, if not already present.

Long-Term Complications
- Prevalence and severity of long-term complications not yet known in adolescents.
- Youth may already have dyslipidemia or hypertension at time of diagnosis.
- Monitor early signs of complications aggressively: at least annual assessments of dyslipidemia, retinopathy, and microalbuminuria.

OTHER TYPES OF DIABETES

MATURITY ONSET DIABETES OF YOUTH (MODY)

- Monogenic disorders: (a) Often present before 30–40 years of age in multiple generations. (b) At least six types of MODY. Except for MODY2, all involve mutations of transcription factors.
- MODY2: Glucokinase mutations, mild course. Commonly no medication required.
- MODY1: Hepatic nuclear factor 1 alpha. May require oral medications as well as insulin. Risk of traditional complications.

MEDICATION INDUCED

- Treat with insulin for persistent hyperglycemia with glycosuria.
- Usually resolves after medication is withdrawn, but not 100%.
- Consider obtaining diabetes autoimmune panel and fasting insulin or c-peptide to better investigate contributing factors to hyperglycemia.
- Implicated medications:
    1. L-Asparaginase: May cause problems with insulin production.
    2. Steroids: Increases hepatic gluconeogenesis and insulin resistance.
    3. Tacrolimus (FK-506): Leads to impaired insulin secretion and increased insulin resistance.

CYSTIC FIBROSIS-RELATED DIABETES (CFRD)

- Unique form of diabetes with features of both type 1 (i.e., impairment of insulin secretion) and type 2 diabetes (i.e., amyloid deposits).
- Increasing evidence supporting the association of glycemic control and pulmonary function.
- Some individuals require insulin only while on steroids. Others all the time.
- Basal-bolus is most effective given the need to encourage PO intake, yet also most labor and time intensive for individuals who are already on intensive pulmonary therapy.

NEONATAL

- Defined as persistent hyperglycemia during the first months of life lasting at least 2 weeks and requiring insulin therapy.
- Associated clinical features may include small-for-gestational age (SGA), failure to thrive, and dehydration from osmotic polyuria.
- Wolcott-Rallison syndrome in presence of epiphyseal dysplasia and renal impairment as well as the diabetes.
- Transient vs. Permanent: (a) One-third transient diabetes which resolves over several months, (b) one-fourth transient diabetes; however, the diabetes reoccurs 7–20 years later, and (c) just under half have a permanent form of diabetes.
- Treat with insulin as discussed in type 1 diabetes. Regular insulin may need to be diluted.

HYPOGLYCEMIA

DEFINITION

- Plasma glucose concentrations should be ≥60 mg/dL (for neonates, see below).
- Whole blood glucose concentrations are 10–15% lower than plasma.
- Any blood glucose concentration ≤50 mg/dL indicates need for evaluation of hypoglycemia, even if at time of illness and decreased food intake. Some glucose concentrations, 51–59 mg/dL may warrant further evaluation.

CLINICAL SIGNS OF HYPOGLYCEMIA

ADRENERGIC
- Sweating, shakiness, tachycardia, anxiety, weakness, hunger, nausea, and vomiting.

NEUROPENIC (DECREASED CEREBRAL GLUCOSE UTILIZATION)
- Headache, visual changes, lethargy, confusion, hypothermia, somnolence, twitching, seizures, unconsciousness, behavior changes, and psychologic changes.

PHYSIOLOGY

- As an infant/young child, endogenous glucose production matches glucose utilization needs of the brain. With increased muscle mass providing precursors for gluconeogenesis and increased hepatic and muscle glycogen stores, children have the ability to fast for longer periods of time as they grow.
- Basal glucose production: 2–3 mg/kg/minute in adults and 4–7 mg/kg/minute in neonates.
- Length of time a normal child can fast without developing hypoglycemia varies with age.
  1. 1 week old to 1 year old: 12–16 hours
  2. 1 year old: 24 hours
  3. 5 year old: 36 hours
  4. Teen/adult: 72 hours
- Glucose homeostasis is tightly controlled. The teleology includes prevention of damaging hypoglycemia, especially to developing brain.
- Insulin promotes lowering serum glucose concentrations and storage of fats.
  1. Insulin inhibits: Glycogenolysis, gluconeogenesis, lipolysis, and ketogenesis.
  2. Insulin stimulates: (a) Glycogenesis and (b) peripheral glucose uptake.
- Counterregulatory hormones promote increasing serum glucose and fatty acid concentrations.
  1. Cortisol stimulates hepatic gluconeogenesis.
  2. Growth hormone stimulates lipolysis.
  3. Glucagon stimulates hepatic glycogenolysis and ketogenesis.
  4. Epinephrine stimulates hepatic glycogenolysis, gluconeogenesis, lipolysis, and ketogenesis.
- The fed state
  1. Glucose absorption from the intestines (based primarily on carbohydrate intake and rate of gastric emptying).
  2. Glucose, gastric inhibitory polypeptide, and glucagon-like peptide.
     a. Stimulate insulin secretion.
     b. Inhibit glucagon release.
  3. Insulin secretion leads to
     a. Increased translocation of GLUT-4 transporters which, in turn, increase glucose uptake by muscle and fat.
     b. Inhibition of glycogenolysis and gluconeogenesis.
     c. Stimulation of glycogen synthesis and lipid synthesis.

- The fasting state:
  1. Glycogenolysis is stimulated and is the major source of glucose early in the fasting state.
  2. With further fasting, glycogen stores are depleted and gluconeogenesis accounts for more of the glucose needs. Main precursors for gluconeogenesis are alanine and glutamine, derived from muscle.
  3. With fasting, lipolysis occurs, leading to free fatty acid and glycerol production which are processed to ketone bodies and glucose.
  4. Ketone bodies serve as a source of energy for brain (which cannot use fatty acids) and for muscle, allowing for decreased glucose utilization by these tissues.
- Insulin secretion from the islet-cell (see Fig. 64-1):
  1. Increased glucose uptake, increased glucose conversion to glucose 6 phosphate by glucokinase.
  2. Glucose is oxidized and ATP is produced.
  3. Increased ATP/ADP ratio promotes closure of potassium channel.
  4. The K+-ATP channel is the main regulator of beta-cell insulin secretion: K+-ATP channel is encoded by the Kir6.2 gene and is regulated by the sulfonylurea receptor encoded by SUR1.

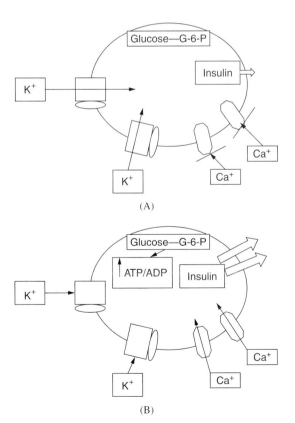

FIG. 64-1 Insulin secretion from the beta-cell. (A) Resting state. (B) Fed state.

5. Closing of the K+-ATP channel depolarizes the cell.
6. Leading to influx of calcium.
7. Resulting in insulin secretion (Fig. 64-1a and b).

DIAGNOSIS

- At time of hypoglycemia:
  1. Obtain critical sample
     a. First priority:
        1. Serum: Insulin, cortisol, growth hormone (GH), electrolytes, glucose, and c-peptide.
        2. Urine: Ketones
     b. Second priority:
        1. Serum: Beta-hydroxybutyrate, free fatty acids, amino acids, acyl-carnitine profile, quantitative carnitine, lactic acid, and pyruvic acid.
        2. Urine: Organic acids
  2. Perform glucagon stimulation test
     a. After obtaining diagnostic labs, but prior to giving dextrose containing fluids or PO foods.
     b. Obtain baseline accucheck (have baseline serum from above).
     c. Give glucagon 1 mg subcutaneously (if infant, 0.03 mg/kg).
     d. Check bedside glucose at 5, 10, 15, 20, and 30 minutes and growth hormone and lactate at 15 and 30 minutes.
     e. Attempt serum glucose at 20 minutes.
     f. Change in glucose concentration of over 30 mg/dL is suggestive of hyperinsulinemia.
     g. If blood glucose does not rise, give oral glucose such as juice or intravenous dextrose as discussed below, if needed.
- History of hypoglycemia
  1. If laboratory data are not available or not diagnostic from episode of hypoglycemia, hypoglycemia will need to be induced. This is done by performing a diagnostic fast. When hypoglycemia develops then laboratory and urine studies and glucagon stimulation test should be done as described above. Fasting a patient with fatty acid oxidation disorder can lead to fatalities. *Do not fast a child until preliminary tests for fatty acid oxidation disorders are normal (acylcarnitine profile and quantitative carnitine).*

ACUTE TREATMENT OF HYPOGLYCEMIA

- If conscious
  1. Give oral glucose, i.e., orange juice, glucose gel, or glucose tablets.
  2. Recheck glucose in 10–15 minutes and repeat oral glucose as needed.

- If not conscious
  1. Give intravenous dextrose.
  2. Dextrose 0.5 g/kg over 5 minutes.
  3. Start D_5 with lytes at maintenance.
  4. Recheck blood glucose in 10 minutes. Increase rate and dextrose concentration as needed to maintain euglycemia. ($D_{12.5}$ should be the most concentrated fluid given through a peripheral line).
  5. Give second bolus of dextrose if needed.
- In patients with hyperinsulinemia or diabetes, glucagon can be given to resolve hypoglycemia at dose of 1 mg subcutaneously (0.5 mg for neonates/infants). Nausea may result. Hypoglycemia itself may also lead to nausea and emesis. Note that glucagons will not increase glucose in hypoglycemia due to most other etiologies.

DIFFERENTIAL

- Non-ketotic hypoglycemia
  1. Hyperinsulinemia
  2. Fatty acid oxidation disorders (may be ketotic in short chain disorders)
- Ketotic hypoglycemia
  1. Hormonal deficiencies (panhypopituitarism, primary adrenal insufficiency)
  2. Benign ketotic hypoglycemia
  3. Glycogen storage diseases
  4. Abnormalities of gluconeogenesis
  5. Miscellaneous

NON-KETOTIC HYPOGLYCEMIA

HYPERINSULINEMIA

- Hyperinsulinemia is present in each of the following disorders. Diagnosis of hyperinsulinemia is made by
  1. Insulin concentration >2 uIU/mL at time of hypoglycemia.
  2. Glucagon stimulation test: Change in glucose >30 mg/dL.
  3. Low free fatty acids.
  4. Low serum beta–hydroxybutyrate.
- Further history, clinical symptoms, and laboratory tests can distinguish the following etiologies of hyperinsulinemia as described below.

CONGENITAL HYPERINSULINEMIA OF INFANCY

Pathophysiology

- Most common reason for hypoglycemia in newborn/infant time period.
- Genetic mutation(s) of the K+-ATP channel or of the sulfonylurea receptor which cause closing of the channel, depolarization, and therefore calcium influx and insulin secretion.

- Autosomal recessive:
  1. Inheritance of abnormal allele from mother and abnormal allele from father.
  2. Histopathology often consistent with diffuse islet-cell hyperplasia.
- Uniparental disomy (loss of maternal heterozygosity):
  1. Loss of maternal normal allele, maintain paternal abnormal allele.
  2. Histopathology often consistent with focal islet-cell hyperplasia.
- Autosomal dominant

Clinical Presentation

- May present in first couple of days of life or after several months, usually when time between feedings is lengthened.
- Presentation may range from mild hypoglycemia to seizures.
- Neonates are sometimes large for gestational age. May have the same appearance as infants of diabetic mothers.
- Infants are sometimes heavy for age because of frequent feeds to counteract hypoglycemia.

Diagnosis

- Hyperinsulinemia as discussed above.
- Genetic testing.
- Its advantageous to discern the focal form from the diffuse form, because partial pancreatic resection may be curative in the focal form.
- Clinically this remains difficult to do; see surgical section.
- Currently focal lesions have not been visualized by traditional imaging techniques.

Treatment
- **Medical:**
  1. Diazoxide
     a. Keeps K+-ATP channel open, therefore decreasing insulin secretion.
     b. Not always effective, especially if one of the gene(s) coding for the channel is mutated.
     c. May protect from hypoglycemia in milder forms.
     d. Therapeutic dose 8–15 mg/kg/day divided tid.
     e. Complications
        1. Hirsutism
        2. Cardiac failure, possibly causing sudden death in the past: (a) Insidious onset of fluid and sodium retention. (b) If high doses are to be used, consider diuretic.
  2. Octreotide
     a. Blocks calcium channel of the islet cells, blocking influx of calcium, and therefore decreasing insulin secretion.

b. Can be given as CSI with an insulin pump.
c. Can be given as injections q 4–6 hours.
  1. Start at 5–10 μg/kg/day
  2. Painful
  3. Causes transient hyperglycemia with each injection
3. CSI dose: Start at 5 μg/kg/day divided hourly: Even glucose regulation.
4. Complications
  a. Tachyphylaxis
  b. Transient diarrhea at onset of medication
  c. Theoretical decrease in growth hormone secretion
  d. Possible cholelithiasis or sludge
5. Calcium channel blockers: Theoretically should block calcium influx and then decrease insulin secretion; however, clinical application has been less successful than expected to date.
• Continuous feeds: Anecdotally, if optimal glucose regulation is not obtained with the above medications, continuous g-tube feeds are possible; however, if control is so poor that continuous feeds are required, may need to consider surgical intervention.
• Several of our patients have had poor feeding once diagnosed and treatment started. May be due to medications/hypoglycemia.
  1. Avoid nasogastric (NG) feeds when possible.
  2. Introduce speech therapy early.
• Surgical
  1. When medical treatment fails, surgical treatment is needed.
  2. Unfortunately to date, there is no easy way to distinguish focal from diffuse hyperinsulinemia of infancy.
  3. Arterial calcium stimulation, venous sampling, and intraoperative histopathology are being explored as ways to localize focal lesions, yet methods are difficult and not conclusive.
  4. Every effort should be made to locate a lesion intraoperatively based on gross appearance, palpation, and biopsy.
  5. If a focal lesion is suspected, a partial pancreatectomy can be curative and decrease the chances of diabetes developing in the future.
  6. If a diffuse lesion is suspected, a partial pancreatectomy may not be sufficient to prevent hypoglycemia.
  7. If near total pancreatectomy is performed, diabetes mellitus may develop postoperatively or in the future.
  8. If pancreatectomy has been performed and hypoglycemia persists, medical therapy with octreotide may provide sufficient glucose control without performing further pancreatic resection.

HYPERINSULINEMIA-HYPERAMMONEMIA SYNDROME

Pathophysiology
• Activating mutation of glutamate dehydrogenase.
• In the pancreas, glucose independent ATP formation, leading to increased insulin secretion.
• In the liver, increased ammonia production, but decreased urea production.

Clinical symptoms
• Mildly increased ammonia.
• Autosomal dominant or spontaneous mutation.
• Milder presentation, usually as infant or child.

Diagnosis
• Hyperinsulinemia
• Mildly elevated ammonia

Treatment
• Diazoxide often works well, since K+-ATP channel is intact.

INFANT OF DIABETIC MOTHER

Pathophysiology
• Hyperglycemia present in mother with diabetes.
• Fetal insulin overproduced in order to maintain euglycemia in fetus.
• After birth, hyperglycemia no longer present, but islet cells take longer to adjust to new milieu.
• Infant hyperinsulinemia may lead to hypoglycemia, without glucose that had previously been provided by mother.

Clinical symptoms
• Hypoglycemia as above, in addition to other features of infants of diabetic mothers, a few of which include the following:
  1. Large for gestational age
  2. Hypocalcemic
  3. Congenital anomalies
  4. Polycythemia

Diagnosis
• Maternal history of hyperglycemia/diabetes during pregnancy.

Treatment
• Supplemental intravenous dextrose.
• Wean dextrose as tolerated, slowly.

Beckwith Wiedemann
• Imprinting: Paternal duplication of region of chromosome 11p15. Paternal uniparental disomy.
• Hyperinsulinemia: (a) Usually self-limiting, but may be severe. (b) Treat as one would congenital hyperinsulinemia.
• Associated symptoms: (a) Omphalocoele, (b) muscular macroglossia, and (c) visceromegaly.

Transient Hyperinsulinemia
- Birth asphyxia/perinatal stress.

Factitious Hyperinsulinemia
- Exogenous administration of insulin: (a) C-peptide is low. (b) Insulin is elevated.
- Oral ingestion of sulfonylureas: (a) Insulin release is glucose dependent. (b) As glucose is given to correct hypoglycemia, hypoglycemia may actually worsen. (c) C-peptide and insulin are elevated.

ISLET-CELL TUMORS—RARE

Pathophysiology
- Islet cells secrete insulin unregulated.
- Usually progress in severity and frequency.

Clinical Symptoms
- Unexplained hypoglycemia.
- Rare, yet more likely in adolescents and adults.
- May be part of multiple endocrine neoplasia I.
  a. Hyperparathyroidism
  b. Pituitary tumors
  c. Pancreatic tumors

Diagnosis
- Once hyperinsulinemia is established as above.
- Locate pancreatic tumor:
  a. CT
  b. Magnetic resonance imaging (MRI)
  c. Endocscopic ultrasound

Treatment
- Surgical resection.

FATTY ACID OXIDATION DISORDERS AND CARNITINE METABOLISM DEFECTS

Pathophysiology
- Inability to process free fatty acids to ketone bodies and to ATP, H_2O, and CO_2.
- Usually affects short, middle (most commonly), or long chain fatty acids.

Clinical Symptoms
- Increased fatigue, encephalopathy with fasting.
- Absent or low ketone production.
- Has been associated with sudden death.
- More common than previously thought.
- Hypoglycemia
- Some types associated with cardiomyopathy, myopathy, neuropathy, Reye syndrome

Diagnosis
- Quantitative carnitine
- Abnormal acylcarnitine profile
- Urine organic acids

Treatment
- Depends on particular defect.

- Avoid prolonged fast.
- Provide exogenous carbohydrate to decrease need to process fatty acids and ketones for energy.
- *Uncooked cornstarch*: 1–2 g/kg/dose, suspended in cold sugar-containing fluid, may not be absorbed well in infant.
- *Carnitine* supplementation may be needed (100 mg/kg/day).

CONGENITAL DISORDERS OF GLYCOSYLATION
- Hypoglycemia, possibly from hyperinsulinemia.
- Associated with coagulopathy and liver dysfunction.
- Measure transferrin (detects underglycosylation).

KETOTIC HYPOGLYCEMIA

HORMONAL DEFICIENCIES

Pituitary Dysfunction
Pathophysiology
- Growth hormone and/or adrenocorticotropic hormone (ACTH) deficiency can contribute to hypoglycemia.
- Isolated hormone deficiency possible or multiple hormone deficiencies.
- Congenital hypopituitarism
  1. Genetic mutations (Pit1, PROP1, HESX1)
  2. Idiopathic
  3. Congenital infection
- Acquired hypopituitarism
  1. Infection
  2. Infiltrative disease
  3. Tumor
  4. Secondary to tumor resection

Clinical Symptoms
- Cortisol deficiency: Fatigue, hypothermia, hypotension, hypoglycemia, emesis, and hyponatremia.
- Growth hormone deficiency: Poor growth, hypoglycemia, increased abdominal adiposity, and high voice.
- Congenital (other pituitary dysfunction)
  1. Microphallus and undescended testes from decreased/absent luteinizing hormone (LH) secretion.
  2. Diabetes insipidus and absent posterior bright spot on MRI.
  3. Giant cell hepatitis
  4. Septo-optic dysplasia: Absent septum pellucidum, optic nerve hypoplasia.
- Acquired (symptoms of tumor or other pituitary dysfunction): Poor growth, headaches, delayed puberty, and diabetes insipidus.

Diagnosis
- Laboratory testing:
  1. Growth Hormone: (a) Neonate: Random growth hormone testing (b) Infants and children: Insulin-like

growth factor (IGF)-1, insulin-like growth factor binding protein (IGFBP)-3, consider GH stimulation testing.

2. Cortisol: (a) Neonate: Random cortisol testing. (b) Infants and children: First morning cortisol, ACTH stimulation test (give cortrosyn 0.25 µg/m^2 IV, check cortisol 0, 30, and 60 minutes later).

• MRI

Treatment

• Hormonal replacement: Growth hormone: If hypoglycemia exists: 0.3 mg/kg/week divided into seven daily doses.

• Cortisol:

1. Hydrocortisone: 8–12.5 mg/m^2/day divided into three daily doses.

2. Increased doses (stress doses) required when ill or stressed. A couple of examples follow: (a) With fever: 25–37.5 mg/m^2/day. (b) For surgery: 100 mg/m^2 × 1 on call to the OR. (c) For emesis: hydrocortisone should be given IM.

ISOLATED PRIMARY CORTISOL DEFICIENCY

Pathophysiology

• Abnormality of the adrenal glands.

• Neonatal: Adrenal hemorrhage, congenital adrenal hyperplasia.

• Acquired: Infection, hemorrhage, autoimmune.

Clinical Symptoms

• Hypoglycemia, hyponatremia as above.

• Bronzing of the skin from increased ACTH.

• Possibly evidence of mineralocorticoid deficiency (salt wasting).

• Salt cravings

• Hyponatremia and hyperkalemia

Diagnosis

• As listed above for cortisol.

• Ultrasound of adrenal glands.

• If suspicious for congenital adrenal hyperplasia (CAH): Obtain testosterone, 17-hydroxyprogesterone, and other intermediates as needed.

• For mineralocorticoid deficiency:

• Renin activity, aldosterone, electrolytes

Treatment

• Hydrocortisone, as above, may need higher dose in CAH.

• For mineralocorticoid: Florinef, free access to salt. For CAH, neonates may need additional salt supplements as well.

BENIGN KETOTIC HYPOGLYCEMIA

Pathophysiology

• Proposed etiology: Decreased alanine and therefore decreased substrate for gluconeogenesis, possibly due to epinephrine deficiency.

• Age range usually 18 months to 5–6 years.

• Most often presents during illness, at which time PO intake is decreased.

• Ketogenesis is accelerated.

• Rarely is associated with acidosis.

Clinical Symptoms

• Signs of hypoglycemia

• Signs of ketosis (i.e., sweetness to breath and ketonuria)

Diagnosis

• Diagnosis of exclusion.

Treatment

• Minimize length of fasting.

• Increased awareness during intercurrent illnesses (Fig. 64-2).

• Monitor ketonuria and capillary glucose.

GLYCOGEN STORAGE DISEASES

Glucose 6-Phosphatase Deficiency (Type I GSD)

Pathophysiology

• Last step of glycogenolysis and gluconeogenesis blocked: Glucose 6-P cannot be converted to glucose.

• Type 1A: 1:100,000; deficiency of glucose 6–phosphatase.

• Type 1B: Deficiency of translocase T1.

Clinical Symptoms

• Type 1A: Hepatomegaly, eruptive xanthomas, hyperuricemia, acidosis, hypertriglyceridemia, and growth failure.

• Type 1B: As in type 1A + oral lesions, neutrophil deficiency, perianal abscess, and enteritis.

Diagnosis

• Glucagon stimulation test in post-absorptive state: No increase in glucose production.

• Liver biopsy

Treatment

• Feedings every 2 hours with continuous feeds overnight.

• Uncooked cornstarch in some children.

DEBRANCHER DEFICIENCY (TYPE III GSD)

Pathophysiology

• Incomplete glycogenolysis, since glycogen cannot be degraded past 1:4/1:6 branch point.

• Gluconeogenesis persists without hinderance.

Clinical Symptoms

• Hepatomegaly, fasting hypoglycemia, ± muscle and leukocyte involvement.

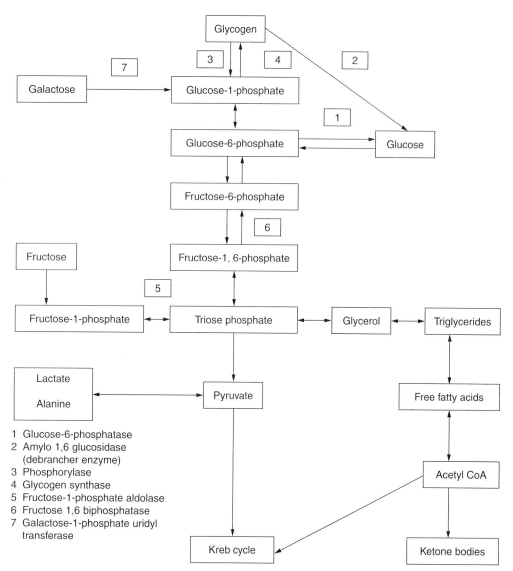

FIG. 64-2 Glucose metabolism.

Diagnosis
- Liver biopsy
- Glucagon response normal in fed state, diminished in fasting state.

Treatment
- Frequent feeds, uncooked cornstarch, avoid prolonged feeds.
- If muscle involved some advocate high protein, low carbohydrate meal.

LIVER PHOSPHORYLASE DEFICIENCY (TYPES VI, IX GSD)

Pathophysiology
- Incomplete glycogenolysis, since glycogen cannot be degraded properly.

Clinical Symptoms
- Hepatomegaly, excessive glycogen deposition in liver, growth retardation, occasional symptomatic hypoglycemia.

Diagnosis
- Liver biopsy

Treatment
- As in GSD III

GLYCOGEN SYNTHETASE DEFICIENCY

Pathophysiology
- Glycogen synthetase activity is low in liver, but normal in muscle.
- Inability to make glycogen in the liver.
- Extremely rare.

Clinical Symptoms
- Hypoglycemia and ketonemia with fasting
- Hyperglycemia and glycosuria after meals
- No hepatomegaly

Diagnosis
- Liver biopsy, genetics
- Glucagon response only shortly after meals.

Treatment
- Frequent protein-rich feedings possibly.

ABNORMALITIES OF GLUCONEOGENESIS

Hereditary Fructose Intolerance (Fructoaldolase Deficiency)
Pathophysiology
- Fructose is ingested, converted to fructose 1-phosphate (1-P).
- Fructose 1-P cannot be converted to glyceraldehyde, causing impaired processing of fructose to glucose.
- Creates build up of fructose-1-P.

Clinical Symptoms
- Begins with introduction of fructose into diet.
- Aversion to fructose often develops.
- Increased intake: Worse symptoms.
- Failure to thrive, renal and liver failure, vomiting, diarrhea, hypoglycemia, and shock.

Diagnosis
- Resolution of symptoms with avoidance of fructose.
- DNA mutational analysis.
- Treatment
- Avoidance

FRUCTOSE 1,6-DIPHOSPHATASE (FDPASE) DEFICIENCY

Pathophysiology
- FDPase is needed to convert fructose-1,6-P to fructose 6-P.
- Deficiency causes impairment of gluconeogenesis from alanine, glycerol, and lactate.

Clinical Symptoms
- Onset at birth or older.
- Hepatomegaly, hypoglycemia, lactic acidosis, and ketoacidosis.
- Worse with fasting and intercurrent illness.

Diagnosis
- Liver biopsy, enzyme studies.

Treatment
- Avoid prolonged fasting.
- Avoid fructose.

MISCELLANEOUS
- Respiratory chain defects.
- Glucose transporter disorders.
  1. Defect in blood-brain glucose transporter: GLUT-1.
  2. At normal plasma glucose, low cerebrospinal glucose concentrations.
  3. Seizure disorder, acquired microcephaly, and developmental delay.
  4. Treat with ketogenic diet.
- Galactosemia
  1. Urine: Positive for reducing substance, negative for glucose.
  2. Other symptoms may include *E. coli* sepsis, diarrhea, vomiting, cataracts, hepatomegaly, and mental retardation.
- Alcohol induced (rubbing alcohol, mouthwash intoxication, or ethanol)
  1. Impaired gluconeogenesis
- Salicylate intoxication
  2. Increased glucose utilization and possibly impaired gluconeogenesis
- Late dumping syndrome
- Sepsis

NEONATAL CONSIDERATIONS

- The lower limit of normal glucose concentrations is controversial.
- More frequent hypoglycemia has been reported in the first 24 hours of life
- Immaturity of enzymes can lead to impaired gluconeogenesis and ketogenesis, especially during the first 24 hours of life, leading to fasting hypoglycemia.
- Evaluation of hypoglycemia can lead to anemia. Commonly infants will require a transfusion if symptomatic anemia develops
- Neonates who are SGA are more likely to have hypoglycemia with fasting
- RH incompatibility and exchange transfusions can lead to hypoglycemia
- When hyperinsulinemia is diagnosed in the newborn, it may be transient (from factors discussed above) or permanent. If hypoglycemia persists after 5–7 days, further evaluation is needed; however, transient forms of hyperinsulinemia may persist after 7 days.

CARE OF CHILD WITH HYPOGLYCEMIA AND INTERCURRENT ILLNESS

- Minimize fasting.
- Frequent blood glucose monitoring where appropriate.

- Goal: Blood glucose concentrations over 60 mg/dL.
- Often will need hospitalization for dextrose containing fluids. Begin D_{10} with electrolytes at maintenance. Adjust dextrose and volume as needed.

PREPARATION OF CHILD WITH HYPOGLYCEMIA FOR SURGERY OR SEDATION

- When child is not able to take food or is not conscious of revealing symptoms of low blood glucose, hospitalization is appropriate.
- Monitor blood glucose frequently, i.e., every 2 hours.
- Provide supplemental intravenous dextrose while NPO and sedated.
- If child is on medications that cannot be given while NPO, i.e., diazoxide, increased IV dextrose may be needed.
- To avoid fluid overload, use most concentrated dextrose possible (no more than $D_{12.5}$ through peripheral line, rarely children will need central access for more concentrated dextrose).

REFERENCES

American Diabetes Association. *Diabetes Care* 2003;26: 3160–3167.

Arslanian SA. Metabolic differences between Caucasian and African-American children and the relationship to type 2 diabetes mellitus. *J Pediatr Endocrinol Metab* 2002;15(Suppl. 1): 509–517.

Bennett ST, Lucassen AM, Gough SC, et al. Susceptibility to Human type 1 diabetes at IDDM2 is determined by tandem repeat variation at the insulin gene minisatellite locus. *Nat Genet* 1995;9:284–292.

Chase HP, Cuthbertson DD, Dolan L, et al. First-phase insulin release during the intravenous glucose tolerance test as a risk factor for type 1 diabetes. *J Pediatr* 2001;138:244–249.

Dabelea D, Hanson RL, Bennett PH, et al. Increasing prevalence of type II diabetes in American Indian children. *Diabetologia* 1998;41:904–910.

Elbein SC, Wegner K, Kahn SE. Reduced beta-cell compensation to the insulin resistance associated with obesity in members of Caucasian familial type 2 diabetic kindreds. *Diabetes Care* 2000;23:221–227.

Fagot-Campagna A, Pettitt DJ, Engelgau MM, et al. Type 2 diabetes among North American children and adolescents: an epidemiologic review and a public health perspective. *J Pediatr* 2000;136:664–672.

Goran MI, Bergman RN, Cruz ML, et al. Insulin resistance and associated compensatory responses in African-American and Hispanic children. *Diabetes Care* 2002;25:2184–2190.

Hollander AS, Olney RC, Blackett PR, et al. Fatal malignant hyperthermia-like syndrome with rhabdomyolysis complicating the presentation of diabetes mellitus in adolescent males. *Pediatrics* 2003;111(6 Part 1):1447–1452.

LaPorte RE, Matsushim M, Chang YF. Prevalence and incidence of insulin-dependent diabetes. In: Harris MI, et al. (eds.), *Diabetes in America*, 2nd ed. National Diabetes Data Group, NIH, NIDDK, NIH Publication No. 95–1468, 1995, pp. 37–45.

Ogden CL, Flegal DM, Carroll MD, et al. Prevalence and trends in overweight among US children and adolescents, 1999–2000. *JAMA* 2002;288:1728–1732.

Sinha R, Fisch G, Teague B, et al. Prevalence of impaired glucose tolerance among children and adolescents with marked obesity. *N Engl J Med* 2002;346:802–810.

Verge CF, Gianani R, Kawasaki E, et al. Prediction of typed 1 diabetes in first-degree relatives using a combination of insulin, GAD, and ICA512abc/IA-2 autoantibodies. *Diabetes* 1996;45:926–933.

BIBLIOGRAPHY

Farrag HM, Cowett RM. Hypoglycemia in the newborn, including the infant of a diabetic mother. In: Lifshiz F (ed.), *Pediatric Endocrinology*, 4th ed. New York, NY: Marcel Dekker, 2003, pp. 541–574.

LeRoith D, Taylor SI, Olefsky JM (eds.), *Diabetes Mellitus: A Fundamental and Clinical Text.* New York, NY: Lippincott Williams & Wilkins, 2000. Also available at www.diabetes.org (the official site of American Diabetes Association). Congenital Hyperinsulinism: *http://www.chop.edu/consumer/jsp/division/generic.jsp?id=71057.* Pituitary Abnormalities: *www.magic-foundation.org*

Sperling MA (ed.), *Pediatric Endocrinology.* New York, NY: W.B. Saunders, 2002.

Stanley CA, Thornton PA, Finegold DN, Sperling MA. Hypoglycemia in neonates and infants. In: Sperling MA (ed.), *Pediatric Endocrinology*, 2nd ed. Philadelphia, PA: W.B. Saunders, 2002, pp. 135–159.

Stanley CA, Thornton PS, Ganguly A, et al. Preoperative evaluation of infants with focal or diffuse congenital hyperinsulinism by intravenous acute insulin response tests and selective pancreatic arterial calcium stimulation. *J Clin Endocrinol Metab* 2004;89(1):288–296.

Thornton PA, Finegold DN, Stanley CA, Sperling MA. Hypoglycemia in the infant and child. In: Sperling MA (ed.), *Pediatric Endocrinology*, 2nd ed. Philadelphia, PA: W.B. Saunders, 2002, pp. 367–384.

Wolsdorf JI, Weinstein DA. Hypoglycemia in children. In: Lifshiz F (ed.), *Pediatric Endocrinology*, 4th ed. New York, NY: Marcel Dekker, 2003, pp. 575–610.

65 GROWTH DISORDERS

Donald Zimmerman, Reema L. Habiby, and Wendy J. Brickman

- Childhood is a time marked by remarkable growth. Growth is common to all multicellular organisms and the outcome is determined by genetic, psychosocial, and economic factors. Despite this complexity, children grow in a remarkably predictable manner.
- Deviation from a normal growth pattern can be the first manifestation of a wide variety of disease processes. Therefore, frequent and accurate assessment of growth is extremely important for health professionals caring for children. Data should be recorded properly for the correct age and on the correct growth charts for sex and the proper equipment should be used. Infants <2 years of age should be measured lying down. When obtaining a standing height, it is best to use a wall-mounted stadiometer.
- Skeletal maturation can be evaluated by obtaining a bone age film (radiograph of left hand and wrist). This can be used to assess progression of ossification within the epiphyses.

NORMAL GROWTH

- Normal growth patterns can be categorized as occurring in three different phases: the *fetal phase*, the *phase of infancy and childhood*, and the *adolescent phase*.

FETAL PHASE

- Fetal growth is remarkably fast. At midgestation, a fetus grows an average of 2.5 cm per week. Though the endocrine system is critical for postnatal growth, normal intrauterine growth is largely independent of the fetal pituitary gland.
- The major influence on fetal growth is the capacity of the *uteroplacental unit* to supply oxygen and nutrients to the fetus. Any compromise of this function may affect fetal growth. This can include placental abnormalities such as abnormal implantation, vascular insufficiency, or infarction.
- Maternal influences such as malnutrition, hypertension, and drug ingestion (especially cocaine, alcohol, and tobacco) also affect fetal growth.
- The endocrine system is of secondary importance, but does play a role in fetal growth.

- The major endocrine regulator of growth is *insulin*. Infants born to diabetic mothers are generally born large for gestational age. In utero, these fetuses have higher insulin levels to accommodate the higher glucose milieu. Conversely, infants with the syndrome of Leprechaunism are lacking a functional insulin receptor. They are born with severe intrauterine growth retardation.
- Thyroid hormone and growth hormone (GH) do not play a significant role prenatally. Infants born with congenital hypothyroidism or growth hormone deficiency are generally of normal size.
- Local production of the insulin-like growth factors (IGF-I, IGF-II) also appears to be critical for normal intrauterine growth, at least in the mouse model. Mice with knockouts of the gene for IGF-I or IGF-II have birth weights that are 60% of normal.

PHASE OF INFANCY AND CHILDHOOD

- Postnatal growth is the result of the interaction of genetic makeup, nutritional factors, hormones, and psychosocial factors.
- The major endocrine regulators of growth in infancy and childhood are *thyroid hormone* and *GH*. Thyroid hormone appears to have a direct effect on epiphyseal cartilage as well as a permissive effect on growth hormone secretion.
- Growth hormone has multiple sites of action. In the bone, GH increases osteoclast differentiation and activity, increases osteoblast activity, and increases bone mass by endochondral bone formation. GH leads to linear growth by promoting epiphyseal growth and stimulating differentiation of prechondrocytes and local expression of IGF-I. In the muscle, GH increases amino acid transport, increases nitrogen retention, and increases lean tissue. In adipose tissue, GH increases lipolysis and decreases lipogenesis.
- Normal regulation of GH involves a complex interplay of hormones and feedback systems collectively called the GH/IGF-I axis.
- Molecules within this axis are growth hormone releasing hormone (GHRH), somatostatin, ghrelin, GH, growth hormone binding protein (GHBP), GH receptors, IGF-I, IGF binding proteins, and the IGF-I receptor.
- Metabolic signals such as exercise, sleep, and other neural signals stimulate the hypothalamus to secrete GHRH and somatostatin.
- GHRH and ghrelin stimulate and somatostatin inhibits GH secretion by the pituitary gland.
- When GH binds to the GH receptors, this stimulates production of IGF-I. As with GH, IGF-I is associated with binding proteins, which enhance or inhibit their bioactivity.

- Most IGF-I in the serum is bound to IGFBP-3. IGF-I binds to the IGF-I receptor where it stimulates amino acid uptake, protein synthesis, and cell growth.
- Growth in infancy is a transition time and correlation between birth height and adult height is poor. Approximately two-thirds of all children will cross growth centiles in the first 2 years of life. Growth rate in infancy is rapid (10–25 cm per year), then drops to 5–7 cm per year until puberty. *After 2–3 years of age, any deviation of height percentile upward or downward should alert the practitioner to a potential problem.*

ADOLESCENT PHASE

- This phase is characterized by the onset of puberty.
- Puberty is regulated by the hypothalamic-pituitary-gonadal axis.
- Gonadotropin releasing hormone (GnRH) is secreted in a pulsatile fashion from the hypothalamus. This stimulates secretion of luteinizing hormone (LH) and follicle-stimulating hormone (FSH) from the pituitary.
- LH and FSH stimulate gonadal production of the sex steroids estradiol and testosterone (as well as ovulation and spermatogenesis). These sex steroids produce the physical changes of puberty.
- During the pubertal growth spurt, growth reaches 6–11 cm per year in girls and 7–13 cm per year in boys. The pubertal growth spurt generally lasts about 2 years.

DISORDERS OF ABNORMAL GROWTH

- Growth disorders can be classified as *primary growth abnormalities*, where the underlying defect is intrinsic to the growth plate, and *secondary growth abnormalities*, in which poor growth results from chronic disease states or endocrine disorders. Overlap between categories can certainly occur. In primary growth disorders, the bone age is usually equal to the chronological age. In secondary growth disorders, the bone age is usually delayed when compared to the chronological age.

PRIMARY GROWTH DISORDERS

OSTEOCHONDRODYSPLASIAS
- Achondroplasia
- Hypochondroplasia

CHROMOSOMAL ABNORMALITIES
- Turner syndrome
- Down syndrome

INTRAUTERINE GROWTH RETARDATION
- Intrinsic to fetus—e.g., Russell-Silver Syndrome, Prader-Willi syndrome, Cockayne, Bloom, Seckel, Noonan, Progeria, Rubinstein-Taybi, congenital infections.
- Placental insufficiency.
- Maternal factors—malnutrition, vascular disorders, uterine malformations, drug ingestions.

GENETIC SHORT STATURE

SECONDARY GROWTH DISORDERS

- Malnutrition
- Cardiovascular disease
- Malabsorption
- Renal disease
- Hematologic disease
- Diabetes mellitus
- Pulmonary disease
- Inborn errors of metabolism

ENDOCRINE DISORDERS

HYPOTHYROIDISM

- In childhood, primary hypothyroidism is most commonly caused by Hashimoto's thyroiditis.
- *Clinical features*: Growth failure in childhood is a common manifestation and the growth failure can be severe. Other features: thyromegaly, weakness, lethargy, decreased appetite, constipation, cold intolerance, dry skin, mild obesity.
- *Diagnosis*: Low total or free T4 level, elevated thyroid stimulating hormone (TSH). Antithyroid antibodies present in the majority of children with Hashimoto's thyroiditis.
- *Treatment*: Replacement L-thyroxine.

CUSHING SYNDROME

- Glucocorticoid excess, regardless of the etiology, can lead to profound growth failure. This syndrome may result from glucocorticoid therapy, an adrenal tumor, or an adrenocorticotropic hormone (ACTH) secreting tumor.
- *Clinical features*: growth failure, truncal obesity, decreased muscle mass, striae, easy bruising, and osteoporosis.
- *Diagnosis*: Increased 24-hour urinary free cortisol, loss of normal diurnal cortisol variation (see adrenal chapter for further details regarding workup and treatment).

PSEUDOHYPOPARATHYROIDISM

- *Clinical features*: short stature, obesity, round facies, short metacarpals, subcutaneous calcifications, decreased mentation.
- *Diagnosis*: In the classic form, expect hypocalcemia, hyperphosphatemia, and elevated parathormone (PTH) level.

RICKETS

- Vitamin D deficiency is the most common cause of rickets.
- *Clinical features*: growth failure, bowing of the legs, frontal bossing, rachitic rosary, and craniotabes.
- *Diagnosis*: 25-OH Vit D low, 1,25-OH Vit D low, normal or high, PTH high, alkaline phosphatase elevated. On x-ray, cupped, widened, and frayed distal metaphyses.
- *Treatment*: Vitamin D replacement.

DISORDERS OF THE GH/IGF-I AXIS

HYPOTHALAMIC DYSFUNCTION

- *Causes*: Congenital malformations of the brain or hypothalamus (e.g., septo-optic dysplasia, holoprosencephaly), trauma, infections, sarcoidosis, tumors, cranial irradiation.
- *Clinical features*: short stature, decreased growth velocity, increased adiposity, frontal bossing, and high-pitched voice.
- *Diagnosis*: low IGF-I, IGFBP-3, delayed bone age, inadequate GH response to provocative stimulation, abnormal magnetic resonance imaging (MRI) with malformations, tumors, or infiltrative diseases.
- *Treatment*: growth hormone replacement therapy as well as replacement of any associated hormone deficiencies.
- *GHRH receptor defects*.
- *Pituitary dysfunction*: Can be difficult in many instances to differentiate between hypothalamic and pituitary dysfunction.
- *Causes*: Idiopathic GH deficiency, genetic defects (*Pit-1* gene), congenital absence or hypoplasia of the pituitary, tumors (craniopharyngioma, histiocytosis X).
- *Clinical features*: same as with hypothalamic dysfunction.
- *Diagnosis*: low IGF-I, IGFBP-3, delayed bone age, inadequate GH response to provocative stimulation, abnormal MRI with malformations, tumors, or infiltrative diseases.
- *Treatment*: GH replacement therapy.

GH INSENSITIVITY SYNDROMES

- *Causes*: can be primary, that is, because of GH receptor or postreceptor defects (Laron dwarfism), or secondary to acquired conditions (malnutrition, liver disease, GH receptor antibodies, circulating antibodies that inhibit GH).
- *Clinical features*: same phenotype as in GH deficiency.
- *Diagnosis*: low IGF-I, low IGFBP-3, normal or elevated GH level, most have decreased GHBP levels though a normal level does not exclude this disorder, delayed bone age.
- *Treatment*: IGF-1 has been used experimentally in patients with genetic GH receptor defects.

CONSTITUTIONAL DELAY OF GROWTH AND MATURITY

- *Clinical features*: A normal variant of growth with short stature but a relatively normal growth rate during childhood, delayed onset of puberty.
  1. Often a family history of delayed puberty.
  2. No evidence of systemic illness.
  3. Achieve a normal adult height.
- *Diagnosis*: Normal IGF-1, IGFBP-3, delayed bone age.
- *Treatment*: Observation, can consider short-term sex steroids.

GENERAL EVALUATION OF THE SHORT OR POORLY GROWING CHILD

CRITERIA FOR EVALUATION

- Severe short stature (height >−3 SD below mean).
- Moderate short stature (height −2 to −3 SD) and growth deceleration.
- Significant growth deceleration.
- Predisposing conditions and growth deceleration.

LABS/RADIOLOGIC STUDIES

- Chemistry panel
- Complete blood count (CBC)
- Thyroid function tests (T4 or free T4, TSH)
- IGF-I and IGFBP-3
- Bone age
- Consider chromosomes
- Consider provocative GH testing if low IGF-I, IGFBP-3
- MRI of the hypothalamus/pituitary if indicated

TALL STATURE

FETAL OVERGROWTH
- Infants of mothers with gestational diabetes.
- Cerebral gigantism (Soto syndrome): Above 90th percentile for height and weight at birth. Prominent forehead, dolicocephaly, macrocephaly, high arched palate, hypertelorism, unusual slant to eyes, prominent jaw, chin, and ears. Mental retardation and poor gross motor coordination.
- Beckwith-Wiedemann syndrome: fetal macrosomia with omphalocele. Organomegaly, macroglossia, neonatal hypoglycemia.

OVERGROWTH IN CHILDHOOD AND ADOLESCENCE
- Familial tall stature: In rare cases of excessive tall stature (predicted adult heights of greater than 6 ft 6 in. in males, greater than 6 ft in females), can consider high-dose estrogen in girls, androgens in males. The use of high-dose sex steroid therapy must be weighed against the known risks which include nausea, weight gain, edema, and hypertension. Thromboembolism, cystic hyperplasia of the breasts, endometrial hyperplasia, and cancer also potential risks.
- Exogenous obesity: rapid skeletal growth and early puberty.
- Precocious puberty (see chapter on Puberty)
- Hyperthyroidism
- GH excess: Very rare. Usually because of GH secreting pituitary adenomas. Rapid growth. Can also see soft tissue swelling, coarse facial features, large hands and feet, galactorrhea, menstrual irregularity.
- Marfan syndrome: Moderate tall stature, hyperextensible joints, dislocation of the lens, arachnodactyly, abnormally long arms and legs, dissecting aortic aneurysm, kyphoscoliosis.
- Homocystinuria

BIBLIOGRAPHY

Gharib H, Cook DM, Saenger PH, Bengtsson BA, et al. American Association of Clinical Endocrinologists medical guidelines for clinical practice for growth hormone use in adults and children—2003 update. *Endocr Pract* 2003;9:64–76.

Pandian R, Nakamoto JM. Rational use of the laboratory for childhood and adult growth hormone deficiency. Clin Lab Med 2004;24:141–174.

Reiter EO, Rosenfeld RG. Normal and aberrant growth. In Larsen PR, Kronenberg HM, Melmed S, Colonsky KS. *Williams Textbook of Endocrinology*, 10th ed. Philadelphia: W.B. Saunders; 2003:1003–1079.

66 THYROID DISEASES

Donald Zimmerman, Reema L. Habiby, and Wendy J. Brickman

EMBRYOLOGY OF THE THYROID GLAND

- The thyroid may be first identified in the 17-day embryo. The main portion of this gland arises as a thickening in the epithelium of the anterior pharyngeal floor. This thickening is between brachial arches 1 and 2. It begins on the 10th day of embryonic life. By the 20th day of embryonic life this median anlage of the thyroid begins caudal migration from its position immediately behind the tongue to a final position in the lower part of the anterior neck. The gland descends along a duct which maintains its connection to the pharynx (the thyroglossal duct). Early in the 7th week of gestation the lateral anlage of the thyroid develop as derivatives of the neural crest. They form ultimobranchial bodies as caudal projections from the fourth or fifth pharyngeal pouches. By approximately the 50th day of gestation the thyroid gland reaches its final location low in the neck. By the 8th week of gestation the lateral anlagen fuse with the median anlage. Following completion of migration and fusion of the components of the thyroid, the thyroid follicular cells express genes needed for thyroid hormone synthesis. These genes include genes for the thyroid stimulating hormone (TSH) receptor, the sodium-iodide symporter, thyroperoxidase, thyroglobulin, and thyroid oxidase. Thyroid hormone receptors are detectable in the brain by approximately the 10th week of gestation, and by the 11th week thyroid hormone is detectable.
- The hypothalamus produces thyrotropin releasing hormone by 9 weeks of gestation and the pituitary is able to make thyroid stimulating hormone by the 13th week of gestation.
- A number of transcription factors are known to be involved in the development of the thyroid gland. These transcription factors include the paired box transcription factor PAX8. Other transcription factors that play a role include thyroid transcription factor 1, a homeobox domain transcription factor of the NKX2 family and thyroid transcription factor 2, a forkhead/winged-helix domain transcription factor.
- The mature thyroid gland is directed by the hypothalamus and pituitary. Hypothalamic thyrotropin releasing hormone is stimulated by pituitary secretion of thyroid stimulating hormone. Thyroid stimulating

hormone acts on thyroid cells to activate thyroid hormone and thyroid hormone synthesis and secretion. Thyroid stimulating hormone also triggers production of growth factors within the thyroid leading to growth of the thyroid gland.

- While thyroid hormone is detectable in fetal blood between 10 and 11 weeks of age, the pituitary gland only produces TSH by 13 weeks of gestation, and TSH is measurable in the fetal serum by this time. There is substantial increase in both TSH and thyroxine beginning at approximately 18 weeks of gestation, while fetal levels of triidothyronine or T3 are quite low until a slow rise in circulating levels begins at 30 weeks gestation. A robust elevation of TSH occurs at birth, largely in response to exposure of the newborn to ambient temperatures lower than the maternal body temperature. Thus, TSH peaks at approximately half hour of life at approximately 70 uIU/mL. T4 and T3 peak at 24–36 hours of life and are still higher at 1 week of age than at 1 month of age. This rapidly changing system must be assessed using normal values for the precise postnatal age. It is noteworthy that premature infants have thyroxine and triidothyronine levels considerably lower than levels found in full-term infants. Thyroid stimulating hormone levels are likewise lower in premature infants.

CONGENITAL HYPOTHYROIDISM

- Congenital hypothyroidism occurs in 1 in 4000 to 1 in 3000 newborns and is more common in Hispanics than in Caucasians. It is also more common in Caucasians than in African-Americans. These prevalences are predicated on iodine sufficiency, since the incidence of congenital hypothyroidism is much higher in iodine-deficient areas. Approximately 85–90% of congenitally hypothyroid infants have thyroid dysgenesis (*athyrosis*, ectopia, or hypogenesis). Approximately 10% of congenitally hypothyroid infants have a defect in one of the steps of thyroid hormone synthesis and may develop goitrous hypothyroidism if untreated. Approximately 5% of congenitally hypothyroid infants have deficiency in pituitary TSH secretion as the cause for their hypothyroidism. Finally, perhaps as many as 10% of infants initially thought to have congenital hypothyroidism have a transient condition which may be due to transport of maternal medicines or antibodies across the placenta. Heterozygotes for one of the steps in thyroid hormone synthesis, generation of hydrogen peroxide through one of the nicotinamide adenine dinucleotide phosphate (NADPH) oxidases, THOX2, may also have transient hypothyroidism.

- *Diagnosis*: Most industrial countries have mandatory screening for congenital hypothyroidism. There is a substantial frequency of false positive results, especially in light of early hospital discharge after birth prompting obtaining blood specimens in the midst of the postnatal TSH surge. Confirmation studies should include free thyroxine and TSH measurements. Further delineation of the cause of primary hypothyroidism with ultrasound studies, thyroid scintigraphy, and measurements of thyroglobulin are carried out in some programs and not in others.

- *Treatment*: Treatment should be initiated as soon as possible in order to optimize the prognosis for normal psychomotor development. L-Thyroxine doses should begin at 10–15 µg/kg/day. Initially, serum levels of free thyroxine and TSH should be measured within approximately 1 week. If levels are not normalizing, additional studies should be performed at 14 and 28 days of therapy. It is important to note that TSH values may continue to be high in a significant fraction of congenitally hypothyroid infants despite ample levels of free thyroxine. Thus, sufficient thyroxine treatment should be given to produce L-thyroxine levels in the normal range. If levels of TSH are elevated, a higher dose of L-thyroxine may be given with the caveat that circulating free thyroxine should not be boosted above the upper limit of normal for age to suppress TSH to the normal range. If free thyroxine levels are at the upper part of the normal range, then the L-thyroxine dose should not be boosted further to normalize thyroid stimulating hormone levels.

- The patients should be tested at monthly intervals the first 6 months and at 3 monthly intervals to age 2 years. Soybean formula, iron, and calcium-containing medications may interfere with L-thyroxine absorption and may account for the apparent need for high doses of L-thyroxine. Since the infant brain depends on adequate amounts of thyroid hormone for its development, a conservative approach to treating infants who may have transient hypothyroidism (for example, due to transplacental passage of maternal antibody or drugs) is to continue this treatment until 2 years of age at which time free T4 and TSH are measured following 6 weeks off thyroid hormone treatment.

ACQUIRED HYPOTHYROIDISM

- Acquired hypothyroidism in children and adolescents is most commonly the result of chronic lymphocytic thyroiditis (Hashimoto thyroiditis). Less frequently, medications such as lithium, amiodarone, high doses of iodine, and phenytoin may produce hypothyroidism. Some congenital defects in thyroid hormone synthesis may produce acquired rather than congenital hypothyroidism. One such form is Pendred syndrome which also includes sensorineural hearing loss. The other major cause of hypothyroidism is deficiency of TSH secretion due to disease of the hypothalamus and pituitary.

- *Diagnosis*: The symptoms which suggest hypothyroidism include poor growth, dry hair and skin, decreased energy, cold intolerance, constipation, and abnormalities in the reproductive system which may include precocious puberty in younger children and menorrhagia in postmenarcheal adolescent females.
- *Laboratory diagnosis*: Under most circumstances, measurement of free thyroxine is more informative than is measurement of total thyroxine. Measurement of free thyroxine comprises measurement of the biologically active component of circulating thyroid hormone. When free thyroxine levels are low and thyroid stimulating hormone levels are elevated, hypothyroidism is due to primary thyroid disease. When free thyroxine is low in association with low levels of thyroid stimulating hormone, then the pituitary gland is undersecreting thyroid stimulating hormone and thereby producing hypothyroidism. When hypothyroidism results from primary thyroid failure, thyroid antibodies should be measured in order to determine whether hypothyroidism is a result of thyroiditis. If TSH levels are nonelevated in association with low free thyroxine levels, then other pituitary axes should be studied and magnetic resonance (MR) scanning of the pituitary and hypothalamus should be pursued.
- *Treatment*: Patients with severe and prolonged hypothyroidism should be treated with small doses of L-thyroxine beginning with approximately 25 µg/m²/day. The dose should be gradually increased over months to the dose of approximately 100 µg/m²/day. The dose of L-thyroxine should be adjusted in accordance with circulating levels of free thyroxine and circulating levels of TSH. Both L-thyroxine and TSH levels should be brought into the normal range. Since, in older children, adolescents, and adults the half-life of L-thyroxine is 1 week, the level of L-thyroxine and TSH should be determined after at least 5 half-lives of L-thyroxine (5–6 weeks).
- A number of problems may occur in the midst of L-thyroxine treatment of hypothyroidism. Patients may be made hyperthyroid. Additionally, some individuals who have prolonged and severe hypothyroidism and are treated with L-thyroxine develop pseudotumor cerebri associated with headache and visual blurring. Other potentially alarming effects of L-thyroxine treatment include desquamation of skin—particularly around fingernails. In addition, patients may experience myalgia. Another quite common

effect of L-thyroxine treatment is hair loss caused by telogen effluvium. Finally, L-thyroxine treatment may be associated with attention deficit and school problems. Reexamination of thyroid function should be repeated at approximately 6-month intervals once hypothyroid individuals are rendered euthyroid.

HYPERTHYROIDISM

- *Etiology*: The most common cause for hyperthyroidism in children is Graves disease. This condition results from autoimmune thyroid disease in which patients produce stimulatory antibodies directed against the thyroid stimulating hormone receptor. Patients with thyroiditis may experience sufficient inflammation to disrupt the integrity of the thyroid follicle causing the contents of the follicle (thyroid hormones and thyroglobulin) to be released into the circulation. This mechanism may occur in patients with subacute lymphocytic thyroiditis (silent thyroiditis), patients with tender granulomatous thyroiditis (deQuervain's thyroiditis), or suppurative thyroiditis. The latter is associated with marked erythema overlying the thyroid gland and with fever. These forms of thyroiditis may be associated with a hyperthyroid phase lasting for weeks to months. Subsequently there is a hypothyroid phase lasting 2–7 months. Thereafter, patients tend to be euthyroid. A third cause of hyperthyroidism in children is autonomously active thyroid adenomas. Finally, hyperthyroidism may be caused by thyroid hyperstimulation by thyroid stimulating hormone. This may be caused by a thyroid stimulating hormone secreting pituitary tumor or by central insensitivity to thyroid hormone causing the hypothalamus and pituitary to hypersecrete TSH in the absence of a pituitary tumor.
- *Diagnosis*: The symptoms of hyperthyroidism include heat intolerance, palpitations, tremor, insomnia and restless sleep, attention deficit and school difficulty, irritability, hyperdefecation, scant menses in postmenarcheal females, hair loss, polyuria and polydipsia, and muscle weakness. If the thyroid gland is quite large, there may be difficulty with swallowing and breathing. All patients with hyperthyroidism may have lid lag and globe lag on examination of the eyes. Patients with Graves disease may have exophthalmos which may be complicated by extraocular movement restriction, periorbital edema, and optic nerve dysfunction.
- *Laboratory evaluation*: This includes measurement of free thyroxine which is typically increased in hyperthyroidism. Some patients with autonomously overactive thyroid adenoma have normal free thyroxine

levels but elevated triidothyronine levels. In patients with Graves disease or thyroid adenomas or thyroiditis, the elevated thyroid hormone levels are accompanied by suppressed levels of thyroid stimulating hormone. When thyroid stimulating hormone levels are not suppressed in association with elevated circulating levels thyroid hormone, pituitary and/or hypothalamic hypersecretion is suspected. In order to establish the diagnosis of Graves disease, thyroid stimulating immunoglobulins are measured and should be elevated. Thyroidal radioiodine uptake tends to be markedly increased in Graves disease but decreased in subacute thyroiditis associated with hyperthyroidism. Thyroid scans of patients with autonomous reactive thyroid nodules show marked radioiodine uptake over the nodule with little radioiodine uptake in the remainder of the thyroid gland. Patients with subacute thyroiditis may have mild elevations of thyroid antibodies. In these patients thyroid stimulating immunoglobulins are typically absent and radioiodine uptake is suppressed.

- *Treatment*: The treatment of Graves disease continues to comprise one of three modalities. The first modality is antithyroid drugs (thionamides). These medications inhibit synthesis of thyroid hormone at the level of activities of the peroxidase enzyme. Thus, attachment of iodine to tyrosine molecules and coupling of tyrosine molecules within thyroglobulin are inhibited. Thyroid hormone secretion, however, is not decreased. Thus, many weeks may pass before propylthiouracil or methimazole are able to normalize thyroid hormone levels. The main advantage of the use of these thyroid medicines is that permanent ablative treatments of the thyroid gland are avoided. This is particularly salutary since the immune stimulation of the thyroid may be transient. Approximately 50% of children go into remission from Graves disease after 4 years. Those individuals who remit are able to enjoy normal thyroid function at least for a period of time. Thioamide drugs, however, may produce side effects such as skin rash, liver dysfunction, granulocytopenia, or arthritis. Prolonged follow-up of thionamide-treated patients has revealed an excess of deaths due to mouth and brain cancers. Propylthiouracil is used in a dose of 5–10 mg/kg/day while methimazole is used in doses of 0.5–1 mg/kg/day. Symptomatic relief may be achieved with concomitant use of propranolol. This may be particularly useful since the onset of action of antithyroid drugs may be delayed for 5–6 weeks.
- Patients with very large thyroid glands or those with extremely severe hyperthyroidism may benefit from the more prompt relief afforded by thyroidectomy. Thyroidectomy, however, may produce hypoparathyroidism and/or disruption of the recurrent laryngeal nerve with resulting vocal cord dysfunction. Finally, Graves disease may be treated with 131-iodine. Typically, this is given in a dose of 150–250 μCi/g of thyroid tissue corrected for radioiodine uptake. The advantage of radioiodine treatment is that it comprises nearly a "magic bullet". No other tissue does both: take up radioiodine and store it. On the other hand, radioiodine may over the long term predispose to thyroid carcinoma and may produce salivary gland dysfunction.
- Patients with subacute thyroiditis typically may respond to beta-adrenergic blockers since the hyperthyroidism is not as severe as that of Graves disease and since the hyperthyroidism is transient. Patients with autonomous hyperfunctioning thyroid nodules are best treated in childhood with surgical resection of the thyroid nodules.
- *Congenital hyperthyroidism*: Congenital hyperthyroidism is most commonly caused by neonatal Graves disease. This condition has been estimated to occur in 1 of 70 cases in which the mother has thyrotoxicosis. Mothers who have had Graves disease but have ablative treatments may still produce antibodies that can be transported across the placenta to the infant.
- Neonatal Graves disease may produce tachycardia, poor weight gain, thyromegaly, hepatosplenomegaly with jaundice and hypoprothrombinemia, and craniosynostosis. Neonatal Graves disease may last only a few weeks but could last many months.
- Treatment of neonatal Graves disease comprises iodide such as Lugol's solution or supersaturated potassium iodine, methimazole, or propylthiouracil in the usual dose, propranolol 1–2 mg/kg/day, and potentially sodium ipodate 100 mg/day or 0.3–0.5 g over 2–3 days. Less frequently hyperthyroidism is due to activating mutations of the thyroid stimulating hormone receptor. Antithyroid drugs may be used for transient control. Total thyroidectomy is a more definitive treatment. Patients with TSH-secreting pituitary tumors should undergo transsphenoidal surgery for removal of the tumor. At times, radiotherapy is needed as an adjunctive treatment.

NODULAR THYROID DISEASE

- When patients present with thyroid nodules and are euthyroid, the major concern is the possibility that such patients might have thyroid cancer. A number of studies have been recommended to distinguish benign from malignant thyroid nodules. These include nuclide scanning (*cold* nodules are more likely to be malignant than warm nodules). Additionally, ultrasound may help delineate nodules that are strictly cystic and which are therefore very unlikely to be malignant. Generally, determination of the status of the thyroid nodule is best accomplished by either fine needle aspiration or surgical resection of the nodule.

- Thyroid cancers may have a number of morphologies. The most common thyroid cancer is papillary thyroid cancer which tends to be unencapsulated and to spread through the lymphangitic route. Papillary thyroid cancers are not infrequently multifocal and bilateral. Follicular thyroid cancers tend to be somewhat more aggressive than are papillary cancers and tend to spread by the hematogenous route. They are commonly encapsulated and are overwhelmingly unifocal. Medullary thyroid cancers in childhood and adolescence tend to occur in the setting of multiple endocrine neoplasia, type 2. In this setting, the tumors are bilateral and multifocal.
- Treatment of thyroid cancer comprises total thyroidectomy. Patients who are at risk of distant metastases should undergo ablation of the normal thyroid remnant with radioactive iodine. Patients with papillary carcinoma and follicular carcinoma may have distant metastases which are often treatable with radioactive iodine as well.

GENERALIZED THYROID HORMONE RESISTANCE

- Patients with this condition present with thyromegaly as well as elevated levels of total and free thyroxine and triiodothyronine. Thyroid stimulating hormone levels are non-suppressed. Some patients have tachycardia, tremor, anxiety and hyperactivity. This condition is caused by mutations in the DNA binding portion of the beta thyroid hormone receptor. Those patients with tachycardia and/or hyperactivity may benefit from treatment with beta blockers such as propranolol.

BIBLIOGRAPHY

Foley TP Jr. Hypothyroidism. *Ped Rev* 2004;25:94–100.

Glaser NS, Styne DM. Predictors of early remission of hyperthyroidism in children. *J Clin Endocrinol Metab* 1997;82: 1719–1726.

Kopp P. Perspective: genetic defects in the etiology of congenital hypothyroidism. *Endocrinol* 2002;143:209–224.

Ron E, Doody MM, Becker DV, Brill AB et al. Cancer mortality following treatment for adult hyperthyroidism. Cooperative thyrotoxicosis therapy follow-up study group. *JAMA* 1998;280: 347–355.

Zimmerman D. Fetal and neonatal hyperthyroidism. *Thyroid* 1999;9:727–733.

Zimmerman D, Lteif AN. Thyrotoxicosis in children. *Endocrinol Metab Clin North Am* 1998;21:109–126.

67 ADRENAL DISEASE AND ADRENAL STEROID USE

Donald Zimmerman, Reema L. Habiby, and Wendy J. Brickman

PHYSIOLOGY

- The adrenal is made up of two parts, the cortex and the medulla. The adrenal cortex has three distinct zones: the zona glomerulosa, responsible for the production of mineralocorticoids; the zona fasciculata and the zona reticularis, responsible for the production of glucocorticoids; and adrenal androgens. The adrenal cortex forms very early embryologically and is actively secreting steroids by 6 weeks' gestation. The fetal adrenal cortex arises from mesodermal cells migrating from the coelomic epithelium. The permanent adult cortex arises from a second migration of cells which forms a rim around the fetal cortex. The permanent adult cortex becomes active after the fetal cortex involutes in the neonatal period. The adrenal medulla secretes catecholamines.
- Cholesterol is the precursor of all steroid production. A simplified scheme of the steroid biosynthetic pathway is shown in Fig. 67-1. A series of cytochrome P450 enzymes are required for conversion of cholesterol to the various steroid hormones. The pituitary gland regulates adrenal steroidogenesis through adrenocorticotropic hormone (ACTH). Circulating cortisol levels exert negative feedback on ACTH secretion. Corticotropin releasing hormone (CRH) regulates ACTH secretion. Plasma cortisol levels are highest in the early morning (between 4 and 6 a.m.) and are the lowest in the evening and during the night.
- Aldosterone secretion is regulated by the renin angiotensin system.

DISORDERS OF PRIMARY ADRENOCORTICAL INSUFFICIENCY

CONGENITAL

CONGENITAL ADRENAL HYPERPLASIA (CAH)

- A class of inherited disorders of adrenal steroidogenesis. Each form of CAH results from deficiency of one of the enzymes involved in production of adrenal steroids (see Fig. 67-1). When an enzyme deficiency is present, there is an accumulation of steroid precursors behind the blockage. Because there is insufficient

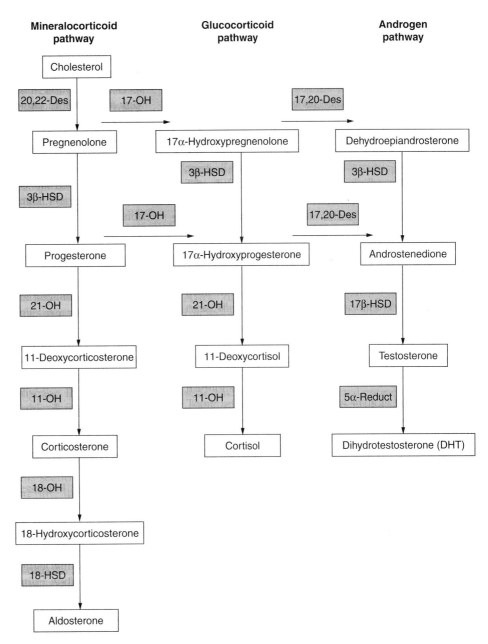

FIG. 67-1 A simplified scheme of the steroid biosynthetic pathway.

production of cortisol, ACTH secretion increases. This leads to hyperplasia of the adrenal gland and stimulates overproduction of the adrenal steroid hormones that are unimpaired by the enzyme deficiency.

21-Hydroxylase Deficiency
• The most common form of CAH. Classic and nonclassic phenotypes.
• *Classic CAH*: Inherited as autosomal recessive condition. Deletions or smaller mutations in CYP21 gene (gene encoding cytochrome P450 enzyme specific for 21-hydroxylation, chromosome 6).

• *Disease frequency*: 1/15,000 to 1/12,000
• *Clinical features*: Prenatal virilization in females and postnatal virilization in males and females. Genital ambiguity in girls results from exposure to excessive adrenal androgens during differentiation of the external genitalia (8–12 weeks gestation).
• The genital ambiguity ranges to mild virilization (e.g., clitoromegaly) to complete virilization with a penile urethra.
• Internal structures (uterus, fallopian tubes, ovaries) unaffected.
• Boys do not show genital abnormalities at birth.

- Postnatally, if untreated, males and females will have clitoral or penile enlargement, pubic, axillary, facial hair, acne, rapid linear growth, and advanced skeletal maturation.
- In 75%, salt wasting occurs. Early, life-threatening, salt-wasting crisis with hyponatremia, hyperkalemia, and shock. In 25%, adrenal crisis does not occur, and the phenotype is "simple virilizing."
- *Diagnosis*: Elevated 17-hydroxyprogesterone level (17-OHP). Low aldosterone, elevated renin in salt-wasting form. Newborn screening with filter paper measurement of 17-OHP performed in several states.
- *Treatment*: Correction of shock with isotonic fluids (0.9 NS or D5 0.9 NS), glucocorticoids (hydrocortisone) as well as mineralocorticoids (9α-fluorohydrocortisone) replacement for salt-wasting form.
- *Nonclassic CAH*: Same inheritance pattern.
- *Disease frequency*: Heterogeneous New York population 1/100. Among Ashkenazic Jews 1/27.
- *Clinical features*: Variable, can present at any age. Premature adrenarche, accelerated linear growth, advanced skeletal maturation in children. In women, irregular menses, hirsutism, acne, and polycystic ovary syndrome (PCOS). Reduced fertility, short stature in adult men and women.
- *Diagnosis*: Measurement of 17-OHP before and 60 minutes after synthetic ACTH administration. Usually have intermediate baseline levels and elevated stimulated values.
- *Treatment*: Glucocorticoids. Can give dexamethasone 0.25 mg at bedtime in adults (Table 67-1).

X-LINKED ADRENAL HYPOPLASIA CONGENITA

- Occurs due to defects in the *DAX-1* gene (dosage-sensitive sex reversal critical region on the X chromosome, gene 1). It can occur as part of a contiguous gene deletion syndrome with Duchenne muscular dystrophy and glycerol kinase deficiency.

- *Clinical features*: Generally severe salt wasting in the neonatal period, hyponatremia, hyperkalemia, hypoglycemia; dehydration, and shock. In some cases, adrenal insufficiency may not present until later in childhood. Associated with hypogonadotropic hypogonadism; may have microphallus or cryptorchidism.
- *Diagnosis*: Absent steroid hormone elevations characteristic of congenital adrenal hyperplasia, abnormal *DAX-1* gene.
- *Treatment*: Glucocorticoid and mineralocorticoid replacement.

AUTOSOMAL RECESSIVE ADRENAL HYPOPLASIA CONGENITA

- Also presents with salt wasting in the newborn period, associated with cerebral malformations.

ACTH UNRESPONSIVENESS

- Due to defects in the ACTH receptor.
- *Clinical features*: Symptoms of adrenal insufficiency, without symptoms mineralocorticoid deficiency. May have recurring episodes of hypoglycemia or seizures caused by unrecognized hypoglycemia. Marked skin hyperpigmentation caused by very high ACTH levels.
- When associated with achalasia and alacrima, referred to as the triple A or Allgrove syndrome.
- *Diagnosis*: Very low plasma cortisol levels, extremely elevated ACTH levels.
- *Treatment*: Glucocorticoid replacement.

ALDOSTERONE DEFICIENCY

- Usually due to impaired conversion of 18-hydroxycorticosterone to aldosterone.
- *Clinical features*: Hyponatremia, hyperkalemia, metabolic acidosis.
- *Diagnosis*: Low aldosterone level, markedly elevated renin.
- *Treatment*: Mineralocorticoid replacement.

TABLE 67-1   Other Forms of CAH

DEFICIENCY	SYNDROME	AMBIGUOUS GENITALIA	POSTNATAL VIRILZATION	SALT METABOLISM
Cholesterol desmolase	Lipoid hyperplasia	Males (undervirilized)	No	Salt wasting
3β-OH steroid dehydrogenase	Classic	Males	Yes	Salt wasting
	Nonclassic	No	Yes	Normal
17α-hydroxylase		Males	No	Hypertension
11-hydroxylase	Classic	Females	Yes	Hypertension
	Nonclassic	No	Yes	Normal
Corticosterone methyloxidase type II	Salt wasting	No	No	Salt wasting

SOURCE: Adapted from M. Sperling, *Pediatric Endocrinology*.

PSEUDOHYPOALDOSTERONISM

- End-organ unresponsiveness to aldosterone. Autosomal dominant or autosomal recessive modes of inheritance. Those with the autosomal dominant form have a milder course and spontaneous remissions over time; they have inactivating mutations in the mineralocorticoid receptor. Those with the autosomal recessive form may have mineralocorticoid unresponsiveness in multiple target tissues, including the sweat and salivary glands, and the colonic epithelium; they may have recurrent pulmonary disease and have inactivating mutations in the epithelial sodium channel.
- *Clinical features*: Hyponatremia, hyperkalemia, metabolic acidosis.
- *Diagnosis*: Aldosterone and renin levels are markedly elevated.
- *Treatment*: Do not respond to mineralocorticoid replacement. Sodium and bicarbonate supplementation required.

ADRENOLEUKODYSTROPHY

- X-linked recessive disorder, presents in the latter part of the first decade of life.
- *Clinical features*: Progressive central demyelination leading to blindness, deafness, dementia, quadriparesis, and death. Occasionally, Addison disease is the only manifestation of the disease.
- *Diagnosis*: Elevated levels of very long-chain fatty acids (VLCFAs).
- *Treatment*: Replacement of hydrocortisone. Neurologic features ameliorated by bone marrow transplant.

WOLMAN DISEASE

- Autosomal recessive lysosomal disorder, caused by deficiency of acid lipase.
- *Clinical features*: Presents in the first few weeks of life with failure to thrive, vomiting, abdominal distention, hepatosplenomegaly, and adrenal calcifications. Death usually occurs within 6 months of life.

ACQUIRED ADRENAL INSUFFICIENCY

ADDISON DISEASE

- Most cases due to autoimmune adrenalitis or idiopathic. Tuberculosis is a less common cause. Other autoimmune disorders occur with increased frequency, including diabetes mellitus, Hashimoto's thyroiditis, Graves' disease, vitiligo, pernicious anemia, celiac disease, hypoparathyroidism, and myasthenia gravis.
- *Clinical features*: Signs and symptoms may be acute or chronic onset. Acute onset signs include weakness, dehydration, hypotension, shock, fever, and symptoms of hypoglycemia. Chronic symptoms include fatigue, weakness, and anorexia and weight loss. Increased appetite for salt. Physical finds may include hyperpigmentation of skin, especially at lip borders, buccal mucosa, nipples, scars, in palmar, axillary, and groin creases, and over bony prominences. Blood pressure may be low.
- *Diagnosis*: Hyponatremia, hyperkalemia, hypoglycemia, neutropenia with eosinophilia, elevated ACTH level, and low cortisol level basally and following synthetic ACTH administration.
- *Treatment*: D5 0.9 NS to reverse shock, glucocorticoid, and mineralocorticoid replacement.

AUTOIMMUNE POLYGLANDULAR SYNDROME TYPE I

- Autoimmune adrenal insufficiency accompanied by mucocutaneous candidiasis, hypoparathyroidism, and gonadal failure. Diabetes mellitus, thyroid hormone deficiency, autoimmune hepatitis, alopecia, and malabsorption can also occur. Autosomal recessive due to mutations in the AIRE (autoimmune regulator) gene.

AUTOIMMUNE POLYGLANDULAR SYNDROME TYPE II

- Autoimmune adrenal insufficiency accompanied by insulin dependent diabetes mellitus, thyroid disorders, or both.

OTHER CAUSES

- Fulminant meningococcemia accompanied by adrenal hemorrhage (Waterhouse-Friderichsen syndrome), sarcoidosis, amyloidosis, neonatal adrenal hemorrhage secondary to traumatic delivery, and drugs.

SECONDARY ADRENAL INSUFFICIENCY

- Congenital pituitary or hypothalamic defects can result in secondary adrenal insufficiency. Acquired pituitary defects such as autoimmune hypophysitis, tumors (e.g., craniopharyngioma), and trauma. *Most common cause of secondary adrenal insufficiency is use of exogenous steroids.*

DISORDERS OF ADRENOCORTICAL HYPERFUNCTION

CUSHING SYNDROME

- Term used to describe the clinical characteristics associated with excess glucocorticoids, regardless of the source (exogenous or endogenous). Causes include exogenous use of steroids, ectopic ACTH production by tumors, adrenal adenoma, or carcinoma.
- *Cushing disease*: Term which specifically describes excessive glucocorticoid production caused by increased ACTH secretion from a pituitary basophilic adenoma.

- *Clinical Features*: Very rare in childhood.
  1. Most common characteristic is weight gain and linear growth retardation with delayed skeletal maturation. Most children with exogenous obesity have accelerated linear growth and advanced skeletal maturation.
  2. Fat distribution in face neck, trunk, and abdomen.
  3. Extremities appear wasted, loss of muscle mass, though this finding may be absent in children.
  4. Rounded facies, chubby cheeks.
  5. Plethora
  6. Hypertrophy of supraclavicular and posterior cervical fat pad.
  7. Hypertension
  8. Muscle weakness
  9. Osteoporosis
  10. Thin skin with purple striae on abdomen, buttocks, thighs, and axillae.
  11. Easy bruising.
  12. Excessive hair growth, low hairline over the front and temples.
  13. Premature pubic hair and acne can occur.
  14. Impaired immune function.
  15. Impaired glucose tolerance.
  16. Psychologic disturbances.
- *Diagnosis*: Hemoglobin, hematocrit, RBC high normal. Lymphopenia and eosinopenia common. Hyperinsulinemia, elevated lipoproteins.
  1. No hormonal test has 100% sensitivity or specificity.
  2. Loss of diurnal variation of plasma cortisol concentration, normally highest in the early morning, dropping in the late evening (11 p.m. to 12 midnight).
  3. Elevated 24-hour urinary free cortisol.
  4. Once hypercortisolism established, must distinguish between a pituitary or adrenal source.
  5. Proceed with *low dose dexamethasone suppression test (20 μg/kg/day × 2 days)*. If cortisol suppresses, there is no Cushing syndrome. If it does not suppress, proceed to *high dose dexamethasone suppression test (80 μg/kg/day × 2 days)*:
     a. If ACTH low and cortisol not suppressed, suggests adrenal tumor. Proceed with adrenal computed tomography (CT).
     b. If ACTH normal or high, and cortisol is suppressed, Cushing disease. Proceed with magnetic resonance imaging (MRI) of pituitary. If scan normal, may need inferior petrosal ACTH sampling after corticotropin-releasing hormone (CRF) stimulation.
     c. If ACTH is elevated with no suppression of cortisol, ectopic ACTH secretion. Need to locate site of the tumor.

TREATMENT

Cushing syndrome: Removal of adrenal adenoma or carcinoma, and replacement of glucocorticoids until the contralateral gland has recovered function (has been suppressed by the tumor). Malignant tumors often present with metastases and have a poor prognosis.

Cushing disease: Transsphenoidal microsurgery (treatment of choice) or pituitary irradiation.

Exogenous glucocorticoids: Prolonged exposure to supraphysiologic doses of glucocorticoids will result in suppression of the hypothalamic-pituitary-adrenal axis. If signs of Cushing syndrome are seen, adrenal suppression is present. If exposure is less than 1–2 weeks, suppression is unlikely. Beyond that time, the degree of adrenal suppression is variable and must be considered possible. Exogenous glucocorticoids should be decreased as dictated by the needs of the disease for which they were used. If the patient is not stressed, the dose can be provisionally decreased to physiologic replacement [hydrocortisone 10 mg/mL BSA(d)]. Periodic (e.g. monthly) determinations of morning cortisol can direct discontinuation.

ADRENAL MEDULLA

PHEOCHROMOCYTOMA

- Catecholamine producing tumors that usually arise from chromaffin cells of the adrenal medulla. Can also arise anywhere along the sympathetic chain. Very rare, ~1 case per 100,000 patient years. In children, 70% are unilateral, 70% are found only in the adrenal gland, and association with familial syndromes is more likely than in adults.
- Occur in the following familial syndromes:
  1. MEN 2A (medullary thyroid cancer, parathyroid hyperplasia, pheochromocytoma).
  2. MEN 2B (medullary thyroid cancer, pheochromocytoma, mucosal neuromas).
  3. Von Hippel-Lindau syndrome
  4. Neurofibromatosis
- *Clinical features*: Highly variable
  1. Hypertension, usually sustained.
  2. Headache
  3. Perspiration
  4. Nausea and vomiting
  5. Weight loss
- *Diagnosis*: Document increased catecholamine secretion. Can measure plasma free metanephrines. Patient must be in calm, basal state. Can measure urinary epinephrine, norepinephrine, metanephrines, and homovanillic acid. Plasma free metanephrines, when obtained properly, offer more sensitivity than urinary catecholamines but yield more false positives. This may

be preferred test in familial syndromes where risk of pheochromocytoma is high.
- Localize tumor by CT or MRI. Can use radioactive iodine metaidobenzoguanidine (I-MIBG) scanning to locate extraadrenal pheochromocytoma.
- *Treatment*: Surgical removal of tumor. Hypertensive crises, myocardial dysfunction, arrhythmias, hypotension, and shock can occur perioperatively. Preoperative α-blockade with phenoxybenzamine 1–2 weeks prior to surgery is indicated.

BIBLIOGRAPHY

Arnaldi G. Diagnosis and complications of Cushing's Syndrome. A consensus statement. *J Clin Endocrinol Metab* 2003;88: 5593–5602.

Speiser PW, White PC. Congenital adrenal hyperplasia. *N Engl J Med* 2003;349:776–788.

Storr HL, Savage MO, Clark AJ. Advance in the understanding of the genetic basis of adrenal insufficiency. *J Pediatr Endocrinol Metab* 2002;15S5:1323–1328.

Weise M, Merke DP, Pacak K, Walther MM, Eisenhofer G. Utility of plasma free metanephrines for detecting childhood pneochromocytoma. *J Clin Endocrinol Metab* 2002;87: 1955–1960.

68 ABNORMALITIES OF PUBERTY

Donald Zimmerman, Reema L. Habiby, and Wendy J. Brickman

NORMAL PUBERTY

- Puberty is the stage of human development that marks the transition from childhood to a sexually mature adult capable of reproduction. The hallmarks of puberty are rapid growth, development of secondary sexual characteristics, and the onset of menstruation, ovulation, and spermatogenesis. Puberty is regulated by the hypothalamic-pituitary-gonadal axis (Fig. 68-1). The sex steroids, estrogens and androgens, produce the physical changes of puberty.
- During childhood, this system is downregulated, as gonadotropin releasing hormone (GnRH) secretion is minimal. This axis is inhibited by higher central nervous system (CNS) systems during this time. At the onset of puberty, GnRH is released in a pulsatile fashion, with

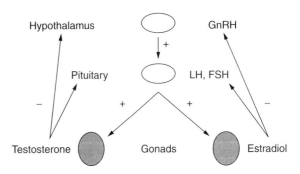

FIG. 68-1 Hypothalamic-pituitary-gonadal axis.

subsequent pulsatile release of luteinizing hormone (LH) and follicle-stimulating hormone (FSH). These pulses first occur during sleep then increase in frequency and amplitude throughout the day. Control of the timing of puberty still remains incompletely understood. Tanner staging is used to describe breast and pubic hair development in girls, genital and pubic hair development and testicular size in males (Table 68-1).

FEMALES

- Thelarche, or the onset of breast development, is usually the first manifestation of puberty in girls, though in some cases (~10%) it can be preceded by adrenarche (onset of pubic hair).
  1. Mean age of onset of breast development is 9.5–10 years.
  2. On average, African-American girls develop breasts and pubic hair earlier than Caucasian girls.
  3. Average duration of puberty is 3–4 years.
  4. Mean age of menarche is 12.7 + 1.0 years.
  5. Growth spurt occurs early in puberty, corresponding best with Tanner stage II breast development.

MALES

- Increased testicular volume (4 cc or 2.5 cm long) is the first manifestation of puberty in males.
  1. Increased testicular volume occurs on average at 12 years but can start as early as 9.5 years.
  2. Growth spurt occurs in midpuberty, generally between Tanner stages III and IV.
  3. Onset of spermarche generally at Tanner III.

PRECOCIOUS PUBERTY

- Sexual development prior to the age of 8 years in girls and 9 years in boys is considered precocious.

TABLE 68-1   Tanner Staging

STAGE	PUBIC HAIR STAGING	TESTICULAR VOLUME OR LENGTH
Girls: breast		
Prepubertal	Prepubertal	
Budding; larger areolae; palpable and larger contour	Pigmented downy hair, mainly labial	
Enlargement of the breast and areola	Coarser, spread over mons	
Secondary mound of areola and papilla	Adult type but smaller area	
Mature	Mature distribution, spread to medial thighs	
Boys: genital size		
Prepubertal	Prepubertal	<3 cc, <2.5 cm
Early testicular, penile, and scrotal growth	Pigmented downy hair, mainly at the base of penis	3–6 cc or >2.5–3.0 cm
Increased penile length and width, scrotal, and testicular growth	Dark, coarse, curly hair, extends midline above penis	6–10 cc or >3.0–3.5 cm
Increased penile size, including breadth, pigmented scrotum	Adult type but smaller area	10–15 cc or >3.5–4.0 cm
Mature	Mature distribution, spread to medial thighs or beyond	>15 mL or >4.0 cm

SOURCE: Adapted from Lee PA. Puberty and its disorders. In: Lifshitz F (ed.), *Pediatric Endocrinology*, 4th ed.

CENTRAL PRECOCIOUS PUBERTY (CPP)/GONADOTROPIN-DEPENDENT

* Central or gonadotropin-dependent precocious puberty indicates premature activation of the hypothalamic-pituitary-gonadal axis. Any event which interferes with normal tonic CNS inhibition of this axis can lead to precocious puberty; however, the majority of girls with CPP have no demonstrable CNS abnormality (Table 68-2).

DIAGNOSTIC EVALUATION

* *History and physical examination*: History should be taken with care to uncover underlying abnormalities that may be associated with precocious puberty, family history of pubertal developments, and exposure to exogenous sex steroids. Height, weight, arm span, upper/lower segment ratio, skin, hair, thyroid, neurologic findings, Tanner staging, and visualization of the vaginal mucosa.

TABLE 68-2   Causes of Central Precocious Puberty

Idiopathic
Central nervous system abnormalities
  Congenital anomalies: Hydrocephalus, arachnoid cysts, hypothalamic hamartomas, septo-optic dysplasia
  Acquired: Cranial irradiation, trauma, surgical, abscesses, granulomas
  Tumors: Astrocytoma, glioma (often associated with neurofibromatosis type 1), craniopharyngioma, ependymoma, LH secreting adenoma
  Secondary to chronic exposure to sex steroids as in congenital adrenal hyperplasia, gonadotropin-independent PP

* *Laboratory evaluation*: Serum LH, FSH, estradiol (girls), and testosterone (boys). Thyroid function tests. If LH, FSH, estradiol, testosterone are not pubertal, may need GnRH stimulation test. Bone age for assessment of skeletal maturation. Magnetic resonance imaging (MRI) of the head with attention to the hypothalamus and pituitary to evaluate for intracranial abnormalities.
* *Treatment*: If an underlying treatable cause is found, this should be treated. Temporary suppression of the hypothalamic-pituitary-gonadal axis with GnRH analog therapy can be used in carefully selected patients where cessation of pubertal progression or menses is necessary or when growth potential is significantly compromised.

PERIPHERAL PRECOCIOUS PUBERTY/ GONADOTROPIN-INDEPENDENT

* The physical changes of puberty can occur due to sex steroid secretion that is independent of the pituitary gonadotropins. The source of the sex steroids can be endogenous or exogenous, come from the gonads or elsewhere, and may be produced autonomously (Table 68-3).

DIAGNOSTIC EVALUATION

* *History and physical examination*: Same. Search for exogenous sex steroid use.
* *Laboratory evaluation*: Serum LH, FSH, estradiol (girls), and testosterone (boys). Expect estradiol or

TABLE 68-3   Causes of Gonadotropin-Independent Precocious Puberty

Genetic disorders
  LH receptor activating mutations (familial, male limited, gonadotropin-independent precocious puberty)
  McCune-Albright syndrome (café-au lait macules, polyostotic fibrous dysplasia, precocious puberty) due to an activating missense mutation in the gene for alpha subunit of the Gs protein
    Congenital virilizing adrenal hyperplasia
Tumors
  Ovarian (granulosa cell, theca cell)
  Testicular (Leydig cell)
  Adrenal sex steroid producing tumor (adenoma or carcinoma)
  Gonadotropin producing (dysgerminoma, choriocarcinoma, hepatoblastoma)
Chronic primary hypothyroidism
Ovarian cysts
Exogenous sex steroids

testosterone to be elevated, gonadotropins low. Thyroid function tests. Bone age, ovarian or testicular ultrasound, consider computed tomography (CT) adrenals.

- *Treatment*: If an underlying treatable cause is found, this should be treated. In the case of autonomous gonadal production of sex steroids, therapy is aimed at reducing sex steroid production and effect. Agents such as steroid synthesis inhibitors (ketoconazole), aromatase inhibitors (testolactone, anastrazole), and estrogen receptor antagonists have been used with variable responses.

DELAYED PUBERTY

- Delayed puberty is defined as the absence of physical changes of puberty by age 13 years in girls and 14 years in boys. In addition, if greater than 5 years has elapsed since the first signs of puberty and menarche in girls or completion of genital growth in boys, this may signify a problem that warrants a complete evaluation. Delayed puberty may be the result of a nonpathologic delay in the maturation of the hypothalamic-pituitary-gonadal axis, or it may be the result of an underlying abnormality.

HYPERGONADOTROPIC HYPOGONADISM

- Hypergonadotropic hypogonadism (elevated LH, FSH, low estradiol, or testosterone) indicates gonadal failure. In the pediatric setting, this is commonly acquired due to chemotherapy and irradiation for malignancies. Chromosomal and genetic disorders (such as Klinefelter syndrome, Turner syndrome,

gonadal dysgenesis androgen insensitivity syndrome, 5-alpha reductase deficiency, galactosemia, and vanishing testes syndrome) can also be a cause as well as trauma, infections, and autoimmune etiologies.

- *Laboratory evaluation*: Serum LH, FSH, estradiol (girls), and testosterone (boys). Expect estradiol or testosterone to be low, gonadotropins high. Karyotype is indicated.
- *Treatment*: See treatment of delayed puberty below.

HYPOGONADOTROPIC HYPOGONADISM

- *Constitutional delay of growth and maturity*: This is a temporary form of delayed puberty in which there is a delayed tempo of pubertal maturation for chronological age. It can be difficult to differentiate constitutional delay of puberty from permanent hypogonadotropic hypogonadism; however, the child with constitutional delay will eventually enter puberty.
- *History and physical examination*: Often a family history of delayed puberty. Generally, height remains below the 5th percentile but growth velocity is normal for the skeletal age. Patients with true hypogonadism may have eunuchoid habitus (arm span > 4 cm longer than height and abnormally low ratio of upper to lower segments).
- *Laboratory evaluation*: Serum LH, FSH, estradiol (girls), and testosterone (boys). Expect estradiol or testosterone to be low, gonadotropins low. Bone age is delayed throughout childhood.
- *Treatment*: If treatment is desired (more often requested in boys), a 3–4-month course of testosterone enanthate (50–150 mg IM each month) can be administered if they are ≥14 years old. This should increase the linear growth velocity as well as induce some secondary sexual characteristic development.

PERMANENT HYPOGONADOTROPIC HYPOGONADISM
- This condition can be caused by a variety of hypothalamic or pituitary disorders, and can be partial or complete.

Isolated Gonadotropin Deficiency
- Can be caused by genetic mutations in the GnRH receptor, the KAL gene (Kallmann syndrome) the β-subunits of LH and FSH, and X-linked adrenal hypoplasia congenita (DAX-1 mutations).
- Kallmann syndrome: Prevalence is 1:10,000 births.
- Clinical features: Hypogonadotropic hypogonadism, hyposmia, or anosmia due to aplasia or hypoplasia of olfactory lobes, midline facial defects such as cleft lip and palate, abnormalities of kidney formation, pes cavus, sensorineural deafness, and synkinesia (mirror movements).

- Etiology: In the X-linked form, it has been found to be due to defects in the KAL gene that codes for an adhesion molecule that allows migration of the GnRH neurons and olfactory neurons from the olfactory placode to the brain.

Anatomic Abnormalities of the Hypothalamus or Pituitary
- Craniopharyngiomas, germinomas, prolactinomas, gliomas histiocytosis X, congenital hypopituitarism, septo-optic dysplasia, can cause GnRH or gonadotropin deficiencies, often in association with other pituitary hormone deficiencies.

Syndromes Associated with Hypogonadotropic Hypogonadism
- Laurence-Moon-Biedl (retinitis pigmentosa, obesity, polydactyly, mental retardation), Prader-Willi syndrome (infantile hypotonia, short stature, obesity, lack of satiety, almond shaped eyes, moderate mental retardation).
- Cranial irradiation
- Chronic disease states
- Anorexia nervosa
- High level of athletic activity in females.
- Hypothyroidism
- Prolactinoma

DIAGNOSTIC EVALUATION

- *History and physical examination*: History should focus on attention to chronic illness, nutritional disorders, head trauma, presence of headaches or visual changes, age of onset of puberty in family members. Physical examination should include assessment of linear growth velocity, accurate heights and weight, upper-to-lower segment ratios and arm span, search for evidence of chronic illness or malnutrition, signs of puberty should be noted, complete neurologic examination with visualization of optic disks and assessment of visual fields, and sense of smell should be tested.
- *Laboratory evaluation*: Serum LH, FSH, estradiol (girls), and testosterone (boys). Expect estradiol or testosterone to be low, gonadotropins low. Screening chemistries, thyroid function tests, consider prolactin level. Bone age is delayed throughout childhood.
- A GnRH stimulation test will show that the hypothalamic-pituitary-gonadal axis is inactive. As mentioned previously, it can be difficult to distinguish permanent hypogonadotropic hypogonadism from constitutional delay. These patients may need to be observed over several years to differentiate these entities.
- *Treatment*: Permanent hypogonadism requires long-term therapy. In boys, this can be accomplished with

intramuscular testosterone enanthate or transdermal androgen therapy. In the case of Kallmann syndrome, pulsatile GnRH therapy can be successful.
- In girls, following initiation of daily, low-dose estrogen therapy, cyclic estrogen-progesterone therapy will be needed.

BIBLIOGRAPHY

Eugster EA, Pescovitz OH. Advances in the treatment of precocious puberty. *Expert Opin Investig Drugs.* 2001;10:1623–1630.
Grumbach MM. The neuro endocrinology of human puberty revisited. *Horm Res* 2002,57S2:2–14.
Herman–Giddens ME, Slora EJ, Wasserman RC, Bourdony CJ, Bhapkar MV, Koch GG, Hasemeier CM. Secondary sexual characteristics and menses in young girls seen in office practice: a study from the Pediatric Research in Office Settings network. *Pediatrics* 1997;99:505–512.
Reiter EO. Delayed puberty. *Adolesc Med* 2002;13:101–118.
Wang Y. Is obesity associated with early sexual maturation? A comparison of the association in American boys versus girls. *Pediatrics* 2002;110–903–910.

69 HYPOTHALAMIC AND PITUITARY DISORDERS
Donald Zimmerman, Reema L. Habiby, and Wendy J. Brickman

THE HYPOTHALAMUS

- The two major mechanisms by which the hypothalamus controls pituitary hormone secretion include production of hormones within cell bodies of neurons located in the hypothalamus and then transport of these hormones down axons which end in the posterior lobe of the pituitary gland. These hormones are then released into the general circulation from nerve endings in the posterior pituitary gland. A second mechanism by which the hypothalamus controls pituitary hormone secretion is by hypothalamic neurons producing signaling molecules (either peptides or biogenic amines) and secreting these molecules into capillary loops which coalesce the portal veins. These veins carry the hypothalamic stimulating hormones to the pars distalis of the pituitary gland. In this area the veins give rise to a second bed of capillaries (sinusoids) which facilitate transport of signaling molecules from the hypothalamus into pituitary cells. The hypothalamus produces gonadotropin-releasing hormone which regulates pituitary production and secretion of luteinizing hormone (LH) and follicle-stimulating hormone (FSH). It also produces growth hormone releasing hormone which stimulates pituitary growth hormone production and release, and somatostatin inhibits pituitary growth hormone production and release. The hypothalamus produces ghrelin which also stimulates pituitary growth hormone production release. A large amount of ghrelin is also produced by the stomach. The hypothalamus produces thyrotropin releasing hormone which stimulates pituitary production and release of thyroid stimulating hormone (TSH) and also of prolactin. Additionally, the hypothalamus secretes dopamine which inhibits pituitary production and release of prolactin; the dominant effect of the hypothalamus on pituitary prolactin secretion is inhibitory. Finally, the hypothalamus produces corticotropin-releasing hormone which stimulates pituitary production and release of adrenocorticotropic hormone (ACTH). Another stimulant of pituitary production of adrenocorticotropic hormone is vasopressin.

VASOPRESSIN OR ANTIDIURETIC HORMONE

- Vasopressin is secreted by the posterior pituitary gland in response to hyperosmolality of the blood and in response to decreased blood pressure and decreased blood volume.

VASOPRESSIN EXCESS OR SYNDROME OF INAPPROPRIATE ANTIDIURETIC HORMONE SECRETION

- The syndrome of inappropriate antidiuretic hormone secretion (SIADH) is the most common cause of hypoosmolality in individuals with normal blood volume.

Diagnostic Criteria
- Low plasma osmolality (less than 275 mOsm/kg).
- Inappropriately elevated urinary concentration (greater than 100 mOsm/kg).
- Normal plasma volume.
- Increased urine sodium excretion in the face of normal intake of salt and water.
- Absence of other causes of hypoosmolality in the setting of normal blood volume such as hypothyroidism, hypocortisolism, and diuretic use.
- Serum uric acid level less than 4 mg/dL.

Causes
- Medications (carbamazepine and oxcarbazepine, omeprazole, serotonin reuptake inhibitors, vincristine,

angiotensin converting enzyme inhibitors, phenothiazines, and of course, desmopresson [DDAVP]).
- Pulmonary infections and mechanical ventilation.
- Central nervous system (CNS) abnormalities (path lesions, inflammatory diseases, degenerative or demyelinating diseases, subarachnoid hemorrhage, and head trauma).
- Non-CNS tumors (lung tumor, nasopharyngeal carcinoma, and leukemia).
- When central nervous system abnormalities are considered, cerebral salt wasting must be considered as a possible explanation. In cerebral salt wasting, patients have evidence of hypovolemia. Thus, elevated vasopressin in this setting is appropriate rather than inappropriate.

Treatment
- The treatment of syndrome of inappropriate antidiuretic hormone secretion depends on the severity of the manifestations.
  1. In patients who have mild-to-moderate hyponatremia and no central nervous system dysfunction, simple fluid restriction may be considered. Fluid restriction may comprise replacing only 90% of a patient's insensible loss plus urine output each hour. In order to estimate insensible loss, it is reasonable to use 25–30% of calculated maintenance requirements.
  2. If patients have severe central nervous system dysfunction thought likely due to hyponatremia, then one can give 3% sodium chloride. An infusion rate of 0.05 mL/kg/min will increase the serum sodium by approximately 2 mEq per hour.
  3. Finally, in patients with rather severe hyponatremia (less than 125 meq/L) but no acute neurologic dysfunction, one can use Lasix in a dose of 1 mg/kg every 6–12 hours in association with intravenous infusion of normal saline. In patients with normal renal function, 30–60 meq/L of potassium chloride should be added to the normal saline. If one is replacing these patients with the normal saline with potassium chloride, one gives an estimate of insensible loss which may be 0.3 times the calculated replacement plus 1/2 cc of fluid for every 1 cc of urine calculated each hour.
- With all techniques of raising low serum sodium levels, once the patient's sodium is sufficiently high that the patient is no longer having neurologic symptoms, there is value in continuing the increase in serum sodium at a slow rate of 1 meq/L every 2 hours. Slow correction of hyponatremia minimizes the risk of central pontine myelinolysis. A number of vasopressin antagonists are becoming available which will have increasing utility in treatment of patients with syndrome of inappropriate antidiuretic hormone secretion. These medications may become particularly useful in patients with chronic SIADH.

Currently, chronic SIADH is treated mostly with fluid restriction and, in some instances, with demeclocycline in a dose of 300 mg by mouth twice daily to four times daily for adult-sized individuals and in proportionately lower doses for children. It is important to note that children less than 8 years of age are susceptible to abnormalities of dental enamel with use of tetracyclines.

DIABETES INSIPIDUS

- Diabetes insipidus results from inability to secrete vasopressin or antidiuretic hormone or from inability to respond to vasopressin.

Symptoms

- Polyuria
- Polydipsia
- Nocturia
- Preference for ice water
- Failure to thrive and fever in infants
- Severe and prolonged hypernatremia may result in central nervous system dysfunction. It is noteworthy that many patients with central diabetes insipidus have associated conditions that also can contribute to their symptomatology.

Associated Conditions

- Brain tumors (with headaches, vision disturbance, deficiencies in other hypothalamic pituitary axes, hydrocephalus, and seizures).
- Diabetes insipidus occurring in the setting of Langerhans cell histiocytosis.
- Sarcoidosis
- Septo-optic dysplasia (associated with optic nerve hypoplasia, occasionally with developmental delay, and with various pituitary hormone deficiencies).
- Wolfram syndrome (diabetes mellitus, sensorineural deafness, optic atrophy).
- Nephrogenic diabetes insipidus may occur from genetic causes which may be X-linked, autosomal dominant, or autosomal recessive. It may also occur in the setting of medullary cystic disease of the kidneys or in the setting of hydronephrosis from a number of causes.

Diagnosis

- The diagnosis of diabetes insipidus depends on the demonstration of increased plasma osmolality in association with inability to concentrate the urine. In some patients, the diagnosis may be made by checking the osmolality or specific gravity of a first-voided morning urine in association with serum electrolytes and/or serum osmolality. If plasma osmolality is increased to more than 295 mOsm/kg or if serum sodium is increased to above 145 meq/L

TABLE 69-1 Diagnosis of Diabetes Insipidus

URINE OSMOLALITY AFTER FLUID DEPRIVATION	URINE OSMOLALITY AFTER ADMINISTRATION OF DESMOPRESSIN 0.3 mg IM OR 5 mg INTRANASALLY	DIAGNOSIS
<300	>750	Central diabetes insipidus
<300	<300	Nephrogenic diabetes insipidus
>750	>750	Primary polydipsia
300–750	<750	Indeterminate

with urine osmolality remaining below 300 mOsm/kg or urine specific gravity remaining below 1.010, then diabetes insipidus is present. In many instances, fasting serum osmolality and/or sodium are not increased. Under these circumstances, a water deprivation study is indicated. During this test, the patient is weighed hourly and the test is terminated if 5% or more of the body weight is lost. When serum osmolality rises above 295 mOsm/kg, blood is drawn for vasopressin levels and urine is obtained to examine concentrating ability. The values may be interpreted in the following manner (see Table 69-1).

- For patients who have indeterminate results, 5% saline (850 mmol/L) may be given at a rate of 0.05 mL/kg/hour over a period of 2 hours or until plasma osmolality is greater than or equal to 300 mOsm/kg. The plasma vasopressin level is drawn in levels compared with appropriate standards.

Treatment >1–2 Years of Age

- The standard treatment for diabetes insipidus in individuals older than 1–2 years is desmopressin or DDAVP. The responsiveness that patients manifest to vasopressin is extremely variable. For this reason, doses are empiric. Typically, treatment is begun with low doses orally of 100 µg twice daily or 2–10 µg intranasally 1–2 times daily. If treatment is initiated subcutaneously the treatment is usually begun with 0.1–0.2 µg subcutaneously each day.
- In patients who are found to have diabetes insipidus that does not respond to administration of desmopressin, the diagnosis of nephrogenic diabetes is made. In these individuals, it is important to study the kidneys to learn whether a specific kidney disease is responsible for the problem. Of particular interest is whether such individuals might have hydronephrosis. Individuals who have normal renal function and normal structure on ultrasound study of the kidneys may have genetic cause for nephrogenic diabetes insipidus or may have this condition on the basis of administration of medication. Medications known to

produce this include lithium, demeclocycline, and methoxyflurane. Nephrogenic diabetes insipidus may also be caused by hypokalemia and hypercalcemia. In all of these circumstances, one should consider either removing the offending drug or correcting the metabolic disturbance producing diabetes insipidus.

Treatment in Infants

• Diabetes insipidus in infants may be treated by administering hydrochlorothiazide in a dose of 2–4 mg/kg/day. These medications may be used with potassium sparing diuretics such as amiloride, 20 mg/1.73 m²/day. In patients with nephrogenic diabetes insipidus, prostaglandin synthesis inhibitors such as indomethacin may be used in addition to hydrochlorothiazide in doses of 2 mg/kg/day.

ACTH

• Excessive secretion of ACTH produces Cushing disease. Cushing syndrome is the clinical condition resulting from glucocorticoid excess. When excessive secretion of ACTH by the pituitary causes adrenal hypersecretion of cortisol, the condition is termed "Cushing disease." ACTH hypersecretion typically results from a pituitary adenoma but may at times result from hypothalamic hypersecretion of corticotrophin releasing hormone. Pituitary hypersecretion of ACTH is not autonomous. Rather, it reflects a higher set point of circulating cortisol.
• The clinical features of Cushing disease are outlined in Table 69-2.

TABLE 69-2 Clinical Features of Cushing Disease

SYMPTOM/SIGN	FREQUENCY (%)
Weight gain	90
Growth retardation	83
Menstrual irregularity	81
Hirsutism or hypertrichosis	81
Obesity (BMI >85th percentile)	73
Violaceous kin striae	63
Acne	52
Hypertension	51
Fatigue and weakness	45
Early puberty	41
Bruising	27
Mental changes	18
Delayed bone age	14
Hyperpigmentation	13
Muscle weakness	13
Acanthosis nigricans	10
Accelerated bone age	10
Sleep disturbance	7
Pubertal delay	7

ABBREVIATION: BMI, body mass index.

• The diagnosis of Cushing disease is established by demonstrating hypercortisolism. A 24-hour urine collection is made from measurement of free cortisol and creatinine (the latter to demonstrate a complete urine collection). Age-related normals should be obtained from the laboratory since techniques vary considerably. A second technique of demonstrating hypercortisolism is determining cortisol levels in plasma or saliva at the time of the diurnal nadir (between 11 p.m. and midnight). Plasma cortisol levels at this time fall below 5 µg/dL. Of course, the act of drawing blood at midnight is likely stressful particularly in younger children. Thus, stress responses in this age group may produce false positive test results. Midnight salivary cortisol levels have been studied and appear to have diagnostic accuracy and predictive values similar to those of midnight plasma cortisol levels. A precise diagnostic cutoff level is likely laboratory-dependent. A recent report showed excellent diagnostic utility of a salivary cortisol level of 0.35 µg/dL. Another technique for establishing baseline cortisol excess is the low-dose overnight dexamethasone suppression test. A dose of 1 mg of dexamethasone per 1.73 m² is administered at 11 p.m. The following morning, cortisol levels greater than 5 µg/dL indicate hypercortisolemia. Confirmation of hypercortisolemia may require repeat determinations of 11 p.m. to midnight salivary cortisol or repeat urine free cortisol determinations. This is particularly important since approximately 10% of individuals with Cushing syndrome have a periodic rather than continuous cortisol hypersecretion.
• The standard dexamethasone suppression test is neither more sensitive nor more specific than the overnight test, nor than the midnight plasma or salivary cortisol test. Typically this test includes two baseline days during which 24-hour urines are collected and morning and evening plasma cortisols are measured. Low-dose dexamethasone is then administered over a 2-day period (20 µg/kg/day divided into three or four doses). Urines and bloods are again obtained as on the baseline days. Plasma cortisol should fall below 2 µg/dL by the second day and urine 17-hydroxycorticosteroids should decrease by a factor of 50% and urine-free cortisol should fall below 20 µg/24 hours in adult-size individuals. In order to distinguish between hypercortisolism due to excessive production of ACTH and that due to autonomous adrenal overproduction of cortisol, ACTH levels are typically suppressed (when two-site immunometric assays are employed) in primary adrenal causes of hypercortisolism but are within the normal range or higher in ACTH-dependent Cushing patients. ACTH levels that are greater than 20 pg/mL

are strong indicators of an ACTH-dependent mechanism. If the ACTH level does not clearly delineate the involvement or the lack of involvement of ACTH in the mechanism of the patient's disease, then a high-dose dexamethasone suppression test may be employed. Eighty μg/kg of dexamethasone are administered and urine is collected for 2 days for measurement of 17-hydroxycorticosteroid and urine free cortisol as well as for creatinine. Blood is drawn for cortisol and ACTH. Typically both urine-free cortisol and serum cortisol are 50% of the baseline or less following 2 days of high-dose dexamethasone administration.

- ACTH excess may result from ectopic secretion of ACTH by a number of tumors. While ACTH production in many of these tumors remains high despite administration of high doses of dexamethasone, a number of cases of ectopic ACTH syndrome demonstrate dexamethasone suppressability. The most reliable method of distinguishing between pituitary and ectopic ACTH production is the inferior petrosal sinus sampling test. An experienced radiologist catheterizes each of the two inferior petrosal sinuses. Blood is drawn in the basal state and 2, 5, and 10 minutes after administration of corticotropin-releasing hormone (CRH) (1 μg/kg). Samples are drawn at those times from a peripheral venous site as well. ACTH levels are measured centrally and peripherally. If the ratio of the petrosal sinus sample to the periphery is greater than 3 following CRH administration then a pituitary source of ACTH is established. If ratios are consistently less than 2, then an ectopic source of ACTH is established.

- Magnetic resonance imaging (MRI) will detect pituitary ACTH-producing tumors between 35 and 60% of patients with Cushing disease. It is important to interpret results of MR scanning in light of data indicating the presence of incidental pituitary tumors in at least 10% of normal individuals between 20 and 40 years of age.

Treatment

- Treatment of pituitary Cushing disease consists of transsphenoidal pituitary resection of the corticotrophic tumor. Since these tumors are not visible on MR scans in approximately 50% of patients, some centers employ inferior petrosal sinus sampling to localize the tumors. The criterion often employed is an ACTH ratio of at least 1.4 in comparison with the contralateral petrosal sinus ACTH level. On occasion, the pituitary tumor is not found, and Cushing disease persists. Under these circumstances, pituitary irradiation may be considered. Alternatively, bilateral adrenalectomy is an option. In the recent past, laparoscopic adrenalectomy has reduced the time of recuperation from surgery. If bilateral adrenalectomy is chosen, then the patient must be monitored carefully for rapid growth of the pituitary tumor (Nelson syndrome). Serial MR scanning and determination of ACTH are helpful in such monitoring.

ACTH DEFICIENCY

- ACTH deficiency may result from congenital abnormalities of the hypothalamus such as septo-optic dysplasia and holoprosencephaly, congenital abnormalities of the pituitary gland such as mutations in PROP-1, PIT-1 mutations, and mutations in Tbx 19. ACTH deficiency may result from hypothalamic and pituitary tumors, trauma and hemorrhage as well as granulomatous disease and radiation therapy. Finally, hypothalamic and pituitary corticotrophic axis suppression can be induced by a history of glucocorticoid treatment.

- The symptoms of deficient ACTH include hypoglycemia, prostration with intercurrent illness, decreased energy and endurance, orthostatic faintness, anorexia, nausea, vomiting, and skin hypopigmentation.

- Low levels of plasma cortisol at 8 a.m. in association with nonelevated ACTH levels suggest ACTH deficiency. This diagnosis can be confirmed using an insulin tolerance test. Regular insulin, 0.1 unit/kg body weight, is given intravenously. Blood glucose is monitored at 15–30-minute intervals. Cortisol levels are measured at 30-minute intervals. With sufficient lowering of blood glucose (50% of the basal level), cortisol should rise to at least 18 μg/dL. Two other tests that may be used are the metyrapone test in which metyrapone is given in a dose of 30 mg/kg at midnight and plasma cortisol and 11-deoxycortisol are measured at 8 a.m. A normal morning 11-deoxycortisol is greater than 7 μg/dL. Plasma cortisol should be unstimulated (less than 5 μg/dL). Another test that may be used is the corticotropin-releasing hormone stimulation test. Bovine CRH is given in a dose of 1 μg/kg intravenously. Levels of cortisol and ACTH are measured at 15, 30, and 60 minutes. Cortisol levels should exceed 20 μg/dL and ACTH levels should exceed 27 pg/mL.

Treatment

- Treatment of ACTH deficiency consists of administration of hydrocortisone in a dose of 7–10 mg/m^2/day. In children, this medication is typically divided into doses given three times daily. Typically, the dose given in the morning is the largest dose and that given in the evening is the smallest dose. The adequacy of the dose is typically judged on the basis of the patient's symptoms of energy and presence or absence of symptoms of hypoglycemia.

THYROID STIMULATING HORMONE

- Thyroid stimulating hormone stimulates thyroid hormone synthesis and secretion by the thyroid gland. It is secreted by the anterior pituitary gland in response to stimulation by the hypothalamic hormone, thyrotropin releasing hormone. Increased thyrotropin releasing hormone occurs in association with central thyroid hormone resistance. Pituitary hypersecretion of thyroid stimulating hormone may also be produced by TSH secreting tumors. The most sensitive test for identification of TSH secreting pituitary adenomas is an elevation of the ratio of serum levels of the alpha-subunit of pituitary glycoprotein hormones to serum TSH levels. This ratio is below 5.7 in patients with normal levels of gonadotropin. These patients also have elevations in the absolute level of alpha-subunit. Normal values for alpha-subunit are less than 3 µg/L.
- In response to infusion of thyrotropin releasing hormone 500 µg intravenously, patients with TSH secreting tumors increase TSH by less than 220% while normal individuals increase TSH by more than 750%.
- In order to confidently diagnose inappropriately elevated TSH, it is important to exclude elevated levels of thyroxine-binding proteins. When levels of thyroxine-binding proteins are elevated, individuals may have hypothyroidism with low levels of free thyroxine but normal or high levels of total thyroxine. Under these circumstances, elevated TSH is an appropriate response to low levels of free thyroxine.
- Individuals with TSH excess producing hyperthyroidism have the usual hyperthyroid symptoms such as heat intolerance, tremulousness, insomnia, tachycardia and palpitations, hypersudation, hyperdefecation, attention deficit, hyperphagia, and menstrual abnormalities in women.
- Treatment of TSH secreting tumors consists of an attempt at removal of the tumor by transsphenoidal surgery. In patients in whom surgical treatment is not curative, external irradiation may be employed. Medical treatment may include octreotide which is often effective at doses of 100–1500 µg daily.
- TSH deficiency may be caused by congenital or genetic abnormalities of the hypothalamus and pituitary such as septo-optic dysplasia and holoprosencephaly. Mutations of Pit-1 or PROP-1 may contribute to multiple pituitary hormone deficiencies including deficiency of TSH. TSH deficiency may also be caused by mutations in the TSH beta-subunit gene.

Symptoms
- Hypothyroid symptoms (decreased energy, cold intolerance, dry hair and skin, decreased appetite, constipation, growth delay in children, and menstrual abnormalities in mature women).
- In infants, TSH deficiency can give rise to psychomotor delay.
- TSH/TRH deficiency may result from tumors, trauma and hemorrhage as well as from granulomatous diseases and other infiltrative conditions.

Diagnosis
- Diagnosis of TSH deficiency is made by finding a low-free thyroxine level in association with a nonelevated level of thyroid stimulating hormone. It is noteworthy that some patients with thyroid releasing hormone (TRH) deficiency manifest a very slight elevation of immunoassayable thyroid stimulating hormone. Studies of TSH in these individuals have shown decreased glycosylation giving rise to decreased bioactivity of the thyroid stimulating hormone.
- Treatment of TSH deficiency comprises administration of L-thyroxine. In infants, L-thyroxine should be given in relatively high doses of 10–15 µg/kg/day. The dose should then be rechecked at 1–2-week intervals to normalize free thyroxine. In individuals older than 2 years, L-thyroxine should be started slowly—particularly in individuals with rather severe hypothyroidism. In children replaced with L-thyroxine excessively rapidly, hyperthyroid symptoms may occur in association with increased intracranial pressure. In adults, patients may develop hyperthyroid symptoms in association with symptoms of ischemic cardiac disease. Thus, treatment may be initiated in doses of 25 µg daily and slowly increased to achieve normal levels of free thyroxine. It is important to recheck levels of L-thyroxine 5–6 weeks after making a change in the dose so that an equilibrium level of circulating hormone can be reached.

PITUITARY GONADOTROPINS LSH AND FSH

- These hormones are secreted in response to hypothalamic secretion of pulses of gonadotropin-releasing hormone. Faster pulsations of hypothalamic gonadotropin releasing hormone (GnRH) induce greater LH than FSH secretion from gonadotropes. Conversely, slower frequencies of hypothalamic GnRH pulsation favor FSH synthesis and secretion. Additionally, the gonadal steroids estradiol and testosterone contribute to determining levels of pituitary LH and FSH secretion. Testosterone decreases gonadotrope production of LH but does not affect gonadotrope production of FSH. A large percentage of the negative feedback by testosterone occurs at the level of the hypothalamus. Much of the negative feedback of estradiol occurs at the level of the pituitary gonadotrope. Estradiol may also have a positive feedback at both the hypothalamus and pituitary gland. This occurs when estradiol levels are maintained at 500 pg/mL for a period of 36 hours. Pituitary gonadotropins are also regulated by inhibins produced by follicular and luteal cells in the ovary and by the sertoli cells in the testes. Inhibins specifically suppress pituitary production of FSH without affecting pituitary production of LH.

- Overactivity of the hypothalamic-pituitary-gonadal axis may be produced by abnormal migration of the neurons which produce gonadotropin-releasing hormone. These neurons originate in the olfactory placode and migrate to both the preoptic area and to the medial basal portion of the hypothalamus. The GnRH secreting neurons are constitutively active. When these neurons are appropriately situated in the hypothalamus, axons from other neurons exert largely inhibitory actions. This inhibition is evident at midgestation as well as in the latter part of infancy. Inhibition is released at the time of puberty. If gonadotropin-releasing hormone neurons are located ectopically (forming hamartomas), then inhibitory influences are absent, and early puberty occurs. Other mechanisms by which inhibitors of gonadotropin-releasing hormone are disturbed include central nervous system tumor, hydrocephalus, and a number of conditions such as Rett syndrome, trauma, and hemorrhage. Some individuals with malformations of the brain such as septo-optic dysplasia or agenesis of the corpus callosum may experience early puberty on this basis. Finally, on very rare occasions, pituitary adenomas consisting of gonadotropes may produce early puberty.

- Recently, loss of the function mutations in a g-protein coupled receptor, GPR54, have been associated with hypogonadotropic hypogonadism. This receptor is apparently activated by peptides derived from a precursor protein, kisspeptin-1. Patients with X-linked congenital adrenal hypoplasia have hypogonadotropic hypogonadism because of loss of function mutations in the gene for DAX-1. This gene is active at both the hypothalamic and pituitary levels. Patients with juvenile hemochromatosis develop iron deposition in pituitary gonadotropes in association with hypogonadotropic hypogonadism. Patients with inactivating mutations of KAL-1 have failure of migration of gonadotropin-releasing hormone neurons from their origin in the olfactory placode to the appropriate places within the hypothalamus. While these neurons make gonadotropin-releasing hormone in the region of the olfactory placode, the concentration of gonadotropin-releasing hormone in blood reaching the anterior pituitary gland is too low to stimulate gonadotrope activity. Patients with septo-optic dysplasia (sometimes associated with mutations in transcription factor HESX1 or LHX3) may have delayed puberty. Mutations may also occur in the gonadotropin-releasing hormone receptor on pituitary gonadotrope. The pituitary transcription factor PROP-1 and the orphan nuclear receptor SF-1 may be mutated and thereby produce hypogonadotropic hypogonadism. Loss of leptin function due to loss of function mutations in the leptin gene, in the leptin receptor gene, or in prohormone convertase 1 may produce hypogonadotropic hypogonadism. Central nervous system tumors, hydrocephalus, cranial irradiation, hemorrhage, and infiltrative diseases may also produce hypogonadotropic hypogonadism. Finally, undernutrition and extremely vigorous activity are associated with hypogonadotropic hypogonadism, perhaps in part because of lower levels of leptin in these individuals.

- The clinical presentation varies largely with the severity of the hypogonadism. Some males manifest hypogenitalism at the time of birth. It is noteworthy that patients with hypogonadotropic hypogonadism may have small phalluses but most commonly do not have hypospadias. Some hypogonadotropic boys manifest cryptorchidism. If hypogonadotropic hypogonadism has occurred by the time of expected puberty, then secondary sexual characteristics will be either totally absent (particularly in individuals with congenital adrenal hypoplasia in whom even adrenal androgens are absent giving rise to total absence of sex hair), or secondary sexual characteristics are underdeveloped. Frequently, individuals will manifest eunuchoid proportions. At times, hypogonadal males will have a degree of gynecomastia. Sexual function may be decreased in proportion to the completeness of the defect. Infertility is also a major problem.

- In infants with micropenis, evaluation depends on the precise timing of the patient's presentation. Male infants tend to have minipuberty beginning at 1 week of life and peaking at 2 months of life. By 6–7 months, these individuals manifest little measurable activity of the hypothalamic-pituitary-gonadal axis. If examined within the first 2–3 months of life, the basal levels of testosterone and gonadotropins should reflect minipuberty with FSH levels ranging from 0.16 to 4.1 mIU/mL in boys from 0.24 to 14 mIU/mL in girls. LH levels range from 0.02 to 7.0 mIU/mL for the first 2 months. Testosterone levels rise from approximately 20–50 ng/dL to 60–400 mg/dL between the first week and 2 months of life in infant boys. In infant girls, estradiol levels increase to between 0.5 and 5 ng/dL between 1 and 2 months of age and then decline to less than 1.5 ng/dL over the first year of life.

- If levels of both sex steroids and gonadotropins are low, this suggests hypogonadotropic hypogonadism. This diagnosis can be bolstered by measuring sex steroid levels following treatment with human chorionic gonadotropin. A frequently used regimen in boys is human chorionic gonadotropin 33 units/lb given three times weekly for 3 weeks. Testosterone and dihydrotestosterone may be measured on the day following the final injection. This fairly extensive regimen allows assessment of gonadal responsiveness to human chorionic gonadotropin and, in addition, end-organ responsiveness to testosterone and dihydrotestosterone.

- In prepubertal individuals, it is impossible to distinguish between patients with hypogonadotropic hypogonadism and normal children with basal hormone levels (testosterone, LH, FSH, estradiol) or with use of gonadotropin-releasing hormone testing. At the expected time of puberty, individuals with hypogonadotropic hypogonadism may be difficult to distinguish from those with constitutional delay of growth and development. Both will have prepubertal levels of LH, FSH, and sex steroids. Both will have prepubertal responses to gonadotropin-releasing hormone. In somewhat older individuals, measurement of body proportions may be useful since teenagers with hypogonadotropic hypogonadism ultimately develop eunuchoid proportions while those with constitutional delay of growth and development do not. Quite frequently, boys who have not begun puberty by 14 years of age and girls who have not begun puberty by 13 years of age may need evaluation unless there is a strong family history of pubertal delay. Since hypogonadotropic hypogonadism and constitutional delay of growth and development are difficult to distinguish, it is important to perform MR scans of the head in order to rule out intracranial pathology. This may be less urgent in patients who have a history of marked weight loss or very high activity level, or in those who have anosmia potentially associated with Kalmann syndrome.

- Because of the difficulty in distinguishing constitutional delay of growth and development from hypogonadotropic hypogonadism, it is common to initiate treatment in individuals with marked pubertal delay. Treatment in boys typically consists of testosterone enanthate, cypionate, or cyclopropionate. Typically this is begun in a dose of approximately 50 mg intramuscularly every 4 weeks. Transdermal testosterone may also be given. A dose of 2.5 mg every other night may be useful for the starting dose and then adjusted once testosterone levels are measured. Very often, this treatment is given for 4–6 months and then discontinued to once again evaluate the patient's spontaneous puberty. If, within 4 months, the patient is still prepubertal, testosterone treatment can be resumed with a gradual increase in testosterone enanthate doses to 100 and then 200 mg each month. The adult dose of testosterone enanthate is in the range of 200 mg intra-

muscularly every 2 weeks. This dose can be altered on the basis of circulating levels of testosterone measured 1 week after the injection. Alternatively, transdermal testosterone gel may be used with increasing doses from 2.5 g every day, increasing if needed to 5 g every day and at times 7.5 g every day based on measurement of circulating testosterone levels. Boys who receive testosterone treatment in the setting of constitutional delay of growth and development may also be given an aromatase inhibitor to prevent excessively rapid advancement of skeletal age. This is particularly important for those boys with constitutional delay who also have an element of short stature. Treatment in girls may begin with estradiol in a dose of 0.5 μg daily, ethinyl estradiol in a dose of 5 mg daily, or conjugated estrogens in a dose of 0.3 mg daily. This treatment may be given for a period of 4–6 months and then discontinued if it appears that the patient may be entering spontaneous puberty. If, over the ensuing 4 months there is no evidence of spontaneous puberty, and if skeletal age is not advancing excessively, then treatment may be restarted with a gradual increase in dose. It should be noted that as the estradiol increases to 1 mg daily or the conjugated estrogen dose increases to 0.625 mg daily, or the ethinyl estradiol dose to 10 μg daily, then it is necessary to add a progestin such as medroxyprogesterone in a dose of 5 mg daily for the first 12 days of each month in order to induce appropriate menstrual flow. The induction of menses is critical in avoidance of endometrial hyperplasia. Subsequently, doses of ethinyl estradiol may be increased to 2 mg daily if circulating levels of estradiol are not within the normal range for late puberty. Similarly, conjugated estrogens may be increased to 1.25 mg daily. If menstruation is not induced with medroxyprogesterone 5 mg daily, despite increasing the estrogen dose, then a trial of higher doses of medroxyprogesterone such as 10 mg daily should be considered.

BIBLIOGRAPHY

Arnaldi G, Angeli A, Atkinson AB, Bertagna X, et al. Diagnosis and complications of Cushing's Syndrome: a consensus statement. *J Clin Endocrinol Metab* 2003;88:5593–5602.

Brucker-Davis F, Oldfield EH, Skarulis MC, Doppman JL, Weintraub BD. Thyrotropin-secreting pituitary tumors: diagnostic criteria, thyroid hormone sensitivity and treatment outcome in 25 patients followed at the National Institutes of Health. *J Clin Endocrinol Metab* 1999;84:476–480.

Findling JW, Raff H, Aron DC. The low-dose dexamethasone suppression test: a reevaluation in patients with Cushing's Syndrome. *J Clin Endocrinol Metab* 2004;89:1222–1226.

Reiter EO, Lee PA. Delayed puberty. *Adolesc Med* 2002;13: 101–118.

Robertson GL. Antidiuretic hormone. Normal and disordered function. *Endocrinol Metab Clin* 2001;30:671–694.

70 ABNORMALITIES OF SEXUAL DIFFERENTIATION

Donald Zimmerman, Reema L. Habiby, and Wendy J. Brickman

NORMAL SEXUAL DEVELOPMENT

- Normal sexual development is the sequential process that successively establishes *chromosomal sex, gonadal sex*, and *phenotypic sex*. It is a complicated phenomenon, which is incompletely understood. Sexual differentiation begins in utero and ultimately results in a sexually mature individual capable of reproduction.

- The establishment of *chromosomal sex* is the first step in sexual differentiation. The genetic sex is determined at the time of fertilization by the constitution of the sex chromosome (i.e., 46,XX, 46,XY). In the presence of a Y chromosome, testis formation will occur, even in the presence of multiple X chromosomes (e.g., 47,XXY).

- *Gonadal sex* refers to the development of gonadal tissue as an ovary or testis. Genetic information determines that the undifferentiated, bipotential gonad develops into testis or ovary. In the presence of a Y chromosome, fetal gonads differentiate into testes under the influence of SRY (sex-related gene on the Y chromosome). Many other genes are necessary to sustain testis development, including *WT1, SF-1, SOX9*, and *DAX-1*. Ovarian development appears to occur in the absence of testis determining genes.

- *Phenotypic sex* refers to the nature of the internal sex ducts and the external genitalia. The internal sex ducts in the fetus include both *Wolffian ducts* and *Mullerian ducts*.

- In the male fetus, the Wolffian ducts become the epididymis, seminal vesicles, and vas deferens. Development of the Wolffian structures requires the presence of testosterone, secreted by fetal testicular Leydig cells. In its absence, the Wolffian ducts regress. The Mullerian ducts differentiate into the fallopian tubes, uterus, and posterior two-thirds of the vagina. In the presence of anti-Mullerian hormone (AMH), secreted by fetal testicular Sertoli cells, the Mullerian ducts regress.

- The external genitalia in male and female fetuses are identical until 8 weeks' gestation. In the presence of androgen, most specifically dihydrotestosterone (DHT), the external genitalia differentiate into a penis and scrotum. The urogenital sinus develops into the prostate and prostatic urethra in males and the urethra and anterior one-third of the vagina in the female. The genital tubercle develops into the glans penis in the male and the clitoris in the female. The urogenital swelling becomes the scrotum in males, the labia majora in females, and the urethral folds fuse to form the shaft of the penis and the urethra in males, the labia minora in females. In the absence of androgen, the external genitalia appear female.

DISORDERS OF SEXUAL DIFFERENTIATION

- It is extremely important to recognize disorders of sexual differentiation as early as possible and not to delay the etiologic diagnosis. Assignment of gender of rearing should be made as quickly as possible. Clear and compassionate communication with the parents regarding the diagnosis, prognosis, and treatment options is of utmost importance. Parents should actively participate in the decision-making process.

ABNORMAL CHROMOSOMAL SEX

KLINEFELTER SYNDROME (47,XXY AND MOSAIC VARIANTS)
- Classic form arises from nondisjunction during the first or second meiotic division of maternal gametogenesis.
- *Clinical features*: No particular stigmata at birth. Postpubertally, small firm testes (<3 cm in length), seminiferous tubule dysgenesis, and azospermia. Gynecomastia is common. Increased risk of breast tumors. Taller than average stature as a result of increased leg length (upper-to-lower segment ratio decreased). Learning disabilities, behavior disorders can be present.
- *Frequency*: Incidence 1:500–1000 men.
- *Diagnosis*: Obtain chromosomes (labs??)
- *Treatment*: Gynecomastia can be treated with surgical reduction. Androgen supplementation may improve virilization, libido, and bone mineralization. Fertility has been reported with intracytoplasmic

sperm injection when sperm can be obtained from testicular biopsy.

TURNER SYNDROME (45,XO GONADAL DYSGENESIS AND MOSAIC VARIANTS)

- Majority of girls with Turner syndrome have a 45,XO karyotype. Others have a 46,XX/45,XO mosaicism or structural abnormalities of the X chromosome such as isochromosomes or rings. Occurs due to nondisjunction either before zygotic formation or in the first or second postzygotic division.
- *Clinical features*: Short stature, short, thick, and webbed neck, high-arched palate, low posterior hairline, posteriorly rotated ears, ptosis, shield-like chest, congenital lymphedema, cubitus valgus, short fourth metacarpals, multiple pigmented nevi, dysplastic fingernails, frequent otitis media, keloid formation, cardiovascular anomalies (bicuspid aortic valve, aortic coarctation, aortic root dilatation), kidney anomalies, specific deficits in spatial abilities, limited or absent pubertal development, amenorrhea, and infertility.
- *Frequency*: Affects approximately 1:2000 live female births. Loss of 45,XO fetuses common. Approximately 7% spontaneous abortuses are 45,XO.
- *Diagnosis*: Should be considered in any girl with unexplained short stature or delayed puberty. Obtain chromosomes. Luteinizing hormone (LH) and follicle-stimulating hormone (FSH) usually increased peripubertally.
- *Treatment*: Detailed cardiac and renal evaluation (echocardiogram, renal ultrasound) at diagnosis. Antibiotic prophylaxis for dental/surgical procedures if heart defects present. Serial ECHOs for aortic root dimensions. Periodic evaluation of thyroid function, hearing, and scoliosis screening. Counseling regarding growth and fertility.
- Recombinant human growth hormone promotes linear growth in most girls.
- Ovarian failure requires estrogen replacement therapy to induce breast and uterine development as well as bone mineralization.

GONADAL DYSGENESIS (45,XO/46,XY AND VARIANTS)

- There is a variable phenotype ranging from phenotypic females to individuals with ambiguous genitalia to a completely normal male phenotype. The gonads range from streak gonads in phenotypic females to dysgenetic testes in phenotypic males. Normal testes as well as fertility have also been described in phenotypic males. Approximately 90% of individuals diagnosed prenatally by amniocentesis have normal male genitalia. Short stature is an associated finding.

TRUE HERMAPHRODITISM

- Occurs when both ovarian and testicular tissue are present in the same gonad or in opposite gonads. The karyotype is most commonly 46,XX. The remainder are 46,XY or mosaics. The phenotype is variable, with ambiguous genitalia usually present.

ABNORMAL GONADAL DIFFERENTIATION

- *Denys-Drash syndrome*: Usually present at birth with ambiguous genitalia, though a normal female or male phenotype can be seen. The karyotype is usually 46, XY. Diffuse mesangial sclerosis is seen on renal biopsy and leads to renal failure. Wilms tumor occurs in the first decade of life. The dysgenetic gonads are at increased risk for gonadoblastoma formation. Mutations in *WT1* (Wilms tumor suppressor gene) are found in these patients.
- *Frasier syndrome*: XY females with gonadal dysgenesis, glomerulopathy, and increased risk of gonadoblastoma.
- *Campomelic dysplasia*: 46,XY individuals with female phenotype. Severe skeletal dysplasia. Death usually occurs in the neonatal period caused by respiratory distress. Mutations of *SOX9* gene cause this syndrome.
- *Pure gonadal dysgenesis*: 46,XX or 46,XY. Female phenotype, streak gonads, female internal genitalia, and sexual infantilism with primary amenorrhea. Genetically heterogeneous, can be sporadic or familial (X-linked recessive, sex limited dominant autosomal transmission). In 46,XY individuals can be due to a deletion or mutation of *SRY*, rearranged Y chromosome or deletion of short arm of Y. At risk for gonadal tumors.
- *46, XX males*: In most 46,XX males, Y chromosomal sequences, such as the *SRY* gene can be detected. In those who are *SRY* negative, mutations in other genes affecting the regulation of sexual differentiation may be involved.
  1. *Clinical features*: Male phenotype, postpubertally having varying degrees of gynecomastia, small testes with azoospermia. Adult height shorter than normal males. Hypospadias present in ~10%.
  2. *Frequency*: ~1:20,000 male infants.
  3. *Diagnosis*: LH, FSH levels elevated, testosterone levels decreased.
- *Vanishing testes syndrome*
  1. 46,XY individuals with varying degrees of under-virilization.
  2. Absent or rudimentary testes. In the neonatal period, testosterone levels are low, LH, FSH levels elevated. Need to treat with exogenous testosterone therapy to induce pubertal changes. Prosthetic testes can be placed.

ABNORMAL GENITAL DIFFERENTIATION

- Disorders of phenotypic sex can be divided into *undervirilized males* and *virilized females*.

UNDERVIRILIZED MALES

Inborn Errors of Testosterone Synthesis

- Congenital adrenal hyperplasia
- See chapter on Adrenal disorders.
- Common features: All inherited as autosomal recessive trait.
- P450scc (StAR mutations)
- 3-Beta-hydroxysteroid dehydrogenase deficiency.
- 17-alpha-hydroxylase/17,20desmolase deficiency.
- 17-beta-hydroxysteroid dehydrogenase-3 deficiency.

Leydig cell hypoplasia

- Reduced number of Leydig cells or LH receptors on Leydig cells leads to decreased testosterone production.
- Testosterone levels low. LH levels elevated. FSH levels normal LH receptor gene defects have been identified.

IMPAIRED METABOLISM OF TESTOSTERONE

Steroid 5-alpha-Reductase Deficiency

- Reduced 5-alpha-reductase activity impairs conversion of testosterone to dihydrotestosterone. This leads to undervirilization. Because of a second normal 5-alpha-reductase gene, virilization occurs at the time of puberty. A large number of affected individuals are described in the Dominican Republic, Turkey, and the New Guinea Highlands.
- Elevated testosterone to dihydrotestosterone ratio before or after human chorionic gonadotropin (hCG) administration.

ANDROGEN RECEPTOR DEFECTS

- Syndromes of androgen resistance
- Range from complete androgen insensitivity with female external genitalia, absent uterus, and absent sexual hair, to partial forms of this disorder ranging from predominantly female phenotype with some virilization to a male phenotype with gynecomastia and infertility.
- In complete androgen insensitivity, usually present with inguinal hernias containing testis or with primary amenorrhea. Spontaneous breast development occurs when the gonads are not removed until after puberty. Sparse axillary and pubic hair is sometimes present.
- Gonadal tumors, including carcinoma in situ, seminomas, and germ cell tumors occur with increased frequency after puberty.
- LH and testosterone levels are elevated.
- Inheritance is X-linked recessive. Several mutations in the androgen receptor gene have been identified.

VIRILIZED FEMALES

Excessive Production of Androgens by the Fetal Adrenal

- Congenital adrenal hyperplasia
- See chapter on Adrenal disorders.
  1. 21-hydroxylase deficiency.
  2. 11-beta-hydroxylase deficiency.
  3. 3-beta-hydroxysteroid dehydrogenase deficiency.
- Main characteristics (in females): varying degrees of virilization of the external genitalia, normal internal female genitalia, ±salt wasting.
- Placental aromatase deficiency (include?)
- Maternal over-production of or exposure to androgens
- Maternal hyperandrogenism, regardless of cause, can lead to virilization of a female fetus.
- Causes include maternal congenital adrenal hyperplasia, adrenal tumors, ovarian tumors, luteomas of pregnancy, and exogenous use of androgenic hormones.

OTHER

PERSISTENT MULLERIAN DUCT SYNDROME

- Phenotypically normal males.
- Fallopian tube and uterus may be encountered during hernia repair, orchiopexy, or abdominal surgery.
- Results from failure of testes to synthesize or secrete AMH or failure to respond to AMH due to an AMH receptor defect.

MAYER-ROKITANSKY-KÜSTER-HAUSER SYNDROME

- Congenital absence of the vagina with abnormal or absent Mullerian structures.
- 1/5000 female births.
- Primary amenorrhea in a female with well-developed secondary sex characteristics.
- Absent or hypoplastic vagina, Mullerian structures range from a normal uterus to bicornuate uterus to absent uterus.
- Ovarian function usually normal.

BIBLIOGRAPHY

Frias JL, Davenport ML. Committee on Genetics and Section on Endocrinology. Health supervision for children with Turner syndrome. *Pediatrics* 2003;111:692–702.

Imperato-McGinley J, Zhu YS. Androgens and male physiology. The syndrome of 5-alpha-reductase deficiency. *Mol Cell Endocrinol* 2002;198:51–59.

MacLaughlin DT, Donahue PK. Sex determination and differentiation *N Engl J Med* 2004;350:367–378.

McPhaul MJ. Androgen receptor mutations and androgen insensitivity. *Mol Cell Endocrinol* 2002; 61–67.

71 GASTROESOPHAGEAL REFLUX

Bhanu Sunku and B U.K. Li

EPIDEMIOLOGY

- Gastroesophageal reflux (GER) is one of the most common gastrointestinal (GI) disorders affecting children. GER refers to the retrograde passage of gastric contents into the esophagus. Most episodes of GER are silent and asymptomatic. GER is especially common in healthy infants usually manifested as regurgitation (passive reflux) and vomiting (forceful reflux). When complications of GER affect quality of life, it is termed gastroesophageal reflux disease (GERD). GER affects approximately 50% of infants under 3 months of age; its prevalence peaks in 4–month olds and declines to 5–10% of 1–year olds. Little is known about the natural history or prevalence of GERD in children and adolescents (Table 71-1).

PATHOPHYSIOLOGY

- Several factors play a role in the pathogenesis of GERD including an increased frequency and duration of reflux, increased gastric acidity, delayed gastric emptying, damaged esophageal mucosal barrier, and refluxate reaching the airway. Current data indicate that the lower esophageal sphincter (LES), a tonically contracted smooth muscle at the distal end of the esophagus, undergoes transient relaxations that allow gastric contents to reach the esophagus.

CLINICAL FEATURES

- The majority of infants with GER who are otherwise thriving and growing are referred to as "happy spitters." This problem presents during the first few months of life, peaks by 4–5 months, and usually resolves by 12–24 months of age (90% by 18 months of age). Although older children and adolescents report symptomatic heartburn, infants often present more subtlety with postprandial irritability, poor growth, or respiratory involvement. Weight loss may result from both caloric loss from emesis and anorexia presumably due to an adversive conditioned response to heartburn. Some important long-term complications of GERD include peptic strictures and Barrett esophagus, precancerous metaplasia of the esophagus (Table 71-1).
- Bronchospasm and laryngospasm can result from direct aspiration of esophageal contents or via an indirect vagally-mediated reflex from esophageal irritation. Both types of GER-induced respiratory symptoms respond to acid suppression. It is important to consider GERD when evaluating infants who present with ALTE (apparent life-threatening event) and in those with refractory lower respiratory tract symptoms including asthma, bronchitis, and pneumonia; however, the presence of an abnormal pH test in a child with respiratory symptoms does not always necessarily indicate that GER is the cause of the pulmonary problems; a causal connection is best established by the cessation of symptoms in response to treatment (i.e., outcomes).

DIAGNOSIS

- A detailed history and physical examination are usually sufficient to reliably diagnose GER, begin therapy, and recognize complications. Though an

TABLE 71-1 Complications of GERD

SYSTEM	SYMPTOM
Growth	FTT, poor growth
Pain symptoms	Pain, irritability (heartburn), Sandifer syndrome (GER with torticollis)
GI symptoms	Dysphagia, feeding refusal, anemia, GI bleeding, protein loss, peptic stricture, Barrett esophagus
Respiratory symptoms	Wheezing, aspiration, pneumonia, apnea, ALTE

upper gastrointestinal series is neither specific nor sensitive for the diagnosis of GER, it is useful in identifying anatomical abnormalities in infants with persistent reflux (Table 71-2). Although esophageal pH monitoring reliably quantifies the amount of acid reflux, in most cases it is not needed to diagnose GER; however, it is useful to establish a temporal relation between silent (without vomiting) reflux and symptoms (e.g., pain, wheezing, and ALTE) and to assess response to therapy.

• Although scintigraphic (99m technetium-labeled meal) evaluation can be used to detect both pulmonary aspiration of gastric contents and to assess the rate of gastric emptying, it is not very sensitive in detecting reflux. Endoscopy with biopsy is useful to evaluate the severity of esophageal injury, document potential complications, and exclude confounding disorders. Endoscopic appearance and biopsies can identify erosions, ulcerations, strictures, and Barrett esophagus related to GERD as well as eosinophilic esophagitis, *Helicobacter pylori* infection, and Crohn disease. Eosinophilic esophagitis can mimic refractory GERD and is being identified with increasing frequency (refer to allergic bowel disease section) (Table 71-2).

TABLE 71-2 Differential Diagnosis

GI	Formula protein sensitivity, eosinophilic esophagitis/gastroenteritis, *Helicobacter pylori* infection, NSAID gastritis, inflammatory bowel disease, cyclic vomiting syndrome, anatomic obstructions (e.g., malrotation, volvulus, pyloric stenosis, intussusception, T-E fistula, annular pancreas), pancreatitis, foreign body
Neurologic	Hydrocephalus, mass lesion (brainstem glioma, medulloblastoma), Chiari malformation
Renal	Hydronephrosis, renal insufficiency
Metabolic	Urea cycle defects, amino and organic acidemias, congenital adrenal hyperplasia
Infectious	Sepsis, meningitis, otitis media, urinary tract infection, pneumonia, sinusitis
Toxic	Lead, medications, food poisoning

ABBREVIATIONS: NSAID, nonsteroidal anti-inflammatory drug; T-E, tracheo-esophageal

TREATMENT

• *Parental reassurance* is a key educational approach to inform them of the high likelihood that the complications can be controlled by measures and medications, and that the disorder will resolve with growth and maturity. Important *measures* include avoiding seated and supine positions while encouraging use of prone positioning especially in the immediate postprandial period; however, one must carefully adhere to the current American Academy of Pediatrics (AAP) recommendations to avoid the prone sleeping position because of its association with an increased incidence of sudden infant death syndrome. Thickening the formula with rice or barley cereal and decreasing the volume of each feeding can reduce the number of emeses, and may improve weight gain through increasing the caloric content. In older children and adolescents, left side down positioning during sleep and elevation of the head of the bed can help. Older children should avoid foods that lower LES tone or exacerbate symptoms including acidic foods, carbonated beverages, coffee, alcohol, and tobacco smoke. Weight reduction in obese children and fasting several hours before bedtime may also be of benefit.

• *Acid suppression therapy* is the initial pharmacologic approach because there are no effective prokinetic agents since the removal of cisapride from the market. Histamine$_2$-receptor antagonists are the first line but proton pump inhibitors provide greater acid suppression (Table 71-3). *Prokinetic agents* such as metoclopramide have not been shown to be effective. Surgery is occasionally considered for patients refractory to maximal medical management or with life-threatening complications of GERD such as failure to thrive (FTT) or aspiration pneumonias. The *Nissen fundoplication*, which involves a 360° wrap of the fundus around the distal esophagus to increase LES pressure, is the most common surgical procedure for GERD with efficacy rates ranging from 60–90%. Unfortunately,

TABLE 71-3 Treatment of GE Reflux

Education	Reassurance regarding efficacy of medication and natural history
Measures	Thickening feeds (1–2 tbsp of rice cereal/8 oz bottle), prone positioning, weight reduction, and avoidance of caffeine, tobacco in older patients
Medications	H$_2$-blockers: Ranitidine (2–3 mg/kg/dose given tid), cimetidine (10 mg/kg/dose given tid-qid), famotidine (0.5 mg/kg/dose bid) PPI: Omeprazole (1.0 mg/kg/day), lanzoprazole (15–30 mg/day) Prokinetics: Metoclopramide (0.1–0.2 mg/kg/dose qid)
Surgery	Nissen fundoplication, pyloroplasty

the surgical outcomes in those with either neurologic impairment (persistent postop retching) or pulmonary complications (breakdown of fundoplication from coughing) are poor. In situations where delayed gastric emptying contributes to the GERD, a pyloroplasty may be combined with the fundoplication (Table 71-3).

PROGNOSIS

- There is a high probability that the child's GER will resolve completely by 1–2 years of age. Because of this natural history, most children will neither require long-term medication nor surgical fundoplication. In general, GERD is a common disorder in children that can usually be managed empirically without extensive diagnostic testing, risk of serious complication, or need of surgical intervention.

BIBLIOGRAPHY

Hassall E. Wrap session: Is the Nissen slipping? Can medical treatment replace surgery for severe gastroesophageal reflux disease in children? *Am J Gastroenterol* 1995:90:1212–1220.

Hillemeier CA. Gastroesophageal reflux, diagnostic and therapeutic approaches. *Pediatr Clin North Am* 1999:43:197–212.

Orenstein SR. Management of supraesophageal complications of gastroesophageal reflux disease in infants and children. *Am J Med* 2000:108:139s–143s.

Orenstein SR, Izadnia F, Khan S. Gastroesophageal reflux disease in children. *Gastroenterol Clin North Am* 1999:28:947–969.

Rudolph CD. Probing questions: When is gastroesophageal reflux the cause of symptoms? *J Pediatr Gastroenterol Nutr* 2000:30:3–4.

Rudolph CD, et al. Guidelines for evaluation and treatment of gastroesophageal reflux in infants and children: Recommendations of the North American Society for Pediatric Gastroenterology and Nutrition. *J Pediatr Gastroenterol Nutr* 2001;32(Suppl. 2):S1–S31.

72 PEPTIC DISEASE AND *HELICOBACTER PYLORI*

Jeffrey B. Brown and B U.K. Li

- Peptic disease refers to histologic evidence of acid-peptic induced inflammation involving esophageal, gastric, or duodenal mucosa with or without ulceration.

Esophageal peptic disease has been covered elsewhere. The predominant cause of gastric and duodenal peptic disease was identified in 1983 as infection with *Helicobacter pylori*, a gram-negative, spiral, and flagellated bacterium. Secondary peptic disease can be due to many causes, including drugs or toxins (nonsteroidal anti-inflammatory drugs [NSAIDs], corticosteroids, ethanol, and ingestion of corrosives), stress (burns, head trauma, surgery, and sepsis), Crohn disease, and bile reflux. Drug, toxin, bile reflux, and stress-induced gastritis are primarily healed with acid-suppression therapy (e.g., a H_2-receptor antagonist or proton pump inhibitor) and are unlikely to recur after removal of the inciting factor. This chapter will focus on *H. pylori*-associated disease.

EPIDEMIOLOGY

- *H. pylori* infection is most often acquired in childhood, usually before 5 years of age. In developed countries, there is a 10% prevalence rate by the age of 10 years. In developing countries, two-thirds of children are infected by age 2 years with prevalence rates exceeding 80% in middle-aged adults. Infection is also clustered in families with large numbers of siblings and the practice of bed sharing. Although domestic cats and nonhuman primates can also harbor *H. pylori*, based on positive cultures from saliva, vomitus, and stool, it appears to be transmitted human-to-human, likely via fecal-oral or oral-oral routes.

PATHOPHYSIOLOGY

- *H. pylori* possess multiple features that facilitate its adaptation and colonization to the acid-peptic environment. It produces urease, an enzyme that hydrolyzes urea to form ammonia and results in an alkalinized microenvironment to protect itself against gastric acid. In addition, ammonia is directly toxic to gastric epithelium. Flagella allow penetration through the gastric mucous layer for attachment to epithelial cells via BabA, a bacterial surface adhesion molecule. Two identified toxins play a role in disease pathogenesis: the protein CagA has been associated with more virulent bacterial strains and the VacA toxin appears to enhance production of bacterial nutrients; however, the precise role these toxins play in pediatric disease is less clear. After colonization, there is a persistent cell- and humoral-mediated inflammatory response accompanied by altered acid secretory apparatus (elevated gastrin:somatostatin ratios). In many children, the infection persists into adulthood; however, there is a spontaneous clearance rate of 2% per year in children.

CLINICAL PRESENTATION

• The relationship between *H. pylori* gastritis and symptoms of recurring abdominal pain (RAP) remains controversial. Serologically-identified and histologically-confirmed *H. pylori* gastritis frequently occurs in asymptomatic children; however, those with confirmed *H. pylori* gastritis and symptoms of RAP undergoing eradication usually improve symptomatically, especially if associated with duodenal ulcer disease. Therefore, there is no clear clinical description of symptomatology in nonulcer *H. pylori* gastritis. When present, duodenal ulcer disease presents with chronic or recurrent symptoms. Episodic epigastric pain is identified in 90% of children and is the sole symptom in 55%. Pain often results in nocturnal awakening and may be accompanied by emesis (or hematemesis), melena, and rare perforation.

DIAGNOSTIC TESTING

• Due to the lack of consistent evidence linking *H. pylori* infection to recurrent abdominal pain, indications on who to evaluate are evolving. Suspected peptic disease,

failure to respond to acid suppression, and severe epigastric symptoms are indications for endoscopic evaluation. Although both invasive and noninvasive testing exist (see Table 72-1), esophagogastroduodenoscopy (EGD) is the gold standard method to confirm both the infection and mucosal injury, as well as exclude eosinophilic esophagitis and gastroenteropathy, celiac disease, and Crohn disease. Endoscopic biopsies may be subjected to rapid (within 24 hours) colorimetric urease testing. Each noninvasive method including serologic evaluation, ^{13}C-urea breath testing (UBT), *H. pylori* stool antigen (HpSA) testing, has limitations. Because of possible spontaneous clearance in children, frequent use of antibiotics, and inconsistent interlaboratory reproducibility, positive immunoglobulin G (IgG) serology does not discriminate actual from prior infection and should be interpreted cautiously. Both UBT and HpSA testing do not evaluate the extent of mucosal injury but can confirm eradication after treatment. UBT has a sensitivity and specificity greater than 90% and is best performed off antibiotics and proton pump inhibitors (PPIs) at least 4 weeks after completion of therapy. The test is based on intragastric hydrolysis of ingested ^{13}C-urea (a naturally occurring stable isotope) to labeled, expired $^{13}CO_2$. The main difficulty is collecting adequate breath samples in toddlers. Early studies on HpSA testing suggest comparable utility and sensitivity to UBT.

TABLE 72-1 Invasive and Noninvasive Testing

TEST	INDICATION	PROS	CONS
EGD (with rapid urease testing)	Initial diagnosis Collection of tissue for culture when resistant to standard antibiotics	Gold standard Assess extent of gastritis and PUD Exclusion of other disorders	Invasive Requires anesthesia High cost
^{13}C-urea breath test (UBT)	Confirmation of eradication Initial diagnosis if EGD contraindicated	Noninvasive Good sensitivity, specificity	Technically difficult in toddlers No correlation with extent of mucosal injury High cost
Hp stool antigen	Confirmation of eradication	Noninvasive Simple to perform	No correlation with extent of mucosal injury Unclear reliability in children
Serology (IgG)	None in children	Simple to perform	No discrimination between active and cleared infection Poor reproducibility in children No correlation with extent of mucosal injury

TREATMENT

• Effective therapy to eradicate *H. pylori* is available, but is not standardized. If peptic ulcer disease (PUD) is identified on EGD, triple therapy should be instituted. If *H. pylori* gastritis is identified, therapy should be offered to the family after discussing the potential long-term risks of infection, the risks of therapy, and the fact that eradication may not resolve symptoms. A triple regimen consisting of a PPI with two antibiotics is recommended to achieve eradication rates above 80% and limit development of selective antibiotic resistance. One week of dual antibiotic therapy with bid dosing maximizes compliance in children: amoxicillin with either clarithromycin or metronidazole. Because the latter two carry resistance rates of 20–50 and 4–20% in the United States, respectively, clarithromycin and metronidazole should not be used together. After therapy, eradication should be confirmed with noninvasive testing such as ^{13}C-UBT or HpSA testing. Although there is no consensus on second-line therapies in failed eradication, a repeated triple regimen for 2 weeks with a change in antibiotics is recommended before quadruple therapy with an additional antibiotic. After two failures, repeat EGD with culture of biopsies to obtain antibiotic sensitivities is recommended.

PROGNOSIS

• Eradication greatly reduces the risk of recurrent duodenal ulcer disease in adults. Because the World Health Organization has classified *H. pylori* as a type I gastric carcinogen, eradication therapy is recommended despite the unknown long-term risks of asymptomatic childhood infection. Currently, there are only four cases of mucosa-associated lymphatic tissue (MALT) lymphomas in children in the literature. Numerous clinical studies are in progress to better define this long-term risk. In adults with gastric MALT lymphomas associated with *H. pylori* (72–98%) treated with an eradication regimen, 70–80% regressed. Laboratory trials of vaccines to prevent infection are promising in animal models, and hold potential promise for future human use.

BIBLIOGRAPHY

Czinn SJ. Serodiagnosis of *Helicobacter pylori* in pediatric patients. *J Pediatr Gastroenterol Nutr* 1999;28:132–134.

Drumm B, Koletzko S, Oderda G, et al. *Helicobacter pylori* infection in children: A consensus statement. *J Pediatr Gastroenterol Nutr* 2000;30:207–213.

Rowland M, Bourke B, Drumm B. Gastritis and peptic ulcer disease. In: Walker WA, Durie PR, Hamilton JR, Walker-Smith JA, Watkins JB (eds.), *Pediatric Gastrointestinal Disease*. Hamilton, ON: BC Decker, 2000, pp. 384–404.

Sherman P, Czinn S, Drumm B, et al. *Helicobacter pylori* infection in children and adolescents: Working Group Report of the First World Congress of Pediatric Gastroenterology, Hepatology, and Nutrition. *J Pediatr Gastroenterol Nutr* 2002;35:S128–S133.

Suerbaum S, Michetti P. *Helicobacter pylori* infection. *N Engl J Med* 2002;347(15):1175–1186.

Tindberg Y, Blennow M, Granstrom M. Clinical symptoms and social factors in a cohort of children spontaneously clearing *Helicobacter pylori* infection. *Acta Pediatr* 1999;88:631–635.

73 ALLERGIC BOWEL DISEASES
Bhanu Sunku and B U.K. Li

EPIDEMIOLOGY

• Allergic gastrointestinal disease encompasses a variety of disorders including allergic colitis, milk protein-induced enteropathy, immunoglobulin E (IgE)-mediated anaphylactic reactions, eosinophilic esophagitis (EE), and gastroenteropathy (EG). Although food allergy is seen commonly in children, the prevalence has been difficult to establish due to varying definitions of food allergy-induced gastrointestinal (GI) disorders, lack of established testing, and the natural history that many outgrow their allergies with age. Prospective studies of cow's milk-induced allergy in infants have reported incidence rates varying from 1.9 to 7.5%. Among the various disorders, eosinophilic esophagitis has been the fastest rising recognized cause of allergic bowel disease.

ALLERGIC COLITIS

• Allergic colitis presents in the first 2–3 months of life with blood and mucus covering normal or loose stools in an otherwise thriving infant. This can be associated with cow's milk or soy milk formulas and even breast-feeds. Because the main differential diagnosis includes infectious colitis, bacterial cultures are indicated. Therapeutically, the formula protein can be switched to a protein-hydrolysate formula, or cow's milk protein removed from the maternal diet in breast-fed infants. If there is no response to formula protein change in 2–3 weeks, sigmoidoscopy can document the presence of eosinophilic inflammation as well as exclude other disorders.

MILK PROTEIN-INDUCED ENTEROPATHY

- Milk protein-induced enteropathy typically occurs in infants fed cow's milk formula although it has also been described in soy protein- and breast-fed infants. In the latter, transmission of maternal dietary antigens through breast milk has been conjectured. The primary symptoms of vomiting, diarrhea, and growth failure usually begin soon after birth (Table 73-1).
- Small bowel injury can present with vomiting, diarrhea, anemia, poor growth from malabsorption, and protein-losing enteropathy. Peripheral eosinophilia can be a clue, and histologic villous atrophy and intraepithelial lymphocytes help to confirm the diagnosis. A higher prevalence of atopic dermatitis has been reported. Some studies have shown that atopy can be circumvented if predisposed infants are fed breast milk or hydrolysate formulas and introduction of high-risk food antigens (milk, soy, egg, gluten, and peanut) is delayed.
- Traditional tests for allergy such as IgE-RAST (radioallergosorbent test) and skin prick testing are generally not useful in allergic bowel disorders. Avoidance of intact cow's milk protein through a switch to soy protein or protein-hydrolysate formulas is effective in the majority of infants; if successful it can obviate the need for further evaluation. Because up to 35% of infants with cow's milk sensitivity have a concomitant soy allergy, soy formulas are not always effective. Those who do not respond to hydrolysate formulas (hexapeptide) may require more complete elimination of cow's milk antigens in peptide (tripeptides) or amino acid-based formulas.
- Most affected infants will require cow's milk protein elimination for the first year of life and outgrow the intolerance by 1–2 years of age. A cow's milk protein challenge may be attempted after a year of age with appropriate monitoring in a medical setting.

EOSINOPHILIC ESOPHAGITIS AND GASTROENTEROPATHY

- EE is a distinct clinical entity with a gastroesophageal reflux disease (GERD)-like presentation whereas eosinophilic gastroenteropathy (EG) presents more like gastritis. EE is characterized by severe eosinophilic inflammation of the esophageal mucosa presumably due to multiple food allergies (Table 73-2). EG is characterized by eosinophilic infiltration of the gastric antrum, duodenum, and other distal parts of the GI tract. It is less common yet more difficult to treat than EE. EE has a bimodal distribution peaking in toddlers and teenagers.
- EE should be considered when patients with refractory "GERD" fail maximal acid suppression and have normal 24-hour pH studies. Suggestive esophageal findings include erythema and edema, furrowing, nodularity, rings, strictures, adherent white plaques, and ulcerations more commonly in the mid than distal esophagus. This is confirmed by a higher density of mucosal eosinophils ($\geq$20/hpf) compared to GERD. Unfortunately, identifying the offending food antigens can be problematic. Only some patients can identify food antigens based on symptoms but IgE-RAST and skin testing are typically normal.
- Although dietary elimination for EE can be guided by symptoms and allergy testing results, the absence of identifiable food antigens necessitates a complete elimination diet consisting of an elemental (amino acid) formula. In most cases, there is symptomatic and pathologic resolution; however, because of difficulties associated with the poor tasting formula, lack of food, and nasogastric tube feeds, some opt for short-term systemic corticosteriod therapy or medium-term topical (swallowed) steroids. In EG, systemic corticosteriod therapy is generally required but, because the effect is not sustained, it often has to be repeated.

TABLE 73-1 Symptoms and Presentation of Cow's Milk Protein Allergy

SYMPTOMS	PRESENTATION
Emesis	Anemia
Diarrhea	Hypoalbuminemia
Failure to thrive (FTT)	Protein-losing enteropathy
Abdominal distention	Atopic dermatitis
Hematochezia	
Irritability/colic	

TABLE 73-2 Symptoms and Findings of Eosinophilic Esophagitis (EE) and Eosinophilic Gastroenteropathy (EG)

SYMPTOMS	FINDINGS
Emesis (often mucoid)	Male preponderance
Nausea	Poor growth
Abdominal pain	Food allergy
Anorexia	Concurrent asthma
Allergy in first-degree relative	Peripheral eosinophilia
Dysphagia (EE)	Elevated IgE
	Esophageal stricture (EE)
	Gastric outlet obstruction (EG)
	Hypoalbuminemia (EG)
	Refractory to therapy (EG)
	Ascites (EG)
(EE): Specific for EE only	(EG): Specific for EG only

TABLE 73-3 Presentations of IgE-Mediated Food Allergy

GENERALIZED	GI	RESPIRATORY
Anaphylaxis	Vomiting	Rhinitis
Urticaria	Diarrhea	Wheezing
Orofacial edema	Malabsorption	Stridor
Atopic dermatitis	GI bleeding	Upper airway obstruction

IgE-MEDIATED ANAPHYLAXIS

• Anaphylactic reactions to food antigens can be life-threatening events. These are typically IgE-mediated reactions that cause immediate and potentially life-threatening symptoms with the most serious being upper airway obstruction (Table 73-3). Evaluation of suspected foods including common food allergens (milk, soy, egg white, peanut, shellfish, and wheat) should be tested by skin prick that carries a greater than 90% sensitivity. IgE-RAST testing may also be helpful in identifying the offending agent. In non-IgE-mediated hypersensitivities, symptoms are usually delayed. Treatment consists of eliminating the offending food from the diet and supplying the patient with injectable epinephrine for emergency use.

BIBLIOGRAPHY

Furuta GT. Clinicopathologic features of esophagitis in children. *Gastrointest Endosc Clin N Am* 2001;11(4):683–715.

Kelly KJ, et al. Eosinophilic esophagitis attributed to gastroesophageal reflux: Improvement with an amino acid-based formula. *Gastroenterology* 1995;109:1503–1512.

Orenstein SR, et al. The spectrum of pediatric eosinophilic esophagitis beyond infancy: A clinical series of 30 children. *Am J Gastroenterol* 2000;95:1422–1430.

74 DIARRHEA AND MALABSORPTION SYNDROMES

Rohit Kohli and B U.K. Li

EPIDEMIOLOGY

• Childhood diarrhea is a common but lethal problem in the United States, with 170,000 hospitalizations and up to 300 deaths a year. Worldwide it plays a central role in the vicious cycle of nutrient malabsorption, ensuing malnutrition and susceptibility to systemic infections such as measles. It is particularly problematic in infants because of their propensity to undergo acute volume and nutrient depletion during a phase of rapid somatic and brain growth. Diarrhea represents an excessive loss of fluid and electrolytes in stool and is defined quantitatively as a total daily volume exceeding 20 g/kg.

ACUTE DIARRHEA

• Acute diarrheal illnesses generally last less than 2 weeks and are caused by viral, bacterial, and parasitic infections (Table 74-1). Viral diarrheas usually produce small bowel mucosal injury that results in carbohydrate malabsorption and osmotic loss of fluids and electrolytes. In contrast, bacterial pathogens often produce toxins (e.g., cholera and verotoxins) that stimulate intestinal chloride secretion via second messenger pathways (e.g., cAMP and cGMP). In *osmotic* diarrheas, fasting eliminates the osmotic load from luminal carbohydrates and thus reduces fluid loss. In *secretory* diarrheas, fasting does not eliminate toxins that act as secretagogues and fluid loss continues unchanged (Table 74-2).

• A positive effect has been seen on both diarrhea and short-term weight gain with early refeeding of soy-based or low-lactose formulas following 6 hours of oral or parenteral rehydration. Oral probiotic and zinc supplementation have also had positive effects on recovery.

TABLE 74-1 Etiologies of Acute Diarrhea

VIRUS	BACTERIA	PROTOZOA
Rotavirus	*Shigella*	*Giardia*
Enteric adenovirus	*Salmonella*	*Cryptosporidia*
Norwalk virus	*Campylobacter*	*Entamoeba*
Calcivirus	*Yersinia*	
Astrovirus	*E. coli*	

TABLE 74-2 Osmotic vs. Secretory Diarrhea

	NORMAL	OSMOTIC	SECRETORY
Etiology		Rotavirus	Cholera
Response to IV/NPO		Stops	Persists
Stool volume mL/kg/day	5–10	20–30	>50
Stool Na⁺ (meq/L)	40	20	120
Stool K⁺ (meq/L)	80	40	10
Stool osmotic gap (mOsm/L)	40	160	20

VIRAL DIARRHEAS

• Viral-induced diarrheas are self-limited illnesses that produce watery, nonbloody diarrhea. Most are osmotic in mechanism, driven by unabsorbed luminal carbohydrates that can be detected by a high osmotic gap [stool osmolality $\approx$ 280 – (stool $[Na^+]$ + $[K^+]$) × 2; normal <50 mOsm)], positive reducing substances and a low pH ≤5.5. Rotavirus is the most common viral cause with a characteristic winter peak. Day care centers are common sources of outbreaks in toddlers and Norwalk-like viruses have been implicated in confined community outbreaks.

BACTERIAL DIARRHEAS

• Bacterial diarrheas usually cause a colitis manifested by bloody, mucousy diarrhea associated with cramping and tenesmus. Because the yield from stool cultures is often low some advocate screening with stool leukocyte smears or fecal lactoferrin assays. *Salmonella* has been associated with pet turtles and *Shigella* outbreaks with public swimming pools. The following bacteria are associated with specific foods: *Yersinia*—pork; *Campylobacter*—dairy, poultry; *E. coli* 0157:H7—ground beef; and *Salmonella*—dairy, eggs, or meat.

• Recent travel to endemic areas merits multiple samples for *Giardia*, *Cryptosporidia*, and other ova and parasites. Antibiotic use in children over a year of age should always prompt testing for *Clostridium* difficile toxin.

COMPLICATIONS

• Although dehydration is the principal complication of acute diarrhea, many other complications can occur (Table 74-3). Infants and toddlers are more susceptible because of their heightened intestinal secretory response to enterotoxins, incomplete colonic fluid reabsorption, and larger mucosal surface area relative to body fluid volume. Clinical confirmation of dehydration is made by the presence of lethargy, depressed anterior fontanel, sunken eyes,

dry mucous membranes, skin tenting, and delayed capillary refill.

CHRONIC DIARRHEAS

• Chronic or persistent diarrhea is a label applied when symptoms last longer than 4 weeks and is responsible for the largest share (c.f. acute diarrhea) of the diarrhea-associated mortality in developing countries. It is especially important in immunocompromised patients (e.g., human immunodeficiency virus/acquired immunodeficiency syndrome [HIV/AIDS] patients) who have an increased risk of chronic diarrhea from microsporidium, blastocystis, cyclospora, isospora, and the like.

ETIOLOGIES

• The etiology of chronic diarrhea changes significantly with age (Table 74-4). In early infancy, formula protein sensitivities are common causes. Congenital transport defects of amino acids (Hartnup disease), carbohydrate (glucose-galactose malabsorption), fat (lipase deficiency), and electrolytes (chloride-losing diarrhea) are rare. In toddlers, toddler's diarrhea (chronic nonspecific diarrhea of infancy) and "day care giardiasis" are common. In the school age child and adolescent, irritable bowel syndrome and acquired lactase deficiency are common whereas inflammatory bowel disease is the most serious. Acquired lactase deficiency is very common and affects 80–90% of African- and Asian-Americans as lactase activity is downregulated after weaning. Sexually active adolescents have an increased incidence of proctocolitis caused by *Campylobacter*, *Shigella*, and *Chlamydia*.

MALABSORPTION

• Malabsorptive disorders result from impaired digestion (intraluminal defects) and/or impaired absorption (mucosal defects) of nutrients (fat, carbohydrate, and proteins) that result in impaired growth. Because both

TABLE 74-3 Specific Complications of Pathogens Causing Diarrhea

ORGANISM	COMPLICATIONS
Shigella	Seizures, hemolytic anemia, meningitis, reactive arthritis
Salmonella	Sepsis, pneumonia, meningitis, osteomyelitis, cholelithiasis
Campylobacter	Meningitis, pneumonia, Guillain-Barré syndrome
Yersinia	Intussusception, peritonitis, Reiter syndrome
Enterohemorragic *E. Coli*	Hemolytic uremic syndrome, thrombotic thrombocytopenic purpura

TABLE 74-4 Etiologies of Chronic Diarrhea

INFANCY	TODDLERS	SCHOOL AGE
Cow's milk protein sensitivity	Irritable bowel syndrome	Irritable bowel syndrome
Soy protein sensitivity	Giardiasis	Acquired lactase deficiency
Congenital transport defects	Sorbitol and fructose excess	Inflammatory bowel disease
Microvillous inclusion disease	Celiac disease	Encopresis (not true diarrhea)

TABLE 74-5 Etiologies of Malabsorption

INTRALUMINAL	MUCOSAL	OTHER
Cystic fibrosis	Celiac disease	Intestinal lymphangiectasia
Schwachman-Diamond	Cow or soy milk enteropathy	Congenital Cl⁻ diarrhea
Zollinger-Ellison syndome	Crohn disease	Glucose-galactose malabsorption
Cholestatic liver disease	Microvillus inclusion disease	Hartnup (amino acid transport)

are not degraded by colonic bacteria, fat and α_1-antitrypsin are the best markers of luminal nutrient loss and endogenous (serum) protein loss, respectively. *Intraluminal defects* include insufficient secretion of pancreatic enzymes and bile salts in cholestatic disorders that lead to maldigestion and impaired emulsification of fat, respectively (Table 74-5). *Mucosal defects* include loss of surface area in celiac disease that leads to impaired nutrient absorption (Table 74-6).

ETIOLOGIES

- Based on the gene frequency in Caucasians, the most common cause of malabsorption in the United States is cystic fibrosis (CF), an *intraluminal defect*. CF constitutes 95% of pancreatic insufficiency while Schwachman-Diamond comprises 3%. The most common global *mucosal defect* is celiac disease, gluten-sensitive enteropathy, but includes rare disorders such as microvillous inclusion disease. A third mechanism includes impaired removal of dietary long-chain fats through the lymphatic system in intestinal lympangiectasia.

DIAGNOSIS

- A detailed dietary *history* is important as to age of onset, number, and character of stools, relation to dietary intake, associated symptoms (pulmonary), and growth parameters. The growth curve is the most important data and, if normal, can exclude chronic severe malabsorption.
- *Initial screening* should include a complete blood count, sedimentation rate, albumin, D-xylose absorption, and stool for ova and parasites, blood, leukocytes, fat stain

(free fatty acids or split fat = poor absorption; neutral or large droplets = poor digestion) or steatocrit, pH and reducing substances (carbohydrate). Reflecting the jejunal surface area, the D-xylose absorption requires a 1-hour serum level after an oral load 14.5 g/m² or 0.3 g/kg in 10% solution following a 4-hour fast. Pancreatic insufficiency can now be suspected based on low-serum trypsinogen and elevated fecal elastase.

- *Definitive testing* includes quantitative fat analysis, CF testing, celiac serology, and endoscopy with biopsies. The 72-hour fecal fat, expressed as the coefficient of fat absorption ($\geq$95%) = (dietary fat intake – stool fat output)/(dietary fat intake) $\times$ 100%, is difficult to complete in infants and toddlers. In CF, an abnormal quantitative sweat Cl⁻ (>60 mmol/L) can be confirmed by the Δ508 mutation on CF transmembrane conductance regulator (CFTR) gene analysis. In Shwachman syndrome, neutropenia and skeletal metaphyseal dysostoses accompany exocrine pancreatic insufficiency. The celiac serology includes the highly specific IgA class antiendomysial and antitissue transglutaminase antibodies; however, endoscopic biopsies must be performed to confirm the inflammatory loss of villi and to exclude disorders such as eosinophilic gastroenteritis. Celiac disease is an immune-mediated inflammatory response to gluten in wheat, barley, and rye and is associated with type I diabetes, Down syndrome, and other autoimmune disorders.

TABLE 74-6 Comparison of Celiac Disease and Cystic Fibrosis

CHARACTERISTIC	CELIAC	CYSTIC FIBROSIS
Defect	Mucosal	Intraluminal
Qualitative stool fat	↑ free fatty acids	↑ neutral fat
Quantitative stool fat	CFA <95%	CFA ≪95%
D-Xylose (mg%)	<20	>20
Serum trypsinogen and fecal elastase	both normal	both ↓
Sweat Cl⁻ (meq/L)	<60	≥60
Celiac antibodies	↑ anti-EMA, anti-TTG	normal
Endoscopy	flat villi, inflammation	normal

BIBLIOGRAPHY

Dennison BA. Fruit juice consumption by infants and children: A review. *J Am Coll Nutr* 1996;15(Suppl. 5):4S–11S.

Fayad IM, Hashem M, Hussein A, et al. Comparison of soy-based formulas with lactose and with sucrose in the treatment of acute diarrhea in infants. *Arch Pediatr Adolesc Med* 1999;153:675–680.

Rothbaum R. Shwachman-Diamond syndrome: report from an international conference. *J Pediatr* 2002;141:266–270.

Saavedra JM. Clinical applications of probiotics agents. *Am J Clin Nutr* 2001;73:1147S–1151S.

Santosham M, Keenan EM, Tulloch J, Broun D, Glass R. Oral rehydration therapy for diarrhea: An example of reverse transfer of technology. *Pediatrics* 1997;100:e10.

Sherman PM, Petric M, Cohen MB. Infectious gastroenterocoli-
tides in children: An update on emerging pathogens. *Pediatr
Clin North Am* 1996;43:391–407.

75 RECURRENT ABDOMINAL PAIN AND IRRITABLE BOWEL SYNDROME

B U.K. Li

RECURRENT ABDOMINAL PAIN

- Recurrent abdominal pain (RAP) is a descriptive term currently defined as three episodes of abdominal pain recurring over a 3-month period sufficiently severe to disrupt usual activities. This symptom pattern affects 10–15% of children ages 5–14 years, it is the most common chronic complaint evaluated by pediatricians. Due to the advent of endoscopic assessment of upper gastrointestinal (GI) tract and hepatobiliary tree, and radiographic evaluation of GI tract and abdominal viscera by barium contrast, ultrasound, computerized tomography, magnetic resonance imaging, and scintigraphy, the prevalence of identified underlying causes has increased sharply. In the 1960s, based on history, physical examination, complete blood counts, and urinalyses, Apley found only 5% of children to have a specific organic etiology, whereas in 1995, Hyams et al. found 33% to have an organic basis (Table 75-1).
- The majority of pediatric abdominal pain is functional rather than structural in origin. The clinical challenge is to differentiate—by history, red flags, laboratory screening, and response to empiric therapy—those with functional disorders (e.g., irritable bowel syndrome) in need of less testing from those having an organic disorder (e.g., peptic esophagitis) that requires further testing and GI consultation (Table 75-2). This challenge is compounded by the fact that the abdomen is targeted not only by GI disorders, but also by extraintestinal diseases (e.g., hydronephrosis) and psychologic stress. In addition, most children under 9 years of age localize pain to the umbilicus, wherever the actual origin, because of an undeveloped body image. In Table 75-3, specific red flags that warrant consideration of organic disorders and further testing are listed.
- The most common disorders causing epigastric pain include peptic, allergic, and infectious disorders or injuries in the upper GI tract (Table 75-4). Functional dyspepsia is defined as epigastric pain, nausea, satiety, and bloating associated with eating in the absence of laboratory findings. The most common functional disorders involving the lower abdomen include motility disorders of the colon such as constipation and irritable bowel syndrome, causing paroxysmal, midline pain, abdominal migraine is common and characterized by sudden onset/offset, stereotypical pattern (e.g., time of onset, length, symptoms) that includes nausea, pallor and lethargy, and a family history of migraine. Other underappreciated disorders causing abdominal pain include peptic disease associated with endoscopically-confirmed *H. pylori* gastritis that requires triple therapy, giardiasis associated with anorexia, nausea, vomiting, halitosis, and bloating without diarrhea in 50% of cases; and gallbladder dyskinesia diagnosed by scintigraphy (<40% emptying following cholecystokinin stimulation) characterized by right upper quadrant pain, nausea, fatty food intolerance, and a clinical response to laparoscopic cholecystectomy.
- Empiric therapy of undifferentiated recurring abdominal pain in the absence of red flags is an appropriate initial approach in both primary and tertiary care settings (Table 75-5). In the case of epigastric pain related to meals or dyspepsia, an initial 2–4-week trial of H_2-receptor antagonists is warranted. If lower abdominal or right lower quadrant pain and increased stool is detected on rectal, a trial of stool softeners or laxatives is warranted. If the pattern fulfills the criteria for irritable bowel syndrome, those with pain and/or diarrhea can be treated with antispasmodics. Suspected lactose intolerance can be treated with lactose elimination or lactase enzyme supplements.

TABLE 75-1   Rome Criteria for Functional Abdominal Pain and Irritable Bowel Syndrome

- Recurrent abdominal pain—three episodes of pain over a 3-month period, causing disruption in daily activities
- Functional abdominal pain—6 months of nearly continuous pain, little relationship to eating or defecation, some loss of daily function, and no other functional GI disorder to explain symptoms
- IBS—≥12 weeks of pain over 1 year mos plus two of three symptoms (relief by defecation, associated change in stool frequency or stool form) and no structural or metabolic abnormalities to explain symptoms.

TABLE 75-2   Clinical Features to Help Differentiate Functional from Organic Disorders

	FUNCTIONAL	ORGANIC
Age <5 years	−	+
Eccentric pain	Less likely	More likely
Nocturnal pain	Less likely	More likely
Upper abdominal pain	Dyspepsia	GE reflux disease
Lower abdominal pain	Constipation and IBS	−

TABLE 75-3 Red Flags for Organic Disease

SYMPTOMS	CONSIDER
Eccentric pain, pain that radiates to shoulder, back, side	GI and hepatobiliary and pancreatic causes
Constitutional symptoms—fever, malaise, arthralgias	Infectious, inflammatory disorders e.g., IBD
Vomiting, diarrhea	Peptic/*H. pylori*, allergic, infectious, celiac disease, IBD
Pain related to meals	Peptic disorders, allergic, GB and pancreatic disorders, IBS, lactose intolerance
Constipation, rectal bleeding	Functional constipation, IBD, intussception
Weight loss or growth failure	Celiac disease, IBD
Nocturnal occurrence	Peptic and migraine disorders
Progressive symptoms over time	Celiac disease, IBD
Family history of peptic ulcer disease	Peptic disease/*H. pylori*
Family history of inflammatory bowel disease	IBD
School absenteeism	Dysability, school phobia

ABBREVIATION: IBD, inflammatory bowel disease.

TABLE 75-4 Differential Diagnosis—Organic Causes

Dyspepsia or epigastric pain

Disorders	GERD, eosinophilic esophagitis, peptic ulcer (±*H. pylori*), giardiasis, celiac disease, Crohn, chronic hepatitis, cholecystitis, biliary dyskinesia, chronic pancreatitis
Screening tests	CBC, ESR, hepatic and pancreatic enzymes, celiac screening, IBD serology
Definitive tests	small bowel radiography, endoscopy, ultrasound, GB scintigraphy (with CCK stimulation)

Periumbilical/lower abdominal pain

Disorders	Hydronephrosis, malrotation, intussception, Crohn, ulcerative colitis, chronic appendicitis, lactose intolerance, abdominal migraine, constipation, gynecologic disorders, acute intermittent porphyria, musculoskeletal pain
Screening tests	CBC, ESR, lactose breath hydrogen, flat plate
Definitive tests	Small bowel radiography, ultrasound, computerized tomography, barium enema, colonoscopy, gynecology consult

ABBREVIATIONS: GERD, gastroesophageal reflux disease; CBC, complete blood count; ESR, erythrocyte sedimentation rate; CCK, cholecystokinin.

TABLE 75-5 Initial Therapy of Undifferentiated Abdominal Pain

POTENTIAL CAUSE	THERAPY	GOAL
Acid-peptic disorder	H_2 blockers, proton pump inhibitors	Acid suppression
Constipation	Milk of magnesia, PEG 3350	Laxation
Irritable bowel syndrome	Antispasmodics	Reduce colonic spasm
Lactose intolerance	Lactose elimination	Stop lactose malabsorption

NOTE: Do *not* treat *H. pylori* gastritis empirically.

TABLE 75-6   Therapy of Irritable Bowel Syndrome

	MEASURES	MEDICATIONS
Pain-predominant	Stress management	Antispasmodics
Diarrhea-dominant	Reduce fructose, sorbitol,	Antidiarrheals, tricyclic antidepressants, alosetron (in adult women only)
Constipation-dominant	Stool softeners, fiber	Laxatives, tegasarod (in adult women)

IRRITABLE BOWEL SYNDROME

- Based on studies by Hyams et al. (1995, 1996, 1998), half of those who present with recurrent abdominal pain meet the criteria for irritable bowel syndrome. The current pathophysiologic understanding involves a triad of triggering psychologic or physiologic stress, altered GI motility (i.e., cramping or spasm) and intensified sensation, so-called visceral hypersensitivity. There are three main patterns of irritable bowel syndrome (IBS) that are found in children including pain-, diarrhea-, constipation-predominant whereas alternating diarrhea and constipation tends to affect adults. The two most common triggers in children include psychologic stress and high-fat foods (e.g., fast foods).

- Treatment can be directed toward any part of the triad including relief of stress through use of stress management techniques or anxiolytics, reduced colonic spasm with fiber and antispasmodics, and attenuation of afferent pain transmission by tricyclic antidepressants and alosetron (Table 75-6). In infants, in whom the primary manifestation is diarrhea, so-called toddler's diarrhea or chronic nonspecific diarrhea of infancy, it is important to reduce intake of poorly absorbed sugars in fruit juices and to normalize the dietary fat and fiber content.

REFERENCES

Hyams JS, Burke G, Davis P, et al. Abdominal pain and IBS in adolescents: A community-based study. *J Pediatr* [Demonstrates the real population-based prevalence of IBS] 1996;129:220–226.

Hyams JS, Hyman PE. RAP and the biopsychosocial model of medical practice. *J Pediatr* 1998;133:473–478.

Hyams JS, Treem WR, Justinich CJ, et al. Characterization of symptoms in children with RAP: Resemblance to IBS. *J Pediatr Gastroenterol Nutr* [Delineates the overlap between RAP and IBS—outstanding article] 1995;20:209–214.

Macarthur C, Saunders N, Feldman W. *Helicobacter pylori*, gastroduodenal disease and recurrent abdominal pain in children. *JAMA* [The causal relationship between Hp abdominal pain is unclear] 1995;273:729–734.

Rasquin-Weber A, Hyman PE, Cucchiara S, et al. Childhood functional GI disorders. *Gut* [Includes Rome criteria for pediatric IBS] 1999;45(Suppl. II):II60– II68.

76 INFLAMMATORY BOWEL DISEASE

Jeffrey B. Brown and B U.K. Li

EPIDEMIOLOGY

- Inflammatory bowel disease (IBD) refers to two specific disorders, Crohn disease (CD) and ulcerative colitis (UC), but more realistically describes a continuum of chronic intestinal inflammatory disease. Although the etiology remains unclear, these disorders are thought to represent an aberrant mucosal immune response to normal enteric bacteria in genetically susceptible individuals. The majority of IBD is acquired during two periods, the mid-to-late teens and during the fourth and fifth decades of life. Relevant to pediatrics, 25% of all cases are diagnosed before 20 years of age. Males and females are evenly affected and carry a lifetime risk of 0.5% in North America and Western Europe. Although the onset of disease is rare before 5 years of age, it has been described in infants.

PATHOPHYSIOLOGY

- Although there is no Mendelian pattern of inheritance, genetics play an important role in susceptibility. IBD is clustered in families with first-degree relatives carrying a 4–20-fold increased risk of disease vs. the general population that has an absolute risk of 5–9%. Monozygotic twins carry a higher rate of concordance than do dizygotic twins. Among populations, Whites and Jews (especially Ashkenazi) have a higher prevalence than non-Whites and non-Jews, respectively.

Work in progress has identified patients carrying mutations within chromosome 16, termed the *IBD 1* locus (NOD2 gene). Finally, numerous genetically-altered animal models spontaneously develop colitis that is similar to human Crohn disease. Additional factors important to the development of IBD include the environment, luminal flora, and a dysregulated immune response. Environmental factors include the use of nonsteroidal agents that can exacerbate disease, and smoking, which increases the risk of CD while apparently acting protectively in UC. The fact that susceptible mice remain healthy in germ-free environments and only develop colitis when colonized with normal bacteria suggests that enteric flora is necessary for disease to occur. Finally, there is a sustained, chronic activation of the mucosal immune system that is a target of evolving therapies. Whether this activation results from enhanced mucosal permeability to bacterial antigens, inappropriate presentation of antigen to lymphocytes, or an aberrant T-cell response is not clear.

CLINICAL PRESENTATION

DIAGNOSTIC TESTING

- The suspicion of IBD is based on combinations of the clinical features described in Table 76-1 and laboratory findings of anemia, elevated sedimentation rate, and low albumin. The radiographic and endoscopic evaluations are necessary to evaluate macroscopic distribution, appearance of disease, and histopathologic findings.
- Infectious colitis must be ruled out prior to making a definitive diagnosis. These include bacterial and parasitic infections (e.g., *C. difficile*, *Yersinia*, *Shigella*, *Salmonella*, *Entamoeba*, and *Giardia*) as well as viral and fungal infections in the immunocompromised. Endoscopic evaluation helps to exclude other diseases such as allergic colitis, eosinophilic gastroenteropathy, vasculitis (e.g., HSP, SLE), and chronic granulomatous disease. Up to 10% of children with disease confined to the colon remain difficult to categorize and are labeled "indeterminate colitis." Even under the best diagnostic

TABLE 76-1   Comparison of Clinical Features of Ulcerative Colitis and Crohn Disease

	ULCERATIVE COLITIS	CROHN'S DISEASE
Clinical features	Diarrhea, often bloody Lower crampy abdominal pain, especially with defecation Weight loss Fever Arthralgia, arthritis Chronic anemia Anorexia Pyoderma gangrenosum	Abdominal pain, often RLQ ± palpable mass Diarrhea, can be bloody Weight loss Growth failure Fever Fatigue Perianal disease Arthralgia, arthritis Chronic anemia Anorexia Nephrolithiasis Protein-losing enteropathy Erythema nodosum
Anatomic location	Limited to the colon with nearly 100% rectal involvement	Ileal disease in two-thirds Colonic disease in two-thirds Upper GI disease in one-third
Endoscopic findings	Continuous involvement from the rectum Friable mucosa Pseudopolyps	Rectum often spared Discontinuous lesions Aphthous lesions and linear ulceration Cobblestoning
Microscopic description	Mucosal/submucosal inflammation Cryptitis with crypt abscesses Distorted crypt architecture	Transmural inflammation Distorted crypt architecture Noncaseating granulomas
Radiologic findings	Continuous involvement Loss of haustra	Segmental involvement with skip lesions Stenotic areas, ileal string sign
Complications	Perforation Toxic megacolon Sclerosing cholangitis Colon cancer	Intestinal strictures Fistulizing disease Colon cancer

ABBREVIATION: RLQ, right lower quadrant.

approach, 15% initially diagnosed as UC may be rediagnosed as CD based on the course or subsequent testing. Adjunct serologic screening currently available includes testing to detect serum antibodies pANCA, present in about 65% of UC, and ASCA, present in about 50% of CD. Because these antibodies are relatively insensitive markers that are even less reliable in children, they must be cautiously interpreted in relation to the larger clinical picture and should not be used routinely to diagnose IBD.

TREATMENT

- The treatment of IBD is complex and not standardized. The current medical therapies for IBD, their mechanism of action, indications, and side effects are summarized in Table 76-2. Good nutrition is critical to treatment and achieving optimal linear growth potential of affected adolescents. Occasionally, the severity of growth retardation and anorexia necessitates temporary parenteral nutrition. An elemental diet can be

TABLE 76-2   Current Medical Therapy of Inflammatory Bowel Disease

DRUG	MECHANISM OF ACTION	INDICATION	SIDE EFFECTS
5-aminosalicyclic acid (5-ASA) compounds (Mesalamine*)	Likely block action of prostaglandins and leukotrienes; inhibit neutrophil chemotaxis; inhibit activation of nuclear factor-κB	Induction and maintenance of mild-to-moderate UC and CD. Can be given orally or rectally for isolated left colon disease	Nausea, vomiting, anorexia, headache, fever, rash, and abdominal pain
Corticosteroids** (Prednisone)	Nonspecific, broad anti-inflammatory action	Induction therapy orally for moderate-to-severe UC and CD, or IV when ill enough to be hospitalized, followed by prescribed taper	Cushingoid appearance, obesity, growth inhibition, osteoporosis, hypertension, diabetes, cataracts
Azathioprine/6-MP	Antagonizes purine metabolism, possibly resulting in a suppressive effect on T cells	Maintenance therapy in moderate-to-severe or corticosteroid-dependent UC and CD or CD problematic in the upper GI tract	Bone marrow suppression, hepatitis, pancreatitis Blood levels can be measured
Methotrexate	Antimetabolite with nonspecific immunosuppressive T-cell effects	Maintenance therapy in moderate-to-severe or corticosteroid-dependent UC and CD or CD problematic in the upper GI tract	Bone marrow suppression, interstitial pneumonitis, hepatic fibrosis
Cyclosporin	Calcineurin inhibitor (inhibits production and release of IL-2)	Severe/fulminant colitis refractory to high-dose IV corticosteroids	Nephrotoxicity, hypertension, hirsuitism, gingival hyperplasia, seizures, infection susceptibility
Infliximab	Chimeric monoclonal antibody with anti-TNFα effects	Fistulizing or moderate-to-severe CD refractory to conventional therapy	Hypersensitivity, infection susceptibility
Antibiotics (e.g., Metronidazole)	Antibacterial or undescribed immunosuppressive effect	Bacterial overgrowth in CD; perianal CD; broad spectrum antibiotics for CD-related abscesses or with fulminant colitis	Peripheral neuropathy

ABBREVIATIONS: TNF, tumor necrosis factor; IL-2, interleukin2.
*Numerous preparations exist to enhance delivery to specific areas of the intestine and colon.
**Oral budesonide is available for isolated ileal/right colon disease with high first-pass metabolism limiting many side effects; however, long-term use may result in growth suppression similar to prednisone.

efficacious short-term therapy by itself, but compliance limits its practicality (Table 76-2).

- When initially diagnosed or during flare-ups in disease, induction therapy is necessary to bring the inflammation under rapid control and is followed by chronic maintenance therapy. Oral or parenteral high-dose corticosteroids are the most effective induction, but the myriad of side effects limits their long-term use. Mild disease may be maintained on oral or topical (enema or suppository) 5-aminosalicylate preparations and moderate-to-severe disease is currently managed by azathioprine or 6-mercaptopurine. Numerous other therapies are under investigation including probiotics, short-chain fatty acids, growth hormone, thalidomide, tacrolimus, various antibodies to interleukins, mycophenolate mofetil, and stem-cell transplantation.

- Although a detailed discussion is beyond the scope of this chapter, surgical intervention may be necessary. Ultimately, total colectomy is curative for refractory UC or in those with evidence of colonic dysplasia. Indications for resection in CD include fixed strictures, refractory fistulous tracts, and rarely fulminant colitis. Surgery is generally avoided with CD until other interventions have been exhausted due to the possibility of disease recurrence at sites proximal to the resection. In spite of this, the majority of CD patients will need some surgical intervention by 20 years of disease duration.

PROGNOSIS

- Normal quality of life, good nutritional status, optimal growth, prevention of osteoporosis, and limitation of drug-related side effects remain the goals of therapy for childhood IBD. Because development of dysplasia is rare in childhood, there is a limited role for surveillance colonoscopy until 10 years of disease duration. For UC, the lifetime risk of colon cancer after 10 years is 1–2% per patient per year. The risk in CD is lower but less clear. In addition, 2–3% of patients with UC will develop hepatic involvement with sclerosing cholangitis. Although severe cases of IBD carry the risk of significant morbidity, most children with IBD who receive and take appropriate therapy are expected to live full, productive lives.

BIBLIOGRAPHY

Griffiths AM, Buller HB. Inflammatory bowel disease. In: Walker WA, Durie PR, Hamilton JR, Walker-Smith JA, Watkins JB (eds.), *Pediatric Gastrointestinal Disease.* Hamilton, ON: BC Decker, 2000, pp. 613–651.

Markowitz J, Grancher K, Kohn N, et al. A multicenter trial of 6-mercaptopurine and prednisone in children with newly diagnosed Crohn's disease. *Gastroenterology* 2000;119: 895–902.

Podolsky DK. Inflammatory bowel disease. *N Engl J Med* 2002;347(6):417–429.

Sentongo TA, Semeao EJ, Piccoli DA, et al. Growth, body composition, and nutritional status in children and adolescents with Crohn's disease. *J Pediatr Gastroenterol Nutr* 2000;31:33–40.

Stephens MC, Shepanski MA, Mamula P, et al. Safety and steroid-sparing experience using infliximab for Crohn's disease at a pediatric inflammatory bowel disease center. *Am J Gastroenterol* 2003;98(1):104–111.

77 CONSTIPATION
Ruba Azzam and B U.K. Li

EPIDEMIOLOGY

- Functional constipation in childhood is currently defined by the Rome criteria as 12 weeks over 12 months of straining with bowel movements, hard stools, or fewer than three defecations per week (Table 77-1). As many as 10% of children are brought to medical attention because of a defecation disorder. Most suffer from functional (nonanatomic) constipation. Functional constipation is a common problem and comprises 3–5% of all visits to pediatricians and up to 25% of referrals to pediatric gastroenterologists.

PHYSIOLOGY

- Normal defecation is a complex and coordinated action involving the pelvic floor musculature, the

TABLE 77-1   Rome Criteria for Constipation

At least 12 weeks, which need not be consecutive, in the preceding 12 months, of two or more of:

Straining $>^1/_4$ of defecations
Lumpy or hard stools $>^1/_4$ of defecations
Sensation of incomplete evacuation $>^1/_4$ of defecations
Sensation of anorectal obstruction/blockage $>^1/_4$ of defecations
Manual maneuvers to facilitate $>^1/_4$ of defecations (e.g., digital evacuation, support of the pelvic floor)
<3 Defecations per week
Loose stools are not present, and there are insufficient criteria for irritable bowel syndrome (IBS).

TABLE 77-2 Key History Points

Family interpretation	What do they mean by constipation (consistency, frequency, discomfort?)
Early history	Delayed passage of meconium, age of onset of constipation (during infancy?)
Stool pattern	Frequency, diameter, and consistency of stools
Associated symptoms	Pain on defecation, soiling (encopresis), hematochezia, abdominal pain, vomiting
Toilet training pattern	Difficulties
Treatment	Diet history (fiber, fluid), response to prior medications
Psychosocial history	Birth of siblings, stressors

TABLE 77-3 History and Physical Findings in Constipation

	FUNCTIONAL CONSTIPATION	HIRSCHSPRUNG DISEASE
Delayed passage of meconium	–	+
Early onset as neonate	–	+
<1 BM/week	–	+
Large diameter stools	+	–
Withholding behavior	+	–
Associated encopresis	+	–
Abdominal mass	+/–	+
Increased sphincter tone	+	–
Narrowed rectal ampulla	–	+
Dilated vault	+	–

ABBREVIATION: BM, bowel movements.

autonomic and somatic nervous systems, and the groups of muscles comprising the internal and external anal sphincters. Although breast-fed infants are less likely to develop constipation than those fed cow milk-based formulas, their normal stool frequency can vary widely from seven per day to one every 7 days. Normal stool frequency ranges from an average of four per day during the neonatal period to two per day by 1 year of age. The normal adult range is three per day to three per week.

• Functional constipation is a clinical diagnosis that can generally be made on the basis of a typical history and an essentially normal physical examination (Table 77-2).

• A thorough physical examination, including one of the rectal vault is a key part of the initial evaluation. The abdomen is often mildly distended and a fecal mass is palpated in the left lower quadrant in 40% of children. The lumbosacral region should be assessed for myelodysplasia and sacral deformities (e.g., pilonidal dimple). A neurologic examination of deep tendon reflexes and perianal sensitivity is recommended. The perianal area should be inspected for ectopic placement of the anus, the presence of fissures, signs of perianal infection (e.g., *Candida* or *Streptococcus*), or anal trauma. A digital examination of the anorectum will assess sphincter tone, potential narrowing or dilation of the rectal vault, stool consistency and volume, and guaiac positivity of stools. A narrowed, empty rectum in the presence of a palpable fecal abdominal mass is suggestive of Hirschsprung disease (Table 77-3).

• Most patients with chronic constipation do not require laboratory investigation initially; however, an abdominal radiograph may be necessary to establish a fecal impaction in the patient who refuses a rectal examination, in the obese child whose abdominal and rectal examinations are suboptimal, or to confirm the adequacy of the prescribed cleanout.

TREATMENT

• The treatment is largely empiric rather than evidence-based. It involves education, initial disimpaction, maintenance laxation, and behavioral approaches (Table 77-4). Education involves a clear explanation of the disorder to the parents and noting that soiling usually indicates overflow leakage of stool around an impaction rather than a psychologic disturbance. Initial disimpaction is critical to the success of

TABLE 77-4 Treatment Approaches to Functional Constipation

Education: Explain mechanisms of constipation, identify its clinical manifestations, and note that soiling is rarely a willful act

Disimpaction:
Oral PEG 3350 powder: 1.5–2.0 g/kg/day for 2–4 successive days
Oral magnesium citrate: <6 years: 1–3 cc/kg/day
                  6–12 years: 100–150 cc/day
                  >12 years: 150–300 cc/day

Phosphate soda enemas
Oral or nasogastric PEG lavage: 10–40 mL/kg/hour (total 50–200 mL/kg) until stool clear

Maintenance therapy:
For anal fissures: Topical hemorrhoidal ointments or 1% hydrocortisone + stool softeners

Laxatives:

Stool softeners: Mineral oil 1–4 cc/kg Q day or bid for ages >12 months and normal swallowing
                  PEG 3350 powder 1 g/kg/day
Osmotic agents: Lactulose 1–3 cc/kg/day in divided doses
                  Milk of magnesia 1–3 cc/kg/day in 2–3 divided doses
Stimulants: Docusate or senna: ages 2–6: 2.5–7.5 cc/day
                  ages 6–12: 5–15 cc/day

maintenance therapy and may be administered either orally or rectally. Oral polyethylene glycol is better tolerated if administered with metoclopramide to enhance gastric emptying. Maintenance therapy helps to reestablish a regular bowel pattern, regain a normal colonic diameter and tone, and prevent reimpaction. It can be administered as osmotic or surface-active stool softeners, and less frequently requires stimulant laxatives.

BEHAVIORAL THERAPY

- Dietary intervention: Encourage increased consumption of water and fiber intake.
- Behavioral modification: Sit on the toilet after meals, positive reinforcement for sitting on toilet.
- For initial maintenance therapy, we most often use milk of magnesia or lactulose in infants, PEG 3350 or mineral oil in toddlers, and PEG 3350 in school-age children and adolescents. The dose is titrated according to treatment response. If the response is suboptimal on high doses, a stimulant may be added to the regimen. In order to reestablish colorectal tone and sensitivity, maintenance therapy is often required for 4–6 months.
- The child who fails to respond despite compliance with therapy requires testing to exclude organic disease (Table 77-5). A serum thyroxine/thyroid stimulating hormone (T4/TSH), electrolytes, Ca++, and celiac panel should be assayed. If all are normal, anorectal manometry or suction rectal biopsy should be performed to exclude Hirschsprung disease. If these are still negative, magnetic resonance imaging (MRI) of the spine should be considered.

TABLE 77-5 Differential Diagnosis of Constipation

Nonorganic (Functional)

Situational	Coercive toilet training, toilet phobia, school bathroom avoidance
Constitutional	Genetic predisposition
Reduced stool volume	Low fiber diet, malnutrition, dehydration

Organic

Intestinal	Hirschsprung disease, anal stenosis, anterior anal placement
Food intolerance	Cow's milk protein intolerance, celiac disease
Metabolic	Hypothyroidism, hypercalcemia, hypokalemia, cystic fibrosis
Neuromuscular	Psychomotor retardation, spinal cord lesions, static encephalopathy, visceral neuromyopathies (pseudoobstruction)
Drugs	Lead toxicity, narcotics, antidepressants, sucralfate, pure aluminum antacids, anticholinergics

BIBLIOGRAPHY

Baker SS, Liptak GS, Colletti RB, Croffie JM, DiLorenzo C, Ector W, Nurko S. Constipation in infants and children: Evaluation and treatment. A medical position statement of the North American Society for Pediatric Gastroenterology and Nutrition. *J Pediatr Gastroenterol Nutr* 1999;29:612–626.

DiLorenzo C. Childhood constipation: Finally some hard data about hard stools. *J Pediatr* 2000;136:4–7.

Hyman PE, Fleisher DR. A classification of disorders of defecation in infants and children. *Semin Gastrointest Dis* 1994;5:20–23.

Loening-Baucke V. Biofeedback training in children with functional constipation. A critical review. *Dig Dis Sci* 1996;41:65–71.

Loening-Baucke V. Encopresis and soiling. *Pediatr Clin North Am* 1996;43:279–298.

78 HIRSCHSPRUNG DISEASE
Ruba Azzam and B U.K. Li

- Hirschsprung disease, a neurocristopathy, results from the failure of craniocaudal migration of ganglion cell precursors along the gastrointestinal (GI) tract early during the first trimester of gestation. The resulting aganglionosis yields a hypercontracted segment secondary to the inhibition of the parasympathetic nerves in the myenteric plexus. These aganglionic segments have a higher content of acetylcholinesterinase and reduced amounts of nitric oxide synthase.

EPIDEMIOLOGY

- The incidence of the disease is estimated to be 1:5000 live births. The male to female ratio is 3.8:1 and there is no racial predilection. A family history is present in 7% of cases and increases to 21% for pancolonic (long-segment) involvement. Although early diagnosis in infancy occurs in 80%, short-segment (<10 cm) involvement may be recognized in adolescents in 8%. Children (3–10%) with Down syndrome carry added risk for Hirschsprung disease.

CLINICAL PRESENTATION

- Delayed passage of meconium beyond the first 48 hours of life, bilious vomiting and abdominal distension are typical neonatal presentations. Older infants and children may present with severe constipation from birth associated with growth failure, abdominal distension, and an empty ampulla on physical examination. Fecal soiling is unusual in older children with Hirschsprung (3%). Enterocolitis is a serious complication manifested by fever, abdominal distension, explosive watery diarrhea, hematochezia, and risk of colonic perforation and mortality.

DIAGNOSIS AND TREATMENT

• The barium enema is preferably performed unprepped to detect the transition zone between the contracted aganglionic segment and dilated hypertrophied colonic. Anal manometry detects approximately 95% of patients with aganglionosis. Rectal biopsy demonstrates absence of the ganglion cells in the submucosal (Meissner) and myenteric (Auerbach) plexus, hypertrophied nerve trunks, and excess mucosal acetylcholinesterase.
• The therapy of Hirschsprung disease is surgical including the Swenson, Duhamel, and Soave procedures that perform side-to-side anastomosis, excision of segment with side-to-side anastomosis, and pulling-through of ganglionated segment through the aganglionic segment.

REFERENCE

Swenson O. Hirschsprung's disease: A review. *Pediatrics* 2002;109:914–918.

79 UPPER AND LOWER TRACT GASTROINTESTINAL BLEEDING

Shikha S. Sundaram and B U.K. Li

• Gastrointestinal (GI) bleeding is an uncommon, though alarming problem in children. Clinically, GI bleeding may be subdivided into upper and lower tract bleeding.

UPPER GI TRACT HEMORRHAGE

CLINICAL PRESENTATION

• Upper GI tract hemorrhage is defined as bleeding proximal to the ligament of Trietz and typically presents with hematemesis or melena. In neonates and young infants, however, it may be manifested as bright red blood per rectum due to rapid GI transit. Several causes of upper GI bleeding are unique to the neonate, including swallowed maternal blood during birth or while nursing from a bleeding nipple (Table 79-1). Although hemorrhagic disease of the newborn has essentially been eliminated by the introduction of routine vitamin K administration, it can cause GI bleeding. Coagulopathy may also result from overwhelming infection (disseminated intravascular coagulopathy) or liver failure. Hematemesis may also be a manifestation of peptic esophagitis, cow's milk or soy protein allergy, or gastritis in the stressed or septic neonate. Although infants and children uncommonly develop gastritis and gastroduodenal ulcers to the point of bleeding, children with burns, infections, surgery, or multiorgan failure are particularly susceptible. Gastric and duodenal erosions and ulcerations can occur from *Helicobacter pylori* infection as well as drugs such as aspirin, nonsteroidal anti-inflammatory drugs (NSAIDs), or corticosteroids. Bleeding esophagitis can result from severe gastroesophageal reflux, eosinophilic esophagitis, medications, and ingestion of foreign bodies or caustic chemicals. Patients may present with hematemesis after repeated emesis or retching that leads to prolapse gastropathy (cardia herniating through the gastroesophageal [GE] junction) or a Mallory-Weiss tear. Upper GI bleeding can occasionally be the presenting sign of portal hypertension from extrahepatic portal vein thrombosis or intrahepatic cirrhosis due to entities such as biliary atresia. Finally, one must consider vascular anomalies including hemangiomas and hereditary hemorrhagic telangectasias.

TABLE 79-1 Causes of Upper GI Tract Bleeding

NEONATE	INFANTS AND CHILDREN
Swallowed maternal blood	Gastritis (stress/medication/ingestion)
Gastritis (stress/sepsis)	Esophagitis
Milk/soy protein intolerance	Gastroduodenal ulcer
Coagulation disorder	Mallory-Weiss tear
Vitamin K deficiency	Varices
Esophagitis	Intestinal duplication
Vascular anomaly	Vascular anomaly
Necrotizing enterocolitis	Varices
Gastroduodenal ulcer	Epistaxis

DIAGNOSIS

- The etiology of an upper GI bleed can often be elucidated by careful history taking, e.g., of recurrent retching and vomiting. Tachycardia is the most sensitive indicator of acute, severe blood loss in children, whereas hypotension and delayed capillary refill are late and ominous clinical signs. One should carefully exclude nasopharyngeal sources of bleeding and also look for signs of a generalized vascular disorder or chronic liver disease.

- Emesis or stool samples should be tested by Gastroccult or Hemoccult, respectively. Because of confounding red or black appearing foods, antibiotics (Omnicef, iron, and Peptobismol) and food coloring, bleeding must be confirmed chemically. A maternal source of blood can be evaluated in neonates using the Apt/Downey test. By mixing the blood with NaOH, more alkaline resistant fetal blood remains pink whereas maternal blood turns brown. Nasogastric lavage with saline should be performed to confirm the presence and assess the extent of bleeding. To assess the amount of bleeding, risk factors, and prepare for replacement, hemoglobin, platelet count, coagulation studies, type and cross for blood, urea nitrogen/creatinine, electrolytes, and tests of liver function should be performed. Standard radiologic studies are of limited utility in upper GI bleeding.

- Endoscopy is the preferred diagnostic approach to upper GI bleeding and has the added potential benefit of intervention. Occasionally, upper GI hemorrhage will require arteriography or nuclear medicine studies using radiolabeled red blood cells to identify the source of bleeding. Although these studies may be successful, they require brisk bleeding at rates of 0.5–1 mL/minute.

TREATMENT

- The initial treatment focuses on basic stabilization including adequate oxygen delivery, aggressive fluid resuscitation, and correction of anemia and coagulopathy. Adequate venous access, optimally two large bore intravenous lines, are essential to this process. Additionally, early use of empiric acid suppressive therapy is often warranted. Both ranitidine and omeprazole may be used. If variceal bleeding is suspected, one may consider visceral vasoconstrictors such as vasopressin or octreotide. Finally, endoscopy therapy using thermal probes, vasopressin therapy, sclerotherapy, or banding may be indicated. These procedures are not without risk and may result in perforation or aggravation of bleeding. Thus, surgical backup should be available.

LOWER GI TRACT HEMORRHAGE

CLINICAL PRESENTATION

- As in the case of upper GI bleeding, it is important to confirm that blood is being passed. Several foods (flavored gelatin and beets) and medications (iron, bismuth preparations, and Omnicef) may give the false appearance of bright red or melanotic blood. Bright red color indicates a more distal colonic source, black appearance a bleeding site above the ligament of Trietz, and maroon a site in between. Bright red (hematochezia), maroon, or dark black and tarry (melena) appearance can suggest either colonic (e.g., polyps), distal small bowel (e.g., Meckel diverticulum) or gastroduodenal (e.g., stress gastritis) sources of bleeding respectively. The irritant effect of blood, however, may shorten intestinal transit and allow upper tract bleeding to present as hematochezia. Bright red blood coating the outside of stool likely indicates anorectal bleeding.

DIAGNOSIS

- Causes of bleeding can be classified by age of occurrence (Table 79-2). Several causes of bleeding are unique to the neonate or young infant such as

TABLE 79-2   Causes of Lower GI Tract Bleeding by Age

NEONATE	TODDLER	SCHOOL AGE	ADOLESCENTS
Swallowed maternal blood	Anal fissure	Anal fissure	Anal fissure
Allergic colitis	Juvenile polyp	Infectious colitis	Juvenile polyp
NEC	Infectious colitis	Juvenile polyp	Infectious colitis
Coagulopathy	Intussusception	Inflammatory bowel disease	Inflammatory bowel disease
Hirschprung disease	Meckel diverticulum	Meckel diverticulum	Hemorrhoids
Upper GI bleed	Intestinal duplication	Hemolytic uremic syndrome	Vasculitis
Malrotation with volvulus	Upper GI bleed	Henoch-Schonlein Purpura	

necrotizing enterocolitis (NEC). Though typically seen in the premature infant, cases in full-term babies are well described. NEC should be suspected in neonates with grossly bloody stools, feeding intolerance, and signs of systemic instability. In the newborn, *Hirschsprung disease with enterocolitis* may present with bloody stools associated with abdominal distension, diarrhea, and fever. Because typical marked dilation above the aganglionic segment of bowel may not have developed in this age group, a barium enema can be misleading and a suction rectal biopsy is recommended. *Malrotation with midgut volvulus*, a surgical emergency, may present with melena accompanying bilious emesis and abdominal distension. Radiographs may show paucity of bowel gas and abnormal location of the jejunum on barium contrast. Swallowed maternal blood or vitamin K deficiency can present in the neonatal period with lower GI bleeding. Finally, milk protein allergy may present with blood in stools with concurrent emesis, diarrhea, or growth failure.

• Toddlers also have several unique causes of GI bleeding, some of which overlap with older children. *Anal fissures* related to constipation are the most common etiology of lower bleeding in this age group. Painless rectal bleeding in an otherwise healthy child should prompt suspicion of a polyp. *Polyps* are found in children 2–8 years of age, with a peak at 3–4 years of age. Most are solitary juvenile polyps, located in the rectosigmoid area, and carry no malignant potential. A full diagnostic colonoscopy with endoscopic polypectomy is recommended.

• The most serious cause of lower GI bleeding is an *intussusception* (telescoping), with what is often described as "currant jelly stools" because of the mixture of blood and mucus. This classic description, however, is not consistently present and more often is replaced by recurrent severe colicky abdominal pain causing children to draw up their legs. The majority of intussusceptions occurs in the ileocecal area and, in older children, can be initiated by polyps or lymphonodular hyperplasia. A diagnostic barium enema may also be therapeutic. Although a *Meckels diverticulum* is usually asymptomatic, it may present with painless, large volume, maroon-colored GI hemorrhage. Ectopic gastric mucosa in the diverticulum (a remnant of the omphalomesenteric duct), located within 100 cm of the ileocecal valve can be confirmed using a ^{99}Tc scan after H_2-receptor blockade. Once confirmed, the diverticulum is surgically excised.

• Although it may affect a child of any age, *infectious enterocolitis* is a major cause of lower GI bleeding in the school-aged child. Important bacterial pathogens are *Salmonella, Shigella, Campylobacter, Yersinia*

enterocolitica, Clostridium difficile, and *Escheria coli. Entamoeba histolytica* is the most important parasitic infection causing bloody stools. With the exception of immunocompromised hosts, viral infections do not cause grossly bloody stools. Systemic diseases may also present with lower GI bleeding in children. Patients with inflammatory bowel disease may present with diarrhea with or without blood, along with anorexia, weight loss, arthralgias, and fatigue. Hematochezia may be the initial symptom of hemolytic uremic syndrome related to *E. coli* 0157. Finally, melena or bloody diarrhea may be the presenting signs of Henoch-Schonlein purpura, with abdominal pain preceding the rash in up to 20% of cases.

DIAGNOSIS

• The diagnostic approach begins with a thorough history and physical examination, which may yield clues to the source and etiology of bleeding. Nasogastric lavage may help to rapidly differentiate upper tract from lower GI tract bleeding. Clinical symptoms such as fever, vomiting, and diarrhea may point to an infectious etiology. Systemic complaints may indicate processes such as inflammatory bowel disease or vasculitis. A complete blood count with platelets, erythrocyte sedimentation rate (ESR), blood urea nitrogen (BUN), creatinine, and urinalysis may assist in screening for systemic diseases. Stool cultures and ova and parasite examinations may identify infectious causes. Plain abdominal films looking for abnormal bowel gas patterns may suggest an obstruction. Barium contrast for intussusception or malrotation can be useful both diagnostically and therapeutically. Colonoscopy remains the preferred diagnostic modality, after a suitable bowel preparation, for maximal visualization and potential intervention.

TREATMENT

• As with upper GI bleeding, primary therapy is focused on stabilization and resuscitation of the patient. Further therapy is then directed toward the specific cause of bleeding. Treatment of constipation with stool softeners will result in resolution of bleeding related to anal fissures. In allergic colitis, protein hydrolysate formulas may resolve symptoms. Antibiotics and anti-inflammatory therapy are used for infections and inflammatory bowel diseases. Endoscopic diagnosis and removal of polyps will stop bleeding. NEC is treated with decompression, treatment of superimposed enteric infections, and may constitute a surgical emergency. Surgical intervention may be necessary to control and resolve the bleeding in diseases such as intussception, Meckel diverticulum, Hirschsprung disease, and malrotation with volvulus.

BIBLIOGRAPHY

Arain Z, Rossi TM. Gastrointestinal bleeding in children: An overview of conditions requiring non-operative management. *Semin Pediatr Surg* 1999;8:172–180.

Fox VL. Gastrointestinal bleeding in infancy and childhood. *Gastroenterol Clin North Am* 2000;29:37–66.

Hyer W, Beveridge I, Domizio P, Phillips R. Clinical management and genetics of gastrointestinal polyps in children. *J Pediatr Gastroenterol Nutr* 2000;31:469–479.

Lawrence WW, Wright JL. Causes of rectal bleeding in children. *Pediatr Rev* 2001;22:394–395.

Squires RH. Gastrointestinal bleeding. *Pediatr Rev* 1999; 20:95–101.

80 PANCREATIC DISORDERS

Ruba Azzam and B U.K. Li

- Pancreatic diseases are relatively uncommon in the pediatric age group. The three major exocrine pancreatic diseases include pancreatitis, pancreatic insufficiency, and congenital or inherited disorders.

ACUTE PANCREATITIS

- Acute pancreatitis is an acute inflammatory process of the pancreas with variable involvement of adjacent tissues and remote systems. It can be classified into mild (interstitial or edematous) or severe (necrotizing or hemorrhagic) according to the extent of local and systemic features.
- Pancreatitis results from an uncontrolled intracellular activation of pancreatic enzymes. Although the exact initiating factors remain unknown, several mechanisms have been proposed. The "common channel" theory proposes that obstruction of the ampulla of Vater leads

TABLE 80-1   Conditions Associated with Pancreatitis

SYSTEMIC DISEASES

Infections	
Bacterial	Typhoid fever, toxigenic *E. coli*, mycoplasma, leptospirosis
Viral	Mumps, coxackie b, echovirus, influenza A and B, varicella, EBV, rubeola, hepatitis A and B, rubella
Parasites	Malaria, ascariasis
Inflammatory	Collagen vascular diseases, Henoch-Schonlein purpura, hemolytic uremic syndrome, Kawasaki disease, inflammatory bowel disease
Sepsis/peritonitis/ shock	
Transplantation	
Mechanical/structural	
Trauma	Blunt injury, child abuse, ERCP
Perforation	Duodenal ulcer
Anomalies	Pancreas divisum, choledochal cyst, stenosis, other anomalies
Obstruction	Stones, parasites, tumors
Metabolic and toxic factors	Hyperlipidemia, hypercalcemia, cystic fibrosis, malnutrition (refeeding), diabetes mellitus (ketoacidosis), organic acidemia
Drugs/toxins	Valproic acid, azathioprine/6-mercaptopurine, corticosteroids, l-asparaginase, metronidazole, tetracycline, acetaminophen overdose, organophosphates

to reflux of bile and/or duodenal contents into the pancreatic ductal tree leading to intraductal flux of zymogen. Once activated, the proteolytic trypsin triggers a cascade mediated by cytokines and vasoactive peptides that lead to inflammation, necrosis, and edema, and in severe cases, extensive necrosis, hemorrhage, thrombosis, and ischemia that can spread into the peripancreatic tissues as well.

- Different from adults, acute pancreatitis in children is most commonly caused by trauma, medications, and viral infections (Table 80-1).

CLINICAL PRESENTATION

- The most frequent symptom is epigastric abdominal pain of variable intensity and duration that often radiates to the back, lower abdomen, or chest. It is frequently associated with anorexia, nausea, and vomiting aggravated by food intake. The patient appears acutely ill and uncomfortable, often curled in a knee-chest position, and may have mild jaundice, low-grade fever, and tachycardia. The abdomen may be distended with rebound tenderness and guarding localized to the upper abdomen, and bowel sounds are decreased or absent. Evidence of complications include left-sided pleural effusion, Cullen sign (bluish periumbilical discoloration), and Grey-Turner sign (bluish discoloration in the flanks) in severe necrotizing

TABLE 80-2 Lab Testing in Pancreatitis

TEST/RESULT	MECHANISM
↑ Hgb	Hemoconcentration
↑ WBC	Cytokine release
↑ Glucose	Excess glycogen release
↓ Calcium	Ca^{++} soap formation
↑ Bilirubinemia	Compression of the intrapancreatic portion of the common bile duct
↑ Alk phos and GGT	Obstruction of the biliary tree by gallstones
↓ Hypoalbuminemia	Protein loss

TABLE 80-3 Treatment of Pancreatitis

TREATMENT	GOAL
Monitor	Amylase, Hgb, glucose, electrolytes, Ca^{++}
NPO and bowel rest	Avoid food-induced (CCK and secretin) stimulation of pancreas
NG suction	When vomiting or with ileus (or sentinel loop)
Fluids and electrolytes	Avoid hypokalemia, hypocalcemia
Analgesia	Meperidine or fentanyl
Other	Restart low-fat/protein diet when pain subsides and serum amylase close to normal. Start parenteral nutrition or jejunal feedings if inadequate calories are given longer than 5 days.

(hemorrhagic) pancreatitis. In severe cases, the clinical picture may be dominated by multisystem deterioration including shock and respiratory distress.

DIAGNOSIS

- The most widely used diagnostic tests for pancreatitis are the serum amylase and lipase. The amylase rises within 2–12 hours, remains elevated for 2–5 days, and reflects the acute course of the disease. Because it is found in other tissues (salivary, intestinal, ovary), total amylase does not necessarily reflect pancreatic origin. The specificity is enhanced when the level is increased at least threefold, there is electrophoretic confirmation (P-type), or urinary amylase clearance is increased. The height of the serum level bears little relation to the severity of pancreatitis. The lipase more specifically reflects pancreatic origin but because it remains elevated for 8–14 days it may not correlate with the course of the disease (Table 80-2).
- Abdominal ultrasound is the most widely used to document increased pancreatic size and decreased pancreatic echogenicity, the more reliable sign; however, the ultrasound either may be normal or obscured by overlying bowel gas in 20–30% of cases confirmed by other studies. It may help detect cholelithiasis and bile duct obstruction. Computed tomography is the imaging method of choice to delineate the extent and severity of pancreatic inflammation, and to detect complications of acute pancreatitis (pseudocyst formation, abscesses, calcifications, duct enlargement, peripancreatic edema, peritoneal exudate, and bowel distension).
- Endoscopic retrograde cholangiopancreatography (ERCP) is warranted when children have acute pancreatitis for 1 month, recurrent pancreatitis (two or more discrete episodes of pancreatitis), and pancreatitis associated with a family history of hereditary pancreatitis, following liver transplantation and in association with cystic fibrosis. Complications of ERCP occur in fewer than 5% of pediatric patients and include transient pancreatitis, pain, cholangitis, ileus, and perforation.

TREATMENT

- The aims of medical therapy are to remove the initiating process when possible, halt the progression of the disease, relieve pain, restore homeostasis, and treat complications. The treatment is largely supportive in nature (Table 80-3).
- Many medications have been tried either in an attempt to put the pancreas to rest (H_2-blockers, atropine, glucagon, somatostatin) or to halt the progression of autodigestion (antiproteases—aprotinin and gabexate), but were of no benefit in clinical trials. The use of antibiotics is indicated only for specific treatment of a specific infection or confirmed abscess.
- Clinical improvement usually occurs in 2–4 days but approximately 15% of patients have a severe, prolonged course associated with necrotizing pancreatitis that carries a substantial mortality. The course of necrotizing pancreatitis is often prolonged and associated with complications of hemorrhage, shock, and respiratory distress. Nutritional support with either total parenteral nutrition (TPN) (IV lipids are safe) or jejunal feedings become extremely important. Currently, in most cases of biliary pancreatitis, endoscopic stone removal rather than surgery is the appropriate treatment in order that cholecystectomy can be performed electively after the acute episode resolves. Surgical indications include exploration in the face of an acute abdomen, suspected disruption of the pancreatic duct by trauma, needed debridement of necrotic tissue, and required drainage of pancreatic fluid collections (e.g., cysts or abscesses).
- Pancreatic pseudocyst is a well-recognized complication of acute pancreatitis and pancreatic trauma. It is delineated by a fibrous wall in the lesser peritoneal sac that may enlarge or extend in almost any direction. Many are asymptomatic and resolve spontaneously especially when the pseudocyst is less than 5 cm in diameter. Complications include spontaneous rupture, infection, internal hemorrhage, erosion into surrounding organs, and biliary or gastric outlet obstruction. Endoscopic, percutaneous, or surgical drainage is

indicated when the pseudocyst exceeds 6 cm in diameter and produces persistent symptoms.

CHRONIC PANCREATITIS

- Chronic pancreatitis results from continuing necrosis and inflammation leading to irreversible scarring of both the acinar and ductular cells. This repeated or ongoing injury can occur from repeated bouts of acute pancreatitis and/or necrotizing pancreatitis. Congenital pancreatic duct anomalites such as pancreas divisum found in 5–15% of the population can lead to chronic pancreatitis if not corrected. It occurs during fetal development when the dorsal and ventral pancreatic ducts fail to fuse leading to the majority of the pancreas being drained through the smaller accessory duct of Santorini rather than via the main duct of Wirsung. It is treated by endoscopic or surgical sphincteroplasty.
- Treatment is directed toward two major problems including pain and malabsorption.
- Pancreatic enzyme preparations are widely used to treat both problems. High protease content preparations appear to be more effective in the treatment of chronic pain whereas high lipase content supplements are aimed at treatment of pancreatic steatorrhea. Oral pancreatic enzymes inhibit pancreatic exocrine secretion through a negative feedback mechanism involving intraduodenal trypsin that suppresses cholecystokinin (CCK) release, inhibits pancreatic enzyme secretion, and prevents reoccurrences of acute pancreatitis.

INHERITED DISEASES OF THE PANCREAS

- Cystic fibrosis is the most common inherited cause of exocrine pancreatic insufficiency among White children. On a worldwide basis, however, acquired and reversible pancreatic dysfunction resulting from severe malnutrition is more prevalent.
- *Schwachman-Diamond syndrome* is the second most common cause of congenital pancreatic insufficiency. It is an autosomal recessive disease occurring in 1 in 10,000–20,000 live births with no sex predilection. Its main features are pancreatic insufficiency with steatorrhea and growth retardation, bone marrow dysfunction with cyclic neutropenia, thrombocytopenia and anemia, and metaphyseal dysostoses affecting the femur, tibia, and ribs. Other findings include dental defects, renal dysfunction, hepatosplenomegaly, abnormal pulmonary function, delayed puberty, and icthiosis. Pathophysiologically, there is extensive fatty replacement of pancreatic acinar tissue with normal ductular architecture.

Most but not all patients have fat maldigestion from birth but approximately 50% of patients exhibit a modest improvement in enzyme secretion with age. Pancreatic enzyme replacement therapy and fat-soluble vitamins are required for these patients.
- *Hereditary pancreatitis* is an autosomal dominant condition with 80% penetrance and variable expressivity. The gene has been recently mapped to the long arm of chromosome 7. The cationic trypsinogen gene or the pancreatic secretory trypsin inhibitor gene (PSTI or SPINK1) create an imbalance in the activation or deactivation of trypsin that allows the pancreatic enzyme cascade to proceed unchecked. In general multiple family members are affected by recurrent bouts of acute pancreatitis.

BIBLIOGRAPHY

Durie PR. Inherited causes of exocrine pancreatic dysfunction. *Can J Gastroenterol* 1997;11:145–152.

Durie PR. Pancreatic aspects of cystic fibrosis and other inherited causes of pancreatic dysfunction. *Med Clin North Am* 2000;84:609–620, ix.

Greenberger NJ. Enzymatic therapy in patients with chronic pancreatitis. *Gastroenterol Clin North Am* 1999;28:687–693.

Lerner A, Branski D, Lebenthal E. Pancreatic diseases in children. *Pediatr Clin North Am* 1996;43:125–156.

Robertson M. Pancreatitis. In: Walker WA, Durie PR, Hamilton JR, Walker-Smith JA, Watkins JB (eds.), *Pediatric Gastrointestinal Disease: Pathophysiology, Diagnosis, Management*, 3rd ed. Hamilton, ON: BC Decker, 2000, pp. 1321–1352.

Stormon MO, Durie PR. Pathophysiologic basis of exocrine pancreatic dysfunction in childhood. *J Pediatr Gastroenterol Nutr* 2002;35:8–21.

81 JAUNDICE

Shikha S. Sundaram and B U.K. Li

PATHOPHYSIOLOGY

- Jaundice results from accumulation of bilirubin pigment in skin and mucous membranes. Hemoglobin and related compounds are sequentially degraded by heme oxygenase to biliverdin, and by biliverdin reductase to bilirubin. At birth, the newborn transitions from placental excretion of bilirubin in utero to independent bilirubin conjugation by hepatocytes, excretion into the biliary system, and elimination through the gastrointestinal (GI) tract. Bilirubin is divided into two components, a direct or conjugated fraction, and an indirect or unconjugated one. A physiologic or pathologic indirect hyperbilirubinemia may result from either increased load from hemolysis or decreased removal through impaired hepatic conjugation. A direct hyperbilirubinemia, defined as a direct bilirubin greater than 1.0 mg/dL or 15% of the total bilirubin, always indicates a pathologic process. In addition, any jaundice presenting in the first day of life is always pathologic.

NEONATAL JAUNDICE

- Neonatal jaundice is observed in 60% of term and 80% of premature infants during the first week of life. Physiologic jaundice typically begins on days 2–3 of life and peaks on days 3–4 at a level of 5–6 mg/dL. This results from both increased degradation of fetal hemoglobin and inability of hepatic conjugation to meet the load. Few newborns exceed an indirect bilirubin of 12 mg/dL. In addition to physiologic jaundice, neonates may experience breast-feeding and/or breast milk jaundice that presents at the end of the first week and peaks in the 2nd to 3rd week of life. The respective mechanisms involve inadequate breast milk intake leading to dehydration and decreased fecal bilirubin excretion, and inherent breast milk substances such as nonesterified long-chain fatty acids that competitively inhibit conjugation activity (Fig. 81-1).

Differential Diagnosis and Evaluation

- The initial diagnostic approach in the neonate should begin with fractionated bilirubin levels to differentiate indirect from direct hyperbilirubinemia, especially when hepatic pathology is suspected. If either the height or timing of the bilirubin level does not fit physiologic,

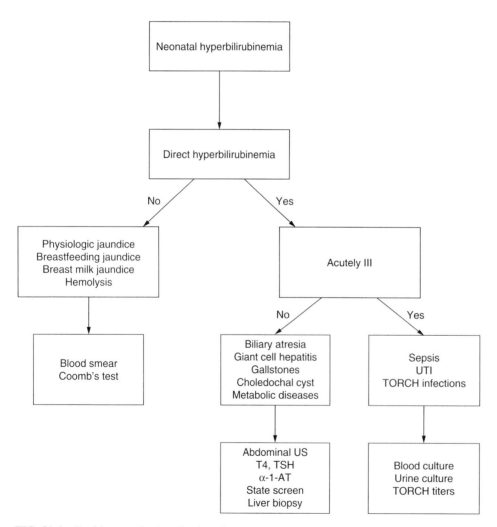

FIG. 81-1 Decision tree for jaundiced newborn.

TABLE 81-1 Differential Diagnosis of Neonatal Direct Hyperbilirubinemia

NEONATAL HEPATITIS	BILE DUCT OBSTRUCTION	METABOLIC DISORDERS	CHOLESTATIC SYNDROMES
Bacterial infection	Biliary atresia	α_1-Antitrypsin deficiency	Progressive familial intrahepatic cholestasis
Viral hepatitis (CMV, HBV)	Choledochal cyst	Galactosemia	Neonatal Dubin-Johnson syndrome
Idiopathic	Alagille syndrome	Hypothyroidism/ hypopituitarism	
Parasitic infection	Neonatal sclerosing cholangitis	Cystic fibrosis	

ABBREVIATIONS: CMV, cytomegalovirus; HBV, hepatitis B virus.

breast-feeding or breast milk jaundice, other potential causes of *indirect hyperbilirubinemia* should be considered. These include excess bilirubin load from various causes of hemolysis: (1) isoimmunization or ABO incompatibility associated with a positive Coombs test; (2) mechanical hemolysis from delayed cord clamping, twin-to-twin transfusion, bruising, or cephalohematoma associated with a negative Coombs test; and (3) inherent defects in red cell morphology such as glucose-6-phosphate dehydrogenase deficiency, pyruvate kinase deficiency, and hereditary spherocytosis or elliptocytosis (Table 81-1). Each of these causes of indirect hyperbilirubinemia can be evaluated with a Coombs test and examination of a blood smear.

- A *direct or conjugated hyperbilirubinemia* is nearly synonymous with cholestasis (impaired bile flow) and is always the result of a pathologic hepatic process. In the neonate, sepsis, urinary tract infection and intrauterine TORCH infections (toxoplasmosis, rubella, cytomegalovirus, herpes, and syphilis) can cause direct hyperbilirubinemia. Affected infants usually have other stigmata of each specific infection. The evaluation of infection should include a urinalysis, blood culture and TORCH titers.

- Giant cell hepatitis and biliary atresia are the two most common causes of direct hyperbilirubinemia and require a diagnostic liver biopsy. Early diagnosis of biliary atresia is crucial to successful surgical management (Kasai procedure). Although hepatobiliary scintigraphy has been used to differentiate biliary atresia from other causes of cholestasis, the results can be misleading. Most patients with direct hyperbilirubinemia will require a liver biopsy for definitive diagnosis. Other extrahepatic causes of biliary obstruction such as gallstones or a choledochal cyst can be detected with Doppler ultrasound screening for anatomic abnormalities. Finally, metabolic conditions that can present with direct hyperbilirubinemia include galactosemia, hypothyroidism, and α_1-antitrypsin deficiency and require a review of the newborn screen for galactosemia, free thyroxine (T4) and thyroid stimulating hormone (TSH) level, and α_1-antitrypsin level or protease inhibitor typing.

THERAPY

- Therapy of hyperbilirubinemia varies with the underlying etiology. Although physiologic jaundice is typically self-limited, high levels may require phototherapy. In full-term newborns, phototherapy is generally initiated for bilirubins greater than 15 mg/dL in the first 48 hours, 18 mg/dL at 48–72 hours, and 20 mg/dL if older than 3 days of age. Phototherapy light at its optimal blue range, 420–470 nm, converts bilirubin in the skin to an ex-cretable water soluble photoisomer. Phototherapy mistakenly used to treat a direct hyperbilirubinemia; however, may result in "bronze baby syndrome." If phototherapy is ineffective in keeping bilirubin levels below 25 mg/dL, an exchange transfusion may be warranted. The goal of these guidelines is to prevent kernicterus, the neurologic consequence (spastic athetosis) of damage from unconjugated bilirubin deposition in the basal ganglia and brain-stem nuclei.

- Breast-feeding jaundice will usually respond to increased feeding frequencies or the temporary addition of supplemental formula. In breast milk jaundice, temporary (24 hours) cessation of breast-feeding with substitution of formula will result in a rapid decline of serum bilirubin.

- An infant with direct hyperbilirubinemia should be referred early on to a pediatric gastroenterologist so that a prompt definitive diagnosis can be made and therapy can be initiated. The success of a Kasai portoenterostomy for biliary atresia depends on early surgery.

JAUNDICE IN THE OLDER CHILD AND ADOLESCENT

- Jaundice occurs much less frequently in older children and adolescents and has distinct causes from neonates.

As in neonates, it is important to distinguish between a direct and indirect hyperbilirubinemia. The most common disorder, Gilbert syndrome, is characterized by a mild indirect hyperbilirubinemia and results from a gene mutation that alters the function of uridine diphosphate (UDP)-glucuronyl transferase. Older children with an indirect hyperbilirubinemia may have a hemolytic process such as hereditary spherocytosis.

• Direct hyperbilirubinemia can result from viral hepatitis, particularly A and less commonly B or C. Metabolic diseases such as Wilson disease, cystic fibrosis, and α_1-antitrypsin deficiency may present similarly. Anatomic lesions of the biliary tree, autoimmune hepatitis, and exposure to hepatotoxic medications may also cause a direct hyperbilirubinemia. Diagnosis begins with a physical examination, fractionated bilirubin, hepatic transaminases, focused viral, autoimmune, and metabolic markers. Potential imaging tests include ultrasound, hepatobiliary iminodiacetic acid (HIDA) excretion, magnetic resonance cholangiogram (MRCP), endoscopic retrograde cholangiopancreatography (ERCP), and transhepatic cholangiography. Treatment relates to the particular etiology of jaundice.

BIBLIOGRAPHY

Bezerra JA, Balisteri WF. Cholestatic syndromes of infancy and childhood. *Semin Gastrointest Dis* 2001;12:54–65.

Dennery PA, Seidman DS, Stevenson DK. Neonatal hyperbilirubinemia. *N Engl J Med* 2001;344:581–590.

Gartner LM, Hershcel M. Jaundice and breastfeeding. *Pediatr Clin North Am* 2001;48:389–399.

Karpen SJ. Update on the etiologies and management of neonatal cholestasis. *Clin Perinatol* 2002;29:159–180.

Pashankar D, Schreiber RA. Jaundice in older children and adolescents. *Pediatr Rev* 2001;22:219–226.

82 LIVER FAILURE

Shikha S. Sundaram and B U.K. Li

EPIDEMIOLOGY

• Fulminant hepatic failure (FHF) is a rare but often fatal event in children and accounts for 10–15% of all pediatric liver transplants. It is broadly defined as accelerated failure of vital hepatic metabolic, synthetic, and excretory function within 8 weeks of the onset of clinical liver disease, e.g., acute viral hepatitis. The etiology of FHF includes viral agents, drug and toxic exposures, and metabolic conditions (Table 82-1). Acute viral hepatitis accounts for over 80% of FHF across all age groups. Drugs and toxins are the second most common etiology of FHF. Autoimmune hepatitis, though usually a chronic disease, also may cause FHF. A careful history can provide clues toward a tentative diagnosis. A history of blood exposures, travel, and risks for hepatitis A and B should be elicited.

CLINICAL PRESENTATION

• The typical patient with FHF is a previously healthy school-aged child with an unremarkable medical past who develops acute viral hepatitis. Unexpectedly, they fail to recover, and worsen to the point of severe jaundice and altered mental status. Patients may have a normal-, large-, or small-sized liver. On examination, they may demonstrate evidence of hemorrhage from the nose, needle puncture sites, and/or the gastrointestinal tract.

• Clinical findings are dominated by potential complications (Table 82-2). Progressive hepatic encephalopathy is often first noted by family members and ranges from personality changes and difficulty concentrating to unresponsiveness and frank coma. Evidence of hepatic encephalopathy requires immediate hospitalization. Ammonia, although not the sole mediator, certainly contributes to and is one marker for hepatic encephalopathy. Failure of hepatic synthesis of clotting and fibrinolytic factors with superimposed platelet dysfunction and disseminated intravascular coagulopathy

TABLE 82-1 Etiologies of Fulminant Hepatic Failure

Viral	Hepatitis A, B, non-A-G, herpesvirus, adenovirus, echovirus
Toxic	Acetaminophen, isoniazid, propylthiouricil, solvents/inhalants, mushrooms
Metabolic	Wilson disease, galactosemia, tyrosinemia, hereditary fructose intolerance
Other	Autoimmune hepatitis, severe asphyxia, malignancy, Budd-Chiari syndrome

TABLE 82-2 Symptoms, Signs, and Laboratory Findings

Symptoms	Fatigue, vomiting, jaundice, abdominal pain
Signs	±Hepatomegaly, bleeding, mental status changes
Laboratory findings	AST/ALT >1000 IU/L, hyperbilirubinemia (10–60 IU/L), prolonged PT (often >20 seconds)

ABBREVIATIONS: AST, aspartate amino transferase; ALT, amino alanine transferase; PT, prothrombin time.

impair hemostasis. Most patients experience renal insufficiency and hypoglycemia secondary to failure of hepatic gluconeogenesis. In addition to these myriad problems, abnormal hemodynamics and ventilatory compromise are universal phenomena.

DIAGNOSIS

- Hepatic necrosis is evidenced by elevated aminotransferases and profound synthetic dysfunction (i.e., prolonged prothrombin time). Serologic studies for acute viral hepatitis (A, B, and C), autoimmune disease (ANA, anti-SM, or anti-LKM), acetaminophen, iron or salicylate levels and serum copper or ceruloplasmin can help identify an etiology. Because the extent and pattern of histopathologic injury varies by etiology and correlates poorly with the degree of cerebral edema and encephalopathy, biopsy is often deferred.

TREATMENT

- Treatment is directed at the array of complications (Table 82-3). Medical support in the intensive care unit and timely referral to a transplant center are critical for patient survival. Placement of adequate arterial and venous access is required for monitoring and treatment. The risk of bleeding can be reduced by prophylactic acid suppression to prevent gastrointestinal bleeding and fresh frozen plasma to correct severe coagulopathy (PT >25 seconds). Treatment of hyperammonemia includes restriction of enteral/parenteral protein and either enteral lactulose or oral neomycin therapy. Lactulose works by acting as a cathartic to remove luminal ammonia whereas neomycin reduces bacterial ureases and proteases that produce luminal ammonia. Management of increased intracranial pressure can be

TABLE 82-3   Complications and Treatment of Fulminant Hepatic Failure

Encephalopathy	Restrict enteral/parenteral protein intake, lactulose, or neomycin
Bleeding	NG to monitor bleeding, acid suppression, FFP for PT >25 seconds
Hypoglycemia	Monitor glucose every 1–2 hours, glucose infusion at 6 mg/kg/minute
Renal insufficiency	Temporary hemodialysis/hemofiltration
Altered hemodynamics	Foley to monitor urine output, volume replacement, diuretics as needed
Acid-base disturbances	Electrolyte replacement
Respiratory failure	Ventilator support
Bacterial/fungal sepsis	Surveillance cultures, antibiotics when indicated

initiated with intravenous mannitol. Over half of patients will require temporary hemodialysis or hemofiltration support. Some will require ventilation for respiratory failure. Currently, liver transplantation is life saving for children in fulminant hepatic failure.

BIBLIOGRAPHY

Bahduri BR, Mieli-Vergani G. Fulminant hepatic failure: Pediatric aspects. *Semin Liver Dis* 1996;16:349–355.

Suchy FJ, Sokol RJ, Balistereri WF (eds.). *Liver Disease in Children*, 2nd ed. Baltimore, MD: Lippincott Williams & Wilkins, 2001.

Treem WR. Fulminant hepatic failure in children. *J Pediatr Gastroenterol Nutr* 2002;35:S33–S38.

Whitington PF, Alonso EM, Piper JB. Pediatric liver transplantation. *Semin Liver Dis* 1994;14:303–317.

Section 11
GENETIC DISEASES

Barbara K. Burton, Section Editor

83 CHROMOSOME ABNORMALITIES

Barbara K. Burton

DOWN SYNDROME

- Down syndrome or trisomy 21 is the most common chromosome anomaly in live-born infants, occurring in approximately 1 in every 800 births. It affects all racial and ethnic populations. The clinical diagnosis can usually be made shortly after birth by identification of a combination of the following features most likely to be present in the neonate:
  1. Hypotonia, poor Moro reflex.
  2. Excess skin folds on the nape of the neck.
  3. Small and anomalous auricles.
  4. Short or incurving fifth fingers, altered palmar creases.
  5. Hyperextensible joints.
- Definitive diagnosis is established by chromosome analysis on a peripheral blood sample.
- Additional significant clinical features include the following:
  1. Congenital heart disease (atrioventricular [AV] canal and ventricular septal defect [VSD] are the most common defects) in 40%.
  2. Mental retardation in 100%.
  3. Hearing loss in 60%.
  4. Refractive errors, strabismus, nystagmus, or cataracts in 70%.
- Many other major anomalies such as duodenal atresia and Hirschsprung disease occur with increased frequency in the neonate. The natural history of the disorder is that muscle tone improves with age while the rate of development slows with age. Growth is relatively slow and short stature is a feature of the disorder. Thyroid disease and leukemia occur with increased frequency during childhood. Early onset Alzheimer disease is common in the adult. All patients with Down syndrome should be enrolled in early intervention programs. In addition, the American Academy of Pediatrics has published guidelines for the health supervision of children with Down syndrome that address their special needs. Ninety-four percent of patients with Down syndrome have standard trisomy 21 with 47 chromosomes. This abnormality results from nondisjunction during meiosis and occurs with increasing frequency with advanced maternal age. When this is observed, it is not necessary to obtain parental chromosome analysis. Empiric data indicate that parents of a child with standard trisomy 21 face a recurrence risk of approximately 1% in future pregnancies of having another affected child. Prenatal diagnosis should be offered. Approximately 5% of patients with Down syndrome have a translocation involving the number 21 chromosome. In such cases, the infant has only 46 chromosomes but has the equivalent of 47 chromosomes since one of these chromosomes is a translocation chromosome involving the number 21 chromosome attached to another chromosome—either a D group (number 13, 14, or 15) or another G group (number 21 or 22) chromosome. When such a translocation is observed in an infant, the parents' chromosomes must be studied since the abnormality may have occurred either de novo or as a result of inheritance from a parent who is a balanced translocation carrier. If a parent is found to be a carrier, the risk of recurrence of Down syndrome will be substantially higher than in the case of standard trisomy 21 and will depend on the type of translocation and which parent is the carrier. In less than 1% of cases of Down

syndrome, mosaicism will be identified, meaning that some cells have a normal chromosomal makeup while others have the extra chromosome. The clinical findings in these rare cases may vary from near normal to indistinguishable from those in nonmosaic Down syndrome.

TRISOMY 13

- Trisomy 13 is a severe pattern of multiple malformations occurring with an incidence of approximately 1 in 5000 births. It is usually suspected at birth in an infant who exhibits a number of the following characteristic clinical features:
  1. Microcephaly
  2. Microphthalmia, anophthalmia, colobomas, or other ocular anomalies
  3. Cleft lip and/or palate
  4. Scalp defects
  5. Polydactyly
  6. Cryptorchidism
- In addition, there may be evidence of congenital heart disease which is present in 80% of affected infants. A significant number of affected infants have holoprosencephaly which is associated with a very characteristic facial appearance including findings such as cyclopia, in its most severe form, and median cleft lip, in its mildest form. A wide variety of other major anomalies including omphalocele and spina bifida may be observed. The prognosis is extremely poor with 80% of affected infants dying within the first month of life, most of these within the first week, regardless of medical intervention. It is generally agreed that aggressive medical therapy is not warranted. Very few affected infants survive beyond 1 year of age and all exhibit severe mental retardation and growth restriction.
- The diagnosis of trisomy 13 is confirmed by chromosome analysis on peripheral blood. Most cases result from nondisjunction during meiosis and occur with increased frequency with advanced maternal age. In such cases the recurrence risk is 1% in future pregnancies. Translocation cases do occur. The genetic principles are the same in these cases as for Down syndrome. See the discussion of that disorder for further information.

TRISOMY 18

- Trisomy 18 is a severe multiple malformation syndrome occurring with an estimated incidence of 1 in 6000 births. It is usually suspected at birth on the basis of a constellation of typical minor dysmorphic features in conjunction with intrauterine growth retardation and an abnormal neurologic examination. Specific findings include the following:
  1. Prominent occiput, short palpebral fissures, small mouth, malformed ears, micrognathia.
  2. Clenched hands with tendency of fingers to overlap, absence of distal flexion creases.
  3. Hypoplasia of nails, especially on fifth fingers and toes, rocker bottom feet.
  4. Short sternum, small pelvis with limited hip abduction.
- In addition to these obvious findings, there is usually evidence of congenital heart disease which is present in over 90% of affected infants. A wide variety of other major anomalies may also be observed. A poor suck, a weak cry, and abnormal muscle tone are often noted. Apneic episodes may occur. The prognosis for survival is extremely poor. Over 90% of affected infants die during the first year of life with most of these deaths occurring during the first 3 months. Some of the deaths are the result of cardiac defects but many are the result of poor neurologic control of normal functions. It is generally agreed that aggressive medical intervention is not warranted for this disorder since it does not alter the outcome. Those few patients who do survive beyond the first year of life are uniformly severely mentally and physically handicapped.
- The diagnosis of trisomy 18 is confirmed by chromosome analysis on a peripheral blood sample. Most cases are associated with 47 chromosomes in the infant and result from a nondisjunctional accident with an increasing incidence with advanced maternal age. Parental chromosome analysis is not necessary in such cases. Parents face a recurrence risk of 1% and should be offered prenatal diagnosis. Translocation cases do occur and the same principles apply as for Down syndrome. See the discussion of that disorder for more details.

TURNER SYNDROME

- Turner syndrome is a sex chromosome anomaly occurring in approximately 1 in every 2000 live-born females. Characteristic clinical findings are as follows:
  1. Short stature
  2. Normal intelligence although specific neuropsychologic deficits are demonstrable on testing, most notably problems with visual-spatial organization.
  3. Ovarian dysgenesis with lack of estrogen production and infertility.

4. Congenital lymphedema with puffy hands and feet.
5. Widely spaced nipples, mild pectus excavatum.
6. Webbed neck, low posterior hairline.
7. Prominent and/or posteriorly rotated ears.
8. Minor renal anomalies, such as horseshoe kidney.
9. Bicuspid aortic valve (30–50%), coarctation of aorta (10%), aortic aneurysm, and dissection in adult life.

• The diagnosis is confirmed by chromosome analysis on peripheral blood. Only about 50–55% of patients with the Turner phenotype have the typical 45,X chromosome makeup. This chromosome abnormality occurs sporadically and is not related to advanced maternal age. The remaining patients are mosaic with a 45,X cell line and a second cell line that is widely variable. The second cell line most commonly contains either two normal X chromosomes or one normal X chromosome and a second structurally abnormal X chromosome such as an isochromosome of the long arm of the X. These karyotypes are designated as 45,X/46,XX and 45,X/46,X,i(Xq). In some cases, a second cell line with a 46,XY complement will be identified. In these cases, the streak gonads must be surgically removed because of the risk of development of gonadoblastoma.

• Treatment of Turner syndrome includes growth hormone treatment for short stature, estrogen replacement therapy for development and maintenance of secondary sexual characteristics, and treatment of congenital heart defects or any other associated anomalies. The American Academy of Pediatrics has published guidelines for the health supervision of children with Turner syndrome that address all of their special health care needs.

KLINEFELTER SYNDROME

• Klinefelter syndrome is a sex chromosome anomaly occurring in approximately 1 in 500 newborn males. Unless the mother has had prenatal diagnosis because of advanced maternal age, the diagnosis is rarely established in the infant or young child. Characteristic clinical findings are as follows:
1. Mean IQ of 85–90 with a wide range from well below normal to well above. Learning disabilities are common. The majority of affected children require some help in school, especially in reading and spelling. Many are able to graduate from college.
2. Height ranging from 25th to 99th percentile with mean at the 75th percentile. There is a tendency to develop a long lean body build with long limbs.

3. Small penis and testes in childhood with the testes remaining small even after puberty. Testosterone production is inadequate and infertility is the rule. Virilization is partial and gynecomastia occurs in about one-third of affected individuals.

• The diagnosis of Klinefelter syndrome is made by chromosome analysis which reveals a 47,XXY karyotype. Treatment includes special education when appropriate and testosterone replacement therapy which promotes normal development of secondary sexual characteristics and normal sexual functioning.

84 SUBMICROSCOPIC CHROMOSOME ANOMALIES (CONTIGUOUS GENE SYNDROMES)

Barbara K. Burton

22q11 DELETION SYNDROME

• The 22q11 deletion syndrome is a recently recognized disorder that has emerged as one of the most common multiple malformation syndromes in pediatrics. It affects at least 1 in every 4000 individuals although the true incidence may be much higher since it is likely that many cases go undiagnosed. The disorder results from a submicroscopic deletion of chromosome 22 detectable in 95% of cases only by fluorescence in situ hybridization (FISH). Characteristic clinical findings include the following:
1. Cardiac defects, most commonly tetralogy of Fallot, interrupted aortic arch, ventricular septal defect (VSD), truncus arteriosus, vascular ring.
2. Altered facial features, such as hooded eyelids, overfolded or protruding ears, a bulbous or prominent nose.
3. Thymic hypoplasia with immune deficiencies.
4. Cleft palate or velopharyngeal insufficiency with hypernasal speech.
5. Hypocalcemia

• The first letters of the above features led initially to the use of the term CATCH-22 to describe the disorder. Certainly any child with one or more of these findings should be tested for the 22q11 deletion; however, it is now clear that there are many more features that may be associated with this deletion. Common ones are listed below

1. Renal anomalies
2. Learning disabilities or mild mental retardation.
3. Short stature with or without growth hormone deficiency.
4. Juvenile rheumatoid arthritis, which is 150 times more common than in the general population.

• The diagnosis of the 22q11 deletion syndrome is established by chromosome analysis with FISH testing using the specific probe for this disorder. In 94% of cases, the disorder occurs de novo in an affected child. In the remaining 6%, it is inherited from an affected parent. Because of the extreme variability observed in clinical manifestations, a parent can be affected with no obvious findings. FISH testing should be performed on the parents of an affected child before concluding that the condition has occurred de novo in any particular case.

WILLIAMS SYNDROME

• Williams syndrome is a contiguous gene syndrome occurring in approximately 1 in every 20,000 infants. The characteristic clinical features are as follows:
1. Cardiovascular disease (elastin arteriopathy). Supravalvular aortic stenosis is the most common cardiovascular lesion and may be progressive. Other vascular stenoses are also observed including peripheral pulmonic stenosis, renal artery stenosis with hypertension, cerebral artery stenoses which may result in stroke, and mesenteric artery stenosis which may cause abdominal pain.
2. Distinctive facies with wide nasal bridge, periorbital puffiness, short nose, stellate iris pattern, long philtrum, and full lips.
3. Short stature
4. Mental retardation, variable in degree, with occasional patients having a low normal IQ.
5. Connective tissue abnormalities such as hernias, bowel/bladder diverticulae, rectal prolapse, and joint laxity.
6. Hypercalcemia and hypercalciuria.
7. Unique cognitive profile with strengths in auditory rote memory and language and extreme weakness in visuospatial construction, independent of IQ.

• The diagnosis of Williams syndrome (WS) is established by FISH using a probe for the WS critical region on chromosome 7. The cardiovascular features of the disorder are the result of deletion of the elastin gene which is located in this region. Additional features of the disorder are thought to result from deletion of additional contiguous genes. In almost all cases, the deletion occurs de novo and recurrence risks are low (1%) after one affected child.

85 AMINO ACID AND ORGANIC ACID

Barbara K. Burton and Joel Charrow

PHENYLKETONURIA

• Classic phenylketonuria (PKU) is among the most common of the inborn errors of metabolism. It occurs in all populations but is most common in Caucasians of western European descent in whom it occurs in approximately 1 in 10,000 births. This autosomal recessive disorder results from a deficiency of the enzyme phenylalanine hydroxylase which is responsible for the conversion of the essential amino acid phenylalanine to tyrosine. Left untreated, patients with PKU develop severe mental retardation, acquired microcephaly, and neurologic symptoms such as hypertonicity, irritability, tremors, hyperactivity, and seizures. Eczema is common and a characteristic mousey odor is present. Skin and hair pigmentation is lighter than that of other family members as a result of insufficient tyrosine for conversion to melanin. Fortunately, these clinical features of PKU are now rarely encountered since the United States and most developed countries include PKU in newborn screening programs and affected infants are diagnosed and treated shortly after birth. The elevated phenylalanine levels experienced by affected infants in the neonatal period are not associated with any clinical symptoms. By the time clinical symptoms such as developmental delay have become apparent, irreversible brain damage has already occurred.

• Not all infants who have an elevated phenylalanine level on newborn screening will be found to have classical PKU. There are milder variants of phenylalanine hydroxylase deficiency that result in less impairment of the normal ability to convert phenylalanine to tyrosine. Patients with these variants are said to have mild or atypical PKU or hyperphenylalaninemia. In addition, a very small number of patients are found to have a defect in the synthesis of tetrahydrobiopterin, a cofactor essential for the phenylalanine hydroxylase reaction.

• Treatment of PKU in the newborn involves the use of a phenylalanine free formula supplemented with prescribed amounts of either breast milk or standard infant formula to provide the infant's requirement for phenylalanine. For optimal outcome, treatment should be initiated within 7–10 days of birth. As the children get older, most of their nutrition comes from the medical food or formula which contains all amino acids except phenylalanine. The diet is very restrictive with no meat or dairy products, no commercial baked goods or pasta, and only measured amounts of fruits and vegetables to provide a prescribed intake of phenylalanine. Patients with PKU must be followed in a metabolic clinic with a nutritionist skilled in the management of PKU. Blood phenylalanine levels should be monitored once a week during the first year and biweekly after that. Frequent diet adjustments are necessary depending on the blood levels. Dietary treatment is continued for life.

- A special problem unique to PKU is that of maternal phenylketonuria. During the 1960s and 1970s, dietary treatment for PKU was typically discontinued at the age of about 6 years. Later evidence revealed that many patients who discontinued dietary therapy experienced loss of IQ points, and changes on neuroimaging. Nonetheless, there were many patients off treatment who were unwilling or unable to resume dietary treatment when advised of this information. As adult women with PKU began having children, it became apparent that high blood phenylalanine levels in the mother were extremely toxic to the fetus. Indeed, the woman with classical PKU who has blood phenylalanine levels in the untreated range has close to a 100% chance of having an infant with mental retardation. Other typical findings associated with the maternal PKU syndrome include microcephaly, intrauterine growth retardation, and congenital heart disease. A wide variety of other congenital malformations can also be observed. It is critically important that girls and women with PKU be counseled to avoid unplanned pregnancies. Blood phenylalanine levels must be very tightly controlled prior to pregnancy and very carefully monitored during pregnancy to assure the best outcome.

HOMOCYSTINURIA

- Excess production of homocysteine and its derivative disulfide, homocystine (denoted together as homocyst(e)ine), occurs in a number of disorders, including vitamin B_{12} deficiency and several inborn errors of metabolism. Cystathionine β-synthase (CBS) deficiency is the most common of the inherited homocystinurias, and demonstrates a characteristic phenotype and laboratory picture.
- CBS deficiency does not cause acute metabolic decompensation, but rather, the chronic hyperhomocyst(e)inemia causes mental retardation, long limbs, osteoporosis, ectopia lentis (with the lenses dislocated downward), and hypercoagulability. Both arterial and venous thrombosis are major causes of long-term morbidity and mortality. Diagnosis is confirmed by detection of excessive homocystine in the urine and blood, associated with a low or undetectable cystathionine and cystine, and elevated methionine in plasma.

- Approximately 50% of patients with CBS deficiency are responsive to pyridoxine, with significant reduction in plasma homocyst(e)ine concentrations following administration of pharmacologic doses. Patients who are not pyridoxine-responsive can be treated with a methionine restricted diet, if the diagnosis is made in the newborn period. After this time, acceptance of the synthetic formula is very poor. Older infants and children with pyridoxine-non-responsive CBS deficiency may be treated with a generalized protein restriction and supplementation with betaine, a methyl donor which increases the remethylation of homocysteine to methionine. If the plasma total homocyst(e)ine concentration can be maintained below 50 µM the incidence of thrombotic events and the other morbidities of the disease are greatly reduced.
- CBS deficiency is an autosomal recessive disorder, with an estimated incidence of 1:200,000–1:335,000. Prenatal diagnosis is possible. Many state newborn screening programs detect CBS deficiency by measurement of elevated methionine levels.

UREA CYCLE DISORDERS

- Infants with complete defects in one of the urea cycle enzymes present in the neonatal period with hyperammonemic encephalopathy. They are normal at birth but after a period of 1–5 days develop symptoms of poor feeding and lethargy, often accompanied by hyperventilation. Sepsis is usually considered to be the likely diagnosis. Initial blood gas measurements typically reveal a respiratory alkalosis. If hyperammonemia is not promptly diagnosed and appropriately treated, lethargy progresses to coma with increased intracranial pressure, seizures, and death. Blood ammonia levels may reach levels higher than 1000 (normal <35). Since the signs and symptoms are similar, a blood ammonia determination should be obtained on any full-term infant, without risk factors, who is being evaluated for sepsis. Significant hyperammonemia represents a medical emergency in the neonate and the differential diagnosis is a limited one. It is illustrated is Fig. 85-1. Although urea cycle disorders are a major cause, organic acidemias and transient hyperammonemia of the newborn can give rise to equally dramatic elevations of the blood ammonia level. In patients with partial urea cycle enzyme deficiencies, the first recognized clinical episode may be delayed for months or years. The hyperammonemia observed in

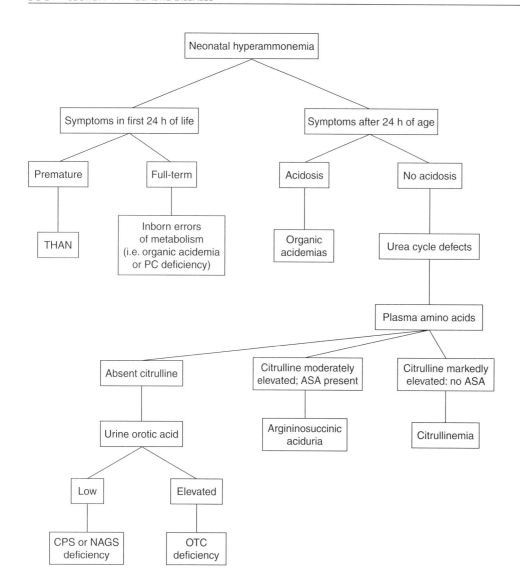

FIG. 85-1 Neonatal hyperammonemia. THAN: transient hyperammonemia of the newborn; PC: pyruvate carboxylase; ASA: argininosuccinic acid; CPS: carbamyl phosphate synthetase; NAGS: *N*-acetyl glutamate synthetase.

older children is typically less severe and the symptoms are more subtle. They may include cyclic vomiting, lethargy, mental status changes, behavioral abnormalities, and hallucinations. The differential diagnosis may include drug intoxication, encephalitis, or a wide range of other neurologic conditions.

• The five major urea cycle disorders likely to be encountered by the pediatrician are *N*-acetyl glutamate synthetase (NAGS) deficiency, carbamyl phosphate synthetase (CPS) deficiency, ornithine transcarbamylase (OTC) deficiency, citrullinemia, and argininosuccinic aciduria. The combined incidence of these disorders is estimated to be about 1 in 30,000 births. OTC deficiency, by far the most common of the group, is an X-linked defect, while the others are inherited in an autosomal recessive pattern. A sixth disorder,

argininemia, is extremely rare and is associated with different symptoms than the other disorders, typically progressive spastic diplegia.

• A urea cycle defect should be suspected when an elevated plasma ammonia level is identified in conjunction with appropriate clinical symptoms. Plasma amino acid analysis will establish the diagnosis of citrullinemia and argininosuccinic aciduria, and will be helpful in the diagnosis of the other two conditions by demonstrating absent or markedly reduced plasma citrulline. Urine orotic acid will be elevated in OTC deficiency. Urine organic acid analysis will rule out organic acid disorders that also lead to significant neonatal hyperammonemia. Liver biopsy may ultimately be necessary in some patients to measure activity of CPS and OTC and establish a definitive diagnosis.

• The treatment of the acutely ill infant with hyperammonemia involves removal of ammonia as quickly as possible. This is best achieved by hemodialysis. Therefore, such infants should be transferred as quickly as possible to a level III neonatal unit with hemodialysis facilities. Protein feedings should be discontinued. Intravenous glucose and fluids should be administered. Long-term management involves dietary therapy with reduced protein intake, treatment with pharmacologic agents that promote nitrogen excretion (ammonia scavengers), and consideration of liver transplantation for patients who have severe CPS or OTC deficiency or who have recurrent symptomatic hyperammonemic episodes despite optimal medical management.

MAPLE SYRUP URINE DISEASE (MSUD; BRANCHED-CHAIN KETOACIDURIA)

• Infants with this disorder typically appear normal at birth, but develop a poor suck and become increasingly disinterested in feeding and lethargic by 4–7 days of life. Onset of symptoms may be delayed in breast-fed infants. If untreated, a progressively downhill course ensues, often culminating in brain edema, seizures, respiratory failure, coma, and death. Untreated survivors are neurologically abnormal, fail to thrive, and typically die in the early months of life from recurrent metabolic crises. Because the initial symptoms are often mistaken as signs of sepsis, definitive diagnosis and treatment may be delayed by failing to recognize the characteristic progression of signs, and the development of an anion-gap acidosis, in a hemodynamically stable infant.

• The diagnosis is often apparent from the maple syrup-like odor of the urine. It is confirmed by demonstrating elevated levels of the branched-chain amino acids leucine, isoleucine, and valine (and the isoleucine derivative alloisoleucine, which is normally undetectable) in plasma or urine.

• Only very small amounts of branched-chain amino acids can be tolerated, and normal infant feeding results in a rapid rise in plasma and brain leucine levels, and leucine toxicity in the brain. Feeding subsequently decreases, catabolism ensues, and the use of endogenous protein stores as a source of energy results in the release of more branched-chain amino acids. Treatment, therefore, involves reversal of the catabolic state by administration of intravenous fluids containing at least 10% dextrose, administration of a lipid emulsion for additional calories, and withholding protein. Hemodialysis is occasionally required to accelerate the clearance of leucine. When the leucine level begins to approach normal, feedings may be reintroduced, using a combination of normal infant formula and a synthetic formula which contains no branched-chain amino acids. The tolerance for natural sources of protein is severely limited, and individuals consume a protein-restricted vegetarian diet, supplemented with a synthetic formula to provide additional amino acids.

• Permanent brain injury and mental retardation are common sequelae of the initial episode of brain edema; however, these may be preventable through early institution of therapy, presumptive or presymptomatic treatment in siblings and prenatally diagnosed cases, and strict adherence to the modified diet, guided by frequent monitoring of plasma amino acid levels.

• MSUD is an autosomal recessive disorder affecting approximately 1 in 185,000 newborns. It is unusually common among the Old Order Mennonites living in Lancaster and Lebanon Counties, Pennsylvania, where the incidence is 1:176. Several variant forms are known, including an intermediate form, an intermittent form, and a thiamine responsive form. Prenatal diagnosis is possible. Many state newborn screening programs detect MSUD through measurement of elevated leucine levels.

ORGANIC ACIDEMIAS AND OTHER INBORN ERRORS OF METABOLISM ASSOCIATED WITH METABOLIC ACIDOSIS

• Methylmalonic acidemia and propionic acidemia are the most common disorders and will be summarized here; others include isovaleric acidemia, 3-methylcrotonyl-CoA carboxylase deficiency, 3-hydroxy-3-methylglutaryl-CoA lyase deficiency, glutaric aciduria, and many others.

• Children with these disorders typically are normal at birth, but in the first few days of life develop profound ketoacidosis, lethargy, refusal to feed, vomiting, and hypotonia. Hyperammonemia and/or leukopenia and thrombocytopenia are found in some infants, and may be severe. Plasma lactate may be elevated. Affected infants are often thought to be septic, despite the profound ketoacidosis and increased anion gap. Infants who survive the initial episode subsequently fail to thrive and experience repeated episodes of metabolic crisis.

• The diagnosis of an organic acid disorder should be suspected in any infant who presents with severe metabolic acidosis accompanied by an increased anion gap. In propionic, methylmalonic, and many other organic acidemias, ketosis is also present. The diagnosis is usually based on identifying the tell-tale metabolite by organic acid analysis of the urine. Confirmation is based on demonstration of the enzyme deficiency in an appropriate tissue, most often cultured skin fibroblasts.

- As with maple syrup urine disease, reversal of the catabolic state is of paramount importance, and can be achieved by administration of intravenous fluids containing 10% dextrose and lipid emulsion. Protein intake should be severely restricted until the diagnosis is made and the acidosis controlled. Administration of alkali will help neutralize the acidosis; peritoneal or hemodialysis are occasionally required. Since secondary carnitine deficiency is common, administration of intravenous L-carnitine (after obtaining blood for measurement of carnitine concentration) is often helpful. Definitive dietary treatment involves restriction of the precursor amino acids, usually achieved by a very low protein (vegetarian) diet supplemented with a formula containing amino acids (minus the relevant precursors) and other essential nutrients.

- Permanent neurologic injury (mental retardation, pyramidal signs, and occasionally seizures), is very common in propionic and methylmalonic acidemias, even with prompt and appropriate therapy; a better prognosis is associated with some of the less common disorders.

- Propionic and methylmalonic acidemias are autosomal recessive, can be prenatally diagnosed, and can be detected by newborn screening by tandem mass spectroscopy.

- Fig. 85-2 illustrates the approach to the infant with metabolic acidosis who is suspected of having an inborn error of metabolism. In addition to organic acidemias, disorders listed include those resulting in significant lactic acidosis with normal organic acids (mitochondrial respiratory chain defects, pyruvate dehydrogenase deficiency, pyruvate carboxylase deficiency), and those associated with hypoglycemia such as glycogen storage disease type I, and fructose-1,6-bisphosphatase deficiency.

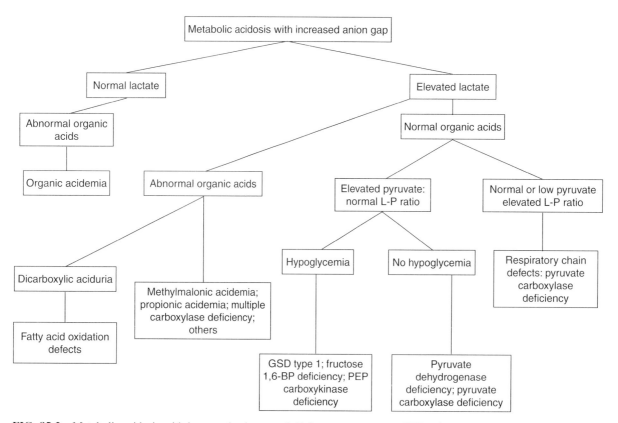

FIG. 85-2 Metabolic acidosis with increased anion gap. L-P: lactate to pyruvate; GSD: glycogen storage disease; BP: bisphosphatase; PEP: phosphoenolpyruvate.

86 CARBOHYDRATE METABOLISM

Barbara K. Burton and Joel Charrow

GALACTOSEMIA

- Classical (transferase deficient) galactosemia results from deficient activity of the enzyme galactose-1-phosphate uridyltransferase, involved in the conversion of galactose to glucose. Several other disorders (galactokinase deficiency, uridine-diphosphate galactose 4-epimerase deficiency) also produce galactosemia, but are much less common, and will not be discussed here.

- Galactose is derived primarily from dietary lactose, which is the major carbohydrate in milk. The pathophysiology of galactosemia is related to excess galactose and its metabolites, especially galactose-1-phosphate, and their toxic effects on numerous tissues, including the liver, erythrocytes, brain, ovaries, and kidneys. The early signs of galactosemia are evident only in infants exposed to galactose, i.e., breast- and formula-fed babies receiving lactose containing formulas (which includes most milk-derived formulas). Failure to thrive and indirect hyperbilirubinemia appear shortly after introduction of feeding. The infant may vomit or have diarrhea, and develop signs of renal injury and proximal tubule dysfunction: hyperchloremic metabolic acidosis, generalized aminoaciduria, and albuminuria. Cataracts may be detected by slit-lamp examination as early as a few days of life, but can be missed on routine direct ophthalmoscopy. Of particular concern is the frequent development of gram-negative sepsis, most commonly related to *E. coli*, in the first few weeks of life. If galactose exposure continues, the hyperbilirubinemia persists, and may be quite marked. It may be accompanied by hemolysis, and a clinical picture resembling erythroblastosis fetalis. Hepatomegaly and hepatocyte injury occur later, and are ultimately followed by ascites, hypoalbuminemia, and cirrhosis, progressing to end-stage liver disease. Lethargy, hypotonia, and later, retarded mental development, are apparent, with language and speech acquisition particularly impaired. Primary ovarian failure (hypergonadotropic hypogonadism) occurs in almost all women.

- The diagnosis should be suspected in any lactose-fed infant with pronounced or prolonged indirect (or mixed) hyperbilirubinemia, failure to thrive, cataracts, or early gram-negative sepsis. The presence of reducing substances in the urine, in the absence of glucose, is suggestive but nonspecific, and the absence of reducing substances provides no reassurance. Definitive diagnosis requires demonstration of deficient transferase activity, typically in erythrocytes. If the infant has been transfused, definitive diagnosis must be postponed, but treatment should be instituted presumptively.

- The pathogenesis of galactosemia can be drastically altered by early introduction and strict adherence to a lactose-free diet. This is easily achieved in infancy by using a lactose- and galactose-free formula, commonly one of the soy-based formulas, although some elemental milk-based formulas are also free of the offending sugars. Treatment becomes more complex with the introduction of solid foods, since milk, milk products, and lactose are found in a variety of foods. Because of the necessary avoidance of dairy products, most children will require a calcium supplement. Treatment is monitored by regularly measuring erythrocyte galactose-1-phosphate concentrations.

- Although the acute toxic effects of galactosemia are ameliorated by a galactose-free diet, treatment has little or no effect on the prevalence of central nervous system disease or ovarian failure. The reason for this is not clear, but may be related to endogenous production of galactose during intrauterine and/or postnatal development. It is not prevented by restricting the mother's galactose intake during pregnancy.

- Galactosemia is an autosomal recessive disorder with an incidence of approximately 1 in 40,000–60,000. Several variant forms are known, some of which have significant residual enzyme activity and do not require lifelong galactose avoidance. For this reason, genotyping and/or electrophoresis of the mutant enzyme should be performed when residual enzyme activity is detected. Galactosemia can be detected by newborn screening based on measurement of galactose and galactose-1-phosphate levels or assay of the transferase in dried blood spots.

GLYCOGEN STORAGE DISEASE (GSD)

- The hepatic glycogenoses result from impaired use of glycogen for the maintenance of normoglycemia. They are all characterized by glycogen storage in the liver (and sometimes kidneys and/or muscle) and fasting hypoglycemia. Only the two most common disorders will be presented: Type Ia (von Gierke disease, glucose-6-phosphate dehydrogenase deficiency) and Type III (Cori or Forbes disease, debrancher enzyme deficiency).

- *Type I GSD* may present in the neonatal period with hypoglycemia and lactic acidosis, but more often is not recognized until 3–4 months of age. Hepatomegaly, hypoglycemia, and ketoacidosis are present. Hypoglycemia occurs after relatively short periods of fasting (as little as 2–3 hours). Liver function is normal, and the transaminases are normal or only slightly elevated. The infants have doll-like facies, central obesity, protuberant abdomens, and short stature. Xanthomas may be present, reflecting the marked hyperlipidemia that is present. Lactic acidemia is always present, and may be marked during periods of hypoglycemia. Hyperuricemia is present, but gout rarely occurs before adulthood. Bruising and epistaxis occur easily, and are associated with a prolonged bleeding time and abnormal platelet aggregation, but otherwise normal coagulation studies. Long-term complications include short stature, gout, nephrolithiasis, and pancreatitis related to the marked hypertriglyceridemia. Hepatic adenomas are common in adulthood, and occasionally hemorrhage or malignant degeneration occur. Albuminuria is common, may herald glomerular hyperfiltration, and later development of impaired renal function.

- Treatment is directed at maintaining normoglycemia at all times, which greatly reduces the morbidity of this disease. In infancy this is achieved by frequent feedings during the day and continuous tube feedings at night. Uncooked cornstarch, which provides a slow release form of glucose, can be used to lengthen the interval between feedings, and in older children may even obviate the need for nighttime feeds. Fructose and galactose (and lactose) intake should be minimized, since these sugars cannot be converted to glucose.
- Diagnosis is suspected in the presence of fasting hypoglycemia, hyperuricemia, hyperlipidemia, and lactic and ketoacidemia in a young child with an enlarged liver. Definitive diagnosis requires demonstration of deficient glucose-6-phosphatase activity in liver.
- GSD Ia is an autosomal recessive condition. It can be prenatally diagnosed if there is a known mutation, or by prenatal liver biopsy. It is not detected by newborn screening.
- *Type III GSD* is characterized by hepatomegaly, fasting hypoglycemia, hyperlipidemia, and elevations of the transaminases. Early in infancy the clinical picture may closely resemble Type I GSD, but is more variable. In contrast to Type I GSD, hyperuricemia and lactic acidemia are usually absent. Most patients (~85%) with Type III GSD also have glycogen accumulation in the skeletal and cardiac muscles as well as liver, and may have varying degrees of the associated myopathies. Serum creatine kinase is typically elevated in the presence of muscle involvement. Hepatic involvement tends to improve with age, and may be absent after puberty. Long-term morbidity is primarily related to the extent and nature of the myopathy.
- Diagnosis is confirmed by demonstration of deficient debrancher enzyme activity in liver, muscle, or cultured skin fibroblasts.

- Type III GSD is an autosomal recessive disorder. It can be diagnosed prenatally, but is not detected by newborn screening.

ESSENTIAL FRUCTOSURIA

- This is a benign, autosomal recessive trait characterized by fructosuria, detected as a reducing substance in the urine. It is of no clinical significance.

HEREDITARY FRUCTOSE INTOLERANCE

- This condition results from deficiency of the enzyme fructose-1-phosphate aldolase, and the consequent excess of fructose-1-phosphate. It is characterized by vomiting and severe hypoglycemia following ingestion of fructose. Continued exposure to fructose (which is present in sucrose or table sugar) leads to poor feeding, diarrhea, hepatomegaly, abdominal distension, failure to thrive, and progressive liver disease. Prolonged exposure in infancy may cause renal and hepatic failures and death. Because fructose is not present in breast milk and most milk-derived formulas, signs of the disorder may not be evident until fruits and vegetables are introduced in the diet. Many patients will develop a strong aversion to fructose containing foods and avoid them. The disorder is completely prevented by avoidance of fructose. The diagnosis may be suggested by the demonstration of fructose and/or glucose in the urine and renal Fanconi syndrome. It is important to note that fructose is present in the urine only following its ingestion. Confirmation of the diagnosis requires demonstration of known mutations in the gene, or if these are not found, an intravenous fructose tolerance test, or demonstration of deficient enzyme activity in liver.
- Hereditary fructose intolerance is an autosomal recessive disorder. Prenatal diagnosis is possible when the mutations are known or by prenatal liver biopsy. It is not detected by newborn screening.

FRUCTOSE 1,6-BISPHOSPHATASE (FBPASE) DEFICIENCY

- This disorder of gluconeogenesis, is characterized by episodic hypoglycemia, and may present as early as the first few weeks of life, or as late as 4 years. Hypoglycemia, triggered by intercurrent illness or dietary exposure to fructose, is accompanied by ketoacidosis and hyperuricemia. Sensitivities to fructose and sorbitol vary, but are generally greater than in hereditary fructose intolerance. Prolonged fasting may induce hypoglycemia, after glycogen stores are depleted, and glucose homeostasis becomes entirely dependent on gluconeogenesis.

- The diagnosis is confirmed by demonstration of deficient enzyme activity in liver. Prenatal diagnosis is possible by fetal liver biopsy. The condition is not detected by newborn screening.

87 FATTY ACID OXIDATION DISORDERS
Barbara K. Burton

- The fatty acid oxidation pathway plays a major role in energy production during periods of fasting or high energy demand, when glycogen stores have been depleted. Over 23 distinct disorders have been described in this pathway. Clinical signs and symptoms may reflect intoxication from the accumulation of toxic substrates or the effects of cellular energy depletion. They vary widely in severity and typically include the following:
  1. Hypoketotic hypoglycemia
  2. Dilated or hypertrophic cardiomyopathy
  3. Transient to fulminant liver disease
  4. Skeletal myopathy
  5. Sudden and unexplained death in early life
- Symptoms appear at any age from birth to adulthood and in various combinations, frequently leading to life-threatening episodes of metabolic decompensation after a period of inadequate caloric intake or intercurrent illness. The most common and best known of the fatty acid oxidation disorders is medium chain acyl CoA dehydrogenase (MCAD) deficiency which occurs with a frequency of about 1 in 15,000 among Caucasians of Northern European descent. It appears to be much less common in other populations. All other fatty acid oxidation disorders are individually rare.
- The biochemical tests most likely to be helpful in the evaluation of the patient suspected of having a fatty acid oxidation disorder are quantitative plasma carnitine, plasma acylcarnitine profile, plasma free fatty acids, and urine organic acids. Enzyme assays on cultured fibroblasts are necessary for definitive diagnosis in some cases. Now that an increasing number of states are using tandem mass spectroscopy for newborn screening, many fatty acid oxidation disorders are being detected a few days after birth, since this

technology allows for the performance of an acylcarnitine profile on the newborn filter paper blood sample.

- Treatment of most fatty acid oxidation disorders involves avoidance of fasting, and careful attention to intercurrent illnesses with oral or intravenous administration of glucose supplements when indicated. Depending on the specific defect, L-carnitine supplementation may also be appropriate. Corn starch supplements can be helpful for the management of hypoglycemia. All of the fatty acid oxidation disorders identified thus far are inherited in an autosomal recessive pattern.

88 LYSOSOMAL STORAGE DISORDERS
Joel Charrow

- Although individually rare, as a group these disorders have an incidence of 1 in 7000–8000. They are all characterized by accumulation of large molecules within the lysosomes, causing cellular dysfunction and enlargement of the involved organ. Only three of the more than 40 known lysosomal storage disorders will be presented.
- The *mucopolysaccharidoses* (MPS) include 10 known enzyme deficiencies which result in the accumulation of the glycosaminoglycans (GAGs, formerly mucopolysaccharides) dermatan sulfate, keratan sulfate, heparan sulfate, and chondroitin sulfate. Six distinct phenotypes are recognized. These are characterized by varying degrees of involvement of five major organ systems: brain, bone, connective tissue, reticuloendothelial tissues, and cornea. Brain involvement is evident as macrocephaly and mental retardation, with progressive loss of skills over time. Boney involvement (dysostosis multiplex) is characterized by abnormal modeling of the bones, widening and shortening of many long bones, and wedge-shaped vertebrae. Progressive joint contractures can create significant functional impairment. Accumulation of GAGs in reticuloendothelial cells causes hepatosplenomegaly; hepatic dysfunction, cirrhosis, and hypersplenism are rare. Corneal clouding is common. Upper airway obstruction, recurrent middle ear effusions, conductive and sensory hearing loss, hydrocephalus, and cardiac valvar insufficiency are common complications. The distinguishing features are summarized in Table 88-1. Unique among these

TABLE 88-1 Characteristics of the Mucopolysaccharidoses

TYPE	NAME	ENZYME DEFICIENCY	MENTAL RETARDATION	GROWTH RETARDATION	COARSE FACIES	BONE DYSPLASIA	CORNEAL CLOUDING	TYPE OF GAG	INHERITANCE
IH	Hurler	α-Iduronidase	+++	++	+++	+++	+	D+H	AR
IS	Scheie	α-Iduronidase	–	–	±	+	+	D+H	AR
IH/S	Hurler-Scheie	α-Iduronidase	–	+	++	++	+	D+H	AR
IIA	Hunter, severe	Iduronate sulfatase	+	+	+	++	±	D+H	X-linked
IIB	Hunter, mild	Iduronate sulfatase	±	+	+	++	±	D+H	X-linked
IIIA	Sanfilippo A	Heparan N-sulfatase	+++	–	+	+	–	H	AR
IIIB	Sanfilippo B	α-N-acetylglucosaminidase	+++	–	+	+	–	H	AR
IIIC	Sanfilippo C	Acetyl-CoA:α-glucosaminide acetyltransferase	+++	–	+	+	–	H	AR
IIID	Sanfilippo D	N-acetylglucosamine-6-sulfatase	+++	–	+	+	–	H	AR
IVA	Morquio A	Galactose-6-sulfatase	–	+++	+	+++	+	K+C	AR
IVB	Morquio B	β-Galactosidase	–	+++	+	+++	+	K	AR
V	Vacant								
VI	Maroteaux-Lamy	Arylsulfatase B	–	++	++	++	+	D	AR
VII	Sly	β-Glucuronidase	+	±	±	+	±	D+H+C	AR

ABBREVIATIONS: D = dermatan sulfate; K = keratan sulfate; H = heparan sulfate; C = chondroitin sulfate.

disorders is MPS IV (Morquio syndrome), which manifests as short-trunk dwarfism (spondylodysplasia) with ligamentous laxity. As with other spondylodysplasias, the odontoid is hypoplastic and there is atlantoaxial instability. Cervical spinal cord injury is common. The other typical features of MPS are absent and intelligence is normal.

- *Gaucher disease* is caused by deficient activity of glucocerebrosidase (acid β-glucosidase), necessary for the intralysosomal catabolism of glucocerebroside (GC), which is derived from phagocytosed cell membranes. It is divided into three types: a nonneuronopathic form (Type I), an acute neuronopathic form (Type II), and a subacute or chronic neuronopathic form (Type III). This discussion will be limited to Type I. Although often referred to as the adult type, this is a misnomer, since nearly 50% of cases are diagnosed before the age of 10 years.

- Deficient glucocerebrosidase activity results in accumulation of GC in the lysosomes of monocyte-derived macrophages in tissues of the reticuloendothelial system. Accumulation in splenic macrophages and in the Kupffer cells of the liver is associated with enlargement of these organs. The resulting hypersplenism produces progressive anemia and thrombocytopenia. Accumulation of GC in bone marrow is associated with osteopenia, lytic lesions, pathologic fractures, chronic bone pain, acute episodes of excruciating bone crisis, bone infarcts, and osteonecrosis. Although anemia and thrombocytopenia may be severe, it is usually the bone disease that results in the greatest morbidity and long-term disability.

- Diagnosis is based on demonstration of deficient glucocerebrosidase activity in peripheral blood leukocytes or cultured skin fibroblasts, or by demonstration of mutations in the gene. Bone marrow aspiration and biopsy may reveal the presence of lipid laden macrophages (Gaucher cells), but this is neither sensitive nor specific, and should not be performed if the diagnosis is suspected. Many children are initially evaluated for leukemia because of the splenomegaly and thrombocytopenia. Gaucher disease is also frequently misdiagnosed as idiopathic thrombocytopenic purpura.

- Type I Gaucher disease responds well to enzyme replacement treatment with purified macrophage-targeted recombinant human glucocerebrosidase. Treatment results in breakdown of stored GC, reduction in liver and spleen size, amelioration or resolution of anemia and thrombocytopenia, decreased bone pain, and increased bone mineralization and remodeling.

- Gaucher disease is an autosomal recessive disorder. It is the most common lysosomal storage disease and the most common genetic disorder among Ashkenazi Jews, among whom the incidence is approximately 1 in 400. Prenatal diagnosis is possible; carrier screening is possible for Ashkenazi Jews. It is not detected by newborn screening.

- *Tay-Sachs disease* (TSD, GM2 gangliosidosis) affects primarily the brain, where ganglioside accumulates in the neuronal and glial elements. Classical or acute infantile TSD is the most common form, but subacute (juvenile) and chronic (late-onset) forms of the disease also occur. This discussion will be limited to the infantile form of the disease. As in most lysosomal storage diseases, the infants appear normal at birth. By 3–6 months of age hypotonia is noted, and there is an exaggerated startle to sudden noises. Progressive weakness and slowing of development are noted, and the neurologic deterioration relentlessly progresses to loss of acquired milestones, and ultimately to a vegetative state, accompanied by blindness, deafness, complete lack of awareness of the environment and inability to suck and swallow. Seizures are common. Death typically occurs by 5 years of age.

- The diagnosis may be suspected based on the clinical course. Macular cherry-red spots strongly support the diagnosis, but can be seen in some other disorders. Definitive diagnosis rests on demonstrating deficient activity of the enzyme hexosaminidase A in peripheral blood leukocytes, serum, or cultured skin fibroblasts. Mutation testing is also available.

- The disorder is autosomal recessive and affects primarily Ashkenazi Jews (1 in 3500 births); 1 in 25 Jews and 1 in 300 non-Jews carry the mutant gene for TSD. Carrier screening is possible for Ashkenazi Jews; when both partners are carriers, prenatal diagnosis should be offered. TSD is not detected by newborn screening.

89 OTHER IMPORTANT SINGLE GENE DISORDERS

Barbara K. Burton and Joel Charrow

MARFAN SYNDROME

- Marfan syndrome is an autosomal dominant disorder occurring in all ethnic groups, with an estimated prevalence of about 1 in 5–10,000. It is a systemic disorder of connective tissue with a high degree of clinical variability. Major clinical manifestations are as follows:

Skeletal system

- Long limbs with a decreased U/L segment ratio and arm span > height.

- Arachnodactyly; joint hyperextensibility.
- Pectus carinatum or excavatum or both; scoliosis.
- High arched palate; dental crowding.

Eye

- Ectopia lentis
- Myopia, often severe, with risk of retinal detachment.

Cardiovascular system

- Dilatation of aorta, most commonly involving the ascending aorta at the level of the sinuses of Valsalva, with risk of dissection. Entire aorta can be involved.
- Mitral valve prolapse with or without regurgitation.
- Dilatation of the main pulmonary artery.

Pulmonary system

- Spontaneous pneumothorax, apical blebs.

Skin

- Striae, recurrent, or incisional herniae.

Dura

- Lumbosacral dural ectasia (ascertained by computed tomography [CT] or magnetic resonance imaging [MRI]).
- The disorder is the result of a mutation in the gene for fibrillin on chromosome 15. Approximately 30% of cases are the result of a new gene mutation. Although molecular testing is available, not all mutations are detectable, so the diagnosis is established on clinical grounds.
- Patients with Marfan syndrome should be followed by a team of specialists including geneticists, cardiologists, ophthalmologists, and orthopedic surgeons. Treatment includes the use of beta-blockers to reduce stress on the aortic wall, exercise restriction, and elective surgery when necessary to replace the aortic valve and ascending aorta and to repair the mitral valve. With appropriate care, the life expectancy for patients with Marfan syndrome now approaches that of individuals in the general population.

EHLERS-DANLOS SYNDROME

- The Ehlers-Danlos syndrome (EDS) is a group of disorders characterized by abnormalities of skin, joints, and other connective tissues. Many different subtypes have been described but those of most importance to the pediatrician are the classical type, the hypermobility type, and the vascular type, all of which are inherited in an autosomal dominant pattern.
- The classical type of EDS is associated with soft, velvety skin that is hyperextensible (can be stretched several centimeters from its attachment sites). It is fragile and there is easy bruising. The skin may tear easily with trauma, and abnormal thin cigarette-paper scars may be present. In areas of repeated trauma, such as the shins, there may be marked pigment deposition. There is hyperextensibility of both small and large joints. Motor development may be delayed because joint hypermobility limits stability until muscle strength is sufficient to overcome ligamentous laxity. Intelligence is normal. All of the characteristics vary widely in severity. Orthopedic complications of the ligamentous laxity may include pes planus and scoliosis. Patients are at increased risk for acute injuries, such as dislocations and sprains, and long term are at risk for early-adult onset osteoarthritis. Cardiovascular complications may also be observed and all patients should have an echocardiogram. A significant percentage have mitral valve prolapse and aortic dilatation may also be observed. Although the diagnosis of the classical type of EDS is made on clinical grounds, it appears that most patients have a mutation in one of the fibrillar collagen genes (COL5A1 or COL5A2). Treatment is symptomatic.
- The hypermobility type of EDS is associated with hypermobility of small and large joints with minimal or no skin findings. There may be a history of recurrent dislocations and pain is often a very prominent complaint, particularly in the adolescent or young adult. The molecular defect in this subtype of EDS has not yet been elucidated. Cardiovascular complications also occur in the hypermobility form so these patients should also have a routine echocardiogram. The classical and hypermobility forms of EDS are both very common. The estimated prevalence of the two combined is 1 in 5000 individuals.
- The vascular form of EDS is much less common but of significance because it may present in a dramatic fashion with arterial rupture or rupture of a hollow organ. Patients with this disorder have thin, translucent skin with a clearly visible venous pattern and easy bruising. Joint laxity is limited to the small joints of the hands. Some patients are recognized in infancy because of the marked bruising and thin skin. Most are diagnosed when they present with an episode of arterial bleeding—hemorrhagic stroke, gastrointestinal bleeding, or even coronary artery dissection. Spontaneous colon rupture can occur in childhood. Surgery is very difficult because of fragility of the blood vessels. Patients with the vascular type of EDS have mutations in the COL3A1 gene. If the diagnosis is suspected clinically, it can be confirmed by demonstration of secretion of abnormal type III collagen by cultured fibroblasts. Treatment is symptomatic. Genetic counseling should be provided.

OSTEOGENESIS IMPERFECTA (OI)

- Osteogenesis imperfecta represents a spectrum of disorders with increased bone fragility as the major morbidity. All forms are caused by abnormalities of type I collagen and result from mutations in either

COL1A1 (the gene encoding the alpha-1 subunit) or COL1A2 (the gene encoding the alpha-2 subunit). The clinical classification system of Sillence is still widely used as a shorthand for describing the features and clinical severity in individual patients. The mildest form (Sillence type I) may be first recognized by the presence of deep blue sclera. Fractures are uncommon in infancy, but occur repeatedly during childhood and adolescence, even with minimal trauma. The fractures heal normally and without deformity. Fractures become less common after puberty, and increase in frequency again in the later decades of life. Stature is normal. Approximately 50% of patients develop progressive hearing loss beginning in late adolescence or early adulthood. X-ray examination reveals generalized osteopenia of otherwise normal appearing bones. In infancy the calvarium appears very thin, and multiple bone islands (Wormian bones) may be noted in the unfused sutures. Studies of collagen synthesis in cultured skin fibroblasts usually reveal decreased synthesis of electrophoretically normal type I collagen.

- The most severe form of OI is Sillence type II, which is associated with multiple intrauterine fractures of the ribs and long bones, marked shortening of the long bones, and respiratory insufficiency and death in the early neonatal period in most cases. The sclera are usually white. X-ray examination reveals marked abnormalities of the bones, including shortening, crumpling, and bowing. Collagen studies usually reveal structurally abnormal collagen.

- Types III and IV OI represent intermediate phenotypes, with type III being more severe. It is associated with white sclera, progressive deformity of the long bones, short stature, and dentinogenesis imperfecta. Type IV OI is also associated with dentinogenesis imperfecta in some patients. The sclera are white, and the skeletal phenotype is intermediate to types I and III.

- The diagnosis of OI is usually evident from the history, physical examination, and x-ray findings. Many children with OI are initially thought to be battered, and in some of the milder cases it may be difficult to distinguish these two possibilities based on the x-ray findings. Two laboratory studies are helpful for confirming the diagnosis, and in particular, for providing a laboratory basis for prenatal diagnosis in future pregnancies: (1) in vitro study of type I collagen synthesis in cultured skin fibroblasts to determine approximate quantity of collagen as well as its electrophoretic mobility; and (2) direct analysis of the genes to detect specific mutations in COL1A1 and COL1A2.

- There is no specific treatment for OI. Most patients will require numerous orthopedic procedures. Rodding of long bones may be appropriate in some cases. Attention has recently been focused on the use of bisphosphonates to improve bone mineralization and density. Several clinical trials have demonstrated a reduction in the frequency of fractures following bisphosphonate use. Their use does not appear to interfere with growth, but because the long term consequences of the use of these agents in young children are unknown, their use should be restricted to patients with more severe disease in whom the benefits clearly outweigh the risks.

- Osteogenesis imperfecta is an autosomal dominant disorder. Although types II and III were previously thought to be recessively inherited, it is now clear that de novo cases in families result from new mutations, and the occasional recurrences observed in families where both parents are normal are the result of germline mosaicism in one of the parents.

NEUROFIBROMATOSIS (NF)

- *Neurofibromatosis-1* (NF-1, von Recklinghausen disease) is the most common type of NF, and is almost always diagnosed during childhood. The diagnosis is clinical, based on the presence of at least 2 of 7 diagnostic criteria:

1. Café-au-lait spots are usually the earliest manifestation, and are frequently present at birth. The presence of at least six, at least 0.5 cm in greatest diameter in prepubertal children (and at least 1.5 cm in diameter after puberty) fulfills the criterion. The location, contour, or intensity of the spots is of no significance.

2. Freckling in the axilla or inguinal region is often the second diagnostic manifestation to appear. The freckles appear like small café-au-lait spots and are not affected by sun exposure.

3. Neurofibromas are frequently not apparent until the teenage years; they may be superficial in the skin, appearing as raised soft nodules, often pink or purplish in color, or may be deeper in the subcutaneous tissue, where they are palpated as firm, sometimes fusiform nodules. Plexiform neurofibromas, which are typically congenital, can be much larger, have an irregular surface, indistinct margins, and may infiltrate or be wrapped around other tissues. Very often the overlying skin is hyperpigmented and has excessive hair growth. These lesions can grow very large and account for the occasional deformities seen in people with NF-1. The presence of two neurofibromas or one plexiform neurofibroma fulfills the diagnostic criterion.

4. Iris Lisch nodules are found in almost all adults with NF-1, but can only be detected reliably by slit-lamp examination. They appear as raised, pigmented

nodules on the surface of the iris, and are of no clinical consequence.

5. There are two distinct, congenital boney lesions seen in children with NF-1: sphenoid wing dysplasia and thinning and bowing of a long bone. These both represent dysplasia of bone, and are not the result of neurofibromas in the regions. Sphenoid dysplasia may not be apparent unless an AP x-ray of the skull is obtained, although pulsating exophthalmos may be apparent if looked for, and represents transmission of the carotid pulse through the deficient posterior wall of the orbit to the globe. This is of no clinical significance. Thinning and bowing of a long bone (most often the tibia) is usually unilateral and mechanically unstable. Fractures are common and heal poorly, resulting in pseudarthrosis; resection of the dysplastic bone segment followed by use of the Ilizarov frame may be necessary to achieve boney union.

6. Optic pathway tumors are common in children with NF-1, found in 15–20% of patients if neuroimaging studies are performed; however, most of these lesions are asymptomatic and do not progress. The lesions may be found anywhere along the optic pathway, although the intraorbital nerve and optic chiasm are the most common sites. Intraorbital lesions may produce proptosis, and chiasmatic lesions are often associated with the development of precocious puberty. Lesions that progress and that have a clearly documented effect on vision can be treated with chemotherapy.

7. The presence of NF-1 in a first-degree relative (parent or child) also serves as a diagnostic criterion. The presence of a more distant relative with NF-1 is not significant, since this is a dominantly inherited disorder with complete penetrance (i.e., it does not skip generations). Because the disorder is so common, occurring in approximately 1 in 3500, and ~50% of the cases arise from new mutations, it is not unusual to discover two unrelated cases in distant branches of a single family.

• The diagnosis of NF-1 remains clinically based. Although there is a laboratory protein-truncation assay available, it has a sensitivity of only ~70%, and therefore has limited use.

• There is no specific treatment for NF-1, and management involves regular examination by a physician experienced with the care of these children. Baseline laboratory and x-ray examinations are discouraged, and should be performed only when there is a specific clinical indication. Malignancies and mental retardation are *not* common in NF-1.

• *Segmental neurofibromatosis* refers to somatic mosaicism for mutations in the NF-1 gene, which results in typical manifestations of NF-1 associated with the affected region of the body. The manifestations (e.g., café-au-lait spots) often end abruptly at the midline. More than one region may be affected. Although segmental NF is never inherited, an individual with segmental NF can have children affected with typical NF-1, if the germ cells possess the mutation.

• *Familial café-au-lait spots* without other manifestations of NF-1, transmitted as a dominant trait, have been observed in a number of pedigrees. Genetic studies in several families have indicated involvement of a gene distinct from the NF-1 gene. The condition is much less common than NF-1.

• *NF-2* (Central NF) is an uncommon condition (incidence 1 in 50,000 to 1 in 100,000), and frequently not diagnosed until early adulthood. It is characterized by bilateral acoustic neuromas, multiple meningiomas, and multiple schwannomas of the nerve roots as they take off from the spinal cord. Neurofibromas and café-au-lait spots are uncommon, and the disorder is not easily confused with NF-1. It is caused by mutations of a tumor suppressor gene located on chromosome 22, distinct from the neurofibromin gene on chromosome 17.

TUBEROUS SCLEROSIS COMPLEX

• Tuberous sclerosis complex is a highly variable multisystem disorder occurring in an estimated 1 in every 5800 individuals. It is inherited in an autosomal dominant pattern. The characteristic clinical manifestations are as follows:

Skin: Hypomelanotic macules or ash leaf spots (95%), facial angiofibromas (85%), shagreen patches (40%), ungual fibromas (50%).

CNS (central nervous system): Subependymal glial nodules (90%), cortical or subcortical tubers on MRI (70%), seizures (80%), mental retardation (50%).

Kidneys: Benign angiomyolipomas (70%), epithelial cysts (20%), malignant angiomyolipoma, or renal cell carcinoma (2%).

Heart: Rhabdomyomas (47%)—typically benign and largest in the neonate. They regress and eventually disappear. May be detected by antenatal ultrasound.

Eye: Hamartomas (75%) usually asymptomatic.

Lung: Lymphangiomyomatosis (1–6%).

• Tuberous sclerosis results from a mutation in one of two genes, TSC1 or TSC2, the function of which are poorly understood. Approximately 70% of cases represent new mutations. Parents of a newly diagnosed child should be thoroughly examined because of the extreme variability in gene expression since a parent may be affected and have only minor skin findings. Treatment of tuberous sclerosis is symptomatic.

FRAGILE X SYNDROME

- The fragile X syndrome is the most common inherited form of mental retardation. It affects approximately 1 in 4000 males and 1 in 8000 females. The disorder typically results in moderate to severe mental retardation in affected males and mild mental retardation in affected females. All children with developmental delay of undetermined cause should be tested for this condition because of its frequency and because of the genetic implications of a positive test result. Males with the fragile X syndrome may have some other phenotypic features but these are often subtle, particularly in early childhood, and cannot be used to select patients for fragile X deoxyribonucleic acid (DNA) testing. Other clinical features that may be present include hyperactivity, elongated face, large ears, prominent jaw, joint hyperextensibility, mitral valve prolapse, and in the postpubertal male, macroorchidism. Affected females rarely exhibit any other phenotypic abnormalities. Some males with fragile X syndrome exhibit autistic characteristics.
- The genetics of the fragile X syndrome are complex. It is caused by a large expansion of a CGG repeat region within the fragile X-linked mental retardation (FMR1) gene on the X chromosome. Large expansions of this region are associated with increased methylation of the region leading to transcriptional silencing of the gene. Such large expansions are referred to as fragile X full mutations. Normal alleles of the FMR1 gene typically contain between 5 and about 55 CGG repeats. Individuals with genes containing 55–200 repeats are said to be fragile X permutation carriers, and are asymptomatic; however, the premutation is very unstable and often expands to over 200 repeats when transmitted by a carrier female. It then becomes hypermethylated and is silenced, thus becoming a full mutation resulting in the fragile X syndrome. Such expansion of the premutation does not occur when it is transmitted by the male, which is why the term normal transmitting male has been used to describe male carriers in families with the fragile X syndrome.
- The appropriate test for a child suspected of having fragile X syndrome is DNA analysis, which should be done in conjunction with chromosome analysis since other conditions may be associated with similar findings. A child diagnosed with fragile X syndrome will always have a carrier mother and many other family members may be at risk. Genetic counseling should

be recommended. There is no specific treatment for the disorder.

90 NEWBORN SCREENING
Barbara K. Burton

- Newborn screening policies and practices are established by individual state health departments and are not uniform throughout the United States. Therefore, pediatricians must become familiar with the newborn screening protocols in the state in which they are practicing. Currently many states are examining their practices and many are moving toward expanded newborn screening using the technology of tandem mass spectrometry. This powerful new technology allows for the measurement of multiple analytes on a single filter paper blood specimen. It is being used in a number of states to perform acylcarnitine profiles for the detection of organic acid and fatty acid oxidation disorders and for amino acid analysis for the detection of amino acid disorders including phenylketonuria (PKU), hereditary tyrosinemia, maple syrup urine disease, and homocystinuria.
- The only disorders that are currently included in the newborn screening panel of all 50 states and the District of Columbia are PKU and congenital hypothyroidism. Hemoglobinopathies and galactosemia are included in most states. Beyond that, the lists are highly variable. Newborn screening is not uniformly performed throughout the world. Pediatricians caring for international adoptees below the age of 3–5 years should send a specimen for screening for metabolic disorders. Even late treatment for disorders such as PKU can be extremely beneficial. In most cases, such tests can be processed through state laboratories like newborn screening specimens.
- Confirmation of positive newborn screening results is always necessary to establish a definitive diagnosis. With every type of screening method, including tandem mass spectroscopy, false-positive test results occur. Each state has developed a system for the evaluation of infants with positive results and the pediatrician should familiarize himself with this follow-up system. The American Academy of Pediatrics (AAP) has also developed fact sheets on each of the disorders that are available on the AAP website (http://www.aap.org/policy/01565.html).
- As newborn screening for metabolic disorders is expanded, an increasing number of inborn errors of

metabolism will be diagnosed presymptomatically. This should not in any way discourage the pediatrician from considering the diagnosis of an inborn error of metabolism in an infant who presents with appropriate signs and symptoms. Some infants with conditions such as galactosemia, maple syrup urine disease, and many of the organic acidemias will become symptomatic before the results of newborn screening tests are available. In addition, there are many important inherited metabolic disorders, such as ornithine transcarbamylase deficiency, that will not be detected by newborn screening, even with tandem mass spectroscopy. Therefore, pediatricians must continue to have a high index of suspicion for metabolic disease in any infant who presents with findings suggestive of such a disorder.

BIBLIOGRAPHY

Jones KL (ed.). *Smith's Recognizable Patterns of Human Malformation*, 5th ed. Philadelphia, PA: WB Saunders, 1997.

Rimoin DL, O'Connor JM, Pyeritz RM, Korf BR (eds.). *Emery and Rimoin's Principles and Practices of Medical Genetics*, 4th ed. London: Churchill Livingstone, 2002.

Scriver CL, Beaudet AL, Sly WS, Valle D (eds.). *The Metabolic and Molecular Bases of Inherited Disease*, 8th ed. New York, NY: McGraw Hill, 2001.

For further reading: www.genetests.org. This is a publicly funded medical genetics information resource developed for physicians and researchers and available at no charge. It includes expert-authored disease reviews, a laboratory directory, a clinic directory, and educational materials.

DISORDERS OF THE BLOOD AND BLOOD CELLS

Alexis A. Thompson, Section Editor

91 ANEMIA OVERVIEW

Alexis A. Thompson

- This section provides a brief, general overview of anemia. More detailed information on specific forms of anemia is covered in subsequent chapters.

DIFFERENTIAL DIAGNOSIS

- Using a mechanistic approach, anemias can be sorted by cause: increased destruction, decreased marrow production, or blood loss. Anemias which fall into these categories are delineated in Table 91-1.

- Under some circumstances, categorizing anemias based on cell morphology provides an important differential (Table 91-2).

BASIC ASSESSMENT

- Important clues to the etiologies of most anemias can be found in a thorough personal history, family history, and physical examination. Essential laboratory studies for evaluating anemia are the following:
  1. Complete blood count (CBC)
  2. Reticulocyte count
  3. Peripheral blood smear
- Other studies that might be useful include the following:
  1. Serum bilirubin
  2. Direct antiglobulin (Coombs) test

TABLE 91-1   Increased Destruction

Intrinsic factors

Membrane defects
   Spherocytosis, elliptocytosis, pyropoikilocytosis
Hemoglobin defects
   Structural/qualitative: Sickle cell disease
   Quantitative: Thalassemias
Enzyme defects
   Hexose monophosphate: G6PD deficiency
   Embden-Meyerhof: Pyruvate kinase deficiency

Extrinsic factors

Immune-mediated
   Transfusion related
   Autoimmune hemolytic anemia
Nonimmune
   Infection related: Parasites, bacterial toxins
   Chemical agents: Heavy metals, oxidants
   Physical trauma: Microangiopathic hemolysis, DIC, HUS/TTP, Waring blender syndrome, burns
Secondary hemolysis
   Acute or chronic infections
   Renal disease

(continued)

TABLE 91-1 *(Continued)*

Chronic inflammatory disorders
Malignancies

Combination

Nutritional deficiencies: Fe, B_{12}, folate
Enzyme defects: G6PD
Membrane defects: PNH

Blood loss

Acute or chronic hemorrhage
    External: Trauma, epistaxis
    Internal: Intracranial, intraabdominal, intramuscular
    Occult: Gastrointestinal or renal

Decreased production

Substrate deficiency
    Primary: Iron, vitamin B_{12}, folate, riboflavin pyridoxine
    Secondary: Chronic inflammation, malabsorption, malignancies

Mechanical interference

Cancer: Leukemias, lymphomas, metastases
    Idiopathic fibrosis
    Myelodysplastic syndrome

Bone marrow failure

Pure red cell aplasia
    Congenital: Blackfan-Diamond
    Acquired: Transient erythroblastopenia of childhood
Generalized marrow hypoplasia
    Congenital: Fanconi, Estren-Dameshek, dyskeratosis congenita
    Acquired: Idiopathic, drug-induced, infections

Ineffective erythropoiesis

Congenital dyserythropoietic anemias
Thalassemias

ABBREVIATIONS: DIC, disseminated intravascular coagulation; HUS/TTP, hemolytic uremic syndrome/thrombotic thrombocytopenic purpura; PNH, paroxysmal nocturnal hemoglobinuria.

3. Blood urea nitrogen (BUN) and creatinine
4. Stool guaiac
5. Hemoglobin electrophoresis
6. Routine urinalysis
• Under some circumstances a bone marrow aspirate is required for diagnosis. More details for the presentation, evaluation, and treatment of specific anemias appear in the chapters that follow this section.

Further information available at www.anemiainstitute. org

TABLE 91-2   **Differential Diagnosis of Microcytic Anemia**

	IRON DEFICIENCY	THALASSEMIA TRAIT	LEAD POISONING
MCV	Decreased	Decreased	Normal/decreased
RDW	Increased	Normal	Normal/increased
Retic count	Decreased	Increased	Decreased
Serum iron	Decreased	Normal	Normal
TIBC	Increased	Normal	Normal
Serum ferritin	Decreased	Normal	Normal
FEP	Increased	Normal	Increased

ABBREVIATIONS: MCV, mean corpuscular volume; RDW, red cell distribution width; TIBC, total iron-binding capacity; FEP, free erythrocyte protoporphyrin.

92 IRON DEFICIENCY

Laurie MacDonald and
Alexis A. Thompson

DEFINITIONS

- Iron deficiency: Absent stores of iron in the bone marrow.
- Iron-deficiency anemia: Also absent stored iron in the marrow, but with consequential hemoglobin (Hgb) or haematocrit (Hct) <5th percentile based on age and sex.

EPIDEMIOLOGY

- Recent studies estimate that 9% of children in the United States between 12 and 36 months of age have iron deficiency, and 3% have iron-deficiency anemia. Those who live at or below the poverty level are at higher risk.
- Reduced incidence in current society secondary to increase in breast-feeding, introduction of iron-fortified formulas, and decreased use of whole milk in the first year of life.

PHYSIOLOGY

- Iron is present in all human cells and serves a variety of functions. It carries oxygen (in the form of Hgb) to tissues from the lungs, it aids in oxygen storage, used in muscle as myoglobin, and it can serve as a transport medium (in the form of cytochromes) for electrons within cells to help various cellular processes.
- When one is not iron-deficient, >70% of the iron found in the body is functional iron (80% of this is found in the red blood cell [RBC] mass as Hgb, and the remainder is in myoglobin and cytochromes). The remainder is stored in the liver, bone marrow, spleen, and skeletal muscle (about 70% as ferritin, much less as hemosiderin) or in transport (by the transferrin protein).
- Two types of dietary iron: Heme iron (10% of dietary iron, primarily from hemoglobin and myoglobin of meat), and nonheme iron (in the form of iron salts in plant-based and iron-fortified food).
- Iron absorption (mainly through the gastrointestinal [GI] tract) is most strongly influenced by the amount of iron stored in the body. Factors causing increased absorption include low total-body iron stores, increased rate of RBC production, ingestion of heme iron (meat, fish, and poultry), and vitamin C.

Decreased iron absorption may be caused by sufficient total-body iron stores ingestion of polyphenols, tannins (in tea), phytates (in bran), and calcium.

- At term, healthy infants are born with adequate iron stores for the first 4 months of life (75 mg/kg). Premature infants have lower total-body iron, but the proportion of iron to body weight is similar to that of term infants.
- Iron losses: Two-thirds from intestinal mucosa, one-third from shedding of skin and urinary tract. This averages 20 µg/kg/day in a healthy term infant.
- Those 9–18 months of age are at greatest risk of iron deficiency because of their rapid rate of growth with an often poor intake of dietary iron. A full-term infant has enough iron stores to meet his needs until about 4–6 months of age; iron-deficiency anemia is usually not seen until 9 months of age. Low birthweight (LBW) and preterm infants are born with lower iron stores and have a more rapid rate of growth in the first year of life, so their iron stores may be depleted by 2–3 months of age.
- Recommendations of Committee on Nutrition of the American Academy of Pediatrics (AAP) = 1 mg/kg/day of iron (maximum 15 mg/day) beginning by 4 months of age until 3 years of age. Low birthweight infants require 2 mg/kg/day (maximum 15 mg/day) beginning by 2 months of age. Infants with birthweight <1000 g require 4 mg/kg/day and it should continue through the first year of life.
- For older children: A more varied diet allows for lower requirement of iron intake. For 4–10 years old = 10 mg/day, and increases to 18 mg/day for those 11 years and older due to accelerated growth during adolescence.
- Iron in breast milk vs. cow's milk: Breast milk contains only about 0.5–1.0 mg of iron per liter, but GI absorption is about 50% and helps make up for its low concentration. Cow's milk has the same concentration of iron as breast milk but only about 10% of this iron is absorbed.

LAB TESTS

- Hgb and Hct: Hgb is more direct and sensitive; it is the concentration of Hgb in the circulating RBCs. Hct is the proportion of whole blood that is occupied by RBCs, so it falls after the Hgb concentration falls. These are good to help detect anemia but are late indicators of iron deficiency. When checking this remember that "milking" blood on a finger/heelstick can yield falsely low readings, as tissue fluid can contaminate the sample.
- Mean cell volume (MCV): Ratio of Hct to RBC count (average volume of the RBCs).

- Microcytic anemias manifest a low MCV; microcytic anemias include iron deficiency, lead poisoning, infection, chronic inflammatory disease, and thalassemia.
- Red blood cell distribution width (RDW): Index of variation in size of the red blood cell population, so may be helpful in detecting subtle anisocytosis.
- This may be the earliest manifestation of iron deficiency, and is more sensitive than ferritin, transferrin, or serum iron. A high RDW is generally >14.0%, but this can be instrument-independent. The RDW is higher in iron deficiency than thalassemia trait/minor, so can be useful when trying to differentiate between the two.
- Red blood cell protoporphyrin: This is the immediate precursor of Hgb, and the concentration increases when there is not enough iron available for RBC production. Elevated RBC protoporphyrin concentration can be seen in iron deficiency, lead poisoning, infection, and inflammation.
- Ferritin: This is the most abundant storage form of iron. Most ferritin is intracellular but there are small circulating amounts in the plasma. It is the earliest (and most specific) indicator of iron store status. Normal value is approximately 30 µg/L for children 6–24 months of age, less than 15 µg/L in those of preschool age or less, can be consistent with iron deficiency. Remember that it is an acute phase reactant, so it may be increased in many medical conditions (which could mask iron deficiency).
- Transferrin: Used for iron transport, so the transferring saturation reflects the percentage of vacant iron-binding sites (and is thus an indicator of iron-deficient erythropoiesis).
- Total binding iron capacity (TIBC): This value is reflective of the availability of iron-binding sites on transferring, and it becomes elevated after iron stores are depleted. May be falsely elevated by pregnancy or oral contraceptives; may be falsely low if malnutrition, inflammation, chronic infection, malignancy, liver disease, or nephrotic syndrome are present.

PATHOLOGY

- Iron deficiency precedes anemia: Iron stores are first lost from the bone marrow (the RDW increases), then transport iron is lost (decreased serum iron), and then erythropoiesis becomes iron-deficient (reduced MCV and increased RBC protoporphyrin) and anemia is seen.
- Moderately severe iron-deficiency anemia: Low MCV, low ferritin, low serum iron, increased iron-binding capacity, increased RBC protoporphyrin, increased RDW, and increase in Hgb after the institution of oral iron therapy.

- For mild iron-deficiency anemia, appropriate history with screening labs such as hemoglobin (ideally supported by elevated RDW, low MCV, and increased RBC protoporphyrin level) and a successful trial of iron therapy may be enough to make the diagnosis. This may be a good screening strategy for full-term infants between 9 and 12 months of age.

CLINICAL PRESENTATION

- Iron-deficiency anemia can present with any of the following manifestations: decreased exercise tolerance, blue sclerae, koilonychia, and alterations in the function of the small bowel (including beeturia, when the urine is pink or red following the ingestion of beets).
- Behavioral effects of iron-deficiency anemia: Iron-deficiency has been associated with decreased performance in mental development examinations in affected students, with severe differences in motor development and mental development in those with Hgb <10.4 g/dL. In those up to 5 years of age, developmental delays and behavioral disturbances (decreased social interaction, attention to tasks, and motor activity). If the iron deficiency is not fully reversed, these delays may persist into school age and beyond. Adolescents with iron deficiency have reported poor exercise performance, decrease in short-term memory, and loss of a sense of well-being.
- Iron deficiency increases susceptibility to lead poisoning due to the GI tract's increased uptake of heavy metals.

DIAGNOSIS AND SCREENING

- Screening Hgb or Hct, then confirm with a repeat. If the results are consistent and the child isn't otherwise sick, presume the diagnosis of iron deficiency and initiate treatment.
- Infants and children
  1. For those at risk of iron-deficiency anemia (low-income families, receiving special supplemental food program for women, infants, and children [WIC], migrant children, or recent refugee arrivals), screen for anemia between 9 and 12 months of age, again 6 months later, and every year thereafter from 2 to 5 years old.
  2. Consider screening preterm or LBW infants not receiving iron-fortified formula.
  3. Question 2–5-year-olds annually for risk of iron-deficiency anemia regarding a low-iron diet, limited access to food secondary to neglect or poverty, or special health-care needs.

4. At 9–12 months and 6 months later assess for the following and screen if applicable:
   a. Preterm or LBW infants.
   b. Non-iron-fortified formula for greater than 2 months.
   c. Introduction to cow's milk prior to 1 year of age.
   d. Breast-fed infants without sufficient supplemental dietary iron after 6 months of age.
   e. Consumption of greater than 24 oz cow's milk per day.
   f. Special health-care needs.
- Adolescent females
  1. Screen nonpregnant females every 5–10 years for anemia.
  2. Screen women with risk factors for iron deficiency including excessive blood loss (including menstrual blood), poor iron intake, or previous diagnosis of iron deficiency.
- School-age children and adolescent males
  1. Screen only those with a history of iron-deficiency anemia, special health-care needs, or an iron-poor diet.

TREATMENT/PROGNOSIS

- Infants and preschool children
  1. Oral iron (ferrous sulfate) trial: 3 mg/kg daily between meals. Oral iron supplementation causes darkening of the stools and can increase constipation. The iron in the stools and supplement may stain clothing. Counsel to increase iron in the diet.
  2. Repeat the screen in 1 month. An increase in Hgb of 1.0 g/dL (or increase in Hct 3%) or more may be considered diagnostic. Then, the iron supplementation should continue for an additional 2 months to fully replete the iron stores. Recheck the Hgb or Hct again at that time, and again 6 months after completion of treatment.
  3. Note that a recent infection may cause a rise in Hgb of 1.0 g/dL, which can cloud the picture. If there is no response seen to the therapeutic iron trial after 1 month (and noncompliance and acute illness have been ruled out) then further assessment of the anemia should be pursued, including lead level, hemoglobin electrophoresis, and serum ferritin.
- School-age children (5–12 years old) and adolescent males
  1. One 60-mg iron tablet daily for school-age children and two 60-mg iron tablets daily for adolescent males. Also include counseling to increase iron in the diet. Follow-up labs are the same as above.

- Adolescent females (nonpregnant)
  1. Oral iron 60–120 mg/day, including counseling about dietary correction of iron deficiency. Follow-up is the same as above.

PREVENTION

- Infancy
  1. Encourage breast-feeding, and provide breast milk for at least 5–6 months if possible. If continuing exclusive breast-feeding beyond 6 months of age, initiate iron supplementation of 1 mg/kg/day.
  2. If not breast-fed, provide iron-fortified formula (12 mg of iron per liter) for the first 12 months of life.
  3. For those who are breast-fed and were preterm or low birthweight, recommend iron drops with 2–4 mg/kg/day (maximum 15 mg/day) from 1 month until 12 months of age.
  4. When introducing solid foods, start with iron-enriched cereal. Two or more servings per day should provide adequate supplementation when initiated at 4–5 months of age.
  5. Avoid providing whole cow's milk during the first year of life.
  6. Around 6 months of age, adding ascorbic acid (vitamin C), meat, fish, and poultry enhance absorption of nonheme iron.
- Toddlers
  1. Preferably no more than 24 oz of milk (cow, goat, soy) per day.

BIBLIOGRAPHY

Oski FA. Iron deficiency in infancy and childhood. *N Engl J Med* 1993;329:190–193.
Recommendations to prevent and control iron deficiency in the United States. *Morb Mortal Wkly Rep* 1998;47:1–36.

93 HEMOLYTIC ANEMIAS
Yasmin Gosiengfiao and Alexis A. Thompson

- Hemolytic anemia should be suspected if normocytic anemia is accompanied by an elevated reticulocyte count in the absence of bleeding or hematinic therapy.

Other evidence of hemolysis includes an elevated fecal urobilinogen, elevated indirect serum bilirubin, hemoglobinuria, and the presence of free hemoglobin in the plasma. Direct assessment of the severity of hemolysis requires measurement of the red cell survival using red cells that are tagged with radioisotope $Na_{251}CrO_4$ (normal half-life = 25–35 days).

• Hemolytic anemias can be divided into two major subgroups: intrinsic and extrinsic hemolytic anemias.

INTRINSIC HEMOLYTIC ANEMIA

MEMBRANE DEFECTS

• Hereditary spherocytosis
1. Epidemiology: This is the most common familial and congenital abnormality of the red blood cell (RBC) membrane, with an incidence of 1:5000 Northern Europeans. It can be autosomal dominant (more common) or autosomal recessive, though 25% arise from new mutations. The most common molecular defect is an abnormality of spectrin: AR—alpha-spectrin, AD—beta-spectrin or protein 3, AD/AR—ankyrin. These defects cause uncoupling of the "vertical" interactions of the lipid bilayer skeleton and loss of membrane microvesicles.
2. Laboratory findings: Normocytic anemia (Hgb 6019 g/dL) with increased mean corpuscular hemoglobin concentration (MCHC), reticulocytosis, and hyperbilirubinemia. (+)Spherocytes in blood smear. Negative Coombs test. Increased incubated osmotic fragility test. Abnormal cytoskeletal protein analysis.
3. Treatment: May need transfusions for severe anemia, poor growth, and aplastic crises. Splenectomy may also be necessary.

• Hereditary elliptocytosis
1. This is an uncommon illness that is transmitted as an autosomal dominant illness. It frequently involves a defect in the horizontal interactions of spectrin, protein 4.1, and glycophorin C. Elliptocytes can be seen on blood smear and the RBCs are mildly heat sensitive.

• Hereditary pyropoikilocytosis
1. A severe form of hereditary elliptocytosis, this also involves abnormalities in the horizontal interactions of alpha-spectrin. There is extreme variation in RBC size and shape on blood smear and fragmentation of RBCs when incubated at 45°C for 15 minutes.

• Paroxysmal nocturnal hemoglobinuria
1. This is a marrow disorder due to mutations in PIG-A gene, wherein the RBCs are unusually sensitive to complement-mediated lysis.

2. Clinical presentation: 60% present with marrow failure while the rest have intermittent or chronic anemia, often with prominent intravascular hemolysis (nocturnal or morning hemoglobinuria if hemolysis is worse during sleep). Lab tests would include Ham test, sucrose lysis test, bone marrow aspirate, and biopsy to assess cellularity and decay accelerating factor (decreased).

ENZYME DEFICIENCIES

• Pyruvate kinase deficiency
1. Epidemiology: Most common glycolytic enzyme defect as a cause of hemolytic anemia. There are 300–400 reported cases. It is transmitted as an autosomal recessive disease (chromosome 1q21).
2. Pathophysiology: There is decreased pyruvate kinase in the RBC or production of abnormal enzyme with decreased activity. Because of this, there is decreased generation of adenosine triphosphate (ATP), decreased pyruvate and nicotinamide adenine dinucleotide (NAD+), and increased 2,3-diphosphoglycerate (2,3-DPG). The RBC thus cannot maintain its K^+ and H_2O content. The cells become rigid and RBC life span decreases.
3. Clinical presentation: Variable: severe neonatal hemolytic anemia to mild, well-compensated hemolysis first noted in adulthood. Hgb 8–12 g/dL, splenomegaly, jaundice.
4. Diagnosis: Decreased pyruvate kinase activity of increased K_m for its substrate, phosphoenolpyruvate. On peripheral blood smear (PBS), polychromatophilia, mild macrocytosis, pyknocytes; no spherocytes. Normal nonincubated osmotic fragility.
5. Treatment: May need exchange transfusion in newborn period. Packed red blood cell (PRBC) transfusion for severe anemia or aplastic crises. Splenectomy.

• Glucose-6-phosphate dehydrogenase (G6PD) deficiency
1. Epidemiology: X-linked disease. More common in males. Two variants known: Type A- in African-American males and B- in Italians, Greeks, Mediterraneans, Middle Easterns, Africans, and Asians.
2. Clinical presentation: Characterized by episodic or induced hemolysis. Symptoms of hemolysis appear 24–48 hours after exposure to an oxidant (see Table 93-1).
3. Diagnosis: Direct or indirect demonstration of decreased G6PD activity in RBCs.
4. Treatment: Prevent hemolysis by avoiding oxidant drugs. May need blood transfusion for severe anemia.

TABLE 93-1   Agents Precipitating Hemolysis in G6PD

MEDICATIONS	OTHERS
Antibacterials	Acetophenetidin
Sulfonamides	Vitamin K analogs
Cotrimoxazole	Methylene blue
Nalidixic Acid	Probenecid
Chloramphenicol	Acetylsalicylic acid
Nitrofurantoin	Phenazopyridine
Antimalarials	Chemicals
Primaquine	Phenylhydrazine
Pamaquine	Benzene
Chloroquine	Naphthalene
Quinacrine	Illness
	DKA
	Hepatitis

ABBREVIATION: DKA, diabetic ketoacidosis.

EXTRINSIC HEMOLYTIC ANEMIA

IMMUNE-MEDIATED

- Alloantibodies: Transfusion of incompatible blood, hemolytic disease of the newborn.
- Autoantibodies:
  1. Warm reactive IgG-mediated.
  2. Primary (idiopathic)
  3. Secondary: Lymphoproliferative disorders, connective tissue disease (systemic lupus erythematosus [SLE]), nonlymphoid neoplasms, chronic inflammatory diseases (ulcerative colitis).
  4. Cold reactive autoantibodies
  5. Primary (idiopathic) cold agglutinin disease.
  6. Secondary cold agglutinin disease: Lymphoproliferative disorders, infections (*Mycoplasma pneumoniae*, infectious mononucleosis).
- Paroxysmal cold hemoglobinuria
- Drug-related antibodies:
  1. Hapten/drug adsorption: Penicillin, cephalosporin
  2. Ternary (immune) complex: Quinine, quinidine
  3. True autoantibody induction: Alpha-methyldopa

MECHANICAL FRAGMENTATION

- Disseminated intravenous coagulation (DIC)
- Thrombotic thrombocytopenic purpura-hemolytic uremic syndrome
- Extracorporeal membrane oxygenation (ECMO)
- Prosthetic heart valve
- Burns, thermal injury
- Hypersplenism

BIBLIOGRAPHY

Gehrs BC, Friedberg RC. Autoimmune hemolytic anemia. *Am J Hematol* 2002;69:258–271.

Nathan DG and Orkin SH (eds.). *Nathan & Oski's Hematology of Infancy and Childhood*, 5th ed. Philadelphia, PA: W.B. Saunders; 2003.

Sackey K. Hemolytic anemia: Part 1. *Peds in Review* 1999;20(5): 152–159.

94   THALASSEMIAS

Alexis A. Thompson

EPIDEMIOLOGY

- The thalassemia syndromes occur in populations that originate from the Mediterranean region, Northern Africa, the Middle East, Southeast Asia, and the Indian subcontinent. The gene frequency varies worldwide. In some areas up to 10% of the population carries one or more defective globin genes. In general, these conditions are inherited in an autosomal recessive manner.

PATHOPHYSIOLOGY

- Thalassemia results from structural defects of the alpha- or beta-globin genes, located on chromosomes 16 and 11, respectively. In general, genetic mutations in thalassemia impair balanced globin synthesis causing ineffective erythropoiesis and chronic hemolysis. Beta-thalassemia results from mutations in both beta-globin alleles. The four alpha-globin genes are organized as paired alleles on each chromosome 16. Loss of function of three of the four alleles results in a condition called hemoglobin H disease and can result in moderate-to-severe anemia. Mutation or deletion of all four alpha-globin alleles causes profound intrauterine anemia, hydrops fetalis, and is often not compatible with life.

CLINICAL PRESENTATION WITH DIFFERENTIAL DIAGNOSIS

- The hallmark of the thalassemic syndromes is a microcytic anemia. Infants with beta-thalassemia may not necessarily have microcytosis immediately because of the relatively high mean corpuscular volume (MCV) in this age group. The severity of the resultant microcytic anemia varies, in part, with the specific mutation inherited. If untreated, compensatory medullary hyperplasia causes classic bony deformities (frontal bossing, maxillary hypertrophy). Extramedullary hematopoiesis persists in the liver and spleen in many patients, causing organomegaly. Other clinical findings in the first year of life include neonatal hyperbilirubinemia, splenomegaly, and poor growth. Older children may also have jaundice, generalized hyperpigmentation, and skeletal deformities.

- The clinical syndromes associated with inheritance of a mutant betaglobin gene include thalassemia major, thalassemia intermedia, and beta-thalassemia trait. Patients who have thalassemia major or Cooley anemia, are homozygous or compound heterozygous for beta-globin gene mutants and are transfusion-dependent from early childhood. Patients who require intermittent or no transfusions have thalassemia intermedia. In general, inheritance of a single mutant allele or thalassemia trait may be associated with microcytosis but is otherwise an asymptomatic condition.

- Deletion or mutation of a single alpha-globin gene results in a silent carrier state. Loss of two functional genes can be associated with a mild microcytic anemia. More serious clinical manifestations of alpha-thalassemia are seen primarily in Asians based on the pattern of gene losses in this population. The three gene deletion or Hemoglobin H disease is characterized by a moderate hemolytic anemia and splenomegaly. An important variant is hemoglobin H/Constant Spring in which a defect in one alpha gene that causes elongation of the globin chains is coinherited with the deletion of two other alpha genes. Patients with this condition have more severe anemia and may be transfusion-dependent.

- The differential diagnosis for microcytic anemia including the thalassemic syndrome is reviewed in Table 91-2.

DIAGNOSIS/LABORATORY FEATURES

- The principal laboratory studies for the diagnosis of thalassemia are a complete blood count (CBC), reticulocyte count, and quantitative hemoglobin electrophoresis. Patients have a microcytic anemia, and most but not all will have an elevated reticulocyte count, reflecting increased red cell turnover. On hemoglobin electropheresis, the predominant adult HgbA is greatly reduced or absent due to impaired alpha- or beta-globin production. HgbA$_2$, a minor adult hemoglobin may be increased. Other laboratory findings include elevated fetal hemoglobin levels, increased nucleated RBCs on peripheral blood smear, and hyperbilirubinemia.

- The majority of states in the United States now have universal newborn screening programs which can identify infants with beta-thalassemia as well as sickle hemoglobinopathies. Accurate diagnosis, genetic counseling, and expectant management can be best achieved with prompt confirmatory testing and consultation with a pediatric hematologist.

TREATMENT

- The mainstay of therapy for patients with severe anemia is chronic RBC transfusions. Transfusions are generally initiated before the age of 1 year in patients with thalassemia major and are given every 3–4 weeks. The goals of transfusion are correction of anemia, improved growth and development, and suppression of endogenous erythropoiesis. Most patients develop some degree of hypersplenism and benefit from splenectomy to reduce transfusion volume requirements.

- Iron-chelating agents such as deferroxime are effective in controlling complications of transfusion-associated iron overload. Iron accumulation in the liver, heart, and endocrine glands causes irreversible damage and can result in hepatic failure, diabetes, hypothyroidism, infertility, and myocardial dysfunction.

Further information available at www.cooleysanemia. org

---

95 THROMBOCYTOPENIA

Joanna L. Weinstein and
Alexis A. Thompson

- Thrombocytopenia is defined as a decrease in the number of circulating platelets. Normal platelet counts ranges from 150,000 to 450,000/mm^3. Platelets, anuclear cytoplasmic fragments originating from bone marrow (BM) megakaryocytes, circulate for 7–10 days until removal by the reticuloendothelial system (RES) or until aggregation at the site of subendothelial injury of a blood vessel.

THROMBOCYTOPENIA DUE TO INCREASED DESTRUCTION

IDIOPATHIC THROMBOCYTOPENIC PURPURA (ITP)

EPIDEMIOLOGY
- Acute ITP, the most common cause of severe thrombocytopenia in the United States, affects approximately 5/100,000 children per year. Approximately 15% of acute cases become chronic, lasting longer than 6 months.

PATHOPHYSIOLOGY
- ITP develops when the host immune system produces antibodies that cross-react with platelet surface antigens. Sometimes a preceding inciting event, such as a viral infection, can be identified. The antibody-coated platelets are removed by the RES, causing thrombocytopenia.

CLINICAL PRESENTATIONS
- ITP is associated with the abrupt onset of bruising or bleeding, including ecchymoses, petechiae, epistaxis, gum bleeding, menorrhagia, or occult or gross bleeding in the stool or urine. Acute ITP tends to occur in healthy, younger children less than 10 years of age, often following a viral illness within weeks. Apart from the bleeding signs listed above, the child has an otherwise normal examination, though mild splenomegaly may be present. In rare instances when thrombocytopenia occurs with Coombs-positive hemolytic anemia, the disorder is called Evans syndrome.

DIAGNOSIS/LABORATORY FEATURES
- Complete blood count (CBC) reveals varying degrees of thrombocytopenia; counts less than 10,000/mm^3 are not uncommon. The rest of the CBC is normal, unless anemia is present after a history of significant bleeding. Peripheral blood smear may reveal large platelets. Immature white blood cells and abnormal red blood cell (RBC) forms, such as fragments, are absent. BM exhibits normal hematopoiesis with normal to increased numbers of megakaryocytes. Sometimes, antiplatelet antibodies are detected.

COMPLICATIONS
- Severe thrombocytopenia may be associated with life-threatening bleeding, namely intracranial hemorrhage (ICH), which fortunately is rare.

TREATMENT
- Some patients with ITP may be observed without therapy. Supportive care includes minimizing physical activities, avoiding products that may affect platelet function, and wearing protective helmets. Pharmacologic options include intravenous immunoglobulin (IVIG), corticosteroids, and anti-D (Rh)-antibody. Refractory cases may require splenectomy or other pharmacologic interventions. Platelet transfusions are not indicated.

ALLOIMMUNE THROMBOCYTOPENIA IN THE NEONATE

EPIDEMIOLOGY
- Alloimmune (isoimmune) thrombocytopenia (AIT) occurs with an estimated frequency of 1/1000 live births. It is a major cause of primary hemorrhagic morbidity and mortality in otherwise well fetuses and newborns.

PATHOPHYSIOLOGY
- AIT results from alloimmunization. Antiplatelet antibodies develop in the maternal serum against paternally-inherited fetal platelet antigens that are absent on the maternal platelet; the antiplatelet antibodies cross the placenta and bind to fetal platelets. The most common platelet incompatibility involves Pl^{A1}, an antigen present on the platelets of 98% of Caucasian persons.

CLINICAL PRESENTATION
- Bleeding, namely intracranial hemorrhage (ICH) may occur in the neonatal period or during gestation. Bleeding, petechiae or ecchymoses may be evident after birth in an otherwise well newborn.

DIAGNOSIS/LABORATORY FEATURES
- Thrombocytopenia of varying degrees is evident by CBC and usually resolves within weeks. Antigen testing is performed on the mother's and father's platelets for diagnostic purposes and for genetic counseling. Maternal platelet count is normal.

COMPLICATIONS
- Thrombocytopenia, which may be severe with an onset early in gestation, can lead to intrauterine or intrapartum ICH. There is a high risk of recurrence in future pregnancies, with more severe symptoms affecting subsequent siblings.

TREATMENT
- Affected neonates are treated with transfusions of maternal platelets, which lack the sensitizing antigen. Other treatments, including IVIG, steroids, exchange transfusion, intrauterine therapies and transfusions, have shown variable results.

ISOIMMUNE THROMBOCYTOPENIA IN THE NEONATE

EPIDEMIOLOGY

- Isoimmune thrombocytopenia is less common than AIT.

PATHOPHYSIOLOGY

- Fetal and neonatal thrombocytopenia occurs because of transplacental transfer of antibodies from a mother with ITP (i.e., passive ITP). Variable degrees of thrombocytopenia may persist for months, paralleling the disappearance of maternal antibodies from the infant's circulation.

CLINICAL PRESENTATION

- Neonates may have bleeding associated with this condition.

DIAGNOSIS

- The maternal history of ITP supports this diagnosis.

COMPLICATIONS

- Neonates should be observed for signs of bleeding.

TREATMENT

- No specific treatment is required.

OTHER THROMBOCYTOPENIAS RELATED TO PERIPHERAL CONSUMPTION

EPIDEMIOLOGY

- Disseminated intravascular coagulation (DIC), hemolytic uremic syndrome (HUS) and thrombotic thrombocytopenic purpura (TTP) cause nonimmune consumptive thrombocytopenia. Some cases of HUS and TTP have familial tendencies.

PATHOPHYSIOLOGY

- The thrombocytopenia of DIC, HUS, and TTP results from platelet consumption in microthrombi related to or triggered by endothelial injury. In hypersplenism, platelets are trapped in an enlarged spleen. Throm-boses, prosthetic valves, and vascular devices can destroy platelets. Heparin occasionally may induce thrombocytopenia via an immunologic mechanism.

CLINICAL PRESENTATION

- DIC in children occurs in the setting of overwhelming infection or sepsis, severe trauma, brain injury, or Kasabach-Meritt syndrome and may be associated with bleeding or thrombosis.
- HUS presents with acute bleeding and bruising, symptoms of thrombocytopenia, with microangiopathic hemolytic anemia and uremia, and may occur after a bout of hemorrhagic colitis.
- TTP is characterized by symptoms of thrombocytopenia, microangiopathic hemolytic anemia, neurologic and renal impairment, and fever.
- Thrombocytopenia occurring in patients with hypersplenism related to portal hypertension and sickle cell disease usually is not associated with bleeding symptoms.
- Heparin-induced thrombocytopenia (HIT), occurring 8–10 days after reexposure to heparin, may be paradoxically associated with arterial thrombosis rather than bleeding symptoms.

DIAGNOSIS/LABORATORY FEATURES

- DIC is characterized by varying degrees of thrombocytopenia along with evidence of consumptive coagulopathy with elevation of prothrombin time (PT), partial thromboplastin time (PTT), fibrin split products, and D-dimers and reduction of fibrinogen.
- In Kasabach-Meritt syndrome, a large vascular lesion is evident with laboratory evidence of the consumptive coagulopathy.
- The peripheral blood smear in TTP and HUS demonstrates thrombocytopenia and RBC fragmentation. Consistent history, physical examination, and bloodwork suggesting of renal insufficiency support the diagnosis.
- Thrombocytopenia due to hypersplenism is a diagnosis of exclusion in a patient with a compatible underlying disorder associated with splenomegaly.
- HIT is diagnosed by detection of heparin-associated antibodies in a patient reexposed to heparin.

TREATMENT

- Treatment is directed at the underlying cause. Platelet transfusions may be indicated for bleeding symptoms. The hematologic manifestations of DIC, HUS, and TTP require supportive care. Plasmapheresis treats the nonhematologic manifestations of TTP. Kasabach-Meritt syndrome may require pharmacologic treatment or embolization of the underlying vascular anomaly. HIT and other drug-induced thrombocytopenias are treated by discontinuation of heparin or the inciting agent.

COMPLICATIONS

- Bleeding can be severe in the consumptive thrombocytopenias, especially if associated with consumption of coagulation proteins. HIT can cause arterial thrombosis.

THROMBOCYTOPENIA DUE TO DECREASED PLATELET PRODUCTION

EPIDEMIOLOGY

- Amegakaryocytic thrombocytopenia (AT), thrombocytopenia-absent radii syndrome (TAR), and its variants are rare congenital disorders with a variable inheritance patterns. Wiskott-Aldrich syndrome typically has an X-linked recessive inheritance. Thrombocytopenia may occur with acquired or inherited bone marrow failure syndromes, such as aplastic anemia and Fanconi anemia, and infiltrative disorders, such as leukemia and myelodysplastic syndrome. Acute or chronic use of some medications can cause bone marrow suppression.

PATHOPHYSIOLOGY

- Thrombocytopenia is caused by defective or ineffective production of platelets in the bone marrow due to genetic defects in thrombocytopoiesis and megakaryocytopoiesis. In infiltrative processes, normal marrow precursors including megakaryocytes are replaced by leukemia or myelodysplastic cells.

CLINICAL PRESENTATIONS

- Thrombocytopenia related to abnormal production may present with bruising and bleeding symptoms. Wiskott-Aldrich syndrome also has features of eczema and recurrent infection related to immunodeficiency. TAR has characteristic deformities of the forearm and thrombocytopenia detected early in life. Aplastic anemia presents with bruising and bleeding or clinical signs of anemia or leukopenia. Infiltrative disorders, including leukemia or myelodysplasia, are characterized by thrombocytopenia associated with pancytopenia, peripheral leukemic blasts, or organomegaly.

DIAGNOSIS/LABORATORY FEATURES

- Varying degrees of thrombocytopenia occur in hypoproductive and infiltrative disorders. The peripheral blood smear typically demonstrates small platelets.

COMPLICATIONS

- Bleeding and bruising symptoms are of variable severity and are related to the degree of the thrombocytopenia.

TREATMENT

- Some of the congenital quantitative platelet syndromes are treated symptomatically with platelet transfusions. In many cases, these disorders are treated with bone marrow transplantation.

THROMBOCYTOPENIA OF NEONATAL SEPSIS AND CONGENITAL INFECTIONS

EPIDEMIOLOGY

- Thrombocytopenia in the neonate commonly occurs in association with infection and sepsis.

PATHOPHYSIOLOGY

- Thrombocytopenia occurs related to overwhelming bone marrow suppression or to peripheral consumption. Congenital infections with cytomegalovirus (CMV), rubella, and toxoplasma may cause impaired marrow production or peripheral consumption related to splenomegaly.

CLINICAL FEATURES

- Neonates with sepsis are commonly febrile, may be hemodynamically unstable, and are generally unwell with signs of thrombocytopenia such as petechiae. Congenital infections are associated with other characteristic symptoms, including fever, lymphadenopathy, and hepatosplenomegaly.

DIAGNOSIS

- Infection-related thrombocytopenia is detected by CBC in a neonate showing other signs of infection. Cultures and serologies may establish an infectious agent.

TREATMENT

- Septic neonates are treated for their underlying infections, with platelet transfusions in situations of bleeding.

BIBLIOGRAPHY

Bussel JB. Alloimmune thrombocytopenia in the fetus and newborn. *Semin Thromb Hemost* 2001;27:245–252.

Dipaola J, Buchanan G. Immune thrombocytopenic purpura. *Pediatr Clin North Am* 2002;49:911–928.

Nathan DG and Orkin SH (eds.). *Nathan & Oski's Hematology of Infancy and Childhood, 5th ed.* Philadelphia, PA: W.B. Saunders; 2003.

96 HEMOPHILIA AND OTHER BLEEDING DISORDERS

Deborah L. Brown

HEMOPHILIA

DEFINITIONS

- Hemophilia is a congenital bleeding disorder caused by the deficiency of Factor VIII (FVIII) (hemophilia A) or Factor IX (FIX) (hemophilia B). Hemophilia A and B are associated with very similar clinical symptoms.

The genes for FVIII and FIX are located on the X chromosome; thus hemophilia is an X-linked disorder affecting primarily males. One in 5000 males is born with hemophilia A and 1 in 30,000 with hemophilia B, incidences that are similar among all studied ethnic groups. Approximately 75% of males with hemophilia have a positive family history, but mutational hotspots within the FVIII and FIX genes lead to a high incidence of sporadic new cases. Forty percent of patients with severe hemophilia have a deletion in intron 22 which causes inversion of the A2 domain.

CLINICAL PRESENTATION

- In coagulation disorders, the initial platelet plug may be adequate, but subsequent fibrin deposition is deficient, resulting in delayed or prolonged bleeding. Common sites of bleeding include mucocutaneous tissues, muscle, joint, gastrointestinal (GI) tract, and genitourinary tract. Hematoma of muscles in the volar forearm or anterior tibialis fascial compartments can cause nerve compression and impairment. Likewise, bleeding in the ileopsoas muscle at the level of the inguinal ligament can cause femoral nerve compression. Recurrent joint bleeding leads to permanent arthropathy and is one of the major causes of long-term morbidity among patients with hemophilia. Intracranial hemorrhage occurs in 10% of patients with hemophilia, often without history of precipitating trauma.

DIAGNOSIS

- The diagnosis of hemophilia A and B is based on a prolonged partial thromboplastin time (PTT) with reduced FVIII or FIX activity in the absence of other coagulation defects (see acquired bleeding disorders below). Coagulation factor activity measurements correlate well with the clinical level of severity, which is indistinguishable between FVIII and FIX deficiency. Patients with factor levels <2% are considered to have severe hemophilia, 2–5% is moderate, and 5–30% is mild. Patients with severe hemophilia average 25 bleeding episodes per year and may bleed with minimal or no trauma, while those with mild hemophilia may have bleeding only with significant trauma or surgery. PTT and factor levels can be obtained from umbilical cord blood in a male baby with a positive family history, as coagulation factors are not transferred across the placenta. Factor IX levels may be lower than adult normal standards in newborns due to vitamin K deficiency and decreased hepatic synthesis. Patients with Factor VIII levels 5–50% should be differentiated from patients with Von Willebrand's disorder (VWD) Type II or III (see below).

TREATMENT

- The treatment of hemophilia consists of replacement of the deficient protein with clotting factor concentrates. Since 1970, the availability of lyophilized factor concentrates has given patients the ability to self-infuse in the home setting. Improvements in the safety of factor replacement therapy have encouraged the use of prophylaxis regimens in which factor is infused on a periodic basis to maintain trough factor levels >1% and prevent bleeding complications. Most are treated with a monoclonal or recombinant antihemophilic product. Up to 30% of patients with severe hemophilia develop inhibiting antibodies to exogenous factor, necessitating high-dose tolerance regimens, and use of "bypass" agents, such as activated prothrombin complexes rFVIIa for treatment of bleeding episodes (Table 96-1).

FACTOR REPLACEMENT THERAPY FOR HEMOPHILIA A
- Dose = % correction desired × weight (kg) × 0.5.

TABLE 96-1 Type of Bleed and Desired Correction

TYPE OF BLEED	FACTOR VIII DEFICIENCY	FACTOR IX DEFICIENCY
Major bleeding episodes		
Head trauma/ICH	80–100%	60–80%
Surgery	80–100% (trough)	60–80% (trough)
Gastrointestinal bleeding	80–100%	60–80%
Throat and neck	80–100%	60–80%
Compartment/iliopsoas	80–100%	60–80%
Minor bleeding episodes		
Target joint bleed	80%	60–80%
Joint or muscle bleed	40%	30%
Epistaxis	30% + local measures	20% + local measures
Hematuria	40% + fluids and bed rest	40% + fluids and bed rest

ABBREVIATION: ICH, intracranial hemorrhage.

**FACTOR REPLACEMENT THERAPY
FOR HEMOPHILIA B**
- Plasma-derived FIX product dose = % correction desired × weight (kg) × 1.0.
- Recombinant FIX product dose = % correction desired × weight (kg) × 1.4 (Table 96-1).

FACTOR XI DEFICIENCY

- Factor XI deficiency is often referred to as hemophilia C. It differs from hemophilia A and B in that it is an autosomal recessive disorder and bleeding symptoms tend to be mild and mainly involve the mucocutaneous tissues. Factor XI activity levels do not correlate well with clinical features, but levels of 40% or higher are considered necessary to insure hemostasis during surgery. Three-point mutations on the FXI gene account for the majority of cases and genotype determination has been shown to predict phenotypic variation to some extent. Approximately 8% of the Ashkenazi Jewish population are carriers. When needed, Factor XI deficiency is treated with fresh frozen plasma.

VON WILLEBRAND DISEASE

DEFINITIONS

- Von Willebrand disease is the most common inherited bleeding disorder, occurring in 1–2% of the population.
- *Type 1 VWD* is the most common form and accounts for 85% of cases. Type 1 VWD is a mild bleeding disorder caused by a partial deficiency of von Willebrand Factor protein. Bleeding symptoms are platelet-type, and usually involve the mucosal membranes, leading to epistaxis, gingival bleeding, and menorrhagia. Definitive laboratory diagnosis is sometimes elusive, as VWF is an acute phase reactant which may be elevated during stress, exercise, and proinflammatory states. PTT and bleeding time are normal in up to 50% of patients with Type 1 VWD, and are therefore inadequate screening tests. Platelet function analyzer (PFA)-100 has emerged as the most sensitive screening test for VWD Type I and has essentially replaced the bleeding time in most laboratories. The laboratory diagnosis of VWD Type 1 is based on proportionally low levels of Von Willebrand protein (VWF:Ag), VWF activity (ristocetin cofactor), and FVIII:coagulant activity (FVIII:c). The clinical diagnosis requires presence of bleeding symptoms as well as a positive family history of bleeding symptoms.

- *Type 2 VWD* is a group of qualitative disorders of Von Willebrand factor characterized by VWF activity which is lower than VWF:Ag. Type 2A is due to inadequate multimerization of VWF with a lack of high molecular weight multimers seen on agarose gel. Type 2B is due to increased VWF binding to the GPIb/IX/V complex on platelets, leading to thrombocytopenia and lack of high molecular weight multimers. Type 2M is caused by defective binding of VWF to GPIb. Type 2N is due to a mutation in the FVIII-binding region of VWF, leading to defective VWF-FVIII binding.
- *Type 3 VWD* is a severe deficiency of VWD in which both VWF:Ag and ristocetin cofactor measurements are undetectable. Patients with Type 3 VWD have FVIII levels less than 10% and may have bleeding symptoms similar to those with hemophilia, such as joint and muscle bleeds.

TREATMENT

- Treatment options for patients with VWD include antifibrinolytic agents, desmopressin acetate (DDAVP), and VWF concentrates. Antifibrinolytic agents impede fibrinolysis in mucosal membranes where endogenous tissue plasminogen activator (TPA) is very active. Epsilon aminocaproic acid (Amicar) or tranexemic acid are available in oral and IV forms and provide a useful adjunct to DDAVP and VWF concentrates. The usual dose of Amicar is 100 mg/kg every 6–8 hours. DDAVP is effective in increasing VWF:Ag, RCF, and FVIII:C levels by greater than threefold in approximately 85% of patients with Type 1 VWD. A DDAVP treatment trial is required to confirm efficacy prior to surgical procedures involving the mucosal membranes, such as tonsillectomy or dental extractions. The usual dose is 0.3 µg/kg IV. Alternatively, DDAVP (Stimate) can be administered intranasally. DDAVP can worsen the thrombocytopenia in patients with Type 2B VWD, and should be used judiciously in this group. It is unlikely to be effective in Type 2A VWD, and has a very short duration of action in Type 2N. The mechanism of action of DDAVP is unknown, but may cause release of stored VWF protein from endothelial cells. VWF concentrates currently available in the United States are derived from intermediate-purity FVIII concentrates which are labeled with ristocetin cofactor units. Maintaining ristocetin cofactor activity >80% appears to provide adequate hemostasis during surgical procedures. Recombinant VWF concentrates are currently in development.

QUALITATIVE PLATELET DISORDERS

- Quantitative platelet disorders (e.g., thrombocytopenia) are discussed elsewhere in this manual. Qualitative platelet disorders can lead to platelet-type bleeding in patients with a normal platelet count. The bleeding time, which is the traditional screening test for platelet disorders, is imprecise and unreliable. The PFA-100, which has been validated for screening Von Willebrand disorder, may be helpful to diagnose most qualitative platelet disorders, but is relatively insensitive to storage pool release defects. Platelet aggregation studies are performed on fresh whole blood or platelet-rich plasma.

GLANZMANN THROMBASTHENIA (GT)

- Glanzmann thrombasthenia is a rare autosomal recessive platelet function disorder caused by a deficient or dysfunctional fibrinogen receptor, GPIIb/IIIa. GT is suspected in a patient with platelet-type bleeding with a normal platelet count. Bleeding time or PFA-100 closure time is prolonged, and platelet aggregation studies show absent aggregation to thrombin, epinephrine, and adenosine diphosphate (ADP), but normal response to ristocetin. GT patients have mucocutaneous bleeding symptoms and are at risk for intracranial hemorrhage, GI bleeding, hematuria, and hemarthrosis. Because of the risk of alloimmunization with exposure to GPIIb/IIIa containing donor platelets, platelet transfusions are reserved for cases of severe or life-threatening bleeding disorders. DDAVP has been shown to partially correct the bleeding time and rFVIIa has decreased bleeding symptoms in several patients with GT.

BERNARD-SOULIER SYNDROME

- Bernard-Soulier syndrome is caused by a deficient or defective platelet VWF receptor, GPIb/IX/V complex. Throm-bocytopenia with large platelets (elevated mean platelet volume [MPV]) is characteristic. The severity of bleeding symptoms is variable.

HERMANSKY-PUDLAK SYNDROME

- Hermansky-Pudlak syndrome is due to abnormal dense granules which can be seen by electron microscopy. Lack of melatonin in the dense granules also causes oculocutaneous albinism.

PLATELET STORAGE POOL RELEASE DEFECTS

- Platelet storage pool release defects, such as *Gray platelet syndrome,* usually result in mild bleeding symptoms, but can cause an abnormal bleeding time or PFA-100 to ADP/collagen.

ACQUIRED COAGULATION DISORDERS

- Acquired bleeding disorders are usually caused by comorbid medical conditions, and may involve coagulation, platelet function, fibrinolysis, or vascular integrity. Acquired coagulation disorders include coagulation inhibitors, disseminated intravascular coagulation, vitamin K deficiency, and liver disease. Coagulation inhibitors are detected if prolongation of PT or PTT is not corrected by the 1:1 mix of normal plasma. The lupus anticoagulant is a coagulation inhibitor in vitro which is prothrombotic in vivo— bleeding symptoms occur only when it is associated with prothrombin deficiency and an abnormal PT. DIC is characterized by a prolonged prothrombin time with elevated D-dimer and thrombocytopenia in a patient with sepsis, trauma, or malignancy. Treatment consists of replacement of blood components including plasma and cryoprecipitate. Vitamin K deficiency may be caused by fat malabsorption, prolonged antibiotic use, or coumadin exposure. Vitamin K deficiency can treated with SC or IV vitamin K replacement, but immediate reversal of the coagulopathy requires plasma infusion. Liver disease can lead to deficiency of the hepatic-synthesized coagulation proteins fibrinogen, prothrombin, FV, VII, FIX, FX, and FXI.

BIBLIOGRAPHY

Colman RW, Hirsh J, et al. *Hemostasis and Thrombosis: Basic Principles and Clinical Practice*, 4th ed. Philadelphia, PA: Lippincott Williams & Wilkins, 2001.

Mann KG. Biochemistry and physiology of blood coagulation. *Thromb Haemost* 1999;82:165–174.

Mannucci PM, Tuddenham EG. The hemophilias—from royal genes to gene therapy. *N Engl J Med* 2001;344:1773–1779.

Sadler JE, Mannucci PM, et al. Impact, diagnosis and treatment of von Willebrand disease. *Thromb Haemost* 2000;84:160–174.

Shapiro AD. Platelet function disorders: World Federation of Hemophilia publications, No. 19, 1999.

Further information available at www.hemophilia.org

97 THROMBOPHILIA

Peter E. Zage and Deborah L. Brown

DEFINITIONS

• Thrombophilia connotes abnormal clotting which may be acquired or inherited. It is an area of intense study as new diagnostic tools and treatments are emerging. Thrombophilia is often suggested by spontaneous thrombi and/or unusual locations.

EPIDEMIOLOGY

• The incidence of thromboses varies with age. The peak risk of thrombosis occurs during the neonatal period, then decreases in infancy and early childhood. The risk increases after puberty with a slow rise during adulthood.
• Children typically have clots that involve large vessels and usually have other predisposing conditions (see next section).
• A variety of factors contribute to increased risk of clotting in neonates. Newborns have a higher hematocrit, increased levels of vWF multimers and increased levels of Factor VIII. Infants have decreased levels of the natural anticoagulants antithrombin III, protein C, protein S, and plasminogen. Healthy full-term infants have markedly reduced levels of Factors II, VII, IX, and X compared to adults and may not reach adult levels until 6–12 months of age.

ETIOLOGY/PATHOPHYSIOLOGY

CONGENITAL

PROTEIN C DEFICIENCY
• Protein C is a natural anticoagulant that is activated by thrombin. Protein S and thrombomodulin act as cofactors. Activated protein C inactivates Factors V and VIII. The inability to inactivate clotting factors results in thrombi formation.

PROTEIN S DEFICIENCY
• Protein S is a cofactor for protein C and, as such, the pathophysiology of protein S deficiency is similar.

ANTITHROMBIN III DEFICIENCY
• Antithrombin III is a serine protease inhibitor that inactivates Factors XIIa, XIa, IXa, Xa, and IIa.

Heparin is an essential cofactor. All individuals who are heterozygous for an ATIII mutation have an increased risk for thrombosis. Homozygotes have lower but detectable levels and tend to have clot formation at an earlier age.

FACTOR V LEIDEN
• A mutation in Factor V that impairs its inactivation by protein C can result in thrombophilia. Approximately 5–8% Caucasians are heterozygous for this mutation and 0.1% are homozygous. The highest prevalence is in Northern Europeans. Factor V Leiden is rare in African-Americans and Asians.

PROTHROMBIN GENE MUTATION
• A G20210A mutation in the 3′ untranslated region of the prothrombin gene results in increased prothrombin production. One to two percent of Caucasians are heterozygous for this mutation.

METHYLTETRAHYDROFOLATE REDUCTASE (MTHFR) DEFICIENCY
• Approximately 10% of the normal population have mutations in the gene which encodes MTHFR. This deficiency may be associated with increased levels of homocysteine and increased risk of myocardial infarctions and strokes in adults. MTHFR deficiency is not associated with hyperhomocysteinemia in children and therefore the risk of thrombosis is unclear in the pediatric population.

ACQUIRED

VENOUS ACCESS DEVICES
• Central venous catheters are the most common acquired risk factor for thrombosis in children. This may be due to vascular obstruction, endothelial irritation by infused medications, or deposition of fibrin and platelets over time from transfused blood products.

ANTIPHOSPHOLIPID SYNDROME
• Primary antiphospholipid syndrome, which is very rare in children, requires the evidence of anticardiolipin or antiphospholipid antibodies in association with a blood clot and in the absence of other conditions. Causes of secondary antiphospholipids syndrome include infections, systemic lupus erythematosis, liver disease, or malignancies.

INFLAMMATORY DISORDERS
• Conditions that are associated with vasculitis, vasculopathies, or platelet activation can induce thromboses.

These include systemic lupus erythematosus (SLE), juvenile rheumatoid arthritis (JRA), diabetes mellitus, and inflammatory bowel disease.

NEPHROTIC SYNDROME
- Proteinuria results in loss of antithrombin III.

MEDICATIONS
- Oral contraceptive use is associated with thrombophilia, particularly in individuals with other thrombotic risk factors.
- l-Asparaginase, a common chemotherapeutic agent, causes diminished protein synthesis in the liver of clotting factors, including antithrombin III.

CLINICAL PRESENTATION

- In general, symptoms associated with thrombosis vary with location. For example, deep vein thromboses (DVT) present with pain, swelling, and reduced perfusion in the affected limb. Pulmonary emboli (PE) may present with tachypnea, shortness of breath, tachycardia, or cyanosis.

DIAGNOSIS

SUSPECTED ACUTE THROMBUS

- Laboratory studies
- D-dimer
- Radiographic studies
  1. Doppler ultrasound with compression.
  2. Venogram for collaterals.
  3. For pulmonary emboli: Spiral computed tomography (CT), ventilation/perfusion (V/Q) scan.

PRIMARY SCREENING

- The purpose of these evaluations is only to determine the need for prophylaxis and for family counseling:
- Complete blood count (CBC)
- ATIII, protein C, protein S
- Factor VIII activity
- Factor V Leiden, prothrombin gene mutation
- Lupus anticoagulant, anticardiolipin Ab
- Hemoglobin electrophoresis
- Homocysteine level

TREATMENT

PROPHYLAXIS

- Routine heparin flushes of venous access devices
- Low-dose warfarin
- Low molecular weight heparin (LMWH)

ACUTE THROMBOSIS

- Anticoagulation
  1. Unfractionated heparin
  2. LMWH
- Thrombolytic therapy
  1. Indications: Large pulmonary embolus, pulmonary embolism (PE) unresponsive to heparin, acute large proximal DVT.
  2. Contraindications: Cerebrovascular accident (CVA), central nervous system (CNS) tumor, recent surgery, hypertension, active bleeding.
- Surgery
  1. Thrombectomy may be considered for large obstructive intracardiac clots.
  2. Intravascular filters are rarely indicated in children and should only be considered for thrombi which fail to respond to medical therapy or when there is an ongoing contraindication to anticoagulation.

SECONDARY PROPHYLAXIS

- Warfarin (coumadin)
- LMWH
- Antiplatelet agents: Aspirin, plavix

DURATION OF PROPHYLAXIS
- For nonidiopathic thrombi (postsurgical, trauma-induced, and catheter-associated): 3 months.
- For idiopathic thrombi: 6–12 months.
- If two or more congenital risk factors: Indefinite.

BIBLIOGRAPHY

Hoppe C and Matsunaga A. Pediatric thrombosis. *Pediatr Clin North Am* 2002;49:1257–83.

Manco-Johnson MJ, Nuss R. Thrombophilia in the infant and child. *Adv in Pediatr* 2001;48:363–84.

Richardson MW, Allen GA, Monahan PE. Thrombosis in children: Current perspective and distinct challenges. *Thrombosis Haemostasis* 2002;88:900–11.

98 NEUTROPENIA

Alexis A. Thompson

- The relative and absolute neutrophil counts (ANC) normally vary with age; however, an absolute neutrophil count of less than 1500/mm^3 should prompt further evaluation. The most important consequence of acute or chronic neutropenia is the risk of bacterial and fungal infections. The following is the formula for calculation for the ANC: % segmented neutrophils + % band forms) × total white blood cell [WBC] count.
- The type and risk of infection increase with the degree of neutropenia:

Mild	ANC	1500–1000	Minimal or no symptoms
Moderate		1000–500	Stomatitis, gingivitis, skin infections
Severe		<500	Pneumonia, abscesses, sepsis

PATHOGENESIS

- The mechanisms for neutropenia are typically one of the following: (1) Bone marrow failure resulting in ineffective granulocyte production; (2) neutrophil destruction; or (3) a combination of both.

TYPES OF NEUTROPENIA

HEREDITARY NEUTROPENIA

- *Severe congenital neutropenia* (Kostmann syndrome, infantile genetic agranulocytosis) is an autosomal recessive condition that usually presents during infancy with omphalitis, delayed umbilical cord separation, or later in childhood with recurrent otitis media, mucosal ulcerations, and skin infections. Bone marrow findings are characterized by myeloid maturational arrest and abundant promyelocytes. In most cases, patients respond to routine injections of granulocyte colony-stimulating factor (G-CSF, filgrastim). Patients with this condition have an increased predisposition for leukemia.
- *Chronic benign neutropenia* is an autosomal dominant disorder that is associated with mild-to-moderate neutropenia. Patients may have recurrent fevers but usually do not have serious infections. *Chronic idiopathic*

neutropenia has a similar presentation and is due to as yet poorly understood defects in myelopoiesis. Spontaneous remissions may occur at age 2–4 years. The relative risk of serious infection is low.

- *Cyclic neutropenia* can be associated with infections during the neutropenic phase. The periodicity of the neutropenic cycles can be 10–21 days. The fundamental defect in this condition is within the G-CSF signal transduction pathway, often associated with mutations in the neutrophil elastase gene. Consequently, administration of recombinant G-CSF can be beneficial in some patients.
- *Pseudoneutropenia* is a common incidental finding in asymptomatic patients, occurring in up to 30–40% African-Americans and 7% of Whites. It results from disproportionate margination of circulating granulocytes, but can be associated with a reduced marrow storage pool. These patients have no increased risk of serious infection and are capable of mounting a normal increased neutrophil count in response to stress.
- Finally, when evaluating patients with neutropenia, it is important to look for associated physical and laboratory findings (Table 98-1).

ACQUIRED NEUTROPENIAS

- *Infections* are the most common conditions associated with acquired neutropenia. Viral, bacterial, fungal, and protozoal infections can induce neutropenia by affecting granulocyte production (marrow suppression, depletion of peripheral storage pools), as well as by enhancing neutrophil consumption, sequestration, and destruction. The severity and duration of neutropenia varies with different organisms. Viruses that cause common childhood illnesses typically result in transient neutropenia. Other viral infections with human immunodeficiency virus (HIV), hepatitis, or parvovirus may result in more protracted neutropenia. Pathogens such as tuberculosis,

TABLE 98-1 Neutropenias Associated with Phenotypic Abnormalities

SYNDROME	OTHER ASSOCIATED FINDINGS
Schwachmann-Diamond	Pancreatic insufficiency, short stature, metaphyseal dysostosis
Chediak-Higashi	Oculocutaneous albinism, rotatory nystagmus, neutrophils with giant intracellular lysosomal granules
Fanconis anemia	Variable pancytopenia, short stature, hyperpigmentation, skeletal or renal abnormalities
Cartilage-hair hypoplasia	Dwarfism, fine hair, impaired cellular immunity
Dyskeratosis congenita	Nail dystrophy, leukoplakia, reticulated hyperpigmented skin

cytomegalovirus, and malaria, which cause chronic splenomegaly, may cause chronic neutropenia due to sequestration. Sepsis causes endotoxin-mediated peripheral destruction, complement driven leukocyte aggregation, and marrow exhaustion. In general, neutropenia associated with gram-negative sepsis resolves rapidly with effective antibiotic therapy.

• *Drug-induced neutropenia* can be idiosyncratic, dose-dependent, or the result of a hypersensitivity reaction. The list of drugs associated with neutropenia is extensive. Antibiotics such as penicillins, sulfonamides, cephalosporins, and chloramphenicol can cause suppression or and immune-mediated destruction which usually begins 1–2 weeks after administration. Anticonvulsants (phenobarbital, carbamazepine, and phenytoin) can cause dose-dependent suppression, immune-mediated destruction, or hypersensitivity reactions. Sedatives such as chlorpromazine and phenothiazines, and anti-inflammatory analgesics such as ibuprofen, indomethacin, and aminopyrines are also associated with neutropenia. Withdrawal of the medication when feasible is often sufficient for reversing the neutropenia.

• Immune-mediated neutropenias can occur at any age. Infants are more likely to have *isoimmune neonatal neutropenia,* while older children and some infants may have *autoimmune neutropenia.* In both instances, patients have circulating granulocyte-specific auto-antibodies which mediate neutrophil destruction by complement-mediated lysis or splenic phagocytosis. Isoimmune neonatal neutropenia results from gestational sensitization to fetal neutrophils and subsequent transplacental transfer of maternal antineutrophil antibodies. Neutropenia can be severe and may be associated with fever and infections. Supportive care including antibiotics is generally sufficient to manage this self-limited condition. Autoimmune neutropenia is less often associated with serious infections. As such, most patients need only supportive care. Effective treatment options include corticosteroids, intravenous immune globulin (IVIG), G-CSF, and rituximab.

• Isolated neutropenia can be the initial indication of marrow replacement, such as myelofibrosis, leukemia, metastases of a solid tumor; however, more often there are other associated findings. Bone pain, fever, anemia, thrombocytopenia, or evidence of an intraabdominal or mediastinal mass are other common presenting signs and symptoms.

• Nutritional deficiencies can also be associated with neutropenia. These include vitamin B_{12}, folic acid, and copper. There may be other hematologic findings such as anemia. The specific diagnosis requires evaluation using serum assays.

• Chemotherapy and radiation therapy have predictable effects on granulocyte production. The time to onset of neutropenia varies with different cytotoxic agents. The risk of serious infection is related to the severity as well as the anticipated duration of neutropenia.

TREATMENT

• For acute or therapy-induced neutropenia one should consider hospitalization for initial management (Fig. 98-1). The use of *oral or IV antibiotics* depends on the severity of neutropenia and the etiology. Evaluation should include appropriate cultures. Initial treatment should be with broad spectrum antibiotics. Antifungal therapy may be needed if still febrile after 5–7 days. Patients with chronic neutropenias warrant site-specific cultures. The choice of antibiotics should cover *Staphylococcus aureus*, pneumococcus, and gram-negative organisms.

• *Granulocyte infusions* are of limited utility in most circumstances. Exchange plasmapheresis and maternal WBC infusion have been used in neonatal isoimmune neutropenia.

• *IVIG* may be efficacious in isoimmune and some cases of autoimmune neutropenia.

• *Corticosteroids* have little benefit in most acute neutropenias. Moreover, the transient increase in circulating neutrophils may be offset by deleterious effect on the overall immune function.

• *Colony-stimulating factors* can be effective in cases which warrant therapy. The efficacy of growth factors in chemotherapy or radiation-induced neutropenia is variable. They can reduce the duration and severity of neutropenia. Some studies report fewer infections when used expectantly in high-risk patients; however, the overall utility of CSFs in the acute management of the febrile neutropenic patient may be limited. Granulocyte-macrophage colony-stimulating factor (GM-CSF) causes a rise in WBC count usually from increased monocytes and eosinophils. The usual dose is 3–30 µg/kg/day given IV or subcutaneously. Toxicities of GM-CSF include pericardial and pleural effusions, phlebitis, fever, and myalgias. Granulocyte colony-stimulating factor (G-CSF) is highly effective in idiopathic, cyclic, and congenital neutropenias with >90% complete response overall (ANC >1500), 50% reduction in incidence and duration of infection-related events and 70% reduction in duration of antibiotics. The optimal dose of G-CSF varies with diagnosis. In general, severe congenital neutropenias will require higher doses of G-CSF.

• Toxicities include mild headache, myalgias, bone pain, and rash (Fig. 98-1).

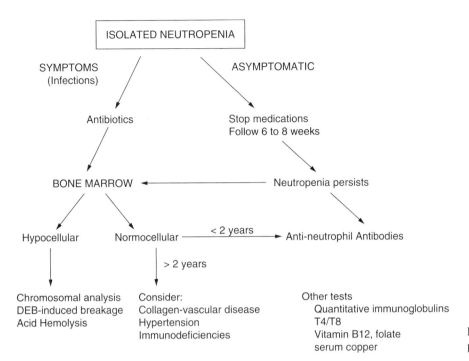

FIG. 98-1 Evaluation of the neutropenic patient.

BIBLIOGRAPHY

Aprikyam AA, Liles WC, Boxer LA, Dale DC. Mutant elastase in pathogenesis of cyclic and severe congenital neutropenia. *J Ped Hematol Oncol* 2002;24:784–86.

Dale DC, Cottle TE, Fier CJ, et al. Severe congenital neutropenia: Treatment and follow up of patients in the severe congenital neutropenia registry. *Am J Hematol* 2003;73:82–93.

Nathan DG and Orkin SH (eds.). *Nathan & Oski's Hematology of Infancy and Childhood, 5th edition,* 2003. W.B. Saunders, Philadelphia, PA.

99 SICKLE CELL DISEASE

Horace E. Smith

• The sickle cell disease comprises a group of hereditary hemoglobin disorders, characterized by red blood cells that undergo a sickle-shaped transformation, when they are deoxygenated. This unusual property is caused by hemoglobin polymerization due to a single nucleotide substitution within the beta-globin gene that results in anemia and vasoocclusive complications. Although intermittent pain crisis is the primary manifestation of vasoocclusion, this process also has the ability to cause damage to every organ system. In addition, patients with a sickling syndrome have functional asplenia and increased susceptibility to infection, primarily with polysaccharide encapsulated organisms.

EPIDEMIOLOGY

• The sickle gene mutation originated in western Africa. Its distribution mimics the areas of the world where *P. falciparum* malaria is endemic, including sub-Saharan Africa, the Mediter-ranean region, and countries in the Middle East. People with sickle cell *trait* infected with the parasite, have a selective advantage over those who do not have the trait. There are approximately 4–5000 births per year in the United States of infants with clinically significant sickling syndromes. This is present in 1/600 African American live births. Sickle trait is present in approximately 9% of persons of African origin in this country. The approximate distribution of the clinically significant sickling disorders in the United States is as follows:
1. Homozygous sickle cell disease 65%
2. Hemoglobin SC disease 25%
3. Sβ^+ Thalassemia 8%
4. Sβ° Thalassemia 2%
5. SHPFH <1%

PATHOPHYSIOLOGY

• The pathophysiology of sickle cell disease is related to the intracellular polymerization of sickle cell hemoglobin, due to the substitution of valine for glutamic acid on the beta-globin chain, and to the abnormal interaction that sickle red cells have with the vascular endothelium as well as other factors. Intracellular polymer formation is an intermittent dynamic process, that is dependent on several factors including the following:
  1. Oxygen tension
  2. Intracellular sickle hemoglobin concentration
  3. Ph
  4. Temperature
  5. Hypertonicity/dehydration

CLINICAL PRESENTATION WITH DIFFERENTIAL DIAGNOSIS

• Hemolytic anemia and clinical signs and symptoms of sickle cell disease are extremely rare before 3 months of age because of the predominance of fetal hemoglobin present in the newborn period. Dactylitis, with swelling of the dorsum of the hands and feet is a common initial presenting sign. Often, the presenting symptom is fever. Parents should be educated about the importance of urgent medical evaluation and treatment of fevers of 101°F or greater. The risk of sepsis is many times that of the general population, with a high risk of mortality in the first 2 years of life. Institution of penicillin prophylaxis no later than 2 months of age, as well as routine pneumococcal vaccines is imperative and greatly reduces the risk of sepsis and death.

DIAGNOSIS/LABORATORY FEATURES

• Forty-four states, the District of Columbia, Puerto Rico, and the Virgin Islands currently provide universal screening for sickling disorders. This has resulted in the early identification of patients and families at risk, and along with penicillin prophylaxis, a dramatic decrease in the incidence of sepsis and mortality. The majority of screening programs use isoelectric focusing (IEF), with a few using high-performance liquid chromatography, (HPLC) or cellulose acetate electrophoresis and the initial screening method. Any high-risk infant not screened at birth should be screened prior to 2 months of age. An abnormal screen must be followed up with definitive testing with citrate agar and cellulose acetate electrophoresis.

Prenatal testing methods are available for expectant parents who desire it.

COMPLICATIONS

• Complications to sickle cell syndromes can be seen in literally every organ system. Acute, common ones include the following:
  1. Vasoocclusive painful episodes
  2. Splenic sequestration episodes
  3. Acute chest syndrome
  4. Infectious syndromes
  5. Central nervous system (stroke)
  6. Aplastic episodes
• Other less common but significant complications include avascular necrosis of the hip, priapism, intrahepatic sickling, poor growth, delayed puberty, and cognitive dysfunction.

TREATMENT

VASOOCCLUSIVE PAINFUL EPISODES

• Painful events in sickle cell disease are intermittent and often unpredictable. Pain commonly occurs in the extremities, chest, abdomen, as well as in other locations. The pain is caused by hypoxia and ischemic tissue injury. Pain can last for hours or several weeks. Effective management of painful episodes has four essential elements:
  1. Identification and treatment of any precipitating or associated events.
  2. Accurate assessment and frequent reassessment of pain.
  3. Appropriate analgesic therapy.
  4. Proper hydration of the patient.
• Parenteral opioids are often required to manage pain, unsuccessfully treated at home. Patient-controlled analgesia (PCA) is often an effective route of administration for opioids. Nonsteroidal anti-inflammatory drugs (NSAIDs) can be used synergistically for effective management.

SPLENIC SEQUESTRATION EPISODE

• The spleen can act as a volume reservoir, dropping the hemoglobin to less than 2 g/dL, and resulting in hypovolemic shock. Early signs of splenic sequestration include abdominal distension or discomfort, anxiety, easy fatigability, and pallor. Prompt packed cell transfusion in small volume is usually effective. Parental education to look for these signs and symptoms can be lifesaving.

ACUTE CHEST SYNDROME

- Acute chest syndrome is the leading cause of death in sickle cell disease and the second leading cause of death in children >5years. It can present with
  1. Fever
  2. Respiratory distress or chest pain
  3. Pulmonary infiltrate
- Acute chest syndrome can be caused by infection and or vasoocclusion. Early recognition is essential to prevent progressive respiratory failure. Tachypnea with increased effort of breathing are signs of progression. Critical measures include oxygen support with decreased oxygen saturation. Early institution of simple packed cell transfusion may avoid the need for exchange transfusion. Proper antibiotic coverage and incentive spirometry may prevent progression of this complication.

INFECTIONS

- Preventative measures are critical in sickle cell disease. They include prophylactic penicillin, immunization with pneumococcal conjugate vaccine during the early newborn period, and using the 23-valent pneumococcal vaccine after age 2 years. Febrile patients should be evaluated in the context of functional asplenia. In a well-appearing child, a temperature of 101°F or greater must be evaluated immediately. Temper-ature of 101°F or greater is an emergency. Laboratory evaluation should include the following:
  1. Complete blood count (CBC) with reticulocyte count.
  2. Blood cultures and other cultures as clinically warranted.
  3. Chest x-ray (CXR) (even if no respiratory symptoms are present).
  4. Treatment with parenteral antibiotics and oral antibiotics to cover culture period (48 hours).
  5. All toxic-appearing children should be admitted for treatment.
- Fevers with a source should be appropriately evaluated and treated. With fever in the presence of bone pain and tenderness, osteomyelitis vs. bone infarction due to vasooclussion can be a difficult differentiation.

CENTRAL NERVOUS SYSTEM

- Patients with homozygous SS disease and $S\beta^\circ$ Thalassemia are at risk for central nervous system (CNS) complications. Other sickling syndromes have a much lower risk. Stroke in the pediatric age group is predominately infarctive or thrombotic in nature. Meningitis and seizures can occur, but are uncommon. Parents are educated to look for "soft" signs of stroke and report them immediately. Computed tomography (CT) or magnetic resonance imaging (MRI) are essential for making this diagnosis. Prompt exchange transfusion to reduce the levels of sickle hemoglobin is indicated in this clinical setting. The risk of stroke can now be predicted by the routine use of Transcranial Doppler (TCD) testing. This should begin at age 2 years and continue serially. Cognitive dysfunction can be subtly present in sickling syndromes early on in life. Guidelines are being developed to prevent, diagnose, and treat this phenomenon.

APLASTIC EPISODES

- Transient red-cell aplasia is usually caused by parvovirus B19. Patients present with increasing anemia and a low reticulocyte count. Inpatient observation is often prudent. Conservative packed red blood cell transfusions are effective to correct severe anemia with signs and symptoms of hypovolemia. Because patients may be viremic at the time of presentation, appropriate isolation measures should be taken.

RECENT ADVANCES

- Recent advances in sickle cell diseases include the following:
  1. Pharmacologic agents (hydroxyurea and other medications)
  2. Bone marrow transplantation
  3. Gene therapy
- Promising research in each of these areas brighten the prognosis for affected patients and their families.

REFERENCES

www.sicklecelldisease.org
www.nhlbi.nih.gov

MALIGNANCIES

Elaine R. Morgan, Section Editor

100 OVERVIEW
Elaine R. Morgan

Pediatric Cancer Is Rare
- Incidence: 150 per 1,000,000 children/year.
- ~12,400 new cases per year in United States.

Prognosis Has Improved Steadily Since 1970
- Survival rates are now 77%.
- Survival after relapse remains poor.

Treatment Is Multidisciplinary
- Children are best treated in large pediatric oncology centers.
- Most children are treated on large group research studies.
- Late effects are common and continue into adulthood.

Long-Term Followup Is Essential
- For optimal patient care.
- For evaluation of treatment protocols and continued progress.

101 CANCER AND GENETICS
*Yasmin Goseingfiao and
David O. Walterhouse*

INTRODUCTION

- Cancer is a clonal disorder. Cells require a series of gene mutations or "hits" to become truly malignant. Mutations may occur during cell proliferation (somatically acquired mutations), or may be inherited as germline mutations, leading to a hereditary predisposition to cancer.

SOMATICALLY ACQUIRED MUTATIONS AND PEDIATRIC CANCERS

- Genes normally involved in promoting cell proliferation (protooncogenes), may become "activated" (*oncogenes*). Mechanisms of activation: Point mutations (leukemia), chromosomal translocations (leukemia, lymphoma, sarcoma), and gene amplification (neuroblastoma).
- Genes normally involved in suppressing cell proliferation, may become "suppressed" (*tumor suppressor genes*); require loss of function of both alleles (*2 hits*). Mechanisms of inactivation: Point mutations and deletions. Tumor suppressor genes in pediatric cancers include retinoblastoma, p53, Wilms tumor (WT), Neurofibromatosis (NF1 and NF2).
- Abnormalities in other cellular functions may also play roles in carcinogenesis.
- Specific oncogene activation in a tumor may be used for diagnosis or as a target for specific treatment (e.g., use of Gleevec to inhibit the BCR-ABL fusion product in chronic myelogenous leukemia).

HEREDITARY PREDISPOSITION TO PEDIATRIC CANCER
- Hereditary predisposition to pediatric cancer may result from a genetic alteration that has been passed on to the child from a parent or that was a new constitutional mutation that occurred in the oocyte or sperm before fertilization (such as trisomy 21 or a de novo mutation in a tumor suppressor gene such as Rb).
- Inherited predisposition to cancer occurs in Down syndrome, Wilms tumor-aniridia-genitourinary

anomalies-mental retardation (WAGR) syndrome, Beckwith-Wiedemann syndrome (associated with Wilms tumor, hepatoblastoma, neuroblastoma, adrenal carcinoma), and type 1 neurofibromatosis.

CLUES THAT CANCER MAY BE INHERITED
- Certain forms of pediatric cancer are frequently inherited: Adrenal cortical carcinoma (50–89% of cases), optic gliomas (approximately 45% of cases), and retinoblastoma (40% of cases).
- Other forms of pediatric cancer have a more modest rate of cases due to hereditary factors including Wilms tumors (3–5% of cases) and leukemia (2.5–5% of cases).
- Certain patterns of cancer in families suggest a hereditary component, including multiple generations affected with cancer, earlier age of onset compared with sporadic cases, increased incidence of multiple or bilateral tumors, and a clustering of a few tumor types in the family (such as leukemia, brain tumors, breast carcinoma, sarcomas, and adrenal cortical carcinoma in families with the Li-Fraumeni familial cancer syndrome).

102 BRAIN TUMORS
Joanna L. Weinstein and Stewart Goldman

EPIDEMIOLOGY
- The second most common group of cancers diagnosed in children in the United States; 2000–3000 new cases diagnosed per year; incidence 3 per 100,000 children.
- Approximately 80% of pediatric brain tumors (BT) occur during the first decade (Table 102-1).
  1. In children <1 year: Supratentorial tumors occur more frequently than infratentorial tumors.
  2. In children 1–11 years: Infratentorial tumors occur more frequently than supratentorial tumors.
  3. In adolescence: Supratentorial = infratentorial lesions.

PATHOPHYSIOLOGY
- Predisposing factors associated with the development of BTs include exposure to ionizing radiation, prior malignancy, immunosuppression, inherited conditions

(neurofibromatosis, Li-Fraumeni syndrome, nevoid basal cell carcinoma [Gorlin] syndrome, and Turcot syndrome).

CLINICAL FEATURES
- Related to the location of tumor or increased intracranial pressure (ICP).

SYMPTOMS
- Increased ICP: Headache, nausea, vomiting, diplopia, papilledema, cranial nerve deficits, decreased sensorium, or posturing.

INFRATENTORIAL MASSES
- Increased ICP or cerebellar signs.

SUPRATENTORIAL MASSES
- Endocrinopathies (diabetes insipidus, growth disorders, precocious puberty), visual changes or field deficits, upward-gaze impairment, hemiparesis, hemisensory loss, hyperreflexia, seizures, personality abnormalities, speech impairments, or deterioration in school performance.

BRAIN STEM LESIONS
- Cranial nerve deficits, diplopia, slurred speech, hearing, swallowing, breathing, or gag impairments.
- *Infants* may present with more global symptoms: Irritability, vomiting, lethargy, loss of milestones, failure to thrive (FTT), an increase in head circumference, diencephalic syndrome (FTT, paradoxical euphoric mood, and pendular nystagmus).

SPINAL CORD INVOLVEMENT
- Radicular pain, bowel or bladder dysfunction, or sensory deficits.

DIAGNOSIS/LABORATORY FEATURES
- Prompt diagnostic neuroimaging of the brain and spine.

GENERAL TREATMENT AND MANAGEMENT
- Definitive treatment depends on primary tumor, location, and age of child and may include surgical resection, chemotherapy, and radiotherapy.

TABLE 102-1 Specific Tumors

TUMOR	SUBTYPES	INCIDENCE (% OF CNS TUMORS)	PEAK AGE (YEARS)	PATHOPHYSIOLOGY	CLINICAL PRESENTATION	R_X MODALITIES	OVERALL SURVIVAL
Medulloblastoma (posterior fossa PNET)	Two risk groups: Average risk = complete resection, age older than 3 years; CSF without tumor cells High risk = >1.5 cm residual disease; young age; CSF positive for tumor cells; metastatic disease	20	5–9	Locally invasive; ventricular and CSF seeding; rare systemic dissemination	Posterior fossa signs; increased ICP	Surgery + craniospinal XRT + adjuvant chemotherapy	50% overall; average risk 85%; poor risk >35%
Supratentorial PNET		3–7	<5	Infiltrate brain; meningeal spread	Supratentorial signs, nonspecific sx	Surgery + craniospinal XRT + adjuvant chemotherapy	35% if completely resected
Ependymoma		5–10	<7	Ependymal lining; infiltrates vital structures	Based on primary site	Surgery ± XRT, chemotherapy	40%
Low-grade glioma (astrocytoma)	Juvenile-pilocytic astrocytoma, oligodendroglioma, and ganglioglioma	25–45		Nonaggressive		Surgery ± chemotherapy, may need multiple surgeries	Prolonged, may recur late
Optic pathway tumorsa	Associated with NF1	5	<5	Low grade; optic nerve chiasm, hypothalamus	Proptosis, vision change	Chemotherapy ± XRT	
High-grade glioma	Anaplastic astrocytoma, glioblastoma multiforme	10–15	~10 (median)	Aggressive, locally invasive	Supratentorial sx; ± spread to neroaxis ± systemic	Surgery. May need multiple surgeries + XRT	30% median survival <1.5 years
Brain stem glioma	Those in patients with NF1 may behave more indolently	10–20		Pontine—very aggressive; medullar and cervicomedullary—more indolent	Cranial nerve deficits, obstructive hydrocephalus	Pons—XRT Medulla—surger + XRT. Midbrain—VP shunt only	
Craniopharyngiomas		6–9	8–10	Predom. suprasellar benign histol may infiltrate locally	Hydrocephalus, behavioral or visual changes Endocrinopathies	Surgery +/- XRT treatment endocrine problems	
Germ cell tumors	Germinoma, teratomas, embryonal, carcinoma, choriocarcinoma, endodermal sinus tumors	1–2	>10	Pineal/suprasellar, may have ↑ CSF, ↑AFP, ↑ beta-hCG	Endocrinopathies, especially DI	Surgery, XRT, chemotherapy	

ABBREVIATIONS: XRzT, irradiation therapy; PNET, primitive neuroectodermal tumor; AFP, alpha fetoprotein; Beta-hCG, beta human chorionic gonadotropin; VP, ventriculoperitoneal shunt; CNS = central nervous system; CSF = cerebrospinal fluid.

- Treatment of tumor-associated increased ICP.
- Dexamethasone, ± mannitol or hyperventilation.
- Ventriculoperitoneal shunting or third ventriculostomy may be required.
- Late effects include neurocognitive morbidity, growth failure, neurobehavioral abnormalities, endocrinopathies, focal neurologic deficits, and psychosocial effects.

103 LEUKEMIA

Elaine R. Morgan

EPIDEMIOLOGY

- Most common childhood extracranial malignancy.
- Incidence 4–6 per 100,000 children.
- Peak age range 3–6.
- M F = increased incidence in identical twin if one child has leukemia (20–50%) within 1 year.

PREDISPOSING CONDITIONS

- Down syndrome—acute lymphocytic leukemia (ALL) and acute nonlymphocytic leukemia (ANLL).
- Human immunodeficiency virus (HIV) infection—ALL
- Ataxia, telangiectasia—T-cell ALL
- Bloom syndrome
- Kostman syndrome
- Fanconi syndrome   AML
- Medically treated AA
- Myelodysplasia
- Prior chemotherapy

INITIAL PRESENTING SYMPTOMS AND SIGNS

- Most common presentations include fever, bone pain, fatigue, pallor, bleeding, and respiratory distress secondary to mediastinum mass.
- Physical findings may include lymphadenopathy and hepatosplenomegaly.
- Rarely may present with central nervous system (CNS) symptoms, mass lesions/testicular involvement, skin lesions, gingival hypertrophy, renal insufficiency, disseminated intravascular coagulation (DIC), and intractable bleeding.

INITIAL WORKUP

- Initial workup includes routine and specialized laboratory studies.
- Laboratory studies: Complete blood count (CBC), chemistry panel, uric acid, coagulation studies, and bacterial cultures.
- Chest x-ray
- LP with cytospin.
- Bone marrow (BM) aspirate.
- Specialized studies for classification include flow cytometry, cytochemical stains, cytogenetics, ± molecular testing for chromosomal abnormalities.

CLASSIFICATION

- One to two percent of childhood leukemias are classic metaphyseal lesions (CML), 15% are ANLL, and 85% are ALL.
- ANLL is subclassified histologically and cytogenetically into eight subtypes ($M_0 \rightarrow M_7$). The M_3 (promyelocytic) subtype is treated differently.
- ALL is subclassified by immunophenotype: B precursor (85%); T cell (13%); mature B cell (1–2%).
- T and B cell types are associated with a worse prognosis.
- B-precursor leukemias can be separated into two to five risk categories (low, standard, high, very high, and infant) based on clinical and laboratory findings.
- Very high-risk features: Chromosomal translocation t 9;22; hypodiploidy; age <1 year.
- High-risk features: Age >10 years, white blood cell (WBC) at diagnosis >50,000, chromosomal translocations t 4;11 t 1;19.
- Low-risk features: Hyperdiploidy; trisomies 4&10; tel/acute myelogenous leukemia (AML) gene rearrangement.
- Possible prognostic findings: Sex, ethinicity, CNS status.
- Patients with rapid initial response have a more favorable prognosis.

INITIAL MANAGEMENT

- Diagnostic workup.
- Transfusions of packed red blood cells (PBRCs) and platelets as needed.
- Hydration.
- Management/prophylaxis of hyperuricemia alkalinization and allopurinol or uricase.
- Preemptive broad spectrum antibiotics if febrile.

CML

- Initial presentation: Splenomegaly, leukocytosis; ±leukostasis (cerebrovascular accident [CVA], pulmonary priaprism).
- Diagnosis confirmed by 9;22 translocation or molecular studies (BCR/abl).
- Treatment: Gleevec PO vs. hydroxyurea ± bone marrow transplant (BMT).
- Survival: Eighty percent with BMT unknown with Gleevec.

ANLL

- Risk analysis limited: (a) Low risk—promyelocytic leukemia (APL), Down syndrome; (b) high risk—secondary leukemia, monosomy 5 or 7; and (c) possible lower risk factors: WBC <25,000; chromosomes: t 8;21, inversion 16.
- CNS disease uncommon.

TREATMENT
- APL—ATRA (all transretinoic acid) + anthracycline + maintenance.
- Down syndrome—Modified
- All patients receive one to two intensive inpatient sequential courses including anthracycline, cytosine arabinoside (AraC) ± other.
- Remission rate: Eighty percent
- Consolidation with either three to five courses of intensive chemotherapy including high-dose Ara-C ± bone marrow transplant.
- Maintenance is controversial.
- Treatment of relapse is difficult.
- Complications: Twenty percent induction death rate due to infection, bleeding, resistant disease, continued risk of infection, and bleeding during consolidation.
- Outcome: APL and Down syndrome 80–90% event free survival (EFS).
- Other: Thirty to forty percent EFS with chemotherapy, 60–70% EFS with BMT.
- Survival after relapse: <20%.

ALL

- B-ALL is treated with short (~6 months) intensive chemotherapy
- EFS 60% (CNS+) to 80% (CNS−).
- Relapse occurs early, usually BM, CNS. Survival after relapse is rare. CNS involvement common.
- T-ALL may be associated with mediastinal mass. A variety of protocols available that use intensive multidrug treatments ± cranial irradiation. Remission rate ~80% EFS—60–70%. Treatment duration ~2 years.

Relapses occur in BM, CNS usually within 2 years of diagnosis. Survival after relapse—poor. CNS involvement more common than B-precursor ALL.
- B-precursor ALL is most common type of leukemia. Treatment with multidrug chemotherapy; risk based. Irradiation is used for CNS disease. Treatment duration 2–3 years. BMT used for very high-risk patients. Remission achieved in 80–95% of patients, usually within 28 days of diagnosis. EFS overall 70–85%. Relapses may occur early or late. Bone marrow most common site; CNS <10%; testicular <5%. Treatment of relapse may be successful. Survival depends on duration of first remission, initial R_x, and site of relapse. Treatment includes alternative chemotherapy ± BMT.

COMPLICATIONS

- Leukostasis secondary to hyperleukocytosis. Metabolic/problems secondary to tumor lysis. Infection—bacterial, fungal, viral, *Pneumocystis carinii* pneumonia (PCP). Bleeding and anemia. Chemotherapy side effects.

104 LYMPHOMA

Elaine R. Morgan and Maureen Haugen

EPIDEMIOLOGY

- Twelve percent of all pediatric cancers; third most common childhood cancer in the United States; 1 per 100,000 children. Forty percent Hodgkin disease and 60% non-Hodgkin lymphoma (NHL).
- Fifty percent of childhood cancers in Africa.

HODGKIN DISEASE

EPIDEMIOLOGY

- Rare under 5 years of age; increased incidence in adolescents and young adults.
- Predisposing conditions: Family history, immunodeficiency.

SIGNS/SYMPTOMS

- Painless, firm lymphadenopathy; cervical supraclavicular 60–90%.

- Respiratory symptoms
- Systemic symptoms: Pruritis "B" symptoms, weight loss, fevers, night sweats 30%.
- Histologic subtypes: *Lymphocytic predominant, nodular sclerosing,* mixed cellularity, lymphocyte depleted.

INITIAL WORKUP

- Chest x-ray (CXR), computed tomography (CT) scan (neck to pelvis).
- Complete blood count (CBC), chemistry panel, erythrocyte sedimentation rate (ESR), copper, ferritin.
- Bone marrow aspirate and biopsy.
- ± Gallium scan or positron emission tomography (PET) scan.

STAGING

- I: Single lymph node region.
- II: Two or more lymph node regions on the same side of the diaphragm.
- III: Lymph node regions/on both sides of the diaphragm.
- IV: Disseminated extra lymphatic sites: Bones, bone marrow, lungs, liver.

TREATMENT

- Combined modality treatment: Chemotherapy and radiation.
- Stem-cell transplant after relapse.
- Prognosis 70–90% 5-year disease free survival (DFS).
- Adverse indicators: Stage III or IV disease, B symptoms, bulky tumor.

NON-HODGKIN LYMPHOMA

EPIDEMIOLOGY

- Rare, less than 2 years of age, peak age is 7–11 years.
- Predisposing conditions: Immunosuppressive therapy, Wiskott-Aldrich syndrome, Chediak-Higashi syndrome, X-linked lymphoproliferative disorder, ataxia-telangiectasia, Epstein-Barr virus (EBV) (African type NHL), human immunodeficiency virus (HIV).

SIGNS/SYMPTOMS

- Respiratory symptoms, chest pain, superior vena cava syndrome.

- Lymphadenopathy, painless.
- Abdominal pain, nausea, vomiting, gastrointestinal (GI) symptoms or bleeding, ascites, abdominal distention.
- Skin/scalp masses, testicular mass.
- Bone pain.
- Renal failure.
- CNS symptoms.

INITIAL WORKUP

- CBC, chemistry panel, uric acid, lactic dehydrogenase (LDH).
- Bone marrow aspirate ± biopsy.
- Lumbar puncture with cytospin.
- CXR, CT scan, bone scan, gallium scan.

HISTOLOGY

- Small, noncleaved, diffuse, poorly differentiated (B cell)
- Lymphoblastic (usually T cell)
- Large cell (B cell, T cell, or non-T; non-B)
- Lymphoproliferative (usually B cell) polyclonal or monoclonal (commonly occurs posttransplant).

STAGING (MURPHY SYSTEM)

- I: Localized
- II: Regional
- III: Above and below diaphragm.
- IV: CNS or BM involvement.

TREATMENT

- Radiation: For emergency relief of symptoms; treatment of CNS disease.
- Chemotherapy: B cell—intensive, repetitive, short duration.
- T cell—similar to ALL for 18–24 months.
- Stem-cell transplant: For refractory or relapsed disease; limited success.
- Lymphoproliferative disease: Reduction in immunosuppressive therapy; consider monoclonal antibody and/or chemotherapy for nonresponsive disease.

PROGNOSIS—80% DFS

- Adverse indicators: Advanced stage, high LDH, Stage IV disease.

105 NEUROBLASTOMA

Susan L. Cohn and Kelly Coyne

EPIDEMIOLOGY

- There are approximately 600 new cases of neuroblastoma (NBL) in the United States each year (1 per 7000 births).
- Most common tumor in children <1-year-old; median 2 years; 90% <5 years.
- Eight to ten percent of all pediatric cancers and 15% of pediatric cancer-related deaths.
- One to two percent familial.

CLINICAL PRESENTATION

- Neural crest origin; adrenal or parasympathetic ganglia.
- Signs and symptoms reflect both the location of the primary tumor and the extent of disease.
- Specific associated findings include paraneoplastic syndromes (opsoclonus-myoclonus; intractable diarrhea secondary to vasoactive intestinal protein (VIP).
- Metastatic disease (approximately 50% of cases).
- Lymphadenopathy, hepatomegaly, pallor, exophthalmos, eyelid ecchymosis, skull mass, bone pain, skin nodules, and purpura.
- Systemic symptoms: Fever, weight loss, fatigue, and hypertension.
- This clinical diversity correlates closely with numerous clinical and biologic factors including tumor stage, patient age, tumor histology, and genetic abnormalities.

DIAGNOSTIC STUDIES AND TESTS

DIAGNOSTIC CONFIRMATION

- Pathologic diagnosis from tumor tissue or bone marrow aspirate with neuroblastoma tumor cells *and* increased urinary catecholamines.
- Clinical *and* biologic studies are critical for risk-group classification (see below).

CLINICAL STUDIES

- Urinary catecholamines—elevated in >90% of those diagnosed.
- Bilateral bone marrow biopsies and aspirates.

- Computed tomography (CT) of the chest, abdomen, and pelvis; ± head CT.
- MIBG (metaiodobenzylguanidine) scan—adrenergic tissue-specific scan.
- Bone scan.
- Magnetic resonance imaging (MRI) if potential intraspinal extension.

TUMOR BIOLOGY STUDIES

- *MYCN* protooncogene copy number.
- Tumor cell ploidy.
- Histopathology.

THE INTERNATIONAL NEUROBLASTOMA STAGING SYSTEM (INSS)

- Stage 1: Localized tumor with complete gross excision.
- Stage 2A: Localized tumor with incomplete gross excision, nonadherent lymph nodes negative.
- Stage 2B: Localized tumor with or without complete gross excision, with nonadherent ipsilateral nodes positive.
- Stage 3: Tumor involvement across the midline.
- Stage 4: Disseminated tumor.
- Stage 4S: Infants <1 year with primary tumor (as defined in Stages I and II) with dissemination limited to skin, liver, and/or bone marrow (<10% tumor cells and MIBG scan negative in the marrow).

RISK-GROUP STRATIFICATION SYSTEM

- Based on clinical and biologic studies.
- Assignment to low-, intermediate-, and high-risk categories based on age at diagnosis, INSS stage, histopathology, *MYCN* amplification status, and *deoxyribonucleic acid* (DNA) index.
- Survival: <30% (high risk) to >90% (low risk).

RISK-BASED TREATMENT

- Low-risk patients.
- Require minimal therapy, perhaps resection alone.
- Newborns and infants with low-risk disease may have spontaneous regression.

INTERMEDIATE RISK PATIENTS

- Tumor biology impacts response to therapy and outcome.

- Treated with moderate intensity chemotherapy, surgery ± irradiation.

HIGH-RISK PATIENTS

- Dose intensity has been shown to correlate strongly with both response and progression-free survival.
- Treatment includes high dose chemotherapy with stem cell rescue.
- Preliminary data suggest that biologic agents may also be clinically effective in the setting of minimal residual disease.
- More effective therapy is needed for high-risk neuroblastoma patients.

106 WILMS TUMOR

Morris Kletzel

EPIDEMIOLOGY

- Affects 1–10,000 children younger than 15 years of age.
- Approximately 400 new cases are reported yearly in the United States.
- Incidence is higher among African-Americans and lower among Asian-Americans.

GENETICS

- Wilms tumor is associated with multiple congenital abnormalities and in some cases with identified syndromes.
  1. Aniridia (1%)
  2. WAGR (Wilms tumor, aniridia, genitourinary malformation, and mental retardation)
  3. Deny Drash syndrome (Wilms tumor, pseudohermaphroditism and glomerulopathy)
  4. Beckwith-Wiedemann syndrome (BWS) (macroglosia, gigantism, umbilical hernia)
  5. Trisomy 18
  6. Genitourinary anomalies (5%)
  7. Hemihypertrophy
- Mutations in the WT1 gene located on chromosome 11p13 and WT2 gene (11p15) result in the development of Wilms tumor.

CLINICAL PRESENTATION

- Mean age at diagnosis is 3.4–4.0 years and for bilateral tumors is 2.5 years.
- Most common presenting symptoms are abdominal mass ± abdominal pain.
- Less frequent symptoms: Hypertension, fever, hematuria, and anemia.
- Acquired Von Willibrand disease has been associated with Wilms tumor.

DIAGNOSTIC IMAGING

- Abdominal ultrasound and/or computed tomography (CT) of the abdomen.
- Chest CT

STAGING

- Stage I: Tumor limited to the kidney and completely excised.
- Stage II: Tumor beyond the kidney but completely excised.
- Stage III: Residual nonhematogenous tumor confined to the abdomen.
- Stage IV: Hematogenous metastases (lung, liver, bone, brain).
- Stage V: Bilateral involvement at diagnosis.

PATHOLOGY

- Subtypes are favorable (trilineage) or unfavorable (anaplasia, sarcoma).

THERAPY

- Highly successful.
- Includes surgery, chemotherapy, and irradiation.
- The treatment is based on the stage and histologic type and over the past 20 years has evolved according to clinical trials develop by the National Wilms Tumor Study Group.

OUTCOME

- Based on the National Wilms Tumor Study #3, the 4-year survivals are Stages I, II, and III with favorable histology: 96.5, 92.2, and 86.8%, respectively; high-risk patients (Stage IV or unfavorable histology): 73%. Stage V (bilateral tumor): 70%.

107 PEDIATRIC BONE TUMORS

Laurie MacDonald, David O. Walterhouse, and Robert L. Satcher

BENIGN BONE TUMORS

STAGING BY PATHOLOGIC AGGRESSIVENESS

- Stage 1 (latent); Stage 2 (active); Stage 3 (aggressive).
- Treatment: Stage 1 (observation); Stage 2 (intralesional excision); Stage 3 (marginal or wide excision).

MALIGNANT BONE TUMORS

OSTEOSARCOMA

- Primary malignant tumor of bone produces osteoid.

EPIDEMIOLOGY
- Four hundred cases/year in children <20 years. Peak incidence occurs in the second decade of life during the adolescent growth spurt.
- Associations: Radiation; retinoblastoma; Li-Fraumeni familial cancer syndrome.

CLINICAL PRESENTATION
- Pain, soft tissue mass.
- Site: Usually metaphyses of long bones (lower extremity more common); other bony sites are rare.
- Fifteen to twenty percent present with metastatic disease; lungs most common.

STAGING WORKUP
- Plain films; magnetic resonance imaging (MRI) of primary.
- Computed tomography (CT) of chest
- Bone scan ± thallium scan ± positron emission tomography (PET) scan.

UNFAVORABLE PROGNOSTIC FACTORS
- Metastasis at presentation.
- Primary site in axial skeleton.
- Tumor size >5 cm.
- Poor initial response to chemotherapy.

TREATMENT
- Chemotherapy generally administered both presurgically (neoadjuvant) and postsurgically.

- Surgery includes amputation (local recurrence <5%) or limb salvage (local recurrence rate 5–10%; more postoperative complications).
- Radiation therapy only for unresectable tumors.

OUTCOME
- ~60–65% disease-free survival with nonmetastatic osteosarcoma of the extremity; 20% with metastatic disease.
- Relapses occur early (<3 years): 85% pulmonary, 15–30% bone; 10–20% of disease-free survival after relapse.

EWING SARCOMA/PNET (PERIPHERAL NEUROECTODERMAL TUMOR)

EPIDEMIOLOGY
- Four hundred new cases/year.
- Ninety-six percent of patients White. Male:Female = 1.3–1.6:1.

BIOLOGY
- Chromosomal translocations: t(11;22)(q24;q12); seen in 85–95% of cases.

PATHOLOGY/DIAGNOSIS
- Small round blue cell tumor.
  1. Ewing sarcoma is a primitive tumor without differentiation; PNET has neural differentiation.

CLINICAL PRESENTATION
- Primary site: (bony or soft tissue) 53% extremities and 47% central (pelvis, chest wall, spine, and head or neck); 74% of PNETs are central, mainly chest.

SIGNS AND SYMPTOMS
- Pain, palpable mass, pathologic fracture; back pain, cord compression.
- Constitutional: Fever, weight loss, increased erythrocyte sedimentation rate (ESR).
- Twenty percent present with metastatic disease: Lung (38%), bone (31%), and bone marrow (11%).

STAGING
- Workup same as osteosarcoma and bone marrow aspirate and biopsy.

UNFAVORABLE PROGNOSTIC FACTORS
- Metastasis at presentation.
- Primary site in axial skeleton.
- Tumor size >10 cm.
- Viable tumor postchemotherapy at time of surgery.

TREATMENT

- Local control with surgery or irradiation.
- Chemotherapy:
  1. All patients require chemotherapy.
  2. The majority of treatment failures are distant.
- Bone marrow transplant: May play a role in high-risk or relapsed patients.

108 SOFT TISSUE SARCOMA

David O. Walterhouse and Peter E. Zage

- Sarcomas are malignant tumors arising from mesenchyme-derived cells.
- Soft tissue sarcomas (STS) include rhabdomyosarcoma (RMS)/undifferentiated sarcoma and nonrhabdomyosarcomatous STS.

RHABDOMYOSARCOMA/UNDIFFERENTIATED SARCOMA

INCIDENCE AND EPIDEMIOLOGY

- RMS is the most common soft tissue sarcoma, accounting for approximately 50% of soft tissue sarcomas in children <15 years old.
- Sixth most common form of cancer during childhood (5–8% of all childhood cancer) with 4.6 cases per million children (less than 15 years of age) per year in the United States or 250–350 new cases diagnosed each year.
- The peak age of onset is <5 years old.
- May occur in Li-Fraumeni familial cancer syndrome, (p53 gene mutation).

BIOLOGY AND PATHOLOGY

- RMS demonstrates some degree of skeletal muscle differentiation.
- Subtypes are embryonal (70%), alveolar (20%), and undifferentiated (10%).
- Chromosomal translocation t(2;13) (q 35; q 14) in alveolar variant.

CLINICAL PRESENTATION

- Most common sites: Head and neck, genitourinary (GU), extremities.
- Usually presents as a mass, ± pain ± organ obstruction ± local invasion.
- Ten to twenty percent of patients present with metastatic disease (bone marrow, lung, lymph nodes, bone, or liver).

WORKUP

- Computed tomography (CT) or magnetic resonance imaging (MRI) of primary tumor, chest and abdominal CT, chest x-ray (CXR), bone scan, bone marrow aspiration and biopsy, lumbar puncture (LP) if parameningeal, and ± regional lymph node sampling.

IMPORTANT PROGNOSTIC FACTORS DEFINE RISK GROUPS

- Site of origin (favorable sites include the head and neck, some genitourinary; unfavorable sites include parameningeal, bladder, prostate, extremities, and trunk).
- Stage (defined by primary site, local invasiveness, regional lymph node involvement, and metastatic spread).
- Group (defined by the extent of tumor remaining after initial surgery).
- Histologic subtype (alveolar and undifferentiated histologies are considered unfavorable).

TREATMENT AND OUTCOME

- Multimodality approach (surgery, radiation therapy, and chemotherapy).
- The Intergroup Rhabdomyosarcoma Study (IRS) Group was formed in 1972 and has conducted sequential therapeutic trials.
- Five-year survival has increased from 55% on the IRS-I protocol (1972–1978) to approximately 71% on the IRS-III (1984–1991) and IRS-IV (1991–1997) protocols.

NONRHABDOMYOSARCOMATOUS SOFT TISSUE SARCOMAS

INCIDENCE, EPIDEMIOLOGY, AND PATHOLOGY

- Fifty percent of STS.
- Subtypes: Synovial sarcoma, fibrosarcoma, malignant peripheral nerve sheath tumor, malignant fibrous histiocytoma, hemangiopericytoma, leiomyosarcoma, alveolar soft part sarcoma, and liposarcoma.

- The peak age of onset is during late adolescence.
- Infants develop a distinctive set of soft tissue sarcomas.
- Associated with the Li-Fraumeni syndrome, neurofibromatosis, and prior irradiation.

CLINICAL PRESENTATION

- Most common sites are the extremities, trunk, head, and neck.
- Metastatic sites most commonly include lungs, lymph nodes, and bones.

WORKUP

- CT or MRI of the primary tumor, CXR, chest and abdominal CT, and bone scan.

IMPORTANT PROGNOSTIC FACTORS

- Resectability or group (complete resection or microscopic residual disease are considered favorable).
- Tumor size (<5 cm has a favorable outcome)
- Tumor pathologic grade; low grade (grades I or II) favorable.

TREATMENT AND OUTCOME

- Surgery represents the mainstay of therapy: Excision may be curative.
- Radiation therapy for local control for patients with residual tumor.
- The role of chemotherapy remains controversial.
- Outcome remains poor for patients with unresectable or metastatic tumors.

109 HEPATIC TUMORS

Howard M. Katzenstein

GENERAL

- 0.5–2% of all pediatric malignancies; tenth most common pediatric malignancy.
- Malignant liver tumors include hepatoblastoma, hepatocellular carcinoma, sarcoma, germ cell tumors, lymphoma, rhabdoid tumor, and metastatic tumors.

- Benign liver tumors include hemangioendothelioma, hemangioma, hamartoma, focal nodular hyperplasia, and adenoma.

EPIDEMIOLOGY

- Hepatoblastoma: Usually less than 3 years of age: Median 1 year.
- Hepatocellular carcinoma has a wide age range at presentation (median 12 years).
- Increased incidence of hepatoblastoma in premature and low birthweight infants with Beckwith-Wiedemann syndrome, familial adenomatous polyposis, and hemihypertrophy.
- Increased incidence of hepatocellular carcinoma is seen in hepatitis B and C; anabolic steroids, tyrosinemia, α-1 antitrypsin deficiency, type I glycogen storage disease, and cirrhosis.

CLINICAL FEATURES

- Liver tumors most commonly present as an asymptomatic abdominal mass.
- Hepatoblastoma is usually unifocal. Additional symptoms include abdominal pain, anorexia, weight loss, emesis isosexual precocious puberty in patients with tumors that secrete β-hCG (3%) and osteopenia.
- Hepatocellular carcinoma often presents as a multifocal lesion and can occur with jaundice (25%), hemoperitoneum, and splenomegaly.
- Metastatic disease: Twenty percent of patients at diagnosis, usually the lungs or lymph nodes.

DIAGNOSTIC WORKUP

- Computed tomography (CT) scan of chest, abdomen, and pelvis.
- Bone scan if clinically indicated.
- Alpha feto-protein (AFP) is elevated in virtually all or the majority of hepatoblastomas and 70% of hepatocellular carcinoma.

STAGING (UNITED STATES SYSTEM)

- Stage I: No metastases, tumor completely resected.
- Stage II: No metastases, tumor grossly resected with microscopic residual disease.
- Stage III: No distant metastases, gross residual tumor or positive lymph nodes.
- Stage IV: Distant metastases, regardless of the extent of liver involvement.

- The PRETEXT staging system for hepatoblastoma used in Europe is based on the extent of liver involvement at diagnosis.

PROGNOSTIC VARIABLES (ADVERSE)

- Metastatic, unresectable or recurrent disease.
- Slow rate of decline of AFP in response to chemotherapy.
- Low AFP (normal) in hepatoblastoma (anaplastic variant).

TREATMENT

- Surgery is essential for cure: At diagnosis 50% of hepatoblastomas and 25% of hepatocellular carcinomas are resectable.
- Liver transplantation used for unresectable liver tumors.
- Chemotherapy effective in the treatment of hepatoblastoma; unproven in hepatocellular carcinoma.
- Radiation therapy used for palliation.

110 LANGERHANS CELL HISTIOCYTOSIS

Elaine R. Morgan and Jacquie Toia

INTRODUCTION

- Spectrum of clinical behaviors ranging from lesions that will spontaneously regress to a multisystem, life-threatening disorder.
- Langerhans cell histiocytosis (LCH) is distinct from both the malignant histiocytic disorders, such as malignant histiocytosis and hemophagocytic lymphohistiocytosis (HLH).
- Pathogenesis is obscure.

NOMENCLATURE

- LCH has had many names during the past decades including the following:
  1. Eosinophilic granuloma
  2. Hand-Schuller-Christian disease
  3. Letterer-Siwe disease
  4. Hashimoto-Pritzker disease
  5. Histiocytosis X (self-healing, pure cutaneous)
  6. Langerhans cell or eosinophilic granulomatosis
  7. Type II histiocytosis
  8. Nonlipid reticuloendotheliosis

EPIDEMIOLOGY

- LCH is rare and sometimes undiagnosed.
- Actual incidence is difficult to establish: It is estimated that four to five children per million under the age of 15 years will be diagnosed with LCH each year.
- LCH may occur at any age; peak incidence 1–3 years.
- Multisystem LCH occurs most often in the first 2 years of life.

CLINICAL PRESENTATION

- Symptoms include fever, weight loss, fatigue, and organ-specific symptoms.
- Many systems involved; skin rash, bone lesions, and chronic otitis are common.

WORKUP

- Biopsy with immunohistochemistry, electron microscopy.
- Skeletal survey; radiographs of involved areas.
- Complete blood count (CBC), liver chemistries.

TREATMENT

- Approaches to treatment of LCH vary widely.
- Localized disease may resolve, be surgically excised or respond to local therapy.
- Multisystem disease requires systemic chemotherapy.

PROGNOSIS

- Disease confined to bone or lymph nodes are associated with a good prognosis.
- Multisystem disease is associated with a poor prognosis.
- Very young infants with extensive disease involving multiple organs statistically have the worst outcomes.
- Recurrence is common and may occur early or late.
- Late effects are more common in patients with multisystem disease, in those that receive long treatment courses and in children diagnosed at an early age.

111 LATE EFFECTS

Elaine R. Morgan

RISK FACTORS FOR LATE EFFECTS

GENETICS, TREATMENT, AGE OF TREATMENT

- Young age may increase organ damage, especially central nervous system (CNS).
- Familial cancer syndromes, genetic predisposition increase second malignant neoplasm (SMN) risk.
- Higher intensity treatment, combination therapy (C, I).
- Increased incidence over time from diagnosis.
- Infertility risk may be higher in children treated after puberty.
- Late effects are drug and modality specific.

SYSTEM-SPECIFIC EFFECTS

HEENT

Cataracts, dry eyes, small orbits (I)
Hearing loss (I, P)
Dry mouth, dental loss, and caries (I)
Facial asymmetry (I)
Cardiopulmonary
Cardiomyopathy (I, A, AA), restrictive pericarditis (I)
Pulmonary fibrosis (C, I, AA), radiation pneumonitis (I)

GI

Hepatitis—medication–induced infections (AM, E)
Hepatic fibrosis/cirrhosis (C)
Malabsorption, radiation enteritis (I)

GU

Bladder fibrosis, incontinence (I)
Hemorrhagic cystitis (AA, I)

RENAL

Renal insufficiency (M, IF, I, P)
Renal Fanconi syndrome, tubular dysfunction (IF, P)

MUSCULOSKELETAL

Scoliosis, kyphosis, musculoskeletal asymmetry (I)
Limb loss (S, I)
Osteomyelitis, osteonecrosis, fracture (I)
Avascular necrosis (S, M)
Osteoporosis (S, M, I)
Breast hypoplasia (I)

METABOLIC

Diabetes mellitus (C, after BMT)
Hyperlipidemia (C, I)
Obesity (C, I)

NEUROLOGIC/NEUROPSYCHIATRIC

Paralysis/paresis secondary to cord compression (D)
Peripheral neuropathy, autonomic dysfunction (C)
Leukoencephalopathy (M, I)
Learning disability (M, I)

ENDOCRINE

Hypo/hyperthyroidism (I)
Growth hormone failure (I)
Precocious puberty (I, C)
Premature menopause (I, AA)
Reproductive
Hormone deficiency (AA, I)
Amenorrhea (AA, I)
Infertility (C, I)

SECONDARY NEOPLASIA

Leukemia, myelodysplasia occur 2–4 years after treatment (AA, T, I)
Sarcomas occur late (I)
Lymphomas—secondary to immunosuppression (C, I, D)
Benign tumors secondary to XRT (I)
Carcinoma—breast most common; also colon, lung (I)

PSYCHOSOCIAL

Cognitive delays
Insurance, employment, military discrimination
Adjustment disorders

ABBREVIATIONS: P = platinum; I = irradiation; C = chemotherapy; A = anthracycline; T = topoisomerose inhibitors; AA = alkylating agents; AM = antimetabolite; IF = ifosfamide; S = steroids; M = methotrexate; S = surgery; D = disease related; BMT = bone marrow transplant; XRT = radiotherapy.

FOLLOW-UP CARE

- Requires multidisciplinary approach including medical specialties, reproductive evaluation, psychosocial, educational, surgical specialties, PT, OT.
- Multidisciplinary follow-up clinics, including adult practitioners are effective.
- Patients require annual medical evaluation into adulthood.
- Preventive medicine is essential.
- Screening tests are disease and treatment specific and may include the following:
  1. Mammograms
  2. Echocardiograms
  3. Organ system evaluation
  4. Metabolic evaluation
  5. Bone mineral density
- Other cancer screening.

BIBLIOGRAPHY

Altman AS, Schwartz AD. *Malignant Diseases of Infancy, Childhood and Adolescence. Renal Tumors.* Philadelphia, PA: W.B. Saunders, 1983, Chap. 16.

Areci RJ. Progress and controversies in the treatment of pediatric acute myelogenous leukemia. *Curr Opin Hematol* 2002;9: 353–360.

Arico M, Egeler RM. Clinical aspects of Langerhan cell histiocytosis. *Hematol Oncol Clin North Am* 1998;12:247–258.

Baggott CR, Patterson-Kelly K, Fochtman D, Foley GV. *Nursing Care of Children and Adolescents with Cancer. Association of Pediatric Oncology Nurses*, 3rd ed. Philadelphia, PA: W.B. Saunders, 2002, Chap. 22, pp. 523–531.

Clericuzio C. Recognition and management of childhood cancer syndromes: a systems approach. *Am J Med Genet* 1999;89: 81–90.

Grier HE. The Ewing family of tumors: Ewing's sarcoma and primitive neuroectodermal tumors. *Pediatr Clin North Am*, 1997;44:991–1004.

Katzenstein HM, Cohn SL. Advances in the diagnosis and treatment of neuroblastoma. *Curr Opin Oncol* 1998;10:43–51.

Medline website: *http://www.nlm.nih.gov/medlineplus/*

Morgan ER, Haugen M. Late effects of cancer therapy. *Cancer Treat Res* 1997;92:343–375

National Institute of Health website: *http://www.health.nih. gov*

Pizzo PA, Poplack DG. *Principles and Practice of Pediatric Oncology*, 4th ed. Philadelphia, PA: Lippincott Williams and Wilkins, 2002.

Provisor AJ, Ettinger LJ, Nachman JB, et al. Treatment of nonmetastatic osteosarcoma of the extremity with preoperative and postoperative chemotherapy: a report from the Children's Cancer Group. *J Clin Oncol* 1997;15:76–84.

Pui CH, Evand WE. Acute lymphoblastic leukemia. *N Engl J Med* 1997;339:605–615.

Raney RB, Anderson JR, Barr FG, Donaldson SS, Pappo AS, Qualman SJ, Weiner ES, Maurer HM, Crisg WM. Rhabdomyosarcoma and undifferentiated sarcoma in the first two decades of life: a selective review of the Intergroup Rhabdomyosarcoma Study Group experience and rational for Intergroup Rhabdomyosarcoma Study V. *J Pediatr Hematol Oncol* 2001;23:215–220.

Rowland J. Molecular genetic diagnosis of pediatric cancer: current and emerging methods. *Pediatr Clin North Am* 2002;49: 1415–1435.

Sandlund JT, Downing JR, Crist WM. Non-Hodgkins lymphoma in childhood. *N Engl J Med* 1996;334:1238–1248.

Spunt SL, Poquette CA, Hurn YS, Cain AM, Rao BN, Merchant TE, Jenkins JJ, Santana VM, Pratt CB, Pappo AS. Prognostic factors for children and adolescents with surgically resected nonrhabdomyosarcoma soft tissue sarcoma: an analysis of 121patients treated at St. Jude Children's Research Hospital. *J Clin Oncol* 1999;17:3697–3705.

Widhe B, Widhe T. Initial symptoms and clinical features of osteosarcoma and Ewing sarcoma. *J Bone Joint Surg Am* 2000;82:667–674.

Tina Q. Tan, Section Editor

112 BACTERIAL INFECTIONS

A. Todd Davis, Alexandra Freeman,
Judith Guzman-Cottrill, Preeti Jaggi,
Stanford T. Shulman, Tina Q. Tan,
Ram Yogev

ACUTE OTITIS MEDIA

EPIDEMIOLOGY AND PATHOGENESIS

- Acute otitis media is an infection of the middle ear chamber caused by bacteria or viruses.
- Otitis media occurs more commonly in males and can occur at any age but it is most frequent during the first 3 years of life with the peak incidence between 6 and 18 months of age. Two out of three children have at least one episode of acute otitis media before their first birthday. The earlier in life an episode of otitis media occurs, the more at risk a child is for recurrent acute or chronic middle ear disease as they grow older.
- Predisposing factors for acute otitis media include abnormal eustachian tube function of any etiology, anatomical abnormality (e.g., cleft palate, craniofacial defects), lower socioeconomic status, day-care attendance, bottle-feeding in the horizontal position, atopy, and certain racial groups.
- There is some evidence that breast-feeding may decrease the incidence of acute otitis media.
- The eustachian tube normally opens and closes multiple times a day, draining fluid secreted by the cells lining the middle ear. When eustachian tube function is impaired by bacterial or viral infections or by allergy, air is trapped in the middle ear. When the

pressure in the middle ear falls below atmospheric pressure the eustachian tube is forced open carrying bacteria from the upper airway into the middle ear. When the eustachian tube closes again, the bacteria become trapped and infection may ensue.

CLINICAL MANIFESTATIONS

- There are multiple clinical presentations of an ear infection most of which are nonspecific. The classic presentation is that of a child with a history of an upper respiratory infection who develops fever, otalgia, irritability or fussiness, and hearing loss. Other nonspecific symptoms include anorexia, loose stools, and scratching or tugging at the ears. Young infants may only present with fever, irritability, and diarrhea. On occasion afebrile seizures may be the presenting symptom.
- The appearance of the tympanic membrane on physical examination is the key to making the diagnosis of acute otitis media. The classic findings include an erythematous, opaque, bulging tympanic membrane with an absent or distorted light reflex, and loss of distinct landmarks that does not move with insufflation. Insufflation by pneumatic otoscopy is a critical part of the examination in order to determine tympanic membrane mobility.

ETIOLOGIC AGENTS

- The most common bacterial agents that cause acute otitis media include *Streptococcus pneumoniae*, nontypeable *Haemophilus influenzae*, *Moraxella catarrhalis*, and less commonly group A streptococcus and *Staphylococcus aureus*. All these organisms have developed some resistance to the antibiotics most commonly used for therapy.

- Viruses also contribute to the burden of this illness with respiratory syncytial virus and influenza viruses being the most common.
- About one-third of middle ear fluid cultures are sterile in patients with acute otitis media.

THERAPY

- Empiric first line therapy is high-dose amoxicillin (80–90 mg/kg/day divided bid) which gram for gram remains the most active drug against the most common organisms that cause otitis media. Second line therapeutic agents include high-dose amoxicillin/clavulanic acid (80–90 mg/kg/day divided bid), oral cefuroxime axetil (30 mg/kg/day divided bid), and oral cefdinir (14 mg/kg/day). Duration of therapy 7–10 days.
- Three doses of intramuscular ceftriaxone (50 mg/kg/dose) given every other day may be used in those patients who are unable to tolerate oral therapy.
- For those patients who are allergic (i.e., hives or anaphylaxis) to the penicillins and cephalosporins, the macrolide and azalide antibiotics may be used.
- At the completion of antibiotic therapy about 80% of children will have residual fluid (effusion) in the middle ear. A half-life curve suggests that by 3 or 4 months after the otitis episode, the middle ear effusion in the vast majority of children will have resolved.
- In children with multiple recurrent episodes of otitis media or chronic middle ear effusions that interfere with hearing and speech, evaluation for placement of pressure equalizing tubes may be warranted.

OTITIS EXTERNAL

EPIDEMIOLOGY AND PATHOGENESIS

- Otitis externa is an infection of the external auditory canal.
- The external auditory canal is normally protected from infection by a squamous epithelial lining which provides a physical barrier and by the acidic pH of the cerumen which provides a chemical barrier.
- Factors that predispose to infection by disruption of these barriers include trauma, high temperature and humidity, and excessive ear cleaning or wetting.
- Infection occurs most commonly in the summer months but may be seen year round in persons who spend a lot of time in swimming pools.

DIAGNOSIS

- Diagnosis is based on clinical signs and symptoms. The most common symptoms are ear pain that is worsened by manipulation of the pinna or tragus, itching, and fullness. Fever is usually absent.

ETIOLOGIC AGENTS

- The infection is frequently polymicrobial. The most common causative agents include *Staphylococcus aureus, Pseudomonas aeruginosa*, other gram-negative bacilli, group A streptococcus, *Aspergillus niger,* and *Candida albicans*.

TREATMENT

- Treatment consists of a combination of good ear hygiene using 3% saline or 2% acetic acid and installation of appropriate antibiotic drops (suspension of polymyxin B-neomycin-hydrocortisone) four times a day for 10–14 days.
- Systemic antibiotic therapy is indicated if the patient is febrile or has associated cervical adenitis or cellulitis of adjacent tissues. Appropriate oral therapy includes amoxicillin-clavulanic acid, cefuroxime axetil, or trimethoprim-sulfamethoxazole.

MASTOIDITIS

EPIDEMIOLOGY AND PATHOGENESIS

- Mastoiditis is a complication of otitis media. It is a bacterial infection of the mastoid air cells that develops when inflammation of the mucoperiosteal lining of the air cells caused by otitis media results in progressive swelling which obstructs the drainage of exudative materials from the mastoid.
- Mastoiditis is uncommon in the modern era of antibiotics but remains a potentially life-threatening disease that requires prompt recognition and treatment.

CLINICAL MANIFESTATIONS

- Otitis media is almost always present. The classic presentation of mastoiditis is that of fever, otalgia, postauricular swelling, and redness. The swelling usually occurs over the mastoid process, displacing the pinna superiorly and laterally. In infants, the swelling may occur above the ear, displacing the pinna inferiorly and laterally. While otherwise a nondescript febrile illness, the presence of ear displacement makes mastoiditis easier to diagnose.

DIAGNOSIS

- Usually made on presence of clinical manifestations.
- Plain-film radiography or computed tomography demonstrating coalescence of mastoid air cells, loss of normal bony trabeculations, or presence of a subperiosteal abscess may be used to aid in the diagnosis.
- A bacteriologic diagnosis should be attempted in all cases of mastoiditis. Specimens may be obtained by tympanocentesis or from the mastoid bone itself. All specimens should be sent for aerobic and anaerobic cultures.

ETIOLOGIC AGENTS

- The most common causative agents of acute mastoiditis include *Streptococcus pneumoniae*, nontypeable *Haemophilus influenzae* group A streptococcus, and *Staphylococcus aureus*. In patients with a history of chronic otitis media, anaerobic organisms (especially *Peptococcus* species, *Actinomyces* species, or *Bacteroides* species) and *Pseudomonas aeruginosa* and other gram-negative bacilli should be considered.

TREATMENT

- Treatment usually consists of myringotomy in combination with parenteral antibiotics. The most common empiric regimen may consist of ampicillin/sulbactam (200–400 mg of the ampicillin component/kg/day divided q 6–8 hours) or a combination of a penicillinase-resistant penicillin (nafcillin or oxacillin) and a third-generation cephalosporin. Minimum duration of therapy is 21 days.
- If complications of mastoiditis develop (e.g., meningitis, brain abscess, epidural abscess, venous sinus thrombosis, subdural empyema, or a subperiosteal abscess) or if there is poor response to intravenous (IV) antibiotic therapy, mastoidectomy, and possibly other surgical interventions may be necessary.

SINUSITIS

CONJUNCTIVITIS

EPIDEMIOLOGY

- The conjunctiva of the eye is a mucous membrane covering the front part of the eye lining the inner surface of the eyelid. It is divided into the bulbar and palpebral portions. Inflammation can be due to viral infections, bacterial infections, allergic causes, or due to vasculitis. It is helpful clinically to divide conjunctivitis into acute (lasting less than 10–14 days) and chronic presentations.

ETIOLOGIC AGENTS

- In the nonneonate, conjunctivitis can be classified into bacterial, viral, allergic, or vasculitic origins.
  1. Allergic conjunctivitis generally causes pruritis and a serous discharge.
  2. Major causes of viral conjunctivitis are adenovirus, herpes simplex virus (HSV), enterovirus, rubella, and rubeola. Major characteristics of each are shown in Table 112-1. Generally, these pathogens cause acute conjunctivitis with a watery discharge, sometimes with bilateral eye involvement. Diagnosis is made clinically, but occasionally viral cultures may need to be sent for confirmation. Treatment is supportive with the exception of herpes simplex virus conjunctivitis, which should be managed with an ophthalmologist. Oral acyclovir may be of benefit in addition to topical ointments for keratitis.
  3. Major bacterial etiologies in the nonneonate include nontypeable *H. influenzae, S. pneumoniae,* and *Moraxella catarrhalis.* Less commonly, infections may be due to *Neisseria gonorrhoeae* and *Neisseria meningitidis.* Erythromycin and bacitracin-polymyxin ointments are commonly used to treat acute conjunctivitis.

TABLE 112-1   Major Viral Etiologies of Conjunctivitis in the Nonneonate

VIRUS (SEROTYPE)	CLINICAL PRESENTATION	PHYSICAL FINDINGS
Adenovirus (3 and 7)	Pharyngoconjunctival fever	Punctate epithelial keratitis, fever, pharyngitis
Adenovirus (8, 19, and 37)	Epidemic keratoconjunctivitis	Punctate epithelial keratitis, lid swelling
Herpes simplex virus	Herpetic keratoconjunctivitis	Vesicles on eyelids, punctate epithelial keratitis
Enterovirus (70), coxsackie virus A24	Acute hemorrhagic conjunctivitis	Punctate epithelial keratitis, often subconjunctival hemorrhage
Rubella, rubeola	Rubella, rubeola (measles)	Punctate epithelial keratitis, fever, diffuse erythema, postauricular lymphadenopathy (rubella), Koplick spots (rubeola)

- Infants with chronic conjunctivitis may have naso-lacrimal duct obstruction. *S. aureus* may cause blephar-itis, a primary infection of the eyelid with a secondary inflammation of the conjunctiva. Topical antibiotics such as erythromycin or bacitracin can be used. Inclusion conjunctivitis from *Chlamydia trachomatis* can occur in sexually active adolescents resulting in mucopurulent discharge, eyelid swelling, ipsilateral preauricular adenopathy, and photophobia. Treatment consists of systemic erythromycin or doxycycline. *Bartonella henselae,* tularemia, tuberculosis, and infec-tious mononucleosis can also cause granulomatous con-junctivitis with ipsilateral lymphadenopathy.
- Children with Kawasaki disease can present with fever and bilateral nonpurulent conjunctivitis among other clinical signs. This diagnosis should be considered in a febrile or irritable child with other signs/symptoms of Kawasaki disease.
- The differential diagnosis of neonatal conjunctivitis (occurring in the first month of life) includes sexually transmitted diseases as well as herpes simplex virus, *S. aureus*, *S. pneumoniae*, and *H. influenzae* species. Viral etiologies, other than herpes simplex virus, are not important pathogens in neonatal conjunctivitis.
- *Chlamydia trachomatis* is the most common cause of neonatal conjunctivitis. It generally occurs 5–14 days after birth. Infants present with swelling of the eyelid, erythema, and uni- or bilateral mucopurulent conjunc-tivitis. Infants may also present with nasal congestion, cough, tachypnea, and rales if a chlamydial pneumonia is present. Diagnosis can be made with direct fluores-cence antibody of conjunctival cells. Treatment is with erythromycin estolate for 14 days.
- *Neisseria gonorrhoeae* was a major cause of blindness before the onset of ocular prophylaxis. Infants present usually within the first week of life with edema of the eyelid and purulent conjunctivitis. Corneal involve-ment can occur which can result in scarring and visual impairment. Diagnosis is made with Gram stain and culture on Thayer-Martin or chocolate agar. The treat-ment of choice is with cefotaxime for 7 days.
- HSV conjunctivitis, usually due to HSV-2, presents within the first 14 days of life; infants typically have unilateral or bilateral conjunctivitis with ipsilateral eyelid edema. Superficial keratitis and geographic ulcers can occur. A cobalt blue examination may be needed to visualize the corneal involvement. Diagnosis is made by culture of vesicles/corneal lesions. Treat-ment for the neonate involves 14 days of parenteral acy-clovir. Topical therapy may also be needed.
- Ocular prophylaxis with silver nitrate, erythromycin ointment, or tetracycline ointment is effective if admin-istered within 1 hour of birth to prevent *N. gonorrhoeae* and *C. trachomatis* infections.

HORDEOLUM

- An external hordeolum, or stye, is a bacterial infection of the glands of Zeis (sebaceous gland) or Moll (sweat gland) associated with a hair follicle of the eyelid. Infection is usually localized in the form of a pustule.
- An internal hordeolum is a bacterial infection of the meibomian gland, a long sebaceous gland whose ori-fice is at the lid margin. A pustule may not always be easily visible without everting the eyelid and examin-ing the tarsal conjunctiva.
- Usually, these infections are caused by *S. aureus*.
- Treatment involves applying bacitracin ointment to the eye to prevent spread of the infection to other fol-licles and warm compresses to facilitate drainage.

PERIORBITAL/ORBITAL CELLULITIS

- Nontraumatic generalized eye swelling may be classi-fied into periorbital or orbital cellulitis based on clin-ical examination. Proptosis, ophthalmoplegia, change in visual acuity, and pain with extraocular movement characterize orbital cellulitis and should be treated as such.
- Periorbital cellulitis is also referred to as preseptal cel-lulitis because it is located anterior to the orbital septum, the continuation of the periosteum from the orbital wall to the tarsal plate. This anatomy acts as a barrier to local spread of infection.
  1. Periorbital cellulitis can be further divided into three etiologies: (1) result of loss of skin integrity and resultant subcutaneous cellulitis (usually caused by *Staphylococcus aureus* or group A strep-tococci), (2) inflammatory edema secondary to sinusitis, or (3) bacteremia without another source in young children less than 3 years old (usually due to *Haemophilus influenzae* b or *S. pneumo-niae*). Those children with disrupted skin barriers usually have an indurated, erythematous swelling emanating from the site of the initial lesion. Children with inflammatory edema have a suba-cute onset of swelling that is usually not tender or indurated. Children that have bacteremia may have mild upper respiratory infections and indurated, tender swelling.
  2. Diagnosis of periorbital cellulitis is based on clini-cal presentation, x-ray or computed tomography of the sinuses, and/or blood culture. For children with a disrupted skin barrier, appropriate treatments include cephalexin, clindamycin, and oxacillin. For those children with sinusitis, anaerobic bacteria should also be covered. Amoxicillin-clavulanate and

clindamycin may be used to cover anaerobes and the common sinusitis organisms, *S. pneumoniae, M. catarrhalis,* and nontypeable *H. influenzae.* For children with suspected bacteremia, lumbar puncture and parenteral therapy is indicated. Initial treatment with ceftriaxone or cefotaxime is appropriate empiric treatment.

• Orbital, or postseptal, cellulitis is a complication of sinusitis. It usually results due to ethmoid sinusitis with a subperiosteal abscess in the thin lamina papyracea bone that separates the ethmoid sinus from the orbit. With further progression, pus can invade into the orbit itself.

1. Orbital cellulitis is characterized by ophthalmoplegia, proptosis, chemosis (edema of the bulbar conjunctiva), and/or decreased visual acuity. If the physical examination is inadequate secondary to eye swelling, an orbital computerized tomography scan should be obtained.

2. Bacterial etiologies include *S. pneumoniae*, nontypeable *H. influenzae*, *M. catarrhalis*, group A *streptococcus, Staphylococcus aureus*, and anaerobes.

3. Treatment requires multispecialty care. Ampicillin/ sulbactam may be used empirically. Ophthalmology should be involved early in the care for an adequate visual examination. Any patient with significant visual impairment or complete ophthalmoplegia should undergo surgical drainage of the abscess and/ or involved sinuses. In addition, any patient that does not respond to treatment in 24–36 hours should also be considered for surgical intervention. Treatment duration depends on the patient's clinical presentation, but is usually needed for 3–4 weeks. The decision to switch to oral therapy should be made by physicians experienced with this clinical entity who can follow the patient's progress.

PHARYNGITIS AND TONSILLITIS

EPIDEMIOLOGY AND ETIOLOGIC AGENTS

• The large majority of acute pharyngitis or tonsillitis is viral in etiology, with Epstein-Barr virus, adenovirus, and enteroviruses most common.

• The most important bacterial cause of acute pharyngitis or tonsillitis, by far, is *Streptococcus pyogenes* (group A beta-hemolytic streptococci), which accounts for 15–20% of episodes, and which can lead to complications like acute rheumatic fever if untreated. Groups C and G beta-streptococci also can cause acute pharyngitis, especially in older children and young adults; this is self-limited and does not require diagnosis and treatment.

CLINICAL MANIFESTATIONS

• Clinical features rarely allow accurate distinction between viral and streptococcal pharyngitis; thus, at least one diagnostic test for group A streptococci (rapid antigen test and/or culture) is indicated unless obvious viral features (especially rhinorrhea, hoarseness, and cough) are present.

• The classic clinical profile of acute streptococcal pharyngitis is a school-age child 5–11 years old in late winter or spring with sudden onset of fever and sore throat. Headache, malaise, abdominal pain, nausea, and vomiting are common, while cough, rhinorrhea, stridor, hoarseness, conjunctivitis, and diarrhea are very infrequent. On examination, pharyngeal erythema with or without exudate, palatal petechiae, tonsillar hypertrophy, hypertrophied tongue papillae, tender enlarged anterior cervical nodes, and a scarlatinal rash may be present.

DIAGNOSIS

• Laboratory confirmation of streptococcal pharyngitis should be by a throat swab that is processed by a rapid antigen detection test and/or culture on sheep blood agar. A positive antigen test is considered diagnostic in the appropriate clinical setting because of its very high specificity. Some believe that a negative antigen test should always be backed up by a throat culture because of the variable sensitivity of antigen tests; opinions vary on this topic.

TREATMENT

• Viral pharyngitis is self-limited and should be treated symptomatically; antibiotics are of no value. Penicillin is the treatment of choice for streptococcal pharyngitis. Recommended therapies include IM benzathine penicillin G (600,000 u for those <27 kg; 1.2 million u for those ≥27 kg); IM benzathine penicillin G plus procaine penicillin G (900,000 u plus 300,000 u); oral penicillin V 250–500 mg bid-tid for 10 days; and oral amoxicillin 50 mg/kg up to 750 mg once daily for 10 days. Shorter courses of some oral cephalosporins (5 days) or azithromycin (3–5 days) are generally effective, but because of cost they should be used only for those allergic to penicillin (avoid cephalosporins in those with anaphylactic hypersensitivity to penicillin).

COMPLICATIONS

• Suppurative complications of streptococcal pharyngitis include retropharyngeal or peritonsillar abscess, cervical adenitis, otitis media, sinusitis, mastoiditis, and rarely bacteremia leading to metastatic infection. Nonsuppurative (immune-mediated) sequelae include acute rheumatic fever, acute glomerulonephritis, and probably poststreptococcal reactive arthritis. The toxin-mediated streptococcal toxic shock syndrome is more often a sequela of cutaneous rather than pharyngeal/respiratory tract streptococcal infection.

SCARLET FEVER

- Caused by *Streptococcus pyogenes* (group A streptococcus) which elaborate erythrogenic exotoxin.
- A person must be hypersensitive to the exotoxin before the person can develop scarlet fever as a manifestation of streptococcal disease.
- Typical clinical presentation includes fever, nausea, vomiting, and abdominal pain which may precede the development of rash by 12–48 hours. Pharyngitis may be absent or mild.
- The rash is an erythematous maculopapular rash which usually begins on the trunk and spreads to cover the entire body within hours to days. The forehead and cheeks are flushed, and the area around the mouth is pale (circumoral pallor). The rash has a sandpaper texture and generally fades on pressure and ultimately desquamates. Deep red, nonblanching, or petechial lesions may be present in the folds of the joints (Pastia's lines) or other parts of the extremities.
- Early in the illness, the dorsum of the tongue may have a white coating, through which the papillae protrude (white strawberry tongue); however, several days later, the white covering desquamates, and the tongue becomes swollen and red (strawberry tongue).
- Penicillin is the drug of choice for the treatment of group A beta-hemolytic streptococcal infections. In patients with a penicillin allergy, erythromycin is the drug of choice.

CHRONIC STREPTOCOCCAL CARRIAGE

- Avoidance of posttreatment follow-up throat cultures in asymptomatic patients and not performing throat swabs in those with obvious viral upper respiratory infections helps to minimize this issue. Studies of chronic carriers show little or no risk of sequelae and little risk of spread to contacts. Antibiotics to terminate carriage can be considered in those with a personal history or a household member with history of rheumatic fever/rheumatic heart disease, those threatened with tonsillectomy, community outbreak of rheumatic fever or acute nephritis, and excessive familial anxiety. When needed, carriage can

be treated with 10 days of oral clindamycin or an injection of benzathine penicillin with 4 days of oral rifampin, with a high rate of clearance.

PNEUMONIA AND EMPYEMA

EPIDEMIOLOGY

- Worldwide, pneumonia or lower respiratory tract infection is a common cause of morbidity and mortality in the pediatric population with an estimated 6.5 million children dying from complications of pneumonia each year.
- Host factors, such as age, underlying disease, and nutritional status, have a great impact on associated morbidity and mortality and also influence the organisms that cause disease.

ETIOLOGIC AGENTS

- Respiratory viruses are the most common cause of pneumonia in pediatric patients. The most common include influenza A and B, adenovirus, respiratory syncytial virus, and enteroviruses.
- *Streptococcus pneumoniae* is the most common bacterial cause of pneumonia. Less common causes include *Staphylococcus aureus* and group A *streptococcus*. In the neonatal period, group B *streptococcus*, *Escherichia coli*, *Listeria monocytogenes*, and other gram-negative bacilli may cause pneumonia.
- *Chlamydia pneumoniae* and *Mycoplasma pneumonia* are the most common causes of "atypical pneumonia," especially in children older than 5 years. *Chlamydia trachomatis* and *Ureaplasma urealyticum* are atypical agents that may cause pneumonia in young infants under 3 months of age.
- *Mycobacterium tuberculosis* (TB) may cause pneumonia at any age and should be thought about in persons with epidemiologic risk factors.
- Fungal pneumonias caused by *Histoplasma capsulatum* (endemic area—eastern and central United States), *Blastomyces dermatitidis* (endemic area—southeastern and midwestern United States), *Coccidioides imitis* (endemic area—southwestern United States) may be seen especially in endemic areas.

CLINICAL MANIFESTATIONS

- The clinical presentation of pneumonia varies depending on the age of the child. Infants may present with only fever and cough. Other symptoms may include ill appearance, apnea, nasal flaring, tachypnea, or decreased oral intake. In many cases these symptoms are preceded by minor upper respiratory tract infection symptoms. Often there is evidence of accessory muscle use and intercostal, subcostal, and suprasternal retractions may be seen.

- Physical examination may demonstrate the presence of rales (crackles), rhonchi, decreased breath sounds, or wheezing over the affected area. Cyanosis or pallor may be seen in children with hypoxemia.

DIAGNOSIS

- Diagnosis of pneumonia in many cases is made based on the presence of clinical signs and symptoms.
- Complete blood count (CBC) may be helpful—total white blood cell counts above 15,000 cells/mL are suggestive of a bacterial etiology. Other tests that may help in defining an etiology include blood culture (positive in up to 30% of bacteremic pneumonias), pleural fluid examination (if present), nasopharyngeal wash for viral culture, *Mycoplasma* titers, *Chlamydia* titers, or *Legionella* titers.
- Chest radiographs are often used to confirm the presence, location, and appearance of pulmonary infiltrates. Bacterial pneumonias are much more likely to have focal infiltrates or consolidation, whereas, viral and atypical pneumonias usually have a more diffuse, bilateral interstitial pattern. Patients with pulmonary tuberculosis may have enlargement of hilar nodes or calcifications and a miliary appearance on chest radiograph. Apical cavitation may also be present, especially in older children and adolescents.
- If pleural fluid is obtained, studies that should be performed include Gram stain and routine bacterial culture, acid-fast stain and culture, and fungal stain and culture; pleural fluid pH, glucose, protein, lactate dehydrogenase, white blood cell count with differential and antigen detection tests. A low pH, low glucose, high protein, elevated lactate dehydrogenase, and an elevated white blood cell (WBC) count with a predominance of neutrophils supports the diagnosis of a pyogenic or bacterial pneumonia with empyema.

COMPLICATIONS

- Up to one-third of patients with bacterial pneumonia will develop a parapneumonic effusion which may evolve into an empyema. Bacterial pneumonias are most commonly associated with this complication. Thoracentesis should be performed in cases of large effusions, for diagnostic purposes and in patients who fail to respond to appropriate antibiotic therapy.
- Other complications of bacterial pneumonia include lung parenchyma abscess formation and pneumatocele formation.

TREATMENT

- In addition to supportive care, the treatment of pneumonia is focused against the most likely suspected pathogen based on age, clinical signs and symptoms and laboratory and radiographic findings. In the neonate, ampicillin and gentamicin is the most common empiric regimen. In older infants and children, high-dose amoxicillin or an oral second generation cephalosporin are often used for empiric outpatient therapy. If an atypical organism is suspected, one of the newer macrolide agents (azithromycin or clarithromycin) is often used.

OCCULT BACTEREMIA

EPIDEMIOLOGY

- Defined as the presence of positive blood cultures for a bacterial agent in children who do not have any focus of infection on clinical examination that would be associated with bacteremia.
- Most commonly seen in children between 3 and 36 months of age, with the highest incidence occurring in children between 6 and 24 months.
- Accounts for 3–6% of bacteremia in highly febrile young children.
- No racial, geographic, or socioeconomic predilection.
- Risk of subsequent meningitis developing in children with occult bacteremia is estimated to be 1 out of 1000–1500 untreated children.

CLINICAL AND LABORATORY FINDINGS

- Patients at highest risk for occult bacteremia usually present with high fever >39.4°C (103°F), total peripheral white blood cell count (per microliter) <5000 or >15,000 and no focus of infection on clinical examination.
- Performance of a urinalysis is indicated in the neonate and in female infants with no other source to explain the fever.
- Performance of a lumbar puncture is based on the child's age, clinical appearance, and degree of fever.

ETIOLOGIC AGENTS

- Most common organisms associated with occult bacteremia: *S. pneumoniae* (responsible for two-thirds to three-fourths of cases), *N. meningitides*, *H. influenzae* type b, and *Salmonella* spp. (history of associated gastroenteritis).

TREATMENT

- Empiric antibiotic therapy is usually given to those patients with risk factors that place them at high risk for occult bacteremia until culture results are available. These include age less than 2 years, fever >40°C (104°F), peripheral white count <5000 or >15,000/mL, toxic appearance, and presence of underlying disease that may predispose to serious bacterial infection.
- Most commonly used agents include amoxicillin (40–60 mg/kg/day divided bid), amoxicillin/clavulanic acid (40–60 mg/kg/day divided bid), oral second- and third-generation cephalosporins, or a single injection of ceftriaxone (50–75 mg/kg) in those patients who cannot tolerate oral therapy.
- Patients need close follow-up and immediate reevaluation if the blood culture yields a pathogen, clinical condition deteriorates, or if signs and symptoms of a serious focal infection develop.

INFECTIVE ENDOCARDITIS

EPIDEMIOLOGY

- Infective endocarditis (IE) occurs significantly less often in children than in adults.
- The underlying risk factors for children with IE have significantly changed. Before the 1970s, up to 50% of cases in the United States were associated with rheumatic heart disease. As the incidence of rheumatic fever has declined, the most common predisposing factors for IE are congenital heart disease and central venous catheters.
- The incidence of neonatal IE is increasing as the survival rate of extremely premature neonates increases. This is primarily a complication of indwelling venous catheters in these patients.
- Up to 12% of IE patients will have no identified predisposing factor.

PATHOPHYSIOLOGY

- Damaged cardiac endothelium induces thrombogenesis, and provides a nidus to which bacteria in the blood can adhere. Thrombogenesis at the eroded site promotes aggregation of platelets, fibrin, and bacterial colonization. As platelets and fibrin accumulate over the organisms, a vegetation forms that increases in size and the bacteria becomes encased within the vegetation.
- In congenital heart disease, endothelial damage can occur as a result of abnormal high-velocity blood flow. Thus, left-sided (high pressure) lesions are more commonly seen. The most common congenital lesions in IE are tetralogy of Fallot and ventricular septal defects.
- In the presence of venous catheters, the catheter itself causes trauma to the valvular or endocardial endothelium. Right-sided IE is typically seen, as central venous catheters are positioned in the right side of the heart.
- In early postoperative endocarditis, vegetation formation occurs in association with damaged endothelium at suture sites. Late postoperative IE occurs after reendothelialization of the cardiac and vascular surfaces.

CLINICAL FEATURES

- IE may present with nonspecific findings such as fever, fatigue, malaise, chills, and myalgias. In children with congenital heart disease or indwelling central venous catheters, IE must be entertained if these symptoms persist without a clear source.
- Children may present with fulminant disease, requiring immediate intervention. These patients include those who present with peripheral embolization to the brain or those who develop congestive heart failure due to valvular damage.
- The physical examination findings in IE are related to bacteremia/fungemia, valvulitis, immunologic responses, and emboli. These signs and their frequency are listed in Table 112-2.

TABLE 112-2   Signs Associated with IE in Children

SIGN	FREQUENCY (%)
Fever	75–100
Splenomegaly	50–75
Petechiae	21–50
Embolic phenomenon	25–50
New/changed murmur	21–50
Clubbing	Rare
Osler nodes	Rare
Roth spots	Rare
Janeway lesions	Rare
Splinter hemorrhages	Rare
Conjunctival hemorrhage	Rare

DIAGNOSIS

- When considering IE, multiple (usually a minimum of 3) blood cultures should be obtained at different times. If the patient is not acutely ill, antibiotics may be withheld while blood cultures are being collected.
- Additional laboratory evaluation includes CBC with differential, erythrocyte sedimentation rate (ESR) and/or C-reactive protein (CRP), rheumatoid factor, and urinalysis.
- In children, transthoracic echocardiography (TTE) is the main modality for evaluating the presence of a vegetation as most children have thin chest walls. Transesophageal echocardiogram (TEE) is usually only required in older children or in cases where TTE does not provide adequate visualization.
- The Duke criteria (Tables 112-3 and 112-4) may also assist in the diagnosis of IE.

POSSIBLE IE
- Findings consistent with IE that fall short of "definite" but "not rejected"

REJECTED
- Firm alternative diagnosis for manifestations of endocarditis, or
- Resolution of manifestations of endocarditis with antibiotic therapy for ≤4 days, or
- No pathologic evidence of IE at surgery or autopsy, after antibiotic therapy for ≤4 days.

ETIOLOGIC AGENTS

- Most common organisms are gram-positive cocci. The viridans group streptococci are the most commonly isolated streptococci. Of the staphylococcal organisms, coagulase-negative staphylococci and *Staphylococcus aureus* are most common.

TABLE 112-3   Duke Clinical Criteria for Diagnosis of IE

DEFINITIVE IE

Pathologic Criteria

Microorganisms: Demonstrated by culture of histology in a vegetation, a vegetation that has embolized, or an intracardiac abscess, or

Pathologic lesions: Vegetation or intracardiac abscess present, confirmed by histology showing active endocarditis

Clinical Criteria as defined in Table 112-3

Two major criteria, or
One major criterion and three minor criteria, or
Five minor criteria

TABLE 112-4   Definitions of Terms Used in the Duke Criteria of the Diagnosis of IE

MAJOR CRITERIA

Positive Blood Culture for IE

Typical microorganism consistent with IE from two separate blood cultures as noted below

Viridans streptococci (includes *Abiotrophia* sp.), *Streptococcus bovis*, or HACEK group, or

Community-acquired *Staphylococcus aureus* or enterococci, in the absence of a primary focus, or

Microorganisms consistent with IE from persistently positive blood cultures defined as

≥2 positive cultures of blood samples drawn >12 hours apart, or

All of 3 or a majority of ≥4 separate cultures of blood (with first and last sample drawn ≥1 hour apart)

Evidence of Endocardial Involvement

Positive echocardiogram for IE defined as

Oscillating intracardiac mass on valve or supporting structures, in the path of regurgitant jets, or on implanted material in the absence of an alternative anatomic explanation, or

Abscess, or

New partial dehiscence of prosthetic valve, or

New valvular regurgitation (worsening or changing of preexisting murmur not sufficient)

MINOR CRITERIA

Predisposition: Predisposing heart condition or IV drug use
Fever: Temperature ≥38.0
Vascular phenomena: Major arterial emboli, septic pulmonary infarcts, mycotic aneurysm, intracranial hemorrhage, conjunctival hemorrhages, and Janeway lesions
Immunologic phenomena: Glomerulonephritis, Osler nodes, Roth spots, and rheumatoid factor
Microbiologic evidence: Positive blood culture but does not meet a major criterion as noted above or serologic evidence of active infection with organism consistent with IE
Echocardiographic findings: Consistent with IE but do not meet a major criterion as noted above

- A group of gram-negative coccobacilli known to cause IE are the HACEK organisms (*Hemophilus aphrophilus, Actinobacillus actinomycetemcomitans, Cardiobacterium hominis, Eikenella corrodens*, and *Kingella kingae*).
- Fungal pathogens (*Candida* and *Aspergillus* sp.) can be seen in catheter- or prosthetic-valve-related IE.
- Blood cultures may be sterile in 5–10% of IE cases.

TREATMENT

- Empiric therapy is based on several factors, including the patient's age, history of cardiac disease, surgical history, and presence of any foreign bodies.
- A prolonged course of antibiotics is required, as the organisms are embedded deep in the fibrin/platelet

matrix at high concentrations. Length of therapy can be anywhere from 2 to 8 weeks.

- Surgical intervention may be necessary if valvular dysfunction, persistence of vegetation, or perivalvular extension occurs.

INTRAABDOMINAL ABSCESS

PATHOGENESIS AND ETIOLOGIC AGENTS

- The most common cause of an intraabdominal abscess is appendicitis. In appendicitis, normal bowel flora infect the appendix, which can then perforate and lead to the formation of an abscess. The abscess is usually located in the right paracolic gutter; however, there can be spread to the left paracolic gutter, the pelvis, or the subphrenic space. *E. coli* is the most common aerobic organism isolated, and *Bacteroides* species are the most common anaerobic organisms.
- Liver abscesses in the United States are typically of a bacterial etiology; however, in many parts of the world, the most common cause is parasitic (usually an amoebic organism). The etiology is dependent on the pathogenesis of the infection since infection can arise from systemic bacteremia, from enteric organisms entering through the portal venous system, from ascension of organisms, from the biliary tract or other adjacent structure, or from trauma. Treatment should be undertaken with surgical and infectious disease consultation. Although *Staphylococcus aureus* liver abscesses can occur in immunocompetent hosts, one should consider the diagnosis of chronic granulomatous disease, as these infections are often a first presentation in these patients. In the preantibiotic era, pylephlebitis (septic thrombophlebitis of the portal vein) was a common cause of liver abscesses with enteric organisms complicating appendicitis in children; this is now a rare complication. Children with underlying malignancies who are on immunosuppressing therapy may develop disseminated fungal (most commonly *Candida* species) infections with multiple liver and splenic abscesses. *Bartonella henselae* (the etiologic agent of cat-scratch disease) can also cause multiple microabscesses of the liver and spleen in the normal host.
- Splenic abscesses are less common than liver abscesses, and result most frequently from bacteremia or fungemia. Immunocompromised hosts (especially those with malignancy or human immunodeficiency virus [HIV]) are the most susceptible to developing splenic abscesses. Etiologic agents are similar to those of liver abscesses, with *Candida* species being the most common etiology in children with malignancies.

CLINICAL AND LABORATORY FEATURES

- Patients with abscess due to a perforated appendix usually present with a persistently draining wound site, high spiking fever, and an elevated peripheral WBC count.
- The symptoms in patients with liver abscess of any etiology tend to be nonspecific. The most prominent symptoms are fever, abdominal pain (usually right upper quadrant), nausea, vomiting, loss of appetite, weakness, malaise, diarrhea, and abdominal distension. Forty to eighty percent of patients will have hepatomegaly.

DIAGNOSIS

- Diagnosis can be made by abdominal ultrasound, computed tomography, or magnetic resonance imaging (MRI) of the abdomen.

TREATMENT

- Antibiotic therapy should be chosen to cover the most common pathogens seen with intraabdominal abscess, as well as any bacteria isolated in culture, taking into consideration the patient's clinical condition and predisposing risk factors. Treatment generally involves a combination of drainage (either percutaneously or surgical) and a prolonged course of intravenous antibiotics. The traditional antibiotic regimen may include a combination of ampicillin, gentamicin, and clindamycin (or metronidazole), a second or third-generation parenteral cephalosporin plus an aminoglycoside or a semisynthetic penicillin plus an aminoglycoside; however, there are many different antibiotic regimens that are appropriate.

LYMPHADENITIS

EPIDEMIOLOGY

- Lymphadenopathy or enlargement of lymph nodes, can by caused by proliferation of normal lymphatic tissue, by invasion of inflammatory cells (lymphadenitis), or by invasion of neoplastic cells. This section will focus on lymphadenitis.
- Cervical lymph nodes may lie in the anterior cervical triangle (anterior to the sternocleidomastoid muscle), the posterior triangle (posterior to the sternocleidomastoid muscle), the submandibular region, the preauricular region, the occipital region, and the supraclavicular region. Palpable, nontender nodes in the supraclavicular region are most commonly associated

with malignancy. Generalized lymphadenopathy, hepatosplenomegaly, and/or radiographic mediastinal lymphadenopathy suggest systemic illness.

PATHOGENESIS OF LYMPHADENITIS/ INFECTIOUS LYMPHADENOPATHY

* Microorganisms reach the infected lymph node via lymphatic flow from an inoculation site or by lymphatic flow from adjacent lymph nodes. Local cytokine release results in neutrophil recruitment, vascular engorgement, and nodal edema. Involvement of the soft tissues adjacent to the node can result in cellulitis and abscess formation. Eventually, the node heals with fibrosis. Microorganisms that cause subacute or chronic inflammatory changes generally produce less of an inflammatory response.
* Generalized infectious lymphadenopathy (usually caused by viral illness) results in nodal hyperplasia without necrosis and resolves spontaneously as the illness resolves.
* A helpful classification in determining the etiology of lymphadenitis is acute unilateral pyogenic lymphadenitis (may be at any site in the body), bilateral cervical lymphadenitis, subacute or chronic cervical lymphadenopathy, and generalized lymphadenopathy.

CLINICAL FEATURES AND ETIOLOGIC AGENTS

* Acute unilateral pyogenic lymphadenitis is usually caused by *S. aureus* or group A *streptococcus* in over 80% of cases. Submandibular and cervical nodes are most frequently involved and occur most commonly in children between 1 and 4 years of age. Concurrent pharyngitis or impetigo of the face suggests group A *streptococcus* as the etiologic agent. In young infants, group B streptococcus is also common. In children with poor dentition, anaerobes should be strongly considered.
* Bilateral cervical lymphadenitis is usually caused by common viruses such as adenovirus, influenza virus, respiratory syncytial virus, Epstein-Barr virus, and cytomegalovirus.
* Subacute or chronic cervical lymphadenitis is usually caused by nontuberculous mycobacterium (*Mycobacterium avium-intracellulare* and *Mycobacterium scrofulaceum* most commonly). If exposure to kittens/cats is elicited in the history, infection with *Bartonella henselae* should be considered. This usually results in a unilateral, chronic, and tender lymphadenitis most commonly in the cervical or axillary region. *B. henselae* infections can be diagnosed by an indirect fluorescent antibody assay,

which correlates well with clinical disease; organisms drained from the lymphadenitis often do not grow in the laboratory and require special media.

* HIV and/or *Mycobacterium tuberculous* (TB) infection should be strongly considered in patients with chronic generalized lymphadenopathy. TB should also be considered in a patient with a persistent unilateral lymphadenitis that fails to respond to appropriate antimicrobial therapy or historically has risk factors for TB exposure.

TREATMENT AND MANAGEMENT

* Children that are well-appearing and have an acute pyogenic lymphadenitis should be treated with oral cephalexin, amoxicillin/clavulanate, or clindamycin (also useful for anaerobic coverage). Consider placing a purified protein derivative (PPD) in those children with risk factors for tuberculosis. If there is no response to the treatment, admission for intravenous therapy and imaging of the node (either ultrasound or contrasted computed tomography) is indicated. In children who are persistently febrile despite appropriate antibiotics and/or imaging, mycobacterial infection, gram-negative infection, fungal lymphadenitis, and noninfectious causes of lymphadenopathy should be explored.
* Children with suspected nontuberculous mycobacterial infection may require a biopsy, recognizing that this can on rare occasion lead to sinus tract formation. Treatment involves node resection or treatment with clarithromycin (a macrolide antibiotic) if surgery is not possible.
* Lymphadenitis from *B. henselae* is often treated supportively, with drainage done to relieve symptoms. Oral azithromycin has shown a modest clinical benefit in shortening the duration of illness.
* Children with acute fungal or gram-negative pyogenic lymphadenitis should be evaluated for chronic granulomatous disease and/or HIV infection.

BACTERIAL MENINGITIS

EPIDEMIOLOGY

* In the last 15 years, two major epidemiological changes occurred. First, in countries where conjugate *Haemophilus influenzae* type b (HIB) vaccines are given, *H. influenzae* (one of the major causes of bacterial meningitis) has almost disappeared. Unfortunately, in many countries, these vaccines are not routinely used and an estimated 500,000 children worldwide die each year from this disease. Second, antimicrobial resistance among the most common bacteria causing meningitis (i.e. *Streptococcus*

pneumoniae, Neisseria meningitidis, and *H. influenzae* type b) is increasing rapidly.

- The estimated incidence of bacterial meningitis in the United States is 30,000–40,000 cases per year. Most of the cases in children occur before 1 year of age.
- Risk factors include racial/genetic differences, low socioeconomic situation, congenital and acquired immunodeficiency, congenital or acquired splenic dysfunction, crowded conditions (e.g., daycares, military or college dormitories), and a neurocutaneous tract or CSF leakage.
- In newborns, *Streptococcus agalactiae* (GBS), *Escherichia coli*, and *Listeria monocytogenes* are the most common pathogens. Young maternal age, heavy colonization, prolonged (>24 hrs) rupture of membranes, and resuscitation of the newborn at birth are some of the risk factors. The increased survival of very premature newborns is associated with increase in nosocomial infection with staphylococci and gram-negative bacteria (e.g., *Enterobacter, Pseudomonas, Citrobacter*).

PATHOGENESIS

- Preceding respiratory viral infection facilitates invasion of colonizing bacteria to the blood. The polysaccharide capsule (a virulence factor of the bacteria) is important for its survival in the bloodstream. The capsule allows the bacteria to evade the complement and phagocytic activity of the polymorpholeukocytes (PMNs) and allows the bacteria to replicate.
- The bacteria most commonly gain access to the meninges by crossing the blood-CSF barrier of the choroid plexus. Once they reach the CSF, they can survive and multiply because host defense mechanisms (e.g., complement, immunoglobulins, and PMNs) are low and ineffective.
- The rapid multiplication of the bacteria releases a cascade of cytokines which induce the inflammatory response. This inflammatory reaction is felt to be the main contributing factor for brain damage seen in bacterial meningitis.

CLINICAL FEATURES

- The classical presentation of bacterial meningitis is fever, headache (or irritability and continuous cry in the very young), and changes in mental status (e.g., lethargy, confusion, delirium). Bulging fontanellae, stiff neck, and positive Kernig and Brudzinski signs are the classic findings during physical examination.
- The clinical presentation differs by age, etiologic agent, and comorbidity. In younger patients the clinical

manifestations are often nonspecific. Patients with immunodeficiency (e.g., neutropenia), post neurosurgery, or head trauma may not exhibit the classic symptoms and/or signs.

- In children, the illness usually starts with nonspecific febrile illness (e.g., upper respiratory infection, otitis media). Within a few days, other nonspecific symptoms (e.g., poor appetite, nausea, vomiting, irritability, continuous cry, listlessness) develop. More severe mental status changes (e.g., lethargy, obtundation, coma, and seizures) may develop. If history raises the possibility of meningitis (e.g., fever with unexplained alteration of mental status) or the patient appears sicker than the potential diagnosis (e.g., URI, OM) a lumbar puncture *must* be done to rule out meningitis.
- In a minority of patients, the signs and symptoms of meningitis may develop rapidly (within hours). This fulminant presentation is ominous and immediate initiation of antibiotic therapy may not affect the outcome. In addition, patients who present with hypotension, altered mental status, and seizures have the worst clinical prognosis (death or permanent neurological sequelae).
- A bulging fontanelle as a sign of meningitis is present in less than 50% of patients with an open fontanelle. Opisthotonus (neck rigidity), Kernig, and Brudzinski signs are also not very sensitive in determining the presence or absence of meningitis. In one-third to one-half of patients, an extrameningeal focus of infection (e.g., URI, OM, pneumonia) is found. Careful evaluation for the possibility of meningitis is required in these cases.

DIFFERENTIAL DIAGNOSIS

- Although the differential diagnosis is very broad, evaluation of the CSF can help in shortening the list.
- Infectious causes include: viruses (e.g., enteroviruses, HSV, HIV, arboviruses, influenza, adenovirus), fungal (e.g., *Cryptococcus, Aspergillus, Candida, Histoplasma*); *Rickettsiaceae* (e.g., *Rickettsieae, Ehrlichieae*), spirochetes (e.g., *Treponema, Borrelia, Leptospira*), protozoa (e.g., *Toxoplasma, Entamoeba, Naegleria, Trypanosoma*), other bacteria (e.g., *Bartonella, Brucella, Chlamydia, Mycobacterium tuberculosis, Mycoplasma*). Other infectious processes such as brain abscess or parameningeal foci (e.g., epidural abscess, subdural empyema, cranial osteomyelitis) can also mimic bacterial meningitis.
- Numerous noninfectious causes can mimic bacterial meningitis. For example, connective tissue disorders (e.g., lupus, rheumatoid arthritis), Kawasaki syndrome, sarcoidosis and serum sickness can cause signs, symptoms, and CSF findings indistinguishable

from bacterial meningitis. Intracranial tumors, leukemia, lymphoma and meningeal carcinomatosis can do the same. In addition, some medications (e.g., sulfa, NSAID carbamozepine, lead, immunoglobulin) and vaccines (e.g., MMR, rabies, pertusis) can cause meningeal inflammation that has to be differentiated from bacterial meningitis.

DIAGNOSIS

- Lumbar puncture (LP) is essential for establishing the diagnosis. A traumatic LP (which occurs in 15%–20% of patients) makes the analysis very difficult in patients with mild pleocytosis (early stages or partially treated meningitis). In these cases the possibility of hemorrhage (e.g., HSV encephalitis, subarachnoid hemorrhage) should be considered. Usually blood from a traumatic tap will be less in the 3rd CSF tube collected. If needed, centrifugation of this tube may help in the differentiation (i.e., clear supernatant suggests traumatic tap, while xanthochromic color suggests hemorrhage).
- Typical CSF findings of bacterial meningitis include: opening pressure of >180 mm H_2O. WBC count greater than 1000 cells/μL with more than 80% of them being neutrophils. Glucose levels are low at <40 mg/dL (and if blood sugar is available the CSF/blood ratio is <0.3) and the protein levels are elevated at >100 mg/dL.
- There is a considerable overlap in the CSF parameters between early or partially treated bacterial meningitis and other causes of infectious or noninfectious meningitis. Up to 15% of neonates with bacterial meningitis may have a normal CSF and 10% of children may have a lymphocytic predominance. Empiric antibiotic therapy is recommended for patients with >300 WBC (>60% polymorphonuclears) and glucose of <30 mg/dL. Elevated C-reactive protein (>20 mg/L for children <6 years of age or >50 mg/L for older children) increases the probability that the child is suffering from bacterial meningitis.
- Other tests that may be helpful in diagnosis include: (1) Gram's stain, which is positive in >80% of childhood bacterial meningitis, but only 50% in meningitis due to *L. monocytogenes* and even less in early and partially-treated meningitis. (2) Rapid CSF antigen tests (e.g., enzyme-linked immunosorbent assays [ELISA], latex agglutination) are more sensitive than the Gram's stain (88% to 100%). These tests are especially helpful in partially-treated cases where the low number of bacteria will cause both the Gram's stain and the culture to be negative. Bacterial antigens should also be tested in the urine, which in some cases increases the yield. (3) Cultures of CSF and blood will

be positive in 70% to 85%. In patients who have received antibiotics, a sample of the CSF can be diluted 1:100 and 1:10,000 (to wash away the WBCs and antibiotic[s]) and then plated (for culture) to help in the recovery of the bacteria.
- CT scan or MRI of the head should be used selectively. They are helpful only if symptoms of intracranial pressure (e.g., abnormal level of consciousness, seizures, detectable neurologic abnormalities, bulging fontanelle, separation of the sutures) are found.

TREATMENT

- There is no direct relationship between prompt administration of antibiotics and the outcome. Therefore, therapy can be delayed for a short period of time (to rule out ICP, await results of the LP to document bacterial etiology or to better tailor the antibiotic therapy).
- If the Gram's stain or rapid antigen tests identify the etiologic agent, specific antibiotic(s) should be given. Otherwise, the initial empiric therapy should be decided by the age of the patient and the known local susceptibilities of the pathogens. In neonates, the combination of cefotaxime with ampicillin or ampicillin with gentamicin (or other aminoglycoside) are the drugs of choice. In children older than 6 weeks, ceftriaxone (or cefotaxine) with vancomycin is the preferred combination. Because vancomycin penetration into the CSF is erratic (especially if corticorteroids are given), rifampin should be considered as an effective alternative. Once the pathogen and its sensitivity is identified, specific antibiotics should be chosen.
- Intravenous dexamethasone (0.6 mg/kg/day QID for 2 days) given before or concomitant with the first antibiotic(s) dose has beneficial effect on the outcome (especially hearing loss) of *H. influenzae* type b meningitis. The use of corticosteroids in patients with *S. pneumoniae* meningitis is controversial and its use, especially when vancomycin is given, should be carefully considered. It is currently not routinely recommended. Dexamethasone has no beneficial effect in patients with *N. meningitides*, neonatal or viral meningitis.
- While inappropriate secretion of antidiuretic hormone has been documented in up to 75% of patients with bacterial meningitis, fluid restriction should be used primarily in patients with increased ICP. Appropriate attention should be given to patients with seizures, shock, hypotension, hyperventilation and coma. Children with these symptoms should be cared for in the ICU setting. Adequate control of fever and pain is also required.
- The duration of therapy depends on the etiologic agent. *H. influenzae* type b meningitis should be

treated for 7 days, *S. pneumoniae* for 10 days, *N. meningitidis* for 5–7 days, and neonatal meningitis for 14 to 21 days. Longer courses of therapy my be needed in complicated cases.

- The mortality rate for bacterial meningitis is 3% to 20% (*N. meningitidis* the lowest and *S. pneumoniae* the highest). The mortality rate for neonatal meningitis is 5% to 20% (GBS the lowest and *E. coli* the highest). The most common complication of bacterial meningitis is neurosensory hearing loss (ranging from 5% for *N. meningitidis* to 30% for *S. pneumonaie*). Other sequelae include: impaired IQ, seizures (especially in children with neurologic sequelae), mental retardation, hemiplegia, quadriplegia and hyperactivity. Other neurologic impairments can occur including ataxia, blindness, and hydrocephalous.
- Prophylactic antibiotics should be given only to those individuals who were in very close contact with the index case of *N. meningitidis* meningitis (e.g., household or day-care members who sleep and eat together).
- Vaccination is the most effective measure to prevent bacterial meningitis. This approach has already been proven to be very effective in the dramatic decrease in *H. influenzae* type b meningitis and preliminary reports suggest that the use of the conjugate pneumococcal vaccine is having the same effect on the incidence of meningitis due to *S. pneumoniae*.

SEPTIC OR INFECTIOUS ARTHRITIS

EPIDEMIOLOGY

- Defined as an acute bacterial infection of the joint space with an estimated annual incidence of 5.5–12 cases per 100,000 children. Infants and children under 2 years of age account for one-third to one-half of the reported cases.
- Predisposing factors include trauma, joint surgery, and surgery or instrumentation of the urinary or intestinal tracts.
- Lower extremity joints involved in over 80% of cases. Most common joints involved in descending order: knee > hip > ankle.

PATHOGENESIS

- There are several ways by which a joint may become infected. Spread of the infection by the hematogenous route is the most common. Other routes of infection include penetrating trauma (including surgery) and contiguous spread from adjacent bone or overlying tissue.

- The blood flow to the synovium of a joint is high relative to its mass. If there is bacteria in the blood, the bacteria enter the synovium and the joint fluid and elicit an inflammatory response in the joint space. Recruitment of white blood cells in response to bacterial products results in fluid accumulation and the development of pain, fever, overlying warmth, and redness of the joint. Swelling of the joint space results in increased pressure which can compromise the blood supply of the head of the femur or the humerus if the hip or shoulder joints are involved.
- Infection of the joint may result in necrosis of the articular cartilage and thickening and scarring of the synovium.

ETIOLOGIC AGENTS

- There are a number of agents that cause septic arthritis depending on the age and immune status of the host. *Staphylococcus aureus* is the most common organism in all age groups followed by group A *Streptococcus* and *Streptococcus pneumoniae*. *H. influenzae* type b may be a cause of disease in unimmunized children under 5 years of age. *Kingella kingae* is an organism that is now being recognized as a more frequent cause of septic arthritis in children.
- Group B *Streptococcus* and *Neisseria gonorrheae* are causes of disease in neonates. *N. gonorrheae* may also be a cause of disease in adolescents.
- Gram-negative enteric organisms and *Pseudomonas* spp. are causes of disease in patients with penetrating trauma or in immunocompromised patients. *Salmonella* spp. may cause disease in patients with hemoglobinopathies and *Pasteurella multocida* may cause disease after an animal bite.

CLINICAL PRESENTATION

- The clinical manifestations of septic arthritis in children are age dependent. In children less than 1 year of age, the disease is usually monoarticular and involves the large joints. The clinical findings may be subtle and include swelling, tenderness, and erythema of the skin overlying the joint. Guarding, limitation of movement of the affected extremity, limp, or pain on passive manipulation may also be found. In the neonate and young infant, pseudoparalysis of the affected limb may be the only clinical manifestation.
- Children over 1 year of age usually present with fever, warmth, redness, swelling, and tenderness of the involved joint.

- Infections involving the shoulder and hip joints may be difficult to diagnose and pain may be referred to the overlying muscle tissue or to the knee. Infants and young children with involvement of the hip joint may hold the affected limb in an abducted and externally rotated position ("frog-leg" position).
- A careful history should be obtained to determine the presence of previous trauma to the affected limb.

DIAGNOSIS

- The diagnosis of septic arthritis requires a high index of suspicion. Aspiration of synovial fluid from the affected joint provides the best specimen to make a tentative diagnosis and to initiate therapy. Once the specimen is obtained it should be sent for Gram stain, cultures, and analysis of cell types and protein/glucose concentrations. Gram stain of the fluid demonstrates an organism in about 50% of cases. Normal synovial fluid is clear and colorless; however, infected fluid is turbid and cloudy. Analysis of the fluid usually shows the presence of a large number of white blood cells (usually over 70,000/mm^3) with over 80% of these being polymorphonuclear cells. The protein concentration is elevated and glucose concentration is depressed. Cultures are positive in about 50–70% of the cases.
- Cultures of blood should also be obtained since they are positive in about 40% of patients. If gonococcal arthritis is suspected, cultures should also be obtained from the cervix, urethra, pharynx, and rectum.
- Radiographic studies add very little to positive physical examination findings. The early radiographic signs of septic arthritis are due to swelling of the joint capsule, which displaces the fat lines. Occasionally increase in joint space size is seen.
- Radiographic evaluation is most useful for the hip joint. The radiographs should be taken with the child in the frog-leg position, as well as with the legs extended at the knee and slightly internally rotated. Findings that are consistent with a septic hip joint include obliteration or lateral displacement of the gluteal fat lines and a laterally displaced femoral head.

THERAPY

- The majority of cases of septic arthritis can be managed medically. Antimicrobial therapy is targeted toward the organisms most likely to cause septic arthritis in the age group of the patient. In neonates and young infants, a combination of intravenous oxacillin or nafcillin and an aminoglycoside provides adequate

initial antibiotic coverage. Cefuroxime covers the most common organisms causing septic arthritis in children between 2 months and 10 years of age and may be used as empiric therapy until an organism is isolated. In children over 10 years of age, monotherapy with oxacillin or nafcillin is adequate empiric therapy given that *S. aureus* is the etiologic agent in the vast majority of cases. Ceftriaxone or cefotaxime may be used as therapy for gonococcal septic arthritis, while combination therapy of a third-generation cephalosporin or a penicillinase-resistant penicillin plus an aminoglycoside may be used as empiric in septic arthritis due to penetrating trauma or in patients with underlying conditions. Duration of therapy ranges from 2 weeks for gonococcal arthritis to 4 weeks for septic arthritis due to *S. aureus*.
- The role of surgical intervention is important in the treatment of septic arthritis of the hip or shoulder where drainage is best achieved by surgical incision and decompression of the joint to preserve the blood supply to the epiphysis.

OSTEOMYELITIS

EPIDEMIOLOGY

- Defined as an inflammation of bone usually caused by a pyogenic organism.
- Occurs in about 1 in 5000 children less than 13 years of age with boys being 2.5 times more likely to develop osteomyelitis than girls, possibly due to an increased incidence of minor trauma.
- Fifty percent of patients with osteomyelitis are less than 5 years of age and one-third are less than 2 years of age.
- The long bones of the legs and arms are the most common sites of involvement, usually affecting the metaphysis of the bones.

PATHOGENESIS

- There are three major ways by which osteomyelitis may develop: (1) hematogenous, which accounts for about 90% of the cases in children under 18 years of age; (2) spread from a contiguous focus including direct inoculation of the bone due to trauma; and (3) vascular insufficiency or peripheral vascular disease.
- Anatomically the nutrient artery that supplies the bones divides into branches and then into a narrow plexus of capillaries that make sharp loops in the area of the epiphyseal plate and then enters a system of large sinusoidal vessels, in which blood flow is sluggish.

Thrombosis of these slow-flowing vessels due to trauma or embolization provides a site for blood-borne bacteria to lodge and proliferate. As the bacteria proliferate, there is accumulation of bacterial products, which stimulate an acute inflammatory response, leading to a change in pH and an influx of polymorphonuclear leukocytes. These factors accumulate under increased pressure, leading to vascular thrombosis, pressure necrosis, and death of small islands of bone. In the absence of therapy, the infection continues to expand involving larger sections of bone and the marrow cavity, and in some cases may rupture into the joint space or through the periosteum into adjacent muscles.

ETIOLOGIC AGENTS

- *S. aureus* is the most common organism causing acute hematogenous osteomyelitis in both children and adults accounting for 80–85% of the cases. Other organisms that are less frequent causes include group A streptococcus, *H. influenzae* type b (in children <2 years of age), and *S. pneumoniae*. In infants less than 2 months of age, group B streptococcus and coagulase-negative staphylococci (especially in premature infants) are frequent causes of osteomyelitis. In children with hemoglobinopathies, organisms such as *Salmonella* species, *Escherichia coli*, *Shigella*, and *Klebsiella* may be the causes of osteomyelitis.
- *S. aureus* and group A streptococcus are the most commonly isolated organisms causing contiguous-focus osteomyelitis, although mixed infections may be seen. In the neonatal period, enteric organisms are a common cause.
- *Pseudomonas aeruginosa* is commonly associated with puncture wounds of the calcaneus, especially in situations of a person stepping on a nail through the bottom of a sneaker.
- Cultures from osteomyelitis due to vascular insufficiency usually involve multiple organisms including staphylococci, streptococci, enterococci, *Enterobacteriaceae*, *Pseudomonas aeruginosa*, and anaerobes.
- Osteomyelitis due to fungi such as *Candida* species and *Aspergillus* most frequently occurs in the immunocompromised host or in the premature infant who have a central venous catheter or are receiving prolonged antimicrobial therapy.

CLINICAL SIGNS AND SYMPTOMS

- In children, the clinical findings of osteomyelitis differ with the age of the patient, the duration of the process, and the location of the infection.

- In newborns and infants, classic findings may be minimal and include slight irritability, low-grade fever, decreased feeding, or the child may appear septic with no focal findings. Physical examination may demonstrate an edematous, red, warm extremity, markedly decreased movement, guarding of the affected extremity (pseudoparalysis), severe irritability with movement or touch of the infected extremity, and regional lymphadenopathy. In neonates with osteomyelitis, up to 50% will have multifocal bone involvement. Osteomyelitis of the skull may be seen in this population as a result of cephalohematomas, scalp monitors, intravenous lines, abscesses, and venipuncture.
- In older children, findings include fever up to 40°C, chills, malaise, anorexia, muscle aches, nausea, and vomiting; edema, swelling, erythema, warmth, and point tenderness are present over the involved bone. There may also be refusal to bear weight on the affected extremity, limp may be present and pain on palpation or active and passive motion may be elicited. Regional adenopathy may also be present. A history of preceding trauma may be elicited in about 50% of the patients.
- In adolescents and adults, the findings are similar to those for older children, but the function of the affected extremity is less restricted and point tenderness over the affected area may be the only finding.

DIAGNOSIS

- In the neonate, physical findings alone are sufficient to make the diagnosis of osteomyelitis. Plain films are usually abnormal when clinical findings are present.
- In the older child and adolescent, radiographic studies can be performed that confirm the diagnosis of osteomyelitis.
- On plain-film radiographs, osteolytic lesions do not become evident until 40–50% of the bone mineral has been destroyed; at least 10 days to 3 weeks are required after the infection begins before bony changes are visible on plain radiographs; however, negative plain films even at 10–14 days do not rule out the presence of osteomyelitis.
- Bone scanning techniques using technetium TC 99m phosphate or diphosphate compounds are more sensitive and can be used earlier in the infection, before bony changes are seen on plain film. Abnormalities can be detected as early as 48 hours from the start of the infection. Increased isotope uptake is seen in areas of infection. The sensitivity of bone scans in neonates and young infants is much lower than in the older infants and children due to the limited amount of mineralization in their bones.

- MRI is useful very early in the infection where bone marrow cellulitis may be seen.

THERAPY

- The optimal management involves a combination of adequate surgical drainage of purulent material from the infected bone and appropriate antimicrobial therapy.
- Empiric therapy must include coverage for *S. aureus* and group A streptococci in all age groups. Initial IV antibiotic therapy usually consists of a penicillinase-resistant semisynthetic penicillin (oxacillin or nafcillin) or a first-generation cephalosporin (cefazolin sodium). For patients with methicillin-resistant *S. aureus* infections or hypersensitivity to the β-lactam class of antibiotics, IV clindamycin or vancomycin should be used if the patient's isolate is susceptible to these agents.
- For children under 2 years of age or in whom immunization status is unknown, coverage for *H. influenzae* type b needs to be included. Therapy with cefuroxime should be considered.
- For patients who are seriously ill and/or immunocompromised and in patients with puncture wounds of the foot, antibiotic therapy should also cover *P. aeruginosa*. Empiric therapy in these cases includes ceftazidime and/or the aminoglycosides.
- For acute osteomyelitis the duration of parenteral antibiotic therapy is a minimum of 4 weeks. Multiple studies have shown up to a 50% failure rate for *S. aureus* osteomyelitis treated for less than 4 weeks. For chronic osteomyelitis the duration of parenteral antibiotic therapy is 6 weeks, followed by 4.5 months of oral therapy.
- For puncture wound osteomyelitis due to *P. aeruginosa*, if the infection is recognized early and management includes aggressive surgical debridement, the duration of therapy is 10–14 days.

SKIN AND SOFT TISSUE INFECTIONS (IMPETIGO, CELLULITIS, ABSCESSES)

EPIDEMIOLOGY AND ETIOLOGIC AGENTS

- Impetigo is an infection of the epidermis. Two forms exist: nonbullous and bullous.
  1. Nonbullous impetigo is more common than bullous impetigo, and occurs at sites of skin trauma. Impetigo lesions initially have a vesicular appearance, but quickly become purulent and rupture leaving a "honey-crusted" exudate. The lesions tend not to be painful, and constitutional symptoms are rare; however, there may be some associated lymphadenopathy. *Staphylococcus aureus* is the most common etiology, with *Streptococcus pyogenes* occurring less frequently; these two etiologic agents cannot be distinguished clinically.
  2. Bullous impetigo occurs more frequently in infants and young children. The lesions occur in areas of intact skin, and the bullae form secondary to local toxin production from *S. aureus*. There tends not to be underlying redness, and the fluid can appear clear or purulent. Lymphadenopathy and systemic symptoms are rare.
- Therapy can be administered topically with mupirocin for limited cases or systemically with antistaphylococcal antibiotics for more widespread cases. Seven days of therapy are usually adequate. Rarely do complications of impetigo occur; deep cellulitis can occur and poststreptococcal glomerulonephritis may follow streptococcal impetigo.
- Staphylococcal scalded skin syndrome (SSSS) is a staphylococcal toxin-mediated (staphylococcal exfoliative exotoxin—exfoliatin) infection most commonly seen in infants with widespread superficial bullae and exfoliation intraepidermally. Nonspecific symptoms such as fever, malaise, and irritability may also be seen. The skin may initially develop an erythematous rash prior to the appearance of the bullae. This rash is accentuated in the flexural creases and the skin is quite tender to the touch. Sheets of skin may peel away in response to minor trauma (Nikolsky sign). There is often extensive associated exfoliation requiring attention to fluid status. Parenteral antibiotics are usually initiated, which are then changed to oral once improvement is apparent.
- Cellulitis is an infection of the dermis and subcutaneous tissues manifested by skin warmth, redness, tenderness, and edema. Cellulitis may or may not be associated with abscess formation. As opposed to impetigo, systemic symptoms such as fever and malaise are common.
- Cellulitis most commonly occurs from the entry of *S. aureus* or *S. pyogenes* through a break in the skin. Less commonly the infection is hematogenously spread from bacteremia with *Streptococcus pneumoniae* or *Haemophilus influenzae* type b. Hematogenously spread infection occurs most frequently on the face and manifests as buccal or preseptal cellulitis. In immunocompromised hosts or diabetics, gram-negative organisms are more frequently seen.
- Erysipelas is a superficial form of cellulitis with lymphatic spread; the onset is often abrupt with fever, chills, and erythema with well-demarcated, elevated edges. The etiology is most frequently *S. pyogenes*.
- Folliculitis results from a superficial infection of the hair follicle and appears as discrete pustules on a red

base. Frequent areas of infection are the scalp, buttocks, or extremities. *S. aureus* is the most common etiologic agent, although *Staphylococcus epidermidis* may also be a cause. Topical antibiotic cleansers are usually adequate therapy, although more severe cases may require systemic antipenicillinase-resistant antibiotics, e.g., cephalexin, dicloxacillin, and clindamycin. Hot tub folliculitis is caused by *Pseudomonas aeruginosa*, and is manifested by red or violaceous papules or pustules; systemic symptoms may be present. Oral antipseudomonal antibiotics may be given if systemic symptoms are pronounced.

- A furuncle is a more suppurative infection of a hair follicle, and a carbuncle results from infection of multiple contiguous follicles with multiple drainage points. The etiologic agent in both is most often *S. aureus*, and infection may be recurrent if *S. aureus* nasal carriage is present. Treatment involves warm compresses to promote drainage and oral antistaphylococcal therapy for more extensive infections or those involving the face.

DIAGNOSIS

- Microbiologic diagnosis for all the entities is possible in about 25% of cases through blood culture, culture and Gram stain of aspirate in the area of inflammation, or skin biopsy culture.

THERAPY

- For all the above entities, therapy in immunocompetent hosts should be directed toward *S. pyogenes* and *S. aureus*. Oral therapy can be initiated if systemic symptoms are minimal and the area of involvement is small. In moderate or severe cellulitis with systemic symptoms, parental therapy is warranted until there is clear improvement.

URINARY TRACT INFECTIONS (UTI) AND PYELONEPHRITIS

EPIDEMIOLOGY

- The prevalence of UTI varies depending on the patient population, the method of collection of the urine, and the diagnostic laboratory tests used. Estimated prevalence in neonates ranges from 2.9% in premature infants to 0.7% in term neonates. Male infants have a greater prevalence of UTI for the first 3 months after birth, after which time the prevalence of UTI in girls far outnumbers that in boys. The prevalence in females between 1 and 5 years old is 1–3%.

- Fever in infants and children may be the only presenting sign of a UTI. The rates among children during a febrile episode range from 1.7 to 7.5%. Younger children, especially infants less than 8 weeks of age, have a higher incidence of UTI associated with a febrile episode. Uncircumcised boys have a higher risk of urinary tract infection than boys who have been circumcised.

- In girls, the incidence of having one UTI increases the risk of a subsequent UTI, especially during the first few months after the infection.

PATHOGENESIS

- Normal colonic flora is in close proximity to the urethra. This anatomical relationship allows microbes to ascend the urethra, bladder, ureters, and kidneys. Normally, the bladder is able to empty the urine contents completely and there is no urostasis. A disruption in this normal pattern predisposes the host to a urinary tract infection. In addition, children with urinary calculi, indwelling urinary catheters, or any other anatomical cause of obstruction (e.g., constipation) will also cause a predisposition to UTIs. Occasionally, hematogenous spread of a microbe can seed the urinary tract, but this occurs much less often than the ascending infection.

- *Cystitis* is defined as an infection of the urethra and bladder. *Pyelonephritis* is defined as an upper urinary tract infection that involves the kidneys. Vesicoureteral reflux is an important risk for developing pyelonephritis, which can result in renal scarring. Vesicoureteral reflux is usually caused by an abnormally shortened ureter as it implants into the bladder wall. This situation allows urine to flow retrogradely back into the ureter and the renal pelvis, especially during micturition.

MICROBIOLOGY

- Gram-negative enteric flora are responsible for most UTIs in children and adults. *E. coli* causes 70–90% of acute bacterial UTIs in children. Other important gram-negative enteric flora are *Klebsiella pneumoniae*, *Proteus mirabilis*, and *Enterobacter* spp. Important gram-positive causes are *Enterococcus* spp. and *Staphylococcus saprophyticus* (a coagulase-negative staphylococcus). *S. saprophyticus* is the most common cause of infection in early female adulthood.

- *Pseudomonas* spp. and yeasts are more common causes of UTI in immunocompromised and/or hospitalized patients.

- It is also important to consider viral cystitis when evaluating patients with UTIs associated with gross hematuria, especially in immunocompromised patients where adenovirus is the most common viral etiology.

CLINICAL FEATURES

- Clinical manifestations of UTI are highly variable with age at presentation and severity of disease affecting the symptoms reported. Many children will present with fever as the only manifestation. Infants may present with decreased activity and poor feeding; jaundice may be present in the neonate. Vomiting with fever is another common manifestation in infants and children. Older children may complain of abdominal pain. Bedwetting, dysuria, and foul-smelling urine may also be signs of UTI. Although costovertebral angle tenderness and high fever may suggest pyelonephritis, it is not possible to reliably differentiate between cystitis and pyelonephritis based on history and physical examination.
- Other noninfectious and infectious etiologies should also be considered in the differential diagnosis of UTI. Other common etiologies are noninfectious urethritis, sexually transmitted disease (especially in the sexually active male), vaginitis/cervicitis, prostatitis, foreign body, and nephrolithiasis.
- Important historical data that should be obtained include prior undiagnosed febrile episodes in the past, foreign body, trauma, and sexual activity. Physical examination should include an accurate blood pressure reading and an examination of the urethral meatus. The presence of suprapubic tenderness and costovertebral angle tenderness should also be assessed.

URINE COLLECTION/LABORATORY DIAGNOSIS

- Urine culture is the gold standard test to confirm the presence of a UTI. It is important to note the method of collection when interpreting results of the urine culture. Four methods have been used: sterile bag collection, midstream urine collection, urethral catheterization, and suprapubic aspiration.
- *Sterile bag* urine collection is often done for convenience because it is noninvasive. It involves placing a sterile bag with adhesive over the perineum in children until urine is present in the bag. In general, this method is discouraged because the only reliable result from this method of collection is a negative urine culture. Any other result is unreliable and may result in a delay of the correct diagnosis. *Midstream* or "clean catch" urine collection can be done in a child who is old enough to initiate the urine stream. After the stream has been initiated, a sterile cup is inserted into the stream to collect a urine specimen. *Urethral catheterization* is done by

TABLE 112-5 Definition of Pyuria and Bacteriuria by Method of Analysis

SAMPLE	WBC	BACTERIA
Uncentrifuged	$\geq 10/mm^3$	Any/10 OIF
Centrifuged	$>5/HPF$	Any/HPF

ABBREVIATIONS: HPF, high power field; OIF, oil immersion field.

cleaning the urethral meatus with Betadine solution and then inserting a small urinary catheter into the urethra. *Suprapubic aspiration* is done on an infant in the supine, frog-leg position by sterile preparation of the area 1–1.5 cm above the symphysis pubis and subsequent insertion of a 1 in., 22 or 23 gauge needle at a 10–20° angle from the perpendicular with gentle suction.

- In general, a positive urine culture is defined as $>10^5$ colony-forming units (CFU)/mL for urine cultures obtained by midstream collection, >50,000 CFU/mL for catheterized specimens, and any number of CFU/mL obtained by suprapubic aspiration is considered to be positive. Urine cultures obtained by bag collection are only helpful if they are negative. Positive cultures by bag collection need to be repeated by another method of urine collection if there is still concern about a UTI.
- Because cultures require 24–48 hours to grow, a urinalysis is often used as a quick test to determine if there are abnormalities present. WBCs in urine, pyuria, can be measured in an uncentrifuged or centrifuged sample. Uncentrifuged samples are considered more sensitive in predicting the presence of a UTI (see Tables 112-5 and 112-6). Nitrites and leukocyte esterase may also be positive in a UTI.

TREATMENT

- Oral antimicrobial agents such as amoxicillin/clavulanic acid, second- or third-generation cephalosporins or trimethoprim-sulfamethoxazole can be used in the treatment of UTI and are generally administered for 10 days. It is important to know the local rates of resistance of *E. coli* to trimethoprim-sulfamethoxazole if using this drug. Parenteral antimicrobial therapy is used in ill-appearing children or in children who

TABLE 112-6 Sensitivity and Specificity of Pyuria and/or Bacteriuria in Predicting UTI by Method of Analysis

	SENSITIVITY (%)	SPECIFICITY
Uncentrifuged	84.5	99.7
Centrifuged	65.6	99.2

cannot tolerate oral medication. Some experts recommend using parenteral therapy for the duration of treatment in young infants (less than 3 months old). A repeat urine culture should be obtained to ensure that the UTI has cleared.
- It is important to obtain imaging of the urinary tract in any male with the first UTI, girls less than 3 years old with their first UTI, girls older than 3 years with the second UTI, or in the case of any extenuating circumstances. Generally an ultrasound of the kidneys can be done during the acute UTI. The voiding cystourethrogram, in which dye fills the bladder and is then visualized radiographically during and before micturition, is done after the UTI is cleared and approximately 1 week has passed.
- Vesicoureteral reflux is graded radiographically. Grade I is urine that flows retrogradely into the ureter without dilatation. Grade II reflux occurs into the distal ureter without dilatation. Grades III, IV, and V reflux into the distal ureter with mild, moderate, and severe dilatation of the renal collecting system, respectively. Any child with any degree of reflux should be placed on antimicrobial prophylaxis, usually nitrofurantoin, trimethoprim-sulfamethoxazole, or amoxicillin until it has been proven that the reflux has resolved or has been surgically corrected.

BACTERIAL CAUSES OF DIARRHEA

- This chapter covers the major causes of bacterial diarrhea in children. With the exception of *Clostridium difficile* enterocolitis, these are usually food-borne illnesses. In these cases, a careful food history (consumption and preparation) may provide helpful clues in the infectious agent. It is important to note that in most instances, however, the responsible food often goes unknown. In all of these illnesses, it is generally recommended not to use antimotility agents in children, as this can prolong the illness and/or colonization with the organism. Treatment, if recommended, is briefly discussed.

BACILLUS CEREUS

- Short incubation period (median incubation period; emesis: 2 hours, diarrhea: 9 hours).
- Illness due to ingestion of a preformed, heat-stable toxin.
- Patients are afebrile, stool is nonbloody. Emesis more significant than diarrhea.
- Diagnosis: History (reheated fried rice), stool culture.
- Treatment: Supportive; no indication for antibiotic therapy.

CAMPYLOBACTER JEJUNI

- Mean incubation period: 48 hours.
- Symptoms include bloody diarrhea, fever, severe cramping, and emesis.
- Patients may develop mesenteric adenitis, mimicking acute appendicitis.
- Diagnosis: History (poultry, raw milk), fecal leukocytes, stool culture.
- Treatment: Antibiotics are usually unnecessary in immunocompetent children.
- Consider antibiotics in patients who have prolonged bloody diarrhea associated with fever and a large number of stools, or in immunosuppressed patients.
- When antibiotic therapy is indicated, a 5–7-day course of erythromycin is recommended (clinical benefit is only seen if erythromycin is given early in illness).

ESCHERICHIA COLI (NONHEMORRHAGIC)

- There are five categories of diarrheagenic *E. coli*; each has a distinct clinical picture and different management recommendations. As enterohemorrhagic *E. coli* (EHEC) are associated with significant morbidity and mortality, it is discussed separately.
- ETEC (enterotoxigenic *E. coli*): Enterotoxin elaborated within the small bowel causes an increased secretion of fluid and electrolytes from the intestine. Stool is watery and nonbloody. Treatment of choice is a 5-day course of trimethoprim-sulfamethoxazole or cefixime.
- EPEC (enteropathogenic *E. coli*): Organism causes a secretory watery diarrhea. Toxin formation is not involved. Antibiotic of choice is a 5-day course of neomycin or trimpethoprim-sulfamethoxazole.
- EAEC (enteroaggregative *E. coli*): Enterotoxin is formed; results in persistent watery diarrhea (can last more than 2 weeks). Antibiotic of choice is unknown.
- EIEC (enteroinvasive *E. coli*): Organism invades the colonic enterocytes, then releases enterotoxins. Stool is watery in nature. Treatment of choice is a 5-day course of trimethoprim-sulfamethoxazole.

EHEC (ENTEROHEMORRHAGIC E. COLI)

- Median incubation period: 96 hours.
- EHEC isolates in the United States are almost all serotype O157:H7.
- Toxins (known as Shiga-like toxins) are elaborated, resulting in colitis with bloody diarrhea. Patients are usually afebrile.
- Two to twenty percent of patients may develop hemolytic uremic syndrome (HUS), which consists of

microangiopathic hemolytic anemia, thrombocytopenia, and acute renal dysfunction.

- Diagnosis: History (undercooked beef and many other vehicles), stool culture, Shiga-like toxin detection assay, and O157:H7 serotyping with agglutination assay.
- Treatment: Correction of dehydration, fluids, and electrolytes is the primary priority. Antibiotic therapy for EHEC is *contraindicated*, as it increases the likelihood of developing HUS; all antimotility agents are also contraindicated.

SALMONELLA SPECIES

- Mean incubation period: 24 hours.
- Symptoms include bloody diarrhea, fever, abdominal cramping, myalgias, and headache. Reactive arthritis can occur in 2% of cases.
- Diagnosis: History (poultry, pork, eggs, dairy products, vegetables, fruit), fecal leukocytes, stool culture.
- Treatment: Supportive care. Antimicrobial treatment can prolong colonization.
- If bacteremia is suspected or documented, patients should be treated with third-generation cephalosporin (e.g., ceftriaxone) while cultures and susceptibilities are pending.

SHIGELLA SPECIES

- Mean incubation period: 24 hours; as few as 10 organisms can cause diarrheal symptoms.
- Symptoms include bloody diarrhea, fever, abdominal cramping, neurologic manifestations (seizure, confusion, hallucinations).
- Diagnosis: History (egg salad, lettuce), fecal leukocytes, stool culture.
- Treatment: Supportive therapy and a 5-day course of antibiotic therapy (cefixime, ceftriaxone, trimethoprim-sulfamethoxazole, ampicillin). Must check sensitivities; antibiotic resistance is an increasing problem, especially with trimethoprim-sulfamethoxazole and ampicillin.

STAPHYLOCOCCUS AUREUS

- Mean incubation period: 3 hours.
- Illness is due to ingestion of preformed enterotoxins; toxin binds to intestinal receptors which stimulate emetic center in the brain.
- Symptoms include acute, forceful emesis, and diarrhea (emesis predominates); patients are afebrile.
- Diagnosis: History (ham, poultry, potato, and egg salad); isolate organism in culture of vomitus, food.
- Treatment: Supportive care; antimicrobial therapy not indicated.

VIBRIO CHOLERAE

- Mean incubation period: 48 hours.
- Toxin-producing strains O1 and O139 are responsible for epidemics; the toxin causes a severe secretory diarrhea.
- Symptoms include voluminous diarrhea (rice-water stools), emesis, and low-grade fever. Shock due to volume depletion can occur in 12 hours; electrolyte derangement is common.
- Diagnosis: History (shellfish), stool, or rectal swab culture.
- Treatment: Rehydration and electrolyte replacement is priority. Antimicrobials for treatment include oral doxycycline, tetracycline, or trimethoprim-sulfamethoxazole.

YERSINIA ENTEROCOLITICA

- Median incubation period: 96 hours.
- Symptoms include diarrhea (bloody in 25% of cases), fever, emesis, abdominal cramping, and pharyngitis. Patients can develop mesenteric adenitis, mimicking acute appendicitis. Adolescents may develop postinfectious arthritis and erythema nodosum.
- Highly associated with consumption of contaminated pork intestine (chitlings).
- Diagnosis: History (pork chitlings), fecal leukocytes, and stool culture.
- Treatment: The benefit of antimicrobial therapy is not established for enterocolitis. In the immunocompromised patient, or if disseminated disease occurs, then treatment is recommended. Recommended antibiotics include trimethoprim-sulfamethoxazole, aminoglycosides, tetracycline, piperacillin, and extended-spectrum cephalosporins. Therapy should be based on susceptibility results.

CLOSTRIDIUM DIFFICILE

- The most important bacterial organism associated with hospital-onset gastrointestinal disease and antibiotic-associated diarrhea.
- Colitis occurs when the usual intestinal flora is altered by antimicrobial therapy. *C. difficile* then proliferates and elaborates toxins A and B.

- Toxins can lead to a broad spectrum of disease, from mild diarrhea to severe pseudomembranous entero-colitis.
- Diagnosis: Definitive diagnosis can be made only by endoscopic examination. Stool assay (enzyme immuno-assay) for toxin or stool culture are the usual diagnostic tests; however, organism and toxin may be present in colon without disease.
- It is important to note that 25–65% of children <12 months of age without diarrhea are colonized with toxin-producing *C. difficile*.

VAGINITIS AND PELVIC INFLAMMATORY DISEASE

VAGINITIS

- Refers to inflammation of the vagina. This discussion focuses on vaginitis in the adolescent population.
- After puberty, the cuboidal vaginal epithelium changes to stratified squamous epithelium. In addition, the vaginal pH decreases from 7.0 to 4.0. As a result, *C. trachomatis* and *N. gonorrhoeae* are unable to infect the vaginal mucosa. Instead, these organisms are common causes of cervicitis and pelvic inflammatory disease (PID) (discussed later).

MICROBIOLOGY

- The three diseases most commonly associated with vaginitis are bacterial vaginosis (due to replacement of the normal flora by *Gardnerella vaginalis*, anaerobes, and genital mycoplasmas), trichomoniasis (*Trichomonas vaginalis*), and candidiasis (*Candida albicans*).

CLINICAL MANIFESTATIONS AND DIAGNOSIS

- Usually characterized by vaginal discharge or vulvar itching and irritation.

- Table 112-7 distinguishes differences in finding of vaginal discharge.

TREATMENT

- Bacterial vaginosis: Metronidazole 500 mg orally twice a day for 7 days, *OR* Metronidazole gel 0.75%, one full applicator (5 g) intravaginally, once a day for 5 days, *OR* Clindamycin cream 2%, one full applicator (5 g) intravaginally at bedtime for 7 days. Alternatives include metronidazole 2 g orally in a single dose, *OR* Clindamycin 300 mg orally twice a day for 7 days, *OR* Clindamycin ovules 100 g intravaginally once at bedtime for 3 days.
- Trichomoniasis: Metronidazole 2 g orally in a single dose. Alternative is Metronidazole 500 mg twice a day for 7 days.
- Candidiasis: Several intravaginal preparations ranging from single dose to 14-day regimens, including Butoconazole cream, Clotrimazole cream, or vaginal tablet, Miconazole cream or suppository, Nystatin vaginal tablet, Tioconazole ointment, or Terconazole cream or suppository. Oral treatment is with Fluconazole 150 mg orally in a single dose.

PELVIC INFLAMMATORY DISEASE (PID)

- PID refers to inflammatory disease of the upper female genital tract.
- Infection can involve the endometrium (endometritis), the fallopian tubes (salpingitis), the pelvic peritoneum (pelvic peritonitis), and contiguous organs (oophoritis and tuboovarian abscess).

MICROBIOLOGY

- The most common causative organisms in acute PID are *Neisseria gonorrhoeae* and *Chlamydia trachomatis*.
- Organisms that comprise the normal vaginal flora are associated with chronic or recurrent infection. These include anaerobes, *Gardnerella vaginalis*, *Haemophilus influenzae*, *Escherichia coli*, and *Streptococcus* sp. Other

TABLE 112-7 Vaginitis in the Adolescent Population: Characteristics of Vaginal Discharge

	BACTERIAL VAGINOSIS	TRICHOMONIASIS	CANDIDIASIS
Discharge	Thin, white, frothy	Heavy, gray or yellow, frothy	Thick, curd-like
pH	>4.5	>4.5	<4.5
KOH	+ Whiff test*	±Whiff test	Hyphae, pseudohyphae
Saline prep	"Clue cells"	Motile organisms	Neutrophils, epithelial cells
Gram stain	Mixed flora	May see trichomonads	Hyphae, pseudohyphae

*Positive whiff test refers to a "fishy," amine odor when the vaginal discharge is mixed with 10% KOH.

organisms such as *Mycoplasma hominis* and *Ureaplasma urealyticum* may be etiologic agents in PID as well.

CLINICAL MANIFESTATIONS AND DIAGNOSIS

MINIMAL CRITERIA
- Lower abdominal tenderness.
- Adnexal tenderness.
- Cervical motion tenderness.

ADDITIONAL CRITERIA
- Fever >38.3°C (101°F).
- Elevated acute phase reactant (ESR or CRP).
- Abnormal cervical or vaginal mucopurulent discharge.
- WBCs seen in microscopic evaluation of vaginal secretions.
- Documentation of *C. trachomatis* or *N. gonorrhoeae* cervical infection.

DEFINITIVE DIAGNOSIS
- Histopathologic evidence on endometrial biopsy.
- Thickened fluid-filled tubes with or without free fluid in pelvis.
- Tuboovarial complex on ultrasonography or other radiologic examination.
- Laproscopic documentation.

TREATMENT

- Consider hospitalization and parenteral therapy if:
  - There are compliance concerns.
  - Evidence of tuboovarial abscess.
  - Pregnant patient.
  - Immunocompromised patient.
  - Cannot exclude a surgical emergency, such as appendicitis.
- Parenteral therapy:
  - Regimen 1: Cefoxitin 2 g IV every 6 hours *OR* cefotetan 2 g IV every 12 hours *AND* doxycycline 100 mg orally or IV every 12 hours.
  - Regimen 2: Clindamycin 900 mg IV every 8 hours, *AND* gentamicin loading dose IV/IM (2 mg/kg) followed by a maintenance dose (1/5 mg/kg) every 8 hours. Single daily dose may be substituted.
- Oral therapy:
  - Regimen 1: Ofloxacin 400 mg orally twice a day for 14 days, *OR* levofloxacin 500 mg orally once daily for 14 days, *with or without* metronidazole 500 mg orally twice a day for 14 days.
  - Regimen B: Ceftriaxone 250 mg IM in a single dose, *OR* cefoxitin 2 g IM in a single dose and probenecid 1 g orally administered concurrently in a single dose, *PLUS* doxycycline 100 mg orally twice a day for 14 days, *with or without* metronidazole 500 mg orally twice a day for 14 days.

PERTUSSIS

- Pertussis is caused by *Bordetella pertussis*, a gram-negative, pleomorphic bacillus. Humans are the only known hosts of this organism. Transmission occurs by close contact via respiratory tract secretions of patients with disease. Incubation period ranges from 6 to 20 days.

EPIDEMIOLOGY

- Disease occurs epidemically with 3–5-year cycles. The epidemiology of disease is changing so that more disease is being seen in adolescents and adults. The clinical manifestations of disease are milder in nature. Disease can occur in all age groups from infants to adults.
- Secondary attack rates of disease in susceptible household contacts may be as high as 90%.

CLINICAL MANIFESTATIONS

- Symptomatic pertussis is generally divided into three stages of varying duration:
  1. Catarrhal stage (1–2 weeks): Symptoms resemble those of a mild upper respiratory tract infection including low-grade fever, rhinorrhea, sore throat, malaise, and cough.
  2. Paroxysmal stage (2–6 weeks): Characterized by repetitive series of coughing paroxysms with whoops, gagging, vomiting, apnea, and copious amount of secretions.
  3. Convalescent stage (1–4 weeks): Cough severity and frequency decreases.
  4. Total duration of disease up to 12 weeks.
- Complications and hospitalizations occur most commonly in the young infant population under 6 months of age and include pneumonia, seizures, acute encephalopathy, and death.
- Symptoms commonly mild and nonspecific in older children, adolescents, and adults making clinical diagnosis more difficult.

DIAGNOSIS

- Confirmation of diagnosis can be made by
  1. Isolation of organism from culture of nasopharyngeal mucus which remains the gold standard. The best yield from culture occurs within the

first 3 weeks of illness. Sensitivity ranges from 50 to 80% and specificity almost 100%.

2. Direct fluorescent antibody (DFA) of nasopharyngeal sections—usually performed in conjunction with cultures. Sensitivity is 60% in best of labs and specificity almost 100%.

3. Polymerase chain reaction (PCR)—highest sensitivity and specificity.

• Negative laboratory confirmation does not rule out pertussis as cause of illness.

TREATMENT

• Treatment most effective if given within first 2 weeks of illness but should be given even after this time to limit spread of organisms to others.

• Infants under 6 months of age and patients with severe disease commonly require hospitalization for complications and to manage apnea, hypoxia, and feeding difficulties.

• Drug of choice is oral erythromycin estolate 40–50 mg/kg/day in four divided doses (maximum 2 g/day) for 14 days.

• Other drugs that may be used include azithromycin dehydrate 10–12 mg/kg/day in one dose for 5–7 days (maximum dose 600 mg/day) and clarithromycin 15–20 mg/kg/day in two divided doses for 7–10 days (maximum dose 1 g/day).

• All household contacts and other close contacts should receive chemoprophylaxis with erythromycin, azithromycin or clarithromycin regardless of age and immunization status.

CONGENITAL SYPHILIS

EPIDEMIOLOGY

• Congenital syphilis is caused by the spirochete *Treponema pallidum* which is contracted from an infected mother via transplacental transmission at any time during pregnancy or at birth.

• In adults, syphilis infection is divided into three stages: primary, secondary, and tertiary or latent. Transmission to the fetus can occur at any stage of the disease. Forty percent of pregnancies among women with untreated early syphilis result in spontaneous abortions. The rate of transmission to the fetus during the secondary stage ranges from 60 to 100% and decreases slowly with time.

• Congenital syphilis is divided into early-onset and late-onset disease. Early-onset disease can appear anytime in the first 2 years of life; 80% of those with early

disease are diagnosed before 3 months of age. Late-onset disease manifests after 2 years of age.

CLINICAL MANIFESTIONS

• Early-onset disease—may or may not be present at birth. Findings include hepatosplenomegaly, snuffles (perfuse nasal discharge that starts clear and may become bloody), generalized lymphadenopathy, mucocutaneous lesions, pneumonia, osteochondritis and other bony radiographic abnormalities (seen in 95% of symptomatic infants and 20% of those with asymptomatic disease), pseudoparalysis, rash (papulosquamous), hemolytic anemia, thrombocytopenia, and abnormal CSF parameters (seen in 50% of symptomatic and 10% of asymptomatic infants).

• Late-onset disease—seen in patients over 2 years of age and findings include malformations in bones (frontal bossing, saddle nose, and saber shins), teeth (Hutchinson peg-shaped, notched central incisors, and mulberry multicusped first molars), and skin (rhagades or linear scars occurring at mucocutaneous junctions) resulting from growth disturbances in these organs; interstitial keratitis; eighth nerve deafness; symmetric chronic, painless swelling of the knees (Clutton joints); and abnormal CSF parameters.

DIAGNOSIS

• Definitive diagnosis is made when spirochetes are identified by microscopic darkfield examination or direct fluorescent antibody tests of lesion exudates or tissue, such as placenta or umbilical cord.

• Presumptive diagnosis most commonly made using nontreponemal and treponemal tests.

• The standard nontreponemal tests for syphilis include the Venereal Disease Research Laboratory (VDRL) slide test and the rapid plasma regain (RPR) test. These tests measure antibody directed against lipoidal antigen from *T. pallidum*, antibody interaction with host tissues, or both. Results may be falsely negative in early primary syphilis, latent acquired syphilis of long duration, and late congenital syphilis. Quantitative results help to define disease activity and monitor response to therapy. Any reactive nontreponemal test must be confirmed by one of the specific treponemal tests to exclude a false-positive result. False-positive results may be caused by certain viral infections (e.g., infectious mononucleosis, hepatitis, varicella, and measles), lymphoma, TB, malaria, endocarditis, connective tissue disease, pregnancy, or IV drug abuse.

- The standard treponemal tests are fluorescent treponemal antibody absorption (FTA-ABS) and *T. pallidum* particle agglutination (TP-PA) tests. Once positive, these tests remain positive for life even after successful therapy. These tests are not 100% specific for syphilis and may be positive in patients with other spirochetal diseases, e.g., yaws, leptospirosis, rat-bite fever, and Lyme disease.
- Other tests that should be done to look for involvement of other organ systems include analysis of CSF parameters and VDRL of CSF, long-bone radiographs, complete blood count and platelet count, and liver function tests.

TREATMENT

- Parenteral penicillin G remains the drug of choice for treatment of syphilis at any stage. Duration of therapy varies depending on the state of disease and the clinical manifestations. This is the only effective therapy for patients with neurosyphilis, congenital syphilis, or syphilis during pregnancy.
- Patients with penicillin hypersensitivity should undergo desensitization.

MYCOBACTERIUM TUBERCULOSIS

- *Mycobacterium tuberculosis* (TB) is an acid-fast bacillus (AFB) with a cell wall high in lipid content. The bacilli are aerobic, nonspore forming, nonmotile, and slightly curved or straight.

EPIDEMIOLOGY

- One-third of the world's population (2 billion people) is infected with TB.
- Approximately 43% of persons with TB in the United States are foreign-born, with six countries (Mexico, Philippines, India, South Korea, Haiti, and China) making up 60% of these cases.
- In addition to being an immigrant, risk factors include incarcerated individuals, HIV infection, homelessness, illicit intravenous drug use, and social and economic disadvantage.

CLINICAL MANIFESTATIONS

- Latent TB infection (LTBI) is when an individual has a positive Mantoux skin test result and a normal chest radiograph. This indicates infection with TB but no active disease.

- Pulmonary disease in children is often asymptomatic or mild (low-grade fever and cough). The radio-graphic hallmark of primary pulmonary TB is enlarged regional lymph nodes in comparison with a small parenchymal focus. Most cases of pulmonary TB in children resolve with or without antituberculous therapy.
- Lymphadenitis due to TB is known as scrofula; it is the most common form of extrapulmonary tuberculosis in children.
- Miliary disease denotes disseminated disease in two or more organs. Lymphohematogenous spread of the tubercle bacilli disseminates to distant anatomic sites. Infants and immunocompromised children are most susceptible to miliary disease.
- Bone and joint infections result from lymphohematogenous spread or contiguous spread from regional lymph nodes or adjacent bones. Pott disease refers to vertebral or paraspinal TB infection.
- Central nervous system TB disease (meningitis) is a result of lymphohematogenous dissemination. The base of the brain is most commonly affected; basilar enhancement is seen on brain imaging (MRI or CT with contrast).
- Renal TB infection is rare. The incubation period from primary infection to symptomatic disease may be several years.

DIAGNOSIS

- The tuberculin skin test (Mantoux) uses 5 tuberculin units (TU) of PPD injected intradermally on the volar service of the forearm. The diameter of induration is determined at 48–72 hours.
- Interpretation of induration diameter is shown in Table 112-8; history of previous bacille Calmette-Guérin

TABLE 112-8 Positive Interpretation of Tuberculin Skin Test

Induration >5 mm in Diameter

Contact of infectious cases
Abnormal chest radiograph
Human immunodeficiency virus infection
Other immunosuppression

Induration >10 mm in Diameter

Foreign-born individual from high-prevalence country
Residents of prison, nursing home, other institution
User of illicit intravenous drugs
Other medical risk (Hodgkin disease, lymphoma, diabetes mellitus, chronic renal failure, malnutrition)

Induration >15 mm in Diameter

Regardless of age or risk factor

(BCG) vaccine is not taken into account in skin test interpretation.

• Once a person is a skin test converter, he should no longer have skin testing done as screening (may remain positive for life). Instead, a chest radiograph is used (only when the person has clinical symptoms suspicious for pulmonary TB or has history of exposure to TB).

• As children are unable to produce sputum, early-morning gastric aspirates (3 separate mornings) are used to obtain specimen for AFB smear and culture. Organism may take 4–6 weeks to grow in vitro.

• Typical cerebrospinal fluid findings in TB meningitis include a markedly low glucose, elevated protein, and an elevated leukocyte count with a lymphocytic predominance. PCR assay can be done on CSF.

TREATMENT

• The recommended regimen for treatment of LTBI (positive skin test, normal chest x-ray [CXR]) in HIV-negative children is a 9-month course of isoniazid as self-administered daily therapy or by twice-weekly directly observed therapy (DOT).

• Treatment for any TB disease beyond LTBI is comprised of multidrug therapy. The number of drugs and length of therapy is dependent on the resistance patterns in the community and the extent of disease. The antituberculosis drugs used in children are listed in Table 112-9. Consultation with an infectious disease specialist is recommended.

LYME DISEASE

EPIDEMIOLOGY

• The etiologic agent of Lyme disease is the spirochete *Borrelia burgdorferi*. It is transmitted by ticks of the Ixodes family; most commonly in the United States by *Ixodes scapularis* (the deer tick) in the northeast and midwest and *Ixodes pacificus* (the western black-legged tick) on the west coast. The nymph tick, which is very small and often undetected, most often transmits Lyme disease.

• Most cases of Lyme disease in the United States occur in the mid-Atlantic states and New England; less commonly, cases occur in Minnesota, Wisconsin, and the northern Pacific states. European cases are typically in Scandinavia and central Europe.

CLINICAL MANIFESTATIONS

• Clinical illness is divided into three stages:

1. Early localized disease occurs typically 1–2 weeks after the tick bite and is characterized by the erythema migrans rash. The rash begins as a red macule or papule that expands over days to weeks to form a large annular erythematous lesion, sometimes with partial clearing, but can be erythematous throughout. The lesion tends to expand to an average diameter of 15 cm, and often persists for 1–2 weeks. Systemic symptoms such as fever, headache, myalgias, and malaise may be present.

2. Early disseminated disease presents 3–10 weeks after the tick bite. Multiple secondary erythema migrans lesions may be present and accompanied by systemic symptoms of fever, headache, myalgias, and malaise. Less commonly, children may present with focal neurologic signs; facial palsy is most frequent. Aseptic meningitis and varying degrees of heart block from carditis may be present at this stage as well.

3. Late disease is characterized typically by monoarticular arthritis. The knee is involved in more than 90% of the cases, and is typically swollen and tender (although less tender than in other bacterial septic arthritidies). Without therapy, the arthritis tends to improve within several weeks, but then will recur.

TABLE 112-9 Common Antituberculosis Drugs Used for Children

DRUG	DAILY DOSE (mg/KG/DAY)	TWICE-WEEKLY DOSE (mg/kg/DOSE)	MAXIMUM DOSE
Isoniazid	10–15	20–40	Daily 300 mg Twice weekly: 900 mg/dose
Rifampin	10–20	10–20	Daily: 600 mg Twice weekly: 600 mg/dose
Pyrazinamide	20–40	50–70	2 g
Streptomycin	20–40 (IM)	20–40 (IM)	1 g
Ethambutol	15–25	50	2.5 g

DIAGNOSIS

• Lyme disease is diagnosed with antibodies tests as the sensitivity of culture is low. Serologic testing for Lyme disease is difficult due to many false positives and should only be undertaken in patients with clear symptoms of disease. Initial screening is by enzyme immunosorbent assay (EIA); Western blot assays are used to confirm positive EIA results. Antibody tests are usually negative in patients with early infection.

TREATMENT

• Erythema migrans and early disseminated disease (including seventh nerve palsy and carditis without third-degree heart block) is treated orally with doxycycline 100 mg bid for 14–21 days (not in children <9 years old) or amoxicillin 50 mg/kg/day (maximum of 500 mg tid) divided tid for 14–21 days. Alternatives are cefuroxime axetil, or erythromycin.
• For meningitis and carditis with third-degree heart block, intravenous ceftriaxone 75–100 mg/kg/day qd for 14–28 days. Alternatives are intravenous cefotaxime or penicillin.
• Arthritis is treated with the oral agents described for erythema migrans, but is continued for 28 days. If a recurrence occurs (about 5–10% of cases), a second oral course or an intravenous course is given.

BIBLIOGRAPHY

Arditi M, Mason E Jr, Bradley J, et al. Three-year multicenter surveillance of pneumococcal meningitis in children: Clinical characteristics, and outcome related to penicillin susceptibility and dexamethasone use. *Pediatrics* 1998;102:1087–1097.

Baraff LJ. Management of fever without source in infants and children. *Ann Emerg Med* 2000;36:602–614.

Baraff LJ, Bass JW, Fleisher GR, et al. Practice guideline for the management of infants and children 0–36 months of age with fever without a source. *Pediatrics* 1993;92:1–12.

Bass JW, et al. The expanding spectrum of Bartonella infections: II. Cat–scratch disease. *Pediatr Infect Dis J* 1997; 16:163–179.

Bayer AS, Bolger AF, Taubert KA, et al. Diagnosis and management of infective endocarditis and its complications. *Circulation* 1998;98:2936–2948.

Berman S. Otitis media in children. *N Engl J Med* 1995;332: 1560–1565.

Cattaneo LA, Edwards KM. *Bordetella pertussis* (whooping cough). *Semin Pediatr Infect Dis* 1995;6:107–118.

Centers for Disease Control and Prevention. Sexually transmitted diseases treatment guidelines 2002. *Morb Mortal Wkly Rep* 2002;51(No. RR–6).

Committee on Infectious Diseases of the American Academy of Pediatrics. Therapy for children with invasive pneumococcal infections. *Pediatrics* 1997;99:289–299.

Craig J. Urinary tract infection: new perspectives on a common disease. *Curr Opin Infect Dis* 2001;14:309–313.

Daoud AS, Batieha A, Al-Sheyyab M, et al. Lack of effectiveness of dexamethasone in neonatal bacterial meningitis. *Eur J Pediatr* 1999;158:230–233.

Ferrieri P, Gewitz MH, Gerber MA, et al. Unique feature of infective endocarditis in childhood. *Circulation* 2002;105: 2115–2127.

Fiore AE, Moroney JF, Farley MM, et al. Clinical outcomes of meningitis caused by *Streptococcus pneumoniae* in the era of antibiotic resistance. *Clin Infec Dis* 2000;30:71–77.

Fliss DM, Leiberman A, Dagan R. Acute and chronic mastoiditis in children. *Adv Pediatr Infect Dis* 1998;13:165–183.

Gerdes LU, Jorgensen PE, Nexo E, et al. C-reactive protein and bacterial meningitis: A meta-analysis. *Scand J Clin Lab Invest* 1998;58:383–393.

Givner LB. Periorbital versus orbital cellulitis. *Pediatr Infect Dis J* 2002;21:1157–1158.

Hoberman A, et al. Enhanced urinalysis as a screening test for urinary tract infection. *Pediatrics* 1993;91:1196–1199.

Hoberman A, et al. Imaging procedures in first febrile urinary tract infection. *N Engl J Med* 2002;348:193–200.

Hughes E, Lee JH. Otitis externa. *Pediatr Rev* 2001;22:191.

Johannson EC, Sifri CD, Madoff LC. Pyogenic liver abscesses. *Infect Dis Clin North Am* 2000;14:547–563.

Kaplan SL. Clinical presentations, diagnosis, and prognostic factors of bacterial meningitis. *Infect Dis Clin North Am* 1999;13:579–594.

Klein JO. Otitis media. *Clin Infect Dis* 1994;19:823–833.

Lew DP, Waldvogel FA. Osteomyelitis. *N Engl J Med* 1997;336:999–1007.

Long SS. *Principles and Practice of Pediatric Infectious Disease.* London: Churchill Livingstone, 2003, pp. 323–328, 333–339, 388–394, 486–498, 509, 791–810.

Lublin M, Bartlett DL, Danforth DN, et al. Hepatic abscesses in patients with chronic granulomatous disease. *Ann Surg* 2002;235:383–391.

Lurie K, Plzak L, Deveney CW. Intra–abdominal abscesses in the 1980s. *Surg Clin North Am* 1987;67:621–632.

Maxson S, Yamauchi T. Acute otitis media. *Pediatr Rev* 1996;17:191–195.

McIntosh K. Community acquired pneumonia in children. *N Engl J Med* 2002;346:429–437.

McIntyre PB, Berkey CS, King SM, et al. Dexamethasone as adjunctive therapy in bacterial meningitis: A meta-analysis of randomized clinical trials since 1988. *JAMA* 1997;278: 925–931.

Montgomery RS, Wilson SE. Intra–abdominal abscesses: image–guided diagnosis and therapy. *Clin Infect Dis* 1996;23(1):28–36.

Novak R, Henriques B, Charpentier E, et al. Emergency of vancomycin tolerance in *Streptococcus pneumoniae*. *Nature* 1999;399:590–593.

Peters TR, Edwards KM. Cervical Lymphadenopahthy and Adenitis. *Pediatr Rev* 2000;21(12):399–404.

Ramaswamy K, Jacobson K. Infectious diarrhea in children. *Gastroenterol Clin North Am* 2001;30:611–624.

Rhody C. Bacterial infections of the skin. *Prim Care* 2000; 27:459–473.

Roy DR. Osteomyelitis. *Pediatr Rev* 1995;16:380–385.

Schuchat A, Robinson K, Wenger JD. Bacterial meningitis in the United States in 1995. *N Engl J Med* 1997;337:970.

Shapiro E, Gerber M. Lyme Disease. *Clin Infect Dis* 2000;31:533–542.

Shapiro ED, et al. Periorbital cellulitis and paranasal sinusitis: a reappraisal. *Pediatr Infect Dis J* 1982;1:91–94.

Small PM, Fujiwara PI. Management of tuberculosis in the United States. *N Engl J Med* 2001;345:3.

Sood S. Lyme Disease. *Pediatr Infect Dis J* 1999;18:913–925.

Stulberg DC. Common bacterial skin infections. *Am Fam Physician* 2002;66:119–124.

Sung L, MacDonald NE. Syphilis: A Pediatric Perspective. *Pediatr Rev* 1998;19:17–22.

Yogev R. Meningitis. In: Jenson HB, Baltimore RS (eds): *Pediatric Infectious Diseases: Principles and Practice.* 2nd ed. W.B. Saunders, 2002;630–650.

113 VIRAL INFECTIONS

A. Todd Davis, Preeti Jaggi, Ben Z. Katz, Ram Yogev

VIRAL EXANTHEMS

- There are a large number of viral exanthems. Only a few have sufficiently distinctive features to allow clinical diagnosis in sporadic cases. Among the recognizable viral illnesses are chicken pox, coxsackie A16, erythema infectiosum, rubella, and rubeola (measles). Epidemics of these diseases tend to occur every few years as the susceptible pool increases.

CHICKENPOX (VARICELLA)

- Chickenpox tends to currently occur every year in the nonimmunized population.
- The typical lesions of chicken pox begin as papules, becoming pustules and finally crusted scabs.
- In contrast to smallpox, the lesions in chickenpox exist simultaneously in varying phases of development.
- The combination of aspirin and chickenpox has been associated with the development of Reyes syndrome (rare).

- One of the more frequent and often fatal complications seen with varicella is streptococcal and staphylococcal skin infections which range in severity from a mild cellulitis to a severe necrotizing fasciitis. Infection, especially with group A streptococcus, has been associated with the development of toxic shock syndrome.
- The varicella vaccine is between 70 and 90% effective.

COXSACKIE A16

- Coxsackie viruses are a group of enteroviruses.
- Outbreaks of these viruses occur during the summertime.
- Only A16 has characteristic findings of papules on the palms, the soles of the feet, and in the mouth—the so-called "hand, foot, and mouth" syndrome.

ERYTHEMA INFECTIOSUM (FIFTH DISEASE)

- Caused by *Parvovirus B19* (PV-B19).
- The characteristic rash of erythema infectiosum, when it occurs, is a lacy rash on the extensor surface of the arms and legs, with an appearance on the face of "slapped cheeks."
- The virus takes up residence in and impairs the function of bone marrow red blood cell (RBC) precursors.
- With cessation of erythrocyte maturation in the bone marrow, patients with hemolytic anemia or bone marrow suppression secondary to chemotherapy are at risk of having an aplastic crisis.
- The anemia associated with impaired bone marrow production of red blood cells may lead to fatal hydrops in the fetus.
- There is no known vaccine to prevent erythema infectiosum.

MEASLES (RUBEOLA)

- Measles generally has a very high attack rate. Outbreaks tend to be relatively explosive and short-lived.
- Begins with respiratory symptoms—cough, conjunctivitis, and coryza—and after 24–48 hours a rash develops on the head and spreads downward.
- The rash often lasts 4–5 days with clearing of the rash at any given site within 2–3 days. Thus, the face may be relatively clear when the rash is fairly intense on the legs.
- As discreet patches of rash coalesce, the resulting pattern is known as morbilliform rash in contrast to a rubelliform rash.

- During the first 24 hours of the measles exanthem a pathognomonic fleeting enanthem may be present. This enanthem is known as Koplik spots—white papules on a red base on the buccal surfaces.
- Worldwide, between 500,000 and 1,000,000 cases of measles occur per year.
- Mental retardation or death is the major sequelae which can be largely prevented by immunization.
- Measles vaccine has an efficacy of 95%.

MUMPS

- Mumps is not as contagious as measles or rubella. Still, outbreaks can stretch over months in a school setting.
- Mumps has a characteristic swelling of the parotid glands. The swollen parotid obscures the angle of the jaw which is the telling distinction on physical examination.
- While sterility is often feared in adult males with mumps, the incidence of infertility appears to be remarkably low.
- Beside the rare case of mumps encephalitis, mumps is otherwise a rather benign disease.

RUBELLA (GERMAN MEASLES)

- In the prevaccine era, rubella outbreaks occurred every 6–9 years.
- The typical clinical course is that of mild constitutional symptoms and low-grade fever.
- A rash, if it occurs at all, is relatively fleeting.
- The rash consists of macules that remain discreet.
- The presence of occipital lymph nodes can be a tip-off to the diagnosis. The presence of joint symptoms (which have to be inquired about—children rarely volunteer the information) is a characteristic feature of rubella outbreaks.
- The major problem with rubella is embryopathy that may occur in the fetuses of mothers who acquire the disease within the first 20 weeks of pregnancy.

VIRAL UPPER RESPIRATORY TRACT INFECTIONS

THE COMMON COLD

EPIDEMIOLOGY
- Children in the United States average three to eight colds per year with over 10% of pediatrician's office visits being for colds.

- More frequent in the winter months with school-aged children serving as the chief reservoir of cold viruses.

ETIOLOGY
- Rhinoviruses account for about one-third of all colds, coronaviruses—15%, adenoviruses and myxoviruses each about 5%.

PATHOPHYSIOLOGY
- Transmitted mainly via hands with inoculation or inhalation into the respiratory epithelium or the conjunctiva. Small- and large-particle aerosols play a more minor role in transmission.

CLINICAL FEATURES
- Symptoms (nasal stuffiness, sore throat, and sneezing) begin 2–3 days following infection. Most cases are generally afebrile.
- Hyperemia and edema of the nasal and pharyngeal mucosa are frequently seen.

TREATMENT
- Symptomatic

ACUTE HERPETIC GINGIVOSTOMATITIS (FEVER BLISTERS, COLD SORES)

ETIOLOGY
- Most cases are due to herpes simplex virus serotype 1 (HSV-1).

TRANSMISSION
- Usually occurs via contact with infected saliva.

CLINICAL FEATURES
- Grouped vesicles on an erythematous base in the *anterior* oropharynx.
- With primary infection, fever, lymphadenopathy, malaise, myalgia, inability to eat, and irritability may also be present.
- In the oropharynx, vesicles can rupture, leading to ulcers, which generally heal without scarring unless they become secondarily infected.
- Recurrences generally become less severe and less frequent with time.
- Those with impaired cell-mediated immunity may experience a protracted infection with severe, painful, and ulcerative stomatitis accompanied by fever and anterior cervical lymphadenopathy. They are also at risk for severe mucocutaneous ulceration and disseminated disease.

- Recurrences can be worse in patients with impaired cellular immunity or eczema, and can be triggered by local stimuli such as injury or sunlight exposure, or systemic conditions such as emotional stress, menstruation, coincident infection, or fevers.

LABORATORY DIAGNOSIS
- Viral culture and direct fluorescent antigen (DFA) detection of the lesions.

TREATMENT
- Acyclovir may be used in immunosuppressed patients and for primary disease in the immunocompetent host.

ACUTE PHARYNGEALCONJUNCTIVAL FEVER

ETIOLOGY
- Adenovirus is the cause of this illness.

CLINICAL FEATURES
- Triad of fever, pharyngitis, and conjunctivitis that is mainly seen in young children.
- Incubation period: 2–4 days.
- Tonsilar and cervical lymph node and adenoidal enlargement may be seen.

TRANSMISSION
- Transmission is sporadic or community-wide in the summer, generally centered around swimming pools or other sources of fomites. Infection occurs via conjunctival inoculation.

LABORATORY DIAGNOSIS
- Isolation of the virus may be done by viral culture.

HERPANGINA

ETIOLOGY
- The enteroviruses (coxsackie A and B, echoviruses) are associated with this illness.

CLINICAL FEATURES
- The classic finding is of vesicular lesions on the *posterior* oropharynx, which can ulcerate.
- Fever, sore throat, headache, and backache may also be present.

TREATMENT
- Supportive

HAND-FOOT-AND-MOUTH SYNDROME

ETIOLOGY
- Most common cause is Coxsakie A16.

CLINICAL FEATURES
- Fever, painful oral lesions (vesicles, ulcers) *anteriorly* in the oropharynx, and vesicles on the hands, feet, and elsewhere is the classic presentation.

LABORATORY DIAGNOSIS
- Diagnosis may be made by viral culture.

TREATMENT
- Supportive

VIRAL MENINGITIS/ENCEPHALITIS

EPIDEMIOLOGY
- Most common during summer and fall (year-round in tropical climates).
- More prevalent in low socioeconomic groups, young children, and immunocompromised hosts.
- Most common mode of transmission is from person to person through fecal-oral route (e.g. enteroviruses) or from mosquitoes (e.g. West Nile, St. Louis) and ticks (e.g. Colorado tick fever). Retrograde neuronal spread is common in cases of HSV and Rabies.

ETIOLOGIC AGENTS
- The most common etiologic agents are the enteroviruses (90%). Other viruses include: arboviruses (e.g. West Nile fever, California or St. Louis encephalitis), *Herpes simplex, adenovirus* and *influenza*. Rare causes include: HHV-6, EBV, HIV, measles, mumps, varicella, rabies and lymphocytic choriomeningitis virus.
- In many cases (>50% of encephalitis) the causative agent is unknown.

PATHOPHYSIOLOGY
- Hematogenous spread of the virus occurs after replication at the site of entry or in regional lymph nodes.
- The virus reaches the CNS after passive transport across the blood-brain-barrier.
- Minimal to moderate involvement of cytokines in the host response.

- Severity of disease depends on viral virulence, viral replication rate, and extent of brain involvement.
- In HSV and rabies, the virus reaches the CNS by migrating along nerves.

CLINICAL FEATURES

- The clinical manifestations are often not specific and do not correspond to a particular agent, especially in infants and young children.
- The most common presentation is fever (with or without upper respiratory tract symptoms) that progresses slowly (i.e., days) to decreased appetite, nausea, and vomiting (without another site of infection to explain these symptoms).
- Listlessness, irritability, sleepiness, and lethargy may also develop. In patients with brain involvement seizures, ataxia, pyramidal tract signs, abnormal reflexes, abnormal movements or behavior can develop. In addition, cranial nerve palsies and hemiparesis can also be seen.
- In older children, headache, photophobia, and generalized malaise are frequent complaints.

DIFFERENTIAL DIAGNOSIS

The differential diagnosis includes:
- Early bacterial meningitis.
- Febrile seizures.
- Tuberculosis, or fungal meningitis.
- Intracranial abscess (e.g. brain, epidural, subdural), CNS tumors.
- Metabolic disorders

DIAGNOSIS

- Lumbar puncture should be performed so that CSF can be examined.
- Usually the CSF is colorless or mildly turbid. Although traumatic tap is common (15%–20% of the times), the possibility of Herpes simplex encephalitis should be considered. To help in differentiating bleeding due to the tap from hemorrhage due to the disease, the bloody CSF should be centrifuged as soon as possible. A clear supernatant suggests a traumatic tap, while xanthochromic/yellowish supernatant suggests the presence of more chronic bleeding (e.g. herpes encephalitis, intracranial hemorrhage).
- The CSF WBC count is usually less than 500 cells/mm^3 with a predominance of mononuclear cells. Early in the infection a predominance of polymorphonuclear cells may be found. In this situation, repeat LP (4 to 6 hours later) will usually show a shift to the more characteristic mononuclear response.

- A lowered CSF glucose is rarely found in viral meningitis and the CSF protein is only mildly elevated (50 to 150 mg%). The Gram's stain and latex agglutination tests are negative.
- Viral cultures, in general, are not recommended unless for epidemiologic purposes. They should be done in cases of encephalitis or in an immunocompromised host. CSF viral cultures are infrequently positive (<25%), while throat and rectal viral cultures are more often positive, and can help in reaching a specific diagnosis.
- Polymerase chain reaction (PCR) techniques are more sensitive and specific and are excellent for detecting HSV and enteroviruses. Acute and convalescent viral titers may also be helpful in making the diagnosis.
- EEG, CT, and MRI of the head should be considered for diagnosis of encephalitis. Brain biopsy may also be helpful in diagnosis, however, it is seldom performed.

TREATMENT

- For most viral meningitis cases, only supportive therapy (e.g. fluids, pain medications) is needed.
- Patients with seizures should receive anticonvulants.
- In patients with focal seizures (and in neonates with all forms of seizures) treatment with IV acyclovir should be considered unless the HSV PCR test is negative. Some physicians prefer to continue acyclovir for at least one week until other tests for HSV (e.g. IgM, EEG and/or MRI) are also negative.
- Corticosteroids are not indicated.

COMPLICATIONS

- Complications of viral meningitis occur rarely and have very little long-term sequelae. In contrast, 2% to 5% of patients with encephalitis die, and patients who present with lethargy, loss of consciousness, or disorientation have a poor prognosis. Poor prognosis is also dependent on the age of the patient (<1 year of age) and the etiologic agent (e.g. HSV, rabies). Severe sequelae include mental retardation, spasticity, paralysis and seizures.

VIRAL GINGIVOSTOMATITIS

EPIDEMIOLOGY

- The two most common forms of viral gingivostomatitis are herpes simplex virus (HSV) and enterovirus infection.
- Herpes gingivostomatitis is not usually seen in children less than 10 months because of the presence of residual maternal antibody.

ETIOLOGIC AGENTS AND CLINICAL PRESENTATION

- The incubation period lasts a few days, and the illness may begin with fever and irritability. Mouth pain follows and vesicular lesions appear on the lips, on the gingival, on the anterior tongue, and on the hard palate; they may also spread around the lips and on the chin. The gingival are usually swollen, ulcerated, and erythematous.
- Cervical and submandibular lymphadenopathy are often present. Lesions evolve over 4–5 days, and then healing occurs for about one more week.
- In adolescents, HSV tends to also present as a posterior exudative pharyngitis with shallow tonsillar ulcers and a gray exudate.
- Enteroviral stomatitis, or herpangina, is differentiated from HSV gingivostomatitis primarily by the location of the lesions. Herpanginal lesions generally are located in the posterior pharynx. Enteroviral stomatitis has a more acute onset, shorter duration, and occurs more during the summer and fall in temperate climates than herpetic gingivostomatitis. Vesicular lesions of the hands and feet (usually bilateral) may be involved with enteroviral illness. Coxsackie viruses are the most common enteroviruses causing herpangina and "hand-foot-mouth" disease.

TREATMENT

- For enteroviral disease, treatment involves supportive care. For HSV disease, acyclovir may be used if the course of illness is unusually severe or prolonged.

VARICELLA

EPIDEMIOLOGY

- Peak age of disease is 5–9 years accounting for 90% of cases.
- Each year varicella results in 11,000 hospitalizations (0.25% of all cases; rate is 2.6 per 100,000, with a rate of 14.6 per 100,000 under 4 years) of which 60% are in children; rate decreased 80% from 1995 to 1999 secondary to vaccination.
- Estimated number of cases per year in the United States prevaccine: 4,000,000.

TRANSMISSION

- Transmission occurs via direct contact with persons with varicella or via airborne or aerosol spread of respiratory secretions.
- Incubation period is 10–21 days following exposure.
- Person is most contagious 2 days before rash appears until rash is completely crusted.

PATHOPHYSIOLOGY

- Infection begins with mucosal inoculation of the virus followed by an incubation period (10–21 days; usually ~14 days) during which time the virus spreads to local lymphatic tissues and initiates a primary viremia.

CLINICAL CHARACTERISTICS

- Patients with varicella usually experience 3–7 days of fever associated with a generalized vesicular eruption appearing in crops, mainly on the trunk and face; lesions are extremely itchy and crust upon healing.
- Patients who have had chickenpox in the past may break out with zoster or shingles which appear as a localized, painful vesicular eruption usually in a dermatomal distribution.

COMPLICATIONS

- Incidence is 2–4 per 1000 unvaccinated children. Incidence is about 3× less for vaccinated children.
- Bacterial superinfection of the skin is the most common, ranging from mild cellulitis around lesion to severe necrotizing fasciitis. Most commonly caused by *Staphylococcus aureus* (e.g., impetigo, fasciitis) or group A *streptococcus* (associated with necrotizing fasciitis and toxic shock syndrome).
- Pneumonia is seen in 8% of hospitalized children and 15% of hospitalized adults. May be severe in adults (mortality rate 10–30%), in the immunocompromised, and in pregnant women.
- Neurologic complications include cerebellar ataxia, aseptic meningitis, postinfectious encephalitis, polyneuropathy, and Bells palsy.
- Less common complications include hepatitis, arthritis, glomerulonephritis, coagulopathies, and Reyes syndrome (associated with aspirin use, rare, and mortality rate 40%).

TREATMENT

- Acyclovir (20 mg/kg/dose qid orally, maximum 800 mg, IV 20 mg/kg q 8 hours).

PREVENTION AND IMMUNOLOGY

- Passive immunity—varicella-zoster immune globulin.
- Active immunity—live, attenuated varicella vaccine, efficacy >95%.
- More than 90% of adults are immune, even those without a documented history of chickenpox, especially those with siblings.
- Immunity is usually lifelong, although documented second cases in healthy individuals do occur.

ADENOVIRAL INFECTIONS

VIROLOGY

- Ubiquitous, double-stranded DNA virus.

- Over 50 serotypes; the lower numbered types generally cause respiratory disease, while the higher numbered types have been associated with diarrhea.
- First isolated from adenoids, hence its name.

EPIDEMIOLOGY
- Spread occurs from the respiratory or gastrointestinal (GI) tracts and environmental surfaces but may also be nosocomially acquired.
- Outbreaks tend to occur in spring and summer.
- Infection is very common in young children, military recruits, and immunocompromised individuals.

CLINICAL MANIFESTATIONS

Illness in the Normal Host
- Very common cause of all types of upper and lower respiratory tract infections.
- Common specific syndromes include the following:
  1. Pertussis-like syndrome (usually adenovirus type 5).
  2. Pharyngoconjunctival fever: Triad of fever, pharyngitis, and conjunctivitis, as its name implies. Conjunctivitis occurs by direct inoculation. Generally a summertime illness most commonly seen in young children with a 2–4-day incubation period. Can be associated with prominent tonsillitis and cervical lymphadenitis. Caused primarily by adenovirus types 3, 4, and 7.
  3. Epidemic keratoconjunctivitis: Mainly seen in adults but can mimic periorbital cellulitis in children. Often associated with preauricular lymphadenopathy and may be associated with pharyngitis.
  4. Rarely adenovirus can cause myocarditis, pericarditis, aseptic meningitis, or encephalitis in previously healthy children.

Clinical Illness in the Immunocompromised Host
- In addition to the above manifestations, hepatitis, hemorrhagic cystitis, colitis, and disseminated infection may be seen. Disease in this population occurs much more commonly with mortality rates that are much higher than that seen in normal children.

DIAGNOSIS
- There are several different methods to make the diagnosis of adenovirus associated disease. These methods include viral culture, rapid viral diagnostic methods (e.g., shell vial assays), and rapid detection of viral nucleic acid (e.g., via polymerase chain reaction [PCR]).

TREATMENT
- There is no proven effective therapy for adenoviral associated disease. In the immune competent host no treatment is usually needed as the illnesses are self-limited.

- Experimental antiviral agents may sometimes be used in immunosuppressed patients.

EPSTEIN-BARR VIRUS (EBV) INFECTIONS

EPIDEMIOLOGY
- Infectious mononucleosis (IM) occurs predominantly in older children and young adults and is characterized by fever, exudative or membranous pharyngitis, generalized lymphadenopathy, and splenomegaly. Characteristically, the peripheral blood shows an absolute increase in the number of atypical lymphocytes, and the serum has a high titer of heterophile antibody. Specific EBV antibodies are detected early in the illness and persist thereafter.
- Although EBV infection is worldwide in distribution, clinical infectious mononucleosis is observed predominantly in developed countries, principally among adolescents and young adults. The modes of transmission are oral-salivary spread in children and close intimate contact (kissing) in young adults.

ETIOLOGY
- EBV is the cause of all heterophile-antibody positive cases of IM and about 50% of the heterophile-antibody negative cases. Other causes of heterophile-antibody negative IM include cytomegalovirus, toxoplasmosis, and other viruses.

CLINICAL MANIFESTATIONS
- The disease usually begins with headache, fever, chills, anorexia, and malaise, followed by lymphadenopathy and severe sore throat. The disease in children is generally mild and may be subclinical; in adults disease is more severe and has a more protracted course. The triad of lymphadenopathy, exudative pharyngitis, and splenomegaly in a febrile patient is typical but not pathognomonic of infectious mononucleosis. Other manifestations of the disease include hepatitis, skin eruptions, pneumonitis, myocarditis, pericarditis, and central nervous system (CNS) involvement.
- There is an increased incidence of skin rashes in patients with infectious mononucleosis who are given ampicillin; the rash is *not* a hypersensitivity reaction to ampicillin.
- Complications include splenic rupture which is a serious but rare complication of infectious mononucleosis. Hematologic complications include thrombocytopenic purpura, hemolytic anemia, aplastic anemia, agranulocytosis, agammaglobulinemia, and acute hemophagocytic syndrome. Neurologic complications include aseptic meningitis, encephalitis, cranial nerve palsies,

optic neuritis, peripheral neuropathy, and transverse myelitis.

DIAGNOSIS

- The diagnosis of infectious mononucleosis is usually made on the basis of (1) suggestive clinical features; (2) atypical lymphocytosis; (3) positive heterophile agglutination antibody test; and (4) ancillary laboratory findings, such as specific antibodies to EBV antigens. Younger children may have EBV infection with symptoms not characteristic of infectious mononucleosis and with negative heterophile-antibody titers. In such instances measurement of specific EBV antibody against EBV antigens is required for diagnosis.

TREATMENT

- Infectious mononucleosis is a self-limited disease, and treatment is chiefly supportive. Contact sports should be avoided until the patient's spleen size has returned to normal.

CMV INFECTIONS

EPIDEMIOLOGY

- Virus is ubiquitous and is transmitted horizontally by direct person-to-person contact with virus-containing secretions, vertically from mother to infant before, during, or after birth, and via transfusions of blood, platelets, and white blood cells (WBCs) from previously infected people. Disease may be primary or recurrent, with recurrent disease most common under conditions of immunosuppression. Prevalence of disease is influenced by multiple factors including socioeconomic status, age, geographic location, and child-bearing practices.

CLINICAL MANIFESTATIONS

- In the normal host most infections are asymptomatic; however, it may present as a heterophile-negative infectious mononucleosis syndrome, hepatitis, and less commonly as myocarditis, thrombocytopenia, hemolytic anemia, vasculitis, hemophagocytic syndrome, and Guillan-Barre syndrome.
- In the immunocompromised host in addition to the above manifestations, other presentations may include interstitial pneumonia (especially posttransplant, human immunodeficiency virus [HIV]), GI disease (esophagitis, colitis) especially in HIV infected patients and retinitis (acquired immunodeficiency syndrome [AIDS]).
- In the congenitally infected infant born to a mother with primary disease, risk of transmission is unrelated to severity of maternal disease. Risk of congenital infection is greatest earlier in pregnancy and disease can be severe.

- Recurrent infection in the mother accounts for the vast majority of congenital cytomegalovirus (CMV) cases. These infections are usually mild or asymptomatic and the infant can be infected perinatally through breast milk.
- The most common findings include hearing loss, thrombocytopenia, jaundice, hepatosplenomegaly (HSM), microcephaly, periventricular calcifications, chorioretinitis, seizures, and pneumonia.

DIAGNOSIS

- For congenital disease, culture of urine, secretions, blood, and buffy coat may be performed.
- Outside the neonatal period, serology—IgM, culture of secretions, blood, PCR, and test for antigenimia are ways to make the diagnosis.

THERAPY

- Most diseases do not require therapy. Therapy is specifically indicated for treatment of serious, life-threatening, or sight-threatening CMV in immunocompromised patients. The agents available include ganciclovir, valganciclovir, foscarnet, and cidofovir.
- A CMV hyperimmune globulin (Cytogam) is available for the prevention of primary or reactivated CMV disease in transplant patients.

HERPES SIMPLEX VIRUS (HSV) INFECTIONS

- Neonatal herpes simplex infection (under 5–6 weeks of age).

EPIDEMIOLOGY

- Source of infection: 55% maternal genital tract, 10% other maternal source, 10% nonmaternal sources, and 25% unknown.
- Seventy percent HSV type 2 (genital).
- Highest incidence in lower socioeconomic groups and with increasing sexual promiscuity.
- Types of infections: encephalitis, disseminated, and skin, eye, mucous membrane (SEM).
- Differential diagnosis: sepsis/meningitis, enteroviral infection (less seizures, fever; more myocarditis, hepatitis usually), varicella-zoster virus (maternal history of chickenpox).

CLINICAL FEATURES

Encephalitis

- Accounts for 33% of cases of neonatal HSV disease.
- Peak incidence at 11–17 days of age (older than other neonatal HSV disease).

- Presenting symptoms include fever, lethargy, and seizures (often but not necessarily focal, as opposed to HSV encephalitis in older children).
- Mortality 15% (40% without therapy), morbidity 70% (seizures most common).

Disseminated Infection
- Accounts for 25% of cases.
- Peak incidence at 7–10 days of age.
- Presenting symptoms include fever, fulminant/non-specific signs of sepsis (e.g., vomiting, jaundice, pneumonia, bleeding).
- Mortality 60% (80% without therapy), morbidity 50%.
- Correlates with primary disease in mom late in gestation.

SEM Disease
- Accounts for 40% of cases.
- Peak incidence at 7–10 days of age.
- Presenting symptoms: Crops of vesicles involving skin, eyes, or mucous membranes.
- Mortality 0%, morbidity up to 20% (CNS involvement) with >3 recurrences (HSV type 2).
- Disease can progress, even while on therapy.

DIAGNOSIS
- Surface cultures and/or direct fluorescent antigen (DFA), after 24–36 hours, and after baby cleaned.
- IgM antibody (more specific than sensitive).
- Imaging study of the head with contrast after about 1 week.
- Electroencephalogram (EEG) (looking for periodic lateral epileptiform discharges [PLEDs]).
- PCR on spinal fluid (75% + for encephalitis [EEG abnormal, LP abnormal + HSV culture from a distant site], 95% + in disseminated disease, 25% + in SEM disease). If PCR remains elevated after therapy the prognosis is worse. Some patients with SEM disease and elevated CSF PCR have neurologic impairment, but the significance of this finding is unclear.

TREATMENT
- Acyclovir 20 mg/kg/q 8 hours, 14–21 days in cases of encephalitis or disseminated disease. Shorter courses may be used for acute outbreaks of SEM disease.
- Ophthalmic antiviral (Viroptic).
- Relapse rate 5–8%.
- Worse prognosis: Disseminated < encephalitis < SEM; semicomatose < lethargic < alert; prematurity < full-term; presence of disseminated intravascular coagulation (DIC), pneumonia, symptoms after acyclovir began.

PREVENTION
- If mother has active lesions (usually primary): Caesarian section delivery
- Isolate baby from anyone with active *oral* lesions.
- Isolate *baby* with active infection/lesions.

CHILDHOOD ENCEPHALITIS (OVER 3 MONTHS OF AGE)

EPIDEMIOLOGY
- Disease occurs through neuronal spread—virus enters through olfactory lobe; usually unrelated to peripheral disease except in the context of primary infection. Accounts for 5–10% of all cases of encephalitis, 40–50% of all deaths due to encephalitis, up to 75% of all diagnoseable cases in some adult series (most common cause of death from encephalitis).
- Most common diagnoseable cause of *focal* encephalitis.
- Patients usually younger than with other forms of encephalitis (average age in one pediatric series around 1 year).
- Usually caused by HSV-1 (as opposed to neonatal).

CLINICAL FEATURES
- Focal gray matter disease.
- Patients present with fever and focal encephalopathy.
- Most common symptoms include nausea, vomiting, and decreased mental status. May also see headache, stiff neck, pyramidal tract signs, focal seizures, ataxia, abnormal reflexes, hemiparesis, and cranial nerve palsies.

DIAGNOSIS
- Lumbar puncture for CSF parameter examination and culture. CSF parameters usually with increased WBC count and protein concentration. Increased RBC count (>50) found in only one-third of cases). Culture usually negative. CSF parameters can be completely normal in up to 25% of cases.
- HSV PCR on CSF has a 98% sensitivity and 94% specificity.
- EEG usually abnormal—but usually only shows focal or generalized slowing, not epileptiform foci, and may be normal in 2–10% of cases.
- Computed tomography (CT) scan of head is the least sensitive of the readily available tests. Seventy percent of cases have normal head CT scans with only one-third of cases having abnormal head CTs.
- Magnetic resonance imaging (MRI)—much more sensitive than CT. Finding of temporal lobe localizing lesion is consistent with HSV encephalitis.
- Brain biopsy is another way to make diagnosis but is rarely done. Performed mainly in patients with focal encephalitis who do not respond to acyclovir therapy.

- Serology—HSV IgG and IgM is not usually helpful unless one is diagnosing primary HSV infection.

TREATMENT

- There is a 70% mortality in untreated cases. Only 2.5% of those infected and untreated will regain normal neurologic function.
- With acyclovir treatment: Mortality 18%; 38% of those treated are either normal or have mild impairment (9% moderate impairment, 35% severe impairment).
- Relapses occur in at least 5% of cases, usually *not* due to resistant HSV and should be retreated with acyclovir. Some data available that indicate that patients treated with higher doses of acyclovir have lower incidence of relapses.
- Dose of acyclovir and duration of therapy same as for neonatal disease.

VIRAL GASTROENTERITIS

EPIDEMIOLOGY

- 40% of all cases of gastroenteritis in the U.S. are caused by viruses; 6 to 10 million episodes occur each year among children under 5 years of age.
- The highest rate of morbidity is between 3 and 24 months of age.
- Two-thirds of the episodes that require hospitalization occur during the winter months and most of them are caused by rotavirus.
- The most common etiologic agents include rotavirus (14 known serotypes), calicivirus (8 serotypes), astrovirus (8 serotypes), adenovirus (2 serotypes), and coronavirus.
- Fecal-oral spread is the most common mode of transmission. Although other mechanisms (e.g. ingestion of contaminated sea products, airborne, and animal source were also suggested.
- In developing countries, viral gastroenteritis is a major cause of death (mostly due to rotavirus). In contrast, less than 100 deaths occur annually in the U.S.

PATHOPHYSIOLOGY

- Viral replication within the enterocytes of the villous epithelium of the jejunum and ileum results in their destruction.
- Enterocyte destruction leads to villous shortening and blunting and transudation of fluid and salts into the lumen.
- Transient malabsorption of carbohydrates and fat results in increased diarrhea.
- Activation of the enteric nervous system results in abnormal gastric and/or intestinal motor function which increased the diarrhea.

- Release of enterotoxins caused efflux of chloride ions which draws more water into the gut and increases the diarrhea volume.
- Severity of disease is affected by the host immune status, pre-existing immunity to the pathogen, size of the inoculum, and virulence of the pathogen.

CLINICAL FEATURES

- Symptoms usually start 1 to 4 days after exposure and last from 3 to 7 days.
- Fever is not common (<40% of cases).
- Vomiting can be a prominent feature (especially in rotavirus infection). In few cases (<10%), fever and vomiting (without diarrhea) may be the only symptoms.
- Multiple episodes of vomiting and diarrhea may lead quickly (within few hours) to dehydration (mostly isotonic).
- Stool is usually watery without mucous or blood.
- Up to 20% of children with rotavirus infection manifest increased hyperemia of the tympanic membrane with loss of landmarks.
- Calicivirus tend to cause a milder but prolonged disease compared to rotavirus.

DIAGNOSIS

- Stool for fecal leukocytes and blood tests usually negative. Stool pH <6 and test for reducing substances is positive.
- Specific laboratory diagnosis is usually unnecessary except when trying to differentiate from a bacterial etiology or for epidemiological investigation during an outbreak.
- Diagnostic tests for rotavirus are available commercially. Research tools (e.g. electron microscopy, EIA, DNA hybridization) can be used to detect other etiologic agents such as enteric adenovirus, caliciviruses or astroviruses.

TREATMENT

- No specific treatment against the various viruses is currently available.
- Fluid and electrolytes management is the most important part of treatment.
- Use of antidiarrheal medications (e.g. bismuth salicilate, probiotics) is rarely, if at all, needed. Antibiotics should never be used.
- Prevention methods include: thorough handwashing, appropriate measures for diaper changing (especially

in daycare center), isolation of ill children, and development of effective and safe vaccines.

VIRAL BRONCHIOLITIS

CROUP (ACUTE LARYNGOTRACHEOBRONCHITIS)

ETIOLOGY
- Most cases caused by parainfluenza virus; however, may also be caused by respiratory syncytial virus (RSV), influenza, rhinovirus, and adenovirus.

EPIDEMIOLOGY
- Most commonly seen in young children (peak age 2 years) with boys outnumbering girls 2:1.
- Attack rate of disease peaks in the late fall and early winter.

CLINICAL FEATURES
- The most common symptoms include coryza, nasal irritation, hoarseness and laryngitis, sore throat, cough and fever, and upper airway obstruction which manifests as a "croupy" cough or stridor.
- Symptoms usually resolve after a few days.
- Important to differentiate from epiglottitis. Differentiating features are shown in Table 113-1.

LABORATORY DIAGNOSIS
- Performance of viral culture may be done to isolate an etiologic agent.

TREATMENT
- Treatment is mostly supportive. If stridor is severe, may need to use racemic epinephrine. And on rare occasions intubation may be required.

TABLE 113-1   Acute Epiglottitis vs. Croup

	EPIGLOTTITIS	CROUP
Usual etiology	Haemophilus influenzae type b	Parainfluenza virus
Usual age	>3 years	<3 years
Onset	Acute	Gradual, nocturnal
Natural history	Progressive	Usually not progressive
Appearance	Toxic	Usually not toxic
Physical examination	Red, edematous epiglottis	Stridor
Chest x ray	Lateral neck: increased size of epiglottis and aryepiglottic folds	Chest: subglottic inflammation and narrowing (*steeple sign*)
Treatment	Antibiotics, intubation	Supportive usually

BRONCHIOLITIS

EPIDEMIOLOGY
- Most commonly seen in infants between 2 and 5 months of age. Annual outbreaks occur and have a duration of 2–5 months occurring primarily from early winter to early spring. Disease severity worse in urban areas. Bronchiolitis due to RSV tends to be more severe than bronchiolitis caused by other viruses.
- Nearly all primary infections occur in the first year of life and are symptomatic.

ETIOLOGY
- Most common due to RSV. Less commonly may be caused by parainfluenza, influenza, rhinovirus, and adenovirus.
- Incubation period 3–4 days.

CLINICAL MANIFESTATIONS
- Most common symptoms include rhinorrhea, low-grade fever, decreased appetite, cough, and wheezing.
- Children at highest risk for developing severe bronchiolitis include those with underlying heart, lung, or renal disease, premature infants, and those with compromised immune systems. Mortality is rare and usually linked to complicating pneumonias.
- In severe cases, cough and wheezing may progress to the point where the child becomes dyspneic with hyperexpansion of the chest, intercostal and subcostal retractions, tachypnea, hypoxemia, and apnea.
- Cyanosis and elevated PCO_2 may be seen in the most severely affected infants.
- Chest x-ray findings include air trapping, peribronchial thickening, interstitial pneumonia, atelectasis, or segmental consolidation.

DIAGNOSIS
- Diagnosis can be made by viral culture of nasopharyngeal secretions or through a rapid RSV antigen test on nasopharyngeal washings.

TREATMENT
- Treatment is supportive; however, nebulized racemic epinephrine, bronchodilators, and steroids may occasionally be useful.
- The antiviral agent ribavirin (aerosolized) can be used early on in the course of the illness in severely ill or high-risk patients.
- To prevent the illness in children at high risk for morbidity and mortality from RSV disease, RSV monoclonal antibody (palivizumab) is administered by IM injection on a monthly basis.

INFLUENZA

EPIDEMIOLOGY

- Influenza is a disease caused by a virus that results in tens of thousands of hospitalizations and up to 40,000 deaths each year. Annual epidemics due to influenza A and B occur during cold weather months in temperate climates. The viruses are constantly undergoing minor genetic changes in their surface glycoproteins. The two most important of these glycoproteins are hemaglutinin and neuramidase. In order to be protected against disease you have to develop an immune response to these glycoproteins; however, the antigenic makeup of these glycoproteins changes from year to year.
- Minor changes = antigenic drift.
- Major changes = antigenic shift, which leads to pandemics, the last one of which was in 1968; only occurs with influenza A.
- Multiple strains of influenza A virus can circulate per season.
- These viruses spread easily from person to person with infants and children being the most efficient transmitters of the viruses because they shed virus for a long time after being infected (>5 days) and at very high viral titers.
- Incubation period 1–3 days.
- There is an increase in the death rate from primary viral pneumonia and bacterial superinfection during influenza epidemics.

ETIOLOGY

- Influenza A and B are responsible for the annual epidemics that occur.

CLINICAL FEATURES

- In adults the most common presentation is the abrupt onset of fever, chills, headache, myalgias, backache, nonproductive cough, rhinorrhea, sore throat, and weakness.
- In children the presentation is very different from that seen in adults. Fever, rhinorrhea, sore throat, vomiting, and diarrhea are the most common symptoms.
- Duration of illness is 1–2 weeks.

COMPLICATIONS

- Most common complications seen in children include acute otitis media, sinusitis, bronchiolitis, and pneumonia. Less common complications include myocarditis, encephalitis, and Reyes syndrome (in conjunction with aspirin use—rare).

DIAGNOSIS

- Diagnosis can be made with rapid antigen tests and through viral cultures.

TREATMENT

- Usually only supportive and symptomatic care necessary. There are four antiviral agents that are effective against influenza virus that may be used in patients at high risk for complications from influenza disease or those who want to shorten duration of illness.
- Amantadine and rimantadine are only effective against influenza A.
- Oseltamivir and zanamivir are effective against both influenza A and B.

PREVENTION

- Yearly influenza vaccination has been shown to be the most effective means for prevention of influenza disease.
- Amantadine, rimantadine, and oseltamivir may be used for prophylaxis in those individuals who are unable to receive the vaccine and for those with high-risk underlying conditions.
- Vaccine should be strongly considered for all healthy children 6–23 months and for all health-care workers.

ROSEOLA

- Caused by human herpesvirus 6 (HHV-6).
- Most frequently occurs in the spring and fall.
- Most commonly affects infants and young children between the ages of 6 months and 3 years, with 80% of the cases occurring before 18 months of age.
- Characteristic clinical presentation is the abrupt onset of high fever (104–105°F) which may persist for 3–4 days with few other clinical findings. Occasionally suboccipital lymphadenopathy, mild erythema of the pharynx, and irritability may be seen. The appearance of the rash of roseola coincides with the abrupt disappearance of the fever. The majority of the cases are either unrecognized or only mildly symptomatic.
- Rash is typically pale pink or rose color with discrete macules or maculopapules seen predominately on the neck and trunk which may persist for several hours to 2 days.
- Febrile seizures are the most common complication seen with roseola.
- Diagnosis can be made by polymerase chain reaction or measurement of serum IgM and IgG antibody titers to HHV-6.
- There is no specific antiviral therapy and treatment is supportive.

BIBLIOGRAPHY

Arav-Boger R, Pass RF. Diagnosis and management of congenital cytomegalovirus infection in the newborn. *Pediatr Ann* 2002;31:719–725.

Arvin AA. Varicella vaccine. *Virology* 2001;284:153–158.

Arvin AM, Prober CG. Herpes simplex virus infections. *Pediatr Infect Dis J* 1990;9:765.

Berlin LF, Rorabaugh ML, Heldrich F, et al. Aseptic meningitis in infants <2 years of age: Diagnosis and etiology. *J Infect Dis* 1993;168:888.

Centers for Disease Control and Prevention. "Norwalk-like viruses." Public Health consequences and outbreak management. *MMWR Morb Mortal Wkly Rep* 2001;50:1–17.

Chang LY, Lin TY, Huang YC, et al. Comparison of enterovirus 71 and coxsackie-virus A16 clinical illnesses during the Taiwan enterovirus epidemic, 1998. *Pediatr Infect Dis J* 1999; 18:1092–1096.

Cohen JI. Epstein–Barr virus infection. *N Engl J Med* 2000; 343:481–492.

Coplan P, et al. Incidence and hospitalization rates of varicella and herpes zoster before varicella vaccine introduction. *Pediatr Infect Dis J* 2001;20:641–645.

Demmler GJ. Adenoviruses. In: Long SS, Pickering LK, Prober CG (eds.), *Principles and Practice of Pediatric Infectious Diseases*, 2nd ed. London: Churchill Livingstone, 2003.

Farthing MJ. Novel targets for the pharmacotherapy of diarrhea: A view for the millennium. *J Gastroenterol Hepatol* 2000; 15:G38–G45.

Gershon AA, et al. Varicella vaccine: The American experience. *J Infect Dis* 1992;166:S63.

Glass RI, Lew JF, Gangarosa RE, et al. Estimates of morbidity and mortality rates for diarrheal diseases in American children. *J Pediatr* 1991;118:27–33.

Grose C. The many faces of infectious mononucleosis: the spectrum of Epstein–Barr virus infection in children. *Pediatr Rev* 1985;7:35–44.

Hammer SM, Connolly KJ. Viral aseptic meningitis in the United States: Clinical features, viral etiologies, and differential diagnosis. *Curr Clin Top Infect Dis* 1992;12:1–25.

Huang CC, Liu CC, Chang YC, et al. Neurologic complications in children with enterovirus 71 infection. *N Engl J Med* 1999; 341:936–942.

Jackson MA, et al. Complications of varicella requiring hospitalization in previously healthy children. *Pediatr Infect Dis J* 1992;11:441–115.

Johnson RT. Acute encephalitis. *Clin Infect Dis* 1996;23:219–226.

Katz BZ. Viral infections of the upper respiratory tract, infectious mononucleosis, and the chronic fatigue syndrome. In: Shulman ST, Phair JP, Peterson LR, Warren JR (eds.), *The Biologic and Clinical Basis of Infectious Diseases*, 5th ed. Philadelphia, PA: W.B. Saunders, 1997.

Kimberlin DW, et al. Natural history of neonatal herpes simplex virus infections in the acyclovir era. *Pediatrics* 2001;108:223.

Kolski H, Ford-Jones EL, Richardson S, et al. Etiology of acute childhood encephalitis at the Hospital for Sick Children, Toronto 1994–1995. *Clin Infect Dis* 1998;26:398.

Lakeman FD, et al. Diagnosis of herpes simplex encephalitis. *J Infect Dis* 1995;171:857–863 [CSF PCR is the state-of-the-art test].

Marfin AA, Gubler DJ. West Nile encephalitis: An emerging disease in the United States. *Clin Infect Dis* 2001;33:1713–1719.

Pang XL, Joensuu J, Vesikari T. Human calicivirus—associated sporadic gastroenterotavirus in Finnish children less than two years of age followed prospectively during a rotavirus vaccine trial. *Pediatr Infect Dis J* 1999;18:420–426.

Pass RF. Cytomegalovirus infection. *Pediatr Rev* 2002;23:163–169.

Peter J, Ray CG. Infectious mononucleosis. *Pediatr Rev* 1998;19: 276–279.

Rautonen J, Koskiniemi M, Vaheri A. Prognostic factors in childhood acute encephalitis. *Pediatr Infect Dis J* 1991;10:441–446.

Reintjes R, Pohle M, Vieth U, et al. Community-wide outbreak of enteroviral illness caused by echovirus 30: A cross-sectional survey and a case-control study. *Pediatr Infect Dis J* 1999;18:104–108.

Rorabaugh ML, Berlin LE, Heldrich F, et al. Relevance of common tests of cerebrospinal fluid in screening for bacterial meningitis in infants younger than 2 years of age: Acute illness and neurologic complications. *Pediatrics* 1993;92:206.

Seward JF. Update on varicella. *Pediatr Infect Dis J* 2001; 20:620–621.

Smalling T, Sefers S, Li HJ, Tang YW. Optimal molecular approaches to detect herpes simplex virus and enteroviruses in the central nervous system. *J Clin Microbiol* 2002;40: 3217–2322.

Subcommittee on Gastroenteritis, American Academy of Pediatrics. Practice parameter: The management of acute gastroenteritis in young children. *Pediatrics* 1996;97:424–436.

Velazquez R, Matson DO, Calva JJ, et al. Rotavirus infection in infants as protection against subsequent infections. *N Engl J Med* 1996;335:1022–1028.

Whitley RJ. Predictors of morbidity and mortality in neonates with herpes simplex virus infections. *N Engl J Med* 1991;324:540.

Wickelgren I. How rotavirus causes diarrhea. *Science* 2000; 287:409–411.

114 FUNGAL INFECTIONS

A. Todd Davis, Alexandra Freeman, Preeti Jaggi, Stanford T. Shulman

TINEA INFECTIONS

EPIDEMIOLOGY

- Skin infections with *Microsporum, Tricophyton*, or *Epidermophyton* fungi are generally designated as "tinea" plus the body site involved (tinea capitis = scalp, tinea pedis = foot, tinea unguium = nail). Generally, the lesions are erythematous and have an area of central clearing that is scale-free.

ETIOLOGIC AGENTS AND CLINICAL MANIFESTATIONS

- Tinea capitis is generally caused by *Tricophyton tonsurans* in North America. It is primarily seen in prepubertal children. Children may present with focal areas scaling with or without alopecia and/or broken hairs in the affected area. A kerion, or soft boggy scalp tumor with overlying pustules may occur if a hypersensitivity reaction develops. "Id reactions are inflammatory autosensitivity reactions of the skin that occur at sites distant from the infection.
- Tinea pedis commonly causes scaling, fissuring, and maceration between toes with erythema surrounding the area of involvement. Vesicles over the instep of the feet may also develop. Occasionally, the entire sole of the foot may be involved.
- Onychomycosis, fungal infection of the nail, is termed tinea unguium when caused by a dermatophyte. Typically, the distal nail is affected with subungual debris and/or a superficial white scaling.
- Tinea versicolor, caused by the yeast Malassezia furfur, is not a dermatophyte infection, although it is termed "tinea." It causes characteristic hypo- or hyperpigmented lesions seen generally over the upper chest, back, face, or neck. Lesions are usually asymptomatic, although some patients have pruritis.

DIAGNOSIS

- Often these infections can be diagnosed clinically, but if the diagnosis is in question, confirmatory examination should be obtained. One can obtain a skin or nail specimen, place it on a glass slide, and apply 10 or 20% potassium hydroxide. After a coverslip is placed over the sample, the epithelial cells will dissipate, and the hyphae and/or spores can be visualized under 20× or 40× objective. If the diagnosis is still in question and/or the potassium hydroxide stain is negative, one should send specimens for fungal culture or skin biopsy.
- Common clinical conditions that can mimic tinea capitis infections are psoriasis, eczema, and seborrheic dermatitis. Kerion infections can often be mistaken for a bacterial abscess. Tinea corporis infections can appear similar to granuloma annulare, but the latter has an indurated border and depressed center. Psoriasis is characterized by silvery-white, loosely adherent scales that, when removed, reveal punctuate bleeding (Auspitz sign).

TREATMENT

- Topical imidazole antifungals are generally safe and effective for localized tinea corporis. Systemic therapy is indicated for tinea capitis, tinea unguium, and for widespread tinea corporis. The drug of choice for tinea capitis is griseofulvin (15–20 mg/kg/day in liquid microsize form or 10 mg/kg/day in ultramicrosize tablet). The treatment should be continued for 8 weeks. There is some resistance to griseofulvin in the community. It is important to continue the full course of this treatment. In the absence of liver disease, no testing of blood counts or liver enzymes is needed.
- Tinea unguium infections can also be treated with oral itraconazole, terbinafine, or ketoconazole, but also require at least 6 weeks. Tinea versicolor can be treated with oral ketoconazole or topical selenium sulfide shampoos three to five times per week for 2–4 weeks.

CANDIDAL INFECTIONS

EPIDEMIOLOGY

- *Candida albicans* accounts for 60–80% of candidal infections, but other important species include *Candida tropicalis*, *Candida krusei*, *Candida* (*Torulopsis*) *glabrata*, *Candida guilliermondii*, and *Candida parapsilosis*. These ubiquitous organisms exist as yeast or pseudohyphae.
- Vertical transmission from mother to infant occurs. Most candidal infections arise from endogenous strains rather than as a result of person-person transmission.

CLINICAL MANIFESTATIONS

- Clinical manifestations of candida infection include superficial mucosal infection, such as oropharyngeal (thrush), glossitis, and chronic otitis externa; cutaneous infection, including diaper dermatitis, intertrigo, nodular folliculitis, and in adults paronychia and onychomycosis. Gastrointestinal candidiasis is usually seen in cancer patients, and candidal esophagitis almost exclusively occurs in immunocompromised hosts (human immunodeficiency virus [HIV], oncology patients). Candidal cystitis occurs most often in hospitalized, instrumented patients, and vulvovaginitis is a common infection in immunocompetent adolescents.
- Hospitalized patients are susceptible to catheter-associated fungemia associated with indwelling vascular lines, intravenous alimentation, urinary catheters, or prolonged neutropenia. *C. albicans* is the most common species. Systemic candidiasis can involve any deep tissue site, with the most common being meningitis, endophthalmitis, endocarditis, hepatosplenic candidiasis, renal microabscesses, and candida arthritis.
- Specific clinical syndromes of serious candidal infection include candida infections in the NICU, which include congenital candidiasis, catheter-related fungemia, and disseminated candidiasis; and candida infections in the neutropenic cancer patient, which manifest as catheter-related fungemia or hepatosplenic candidiasis.

DIAGNOSIS

- Diagnosis of candida infection is supported by potassium hydroxide preparation or Gram stain of lesions, fluids, or biopsy specimens or by culture on standard or fungal media. Typical features on ophthalmologic (fluffy, white, and cotton-like retinal lesions), computed tomography (CT), or magnetic resonance imaging (MRI) (e.g., renal pelvis masses, microabscesses of liver and spleen, and echocardiographic vegetations) examinations support the diagnosis.

TREATMENT

- Treatment is dependent on the site and severity of candida infection. Oral thrush can be treated with Nystatin suspension (1 mL each side qid × 7–10 days) and diaper dermatitis by Nystatin cream 4–6 × per day. More serious infections require parenteral amphotericin B, fluconazole, or the newer agents voriconazole or caspofungin. Lipid formulations of amphotericin can be used at higher doses than amphotericin B with fewer side effects in seriously ill patients with intolerance or renal toxicity. Removal of lines and other foreign bodies is generally required. Certain candidal species are often resistant to selected antifungals: *C. krusei* and *C. glabrata* to fluconazole and itraconazole; *C. lusitaniae* and *C. guillermondi* to amphotericin B.

ASPERGILLUS INFECTIONS

EPIDEMIOLOGY

- *Aspergillus* species are ubiquitous molds which grow on soil, plants, and decomposing organic matter. The most common species is *Aspergillus fumigatus* with *Aspergillus flavus*, *Aspergillus nidulans*, and *Aspergillus terreus* occurring less frequently.
- *Aspergillus* infections are acquired through inhalation of spores. Lung macrophages and neutrophils are the most important lines of defense against infection.

CLINICAL MANIFESTATIONS

Invasive Aspergillosis

- Invasive disease occurs most commonly in patients who are neutropenic due to therapy for malignancies, recipients of bone marrow or solid organ transplantation, or have neutrophil deficiencies or dysfunction (e.g., chronic granulomatous disease).
- Invasive disease most commonly involves the lung, with the sinuses and central nervous system (CNS) also being frequently infected. Skin and bone involvement is less common. Infection can spread to contiguous structures and angioinvasion is common, leading to thrombosis and necrosis or hemorrhage.

- Pulmonary infection often presents with fever not responsive to antibiotics. Respiratory symptoms may be minimal.
- Sinusitis typically presents with fever in a neutropenic patient with headache, sinus pain, epistaxis, or blackish nasal discharge.
- CNS infection most commonly occurs by hematogenous spread or by extension from infected sinuses (although this route is less common). Cerebral aspergillosis can present with single or multiple abscesses, meningitis, an epidural abscess, or a subarachnoid hemorrhage.

Allergic Bronchopulmonary Aspergillosis

- This condition results from colonization of the airways in children with underlying lung disease (most often asthma or cystic fibrosis). This can lead to a syndrome characterized by wheezing, peripheral blood eosinophilia, elevated serum IgE, transient infiltrates on radiographs, and positive skin prick tests to *Aspergillus* antigens. A similar syndrome can occur in patients with chronic sinusitis who have *Aspergillus* colonization of the sinuses.

Aspergilloma

- Aspergilloma develops in preformed pulmonary cavities from fungal disease, tuberculosis, orcystic fibrosis. Chest radiographs show a solid mass within a cavity. Most cases are asymptomatic, but hemoptysis can develop.

Otomycosis

- Otomycosis is a chronic condition manifested by ear discharge, irritation, and discomfort that is most common in tropical or subtropical regions.

DIAGNOSIS

- CT scanning or MRI of the chest and the sinuses is more sensitive than plain radiographs for detecting disease. Classic findings on chest CT include the "halo sign" which are pleural lesions surrounded by an area of low attenuation and the "crescent sign" which is from air at the edge of the nodule. Sinus CT or MRI may show bony destruction or spread of disease into contiguous areas.
- Definitive diagnosis is made by isolation of the organism in culture or by biopsy of a lesion with histologic evidence of hyphae in lung or sinus tissue.
- Patients are often treated presumptively based on clinical findings and imaging study results.

TREATMENT

- Traditional therapy of invasive disease is with amphotericin B. Newer agents such as lipid formulations of amphotericin B, itraconazole, voriconazole, or caspofungin are available and can be used with advice from an infectious disease consultant. Despite appropriate therapy, mortality rates still remain high.

• Treatment for allergic bronchopulmonary aspergillosis is with anti-inflammatory agents and management of asthmatic exacerbations. The role of antifungal therapy remains unclear. For patients with allergic sinus disease, therapy is similar to that of chronic sinusitis and antifungal agents are not warranted.

• In cases of aspergillomas, optimal therapy is still being investigated; however, surgical excision or instillation of antifungals have been used.

• Treatment of otomycosis involves cleaning of the ear canal and instillation of topical antifungal agents.

BLASTOMYCOSIS

ETIOLOGY

• Caused by a dimorphic fungus found in many different parts of North America.

CLINICAL MANIFESTATIONS

• Clinical manifestations are based on the predilection for particular sites of infection: the lungs, skin, and bone.

• The patient may or may not have a systemic symptom such as fever and fatigue.

• With pulmonary involvement, a radiograph may show consolidation similar to that seen in bacterial pneumonia.

• Skin manifestations are herpetic like raised papules. There is nothing characteristic about the skin lesions per se, but in the presence of skin and lung findings, the diagnosis of blastomycosis should be entertained.

• The infection is not communicable from person to person.

• Most patients recover spontaneously.

• On occasion, the severely ill patient may require antifungal therapy.

HISTOPLASMOSIS

EPIDEMIOLOGY

• The endemic areas of histoplasmosis in the United States are principally associated with the Ohio and Mississippi Valleys. The organism can be found in soil. There is a particular predilection for histoplasmosis to be associated with bats although the bats themselves do not become ill.

CLINICAL MANIFESTATIONS

• For those who do become ill, the symptoms are nonspecific: weight loss, fatigue, and anorexia.

• With extensive lung involvement, the patient may complain of chest pain.

• Insofar as the organism concentrates in the reticuloendothelial system, bone marrow aspiration may sometimes yield the diagnosis when puzzled about the cause of pulmonary consolidation.

DIAGNOSIS

• A diagnosis may be made by the demonstration of organisms in body fluids such as bronchial lavage. Skin testing is no longer available.

• The overwhelming majority of people recover without incident.

TREATMENT

• Those that are severely ill, particularly if they are immunocompromised, may require amphotericin B or itraconazole.

COCCIDIOMYCOSIS

EPIDEMIOLOGY

• *Coccidioides imitis* is a dimorphic fungus that causes primary pulmonary infection with frequent lympho-hematogenous dissemination.

• Coccidiomycosis occurs primarily in the southwestern United States, being endemic in southern California, Arizona, New Mexico, and western and southern Texas. It also occurs in areas of Mexico and Central and South America. About 25,000–100,000 new infections occur each year in the United States.

CLINICAL MANIFESTATIONS

• Sixty percent of infections are subclinical. Most symptomatic patients have self-limited pulmonary infection, with pulmonary complications only in <5% and disseminated infection in <1%, especially in immunocompromised hosts, including those with HIV infection.

• The incubation period is usually 10–15 days, and the most common symptoms are fever, chest pain, and malaise, sometimes with cough. Children rarely develop hemoptysis, but an acute diffuse red rash or erythema multiforme are common in children. Erythema nodosum can follow 3–18 days later. Symptoms generally resolve spontaneously in <1 week to 1 month.

• Extrapulmonary dissemination occurs within several months after primary infection, accompanied by persistent fever. Neonates and young infants are among those at increased risk. Sites of dissemination include bones or joints, skin, and meninges (mononuclear pleocytosis in cerebrospinal fluid [CSF]).

DIAGNOSIS

- Diagnosis requires careful travel history and/or chest radiographic findings, with confirmation by direct staining of tissue specimens or culture. Skin testing is of limited value, but IgM antibody indicates recent infection as it is detectable in 75% 1–3 weeks after symptom onset and disappears before 6 months. IgG complement fixation antibody is present in 50% at 4 weeks, 80% at 3 months, and disappears as infection resolves; it is also present in 95% with coccidioidal meningitis.

TREATMENT

- Treatment is not required in >95% of those infected. Those with immunodeficiency, fulminant or extrapulmonary infection, or with prolonged symptoms should be treated. Ketoconazole, fluconazole, or itraconazole is usually employed.

BIBLIOGRAPHY

Chen BA, Friedlander SF. Tinea capitis update: a continuing conflict with an old adversary. *Curr Opin Pediatr* 2001;13:331–335.

Feigin RD, Cherry JD, Demmler GJ, Kaplan SL. *Textbook of Pediatric Infectious Diseases.* Philadelphia: W.B. Saunders, 2004,2569–2579.

Soubani A, Chandrasekar P. The clinical spectrum of pulmonary Aspergillosis. *Chest* 2002;121:1988–1999.

Stevens DA, Kan VL, Judson MA, et al. Practice guidelines for diseases caused by Aspergillosis. Infectious Diseases Society of America. *Clin Infect Dis* 2000;30:696–709.

115 INFECTIONS IN IMMUNOCOMPROMISED HOSTS

Ellen G. Chadwick

CATEGORIES AND CAUSES OF IMMUNE COMPROMISE

CANCER

- Chemotherapy-associated neutropenia, <200–500 neutrophils/dL most significant.
- Prolonged neutropenia associated with oral and gastrointestinal mucositis, which provides portal of entry for anaerobes and gram-negative enteric bacteria.
- Indwelling catheters increase risk of bacteremia.
- Also associated with altered cell-mediated immunity and hypogammaglobulinemia.

TRANSPLANTION

- Bone marrow (BMT): Same as cancer (above) with highest risk occurring in the first 100 days posttransplant and influenced by type of transplant (autologous vs. allogeneic).
- Prior human herpesvirus infections can reactivate to cause disease.
- Graft-vs.-host disease (GVHD) predisposes to increased risk of superinfection.
- Solid organ transplant: Same as BMT plus infection in site of transplant; transplanted organ may carry viral or parasitic pathogens.

SPLENECTOMY

- Functional (sickle cell disease) and malignancy-associated (Non-Hodgkin lymphoma) splenectomies are at highest risk for overwhelming bacteremia with encapsulated organisms.
- Posttraumatic splenectomy at somewhat less risk after the first year postsplenectomy.

HIV/AIDS

- CD4+ T-cell depletion associated with opportunistic infections (*Pneumocystis carinii*, nontuberculous mycobacteria, and so on).
- Neutropenia associated with disease or antiretroviral therapy predisposes to bacterial infections with deficient humoral immunity increasing risk for bacteremia with encapsulated organisms.

CONGENITAL IMMUNE DEFICIENCIES

- Humoral, T-cell, and phagocytic-cell deficiencies also predispose person to a variety of infections.

INFECTIONS BY UNDERLYING CAUSE OF IMMUNOSUPPRESSION/ SYMPTOM COMPLEX

NEUTROPENIC PATIENTS WITH CANCER OR UNDERGOING BONE MARROW TRANSPLANT

- Bacteremia: Gram-positive organisms account for over half of microbiologically proven infections in BMT patients in the United States and western Europe. Coagulase-negative staphylococci in patients with indwelling intravenous devices are most common, as well as *Staphylococcus aureus*, viridans group streptococci, and enterococci. An increasing proportion of staphylococci are methicillin-resistant. *Streptococcus mitis* and other viridans streptococci may be sensitive only to vancomycin. Gram-negative enteric organisms and *Pseudomonas aeruginosa* occur less frequently but are more common than gram-positive organisms in resource-poor nations. Empiric therapy when patients present with fever includes broad-spectrum coverage such as ceftazidime plus or minus clindamycin; meropenem; vancomycin or an aminoglycoside may be added if patient is hypotensive. Therapy should be tailored once an organism is identified.

- Fungemia: Patients with prolonged neutropenia (>10 days) are at highest risk for fungemia, predominantly due to *Candida*, *Aspergillus*, and less commonly, *Fusarium* and *Trichosporon*. Empiric amphotericin B (often liposomal) is added to antibiotics after 5–7 days in patients with fever and neutropenia without an identified source.
- Sinusitis: Routine sinus pathogens (*Streptococcus pneumoniae, Haemophilus influenzae, or Moraxella catarrhalis*), as well as fungi such as *Aspergillus*, *Mucormycosis* (*Mucor* sp., *Rhizopus* sp.), and Pheohyphomycoses (*Curvularia, Bipolaris, Alternaria*) occur in patients with severe and protracted neutropenia.
- Interstitial or nodular pneumonitis most commonly are due to *Candida* or *Aspergillus*. This is often treated with empiric antifungals (amphotericin, caspofungin, or voriconazole).
- Oral, esophageal, or intestinal mucositis, typhlitis are most often due to anaerobic organisms. Treatment should include clindamycin, metronidazole, or ampicillin/sulbactam. Herpesvirus infections may also be the cause of this (herpes simplex virus [HSV], cytomegalovirus [CMV]) and is treated with acyclovir or ganciclovir. *Candida* species is another etiology and is treated most commonly with fluconazole.
- Hepatosplenic nodular lesions (evident in patients recovering from prolonged neutropenia) are most commonly due to *Candida* or *Aspergillus* species and are treated with amphotericin B, voriconazole, or itraconazole alone or in combination.
- Central nervous system (CNS) disease may be due to *Aspergillus* sp., pheohyphyomycotic organisms (see above) and are treated with amphotericin B.
- Cutaneous manifestations include ecthyma gangrenosum caused by *P. aeruginosa* and erythematous papulonodular lesions caused by fungi (*Candida, Aspergillus, Fusarium, Trichosporon*). Specific therapy should be guided by biopsy results.

COMMON INFECTIONS PRESENTING IN THE FIRST 30 DAYS FOLLOWING BONE MARROW TRANSPLANT (BEFORE ENGRAFTMENT)

- Bacteremia and fungemia (see above).
- HSV gingivostomatitis may be difficult to differentiate clinically from mucositis due to other causes. Diagnosis can be made by direct fluorescent antibiotic testing or by culture. Teatment consists of a course of acyclovir.
- Hemorrhagic cystitis may be caused by papovaviruses (BK and JC viruses) and adenovirus. Ribavirin treatment has been used anecdotally; however, efficacy is not proven.
- Enteritis may be caused by a number of viruses including enteric adenovirus, rotavirus, and enteroviruses or *Clostridium difficile*. *C. difficile* disease should be treated with metronidazole.

COMMON INFECTIONS PRESENTING FROM 30 TO 100 DAYS FOLLOWING BONE MARROW TRANSPLANT (EARLY ENGRAFTMENT)

- CMV infections (viremia, pneumonitis, and hepatitis, colitis) are most commonly seen in patients with mismatched transplants (CMV + donor with CMV – recipient). Even though these patients are at the highest risk for disease, incidence of disease has decreased with the use of prophylactic ganciclovir.
- Viral pneumonitis is most commonly caused by adenovirus, respiratory syncytial virus (RSV), parainfluenza, and influenza. Influenza should be treated with amantadine or oseltamivir. In severe cases, adenoviral and RSV disease may be treated with ribavirin.
- Fungemia (as above) often seen complicating GVHD.
- *Pneumocystis carinii* pneumonia (PCP) and CNS toxoplasmosis are opportunistic infections seen in the severely immunocompromised population. Therapy is guided by the results of bronchoalveolar lavage or biopsy, respectively and includes trimethoprim/sulfmethoxazole plus prednisone for PCP and pyrimethamine/sulfadiazine for toxoplasmosis. Duration of therapy may be lifelong.

COMMON INFECTIONS PRESENTING >100 DAYS FOLLOWING BONE MARROW TRANSPLANT (LATE POSTTRANSPLANT PERIOD)

- Bacteremia due to encapsulated organisms. Risk is greatly augmented by the presence of GVHD.
- Varicella-zoster virus infection. The risk for disease is greatly increased by the presence of GVHD. Disease may involve one or more dermatomes or may be disseminated.
- Viral hepatitis caused by hepatitis viruses A, B, C, D, HSV, adenovirus, enterovirus, and papovavirus may be seen during this period posttransplant.

INFECTIONS IN SOLID ORGAN TRANSPLANT RECIPIENTS

- Within the first several weeks following transplant, solid organ transplant recipients are at risk for systemic bacterial infections and postsurgical bacterial infections at the graft site.
- Infections following transplantation of specific organs:
  1. Kidney: (a) Pyelonephritis or peritonitis due to gram-negative bacilli or enterococci is most common. Empiric broad-spectrum therapy is recommended with ceftazidime or piperacillin/tazobactam. (b) Patients with donor-recipient mismatch are at very high risk for systemic CMV infection. These patients should be treated with ganciclovir.
  2. Liver: Ascending cholangitis or liver abscess due to *Pseudomonas*, enteric gram-negative bacilli, or enterococci (including vancomycin-resistant enterococci). Empiric therapy should include ceftazidime and vancomycin.
  3. Lung: Pneumonitis caused by CMV, HSV, adenovirus, and fungi may be seen. Diagnosis can be made with bronchoalveolar lavage or lung biopsy and should guide therapy.
  4. Heart: (a) Causes of pneumonitis are similar to those seen in lung transplant patients. (b) Mediastinitis most commonly is due to staphylococci and skin flora and should be treated with clindamycin or vancomycin until organism sensitivities are available.

ASPLENIC PATIENTS

- These patients are at risk for overwhelming sepsis or meningitis with encapsulated bacteria such as *S. pneumoniae, H. influenzae,* and *Neisseria meningitidis.* Empiric therapy includes ceftriaxone or cefotaxime ± vancomycin until a specific organism is isolated.
- *Capnocytophaga canimorsus* (DF-2 bacillus) can cause fulminant sepsis in this population. If this organism is isolated it should be treated with penicillin or a third generation cephalosporin.
- The intraerythrocytic parasite *Babesia microti* may cause fulminating infection in this population and is associated with hemolysis, which may require exchange transfusion in addition to standard therapy with quinine and clindamycin.

HIV INFECTION/AIDS

- These patients are at increased risk for bacteremia with encapsulated organisms (as above in asplenic patients).

- Patients with severe CD4 depletion (<100 cell/mL) are at high risk for *Mycobacterium avium* complex (MAC) infections. Treatment consists of clarithromycin and ethambutol plus rifabutin or amikacin.
- Patients are predisposed to recurrent episodes of sinusitis and otitis media. Acute infections are caused by the typical bacterial pathogens such as *S. pneumoniae, M. catarrhalis, and H. influenzae* and are treated first line with high-dose amoxicillin or amoxicillin/clavulanatic acid. Chronic infections may be caused by *Pseudomonas aeruginosa* and are treated with ceftazidime or a fluoroquinolone.
- Pneumonitis may be diffuse and is most likely due to *Pneumocystis carinii* and or CMV in the setting of severe CD4 depletion (<50 cells/mm^3). Focal pneumonitis is commonly due to *S. pneumoniae, S. aureus,* group A streptococci, and other common organisms that cause pneumonia. A progressive pneumonitis may be caused by *Pseudomonas* species.
- Disease of the gastrointestinal tract may manifest in different ways: esophagitis is commonly due to *Candida* sp., HSV, or CMV. Enteritis may be due to *Cryptosporidiosis, Microsporidiosis, C. difficile,* MAC, *Giardia, Salmonella, Shigella, Campylobacter, or Yersinia.* Cryptosporidia enteritis is chronic and is treated with nitazoxanide. Microsporidia has been treated with albendazole, clindamycin, metronidazole, or nitazoxanide, but is often poorly responsive.
- Central nervous system disease includes CMV retinitis or encephalitis, cerebral toxoplasmosis, cryptococcal meningitis, and papova virus (JC or BK virus) infection which may cause progressive multifocal leukoencephalopathy. Cryptococcal meningitis should be initially treated with amphotericin followed by fluconazole for prolonged suppressive therapy.
- Mucocutaneous disease includes recurrent oropharyngeal candidiasis, HSV gingivostomatitis or labialis, varicella-zoster virus causing dermatomal or disseminated disease, recurrent or disseminated molluscum contagiosum, and recurrent severe aphthous ulcers.

X-LINKED AGAMMAGLOBULINEMIA (XLA)

- Patients with this disorder present with recurrent pyogenic infections in infancy and early childhood including pneumonia, otitis media, meningitis, and diarrhea. These infections are most commonly due to encapsulated organisms such as *S. pneumoniae* and *H. influenzae* type b and are treated with ceftriaxone or cefotaxime ± vancomycin.
- Patients may also have chronic or recurrent gastrointestinal infections due to rotavirus, *Giardia lamblia* or *Campylobacter jejuni* causing diarrhea, steatorrhea,

or malabsorption. The latter two should be treated with metronidazole or erythromycin, respectively.

- Mycoplasma and ureaplasma may cause infections of the respiratory tract, joints, or urogenital system and may be chronic in nature.
- These patients may also have chronic enteroviral meningoencephalitis which presents with the insidious onset of ataxia, cognitive impairment, and paresthesias. Enteroviral PCR is the more sensitive diagnostic tool than CSF viral culture. Treatment is intravenous immunoglobulin. Pleconoril, an investigational agent, has potential benefit, but is not Food and Drug Administration (FDA) approved for this use.
- Echovirus or more rarely, coxsackie virus infections, may cause a dermatomyositis-like syndrome with muscle weakness, edema of the skin, and a violaceous rash over the extensor surfaces of the joints with or without hepatic enzyme elevation.
- There is an increased risk of vaccine-associated disease with use of live-virus vaccines such as oral polio vaccine, varicella vaccine and measles, mumps, and rubella vaccine.

HYPERIMMUNOGLOBULINEMIA M SYNDROME (HIM)

- These patients usually present with the same recurrent pyogenic infections that are seen in XLA; however, in addition they have a particular predisposition to opportunistic infections. *Pneumocystis carinii* pneumonia is the presenting illness in >40% of cases. Other pulmonary infections include *Cryptococcus* sp., *Histoplasma capsulatum*, nontuberculous mycobacteria including the Calmette-Guerin bacillus, and cytomegalovirus.
- Enteric infections with *Cryptosporidium sp.* and *G. lamblia* cause chronic diarrhea and sclerosing cholangitis associated with cryptosporidia is common.

COMMON VARIABLE IMMUNODEFICIENCY (CVID)

- Patients with CVID present with recurrent bacterial sinopulmonary infections, as seen in XLA, which are often complicated by bronchiectasis.
- Chronic *Giardia lamblia* infections may cause chronic diarrhea.
- Mycoplasma infections of the genitourinary tract, joints, and respiratory tract may be seen.
- Enteroviral infections may result in chronic meningoencephalitis or dermatomyositis-like syndromes albeit less commonly than in XLA.
- CVID patients with hepatitis C infection are more likely to progress to cirrhosis and other chronic complications.

SEVERE COMBINED IMMUNODEFICIENCY (SCID)

- These patients almost always manifest in early infancy with recurrent or prolonged severe viral, fungal, or protozoan infections.
- Rotavirus, adenovirus, or enterovirus may cause chronic diarrhea and failure to thrive.
- Protracted organ-specific infections (lung, CNS, and liver) may be due to adenovirus, parainfluenza, and influenza or herpesviruses (CMV, HSV, Epstein-Barr virus [EBV]).
- These patients are at a greatly increased risk of acquiring vaccine-strain disease from live-virus vaccines.
- Chronic severe mucocutaneous candidiasis or PCP are common presenting symptoms of this disease.
- These patients also develop severe infections with intracellular bacterial pathogens such as *Listeria, Mycobacteria,* and *Salmonella* in addition to gram-negative infections.
- After 6 months of age, when maternally-derived IgG has decayed, systemic infections with encapsulated bacteria become more prominent.
- Because all arms of the immune system are affected, multiple pathogens may simultaneously cause disease and aggressive diagnostic measures such as tissue biopsy (especially lung biopsy for pneumonia) should be considered.

TERMINAL COMPLEMENT (C7-C9) DEFICIENCY

- These patients have a predilection for systemic *Neis-seria* sp. infections including bacteremia, meningitis, and disseminated arthritis. Patients should receive a third-generation cephalosporin for empiric therapy of sepsis or meningitis and meningococcal vaccine should be given after diagnosis is established.

CHRONIC GRANULOMATOUS DISEASE (CGD)

- Patients with CGD have an increased susceptibility to smoldering granulomatous infections, especially abscesses, caused by catalase-positive organisms such as *S. aureus, Serratia marcescens, Burkolderia cepacia, Candida* spp., *Aspergillus* spp., and *Nocardia* spp. The organs most frequently involved are the liver, lymph nodes, lungs, and bones. Incision and drainage or biopsy of the site of infection is important to isolate an organism and to initiate specific anti-infective therapy. Prolonged treatment using agents with efficient tissue penetration is required for cure of infections.

BIBLIOGRAPHY

Adderson EE, Shackelford PG. *Infectious Complications of Antibody Deficiency. Principles and Practice of Pediatric Infectious Diseases*, 2nd ed. Philadelphia, PA: Churchill Livingstone, 2003.

Pizzo P. Fever in immunocompromised patients. *N Engl J Med* 1999;341(12):893.

Shenep JL, Flynn PM. Pulmonary fungal infections in immunocompromised children. *Curr Opin Pediatr* 1997;9:213.

Soldatou A, Davies EG. Respiratory virus infections in the immunocompromised host. *Paediatr Respir Rev* 2003;4:193.

Yogev R, Chadwick EG. *Acquired Immunodeficiency Syndrome (Human Immunodeficiency Virus). Nelson Textbook of Pediatrics*, 17th ed. Philadelphia, PA: W.B. Saunders, 2004.

116 OTHER INFECTIOUS DISEASES

A. Todd Davis and Stanford T. Shulman

KAWASAKI DISEASE

EPIDEMIOLOGY AND CLINICAL MANIFESTATIONS

- Kawasaki disease (KD) was described by T. Kawasaki, a Japanese pediatrician, in 1967. Potentially fatal coronary artery abnormalities were recognized shortly thereafter to be a complication. This illness classically is characterized by fever for ≥5 days with at least 4 of 5 major clinical features: (1) bilateral nonpurulent conjunctival injection, (2) rash, primarily truncal, of many forms but not vesiculobullous, (3) injected lips and oral mucosae, (4) swollen, erythematous hands and feet with later periungual desquamation, and (5) unilateral nonsuppurative cervical lymphadenopathy (≥1.5 cm diameter).
- The etiology of KD is unknown, but clinical and epidemiologic features strongly suggest an infectious cause. One hypothesis is that a ubiquitous respiratory agent triggers an unusual IgA plasma cell response that leads to vasculitis.
- Median age is 18–24 months, with 80% <5 years old. Rarely teenagers can develop this illness. Male:female ratio is 3:2. Untreated, 20–25% develop coronary artery abnormalities, with greatest risk in children (especially boys) <1 year of age and perhaps in older patients (>8 years). The highest attack rate (cases/100,000 children <5 years old per year) occurs in Asian children although in areas with large majorities of non-Asian children, the large majority of KD patients are non-Asian.
- Atypical or incomplete KD refers to patients who do not develop at least four major features but who are at risk for coronary complications. This poses difficult diagnostic and treatment dilemmas.

LABORATORY FINDINGS

- Laboratory findings in acute KD include elevated acute phase reactants (white blood cell [WBC], sedimentation rate, and C-reactive protein), sterile pyuria, late thrombocytosis, and echocardiographic findings. In the first 8–10 days of illness, pericardial effusion or mitral regurgitation may be apparent, while later echocardiograms may show evidence of coronary artery enlargement or aneurysm formation.

TREATMENT

- KD patients ideally should be treated by the 10th illness day with intravenous immunoglobulin (IVIG) at 2 g/kg over 10–12 hours and high-dose aspirin (80–100 mg/kg/day in four divided doses). The latter is continued until the 14th illness day and the patient has been afebrile for at least 3 days, then is decreased to 3–5 mg/kg/day as a single daily dose. Patients who remain febrile or have recurrent fevers 48 hours or more after IVIG treatment may require a second dose of 2 g/kg IVIG. Pulse corticosteroids is another treatment option, which some prefer, rather than repeat IVIG.
- Echocardiographic evaluation at baseline, about 2 weeks and 2 months later is necessary to detect the appearance of coronary abnormalities. If they develop, patients are maintained on low-dose aspirin (3–5 mg/kg/day) at least until the abnormalities resolve. Those with persistent abnormalities should continue aspirin and have periodic echocardiographic monitoring. Patients with more severe abnormalities are generally maintained on coumadin as well.
- A small number of patients with early coronary changes may develop stenotic coronary changes and ultimately ischemia after several years that may necessitate intervention (angioplasty, coronary bypass grafting, or even transplantation).

TOXOPLASMOSIS

EPIDEMIOLOGY

- Toxoplasmosis, caused by the protozoan parasite *Toxoplasma gondii* is universally found with no particular geographic boundaries and infects most species of mammals.
- The organism is most clearly identified in cat feces and excreted eggs become infectious after 3 days.
- Humans become infected through consuming raw or undercooked meat that contains cysts or by accidental ingestion of sporulated oocysts from soil or contaminated food.

- Congenital infection may occur as the result of primary maternal infection during gestation.

CLINICAL MANIFESTATIONS

- There are a wide range of clinical manifestations associated with infection with *T. gondii*. The majority of the infections are asymptomatic. Symptoms of clinically apparent cases mimic a mononucleosis-like illness with fever, malaise, sore throat, myalgia, lymphadenopathy (especially in the cervical region), and a mild hepatitis. The clinical course is usually benign and self-limited.
- Infants with congenital infection are asymptomatic at birth in up to 90% of cases; however, learning disabilities, mental retardation, and visual impairment develop in a large portion of these cases months to years later.

DIAGNOSIS

- Serology (*T. gondii* specific antibodies) is the primary means of diagnosis and should be sent to laboratories with a special expertise in toxoplasma serologic assays and their interpretation. IgM specific antibodies can be detected 2 weeks after infection and achieve peak concentrations in 1 month.

TREATMENT

- Except for the immunocompromised population, people who acquire toxoplasmosis rarely become ill enough to require treatment. Treatment, when indicated, consists of a combination of pyrimethamine and sulfadiazine.

ZOONOSES

- Zoonoses are diseases usually found in nonhuman animals that may spill over into the human population. Diseases in this group include anthrax, borreliosis (relapsing fever), brucellosis, cat-scratch disease, hantavirus, lyme disease, plague, psittacosis, trichinosis, tularemia, and yellow fever.

ANTHRAX

EPIDEMIOLOGY

- Anthrax is caused by the bacteria, *Bacillus anthracis*, and occurs in many rural regions of the world. It has three clinical forms: cutaneous, inhalational, and gastrointestinal. The clinical presentation depends on where the spores are deposited and the size of the spores.
- Infection in humans occurs through contact with infected animals or contaminated animal products e.g., carcasses, hides, hair, wool, meat, and bone meal.

CLINICAL PRESENTATION

- Cutaneous infection begins as a small painless papule or vesicle that goes on to ulcerate and crust over with the formation of a black eschar. There is usually surrounding edema, erythema, and regional lymphadenopathy; however, patients may also develop fever, malaise, and headache.
- Inhalational anthrax is the most lethal form of disease. It begins with fever, chills, nonproductive cough, chest pain, headache, and myalgias. This progresses over the next 2–5 days to a hemorrhagic mediastinal lymphadenitis, hemorrhagic pleural effusion, and bacteremia leading to severe dyspnea, hypoxia, and septic shock.
- Gastrointestinal tract disease may present in two different ways: (1) intestinal and (2) oropharyngeal. Patients with intestinal disease have symptoms of nausea, vomiting, and fever which progresses to severe abdominal pain, ascites, hematemesis, and bloody diarrhea. In oropharyngeal anthrax, patients develop unilateral posterior oropharyngeal ulcers, neck swelling, regional adenopathy, and sepsis.
- Mortality can exceed 50% for both inhalational and gastrointestinal disease.

DIAGNOSIS

- Gram stain and culture should be done on specimens of blood, pleural fluid, cerebrospinal fluid (CSF), and tissue or discharge from cutaneous lesions.
- Additional tests that may be used include immunohistochemistry, real-time polymerase chain reaction (PCR), and an enzyme immunoassay that measures IgG antibodies against *B. anthracis* protective antigen. All are performed at the Centers for Disease Control and Prevention (CDC).

TREATMENT

- Several antibiotics seem to be effective for treatment and include penicillins, macrolides, tetracyclines, and the fluoroquinolones. Multidrug regimens are needed for treating inhalational anthrax, gastrointestinal anthrax, anthrax meningitis, or cutaneous anthrax with systemic signs.

BORRELIOSUS (RELAPSING FEVER)

EPIDEMIOLOGY

- Relapsing fever is caused by spirochetes of the genus *Borrelia*, which are carried worldwide in either ticks or lice.
- In the United States, *Borrelia hermsii* is the most common etiologic agent of borreliosis with ticks being the most common vectors; rodents are the carrying agents. Infections typically result from tick

exposures in rodent-infested mountain cabins in state and national parks or in rodent-infested caves.

CLINICAL CHARACTERISTICS

- Relapsing fever is characterized by the sudden onset of high fever, headache, shaking chills, muscle and joint pains, and progressive weakness. The initial febrile period of borreliosis generally lasts 3–7 days. This episode is followed by an afebrile period of several days to weeks. One or more episodes of fever may recur 5–10 days after the initial febrile period abates.
- Relapses generally become progressively shorter and milder as the afebrile periods lengthen.

DIAGNOSIS

- Dark-field microscopy can be used to observe the presence of spirochetes. Wright, Giemsa, or acridine orange-stained preparations of thin or thick smears of peripheral blood or stained buffy-coat preparations may also be used.
- Spirochetes may also be cultured from blood in special media or by intraperitoneal inoculation of immature laboratory mice.
- Serum antibodies to *Borrelia* species can be detected by enzyme immunoassay and Western immunoblot analysis.

TREATMENT

- Antibiotics such as tetracycline, penicillin, doxycycline, and erythromycin are effective in preventing relapses and in clearing the spirochetes.

BRUCELLOSIS

EPIDEMIOLOGY

- Brucellosis is caused by a variety of *Brucella* species which are gram-negative coccobacilli. The species that infect humans are *Brucella abortis, Brucella melitensis, Brucella suis,* and *Brucella canis.*
- These organisms are dispersed worldwide. Humans are accidental hosts, contracting the disease by direct contact with infected animals and their carcasses or secretions or by ingesting unpasteurized milk or milk products.
- Infections occur by inoculation through breaks in the skin, by inhalation of organisms, by contact with the conjunctival mucosa, or by oral ingestion.

CLINICAL PRESENTATION

- The onset of disease can be acute or insidious. The symptoms are nonspecific including lethargy, weight loss, weakness, fever, arthralgia, myalgia, abdominal pain, night sweats, headache, and hepatosplenomegaly.

- Complications of infection include meningitis, endocarditis, and osteomyelitis.

DIAGNOSIS

- Definitive diagnosis is a positive *Brucella* culture of blood, bone marrow, or other tissues. Cultures must be incubated for a minimum of 4 weeks.
- Serologic testing can also confirm the diagnosis with a fourfold or greater increase in antibody titers in serum specimens collected at least 2 weeks apart.

TREATMENT

- Prolonged antibiotic therapy (4–6 weeks) is necessary to achieve a cure. Shortened durations of therapy are associated with relapses of the disease.
- Doxycycline, tetracycline, and trimethoprim sulfamethoxazole are the drugs of choice; however, combination therapy, with rifampin or gentamicin, is recommended in order to decrease the incidence of relapse and for treatment of serious infection or complications.

CAT-SCRATCH DISEASE

EPIDEMIOLOGY

- Cats are the reservoir for human disease, with most disease typically associated with bacteremia in young kittens. Infection may occur through a bite, scratch, or lick from an infected animal.
- The causative organism of cat-scratch disease is *Bartonella henselae.*

CLINICAL MANIFESTATIONS

- The major manifestation of cat-scratch disease is chronic regional lymphadenopathy. The illness begins as fluid-filled papule at the site of the bite, often associated with regional lymphadenopathy. The skin overlying the affected lymph nodes is tender, warm, erythematous, and indurated and in 30% of cases the affected nodes suppurate.
- Occasionally infection can produce Parinaud oculoglandular syndrome in which inoculation of the conjunctiva results in ipsilateral preauricular or submandibular lymphadenopathy.
- Other less common presentations include aseptic meningitis, encephalitis, hepatitis, granulomata in the liver and spleen, osteolytic bone lesions, pneumonia, and thrombocytopenia purpura.

DIAGNOSIS

- Indirect immunofluorescence antibody assay (IFA) for detection of serum antibodies to antigens of *Bartonella* species is useful in diagnosis.

- If tissue specimens are available, bacilli may be visualized using Warthin-Starry silver stain.
- PCR assays are also available.

TREATMENT
- Disease is usually self-limited and management is symptomatic and supportive.
- Trimethoprim-sulfamethoxazole, rifampin, azithromycin, ciprofloxacin, and gentamicin have been shown to be effective in the treatment of severely ill patients with systemic disease, especially for persons with hepatic or splenic involvement.

HANTAVIRUS

EPIDEMIOLOGY
- Hantavirus infections are caused by viruses in the Bunyaviridae family. Rodents are the natural hosts of the hantavirus. Most commonly, transmission to humans occurs through direct contact between humans and infected rodents, their droppings or nests, or inhalation of aerosolized virus particles from rodent urine, droppings, or saliva. Cases tend to be sporadic, with most occurring during the spring and summer.
- The usual reservoir appears to be the deer mouse, with most cases in the United States occurring in the Four Corners area of the southwest.

CLINICAL MANIFESTATIONS
- Hantavirus infections in humans cause hantavirus pulmonary syndrome (HPS) or hemorrhagic fever with renal syndrome (HFRS).
- The prodrome of HPS is 3–7 days and is characterized by fever, chills, headache, myalgias, nausea, vomiting, diarrhea, and dizziness. This is followed by the abrupt development of pulmonary edema and severe hypoxemia which may be associated with myocardial dysfunction, persistent hypotension, and septic shock. Intubation and assisted ventilation are commonly required.

DIAGNOSIS
- Immunohistochemical staining of capillary endothelial cells may identify the virus.
- Serology for hantavirus-specific immunoglobulin IgG and IgM antibodies and reverse transcriptase PCR of peripheral blood mononuclear cells and other clinical specimens may aid in the diagnosis.

TREATMENT
- Supportive. If given early in the illness, intravenous ribavirin has been shown to decrease morbidity and mortality.

LYME DISEASE (SEE SECTION 1, BACTERIAL INFECTIONS, #19)

PLAGUE

EPIDEMIOLOGY
- Plague is an infection whose reservoir includes rodents, carnivores, and their fleas occurring in many areas of the world. In the United States most cases are seen in rural areas of the western United States and are associated with ground squirrels, prairie dogs, and other wild rodents. The causative organism is *Yersinia pestis*, a pleomorphic, gram-negative coccobacillus.
- Bubonic plague usually is transmitted by bites of infected rodent fleas. Septicemic plague occurs as a complication of bubonic plague but may also result from direct contact with infectious materials or the bite of an infected flea. Primary pneumonic plague is acquired by inhalation of respiratory droplets from a human or animal with respiratory plague. Secondary pneumonic plague occurs from hematogenous seeding of the lungs with *Y. pestis* in patients with bubonic or septicemic plague.

CLINICAL MANIFESTATIONS
- After an incubation period of 2–6 days, patients experience the sudden onset of fever, chills, headache, and rapidly progressive weakness. Additional manifestations depend on the type of plague.
- The bubonic form is the most common manifestation with the acute onset of fever and painful swollen regional lymph nodes (buboes), especially in the inguinal region.
- Septicemic plague also presents with hypotension, acute respiratory distress, and disseminated intravascular coagulation (DIC).
- Pneumonic plague also presents with cough, fever, dyspnea, and hemoptysis.

DIAGNOSIS
- Isolation of organism in culture from affected tissues, especially lymph nodes, spleen, and liver.
- Fluorescent antibody test for the presence of *Y. pestis* in direct smears and cultures of a bulbo aspirate, sputum, CSF, or blood.
- Single serologic test result by passive hemaglutination assay or enzyme immunoassay in an unimmunized patient.

TREATMENT
- Streptomycin or gentamicin is the drug of choice. Alternative agents include doxycycline or tetracycline.

PSITTACOSIS

EPIDEMIOLOGY

- Psittacosis is worldwide in distribution; however, infection is rare in children.
- In the United States, birds (parakeets, parrots, and macaws, especially those imported into this country, pigeons and turkeys) are the major reservoir for the psittacosis causing bacteria, *Chlamydia psittaci*. Transmission of the organism is via the airborne route in fecal dust or secretions. Persons in close proximity to infected birds are at the highest risk of infections, especially workers at poultry slaughter plants, poultry farms, pet shops, pet owners, and laboratory workers.

CLINICAL MANIFESTATIONS

- The most common symptoms are a pronounced nonproductive cough, high fever, chills, malaise, and headache.
- An extensive interstitial pneumonia may be present on chest radiograph with changes more severe than what would be expected on physical examination findings.

DIAGNOSIS

- Serologic testing with a fourfold increase in antibody titer by complement fixation testing between acute and convalescent specimens obtained 2–3 weeks apart or a single titer of 1:32 or greater.

TREATMENT

- Tetracyclines are the drugs of choice. Other agents that may be used include erythromycin and the macrolide agents.

TRICHINOSIS

EPIDEMIOLOGY

- Infection is caused by nematodes (roundworms) of the genus *Trichinella* with *Trichinella spiralis* being the most common species to cause human infection worldwide.
- Infection occurs through ingestion of raw or undercooked meat from infected animals containing encysted larvae. The most common source of infection is pork, but horse meat and wild carnivorous game can also be sources.
- Trichinosis is a self-limiting condition that is often undiagnosed but may also be fatal.

CLINICAL MANIFESTATIONS

- The clinical spectrum of disease ranges from inapparent to fulminant and fatal with the severity of illness proportional to the infective dose. The majority of infections are inapparent.
- Symptoms proceed in stages as the larvae move through the small intestine and into muscle. The symptoms begin as fever, diarrhea, nausea, vomiting, and abdominal pain, and generally terminate as fever, muscle pain, periorbital edema, and urticarial rash.
- In severe infections, myocarditis, neurologic involvement, and pneumonitis may occur.

DIAGNOSIS

- Eosinophilia approaching 70% in conjunction with compatible history and symptoms is highly suggestive of the diagnosis.
- Visualization of encapsulated larvae in skeletal muscle biopsy specimen.
- Serologic titers.

TREATMENT

- Recommended treatment usually involves coadministration of corticosteroids and mebendazole or albendazole.

TULAREMIA

EPIDEMIOLOGY

- Tularemia is a bacterial disease caused by a gram-negative, pleomorphic coccobacillus, *Francisella tularensis*.
- The reservoir for the organism is very large and includes over 100 species of wild mammals and domestic animals. In the United States, rabbits and rodents are the major reservoir with fleas, deer flies, and ticks serving as vectors for infection.
- Persons at the greatest risk for infection are those with occupational or recreational exposure to infected animals or their habitats.

CLINICAL PRESENTATION

- A few days after infection, patients usually develop the abrupt onset of fever, chills, myalgia, and headache. Other symptoms depend on the type of tularemic syndrome the patient has.
- Ulceroglandular syndrome is the most common and is characterized by a painful, maculopapular lesion at site of infection. The papule enlarges and subsequently ulcerates with associated painful regional lymphadenopathy which may drain.
- Glandular syndrome is characterized by regional lymphadenopathy with no ulceration.
- Less common syndromes are oculoglandular, in which there is the presence of severe conjunctivitis and preauricular lymphadenopathy; oropharyngeal,

which is characterized by severe exudative stomatitis, pharyngitis, or tonsillitis and cervical lymphadenopathy; typhoidal, in which there is high fever and hepatosplenomegaly; intestinal, in which there is intestinal pain, vomiting, and diarrhea; and pneumonic characterized by primary pulmonary disease.

DIAGNOSIS

- Diagnosis is made most often by serologic testing using a single serum antibody titer of ≥1:128 determined by microagglutination or of ≥1:160 determined by tube agglutination.
- Can also make the diagnosis by culturing the organism from specimens of blood, skin, ulcers, lymph node drainage, gastric washings, or respiratory secretions.

TREATMENT

- Gentamicin or amikacin are the recommended agents for the treatment of tularemia. Duration of therapy is 10 days or more depending on severity of illness. Alternative agents for treatment include imipenem-cilastatin, doxycycline, and ciprofloxacin.

YELLOW FEVER

EPIDEMIOLOGY

- Yellow fever is an arboviral disease that is caused by a virus that belongs to the family Flaviviridae and is limited to Africa and South America.
- Mosquitoes are both the reservoir and the vector for the disease.

CLINICAL MANIFESTATIONS

- Disease begins with a nonspecific febrile illness with headache, malaise, weakness, nausea, and vomiting and progresses to a hemorrhagic fever with gastrointestinal tract bleeding and hematemesis, jaundice, hemorrhage, cardiovascular instability, myocarditis, and renal dysfunction.

DIAGNOSIS

- Definitive diagnosis is made by serologic testing of CSF or serum or by viral isolation.

TREATMENT

- Supportive. No specific treatment exists; illness resolves itself without difficulty.
- Travelers can be fully protected by immunization.

BIBLIOGRAPHY

Lynfield R, Guerina NG. Toxoplasmosis. *Pediatr Rev* 1997; 18:75–83.

Rowley AH, Shulman ST. Kawasaki syndrome. *Pediatr Clin North Am* 1999;46:313–329.

Weinberg AN. Ecology and epidemiology of zoonotic pathogens. *Infect Dis Clin North Am* 1991;5:1–6.

Section 15
DISEASES OF THE KIDNEY, URETERS, AND BLADDER

Craig B. Langman, Section Editor

117 KIDNEY EMERGENCIES
Craig B. Langman

ACUTE KIDNEY FAILURE

- Heralded by *symptoms* that may include fever, lethargy, malaise, pallor, swelling, reduced urine production (oliguria), abdominal pain, skin rashes, pinpoint, or diffuse bleeding in the skin; by *signs* that may include the following:
  1. Edema (if generalized, termed anasarca)
  2. Gross or microscopic hematuria
  3. Hypertension
  4. Congestive heart failure
  5. Pulmonary edema
  6. Purpuric or other types of skin rashes
- By laboratory abnormalities that may include the following:
  1. Proteinuria (dipstick examination ≥ 100 mg/dL Urinary protein/creatinine ratio ≥ 0.6)
  2. Hematuria
  3. Pyuria
  4. Crystalluria
  5. Bacteriuria
  6. Azotemia
  7. Hyperkalemia
  8. Hypocalcemia
  9. Hyperphosphatemia
  10. Metabolic acidosis
  11. Hypocomplementemia (C_3 and/or C_4)
  12. (+) Serologies for systemic lupus erythematosus, (+) antineutrophilic cytoplasmic antibody (ANCA) titer, anemia, and thrombocytopenia.

DIFFERENTIAL DIAGNOSIS

- Acute glomerular disease; acute tubulointerstitial disease; acute urinary obstruction.

ABCs OF ACUTE KIDNEY FAILURE

- *A*void fluid overload, hyperkalemia, dietary excesses of protein, potassium, phosphate, and nephrotoxic drugs or agents.
- *B*egin immediate diagnostic evaluation with urine, blood studies; electrocardiogram (ECG) and/or echocardiogram; kidney imaging studies.
- *C*onsider need for diagnostic kidney biopsy, acute dialysis, or more conservative treatments of hypertension, hyperkalemia, and deranged metabolic milieu; relief of urinary obstruction.

ACUTE URINARY OBSTRUCTION

- Heralded by *symptoms* that may include the following:
  1. Intense generalized or lower abdominal pain
  2. Dysuria
  3. Urinary frequency
  4. Hesitancy in urination
  5. Fever
  6. Unilateral or bilateral flank pain
- By *signs* that may include any of those for acute kidney failure
- By *laboratory abnormalities* that may include any of those for acute kidney failure.
- The hallmark of acute urinary obstruction is the *radiographic demonstration* of unilateral or bilateral obstruction to urinary flow at the level of the kidneys;

439

bladder outlet obstruction; or more rarely, urethral blockages.

DIFFERENTIAL DIAGNOSIS

- Nephrolithiasis
- Anatomic abnormalities intrinsic to the genitourinary system
- Retroperitoneal masses that prevent urinary flow.

ABCs OF ACUTE URINARY OBSTRUCTION

- *Address* the level of obstruction by obtaining minimally invasive radiographic demonstration.
- *Begin* an orderly plan for relief of the obstruction that generally includes placement of a Foley catheter in the bladder.
- *Consider* the consequences of the relief of obstruction, such as postobstruction diuresis (glomerular-tubular imbalance) with multiple metabolic effects.

HYPERKALEMIA

- Heralded often by the surprising *lack of symptoms*.
  1. *Signs* are generally limited to the cardiovascular effects on conduction times with production of arrhythmias, congestive heart failure, and if present, condition is termed "malignant hyperkalemia."
  2. *Laboratory sign* generally reflects an elevation of serum potassium concentration ≥6 mEq/mL, but sudden rises from lower to higher values may reproduce the cardiac effects.
  3. *Diagnostic finding* of abnormal ECG with peaked T waves in the precordial leads, bizarre QRS complexes with worsening hyperkalemia, leading to eventual ventricular tachycardia and asystole.

DIFFERENTIAL DIAGNOSIS

- Any cause of acute kidney failure can lead to malignant hyperkalemia; tumor lysis syndrome without acute kidney failure; intravenous infusion of excess potassium salts in an otherwise healthy individual can produce malignant hyperkalemia too.

ABCs OF HYPERKALEMIA

- *Albuterol* nebulization immediately to move potassium intracellularly by β-sympathomimetic receptor activation

- *Begin* consideration of Kayexylate exchange resin therapy, calcium infusion, glucose + insulin infusion to stabilize myocardium, and reduce serum potassium levels.
- *Cardiac monitoring* and *Consider* need for acute dialysis for removal of potassium.

HYPERTENSIVE CRISIS

- Sudden or sustained elevations in systemic blood pressure may produce clinical manifestations that are termed "accelerated" if associated with modest organ dysfunction or "malignant" if organ dysfunction is more severe.
- *Symptoms* may include intense headache, photophobia, epistaxis, chest pains typical for coronary artery insufficiency, abdominal pain, facial flushing, tachycardia, palpitations, seizures, coma, loss of central vision or total vision bilaterally, or others related to the setting of causes of acute kidney failure.
- *Signs* may include altered levels of consciousness (low Glasgow coma score), visual field defects, retinal hemorrhages, alteration of retinal blood vessels caliber and course (tortuosity), arrhythmias, congestive heart failure, pronounced tachycardia, in addition to the other signs of acute kidney failure.

DIFFERENTIAL DIAGNOSIS

- Renovascular hypertension from intrinsic or extrinsic compression of the renal artery unilaterally or bilaterally.
- Acute kidney failure.
- End-stage kidney disease.
- Acute intoxications with xenobiotics.
- Excess circulating catecholamines or catecholamine-like agents, such as in pheochromocytoma, neuroblastoma, carcinoid syndrome, VIP-omas, and licorice overdose.
- Malignant hyperthermia syndrome, in response to general anesthetics.
- Rarely, malignant hypertension may be the presenting feature of primary intracranial pathology or severe hypercalcemia.

ABCs OF MALIGNANT HYPERTENSION

- *Always* lower the blood pressure in a graded, monitored manner with infusional agents such as nicardipine, nitroprusside, or others.

- *Begin* a careful assessment of the likely cause, and if pheochromocytoma is a high likelihood, consider use of α-antagonist as primary therapy, *but* otherwise, move to conventional therapies with beta-blockade, calcium-channel blockers, and peripheral vasodilators.
- *Consider* not using angiotension-converting enzyme inhibitors and angiotension-receptor blockers until kidney function and serum potassium levels are known.

RENAL COLIC

- *Symptoms* of intense, writhing abdominal, flank, groin, or testicular pain are most common, and may be associated with nausea, emesis, and fever.
- *Signs* are uncommonly few, and may relate to those for acute kidney failure.
- *Laboratory manifestations* generally reveal an abnormal urinalysis with hematuria, pyuria, crystalluria, or others of acute urinary obstruction and acute kidney failure.
- *Diagnostic imaging* generally reveals evidence of urinary obstruction, either intrinsic to the urinary tract (nephrolithiasis) or extrinsic to it (mass lesion effect). Common modalities of imaging include ultrasound of the abdomen and urinary tract, computed tomography (CT) scan with or without contrast agent.

DIFFERENTIAL DIAGNOSIS

- Nephrolithiasis of any cause. Retroperitoneal masses from any cause. Rarely, extensive tumor lysis (or uric acid *sludge* in a severely catabolic, febrile young child).

ABCs OF RENAL COLIC

- In addition to those for *Acute* urinary obstruction, provide *Ample* pain relief with opiates such as morphine.
- *Begin* vigorous parenteral hydration, without potassium, if unilateral stone is found as cause of renal colic.
- *Catch* a calculus by straining all urine through a tea-strainer, and send it for *crystallographic* (not chemical) analysis. *Consider* removal of offending calculus by percutaneous means such as extracorporeal shock-wave lithotripsy or other procedures. *Counsel* the patient and family to have an appropriate diagnostic evaluation of a stone in the urinary tract after the acute episode.

118 COMMON COMPLAINT REFERABLE TO THE KIDNEY AND UROLOGIC SYSTEMS

Craig B. Langman

- *Hematuria*: Defined by finding ≥5 red blood cells per high-power field in a microscopic examination of the urine. Often coincides with a (+) urine dipstick for blood.
- *Proteinuria*: Defined as finding a random urine protein to creatinine ratio, expressed in the same units as ≥0.3 or a random urine dipstick finding of ≥30 mg/dL, or finding in a 24-hour urine excretion of ≥ 4 mg/m² body surface area/hour. Nephrotic range proteinuria is >40 mg/m²/h BSA.
- *Recurrent urinary tract infection*: Defined by having two or more, time-separated, urinary infections in a calendar year.
- *Hypertension*: Defined by having a systolic and/or diastolic blood pressure ≥95th percentile for age and body mass.
- *Think of kidney diseases with these other complaints: Growth failure (short stature), metabolic acidosis, rickets, anemia, seizures, and the presence of other congenital anomalies or syndromes.*

119 GLOMERULAR DISEASE

Richard A. Cohn and
H. William Schnaper

- The onset of most glomerular disorders is usually heralded by a child developing edema or gross hematuria. Occasionally, however, proteinuria is first noted on a routine urinalysis. It is often useful to classify glomerular diseases into those that typically cause nephrotic syndrome and those that usually do not do so keeping in mind that significant overlap exists.
- Table 119-1 lists those glomerular disorders *with* nephrotic syndrome as a feature, as defined by heavy proteinuria, hypoalbuminemia, hyperlipidemia, and peripheral edema. Within the category of primary kidney disorders, *minimal change nephrotic syndrome* is by far the most common. Its onset is usually between

TABLE 119-1 Glomerular Disorders That Usually Present with Nephrotic Syndrome

Minimal change disease (lipoid nephrosis)
Focal segmental glomerulosclerosis
Mesangial IgM nephropathy
Diffuse mesangial proliferation
Congenital nephrotic syndrome
Membranoproliferative glomerulonephritis
Membranous nephropathy
HIV nephropathy

ages 1 and 8. Kidney function, blood pressure, and C_3 complement levels are normal. Microscopic hematuria may be noted. Response to corticosteroids occurs within 3 weeks in the majority of children who then may continue a relapsing/remitting course for 5–10 years, usually followed by a permanent remission. Potentially serious complications include infections (peritonitis, pneumonia, bacteremia, and meningitis) as well as vascular thromboses. For children with frequent relapses (20–25% of cases) or the minority who do not respond to steroids, other medications that may be useful include cyclophosphamide, cyclosporine, tacrolimus, and mycophenolate mofetil. The cause of minimal change nephrotic syndrome is unknown.

- *Focal segmental glomerular sclerosis* (FSGS) is the second most common glomerular disorder with nephrotic syndrome. Patients with FSGS rarely respond to steroids but may improve with cyclosporine, tacrolimus, cyclophosphamide, or mycophenolate mofetil. Untreated, most children progress from having normal kidney function to end-stage kidney disease and require transplantation. Unfortunately, the condition may recur after transplantation as well, but unlike the disease in native kidneys, it may remit after a course of intensive plasmapheresis.
- *Membranoproliferative glomerulonephritis* (MPGN) *and membranous glomerulonephropathy* (MGN) often present with nephrotic-range proteinuria, often with overt nephrotic syndrome. MPGN may present with or without hematuria and is usually accompanied by profound hypocomplementemia. There are three subtypes of MPGN, each distinguished by kidney biopsy. Treatment with alternate day corticosteroids is often of benefit, particularly when started early in the course of the disease. MGN is uncommon in children and may accompany hepatitis B infection, systemic lupus erythematosus (SLE), or neonatal syphilis. As an idiopathic glomerular disorder, it is often treated with long-term, alternate-day steroids with benefit. Immunosuppressive agents also have been reported to be effective, although no prospective clinical trials have established the efficacy of either treatment in the pediatric age range.

- *Diffuse mesangial proliferative glomerulonephritis* is often diagnosed on kidney biopsy after a nephrotic child remains with unremitting proteinuria after the initial 4–6 weeks of prednisone treatment. The course and prognosis vary, with approximately one-third of children achieving remission with either steroids or other immunosuppressive medications, one-third remaining persistently proteinuric while maintaining excellent glomerular function, and one-third progressing to kidney failure.
- Nephrotic syndrome can accompany systemic childhood diseases as well. *Lupus nephritis* and the *nephritis of Henoch-Schonlein purpura* are the two most common diseases in this category. When accompanied by heavy proteinuria, the kidney biopsy findings are usually abnormal, with extensive glomerular crescents. Treatment of the underlying illness may improve the kidney disease but patients with the most damage on biopsy are the most likely to progress to end-stage kidney disease with the need for transplantation.
- Diseases that less commonly present with nephrotic syndrome include *human immunodeficiency virus (HIV) nephropathy, nephropathy of epithelial cello (solid-organ) malignancies, Hodgkin disease,* and *systemic vasculitis.*
- *Congenital nephrotic syndrome* (CNS) is a rare, autosomal recessive disorder that presents at birth with massive proteinuria and anasarca. It occurs in many ethnic groups, but was first reported in Finland. The disorder results from mutations in the gene coding for nephrin (NPHS1), a transmembrane protein of the glomerular basement membrane. Most, but not all children, develop early kidney failure and require dialysis, bilateral nephrectomy, and kidney transplantation by age 5. Significant accompanying problems are poor nutrition, hypercoagulability, and hypothyroidism. Instead of a nephrin mutation, other children with a congenital form of nephrotic syndrome present with diffuse mesangial sclerosis. This condition is often associated with gonadal abnormalities when related to a mutation in the WT1 Wilms tumor gene.
- Glomerular diseases that present *without* nephrotic syndrome are listed in Table 119-2. These conditions

TABLE 119-2 Glomerular Disorders That Usually Present without Nephrotic Syndrome

IgA nephropathy
Henoch-Schonlein purpura nephritis
Rapidly progressive glomerulonephritis
Acute glomerulonephritis
Alport syndrome
Lupus nephritis

can be separated into ones with an acute presentation and others that are chronic disorders.

- *Acute glomerulonephritis* typically occurs after an acute, systemic viral or bacterial infection. Florid "textbook" cases present with the constellation of coca-cola colored urine, edema, hypertension, oliguria, and hypertension, all following an antecedent infection 10–21 days earlier. While group A beta-hemolytic streptococcus is the most common etiologic agent, other streptococci, Staphylococci, Pneumococcus, Mycoplasma, Leptospira, Meningococci, and viruses such as Varicella, Rubeola, CMV, Herpes simplex, and Epstein-Barr Virus have been reported to cause postinfectious glomerulonephritis. Blood levels of C_3 are very low at presentation in over 90% of cases and normalize within 6 weeks of diagnosis. Treatment is supportive and consists of sodium and water restriction, reduction of blood pressure, diuretics, and regulation of potassium, phosphorus, and acid-base homeostasis. The prognosis for full recovery is very high with almost all children experiencing resolution of proteinuria within 6 months and microscopic hematuria within 18–24 months of onset while maintaining normal kidney function. The few exceptions are children who experienced severe glomerular dysfunction at the onset with crescents on kidney biopsy and nephrotic-range proteinuria beyond 3 months.

- A hypocomplementemic glomerulonephritis can accompany *subacute bacterial endocarditis* and *ventriculoatrial shunt infection*. These nephropathies generally resolve with successful treatment of the underlying infection.

- *Idiopathic crescentic glomerulonephritis* is another acute glomerular disorder occasionally seen in children. Often an antineutrophil cytoplasmic antibody (ANCA) is found and may be useful in both diagnosis and assessing adequacy of treatment. Goodpasture syndrome (antiglomerular basement membrane antibody-mediated nephritis with pulmonary hemorrhage) is extremely rare in children.

- There are a number of chronic glomerular disorders. The most common of these is *IgA nephropathy*, which typically presents in a boy older than age 8 who develops recurrent episodes of gross hematuria coincident with upper respiratory or other nonspecific infections, most often with normal kidney function, blood pressure, and C_3 levels. The diagnosis is established by the presence of IgA antibody within the mesangium of glomeruli on immunofluorescence microscopy. Patients with minimal proteinuria, normal blood pressure, and normal kidney function generally do not progress to more serious kidney disease in childhood.

Definitive treatment of this condition has not been established though clinical trials in adults have suggested benefits from long-term use of omega-3 fish oils and ACE inhibitors.

- *Membranoproliferative glomerulonephritis and membranous glomerulonephropathy* may present without nephrotic syndrome. They are described in the section on glomerular disorders associated with nephrosis.

- *Alport syndrome* is a result of a mutation in the collagen gene responsible for the basement membrane of glomerulus, the cochlea, and the lens of the eye. Most often the mutation is in the alpha-5 chain of type IV collagen, coded on the X chromosome. These boys usually develop progressive glomerular dysfunction and a high-frequency, sensorineural hearing loss by late adolescence. They usually require kidney transplantation.

- Patients with *Henoch-Schonlein purpura* develop hematuria, proteinuria, or kidney dysfunction in approximately 25% of cases. While microscopic hematuria alone carries a favorable prognosis, this may not be the case when heavy proteinuria, hypertension, or kidney dysfunction is present. Kidney biopsy findings may help define the prognosis and best course of treatment, which may consist of steroids and other immunosuppressives.

- *Clinical assessment*: Children who present with a possible glomerular disorder should be differentiated with regard to whether they have hematuria and/or proteinuria.

- Isolated proteinuria greater than 500 mg/m^2/d, or proteinuria of 200 mg/m^2/d when accompanied by hematuria, suggest the presence of a significant glomerular lesion.

- In assessing the history, the physician should, in particular, determine whether the patient has had decreased urine output, headache (a potential sign of hypertension), an antecedent illness, or symptoms of inflammation such as rashes or arthritis.

- A family history of deafness should be sought.

- Physical examination should evaluate the patient for rashes or arthritis, edema, and most importantly for hypertension.

- Initial laboratory evaluation, in addition to urinalysis for blood, protein, and casts, should examine blood urea nitrogen, serum creatinine, serum complement levels, and antinuclear antibody.

- The finding of nephrotic symptoms, decreased renal function, abnormal serum electrolytes, or hypertension should lend some urgency to this referral.

- Referral to a pediatric nephrologist should be considered for any patient with suspected glomerular disease.

BIBLIOGRAPHY

Bhimma R, Coovadia HM, Kramvis A, Adhikari M, Kew MC, Connolly CA. HBV and proteinuria in relatives and contacts of children with hepatitis B virus-associated membranous nephropathy. *Kidney Int* 1999;55:2440–2449.

Braun MC, West CD, Strife CF. Differences between membranoproliferative glomerulonephritis types I and III in long-term response to an alternate-day prednisone regimen. *Am J Kidney Dis* 1999;34:1022–1032.

Niaudet P. Treatment of lupus nephritis in children. *Pediatr Nephrol* 2000;14:158–166.

O'Donoghue DJ, Lawler W, Hunt LP, Acheson EJ, Mallick NP. IgM-associated primary diffuse mesangial proliferative glomerulonephritis: natural history and prognostic indicators. *Q J Med* 1991;79:333–350.

Patrakka J, Kestila M, Wartiovaara J, Ruotsalainen V, Tissari P, Lenkkeri U, et al. Congenital nephrotic syndrome (NPHS1): features resulting from different mutations in Finnish patients. *Kidney Int* 2000;58:972–980.

Ray PE, Rakusan T, Loechelt BJ, Selby DM, Liu XH, Chandra RS. Human immunodeficiency virus (HIV)-associated nephropathy in children from the Washington, DC area: 12 years' experience. *Semin Nephrol* 1998;18–25.

Robson WL, Leung AK. Henoch-Schonlein purpura. *Adv Pediatr* 1994;41:163–194.

Schnaper HW. Focal segmental glomerulosclerosis. In: Neilson EG, Couser WG (eds.), *Immunologic Renal Disease*, 2nd ed. Philadelphia, PA: Lippincott Williams and Wilkins, 2001, pp. 1001–1027.

Schnaper HW, Robson AM. Nephrotic syndrome: minimal change disease, focal glomerulosclerosis, and related disorders. In: Schrier RW, Gottschalk CW (eds.), *Diseases of the Kidney and Urinary Tract*, 7th ed. Philadelphia, PA: Lippincott Williams and Wilkins, 2001, pp. 1773–1831.

120 ACUTE INTERSTITIAL NEPHRITIS

H. William Schnaper

OVERVIEW

- The term acute interstitial nephritis (AIN) refers to inflammation of nonglomerular and nonvascular elements of the renal parenchyma; that is, the tubules and interstitium. It is also referred to as acute tubulointerstitial nephritis. Normally tubules are closely packed with minimal intervening stromal elements. Mediators of inflammation (cytokines, chemoattractants) accompany cellular infiltration of the interstitium surrounding tubules in both the cortex and medulla. It is also

TABLE 120-1 Medications That Cause Acute Interstitial Nephritis

Penicillins
Cephalosporins
Sulfonamides
Quinolones
Thiazides
Furosemide
Allopurinol
Phenytoin
Rifampin

believed that nephrotoxic insults to tubular cells cause injured cells to release inflammatory mediators into the local interstitium, including chemoattractants that stimulate cellular infiltration.

- Acute interstitial nephritis usually presents as the insidious but rapid onset of acute kidney failure. Although it is not commonly encountered in children, when it does occur it is usually as a consequence of a hypersensitivity reaction to a medication; however, in a technical sense, invasive bacterial infection of the renal parenchyma (acute pyelonephritis) is also a form of AIN. Acute transplant rejection is also a form of acute tubulointerstitial nephritis.

ETIOLOGY

- Most instances of AIN encountered in pediatrics are due to immune-mediated acute hypersensitivity reactions to medications. The Table 120-1 lists medications implicated in hypersensitivity-induced AIN.

- The precise mechanisms of immune mediation are under study but are believed to involve both B-cell and T-cell mediated mechanisms. It is possible that an unusual conformational configuration of a ligand-receptor complex functions as a neoantigen triggering an immune reaction. Although mononuclear cells are prominent in the interstitial infiltrate, eosinophils are sometimes seen when AIN is associated with a hypersensitivity reaction to a medication.

CLINICAL PRESENTATION

- The prodrome and onset of overt illness are accompanied by nonspecific symptoms and recognition of impaired kidney function may be delayed. Typical symptoms include malaise, fatigability, nausea, emesis, rash, and fever.

DIAGNOSIS

- The presence of azotemia may be the first evidence of kidney involvement. Acute kidney failure may be either oliguric or nonoliguric. If the inflammatory process is especially active in the kidney medulla with disruption of the countercurrent multiplier mechanism, urine output may not be diminished and the urine concentration may be relatively dilute.

- The urine may not have striking findings although microscopic hematuria, sterile pyuria, and low-grade proteinuria are common; however, since the dipstick is not sensitive to low-molecular mass proteins, the presence of tubular proteinuria may go unrecognized. Subnephrotic-range proteinuria for pediatric-age patients is a random urine protein-creatinine ratio less than 0.5–2.0. AIN associated with a hypersensitivity reaction to nonsteroidal anti-inflammatory drug (NSAID) administration may be accompanied by nephrotic-range proteinuria. Examination of the sediment may reveal eosinophils if an appropriate cellular stain is used. A peripheral blood differential count may show eosinophilia. A definitive diagnosis is established by means of a kidney biopsy.

TREATMENT

- The usual management of acute kidney failure should be implemented, including dialysis if indicated. Prompt cessation of the offending medication will often be followed by rapid reversal of acute kidney failure. If resolution of impaired kidney function is delayed, a course of steroid treatment, for up to several weeks, is often used; however, there are no randomized controlled trials attesting to its efficacy.

121 PROXIMAL AND DISTAL TUBULAR DISEASE

Craig B. Langman

TUBULAR DISEASES

PROXIMAL TUBULE

- The proximal tubule of the kidney is responsible for bulk transport of fluid and all substances that enter after glomerular filtration. Failure of the proximal tubule may be restricted to the efficient movement of bicarbonate out of the urinary filtrate, and is termed proximal renal tubular acidosis (PRTA) (or type II). When the complete resorptive apparatus of the proximal tubule is inefficient, the term renal Fanconi syndrome is applied. The diseases of the proximal tubule may be genetic or acquired, and are listed in Table 121-1.

TABLE 121-1 Causes of Proximal Renal Tubular Acidosis

Primary

Sporadic
  Transient childhood
  Persisting (adult onset)
Genetically determined
  Primary PRTA
  Sporadic transient
  Genetic
    Autosomal dominant
    Autosomal recessive
  Isolated PRTA with mental retardation and occular and dental
    abnormalities
  Pyruvate carboxylase deficiency
  Mitochondrial myopathies
  Osteopetrosis with carbonic anhydrase deficiency
    Sporadic
    Genetic
  Drug-induced (acetazolamide, sulfanilamide, mafenide acetate)

Secondary

Hereditary multiple proximal tubular dysfunction, Fanconi syndrome
  Cystinosis
  Galactosemia
  Glycogen storage disease type 1
  Hereditary fructose intolerance (with fructose exposure)
  Tyrosinemia
  Wilson disease
  Heavy metals
  Drugs and toxins
  Carbonic anhydrase (CA) inhibitors
  6-Mercaptopurine
  Streptozotocin
  Iphosphamide
  Outdated tetracycline
  Sulfonamides
  Mafenide acetate
  Valproic acid
  Heavy metals (Cd, Pb, Hg)

Miscellaneous

- Amyloidosis
- Cyanotic congenital heart disease
- Fallot tetralogy
- Hereditary nephritis
- Hyperkalemia
- Multiple myeloma
- Nephrotic syndrome
- Renal cystic disease
- Renal transplant
- Renal vascular accident
- Sjögren syndrome

Referral to a pediatric kidney diseases specialist is required for confirmation of most cases of proximal tubular dysfunction, as the testing is specialized.

- The symptoms of chronic metabolic acidosis usually prevail, even in a Fanconi syndrome. Such symptoms may include anorexia, nausea, emesis, cachexia, muscle weakness, rickets, and linear growth failure. Signs include those associated with the symptoms listed above. The laboratory evaluation usually reveals a hypokalemic metabolic acidosis and any of the features that would be suggested by a systemic disease listed in the tables.

TABLE 121-2 Causes of Distal Renal Tubular Acidosis

Inability to secrete H+ (secretory defect)

Primary distal RTA (persistent classic syndrome)
  In infancy, associated HCO_3 wasting
  In adolescence, secondary hyperparathyroidism
  Nerve deafness develops in adolescence
  Transient infantile form
  Genetic
  Sporadic
  Endemic

Secondary distal RTA

  Disorders of calcium metabolism with nephrocalcinosis or
    hypercalciuria
  Primary hyperparathyroidism
  Hyperthyroidism
  Vitamin D intoxication
  Genetic
  Idiopathic hypercalciuria
  Hyperthyroidism (with nephrocalcinosis)
  MCD-FJN
  Hereditary fructose intolerance with fructose exposure

Associated with genetically transmitted disease

  CA type 2
  Erythrocyte CA B deficiency
  Ehlers-Danlos syndrome
  Hereditary elliptocytosis
  Marfan syndrome
  Sickle cell anemia
  Osteopetrosis (Type III RTA)

With associated deafness

  Carnitine palmitoyl transferase deficiency type 1

Autoimmune disorders

  Hypergammaglobulinemia
  Sjögren syndrome
  Chronic active hepatitis
  Primary biliary cirrhosis
  Thyroiditis
  Fibrosing alveolitis
  Systemic lupus erythematosis
  Polyarteritis nodosa
  Rheumatoid arthritis

Drug or toxin

  Amphotericin B
  Toluene
  Analgesic abuse
  Lithium
  Cyclamate
  Mercury

Associated with other renal diseases

  Obstructive uropathy
  Pyelonephritis
  Renal transplant rejection
  Sickle cell disease
  Leprosy

Associated with endocrine disease

  Hypothyroidism
  Salt-losing congenital adrenal hyperplasia

Functional RTA (exchange defect)

  Marked volume depletion
  Hyponatremic states (hepatic cirrhosis/nephrotic syndrome)
  Sodium depletion

Increased back-diffusion H+ (gradient defect)

  Amphotericin B

It should be remembered that in proximal tubular acidosis, once the serum bicarbonate is reduced to a level below a certain threshold, and almost always ≥ 14 mEq/L, the kidney stops losing bicarbonate at the level of the proximal tubule, a phenomenon termed "gradient-limited." Under such circumstances, the urinary pH may *not* reflect bicarbonate loss, and is below 6.0.

- The treatment is aimed at both reversal of the extracellular acidosis as well as provision of optimal linear growth. This requires supplemental oral alkali, often in large amounts exceeding 10–15 mEq of base/kg/day.

DISTAL TUBULE

- Unlike the gradient-limited acidosis that occurs with diseases of the proximal tubule, the inability to sustain a hydrogen-ion gradient across the distal renal tubule results in an ongoing, relentlessly severe hypokalemic metabolic acidosis, where the serum bicarbonate level is generally ≤ 10 meq/L, in the untreated state. Table 121-2 lists the causes of distal renal tubular acidosis (RTA). Most are accompanied by hypokalemia, and are termed type I. A few are associated with an inability to excrete potassium, and are termed type IV. Kidney stones or nephrocalcinosis (interstitial deposition of calcium salts) are common in distal renal tubular acidosis, and occur more frequently than in type I disease.

- The treatment is aimed at both restoration of the extracellular acidosis as well as provision of optimal linear growth. This requires supplemental oral alkali, often in large amounts exceeding 10–15 meq of base/kg/day. Thus, the treatments of the two general types of acidosis often do not differ.

122 DISORDERS OF THE COLLECTING DUCT

Ronald J. Kallen

- The kidney collecting duct regulates the final movement of water into and out of the urine, in response to the hormone vasopressin (AVP, also known as antidiuretic hormone, ADH). A disruption of this process produces the inability to adequately conserve water, and is termed nephrogenic diabetes insipidus when the defect is localized to the collecting duct. It is characterized by the presence of elevated, circulating levels of AVP, in comparison to central diabetes insipidus, where there is a failure of pituitary production of the hormone.

In central diabetes insipidus, provision of the hormone restores water balance, as the kidney apparatus remains intact. Searching for the presence of diabetes insipidus should be done carefully and generally by a specialist, as water deprivation, the mainstay of testing, may lead to profound volume depletion in the affected patient, with subsequent vascular collapse, shock, and death.

- The symptoms of nephrogenic diabetes insipidus often start in the very young infant, with recurrent episodes of hypernatremic dehydration, fevers, poor growth, and often have a positive family history associated with the most common form of the disease that is X-linked dominant. The signs of severe volume depletion are evident. The laboratory manifestations include hypernatremia, and inappropriate low urine osmolality at the time of clinical volume depletion, to values often ≤ 100 mOsm/kg H_2O.

- Initial treatment consists of reduction of dietary salt intake to lessen overall urine volume and administration of thiazide-class diuretics to increase proximal tubular water resorption, and/or administration of indome-thacin, to both reduce, mildly, overall glomerular filtration rate, and hence, water filtration, and to sensitize the collecting duct, in some cases, to work a bit more at normalizing a response to the high levels of circulating AVP. Referral to a specialist is mandatory for treatment of this complex water disorder.

123 RENOVASCULAR DISEASE

Jerome C. Lane

EPIDEMIOLOGY

- Kidney and renovascular diseases are the causes of hypertension in approximately 90% of young children with a definable cause of hypertension. Renovascular disease is the etiology of hypertension in 8–10% of children referred for evaluation of hypertension. The incidence of renovascular hypertension is much lower in the adult population (<1%).

ETIOLOGY

- Atherosclerosis comprises 60% of renovascular disease in adults, whereas in children 75–95% of renovascular disease is caused by various forms of arterial dysplasia, the most common of which is fibromuscular dysplasia. Table 123-1 lists the other causes of renovascular hypertension.

TABLE 123-1 Causes of Renovascular Hypertension

Fibromuscular dysplasia
Neurofibromatosis 1
Klippel-Trenaunay-Webber syndrome
Feuerstein-Mimms syndrome
Tuberous sclerosis
Takayasu arteritis
Moyamoya disease
Sarcoidosis
Kawasaki disease
Thromboembolic disease
   Neonatal renal artery thrombosis
   Following angiography
   Following blunt abdominal trauma
Extrinsic compression of the renal artery
   Tumors
   Congenital fibrous bands
   Posttraumatic hematomas
Kidney transplant renal artery stenosis

- *Fibromuscular dysplasia* most often involves the media of kidney vessels. The main renal artery and/or segmental branches are involved. Stenotic lesions followed by post-stenotic dilatation can resemble a "string of beads" appearance on angiography. Involvement of the intima of vessels is occasionally seen, though adventitial involvement is rare. Medial lesions generally are characterized histologically by replacement of normal media with collagen and fibrous matrix, as well as degenerated elastic fibers and displaced smooth muscle cells. Other less common forms of arterial dysplasia include medial fibroplasias, intimal fibroplasia, perimedial fibroplasia, and periarterial fibroplasia. *Neurofibromatosis* (NF-1) has been reported to comprise 10–25% of renovascular disease in some reports. Neurofibromatosis typically involves the intima and often causes lesions close to the origin of the renal arteries from the aortic trunk. Fibromuscular dysplasia, in contrast, typically involves more distal areas of the renal arteries. Renovascular disease most often (70%) occurs bilaterally in patients with neurofibromatosis.

PATHOPHYSIOLOGY

- The common physiologic pathway leading to hypertension in renovascular disease involves activation of the renin-angiotensin-aldosterone axis. In unilateral renovascular disease, the affected kidney, sensing relative arterial hypoperfusion, generates and secretes renin. Renin results in the conversion of angiotensinogen to angiotensin I, which then is converted to angiotensin II by angiotensin converting enzyme (ACE). Angiotensin II is a direct vasoconstrictor, leading to a systemic rise in blood pressure. Angiotensin II also stimulates the release of aldosterone, which leads to tubular retention of sodium and water, also contributing to the rise in blood pressure from an expansion of blood volume.

While the unaffected kidney generally compensates by excreting excess sodium and water, overall fluid and sodium balance remains positive in unilateral disease.

- In bilateral renal artery disease, there also is an initial rise in renin, angiotensin II, and aldosterone, leading to vasoconstriction, tubular sodium and water retention, and expansion of plasma volume; however, since both kidneys are affected, there is no ability of the kidneys to compensate by excreting the excess salt and water. This leads to marked systemic volume expansion and subsequent suppression of the renin response, such that renin levels eventually become normal in bilateral disease.

CLINICAL FEATURES

- The majority of children with renovascular hypertension are asymptomatic. Typical symptoms, when present, are those of accelerated or malignant hypertension (see above). Features of systemic or genetic disease can be present. Features suggestive of renovascular disease include symptoms of genetic or systemic inflammatory disease, hypertension following trauma, severe and/or difficult to control hypertension, and hypertension associated with a change in kidney function.

DIAGNOSIS

- A thorough history and physical examination is the first step in evaluating a child for renovascular disease in the setting of hypertension. A complete neonatal history is essential, as umbilical artery catheterization is an important association with renovascular lesions. A history of *symptoms* associated with hypertension (see Clinical Features) should be sought. Prior history of renal disease, urologic malformation, or urinary tract infection should be elicited. Use of oral contraceptive agents or medications with vasopressor effects (stimulants, illicit drugs, corticosteroids, or anabolic steroids) must be reviewed. Endocrine symptoms also should be investigated, such as weight loss, sweating, flushing, and palpitations. A thorough family history is essential regarding genetic disorders, inflammatory diseases, malignancy, and essential hypertension.
- *Signs* of hypertension should be sought (see above). It is essential to examine for signs of genetic syndromes, such as café au lait spots, lesions of tuberous sclerosis, or phenotypic characteristics of Williams syndrome. The presence of carotid bruits, midline abdominal bruits, or bruits over the renal fossae may suggest the presence of a systemic vascular disease, such as fibromuscular dysplasia, Takayasu arteritis, or Moyamoya disease. Signs of endocrine diseases should be sought, such as hirsutisim, striae, buffalo hump, tremor, fine hair, sweating, or obesity.

- *Initial screening tests* should include the following: urinalysis; urine culture; serum levels of urea nitrogen, creatinine, electrolytes, total carbon dioxide, and calcium; kidney ultrasound with Doppler of the kidney vessels; and echocardiography (to evaluate for end-organ damage, such as left ventricular hypertrophy, as well as cardiac disease). A peripheral plasma renin activity can be useful if hypertension is quite elevated, but a normal result does not rule out renovascular hypertension, since this test can be affected by medications, hydration status, salt intake, and many other factors. A captopril "challenge" test is not recommended.
- *Imaging studies* of the kidney vessels remain an essential, but controversial, part of investigating renovascular disease. The gold standard test for diagnosis of renovascular disease is the conventional renal arteriography with a radiocontrast agent; however, due to the expensive and invasive nature of this test, less invasive methods have been investigated. Kidney ultrasound with Doppler study of the kidney vessels has been reported to have high sensitivity and specificity for renovascular disease is some studies, approaching 90% correlation with renal arteriography; however, this procedure is highly operator-dependent, and up to 20% of studies may be inadequate for diagnosis, even in experienced centers. Captopril renography also has been reported to have high sensitivity and specificity in adult studies. In this procedure, a radionuclide renal scan is performed after a dose of captopril. A reduction in renal function is seen in the kidney affected by renovascular disease; however, pediatric studies have demonstrated a low sensitivity (59%) and specificity (68%) in children, limiting the usefulness of this test. Additionally, since many causes of renovascular disease are bilateral in children, there is a remote risk of producing kidney failure with the use of captopril.
- Newer imaging modalities include magnetic resonance arteriography (MRA) and helical or spiral computed tomography angiography (CTA). MRA can detect lesions effectively in the proximal renal arteries; however, MRA might not be sensitive enough to detect smaller lesions in the distal renal arteries, which are characteristic of fibromuscular dysplasia. CTA might provide better resolution for smaller lesions. The sensitivity and specificity of CTA has been reported to be 98 and 94% in adult studies. Neither MRA nor CTA have been studied in pediatric renovascular disease.
- For those children with a high suspicion of renovascular disease as a cause of their hypertension, conventional renal arteriography remains the most reliable means of diagnosis. This procedure, though invasive, has the added advantage of providing a possible therapeutic intervention, through performance of percutaneous transluminal angioplasty (PTLA) at the time of diagnosis. Renal vein renin sampling can also be performed during

conventional arteriography. Blood is selectively sampled from each renal vein; an elevated plasma renin activity ratio in the affected compared to the unaffected kidney (>1.5) confirms renovascular disease as the etiology of the hypertension. Such studies may be helpful in making therapeutic decisions for surgical cure of the hypertension by performance of a nephrectomy.

TREATMENT

- PTLA can often cure renovascular hypertension in selected patients. Patients who do well with this procedure are those with accessible unilateral main artery or main branch lesions. There is a lower success rate with bilateral and or distal renal arterial disease. Long stenotic lesions and lesions at the origin of the main renal artery also have a lower success rate. Overall success rates in children are reported in the range of 38–90%. About one-third of patients undergoing PTLA will experience a subsequent restenosis. The uses of intravascular stents or baffles have been reported in adults, but have not been studied in children.

- Surgical vascular reconstruction, such as reconstruction of the renal artery or a bypass graft from the aorta to the artery distal to the stenosis, may be performed in those patients in whom PTLA cannot be performed or is unsuccessful. Cure rates are reported in the range of 70–90%, with improvement in a further 19–26%. In patients with complex bilateral disease, the success rate is reported to be approximately 50%, with up to 18% requiring more than one procedure. Nephrectomy can be considered in the case of unilateral disease with a poorly functioning affected kidney (<10% of renal function as measured by radionuclide renography).

- Pharmacotherapy is a critical component in the management of patients with renovascular disease. ACE inhibitors should be used with caution, since they might precipitate renal failure in severe bilateral renovascular disease; however, once the renal lesions have been defined, ACE inhibitors can play a useful role in the treatment of renovascular hypertension, as they directly block the renin-mediated pathophysiologic pathway causing the hypertension. Other useful agents include calcium-channel blockers, beta-blockers, and diuretics.

BIBLIOGRAPHY

Bartosh SM. Childhood hypertension. An update on etiology, diagnosis, and treatment. *Pediatr Clin North Am* 1999; 46:235–252.

Deal JE, Snell MF, Barratt TM, Dillon MJ. Renovascular disease in childhood. *J Pediatr* 1992;121:378–384.

Ingelfinger JR. Renovascular disease in children. *Kidney Int* 1993;43:493–505.

Leung DA, Hagspiel KD, Angle JF, Spinosa DJ, Matsumoto AH, Butty S. MR angiography of the renal arteries. *Radiol Clin North Am* 2002;40:847–865.

McTaggart SJ, Gelati S, Walker RG, Powell HR, Jones CL. Evaluation and long-term outcome of pediatric renovascular hypertension. *Pediatr Nephrol* 2000;14:1022–1029.

Swinford RD, Ingelfinger JR. Evaluation of hypertension in childhood diseases. In: Barratt TM, Avner ED, Harmon WE (eds.), *Pediatric Nephrology*, 4th ed. Baltimore, MD: Lippincott Williams and Wilkins, 1999, pp. 1007–1030.

124 NEPHROLITHIASIS
Craig B. Langman

- A stone may occur in the urinary tract from the renal pelvis collecting system through the tip of the urethra, regardless of its etiology. It may occur as an isolated finding, or point toward a systemic disorder, regardless of a similar crystalline structure. A stone may be innocent, being seen only on an abdominal radiograph, ultrasound, or computed tomography (CT) scan performed for other purposes, or may result abruptly in renal colic (see above). Stones tend to be recurrent problems, and over 90% of children with kidney stones have a definable, metabolic problem that is amenable to therapy. Therefore, the clinician is encouraged to evaluate every child with nephrolithiasis completely in order to ascertain the reason for the stone.

- A simplified evaluation of nephrolithiasis involves collection of several complete, 24-hour urine samples for purposes of quantifying the overexcretion of lithogenic substances (calcium, oxalate, uric acid, phosphate), or the underexcretion of inhibitors of nephrolithiasis (citrate, magnesium). Such collections should be done with a gap from an acute stone event, perhaps several weeks, and when the patients are on their usual diet. Forced-fluid administration is not recommended during such collections, since the usual urinary volume is an important part of the overall evaluation. At the end of three to four collections over a short period of time (i.e., the same 7-day period), it is recommended that a blood comprehensive metabolic profile be obtained, including the measurement of serum uric acid.

- Tables 124-1 through 124-5 list the common causes of each type of stone by primary etiology. The clinician is advised that simultaneous disturbances may coexist, and each deserving of treatment. Successful treatment of nephrolithiasis is judged by the absence of new

TABLE 124-1 Hypercalciuric Conditions Associated with Kidney Stone Formation

ASSOCIATED WITH HYPERCALCEMIA	ASSOCIATED WITH NORMAL SERUM TOTAL CALCIUM
Primary hyperparathyroidism	Idiopathic hypercalciuria
Sarcoid; cat-scratch fever	Mutations in kidney chloride gene CLCN5
Idiopathic infantile hypercalcemia	Immobilization (common)
Immobilization	Associated with prematurity and furosemide therapy
Neonatal Bartter syndrome	Renal distal tubular acidosis, type I
Seyberth syndrome	Glycogen storage disease
Thyrotoxicosis	Hereditary hypophosphatemia with hypercalciuria
	Use of ketogenic diet
	Activating mutation of the extracellular calcium-sensor gene (hypocalcemia)
	Medullary sponge kidney
	Inflammatory diseases, such as juvenile arthritis
	Corticosteroid therapy

TABLE 124-2 Causes of Hyperoxaluria

Primary overproduction of oxalate	Enteric overabsorption
Primary hyperoxaluria	Increased serum bile acid levels
AGXT mutation: type I	Inflammatory bowel disease
GRHPR mutation: type II	Dietary oxalate excess
Secondary overproduction of oxalate	Dietary calcium deficiency
	Small bowed resection
Ethylene glycol poisoning	
Vitamin C excess	
Pyridoxine deficiency	

TABLE 124-3 Conditions Associated with Calcium-Phosphate Kidney Stones

Distal renal tubular acidosis	Urine infection
Alkaline urine	Hereditary hypophosphatemia with hypercalciuria
Calcium-oxalate kidney stones	Primary hyperparathyroidism
Hypocitraturia	

TABLE 124-4 Causes of Hyperuricosuria

INCREASED PRODUCTION	INCREASED EXCRETION
Hemolytic anemia	Proximal tubular defect
Hematologic malignancy	Acidosis
Irradiation or treatment with cytotoxic agents	
Gout	
Lesch-Nyhan syndrome	

TABLE 124-5 Normative Data for Excretion of Selected Lithogenic Substances

SUBSTANCE	REFERENCE RANGE
Calcium	≤4 mg/kg/day for children ≥2 years of age
Citrate	≥0.4 mg/m^2 BSA/day
Oxalate	≤0.5 mmol/m^2/day
Uric acid	Varies with age, up to a maximum of 750 mg/day in adolescence

stones, avoidance of urinary infection, and the absence of stone growth of existing stones. Referral to a specialist in nephrolithiasis is recommended for all children who form a kidney stone.

125 UROLOGIC ANOMALIES
Jerome C. Lane

RENAL ECTOPIA

- As the kidneys develop, they may fail to ascend normally from the pelvis to their usual position in the renal fossae, resulting in renal ectopia. An ectopic kidney may be pelvic, iliac, thoracic, or contralateral. A contralateral ectopic kidney has a ureter that crosses the midline; such a kidney often fuses with the other kidney, a condition known as crossed-fused renal ectopia. Renal ectopia occurs in approximately 1 in 900 individuals. The adrenal gland usually remains in the normal position. Bilateral ectopia is less common (10% of cases).
- Hydronephrosis is seen in 56% of ectopic kidneys, most commonly as a result of obstruction at the ureteropelvic or less commonly at the ureterovesical junctions. Hydronephrosis may also occur as a result of vesicoureteral reflux or malrotation. Vesicoureteral reflux into the ectopic kidney is frequently observed in crossed-fused ectopia. There is a higher incidence of abnormalities in the nonectopic kidney. Approximately 25% of the nonectopic kidneys may exhibit hydronephrosis secondary to obstruction or vesicoureteral reflux. There is also a higher incidence of renal agenesis on the side opposite to the ectopic kidney.
- Patients with renal ectopia have a higher incidence of genital anomalies (15–45% of patients). Women may have one or more of the following anomalies in 20–66% of cases: bicornuate or unicornuate uterus with atresia of one horn, rudimentary or absent uterus and proximal and/or distal vagina, and duplication of the vagina. Approximately 10–20% of men may have anomalies, including undescended testes, duplication of the urethra or hypospadias. Other congenital anomalies are seen in 21% of patients with renal ectopia, most commonly involving the heart or skeletal system. Renal ectopia can be isolated or associated with various syndromes. Some of the more common syndromes include Beckwith-Wiedemann, CHARGE association, infant of a diabetic mother, Denys-Drash, DiGeorge, Fanconi anemia, fetal alcohol, Goldenhar, Turner, VACTERL association, and Williams.

- The majority of ectopic kidneys are asymptomatic and are found serendipitously during imaging of the abdomen or urinary tract for other reasons. The patient with renal ectopia may present with signs of urinary infection due to obstruction of the ectopic kidney, or reflux or obstruction of the contralateral kidney. An obstructing kidney stone leading to renal colic is a common reason for presentation. Ultrasonography, radionuclide renography, excretory urography, or abdominal/pelvic computed tomography (CT) scan all are adequate methods of diagnosing renal ectopia.
- Total renal function generally is normal, although the ectopic kidney often is hypoplastic and may have reduced function. There is no increased risk of malignant transformation in renal ectopia.

HORSESHOE KIDNEY

- A horseshoe kidney arises when fusion of the lower poles of both kidneys occurs across the midline. The kidneys are connected by parenchymal or, less commonly, fibrous tissue. Migration of the horseshoe kidney is usually incomplete and the kidney is situated lower in the abdomen than the usual kidney position. The incidence of horseshoe kidney is approximately 1 in 500 births. Patients with Turner syndrome have a 7% incidence of horseshoe kidney. Some of the syndromes associated with horseshoe kidney include Antley-Bixler; infant of diabetic mother; Fanconi anemia; Roberts; trisomies 13, 18, 21, and 22; Turner; and VACTERL association.
- Congenital anomalies are frequently associated with horseshoe kidney, most commonly involving the skeletal, cardiac, and central nervous systems. Three percent of children with neural tube defects have a horseshoe kidney. Anorectal anomalies are common. Approximately 20% of trisomy 18 patients have horseshoe kidney. Genitourinary anomalies also are more frequent, including hypospadias (4% of male children), cryptorchidism (4%), bicornuate uterus (7% of female children), and septate vagina (7%). Ureteral duplication occurs with an incidence of 10%, occasionally associated with an ectopic ureterocele. Vesicoureteral reflux can be demonstrated in approximately 50% of patients. One-third of patients may have ureteropelvic junction (UPJ) obstruction and hydronephrosis.
- About 30% of patients are asymptomatic. Patients who present with symptoms usually have hydronephrosis, infection, or renal calculi. Horseshoe kidneys are occasionally detected after discovery of an abdominal mass (5–10% of cases). Ultrasonography, radionuclide renography, excretory urography, or abdominal/pelvic CT scan all are adequate methods of diagnosing horseshoe kidney.

- As in renal ectopia, prognosis is related to presence of hydronephrosis, infection, or calculi. The majority of patients who are asymptomatic will remain so. Prognosis is also related to associated anomalies and syndromes.
- Unlike renal ectopia, there is an increased risk of malignancy in the horseshoe kidney. Wilms tumor is two to four times more likely to occur in patients with horseshoe kidney than in the general population. Other reported tumors include renal cell carcinoma, adenocarcinoma, transitional cell carcinoma, malignant teratoma, oncocytoma, angiomyolipoma, and carcinoid.

HYDRONEPHROSIS AND URINARY OBSTRUCTION

- Prenatal hydronephrosis has become a frequent finding with the increasing performance of prenatal ultrasonography. Hydronephrosis is the most commonly detected prenatal urologic abnormality, accounting for 87% of findings. Many cases of prenatal hydronephrosis are not clinically significant and represent a developmental phenomenon. As many as 50% of cases have resolved by the time a postnatal ultrasound is performed. For those infants with postnatal hydronephrosis, the condition will resolve spontaneously over time without intervention in up to 38% of cases. In the remainder of patients, hydronephrosis may be associated with an obstructive or nonobstructive anomaly. The most common anomaly associated with congenital hydronephrosis is ureteropelvic junction obstruction (48% of cases). Other causes include renal duplication and ureterocele, posterior urethral valves, vesicoureteral reflux (see chapter on UTI and vesicoureteral reflux), and prune-belly (Eagle-Barrett) syndrome.

URETEROPELVIC JUNCTION OBSTRUCTION

- As previously mentioned, UPJ obstruction is the most common obstructive lesion associated with hydronephrosis. Most cases are unilateral, with the left kidney most commonly involved (60%). Bilateral UPJ obstruction occurs in 10% of cases. There is a male to female preponderance of 2:1.
- UPJ obstruction in the infant usually presents due to the finding of prenatal hydronephrosis, discovery of an abdominal mass, or urinary tract infection. Older patients usually present with urinary tract infection; abdominal, flank or back pain; or hematuria, especially after minimal trauma.
- Renal ultrasonography usually establishes the diagnosis of hydronephrosis. A diuresis renogram, in which furosemide is given during conventional radionuclide renography, can help identify obstructive vs. nonobstructive hydronephrosis. A diuretic radionuclide renogram also can provide an assessment of the function of the affected kidney and allow differentiation between true hydronephrosis and dysplastic or multicystic-dysplastic kidneys. A voiding cystourethrogram should be performed, due to the increased risk of vesicoureteral reflux in the contralateral kidney.
- Indications and timing of surgical repair for UPJ obstruction are controversial. As previously mentioned, many cases will improve spontaneously over time without surgical intervention. In one study of neonates with unilateral hydronephrosis and UPJ obstruction, after almost 2 years of follow-up, only 7% of the patients required surgical intervention for progression of hydronephrosis or 10% or greater reduction in kidney function on radionuclide renography. The goal of intervention is relief of symptoms, such as pain or urinary infection, and/or improvement in kidney function. Thus, the general indications for surgical intervention include persistent symptoms, such as pain; recurrent urinary infection; initial impairment in overall kidney function; or progressive hydronephrosis or kidney impairment in the affected kidney. Regardless of surgical vs. conservative management, most practitioners would recommend antibiotic prophylaxis against urinary infection in all patients until the hydronephrosis resolves. Surgical repair by pyeloplasty has excellent results in the range of 95% or better. Newer techniques, such as endourologic or laparoscopic repair, also are being explored in adults but have not gained widespread application in children at this time. Nephrectomy also may be considered if the affected kidney has little parenchyma or function (<10% on renogram).

POSTERIOR URETHRAL VALVES

- Posterior urethral valves occur in 1 in 8000 boys and are the most common cause of severe obstructive uropathy in boys. Posterior urethral valves account for approximately 10% of overall hydronephrosis in infants. The most common type of valves (Type I, >95% of cases) is caused by leaflets of tissue which extend from the prostatic urethra to the external urinary sphincter and obstruct urinary flow.
- Clinical presentation of posterior urethral valves varies by age. Newborn infants may come to attention due to a prenatal diagnosis of hydronephrosis or oligohydramnios. In the postnatal period, infants may present with abdominal masses due to massive hydronephrosis; abdominal distention from urinary ascites; respiratory distress from pulmonary hypoplasia and Potter sequence; and/or acute kidney failure.

Older infants and children may present with voiding dysfunction and enuresis, urinary tract infection, and/or signs of kidney insufficiency.

- Prenatal management by vesicoamniotic shunting of the obstructed fetal bladder in utero has been attempted in many cases. Prenatal intervention might increase initial survival by reducing the incidence of oligohydramnios and pulmonary hypoplasia (60% vs. 93% in untreated vs. treated infants, respectively); however, prenatal intervention has not been shown to reduce the overall risk of progression toward end-stage kidney disease (approximately 30%, with rates as high as 70% in some studies). Insufficient studies have been performed to universally recommend prenatal intervention at this time.

- Postnatal management of posterior urethral valves consists of immediate placement of a urinary catheter to relieve the urinary obstruction. A prophylactic antibiotic, such as amoxicillin or a second or third generation cephalosporin, usually is prescribed to reduce the risk of urinary infection and urosepsis. If the infant's serum creatinine improves after several days of bladder drainage, endoscopic ablation of the valves is performed. If the creatinine remains high or increases despite bladder drainage with a small catheter, urinary diversion is usually performed, most often by vesicostomy. Supravesical diversion by ureterostomy might be necessary in the presence of secondary causes of obstruction, such as ureteropelvic or ureterovesical junction obstruction. Endoscopic ablation of the valves and reconstruction of the urinary tract after diversion then can be performed at a later date, after stabilization of the infant and improvement in kidney function. Infants and children can present later in life with infection, kidney insufficiency, electrolyte abnormalities, and/or voiding dysfunction. Treatment at this stage requires management of infection, electrolyte disturbances, and complications of kidney failure; endoscopic ablation of valves then is performed.

- Children with valves, or other types of obstructive uropathy, are at risk for tubular dysfunction. Type 4 renal tubular acidosis and poor urine concentrating ability with polyuria are often present and require careful management. These children are at increased risk of volume depletion, acidosis, and electrolyte disturbances, especially during times of fever or illness. Boys with valves often have persistent enuresis and bladder dysfunction despite adequate valve ablation. Continued urologic care and urodynamic studies are an important part of overall management. Enuresis may improve over time.

- The overall mortality of children with posterior urethral valves has improved considerably with earlier recognition and better management. Current mortality is approximately 2–3%. Early neonatal mortality is usually related to pulmonary hypoplasia and respiratory failure, with mortality approaching 50% in such cases. As mentioned previously, approximately 30% or more of patients with valves will progress to end-stage kidney disease despite adequate early detection and relief of urinary obstruction. Such relentless progression is likely to be related to associated renal dysplasia. Although obstructive uropathy might play a role in the development of renal dysplasia in children with valves, there likely are associated host and genetic factors that contribute to dysplasia apart from the presence of urinary obstruction. Patients with a serum creatinine of 0.81.0 mg/dL or less by the age of 1 year have a favorable prognosis regarding progression of kidney insufficiency, although these patients may continue to have morbidity from bladder or kidney tubular dysfunction.

PRUNE-BELLY SYNDROME

- Prune-belly syndrome, also referred to as Eagle-Barrett syndrome, results from congenital absence, deficiency, or hypoplasia of the abdominal musculature. The syndrome is also called "triad syndrome," because of its effects on the abdominal musculature, urinary tract, and testicles. Although rare cases have been reported in girls, the syndrome almost exclusively affects boys. The incidence of the syndrome is approximately 1 in 35,000 to 1 in 50,000 live births.

- Several theories have been proposed for the etiology of prune-belly syndrome, but the cause of the syndrome is unknown. Obstruction of the fetal urethra may lead to severe dilation of the bladder and urinary tract, which then blocks descent of the abdominal testes and interferes with development of the abdominal wall musculature. An error in mesodermal development also may explain the syndrome, since the urinary tract and the abdominal musculature arise from the paraxial intermediate and lateral plate mesoderm. No definite genetic links or patterns of inheritance have been discovered, and most cases are sporadic and not familial.

- Characteristic clinical features of prune-belly syndrome include deficiency of the abdominal musculature; cryptorchidism; kidney dysplasia and hydronephrosis; massive ureteral dilation; bladder enlargement; vesicoureteral reflux; and megalourethra. Other anomalies include cardiac abnormalities (10% of cases); musculoskeletal defects (50% or more of cases), including limb abnormalities and scoliosis; gastrointestinal defects (31%), such as malrotation, intestinal atresia, or stenosis, volvulus and imperforate anus; and pulmonary abnormalities (55%), most commonly pulmonary hypoplasia. Oligohydramnios and respiratory failure from pulmonary hypoplasia are frequent causes of death in the neonatal period. Diagnosis often is made by prenatal ultrasound, although the appearance of prune-belly syndrome may be difficult to distinguish from severe vesicoureteral reflux or posterior urethral valves. Postnatal diagnosis usually is made by the characteristic constellation of clinical findings.

- The surgical and medical management of prune-belly syndrome is complex and highly individualized, and only a brief summary is provided. Initial management of the infant born with prune-belly syndrome consists of treatment of associated cardiopulmonary complications and management of fluid and electrolyte abnormalities if kidney failure is present. Urinary diversion by means of vesicostomy, ureterostomy, or pyelostomy occasionally is required, especially in the presence of urinary obstruction, intractable urinary infection, and/or deteriorating kidney function. Reconstruction of the abdominal wall musculature by abdominoplasty improves cosmetic appearance, as well as bowel, bladder, and pulmonary function. Reconstruction of the urinary tract is performed where indicated, including cystoplasty, ureteroplasty and reimplantation, orchidopexy, and/or correction of other abnormalities.

- The prognosis of children with prune-belly syndrome is related to the extent of kidney dysplasia and pulmonary hypoplasia. The incidence of stillbirth or death in the first few months of life exceeds 30%. End-stage kidney disease occurs in approximately 30% of patients as a result of dysplasia, infection, and/or reflux. Kidney transplantation can be performed for patients with end-stage kidney failure, often with excellent results.

ECTOPIC URETER

- An ectopic ureter is defined as a ureter that drains into the bladder neck or outside of the bladder. The true incidence is unknown, since many cases are asymptomatic, but autopsy studies in children have estimated the incidence to be approximately 1 in 1900. The condition occurs three times more frequently in girls than in boys. Five to 17% of cases occur bilaterally. The majority of cases in girls are associated with a duplicated collecting system; the ectopic ureter usually drains the upper pole unit of the duplicated system. In boys, an ectopic ureter is usually associated with a single collecting system. In girls, the ureter may drain into the bladder neck (35%), urethrovaginal septum (35%), vagina (25%), or other locations, such as the cervix, uterus, or Gartner duct. In boys, common locations include the posterior urethra (47%), prostatic

utricle (10%), seminal vesicle (33%), ejaculatory duct (5%), and vas deferens (5%). In many cases, the ureter exhibits dilation and poor drainage.

- The clinical presentation in girls is usually urinary incontinence and urinary tract infection. Incontinence usually is not a feature in boys, who present with urinary tract infection or epididymitis. Prenatal ultrasound may demonstrate the nonspecific finding of hydronephrosis. The diagnosis sometimes can be established in girls by physical examination and direct visualization of constant urinary dribbling or the presence of an abnormally located orifice. Postnatal ultrasonography may demonstrate a duplicated kidney (in girls), hydronephrosis, and dilated ureter but normal appearing bladder. Voiding cystourethrography may demonstrate reflux if the ectopic ureter drains into the bladder neck; reflux to the nonectopic ureter of a duplicated system or to the contralateral ureter occasionally may be demonstrated as well. Retrograde pyelography can be performed if an ectopic orifice can be visualized and cannulated. Excretory urography (intravenous pyelogram [IVP]) may be helpful in detecting the presence of a duplicated system. Radionuclide renography should be performed in order to assess the function of the upper and lower moieties of a duplicated system.

- Treatment depends on the function of the affected kidney. In many cases, the function of a nonduplicated kidney, or the upper pole unit of a duplicated system is severely impaired. In this instance, total or heminephrectomy is performed. If kidney function is normal or only modestly impaired, ureteral reimplantation or ureteroureterostomy (joining of the ectopic upper pole ureter to the normal lower pole ureter) is performed.

URETEROCELE

- A ureterocele is a cystic dilatation of the terminal ureter. Ureteroceles are four times more common in girls than in boys and occur almost exclusively in Caucasians. Ten percent of cases are bilateral. The majority of cases arise from the upper pole of a duplicated collecting system. The ureterocele generally causes obstruction and hydronephrosis of the affected kidney and occasionally can be large enough to obstruct the contralateral kidney. The upper segment of the duplicated kidney is often dysplastic and has poor function; the lower segment often has vesicoureteral reflux.

- The presence of a ureterocele may be suspected by the finding of prenatal hydronephrosis and confirmed by postnatal ultrasonography. Cases undetected prenatally usually present later in infancy or childhood with urinary tract infection or urosepsis. Diagnosis usually can be established by ultrasonography, which will demonstrate the ureterocele itself, as well as hydronephrosis and renal duplication. Voiding cystourethrography also may delineate the presence and size of a ureterocele, as well as demonstrate associated reflux. Radionuclide renography or excretory urography should be performed to assess the function of the affected kidney.

- Antibiotic prophylaxis usually is prescribed until a definitive procedure can be performed. Uncomplicated cases may be treated by cystoscopic incision and decompression of the ureterocele. In other cases, excision of the upper duplicated segment and ureter. The surgical management of ureteroceles is complex and must be individualized to the anatomy of each patient.

BIBLIOGRAPHY

Bauer SB. Anomalies of the upper urinary tract. In: Walsh PC, Retik AB, Vaughan ED, Wein AJ (eds.), *Campbell's Urology*, 8th ed. Philadelphia, PA: Elsevier, 2002, pp. 1885–1924.

Elder JS. Congenital anomalies and dysgenesis of the kidneys. In: Behrman RE, Kliegman RM, Jenson HB (eds.), *Nelson Textbook of Pediatrics*, 16th ed. Philadelphia, PA: W.B. Saunders, 2000, pp. 1619–1621.

Elder JS. Obstructions of the urinary tract. In: Behrman RE, Kliegman RM, Jenson HB (eds.), *Nelson Textbook of Pediatrics*, 16th ed. Philadelphia, PA: W.B. Saunders, 2000, pp. 1629–1638.

Gonzales ET. Posterior urethral valves and other urethral anomalies. In: Walsh PC, Retik AB, Vaughan ED, Wein AJ (eds.), *Campbell's Urology*, 8th ed. Philadelphia, PA: Elsevier, 2002, pp. 2207–2230.

Limwongse C, Clarren SK, Cassidy SB. Syndromes and malformations of the urinary tract. In: Barratt TM, Avner ED, Harmon WE (eds.), *Pediatric Nephrology*, 4th ed. Baltimore, MD: Lippincott Williams and Wilkins, 1999, pp. 427–452.

Schlussel RN, Retik AB. Ectopic ureter, ureterocele, and other anomalies of the ureter. In: Walsh PC, Retik AB, Vaughan ED, Wein AJ (eds.), *Campbell's Urology*, 8th ed. Philadelphia, PA: Elsevier, 2002, pp. 2007–2052.

Smith EA, Woodard JR. Prune belly syndrome. In: Walsh PC, Retik AB, Vaughan ED, Wein AJ (eds.), *Campbell's Urology*, 8th ed. Philadelphia, PA: Elsevier, 2002, pp. 2117–2135.

Streem SB, Franke JJ, Smith JA. Management of upper urinary tract obstruction. In: Walsh PC, Retik AB, Vaughan ED, Wein AJ (eds.), *Campbell's Urology*. 8th ed. Philadelphia, PA: Elsevier, 2002, pp. 463–512.

126 URINARY TRACT INFECTIONS

Ronald J. Kallen

- Urinary tract infections (UTIs) are especially common in infants and young children, before and during toilet training. In children 3–4 years of age undergoing the transition from diapers to continence, symptoms such as dysuria and incontinence (after having learned continence) are easily recognized as indicators of a UTI or voiding dysfunction. In fact, voiding dysfunction may be an etiologic factor for UTI in young girls; however, it is during infancy that the risk of adverse sequelae of UTI is high, since symptoms are nonspecific and diagnosis (and treatment) delayed. The recognition of a UTI is critically dependent on the threshold of suspicion, adequacy of history and physical examination, and medical decision-making.

- The youngest of infants, perhaps within 1 month of birth, are at risk of sepsis, originating in the urinary tract. The risk of bacteremia may be as high as 10%. In view of the susceptibility of infants to serious sequelae of UTI, the American Academy of Pediatrics (AAP) published a practice parameter on the diagnosis and management of UTIs in infants between 2 months and 2 years of age. The same general principles of management apply to infants younger than 2 months of age, with the caveat that such infants are at increased risk of systemic illness.

DIAGNOSIS

- All infants less than 2 years of age with unexplained fever should be suspected of having a UTI. They often continue to appear ill and irritable despite measures to reduce fever. In the first few months of life, there is a male preponderance in incidence of UTI; however, after about 4 months of age, a female preponderance supervenes and continues throughout childhood and adolescence. The overall incidence of UTI during infancy is about 6–7%. The prevalence of UTI in infants worked-up for fever-without-source is under 10%. Noncircumcised infants have a much higher risk of UTI, at least during the first 6 months of life, than circumcised infants.

- Although a UTI may be suggested by either a urine dipstick showing a positive test for leukocyte esterase (or rarely, nitrites) or leukocytes in the sediment, the "gold standard" for diagnosis is culture of urine obtained by catheterization (or suprapubic aspiration, although this is rarely done). In children older than 2 years of age, especially if they have become sufficiently verbal, a UTI is suggested by reported symptoms of dysuria, urinary tenesmus, frequent urges, incontinence (either daytime or nocturnal enuresis, after having become continent), and malodorous urine, with or without fever.

• There is no reliable way to distinguish "upper tract" (pyelonephritis) from "lower tract" (cystourethritis) infection; however, ill-appearing, febrile infants are presumed to have pyelonephritis. Although the "gold standard" for documenting acute pyelonephritis is cortical scintigraphy with technetium-90 DMSA, in clinical practice it is not necessary to resort to this invasive study to "prove" the diagnosis of pyelonephritis.

TREATMENT

• For ill-appearing (*toxic*) infants, younger than 2 years of age, antimicrobial therapy (AMT) should begin as soon as the catheterized specimen for urine culture and sensitivity is obtained. A recent study showed that such infants can be treated with oral AMT on an outpatient basis. It is only necessary to hospitalize infants for intravenous AMT if sepsis is suspected or the infant is unable to tolerate or retain orally-administered antimicrobial. Third generation cephalosporins are appropriate medications for initial treatment of UTI, whether administered orally or parenterally. If an infant does not appear acutely ill and close follow-up is assured, AMT may be deferred until the results of the urine culture are reported. The final choice of antimicrobial for older children with UTI should be guided by sensitivity patterns of common gram-negative urinary pathogens in the community.

• The consensus is that a 7 to 10-day course of treatment with an appropriate antimicrobial, as dictated by culture and sensitivity results, is adequate. There are not adequate data supporting a "short" course of treatment. If the expected clinical response fails to occur after 2 days of treatment, the urine culture should be repeated and treatment with an alternative antimicrobial begun.

IMAGING STUDIES

• A UTI may be a harbinger of serious, underlying urinary tract anomalies although, statistically, this is rarely the case. All infants should have a kidney-bladder ultrasound examination to rule out major congenital obstructive anomalies or nonobstructive hydronephrosis. The latter may be the only indication of possible vesicoureteral reflux.

• Vesicoureteral reflux is commonly found during the imaging workup of a UTI, perhaps in up to 40% of cases. It is not considered a major urinary tract anomaly but may represent a risk factor for scarring. Although performing a voiding cystogram (VCG) is a widespread practice, the AAP consensus statement considers the basis in evidence for routine imaging to be only "fair." Decision-making regarding imaging studies depends on a careful and nuanced risk-assessment and is best done by a pediatric nephrologist. The common finding of pelviectasis on an ultrasound study may be a normal variant. Moderate-to-severe bilateral hydronephrosis in a male should be followed by a VCG to rule out posterior urethral valves. Other possible causes of hydronephrosis include uretero-pelvic junction obstruction, ureterovesical junction obstruction, and a duplication anomaly with uretero-cele. Hydronephrosis may be nonobstructive, as in the instance of vesicoureteral reflux.

• The initial VCG in females should use a radionuclide rather than a conventional contrast study, to limit gonadal radiation exposure. Imaging studies are probably not necessary in older female children with typical symptoms of UTI. A kidney ultrasound may disclose attenuated parenchyma which is often attributed to postinfectious scarring. In the context of high-grade reflux, these changes may actually represent kidney dysmorphogenesis early in pregnancy resulting in a hypoplastic or dysplastic kidney, which may be smaller in size and poorly functioning compared to the opposite kidney.

ANTIMICROBIAL PROPHYLAXIS

• All newborns, suspected of hydronephrosis on the basis of prenatal maternal ultrasound, should have antimicrobial prophylaxis until appropriate imaging studies are done shortly after birth. Infants or young children with frequent, closely spaced UTIs may be considered for prophylaxis with a lower dose of antimicrobial, given in the evening; however, there are not sufficient randomized controlled trials supporting such a practice.

PROGNOSIS

• Prompt recognition and treatment of UTI enhances a favorable prognosis for practically all infants and children. Complications such as kidney failure or hypertension are rare and probably occur only in those infants with congenital anomalies, especially if obstructive, or with hypoplastic or dysplastic kidneys.

BIBLIOGRAPHY

Bloomfield P, Hodson EM, Craig JC. Antibiotics for acute pyelonephritis in children. *Cochrane Database Syst Rev* 2003;CD003772.

Coulthard MG. Do kidneys outgrow the risk of reflux nephropathy? *Pediatr Nephrol* 2002;17:477–480.

Michael M, Hodson EM, Craig JC, Martin S, Moyer VA. Short versus standard duration oral antibiotic therapy for acute urinary tract infection in children. *Cochrane Database Syst Rev* 2003;CD003966.

Norton KI. New imaging applications in the evaluation of pediatric renal disease. *Curr Opin Pediatr* 2003;15:186–190.

127 PRIMARY NOCTURNAL ENURESIS

Ronald J. Kallen

OVERVIEW

- Nighttime urinary incontinence in an otherwise healthy child is common and affects up to 20% of 5-year-old children. If continence has never emerged for a sustained length of time by the age of 5–6 years, it is referred to as primary nocturnal enuresis (PNE). These comments presume that the child is otherwise healthy, dry during the day, and does not have a urinary tract infection.

- If enuresis recurs after a sustained period of nighttime continence, for up to 6 months, it is referred to as secondary enuresis. In this context the word, secondary, does not refer to underlying kidney or urinary tract disease.

- Most children succeed in achieving daytime urinary continence by the age of 3 years but many continue to have nighttime wetting for up to a year or more. Nighttime continence is gradually attained in 80% of children by the age of 5 years and in 90% by the age of 8 years. The probability of spontaneous resolution is about 15% per year.

- Since females have a somewhat earlier acquisition of certain developmental milestones, including bladder control, PNE is usually not considered for intervention in girls until the age of 5–5.5 years. Boys older than 6 years with frequent nighttime wetting are considered to have PNE. PNE is more common in boys.

- PNE is not a disease in the usual sense. Rather, it is a delay in maturation of neural mechanisms for nighttime continence. By definition PNE is not associated with underlying kidney or urinary tract pathology. Despite the fact that it rarely portends serious disease, it can be a source of considerable emotional distress to the child and family.

ETIOLOGY

- PNE is a multifactorial disorder and a number of mechanisms have been proposed. It is a benign form of voiding dysfunction, generally attributed to delayed maturation of bladder control. The consensus view is that the neural pathways which perceive bladder fullness and inhibit detrusor activity during the day have not yet developed fully for nocturnal bladder control.

- Many parents describe their enuretic children as "deep sleepers" and are difficult to arouse. Research on this matter has yielded conflicting data; however, recent data suggest that enuretic children have an altered sleep state with an impaired arousal in response to the sensation of bladder distention. It is useful to explain to the family that perception of increasing bladder distention fails to break through a critical threshold of awareness at the subconscious level needed to trigger an inhibitory message. Because of the presumed delayed maturation of both the sensory mechanism perceiving bladder fullness at the subconscious level and the inhibitory neural pathway, the bladder of an enuretic child has infantile characteristics with heightened "hair-trigger" automaticity. As a consequence, uninhibited reflex detrusor contractions occur during sleep as the bladder fills.

- Another view regarding etiology is that the bladder has a reduced functional capacity and is unable to accommodate the usual nocturnal volume, especially if the child tends to drink large quantities of fluid during and after dinner. Since the bladder is a highly compliant structure, capacity is not a static value but represents the net effect of the volume, degree of distention, and the trigger threshold for detrusor contraction.

- Some children with enuresis may be unable to achieve maximal release of endogenous arginine vasopressin and, as a consequence, urinary concentration (osmolality) during sleep is less than maximal. The prevalence of this apparent defect in the general population of enuretic children is not known.

- There is frequent association of enuresis with constipation although the role of the latter in causing delayed acquisition of bladder control is not clear.
- A family history of enuresis during childhood in one or both parents is common. If both parents were affected, there is a 77% chance the child will have enuresis. If one parent had enuresis, there is a 44% chance the child will be similarly affected. This heredofamilial pattern may have a genetic basis with an apparent autosomal dominant inheritance. Candidate gene loci had been mapped to chromosome 13q13-q134.3 (ENUR1), chromosome 12 (ENUR2), and chromosome 22 (ENUR3). Although the function of the putative gene products are not known, presumably they play a role in the maturation of those neural pathways important for bladder control at the conscious and subconscious (during sleep) level.
- On the basis of histories obtained from parents, there are circumstantial data that food sensitivities may play a role. It is not clear if certain foods or additives have a direct effect on the bladder. Caffeine-containing beverages or foods may play a role by increasing the urine volume.

DIAGNOSIS

- Nocturnal enuresis unaccompanied by a urinary tract infection or symptoms suggestive of underlying kidney or urinary tract disease does not call for urinary tract imaging studies or extensive laboratory testing. A dipstick urinalysis test should be done. A questionnaire regarding elimination behavior of both bladder and bowel can be helpful. In selected instances, it is also useful to have the parent complete a 2–3-day voiding diary.

MANAGEMENT

- Persistence of nocturnal enuresis beyond 6–7 years of age calls for intervention. There is no standard definition as to the frequency of wet nights that should prompt intervention; however, if the majority of nights are wet and there is distress for both the child and the family, intervention for a child 6 years of age or older is appropriate.
- General measures, such as restricting fluids after the evening meal or awakening and carrying the child to the bathroom are almost never helpful by themselves. Managing the enuretic child calls for tact and a gentle

approach. The family is counseled that the child does not intentionally wet the bed and does not want to displease his parents. It should be explained that PNE is a maturational problem. Just as some children walk earlier than others, so too is nighttime continence achieved at different rates in individual children. The probability of success of a treatment program is contingent on the maturity and motivation of the child. Intervention is not likely to succeed if the child is relatively immature or unable to understand the goals of treatment.

- If there is a history of constipation or stool withholding, a treatment program for enuresis is unlikely to succeed until the bowel elimination dysfunction is resolved. Treatment of PNE associated with comorbid behavioral disorders, such as attention deficit hyperactivity disorder, has a lower rate of success.
- General measures, such as restricting fluids after the evening meal or awakening by the parent after the child has fallen asleep, are usually not helpful by themselves. Treatment for enuresis is often explained as "training" the bladder as if it were an autonomous organ, detached from the nervous system; however, like all learning, neural pathways become selected and reinforced while others are blocked or inhibited. The desired outcome is not so much a change in arousal state such that the child wakes up during the night to void in the bathroom but, rather, to heighten subconscious awareness of bladder-filling integrated with inhibition of the detrusor muscle so that the child does not need to awaken at all.

MOISTURE ALARM

- The mainstay of treatment is a moisture-sensing alarm that is triggered by a small volume of urine at the beginning of the stream. Several manufacturers produce alarms that provide either an audible or vibratory signal. There is also an alarm that does both. Most alarms have a "hard wired" connection between the moisture sensor in the underwear and the alarm which is attached to the pajama top so that it is close to the ear. There are also wireless alarms which transmit a radiofrequency signal to the alarm-emitting unit.
- The alarm should not be prescribed until there is considerable preparation in terms of education on its proper use, and self-motivation guided by visual imagery of each discrete step in the sequence of behavior, immediately following awakening. This effort must be a joint enterprise by both the parent and the child. The parent must awaken with the child and help him or her get out of bad and go the toilet to complete voiding. Eventually the role of the parent can be faded away. There is about a 66% probability of success in using the alarm, but improvement may

not occur for several weeks. It is not known how the "conditioning" effect of the alarm brings about cessation of enuresis. It is possible that consistent use of the alarm lowers the threshold of subconscious awareness of bladder filling and facilitates inhibition of detrusor activity.

ANTISPASMODICS

• Given that uninhibited reflex detrusor activity plays a central role, an antispasmodic may be used as an adjunct to a moisture alarm; however, when used alone, these medications are rarely successful. A single bedtime dose of oxybutynin chloride, 5 mg, is appropriate. Possible side effects include dry mouth and constipation.

DESMOPRESSIN ACETATE (DDAVP)

• There are data that some enuretic children do not secrete an appropriate amount of endogenous arginine vasopressin and are unable to achieve maximal concentration of urine. If an enuretic child is shown to be unable to elaborate a maximally concentrated urine after 12 hours of fluid restriction, DDAVP may be used as an adjunct to alarm therapy. It is available in tablet form and a single oral bedtime dose, starting at 0.2 mg may be used, eventually titrating up to 0.6 mg, if there is not a response to a lower dose. As a general measure, fluid restriction after the evening meal is advisable but, in the instance of treatment with DDAVP, it should be done assiduously to avoid the risk of hyponatremia.

• Although a good response to treatment has been reported, relapse after discontinuation is common. In some instances, treatment with the alarm may be combined with oxybutynin chloride and DDAVP but care should be taken to control excessive fluid intake that may occur as a consequence of the sensation of dry mouth caused by oxybutynin chloride.

IMIPRAMINE

• Although widely used at one time, the potential cardiotoxicity consequent to accidental or intentional overdosage relegates this medication to a treatment of last resort. It should be stored in such a way that a young child does not have access to it. There is a case report of fatality in a young child receiving imipramine for enuresis who intentionally consumed a large dose believing that the larger dose would provide a cure (*magical thinking*). The starting dose is 25 mg at bedtime.

ASSESSING THE RESPONSE TO TREATMENT

• The response pattern to any of the above treatments is highly individual and it is difficult to make generalizations. The enuresis alarm may take several weeks before improvement is noted. It also requires strict and consistent adherence to a routine that reinforces the motivational component, mental imagery, and continent nights. The parent and child must both be highly motivated and work together as a team. Punishment for a wet night is never appropriate.

• The response to DDAVP may appear "overnight" and, in some instances, suggests a placebo effect. DDAVP may be helpful for occasional use such as sleepovers, while traveling and staying in hotels, or overnight camp.

FOLLOW-UP

• The response to treatment is variable. Some children have a prompt response, sometimes suggesting a placebo effect. Others may not achieve success until after 3 months or more have elapsed. If success has not occurred after 4–6 months despite good compliance, the treatment should be abandoned until the child is somewhat older or more highly motivated. Close follow-up and reinforcement by the physician of the motivational component at each visit is critical to success.

Section 16
NEUROLOGIC DISORDERS

Joshua L. Goldstein, Section Editor

128 NEWBORN NEUROLOGY
David G. Ritacco

- Some features of the perinatal period raise unique issues regarding nervous system assessment and function. These include the shift from intrauterine to extrauterine environment, unique central nervous system (CNS) susceptibility to insults (especially in premature infants), limited information about history (i.e., information about events antenatally), and limited clinical information about function in this age group given paucity of functional skills.

GATHERING INFORMATION—THE NEWBORN PHYSICAL EXAMINATION

- The newborn neurologic examination includes assessments of integrative functions, cranial nerve functions, reflexes, motor functions, and sensory functions. Included here are also crucial components of the general examination, such as measuring head circumference and assessing physical features of the anterior and posterior fontanelles.
- The principle of observation without disturbance of activity that is a significant part of any pediatric physical assessment takes on a larger significance in the neonate, who is unable to be instructed in the usual sense.
- Integrative function refers here to the infant's level of consciousness or state of activity. It includes the infant's overall responsiveness or awareness of changes in surroundings. The degree to which the infant is able to maintain different levels of alertness or different "states" is an indication of the ability to combine activity at different nervous system levels, and may provide a measure of higher level nervous system function in this age group.
- An assessment of spontaneous movement is needed as well as that of response to stimulation, and in the impaired infant this includes an assessment of response to pain.
- Cranial nerve function testing includes assessment of pupillary (and visual) reaction to light. Vision at term includes tracking a bright object, but it may be necessary to present the stimulus within 5–10 cm of the eyes to elicit a response. A face provides a particularly engaging target. The optic fundus of the newborn may be difficult to see because of the small size of the pupil and difficulty opening the eye against resistance, but older infants often gaze in the direction of the ophthalmoscope. Eye movements may be elicited by the oculocephalic reflex (doll's eyes), by which turning the head side to side or up and down results in the eyes moving in the opposite direction (so as to keep the eyes looking at an unmoving target). If head movement is restricted, caloric stimulation may be used. Blink is often elicited by presenting a bright light, but also by corneal reflex. Facial symmetry is best assessed by comparing grimace reflex, and although robust results may be elicited by sharp stimulus to the cheek, when the cheek is not accessible (e.g., the intubated and taped patient) the reflex may be elicited at the inner surface of the nostrils. Hearing can usually be demonstrated by the infant's alerting to sound—cessation of activity sometimes accompanied by widening of the eyes or even a full startle response. A novel stimulus and a quiet setting are helpful. Assessing sucking or biting on the finger or pacifier, gag, and cry completes the cranial nerve assessment (olfactory, taste, and spinal accessory functions need not be routinely checked).

- Deep tendon reflexes are variable in amplitude but are usually easily elicitable in infants. Pectoralis, biceps, brachioradialis, patellar, thigh adductor, and achilles tendon reflexes should all be present and symmetric. Putting a finger on the tendon and striking the finger with the hammer works best for all except the Achilles, which can be activated by tapping the underside of the foot to flex the ankle. Spread may be observed in the normal infant (crossed adductor in the legs, brachioradialis activation with biceps stretch in the arms).

- The response to plantar stimulation (Babinski reflex) is not so reliable in this age group, but symmetry is still a useful screen. Palmar and plantar grasp are easier to interpret, and again they should be bilaterally symmetric.

- Although many other postural reflexes may be tested at different ages, the Moro (a startle triggered by abrupt drop of the head relative to the trunk) is useful for eliciting bilateral stereotyped arm and leg movements that can be checked for symmetry. This reflex should be present at birth and persists for up to 6 months.

- Observation of the resting posture is an important tool, as any evidence of asymmetry at limbs or trunk may reflect disturbance of nervous system activity. The typical flexed posture of limbs when supine provides information about relative muscle strength and activity, and deviations may indicate abnormalities of tone.

- Examination when the infant is asleep, although less hampered by movements, will give a falsely low impression of tone. When the infant is upset (crying), tone is increased. It is also important to be sure that the head is in the midline, as the tonic neck reflex will affect tone and reflex assessments if the head is turned to either side.

- Tone is assessed as the resistance, at rest, to passive movement. The assessment usually involves swinging the arms or legs side to side or up and down and looking for a catch or slowing of movement. The scarf sign is a measure of upper extremity tone, by drawing the hand across the chest toward the opposite shoulder and looking at the position of the elbow with respect to the chest. The elbow does not cross the midline unless hypotonia is present.

- The most sensitive determination of motor function is gathered from observing spontaneous movements. The same is true with regard to facial movements. Sensory assessment in infants, in addition to the activities involved in the reflex assessments listed above, does not usually require more than lightly touching the extremities and observing the infant's response. The lack of distinction between response to noxious and bland stimuli is an indication of disturbed integrative function.

HYPOXIC-ISCHEMIC ENCEPHALOPATHY

- The presentation of the infant with asphyxia in the perinatal period is a syndrome, with a number of features that evolve over time. Markers for hypoxic-ischemic encephalopathy (HIE) include depressed Apgar scores, cord blood acidosis, and seizures. Asphyxia combines a deficit in energy supply (hypoxemia and ischemia) with tissue accumulation of by-products of metabolism (hypercapnea and lactic acidosis). The injury resulting from asphyxia has been divided into two broad patterns—one associated with acute total asphyxia and the other with partial but prolonged asphyxia. HIE requires strict criteria to diagnose. It should be remembered that infants with antenatal brain injuries including CNS malformations may be at greater risk for a secondary intrapartum ischemic event. This has both prognostic and medical-legal implications. For this reason the term neonatal encephalopathy is gaining favor unless hypoxia and ischemia are clearly the only causative factors.

- The pattern of parasaggital cerebral injury results from the acute interruption of perfusion of large regions of the brain, and as such is the pattern most typical of HIE in the full-term infant. The most severely affected areas are in the borderzone or watershed areas of cerebral circulation, thus the name "parasaggital." Involved territories include the parasaggital cortex, with hippocampus, lateral cortex, striatum, and dentate progressively less severely affected.

- The pattern of periventricular leukomalacia is more common in premature infants, but is also seen in full-term infants who are sick or who have cardiac deficits. Damage involves both multifocal (periventricular) as well as diffuse regions of white matter.

- The sequence of clinical features of HIE develops and becomes maximal over the first 72 hours of life. In the first 12 hours, the level of responsiveness of the infant appears depressed. Breathing is often depressed, and spontaneous movement is limited. Tone may be low.

- Seizures may occur in the more severely affected infant. In the next 12 hours, seizures may begin (or worsen, if already begun). Level of consciousness may become more like waking but monotonous (with poor integrative function). Twitchy or jittery movements may be seen. From 24 to 72 hours, stupor becomes deeper. Brainstem impairment is more overt, with loss of brainstem reflexes.

- A determination of prognosis is the most eagerly sought information by the family and care providers for the infant with HIE. The markers mentioned above for the diagnosis of HIE are also indicators of prognosis, to the extent that they indicate severity of injury.

The longer the time to reach an Apgar greater than 7, the more likely will be CNS sequelae. The longer to reach an Apgar greater than 0, of course, the more severe the ischemic insult. Similarly, seizures are an indication of HIE, but burst-suppression pattern on the EEG is an indication of greater severity and more serious CNS injury.

- The major intervention from the perspective of neurologic treatment is the treatment of seizures with anticonvulsants. Phenobarbital is the agent of choice, and there is some data to support treatment of the asphyxiated infant with phenobarbital proactively, before seizures occur. The typical loading dose for seizures is 20 mg/kg, and additional doses of 10 mg/kg may be provided for breakthrough seizures, to total 40–50 mg/kg. Maintenance is 3–5 mg/kg/day. For prophylaxis, a single loading dose of 10–20 mg/kg is typical.

129 NEURODEVELOPMENTAL DISABILITIES

Charles N. Swisher

- Neurodevelopmental disabilities is that area of child neurology that overlaps with many other pediatric subspecialties in the evaluation and overall management of a child who is not demonstrating the usual pattern of developmental progress. Neurodevelopmental issues can present in a "high frequency, limited morbidity" pattern such as children with learning disabilities and attentional problems as well as a "low frequency, high morbidity" picture seen in children with multiple congenital anomalies, prenatal and perinatal problems, and rare neurogenetic disorders. The high frequency group is a very significant proportion of the pediatric age group, with attention deficit/hyperactivity disorder (ADHD) and learning disabilities accounting for 5–8% of the general population.

- Most children with risk factors for developmental disabilities have one, and most children with developmental disabilities have no preexisting risk factors. Most of the commonly used screening tests for developmental disabilities have many false positive tests and miss a considerable number of children with true delay. In evaluation of a child with developmental delay, one should remember the three Ds:
  - Delay: A lag behind expectations for age: Greater than 50% delay in motor development, greater than 75% in language development (allowing for the greater variability in language development).
  - Dissociation: One or more developmental features out of phase (e.g., dyslexia, dyspraxia, dysphasia).
  - Deviance: Nonsequential development, e.g., pervasive developmental disorder, where language and socialization differ from motor development.

- In assessing a child for neurodevelopmental disabilities, one needs to make the distinction between quantitative and qualitative disorders:
  1. Qualitative: The child has spastic diplegia and therefore does not walk until 2 years of age.
  2. Quantitative: The child does not walk at 2 years of age and therefore is about 50% delayed in walking.

- The distinction needs to be made very clearly between global functional delay and an isolated disorder with a neurologic cause. Additionally, it should be recognized that it is very difficult to make conclusive statements of language or cognitive disability until children have reached an age where these delays may be apparent and evaluated.

- Motor function is usually rather well-established and predictable at 2 years of age, language and cognition have a far more variable pattern of development and quantitative evaluation may not be possible until age 5. Therefore it is often more appropriate to speak of the preschooler as a child "at risk" for neurodevelopmental disabilities rather than exhibiting a defined disorder requiring lifetime management. This is dramatically seen in some children who present with pervasive developmental disorders at age 2 which by 5 may have progressed to a pattern of an isolated language disorder with minimal socialization problems.

- Plasticity of the developing nervous system results from a complex pattern of genetic influence and the patterns of dendritic growth and pruning, coupled with the complex effects of the environment. Compared to the higher incidence of children with problems with disorders of dissociation (5–8%), the pattern of global delay occurs in about 1% of children.

- Routine cytogenetic testing and molecular testing. Testing specifically for the fragile X mutation (FMR-1 gene) is recommended for this group, as the yield of this testing is much higher than metabolic testing (Down syndrome and fragile X being the two most common chromosomal causes of mental impairment). The phenotypic stigmata of fragile X include large and low-set ears, macroorchidism, and a prominent jaw. If the results of newborn metabolic screening are not available, these studies should also be obtained. Recognizing the difficulty of determining global delay at an early age, the following algorithm has recently been developed by the Child Neurology Society for appropriate assessment.

- For an overview of the evaluation of developmental delay the reader is referred to the above consensus statement of the American Academy of Neurology in conjunction with the Child Neurology Society (Shevell et al., 2003).
- The role of the pediatrician in assessing a child with neurodevelopmental disabilities is to initially obtain a careful history of possible etiology, recognizing that in the majority of cases there may be no clear cause identified, although frequently a subtle genetic influence is suspected. Information from other specialists is essential. The development of the early intervention (birth to age 3) and early childhood (ages 3–5) programs through governmental mandate has allowed for near-universal assessment of infants and young children by psychology, physical and occupational therapy, and audiology and speech and language pathology.
- With the lack of ability for definitive assessment in the very young child, the focus is on intervention strategies to maximize the opportunity for developmental progress. Clinical studies do not always indicate the efficacy of conventional therapies, but an important advocacy role of the pediatrician in managing children at risk is to guide parents regarding the lack of efficacy demonstrated for some of the more controversial and financially draining unconventional therapies such as hyperbaric oxygen administration, intensive motor "patterning," specialized diets based on hypothesized trace mineral deficits or excesses, and the like.
- Children with neurodevelopmental disabilities are eligible for a special education program based on an IEP, or Individualized Educational Program, under the mandates of the Individuals with Disabilities Education Act of 1997. One paradox of this system is that although there is a long history of federal legislation from 1975 to the present, and although all children are entitled by law to "FAPE" or Free Appropriate Public Education, the legislation largely consists of unfunded mandates, resulting in wide disparities in what is actually provided in a specific school district. The end result is often that parents must resort to expensive private educational therapies for children with learning disabilities.
- Certain specific educational therapies, such as the Orton-Gillingham approaches to reading instruction for children with dyslexia, have proven effectiveness but limited availability in the present school setting. Greater understanding of the educational needs of the dyslexic child needs to be coupled with adequate local school resources.
- Any evaluation of a child with neurodevelopmental disabilities does require an interdisciplinary approach, either within the structure of an early intervention or childhood program or some collaboration between the pediatrician, the school, and the community. The state divisions of services for children with special health care needs are often valuable centers for providing information on specific programs and with some income restrictions, financial assistance for therapy programs.

REFERENCES

Shevell M, Ashwal S, et al. Practice parameter: evaluation of the child with global developmental delay: report of the Quality Standards Subcommittee of the American Academy of Neurology and the Practice committee of the Child Neurology Society. *Neurology* 2003;367–380.

130 EVALUATION AND MANAGEMENT OF CHILDHOOD HEADACHE
Mark S. Wainwright

PATHOPHYSIOLOGY OF HEADACHE

- Head pain requires the stimulation of pain-sensitive intracranial structures including vascular (arterial and venous sinuses), meningeal (particularly the perivascular components of the dura), and neuronal elements (particularly the trigeminal, glossopharyngeal, and vagus nerves). Neurotransmitters implicated in the pathophysiology of headache (May and Goadsby, 1999) include thromboxane A2, nitric oxide, Substance P, glutamate, serotonin, and neuropeptides.

THEORIES OF MIGRAINE PATHOPHYSIOLOGY

- The vascular theory of migraine (Wolff, 1948) proposes an initial phase of vasoconstriction resulting in ischemia and neurologic symptoms (manifest as the aura of migraine). Ischemia is followed by a reactive vasodilatation culminating in head pain. Cerebral blood flow studies have not supported this mechanism and most evidence suggests that vasodilatation occurs secondary to an earlier process in migraine.
- Neurovascular theories of migraine propose that the release of proinflammatory vasoactive peptides into the dural space results in dural inflammation, vasodilatation, and pain transmission to the trigeminal

nucleus caudalis. Other evidence suggests that migraineurs may have a lower threshold for cortical neuron excitation (central nervous system [CNS] *hyperexcitability*). Both clinical and preclinical studies also support the involvement of serotonin, glutamate-mediated neuronal excitation, and nitric oxide in the pathogenesis of migraine. Taken together, this model implies a lowered threshold for neuronal activation in migraineurs associated with genetic susceptibility, glutamate dysfunction, low magnesium, nitric oxide release, or a combination thereof. The precise location of the migraine generator remains to be determined (Welch, 1998) although activation of the trigeminovascular system is a pivotal event in migraine pathophysiology.

EPIDEMIOLOGY OF HEADACHE IN CHILDREN

• Headache and migraine are uncommon before the age of 4. Prevalence of all types of headache increases with age. The classic study of Bille (1962) among 9000 school children demonstrated an equal rate of increase in prevalence of headache in boys and girls up to the ages of 10–12 followed by a faster rate in girls thereafter. Later studies totaling 27,606 children reported a prevalence of headache of 37–51% in 7-year olds, increasing to 57–82% by age 15 years.
• The male:female ratio below age 12 is 1:1, compared to 1:1.5 in teenagers and adults. The prevalence rate of migraine in boys increases from 4% at age 7 to 6.5% at age 13. In girls the prevalence increases from 3.6% at age 7 to 15% at age 13. Seventy percent of children experience headache at least once a year with a prevalence of greater than 90% at ages 12–13. *Most childhood headaches are migraine or tension-type in origin.*
• *Natural history of headache*: The overall prevalence of headache including migraine is increasing. Longitudinal studies of childhood onset headache and migraine show a remission in 70% of cases between 9 and 16 years of age (Congdon and Forsyth, 1979). Forty-year longitudinal follow-up studies (Bille, 1997) show one-third of children headache-free after 6 years and two-thirds headache-free after 16 years.

CLASSIFICATION OF HEADACHES IN CHILDREN

• There is no consensus on the definition and classification of headaches and migraines in children. This reflects unreliability of the clinical diagnosis, deficits in understanding of basic mechanisms of headache in children, and age-dependent differences in causes of headache. The following are acceptable criteria for description and classification for diagnostic purposes.
• Classification may be based on temporal patterns:
  1. Acute
  2. Acute, recurrent
  3. Chronic progressive
  4. Chronic, nonprogressive
  5. Comorbid
• For differential diagnosis, headaches may be classed as
  1. Primary headache disorder (based on the International Headache Society [IHS] criteria)
     a. Migraine
     b. Cluster-type headache
     c. Tension-type headache
  2. Secondary Headache Disorder (implies underlying treatable etiology)

CLASSIFICATION OF MIGRAINE HEADACHES IN CHILDREN

• A set of modified criteria for children with migraine has been proposed (Winner et al., 1995) based on the International Headache Society criteria for migraine (Olesen, 1988) (Fig. 130-1).

PEDIATRIC MIGRAINE WITHOUT AURA DIAGNOSTIC CRITERIA	PEDIATRIC MIGRAINE WITH AURA* DIAGNOSTIC CRITERIA
A. At least five attacks fulfilling B-D B. Headache lasting 1–48 hours C. Headache has at least two of the following 1. Bilateral location (frontal/temporal) or unilateral location 2. Pulsating quality 3. Moderate to severe intensity 4. Aggravation by routine physical activity D. During headache, at least one of the following: 1. Nausea and/or vomiting 2. Photophobia and/or phonophobia	A. At least two attacks fulfilling B B. At least three of the following: 1. One or more fully reversible aura symptoms indicating focal cortical and/or brainstem dysfunction 2. At least one aura developing gradually over more than four minutes, or two or more symptoms occurring in succession 3. No aura symptoms lasting more than sixty minutes 4. Headache follows after less than sixty minutes

*Idiopathic recurring disorder; headache usually lasts 1–48 hours

FIG. 130-1 Proposed revised IHS classification scheme for childhood migraine.

CLINICAL FEATURES OF MIGRAINES IN CHILDREN

- Multiple studies support a genetic component to migraine, which is more robust for migraine with aura than in migraine without aura. *The most common triggers are stress, sleep deprivation, illness, and travel* although more than 50% of migraineurs cannot identify definite triggers for their attacks. *Migraine without aura* represents 70–85% of childhood migraine. A visual aura is not present but autonomic symptoms (pallor, lethargy) may occur. A visual aura is most common in *migraine with aura* and may include bright lights, moving lights, scotomata, or fortification spectra. Aura usually occurs 15–30 minutes antecedent to the headache. Both types may be associated with abdominal pain, nausea, vomiting, photophobia, or phonophobia.
- A number of less common migraine syndromes are also found in children and are summarized below (Fig. 130-2).

COMORBID CONDITIONS WITH HEADACHE IN CHILDREN

- A number of studies report an association with other (often abdominal) aches and pains in children with headache and migraineurs. The prevalence of migraine in children with epilepsy ranges from 8 to 15%. Studies in adults report an increased risk of migraine in patients with major depression or panic disorder. In a series of children diagnosed with a psychiatric disorder, more of these children (21%) reported the occurrence of headaches than in the control population (9%) (Egger et al., 1998).

DIAGNOSTIC CRITERIA FOR TENSION-TYPE HEADACHE

- This can be summarized as a benign condition without underlying cause and without autonomic symptoms. Pain is typically posterior or anterior with a squeezing

SYNDROME	CLINICAL FEATURES
Basilar Artery Migraine	Symptoms are referable to dysfunction of the brainstem, cerebellum, parieto-occipital and inferior temporal cortices Most common subtype of migraine with aura Present in 3–19% of migraineurs Symptoms include visual field defects, paresthesias, vertigo, ataxia, confusion, hemiparesis, loss of consciousness Often associated with occipital headache
Familial Hemiplegic Migraine	Association of recurrent headaches and hemiparesis May have associated visual field defects Sporadic or familial (linked to Chr 19p13 or 1q31)
Ophthalmoplegic Migraine	Associated with complete or incomplete third nerve palsy Pain is unilateral, severe, and located behind the eye Eye moves laterally due to unopposed sixth nerve function Headache lasts hours but opthalmoplegia may last weeks
Retinal Migraine	Patients have ophthalmic symptoms of migraine but without headache Patients often have a family history of migraine and previous migraine attacks
Confusional Migraine	Often a retrospective diagnosis Most common in adolescents with migaine without aura Begins with headache then followed by confusion and agitation
Alice in Wonderland Syndrome	Visual hallucinations and distortions associated with migraine attacks Rare in children
Benign Paroxysmal Vertigo	Recurrent stereotypical bouts of vertigo Usually accompanied by nausea, vomiting, and nystagmus
Cyclic Vomiting Syndrome	Recurrent episodes of severe, sudden, self-limiting nausea, and vomiting Attacks last hours to days Symptoms resolve between attacks
Alternating Hemiplegia	Repeated attacks of hemiplegia affecting both body sides Onset before 18 months Normal at birth but characterized by mental and neurologic deficits after symptom onset
Paroxysmal Torticollis	Benign, intermittent self-limiting episodes of head tilt Spells last from hours to days Start in 1st year and resolve by age 5

FIG. 130-2 Less common presentations of migraine and syndromes related to migraine.

sensation. Neck muscles are often sore. IHS criteria include headache occurring at least 15 times per month and lasting 30 minutes to 7 days without autonomic symptoms.

EVIDENCE-BASED APPROACH TO HEADACHE IN CHILDREN

- Practice parameters are published for children with recurrent headaches (Lewis et al., 2002). This statement (www.aan.com/professionals/practice/guidelines.cfm) relates to children 3–18 years old presenting with recurrent headache unassociated with trauma, fever, or other provocative causes. These recommendations apply therefore principally to children with recurrent migraine, tension-type, and other *primary headache disorders.*

EVALUATION OF CHILDHOOD HEADACHE

- Not surprisingly, differential diagnosis and the need for and selection of diagnostic testing are guided by history and physical examination. *The evaluation needs to determine whether this is a primary or secondary headache.* Guidelines for primary headache evaluation are cited in following sections.
- Salient issues for history taking
  1. How many days of school have you missed?
  2. How many kinds of headache do you have?
  3. What analgesics do you use and how often?
  4. Do headaches wake you up?
  5. Is there a family history of headaches?
  6. What are the associated symptoms?
  7. What is the headache frequency and is it increasing?
  8. What are the triggers?
  9. What is the headache location and does it change?
  10. Medical risk factors (systemic illness, surgery)
  11. Drug exposure
  12. Key elements of the physical examination.
  13. Temperature
  14. Blood pressure
  15. Mental status
  16. Focal neurologic signs
  17. Fundoscopic examination

DIFFERENTIAL DIAGNOSIS FOR SECONDARY HEADACHE

- The principal categories to be considered in the differential diagnosis of children with secondary headache are summarized in Fig. 130-3.

- Secondary, "symptomatic" headache may be readily evident based on the patient's history, examination, and family history. The diagnosis of the underlying cause may be more challenging. A simple method with high predictive value for the diagnosis of headache in children is described by Stafstrom et al. (2002) by asking children to draw a picture of how their headache felt.

DIAGNOSTIC TESTING

- For evaluation of primary recurrent headache (see Practice Parameters).
- There is inadequate evidence to support the value of routine laboratory studies or lumbar puncture in primary recurrent headache.
- Electroencephalogram (EEG) may be normal or show nonspecific abnormalities in children with headache. The evidence does not support the use of EEG to distinguish between migraine and other headache types. There is no evidence to support the use of EEG to determine headache etiology. EEG is *not* recommended in the routine evaluation of children with recurrent headaches.
- Review of six studies with data on 1275 children with recurrent headache found only 14 (2.3%) with CNS lesions requiring surgical treatment. All 14 had abnormalities on neurologic examination. Neuroimaging is *not* recommended in children with recurrent headache and a normal neurologic examination.
- Neuroimaging should be considered for
  1. Children with an abnormal neurologic examination.
  2. Change in headache frequency or intensity.
  3. Change in headache type.
- For evaluation of children with secondary headache.
- The foremost question in this case is when to obtain neuroimaging. There are no practice parameters for secondary headache. A review of the published studies (Whitehouse, 2002) found an incidence imaging abnormalities of 0–0.4% in children referred to a neurology or headache clinic and 6–9% in children evaluated in an emergency room. The decision of whether to obtain imaging must therefore be made on an individual basis according to the risk factors of a given patient. A reasonable approach to headache diagnosis would select from the following studies.
  1. Magnetic resonance imaging (MRI) (where indicated magnetic resonance angiography [MRA] or magnetic resonance venography [MRV])
  2. Computed tomography (CT)
  3. Lumbar puncture (with opening pressure)
  4. Other studies for systemic disease, infection, thrombotic disorders, metabolic disorders, acidosis, and

CATEGORY
Increased intracranial pressure
Tumor: Headache is considered a common presenting symptom of supra and infratentorial tumors
Post-infectious of hemorrhagic blockage of CSF flow
Chiari 1 malformation
Occipital headache precipitated by cough or valsalva
Cerebral edema
Benign intracranial hypertension: Papilledema with or without VI nerve palsy
Vascular
Subarachnoid hemorrhage: Sudden development of severe headache which is not localized
Nausea vomiting and altered mental status common
Diagnosis by CT scan followed by lumbar puncture
Carotid or vertebral dissection
Vasculitis
Arteriovenous malformations: Most common presentation is acute illness with subarachnoid or parenchymal hemorrhage
Stroke: Headache more likely in hemorrhagic than embolic stroke
Epilepsy
Post-ictal
Ictal
Cranial Pathology
Sinusitis
Posttraumatic headache
Dental abcess
Neuralgia
Systemic Illness
Malignant hypertension: Rare; usual etiology is chronic renal disease
Drug use
Analgesic rebound
Drugs of abuse
Psychological
Depression

FIG. 130-3 Differential diagnosis for secondary headache in children.

drug use will be adjusted as indicated by the individual presentation.

5. Ophthalmologic examination with perimetry.
- When is imaging justified?
- For children with acute headache, neuroimaging should be performed and may need to be accompanied by lumbar puncture if the clinical examination shows the following:
1. Nuchal rigidity
2. Lateralizing signs
3. Altered mental status
4. Signs of increased intracranial pressure

TREATMENT

- There are no evidence-based practice parameters for the management of headache or migraine in children. Practice parameters for the treatment of migraine in adults are published (http://www.aan.com/professionals/ practice/guidelines.cfm). Absent pharmacologic treatment, general approaches in the management of headache include
1. Avoidance of triggers.
2. Good sleep hygiene.
3. Identification and reduction of dietary triggers (cheese, chocolate, processed meats, soft drinks, monosodium glutamate, red wine, food additives, and colorings.
4. Biofeedback
5. Acupuncture
6. Self-hypnosis

ACUTE THERAPIES FOR MIGRAINE

- The goal of acute therapy is to reduce or ablate pain, restore the patient's ability to function, and minimize the need for rescue medications. Therapy should (i) begin promptly; (ii) include antiemetics (intravenous if necessary) for patients with vomiting or severe nausea;

(iii) avoid the precipitation of medication-overuse headache in patients who require frequent treatment with abortifacient medications (typically considered in adults to be a frequency of more than twice a week); and (iv) include a self-administered rescue medication for patients who fail initial treatment.

- First line therapy specific to headache should include a nonsteroidal anti-inflammatory (NSAID) agent. *Acetaminophen* (10–15 mg/kg/dose; maximal dose 60 mg/kg/day) has a more rapid onset than *ibuprofen* (10–20 mg/kg/dose; maximal dose 40 mg/kg/day), but ibuprofen has been found more effective in aborting migraine. No other NSAIDs have been investigated in children for acute treatment of migraine.
- Among the triptans (serotonin 1B/1D receptor agonists), *sumitriptan* has been most extensively studied in children (Winner et al., 2000) in a placebo-controlled study of the efficacy of nasal sumitriptan. *Doses of 10 or 20 mg administered by nasal spray are effective.* Other triptans (Naratriptan, Rizitriptan, and Zolmitriptan) are considered safe and appropriate choices for initial treatment of adults with moderate-to-severe migraine (Grade A evidence) but have not been studied in children.
- The *antiemetics* metoclopramide (0.1 mg/kg IV) or prochlorperazine (0.1–0.3 mg/kg PO or rectal) may be administered to reduce nausea or vomiting.

PROPHYLACTIC THERAPIES

- The most commonly used agents for migraine prevention in the United States are propranolol and amitriptyline. Preventive therapy may be indicated for children with headaches occurring more than twice a week or whose headaches are prolonged and debilitating. *Propranolol* (0.5–2 mg/kg/day) may be beneficial in these cases. Patients should be monitored for hypotension or bradycardia. Among the tricyclic antidepressants, *amitriptyline* (0.2–2 mg/kg/day) has been used most extensively in the United States in children. The dose should begin low and escalate gradually as the principal side effect is drowsiness. In both cases, a trial of sufficient duration (6–12 weeks) should be used before the therapy is considered ineffective.
- A number of other classes of drugs including antiepileptics (principally carbamazepine, sodium valproate, gabapentin), calcium-channel blockers, serotonin antagonists (cyproheptadine, methysergide), and vitamins (B$_2$) are used in clinical practice for headache prophylaxis. Each class may be considered for the preventive therapy of headache in children who do not respond to therapy with propranolol or amitriptyline. There is no evidence-based data to guide this selection in children.

WHEN SHOULD A DIAGNOSIS OF PRIMARY HEADACHE BE RECONSIDERED?

- Patients may have multiple headache types and the diagnosis of headache type may not always be readily apparent.

FEATURES WHICH SHOULD CALL A DIAGNOSIS INTO QUESTION

- Recurrent headache that is always in the same location.
- Failure to respond to multiple medical regimens.
- Focal neurologic findings.
- Increasing frequency of headaches.
- Headache awakening from sleep.

131 PERIPHERAL NERVOUS SYSTEM DISORDERS
Wes McRae

- Anatomically the nervous system can be divided into two components, the central nervous system (brain and spinal cord) and the peripheral nervous system (PNS). The PNS, or motor unit, is comprised of (1) the anterior horn cell (AHC); (2) the peripheral nerve; (3) the neuromuscular junction (NMJ); and (4) the muscle. Any PNS or neuromuscular disorder will fit into one of the four anatomical sites.
- Motor impairment is the common symptom seen in all four anatomical sites. This may be seen as weakness, hypotonia (two distinct entities), muscle atrophy, muscle fasciculations, or fatigue. In addition, each anatomical site does show an individual symptom complex which allows refining of the differential diagnosis (Table 131-1). Although exceptions exist, most PNS conditions will fit into this general symptom complex.

TABLE 131-1   AHC Conditions

	AHC	PERIPHERAL NERVE	NMJ	MUSCLE
Sensory symptoms present	No	Yes	No	No
DTRs reduced	Yes	Yes	No	No
Serum CK elevated	No	No	No	Yes >3–5 × normal

ABBREVIATION: DTRs, deep tendon reflexes.

- This section will cover the most common conditions seen in each category. Typically the pediatrician will be the first physician consulted for complaints of weakness or fatigue. In addition to the above symptoms and signs, it is also important to know if the weakness is chronic or acute and the age of presentation.

AHC CONDITIONS

- Spinal muscular atrophy (SMA) is the most common anterior horn cell (AHC) condition seen in children. The most serious type, Type 1 SMA (Werdnig-Hoffman) usually presents with extreme hypotonia with respiratory and feeding difficulties in the neonatal period. Pregnancy history may reveal decreased fetal movements (Table 131-2).
- Children with Type 1 SMA are usually not strong enough to sit, Type 2 SMA are usually strong enough to sit but not walk, and Type 3 SMA (Kugelberg-Welander) may walk for a while, but will progress to being wheelchair bound. If the diagnosis of SMA is suspected based on presentation and clinical symptoms, the diagnostic workup is outlined in Table 131-3. If the genetic study is positive for SMA, electromyography/nerve conduction velocity (EMG/ NCV) testing and muscle biopsy is not necessary.
- Respiratory depression is the most serious complication and the most common cause of mortality. Aggressive and early respiratory toilet and treatment is required. Most Type 1 patients will have severe respiratory compromise and may eventually require assisted ventilation.
- Contractures and significant orthopedic problems will occur without a continuous program of therapy focused on stretching and reducing contractures. Many Type 1 and Type 2 patients do not survive childhood without mechanical ventilation.
- It is well-known that patients with SMA are very intelligent and they should be encouraged to pursue

TABLE 131-2   Spinal Muscular Atrophy (SMA) Fast Facts

*Presentation: neonatal or early infancy in most cases
*Triad of Symptoms:
  Severe hypotonia
  Absent reflexes
  Tongue fasciculations
*Swallowing and breathing weakness present
*Face and eye weakness absent
*Incidence: 10–15 per 100,000 live births
*Autosomal recessive genetics
  Gene location 5q11.2–13.3 or survival motor
  Motor neuron (SMN) gene
*Prognosis: poor

TABLE 131-3   Diagnostic Studies for SMA

Genetic Studies
  Highly sensitive and specific
EMG/NCV
  Normal conduction velocities
  Fibrillations on EMG
Muscle Biopsy
  Classic finding is grouped atrophy

independence and educational objectives wholeheartedly despite their severe motor disabilities.

PERIPHERAL NERVE DISORDERS

- The second anatomical site in the motor unit is the peripheral nerve. There are two unique features present in nerve disorders that distinguish this anatomical category from the other three. First, this is the only type of motor unit disorder in which sensation is effected. Therefore, if the examination confirms sensory loss, the other forms of motor unit disorder can be ruled out immediately. Second, of the four anatomical sites, peripheral neuropathies generally show signs of distal weakness before proximal weakness; therefore, if the majority of symptoms involve the hands and feet, peripheral neuropathy is definitely a possibility.
- Although the differential diagnosis of peripheral neuropathies in childhood is extensive, the majority of causes are extremely rare. The discussion below will focus on the most common acute neuropathy to affect children: acute inflammatory demyelinating polyradiculoneuropathy (AIDP) or Guillain-Barre syndrome (GBS); and the most common chronic neuropathy to affect children, hereditary sensory motor neuropathy (HSMN) or Charcot-Marie-Tooth disease (CMT).
- Table 131-4 lists the features of AIDP. In most cases the symptoms are very acute and the patient may stop walking within a few hours or days. If the symptoms continue, the upper extremities and breathing may be affected. Miller-Fischer variant is the term used for cases in which the cranial nerves are involved.
- Many cases may be associated with an infectious process. Among the pathogens associated with AIDP are *Campylobacter jejuni*, cytomegalovirus (CMV), Epstein-Barr virus (EBV), hepatitis, influenza, mycoplasma, and herpes simplex virus (HSV). *C. jejuni* is a common associated pathogen in cases in China, with up to 74% correlation.
- AIDP must be considered a neurologic emergency when the respiratory or autonomic systems are involved.

TABLE 131-4   Fast Facts AIDP

*Most common cause of rapidly progressive weakness; incidence
  0.6–1.9 per 100,000
*Ascending bilateral paralysis typical, although variation may occur
*May occur at any age
*Reflexes reduced or absent
*2/3 patients report antecedent infection 1–3 weeks prior to symptoms
  starting
*Symptoms may continue to worsen up to 4 weeks
*Medical emergency if respiration or autonomic nervous system
  affected
*"Pins and needles" in hands and feet often described
*Back and hip pain common in children

- If history and clinical examinations are suspicious for AIDP, Table 131-5 lists the diagnostic studies to confirm the diagnosis. It may be difficult to confirm AIDP if symptoms have only been present for a few days, since it may often take up to 1 week for cerebrospinal fluid (CSF) protein to rise and nerve conduction velocities to slow (although electrical studies are not needed for the diagnosis). If these studies are still normal, it may be helpful to obtain magnetic resonance imaging (MRI) looking for nerve root enhancement.
- Management of AIDP is fully dependent on the severity of symptoms and whether the patient has reached the clinical nadir (i.e., worst symptoms). If the patient is in the process of recovery, then treatment may not be necessary.
- There is some controversy regarding the best management strategy; however, a course of either IVIG or plasma exchange is recommended if ventilation is affected and should be considered with a patient who is progressing rapidly and has not reached the nadir. A 4-day course of either IVIG or plasma exchange is usually recommended.
- Prognosis for AIDP is usually good; however, recovery may take weeks to months. Usually recovery is prolonged with more severe symptoms. An ongoing PT/OT program should be initiated until symptoms resolve. Poor prognostic signs include age less than 60 years, rapidly progressive weakness in less than 7 days, assisted ventilation required, and decreased amplitude of responses in the nerve conduction velocity testing (indicating axonal involvement). It is estimated that a good recovery occurs in 75% of patients.

TABLE 131-5   Diagnostic Studies for AIDP

*Nerve conduction velocities show slowing
*CSF shows increase in protein without an increase in WBC count
*MRI may show enhancement of nerve roots
*Consider sending titers for associated pathogens

- The most common chronic neuropathy seen in childhood is HSMN or CMT. Phenotypical variation is very common; however, when this neuropathy is evident in early childhood, the usual complaint is abnormality of gait or feet deformities. Oftentimes patients are referred from orthopedic surgeons. Typically the symptoms present in the second decade and progress slowly over several decades. Usually feet are involved much earlier than hands, and typically the peroneal muscles are the first involved. This causes a typical difficulty with gait in which the patient has a bilateral foot drop or slaps the feet when they walk. It is also difficult for the patient to walk on the heels, and as symptoms progress, the child may become a toe walker.
- On examinations peroneal weakness is usually most prevalent. In addition reflexes may be reduced or absent, usually in the lower extremities before the upper extremities. There may be sensory symptoms and signs present. There may be orthopedic abnormalities of the feet and legs, including high arches and atrophy below the knees.
- Diagnostic studies to confirm HSMN begin with evaluation of nerve conduction velocities. By definition, there must be abnormality of NCVs to confirm HSMN; however, if the child presents very early on (i.e., infancy or preschool), the NCVs may not yet show significant slowing.
- The genetics of HSMN is variable. The most common form (HSMN 1A or CMT 1A) is autosomal dominant, therefore both parents should be examined if possible. The gene locus for HSMN 1A is chromosome 17p11.2, which encodes for peripheral myelin protein 22 (PMP22). Currently there are a total of approximately 22 gene loci abnormalities recognized to occur with hereditary neuropathies. It is estimated that there may be up to 100 gene loci abnormalities associated with different forms of HSMN, and the inheritance may be AD, AR, or X-linked depending on the type.
- Along with NCVs, genetic studies should be done on any child suspected of having a hereditary neuropathy. Currently, only approximately 5–10 forms of HSMN can be confirmed by genetic studies, therefore if the genetic study is normal, this still does not rule out all forms of HSMN.
- Management of the child with HSMN involves an active physical and occupational therapy program. Bracing to accommodate the foot drop often improves the abnormality of gait a great deal. Children usually remain quite stable during childhood; however, many have significant problems with gait as they reach middle age and older. It is still relatively rare for a person with HSMN to become wheelchair dependent with proper care and intervention.

NEUROMUSCULAR JUNCTION DISORDERS

- The most common disorder of the neuromuscular junction in children is myasthenia gravis (MG). There are three forms of MG that can affect children. The autoimmune form of MG is the most common form seen in children; however, this form of MG is much more common in adults. Lambert-Eaton syndrome (LES) is another disorder of the NMJ that may occur in adults, usually as part of a paraneoplastic phenomenon. LES is essentially nonexistent in children.

- The first form of MG that may occur in children is neonatal MG. This is seen as severe generalized hypotonia within the first few hours of life. The mother must have MG, and the cause is transplacental passage of acetylcholine receptor antibodies (ACHRA). Therefore this condition should be very easy to rule out. If mother has not been diagnosed with MG, but has questionable signs, ACHRA should be sent on the mother and possibly the newborn. The condition is usually self-limited over a course of 2–3 days. The newborn may require respiratory and feeding support, but once the ACHRA are cleared the symptoms resolve.

- The second form of MG that may affect children is congenital myasthenic syndromes (CMS). Presentation may be neonatal, infantile, or very early childhood. The pathology is an anatomical or physiologic abnormality of the neuromuscular junction. This may be presynaptic, synaptic, or postsynaptic involving acetylcholine packaging, deficiency of acetylcholinesterase, or abnormalities of the acetylcholine receptor. Several distinct forms have been identified. All forms are extremely rare; however, they deserve mention because it may be very difficult to distinguish CMS from the more common autoimmune form of MG.

- Diagnostic testing for CMS is the same as for autoimmune MG, and the results may look very similar; however, many forms of CMS do not respond well to typical medications used for autoimmune MG. Generally a very specific type of muscle biopsy is required to confirm the diagnosis of CMS, looking at the submicroscopic structure of the NMJ.

- Of the three types of MG that may affect children, the most common is "autoimmune" MG. Autoimmune is in parentheses because this is the presumed pathology to the condition. The presence of (ACHRA) in the serum and thymomas are frequently seen in adult MG; however, many children do not have elevated serum ACHRA, and it is extremely rare to discover a thymoma during the workup for childhood MG. Table 131-6 summarizes the main features of childhood onset MG.

TABLE 131-6   Fast Facts MG

*Symptom onset usually acute/subacute
*Can present at any age
*2 forms recognized:
  isolated ocular
  generalized
*Eye, face weakness present along with bulbar and generalized weakness
*Fatigue usually present with symptoms worse at night.

- Usually MG occurs in an otherwise healthy child. In nearly all cases there is some evidence of eye weakness; therefore, if eye weakness is not present, the differential diagnosis should be widened. Some children present with isolated ocular symptoms, whereas others present with more generalized symptoms including weakness of the cranial nerves and extremities. Occasionally the initial presentation can be extreme and require ventilatory support.

- The typical symptom associated with MG is fatigue, and generally patients are strongest in the morning. If history and clinical examination are consistent with possible MG, diagnostic studies should be pursued (Table 131-7).

- Tensilon testing should be considered if MG is suspected. The patient must have weakness at the time of the test. Potentially there may be life-threatening cholinergic symptoms during a tensilon test; therefore atropine must be drawn and ready. The tensilon test should be done "double blind." That is, the person actually completing the test should not know which syringe the tensilon is in. A duplicate syringe containing normal saline should be used as a placebo. Approximately 20% of the tensilon/normal saline is first given and if no cholinergic symptoms are present, the remainder of the tensilon/normal saline may then be given. Recommended tensilon dosing is 0.04 mg/ kg as test dose with 0.16 mg/kg to follow.

- Long-term care of the child with MG can be challenging. Generally cholinesterase inhibitors (i.e., pyridostigmine or mestinon) are initiated with a beginning dose of 0.5–1 mg/kg per dose q 3–4 hours while awake. Multiple dosage adjustments are required to

TABLE 131-7   Diagnostic Studies for MG

*Serum acetylcholine receptor antibodies (ACHRA); may not be elevated in children. If positive, MG confirmed
*Repetitive stimulation testing/EMG. Typically there is a decremental response of the muscle to repetitive stimulation (=fatigue)
*Edrophonium (tensilon) testing
*CT chest to r/o thymoma; rare in childhood MG
*Consider MRI brain since brainstem tumor may mimic symptoms.

improve symptoms completely. Once on an MG regimen, very careful history is required in follow-up visits to distinguish myasthenic weakness (usually occurring prior to a dose of mestinon) vs. cholinergic weakness (usually worse after a dose of mestinon).

- The parents/patient also need to be taught cholinergic symptoms (increase in lacrimation and salivation, bradycardia, and stomach cramps). Other treatments for MG include plasma exchange, especially for an acute and severe exacerbation with respiratory depression. Also, addition of prednisone at a dosage of 1 mg/kg every other day may be added to the long-term regimen if weakness is not completely resolved with mestinon.
- Thymectomy should be considered for generalized MG. Various studies have shown that thymectomy is beneficial in adults, and it is generally accepted that the same applies to childhood MG.
- Any type of infection can exacerbate myasthenic weakness, as can hot weather, and many different medications, including certain antibiotics.
- Prognosis is variable. Most children with autoimmune MG do relatively well, with occasional flare-up of symptoms. Spontaneous remissions may occur; however, the family should be counseled that if MG begins, it may be present the entire life of the patient. Patients with congenital myasthenic syndrome have a much worse prognosis in general, since symptoms are usually refractory to treatment.

MUSCLE DISORDERS

- By far, the most common muscle disorder seen in clinical practice is Duchenne muscular dystrophy (DMD). Becker muscular dystrophy (BMD) is a genotypically similar condition, and phenotypically slower in progression Table 131-8.
- DMD is the most rapidly progressive of the muscular dystrophies, with death usually occurring in the late teens to early 20s. Prognosis for BMD is much more variable and often patients may live well past middle age. Wheelchair confinement in DMD is usually in the early to mid-teens, BMD patients may continue to ambulate for several decades. In both phenotypes progressive dilated cardiomyopathy occurs, and often end-stage cardiac failure may occur in BMD.
- Weakness continues to progress in both phenotypes and eventual cause of death is usually respiratory compromise secondary to immobility and scoliosis. Therefore paramount in the long-term care of these patients is to preserve ambulation with orthotics as long as possible, and once wheelchair confinement occurs, prevention of scoliosis with a proper fitting wheelchair and spinal fusion if necessary.

TABLE 131-8   Fast Facts DMD/BMD

*Symptoms of proximal weakness: difficulty running, hopping, stair climbing standing from sitting (Gower's sign)
*Legs affected much earlier than arms classic sign is pseudohypertrophy of gastrocnemius muscles which cause toe walking
*Classic gait pattern
 toe walking
 wide based and lordotic to compensate
 for hip weakness
*Symptom onset
 DMD usually preschool
 BMD more variable preschool to
 midschool age
*Face and eye weakness not present
 inheritance X-linked therefore affects boys
*Serum CK extremely elevated (50–100 + X nl)
*Dilated cardiomyopathy eventually affects all patients with DMD/BMD

- With progressive weakness, contractures of joints are also a significant problem. An ongoing course of physical therapy to limit contractures is imperative. Surgical intervention should also be considered when necessary.
- If DMD/BMD is a possibility, Table 131-9 lists the diagnostic workup. It should be noted that the best way to differentiate DMD from BMD is by dystrophin staining on the muscle biopsy. Table 131-10 summarizes the genetics of DMD/BMD and the properties of dystrophin.
- DMD/BMD will be the most common muscular dystrophy seen in clinical practice; however, there are several other less severe muscular dystrophies (limb girdle MD, facioscapulohumeral MD, myotonic MD, Emory Dreifuss MD, and congenital MD, as examples). Since many of these forms are relatively common and many show distinctive signs and symptoms, further reading is encouraged.
- Terminology for muscle disease is often confusing. Muscular dystrophies are only one category of muscle disease. The term "myopathy" is even more

TABLE 131-9   Diagnostic Studies DMD/BMD

*CK levels extremely elevated
*Genetic studies
 cannot differentiate DMD vs BMD completely
 study is positive in 2/3 of patients, & negative in 1/3
*Muscle biopsy
 routine histology: dystrophic process
 dystrophin staining:
  absent in DMD
  reduced in BMD
  nl in other muscle
  disorders

TABLE 131-10 Genetics of DMD/BMD and Dystrophin

*Genetics: X-linked
*Gene location: Xp21
*Gene product: dystrophin
*Dystrophin:
    very large structural membrane protein absent in DMD, reduced in
    BMD present in skeletal and cardiac muscle, and brain dystrophin
    may explain high rate of learning disorders in DMD/BMD several
    other structural proteins associated with dystrophin, found to be
    abnormal in other forms of muscular dystrophy

general and refers to any condition that affects the muscle. Listed below are some other general categories of muscle disease seen with some unique features.

- Congenital myopathies: All present in the neonatal or infant age. Eye, face, bulbar, and generalized weakness present. Serum CK usually 3–5 × elevated. Muscle biopsy required to confirm diagnosis. The prognosis is variable depending on type. Often confused with SMA; however, should not have eye and facial weakness with SMA. Specific types include nemaline myopathy, myotubular myopathy, and mini-core myopathy as examples.
- Inflammatory myopathies: Dermatomyositis most common in children, with elevation of serum CK and typical rash (heliotropic rash over face and other skin changes over extensor surfaces). Immunologic markers, MRI muscle, and muscle biopsy to confirm diagnosis. Treatment usually immunosuppression. Viral myositis is a common self-limited inflammatory myopathy occurring during a viral exanthem such as influenza. Pain and disability may be severe in some children; however, typically self-limited condition.
- Metabolic myopathies: Large number of varieties. May be a problem with mitochondrial function/fat metabolism or may be a problem with glycogenosis. Mitochondrial problems may not only involve muscle but affect other organ systems (including the central nervous system). Symptoms are extremely variable. Muscle biopsy usually required to confirm diagnosis. The syndromes involving glycogenosis are also variable. A common symptom of these disorders is exercise intolerance with weakness and muscle cramping/pain. The most common example is McArdle syndrome. Muscle biopsy is usually required to confirm diagnosis (Table 131-10).
- In summary, the task of pinpointing the specific diagnosis of a peripheral nervous system disorder should not seem overwhelming. By categorizing to a specific location within the motor unit based on the physical examination, and then using other information such as

age of onset, and acuity of symptoms, along with specific diagnostic studies, most conditions can be determined and an appropriate treatment plan initiated. Currently treatment is limited in most disorders; however, with the massive explosion of genetic information in the last several years, families should be encouraged to remain optimistic about future treatment modalities.

132 ATAXIA

Alexander Bassuk

- *Definition*: Refers to a disturbance in the smooth performance of voluntary acts. The most prominent feature of ataxia is usually an abnormal gait, although any disturbance in the fine control of movement (speed, range, force, and timing) may be called ataxia.

ANATOMICAL CONSIDERATIONS

- Generally, ataxia is caused by dysfunction in the cerebellum or from cerebellar afferents, thus the discussion of ataxia requires a basic understanding of the anatomy of the cerebellum and its connections.
- The cerebellum is divided into three lobes: the anterior lobe, the posterior lobe, and the flocculonodular lobe. The primary fissure separates the anterior and posterior lobes. The posterolateral fissure separates the posterior and flocculonodular lobe. The cerebellar peduncles connect the cerebellum to the brain stem. The superior cerebellar peduncle connects to the midbrain, the middle cerebellar peduncle connects to the pons, and the inferior cerebellar peduncle connects the medulla. The cerebellar vermis lies between the two cerebellar hemispheres. The cerebellum receives input from the frontal lobes (which essentially initiate volitional movement), and the spinal cord (which provides proprioceptive input from the periphery).
- There are several signs and symptoms associated with lesions in these anatomical locations.
- *Cerebellar dysarthria*: This term is used to denote the scanning or staccato-like speech that may be seen in patients with cerebellar disease.

- *Tremor*: Cerebellar lesions tend to produce an intention (kinetic) tremor. A postural (static) tremor may also be seen.
- *Ocular motor dysfunction*. Nystagmus is frequently observed in midline cerebellar lesions. Ocular dysmetria (conjugate overshoot and undershoot of a target) may be seen with lateral or midline cerebellar lesions. Many other abnormalities of eye movements may be attributable to cerebellar lesions.
- *Truncal ataxia and titubations* generally suggest a midline cerebellar lesion; dysmetria and hypotonia suggest a lesion of the ipsilateral cerebellar hemisphere.
- *Cautious and/or lurching gait*: Patients with disease of the peripheral nervous system and/or the spinal cord may need to look at their feet in order to know where they are in space. They typically have a high stepping gait, and their gait dysfunction is exacerbated by eye closure. Patients with these lesions may demonstrate the Rhomberg sign.
- Patients with bifrontal disease may have any or all of the above mentioned symptoms; in addition, they may demonstrate difficulty in gait initiation.
- The differential diagnosis of ataxias may be divided into acute, episodic, and chronic or progressive causes. It is important to note the progressive ataxias may be noticed acutely, episodic ataxias are always "acute" when they first present, and patients with episodic ataxias may not always return to baseline following exacerbations, thus demonstrating an "acute or chronic" presentation.

ACUTE ATAXIA

- *Drug ingestion*: History is essential in clarifying this presentation. A toxicology screen should be obtained on all children presenting with acute ataxia. Toxic causes of ataxia include alcohol, benzodiazepines, anticonvulsants (particularly phenytoin), antihistamines, and thallium (occasionally used in pesticides). Treatment depends on the particular toxin. All medications in the home should be noted and accounted for.
- *Postinfectious cerebellitis*: This occurs primarily in children aged 1–3 years and is a diagnosis of exclusion. The condition often follows a viral illness, and is thought to represent an autoimmune phenomenon. Ataxia is typically maximal at onset. CSF analysis is usually normal or shows a mild protein elevation. Ataxia tends to improve in a few weeks but may persist for months. Most patients improve in a few weeks, but symptoms may persist for months. Varicella is thought to be the most common etiology, although in the future the vaccine may diminish its importance.

- *Brainstem encephalitis*: Ataxia may be the first sign of encephalitis. Cranial nerve abnormalities are often coexistent along with other signs of encephalitis (meningismus, change in mental status, and seizures). Diagnosis depends on a cellular cerebrospinal fluid (CSF) response. Treatment is supportive.
- *Metabolic*: Patients with hypoglycemia, hyponatremia, and hyperammonemia may all present with ataxia.
- *Neuroblastoma*: Patients with neuroblastoma may initially present with ataxia or chaotic eye movements. The eye movement abnormality is known as opsoclonus (dancing eyes). Patients may later develop a myoclonic encephalopathy. Typical age of presentation is 1 month to 4 years. The symptoms appear to be the result of a dysimmune state. All patients with opsoclonus should be thoroughly evaluated for occult neuroblastoma, with full body imaging and measurement of urinary homovanillic (HVA) and vanillylmandelic (VMA). Neuroblastoma, if found, should be removed and treated. Adrenocorticotropic hormone (ACTH) and steroids have both been used to treat symptoms. In the future nuclear medicine scans may prove to be the most effective to make this diagnosis.
- *Brain tumors*: Brain tumors usually cause chronic ataxias in children; however, if a tumor bleeds or causes hydrocephalus, the child may present acutely.
- *Trauma*: Ataxia may follow even mild head injuries, and is the most typical postconcussive symptom in small children. The diagnosis depends on the clinical context. Imaging may be normal, or show evidence of axonal injury. Symptoms usually clear within 1–6 months. Trauma to the vertebrobasilar system may occur with sports-related injuries or chiropractic manipulation. Symptoms are noted shortly after injury. History and examination typically reveal signs and symptoms of ipsilateral cerebellar and brainstem disturbance. Imaging may show infarction in the cerebellar hemisphere and medulla.
- *Vascular lesions*: Cerebellar hemorrhage. In the absence of an underlying coagulation disorder cerebellar hemorrhage in children is usually due to an AVM. Cerebellar AVMs may present with headache and ataxia.
- *Kawasaki disease*: Kawasaki disease is a systemic illness that may include multiple brain infarcts, potentially causing ataxia. Diagnosis depends on the appropriate constellation of signs and symptoms.
- *Polyradiculopathy*: As noted above, disease of the peripheral nervous system can cause ataxia. Guillain-Barre syndrome and tick paralysis are two common diseases of children that may present as acute ataxia although most likely as a secondary effect of the overt weakness.

- *Biotinidase deficiency*: Ataxia may be present at any point in the course of a patient with this rare disorder. The initial features are usually seizures and hypotonia. Diagnosis is suspected when ketoacidosis, hyperammonemia, and organic aciduria are present and onset of symptoms is after the newborn period. Diagnosis is confirmed by demonstrating biotinidase deficiency in serum. Treatment is with biotin.

- *Conversion reaction*: Children may manifest a myriad of gait disturbances in response to underlying psychologic stressors. The so-called "hysterical" gait is often quite dramatic, involving extraordinary balance. The physical examination is entirely normal. Diagnosis is made based on history and an otherwise normal physical examination. Treatment is aimed at elucidating the underlying psychologic stressors.

RECURRENT ATAXIAS

- *Basilar migraine*: Ataxia is a relatively common manifestation of migraine in children. Pathophysiologically, migraine manifesting as ataxia is thought to involve the vasculature in the posterior circulation. Gait ataxia occurs in about 50% of patients, but since the posterior circulation also irrigates the cerebellum, brainstem structures, and occipital lobes, children may present with emesis, autonomic disturbances (including arrhythmias and loss of consciousness), and visual changes. Attacks are often accompanied by occipital headache. Attacks usually begin in adolescence but may occur at any age. Many children with recurrent bouts of migraine with ataxia may later present with common or classic migraine. The diagnosis of migraine as a cause of ataxia remains a diagnosis of exclusion. Electroencephalogram (EEG) should be performed to distinguish migraine from benign occipital epilepsy. Basilar migraine should be treated according to standard migraine treatment, although vasoconstricting agents (e.g., triptans) should be avoided in children with life-threatening autonomic disturbances.

- *Multiple sclerosis (MS)*: MS is rare in the pediatric population, but ataxia is one of the most common presentations of MS in children. MS is routinely diagnosed by two clinical attacks of demyelination separated by space and time. New criteria allow for diagnosis based on supplementation by preclinical testing (brainstem and visual evoked potentials) and magnetic resonance imaging (MRI) in some cases. Acute treatment with corticosteroids may decrease length of symptoms but does not affect the progression of the disease. Treatment with immune modula-

tors may be indicated in children to prevent frequency of relapse.

- *Pseudoataxia (epileptic)*: Ataxia is rarely a seizure manifestation. Diagnosis should be suspected in otherwise unexplained episodic ataxias. EEG may show generalized 2–3 Hz spike and wave complexes with frontal predominance. Epileptic ataxia should respond to anticonvulsant treatment.

- *Episodic ataxia type 1 (EA1)*: EA1 is caused by mutations in a potassium-channel gene, KCNA1, on chromosome 12p. Inheritance is autosomal dominant. The onset is between childhood and adolescence. Besides episodic ataxia, clinical manifestations are myokymia (continuous motor unit activity) around the eyes, lips, or fingers. Brief attacks of ataxia and dysarthria usually lasting seconds (but possibly hours) are precipitated by exercise or startle. Myokymia can also be observed between attacks. Diagnosis is based on history and family history. Electromyography (EMG) confirms the presence of myokymia. Treatment with acetazolamide is effective in many patients. Anticonvulsants such as phenytoin have also been used.

- *Episodic ataxia type 2 (EA2)*: EA2 is caused by a mutation in the gene encoding the calcium channel on chromosome 19. Inheritance is autosomal dominant. Mutations in this channel are also associated in spinocerebellar ataxia type 6 (SCA6) and familial hemiplegic migraine. Clinical manifestations of EA2 consist of mild-to-severe intermittent cerebellar dysfunction ± oculomotor abnormalities, including interictal nystagmus, diplopia, and migraine. Symptoms can last minutes to days. Attacks are provoked by stress and exercise but not startle. EA2 may respond to treatment with acetazolamide.

- *Hartnup disease*: Hartnup disease is caused by impaired tryptophan absorption in the kidney and small intestine. Inheritance is autosomal recessive. Affected children are normal at birth, but may show developmental delay. Episodic ataxia is usually precipitated by stress or infection, and may include limb ataxia, mental status changes, and decreased tone. Affected children have a photosensitive pellagra-like skin rash. Diagnosis is made by establishing aminoaciduria involving neutral monoaminocarboxyclin amino acids (alanine, serine, threonine, asparagines, glutamine, valine, leucine, isoleucine, phenylalanine, tyrosine, tryptophan, histidine, and citrulline). Treatment with nicotinamide can prevent the skin rash, and may reverse neurologic manifestations. A high-protein diet supplements lost amino acids.

- *Intermittent maple syrup urine disease*: Maple syrup urine disease is caused by a deficiency in metabolism of branched-chain ketoacid dehydrogenase. Inheritance is autosomal recessive. The intermittent form of this disease is characterized by episodic ataxia ± irritability and lethargy provoked by infection or high-protein meals. During attacks, valine, leucine, and isoleucine are excreted in excess in the urine, and the urine may have a maple syrup odor. Diagnosis is made by demonstrating the enzyme deficiency in fibroblasts. Prophylactic treatment requires a protein-restricted diet. Some children have a thiamine responsive enzyme abnormality and a trial of thiamine (1 g) during attacks should be attempted. If the attacks respond to thiamine, maintenance thiamine should be started. Management during attacks is aimed at reversing ketoacidosis.

• *Pyruvate dehydrogenase deficiency-E1 (PDH-E1)*: PHDE-1 is caused by a mutation in one of the subunits of the pyruvate dehydrogenase complex. Inheritance is X-linked. Development in the first 3 years of life is variable. Episodes of ataxia usually begin in the third year and may be associated with generalized weakness and mental status change. Attacks may be spontaneous or provoked by infection, stress, or high-carbohydrate meals. Metabolic acidosis is usually present. Laboratory evaluation usually reveals a low lactate/pyruvate ratio, with elevated lactate and pyruvate during attacks. Diagnosis is confirmed by analysis of enzyme activity. Treatment with thiamine and a high-fat, low-carbohydrate diet may prevent disease progression in some children.

CHRONIC OR PROGRESSIVE ATAXIA

• *Brain tumors*: Brain tumor should be suspected in any child with progressive ataxia. Brain tumors are the second most common tumors in children, and the most common solid tumors. Between the ages of 1 and 8, posterior fossa tumors are more common than supratentorial tumors in children. Posterior fossa tumors typically present with ataxia, gait disturbance, emesis, and signs and symptoms of increased intracranial pressure. It is important to note that children with supratentorial brain tumors may also present with gait disturbances and ataxia. The most common posterior fossa tumors in children are cerebellar astrocytoma, brainstem glioma, ependymoma, and medulloblastoma. Diagnosis is usually made by computed tomography (CT) and MRI, and treatment is specific for tumor type.

• *Brain malformations*: Several congenital brain malformations may manifest initially or eventually as ataxia. Basilar impression is a disorder of the cran-

iocervical junction in which the odontoid process is displaced posteriorly and displaces the spinal cord or brain stem. Children initially present with head tilt, neck stiffness, or headache, and symptoms may be precipitated by neck trauma. Symptoms may include ataxia. The abnormality is best seen by MRI. Surgical decompression relieves the symptoms.

• Congenital hypoplasia of the cerebellar hemispheres may be unilateral or bilateral, and may present with developmental delay, hypotonia, titubation, ataxia, and tremor. Nystagmus is usually present. Fifty percent of cases with bilateral hypolplasia are associated with an underlying genetic disorder. Diagnosis is made by MRI. Cerebellar vermal aplasia is usually associated with other brain malformations, as can be seen with Joubert syndrome and the Dandy-Walker malformation. Vermal aplasia is typically associated with head and trunk titubation and truncal ataxia. Diagnosis is made by MRI.

• *Chiari malformations*: Chiari type I is defined as displacement of the cerebellar tonsils and posterior vermis of the cerebellum through the foramen magnum, compressing the cervicomedullary junction. Chiari type II is defined by the type I malformation with a dysplastic lower medulla and a lumbosacral meningomyelocele. Chiari type II may not present until adolescence. Presentation is myriad and may include ataxia. Diagnosis is made by MRI. Decompression of the posterior fossa may help alleviate symptoms in some selected patients.

• *Freidrich ataxia (FA)*: Friedrich ataxia is the most common form of hereditary progressive ataxia. The disease is caused by a GAA expansion in a noncoding region of the frataxin gene. Normal alleles contain 6–28 GAA repeats, while affected individuals have 60–1800 repeats. Inheritance is autosomal recessive. The disease is a progressive spinocerebellar degeneration with typical onset before the age of 25 years, especially during childhood or adolescence.

• Pathologic changes in Friedrich ataxia classically include degeneration of the dorsal root ganglia, posterior columns, corticospinal/spinocerebellar tracts, and cerebellum. These pathologic changes give rise to an ataxic gait, classically followed by dysarthria, upper limb ataxia, distal sensory loss, decreased vibration and position sense, and absence of reflexes with extensor plantar responses (up-going toes). Scoliosis and pes cavus also may also be seen.

• The disease (FA) often includes hypertrophic cardiomyopathy, diabetes mellitus, ± hearing loss or optic atrophy. The diagnosis is confirmed by molecular testing. All patients should receive regular electrocardiograms

(ECGs), and should be monitored for development of diabetes.

- *Ataxia telangiectasia (AT)*: AT is caused by mutations in the ataxia telangiectasia mutated (ATM) gene which encoded a protein kinase involved in *deoxyribonucleic acid* (DNA) repair. The mutation leads to exquisite radiation sensitivity in affected individuals.
- Inheritance is autosomal recessive. Gait ataxia is a prominent sign presenting during infancy or childhood. Neurologic symptoms include ocular apraxia, slow horizontal saccades, cerebellar syndrome, dystonic postures, chorea, tics or jerks, dysphagia and choking, and peripheral neuropathy. Other manifestations include telangiectasias (appearing after age 2, usually first in the conjunctivae), premature senile keratosis and graying of the hair, atrophy of thymus and lymphoid tissues, lymphopenia, hypogammaglobulinemia (leading to frequent infections), lymphoma, and leukemia.
- Diagnosis of AT is suspected based on the appropriate constellation of symptoms. Most patients have an elevated alpha-fetoprotein, decreased serum IgA, IgE, and IgG. Treatment includes aggressive treatment of infections and prevention of exposure to radiation.
- *Disorders related to vitamin E deficiency*: Acquired vitamin E deficiency results in spinocerebellar degeneration, peripheral neuropathy, and retinitis pigmentosa. This deficiency is usually secondary to fat absorption. Treatment in acquired deficiency is aimed at underlying etiologies. Several disorders result in hypobetalipoproteinemia, in which patients have relative deficiency of apolipoprotein A and B. Treatment includes administration of DL-alpha-tocopherol. Ataxia with vitamin E deficiency is a rare autosomal recessive disease with slowly progressive gait and limb ataxia. The disease is due to a defect in the TTP1 gene which transfers alpha-tocopherol to the circulating lipoproteins. Abetalipoproteinemia (Bassen-Kornzweig disease [BKD]) is caused in some cases by mutations in the microsomal triglyceride transfer protein (MTP) gene. Inheritance is autosomal recessive. Fat malabsorption results in secondary vitamin E deficiency. BKD presents in infancy with steatorrhoea and fat malabsorption. Diagnosis is confirmed by the absence of apolipoprotein B in plasma. Treatment includes dietary fat restriction and large doses of vitamin E.
- *Spinocerebellar ataxia*: The spinocerebellar ataxias (SCAs) now include over 16 distinct genetic loci with overlapping phenotypes. The majority are autosomal dominant, and many (SCA1, 2, 3, 6, 7, 17, and dentate-rubral-pallidulysian atrophy) are caused by

an expansion of CAG repeats in their respective genes. The mutation in these disorders is an expansion of a naturally occurring CAG repeat in the protein coding region of a specific protein. This leads to an abnormal expanded series of glutamines being translated in that protein. The expansion is unstable over generations leading to progressive lengthening of the repeat. Disease results when the repeat reaches a specific range. Further expansion leads to earlier age of onset. Thus, the CAG repeat size correlates inversely with the age of onset. The mutations for SCA8 and SCA12 are expansions of a CAG/CTG repeat in untranslated regions of the genes. Individuals with SCA10 have an expansion of an intronic ATTCT repeat. The clinical features of the SCAs overlap, and the specific SCAs are best diagnosed by genetic testing. Treatment is symptomatic, and varies according to disease.

RARE FORMS OF CHRONIC OR PROGRESSIVE ATAXIA

- Other rare diseases that may demonstrate ataxia include vanishing white matter disease (progressive hypomyelination on MRI), adrenoleukodystrophy (X-linked, increase very-long chain fatty acids), metachromatic leukodystrophy (deficient arylsulfatase A), refsum disease (increased phytanic acid), Krabbe disease (galactocerebrosidase deficiency), Pelizaeus-Merzbacher syndrome (neonatal tremor and shaking movements of the head, abnormal eye movements, and progression to cerebellar ataxia, dysarthria, and intention tremor of the upper limbs), juvenile GM2 gangliosidosis (decreased alpha- and beta-hexominidase activity in fibroblasts), Ramsay Hunt syndrome (cerebellar ataxia and myoclonus), Marinesco-Sjoren syndrome (bilateral cataracts, progressive cerebellar ataxia, and mental retardation), sea-blue histiocytoses (hepatosplenomegaly and ataxia, evaluate for Niemann-Pick), ataxia with dementia (X-linked, progressive incoordination), recessive ataxia with ocular motor apraxia, spastic ataxia of Charlevoix-Saguenay (autosomal recessive ataxia with axonal neuropathy and progressive spastic quadraparesis), xeroderma pigmentosum (cutaneous cancers), Cockayne syndrome (growth retardation, moderate skin photosensitivity and premature aging, and neuropathy), and Kallman syndrome (hypogonadotrophic hypogonadism and anosmia with associated eye movement abnormalities and cerebellar ataxia).

133 EPILEPSY

Linda C. Laux

OVERVIEW

- A seizure is an alteration of behavior that results from an abnormal and excessive activity of a group of cerebral neurons. Epilepsy is defined as two or more unprovoked seizures. Epilepsy syndromes are a classification of epilepsies based on a cluster of signs and symptoms, including the clinical seizure type, age of onset, electroencephalogram (EEG) pattern, neurologic examination, and neuroimaging.
- The incidence of a single seizure in childhood is 4–6%. The incidence of epilepsy during childhood is approximately 1%. Seventy to 80% of children will eventually "outgrow" their seizure disorder.
- History is the most important tool the clinician has to evaluate a spell. A careful and complete history including what happened immediately prior to the spell, the first indication to the witness that something was wrong, a complete description of the event, the level of responsiveness of the child, the duration of the event, how the episode resolved, and what the child did after the event are important questions to determine if the spell was a seizure and, if so, to classify the seizure/epilepsy syndrome. The EEG and video EEG are adjunctive tests to the history that also may help answer these questions.

PAROXYSMAL SPELLS THAT MAY MIMIC SEIZURES

- *Apnea/acute life-threatening events*: Apnea is the cessation of breathing for greater than 15 seconds. Apnea may be secondary to centrally mediated or obstructive causes. Nonepileptic apnea is usually associated with bradycardia without any other abnormal movements or behaviors. Apnea is rarely the sole manifestation of a seizure.
- *Gastroesophageal reflux*: Infants with GER may have spells of staring, extremity movement/posturing, and opisthotonic posturing (Sandifer syndrome). A careful history will disclose that these episodes are temporally associated with feeds.
- Sleep disorders including benign nocturnal myoclonus, night terrors, sleepwalking, and narcolepsy/cataplexy.
- Migraine and migraine variants including paroxysmal torticollis, benign paroxysmal vertigo, confusional migraine, and hemiplegic migraine.

- *Cyanotic and pallid syncope*: Cyanotic syncope (breath-holding spells) occurs in children aged 6 months to 6 years. Secondary to frustration or minor injury, the child will cry and suddenly stop breathing in expiration and turn blue. If the episode is of sufficient length, the child will lose consciousness and may have a few extremity jerks or stiffness. A similar spell is pallid syncope. Again, the event is provoked by frustration, injury, or fright. In this spell, however, the child initially turns pale prior to losing consciousness and becoming limp. Both types of syncope are benign and typically do not require treatment.
- *Movement disorders*: Nonepileptic movements such as jitteriness, shuddering attacks, tics, Tourette syndrome, choreoathetosis, and dystonia may be paroxysmal and mimc seizures.
- *Inattention/daydreaming spells*: School-age children are commonly evaluated for inattention spells that may represent attention deficit hyperactivity disorder or simply daydreaming behaviors. "Staring episodes" can also be seen in either absence seizures or complex partial seizures; however, nonepileptic staring spells usually occur only during passive activity and can be interrupted by tactile stimulation.
- *Repetitious behaviors*: Children have many behaviors that may mimic seizures. Stereotypies and self-stimulatory behaviors including head banging and body rocking are especially common in the neurologically impaired child. Temper tantrums and "rage attacks" may also mimic seizures; however, in nonepileptic rage attack, the attacks are typically provoked and the anger is usually directed.
- *Pseudoseizures/psychogenic seizures*: Children may have nonepileptic spells that may be difficult to distinguish from seizures in response to an emotional stress. Video EEG monitoring may be required to distinguish these episodes from epileptic seizures. It is important to remember that both epileptic and psychogenic seizures may occur in the same patient.

CLASSIFICATION OF SEIZURES

- The International League Against Epilepsy proposed a classification of all seizures based on clinical seizure semiology and EEG patterns. This classification basically divides seizures into partial (focal/localization-related) vs. generalized seizures.
- A partial seizure is a seizure in which the first clinical or EEG changes indicated that the seizure arises from a group of neurons localized to one area in one hemisphere. If consciousness is preserved throughout the seizure, the seizure is classified as a simple partial

seizure. If consciousness is at all impaired and the patient does not respond appropriately, then the seizure is classified as a complex partial seizure. A seizure may begin as a simple partial seizure and evolve into a complex partial seizure. Either a simple partial seizure or a complex partial seizure may directly progress to a secondarily generalized convulsion. The clinical seizure semiology of partial seizures depends on where in the brain the seizure arises from. Partial seizures may present with abnormal motor signs (unilateral clonic jerking, posturing, twisting, automatisms), sensory symptoms (somatosensory, visual, auditory, olfactory, gustatory, vertiginous), autonomic signs (tachycardia, papillary dilatation, sweating, flushing, rising epigastric sensation), and psychic symptoms (deja vu, distortions, illusions, hallucinations, affective changes).

- With generalized seizures, the first clinical and EEG changes suggest involvement of both hemispheres diffusely. As a result, the seizure semiology of generalized seizures does not have the variability of focal seizures. Generalized seizures include absence seizures (brief staring spells), myoclonic seizures (sudden, quick, nonrhythmic muscle jerks), clonic seizures (generalized rhythmic extremity jerking), tonic seizures (generalized stiffening episodes), tonic-clonic seizures (generalized stiffness followed by rhythmic extremity jerking), and atonic seizures (sudden loss of muscle tone resulting in a head drop or sudden fall to the ground). The EEG correlates to these seizures will be generalized epileptiform discharges often provoked by photic stimulation or hyperventilation.

COMMON EPILEPSY SYNDROMES

- *Benign neonatal familial convulsions*: Seizures begin typically on the second or third day of life after an unremarkable delivery. Seizures are of a mixed type with a combination of apnea, clonic, tonic, autonomic, and oculofacial movements. The neonates are otherwise healthy and head imaging as well as interictal EEG is normal. This disorder is autosomal dominant with a chromosome heterogeneity including chromosomes 20 and 8. The identified gene product is an alpha-subunit of an acetylcholine receptor. This syndrome is benign with seizures that are typically easy to control and resolution of this seizure tendency occurs in the first year of life in the majority of patients.
- *Benign childhood epilepsy with centrotemporal spikes (benign rolandic epilepsy)*: This epilepsy syndrome presents in school-age children, ages 3–13

years, with nocturnal simple partial seizures involving unilateral face and upper extremity. Typically, the child will awaken from sleep with gagging, drooling, and inability to talk although clearly responsive with unilateral face/arm sensations or movements. A small minority of children will have nocturnal convulsions or diurnal episodes. EEG has a characteristic pattern of bilateral independent centrotemporal spikes. Examination, development, and neuroimaging are normal. This syndrome is typically benign with seizures that are infrequent, easily treated, and resolve by adolescence.
- *Childhood absence epilepsy*: This syndrome presents in school-age children with short duration absence seizures often occurring multiple times a day. The patients are otherwise neurologically normal. EEG has a typical 3 Hz spike wave discharge often provoked by photic stimulation and hyperventilation. Rarely are other generalized seizure types (myoclonic, clonic seizures) noted. This syndrome usually resolves by adolescence. This epilepsy syndrome has a presumed genetic predisposition and chromosomal localization to 8q24 and 5q31 has been described.
- *Juvenile absence epilepsy*: This syndrome presents in early adolescence with staring spells that are often longer in duration (minutes) but less frequent than the absence seizures noted in *childhood absence epilepsy*. This epilepsy syndrome has a higher risk for other generalized seizure types and is less likely to spontaneously resolve as is its childhood counterpart. The EEG correlate is a spike wave discharge typically faster than 3 Hz.
- *Juvenile myoclonic epilepsy*: This syndrome is characterized by early morning erratic myoclonic jerks with infrequent generalized tonic-clonic and absence seizures. Seizures are often provoked by sleep deprivation, unexpected arousals, alcohol intake, and photic stimulation. The mean onset is age 14. The EEG correlate is a 4–6 Hz fast spike wave discharge that is quite photic sensitive. While the seizures are often controlled with medication, the chance of relapse is high (~90%) if medications are discontinued. JME shows a strong genetic component with one candidate gene on chromosome 6 identified.
- *Infantile spasms (West syndrome)*: A triad of clinical spasms, hypsarrhythmia pattern on interictal EEG, and developmental delay/regression mark this disorder of infancy. Clinical spasms are quick body jerks with a subtle sustained tonic position for 1–2 seconds. Spasms may be extensor, flexor, or mixed. The seizures tend to cluster while the child is drowsy. The interictal EEG shows a disorganized, discontinuous,

high amplitude pattern with multifocal epileptiform discharges (hypsarrhythmia). This disorder may be secondary to prior clastic brain injury, developmental brain abnormalities, or metabolic disease. The infantile spasms are cryptogenic if no identifiable underlying etiology is identified. Prognosis is poor for both control of the spasms and future cognitive ability.

• *Lennox-Gastaut syndrome*: This syndrome occurs in young children aged 1–8 years with mixed generalized seizure types including tonic, atypical absence, myoclonic, tonic-clonic seizures, as well as partial seizures. The EEG pattern is markedly abnormal with a slow (<2.5 Hz) spike wave discharge. The children typically have significant cognitive impairment/mental retardation. As with infantile spasms, the etiology may be symptomatic or cryptogenic. Prognosis is poor for seizure control.

ETIOLOGY

• *Febrile seizures*: Febrile seizures are seizures provoked by fever in children ages 3 months to 5 years. By definition, these seizures have no other underlying neurologic etiology. Febrile seizures are common and occur in 2–5% of all children. Simple febrile seizures are brief (less than 15 minutes) generalized convulsions that only occur once in the course of an illness. Complex febrile seizures are febrile seizures that are either prolonged, have focal features, or occur multiple times during the course of an illness. Complex febrile seizures increase the risk of future epilepsy. Febrile seizures are considered benign and typically do not require the use of daily antiepileptic medication. If prolonged febrile seizures have occurred, rectal valium (Diastat), 0.4–0.5 mg/kg, can be prescribed to stop the acute seizure. Antipyretic therapy has not been proven to be effective in decreasing the risk of recurrent febrile seizures.

• *Acute symptomatic etiology*: Acute metabolic disorders including hypoglycemia, hypo/hypernatremia, and hypocalcemia may cause seizures. In addition, a direct central nervous system infection such as meningitis or encephalitis, may present with seizures. Other acute etiologies to provoke seizures include toxin, trauma, and stroke. In children with epilepsy, a common reason for sudden increase in seizures is poor drug compliance.

• *Remote symptomatic etiology*: Prior clastic brain lesions including hypoxic ischemic encephalopathy, trauma, infection, and stroke may cause seizures.

Developmental brain abnormalities, especially cortical dysplasias and migration defects, often are associated with seizures. Finally, tumors are an infrequent cause of childhood epilepsy. In remote symptomatic etiology, the seizures appear suddenly although the brain abnormality may have been present for a long time.

• *Neurodegenerative diseases*: Intractable seizures are often one of the signs of neurodegenerative diseases. These diseases typically are associated with cognitive and motor abnormalities as well. Categories of diseases include mitochondrial abnormalities, peroxisomal diseases, lysosomal diseases, amino/organic acid abnormalities, neurocutaneous syndromes, and neuronal ceroid lipofuscinosis to only name of a few. While neurodegenerative diseases are rare, they are devastating to the families.

TREATMENT OF SEIZURES

• The decision to begin an antiepileptic drug (AED) must balance the risks/benefits of therapy vs. the risks of a subsequent seizure. While reports vary, the recurrence risk after the first nonprovoked seizure is approximately 40%. The majority of recurrent seizures occur soon after the first event, with 50% occurring within 6 months. Recurrence risk is increased for children with remote symptomatic etiology, abnormal EEG, prior history of febrile seizures, Todd paralysis, and nocturnal seizures. Factors that do not appear to influence recurrent seizures are age of the patient and duration of the initial seizure. Diagnosis of specific epilepsy syndromes will help determine prognosis and treatment requirements. In general, treatment is often not begun after the first seizure in children although specific individual cases vary.

• The choice of an AED is based on efficacy and adverse side effect profile (Table 133-1). The goal of treatment is to prevent further seizures with no adverse medication effects. Monotherapy is preferable if possible. Other factors involved in choosing an AED may include drug formulation, dosing schedule, drug interactions, and physician comfort.

• Seventy percent of children become seizure-free on monotherapy. Another 15% of children become seizure-free on polypharmacy. Fifteen percent of children have intractable epilepsy.

• Alternative epilepsy treatment (other than medication) includes the following: (1) *The ketogenic diet*: This is a very strict high-fat diet useful for intractable generalized seizures. (2) *The vagal nerve stimulator*: This is a surgically implanted wire around the vagal nerve

TABLE 133-1 Antiepileptic Medications

DRUG	EFFICACY	COMMON SIDE EFFECTS (OFTEN DOSE-DEPENDENT)	RARE/SERIOUS SIDE EFFECTS (OFTEN IDIOSYNCRATIC)
Phenobarbital	Broad spectrum (especially useful in neonates and infants)	Lethargy, dizzy, ataxia Cognitive disturbance Hyperactivity, emotional disturbance Sleep disturbance, headache	Rash Megaloblastic anemia Liver toxicity
Phenytoin (Dilantin)	Partial seizures	Lethargy, dizzy, ataxia, nystagmus Coarse facies, hirsuitism, gingival hyperplasia Osteomalacia	Rash Blood dyscrasias-variable Liver toxicity Lymphadenopathy
Primidone (Mysoline)	Broad spectrum	Lethargy, dizzy, ataxia Behavioral changes	Rash Megaloblastic anemia, leukopenia Systemic lupus-like syndrome
Ethosuximide (Zarontin)	Absence seizures	Lethargy, dizzy, ataxia, headache Behavioral changes Nausea, vomiting, stomach pain, hiccups	Rash Blood dyscrasias-variable (rare)
Carbamazepine (Tegretol, Carbitrol)	Partial seizures	Lethargy, dizzy, ataxia, nystagmus, diploplia Nausea, vomiting, abdominal pain	Rash Blood dyscrasias-variable including aplastic anemia Liver toxicity Pancreatitis Hyponatremia
Valproate (Depakote/ Depakene)	Broad spectrum	Lethargy, dizzy, ataxia, headache Behavioral problems Nausea, vomiting, weight gain or loss Alopecia, tremor	Rash Thrombocytopenia Liver toxicity Pancreatitis
Felbamate (Felbatol)	Broad spectrum	Lethargy, dizzy, ataxia, headache, insomnia Anorexia, abdominal pain	Rash Aplastic anemia Liver toxicity
Gabapentin (Neurontin)	Partial seizures	Lethargy, dizzy, ataxia Behavioral changes Nausea, vomiting, weight gain	Rash
Lamotrigine (Lamictal)	Broad spectrum	Lethargy, dizzy ataxia, diploplia Nausea, vomiting	Rash/ Stevens-Johnson syndrome
Topiramate (Topomax)	Broad spectrum	Lethargy, dizzy, ataxia, nystagmus Cognitive slowing Weight loss Kidney stones (1.5%)	Rash Acute angle glaucoma
Tiagabine (Gabatril)	Partial seizures	Lethargy, dizzy, ataxia Cognitive concerns, poor concentration Tremor, generalized weakness	Rash
Levetiracetam (Keprra)	Broad spectrum	Lethargy, dizzy, ataxia Behavioral changes, psychosis	Rash
Oxcarbazepine (Trileptal)	Partial seizures	Lethargy, dizzy, ataxia, headache Nausea	Rash (30% cross-react with CBZ) Hyponatremia
Zonisamide (Zonegram)	Broad spectrum	Lethargy, dizzy, ataxia Psychomotor slowing, difficulty concentration Nausea, anorexia Kidney stones (4%)	Rash Oligohydrosis/hyperthermia

ABBREVIATION: CBZ, carbamazepine

hooked to a pacemaker device in the chest that is programmed to give intermittent stimulation to the vagal nerve. This device is Food and Drug Administration (FDA) approved as adjunctive therapy for partial seizures in children over 12 years of age; however, efficacy in younger children as well as in children with intractable generalized seizures is suggested in the literature. (3) *Epilepsy surgery*: Some patients, particularly with intractable focal seizures and identifiable lesions on head imaging studies, may be candidates for epilepsy surgery. Different surgical techniques include hemispherectomy, lobectomy, and lesionectomy as well as corpus callosotomy.

134 STATUS EPILEPTICUS

Kent R. Kelley

- Status epilepticus (SE) was defined by the International League Against Epilepsy in 1884 as "a seizure that persists for a sufficient length of time, or is repeated frequently enough that recovery between attacks does not occur" and by convention is any type of seizure lasting more than 30 minutes.
- Status epilepticus occurs in about 100,000–150,000 cases per year and children represent about half of these cases. About 75% of children with onset of epilepsy before 1 year will have at least one episode of SE and it represents about ~5% of all febrile seizures.
- The etiology of SE includes all the causes of seizures and types of seizures seen in children of different ages, including acute symptomatic, febrile, central nervous system infection, and head trauma, known epilepsy or remote symptomatic epilepsy.
- Precipitants of SE include a change in or abrupt termination of medications, fever, infection, toxic ingestions, metabolic derangements and disease, and trauma.
- A significant mortality has been seen in SE of 3–35% depending upon etiology, duration, associated systemic abnormalities, age, and type of treatment. A metaanalysis refractory SE found a mortality of 20% in symptomatic and 4% in idiopathic cases (Gilbert and Galuser, 1999). The mortality and morbidity of SE is lowest in children with idiopathic epilepsy and is increased with more prolonged seizures and depended upon etiology.
- An episode of SE usually begins with overt continuous or intermittent motor activity, progressing to erratic, migratory, asynchronous twitching, subtle convulsive SE, and then evolves into electrographic SE without motor manifestations evolving with periodic discharges (Trieman, 1995).
- While most seizures are brief and last less than 1–2 minutes, DeLorenzo et al. studied seizures lasting 10–29 minutes in 91 children and 135 adults compared to a similar demographic group and found that the seizures stopped spontaneously in 435 and there

was no mortality; 57% were treated and there was a 4.4% mortality in comparison with a 195 mortality in the comparison group with SE (DeLorenzo et al., 1999). Furthermore, Haut et al. examined the characteristics of patients with epilepsy who had clusters of seizures in 76 patients with complex partial epilepsy and found that 28% had a history of SE, 47% had clusters (>2 sizures/24 hours), and 44% of patients with clusters had SE vs. 12% of the patients without a history of clusters (Haut et al., 1999).

- SE is a neurologic emergency because of a failure of the usual mechanisms for seizure termination, and the disruption of the excitatory amino acid, N-methyl-D-aspartate (NMDA) and inhibitory gamma aminobutyric acid (GABA) pathways. Animal data suggest that neuronal injury occurs after more than an hour of SE, even if systemic and metabolic factors are controlled.
- Early appropriate treatment is advantageous, because it is easier to stop SE earlier than later and it reduces morbidity and mortality. More than 50% of patients with convulsive SE respond to the first line agent, while less than 15% in subtle SE respond. Since most seizures last less than 1–2 minutes, it is recommended that acute treatment be initiated for seizures lasting longer than 5 minutes.
- Treatment protocol begins with the ABCs of emergency care and evaluation of vital signs including respiratory rate, heart rate, blood pressure, temperature, and glucose. A focused past medical history with recent changes and symptoms is then evaluated and the patient is examined for level of consciousness and cranial nerve and motor function.
- Laboratory evaluation may include complete blood counts, electrolytes including sodium, calcium, magnesium, blood urea nitrogen (BUN), and glucose, and antiepileptic drug levels. Blood, urine, and cerebrospinal fluid (CSF) cultures may be appropriate. Depending on level of consciousness, O_2 saturation monitoring and arterial blood gases may be required.
- Treatment recommendations for SE generally start with a benzodiazepine, followed by phenytoin, and then Phenobarbital.
- Recommendations of the Epilepsy Foundation of America (1993) are the following:
  1. Diazepam (DZ): 0.1–1.0 mg/kg IV at a maximum of 5 mg/minute or 0.5 mg/kg PR to a maximum of 20 mg, or lorazepam 0.05–0.5 mg/kg at maximum 2 mg/minute (maximum 1–4 mg).
  2. Phenytoin 20 mg/kg at maximum of 50 mg/minute.
  3. Phenobarbital 20 mg/kg at maximum 100 mg/minute as needed. Be prepared to intubate and support respirations (Dodson et al., 1993).
- Recommendations modified from Aicardi (1992) and Berg (1996):

1. DZ: IV 0.25–0.5 mg/kg at maximum of 2 mg/minute, or PR 0.5–0.75 mg/kg with a maximum in infants of 5 mg and in children 1 mg/year to 10 mg.
2. Pyridoxine 100 mg IV should be given for possible B_6 dependency in infants less than 2 years.
3. The dose of diazepam may be repeated.
4. Phenytoin 20–30 mg/kg not faster than 25–50 mg/minute.
5. Phenobarbital 5–20 mg/kg at maximum of 25 mg/minute, consider intubation.

• Our recommendations at the Children's Memorial Hospital/Children's Epilepsy Center for acute management of SE:
1. DZ: IV 0.25–0.5 mg/kg at maximum 2 mg/kg, or PR 0.5 mg/kg. Maximum in infants 5 mg and in children calculate 1 mg/year to 10 mg.
2. IV pyridoxine 100 mg in infants less than 2 years.
3. May repeat diazepam once.
4. Fosphenytoin 20–30 PE/kg not faster than 150 PE/minute. Fosphenytoin produces equivalent plasma free phenytoin concentrations at injection rates of 100–150 PE/kg to 50 mg/kg for phenytoin. Advantages include decreased pain and burning at the infusion site, hypotension is less common, but paresthesias are more common.
5. Depacon IV 20–30 mg/kg loading over an hour (volume of distribution 0.2–0.25 in adults and rate 3–6 mg/kg) (Wheless and Venkataraman, 1999). Volume of distribution 0.20–0.25, safe. Consider carnitine.

BIBLIOGRAPHY

Aicardi J. Disease of the nervous system. In: *Clinics in Developmental Medicine*, No.115/18, London, UK: Mac Keith Press, 1992, p. 955.

Berg BO. *Principles of Child Neurology*. New York: McGraw Hill, 1996, p. 274.

DeLorenzo et al. Comparison of status epilepticus with prolonged seizure episodes lasting from 10–29 minutes. *Epilepsia* 1999;40:164–169.

Dodson WE, et al. Treatment of convulsive status epilepticus: Recommendations of the Epilepsy Foundation of America's Working Group on Status Epilepticus. *JAMA* 1993;270:854–859.

Gilbert DL, Galuser TA. Complications and costs of treatment of refractory generalized convulsive status epilepticus in children. *J Child Neurol* 1999;14:597–601.

Haut SR, et al. The association between seizure clustering and convulsive status epilepticus in patients with intractable complex partial seizures. *Epilepsia* 1999;40:1832–1834.

Trieman DM. Electroclinical features of status epilepticus. *J Neurophysiol* 1995;12:343–362.

Wheless JW, Venkataraman V. New formulations of drugs in epilepsy. *Expert Opin Pharmacother* 1999;1:49–60.

135 ADDITIONAL NEUROLOGIC EMERGENCIES

Joshua L. Goldstein

ACUTE CHANGES IN MENTAL STATUS

• Mental status changes encompass acute confusion to frank coma. For this reason the first step in the evaluation of acute changes in mental status should be to assess the actual level of consciousness via examination. This may often follow the well-documented Glasgow Coma Scale which rates patients in three categories (motor response, verbal response, and eye opening) on a 15-point scale. This is a rough and non-descriptive tool (see Table 135-1).

• When documenting mental status it is preferable to fully describe responses to a variety of stimuli (e.g., patient briefly opens eyes to sternal rub but has neither purposeful movements nor any response to verbal stimuli). Likewise the phrase "oriented times three" is often insufficient. A complete mental status examination should include commentary regarding arousal, attention, memory, orientation, and affect. Not only will good descriptions and documentation assist in the diagnosis, but it will make assessing change over time possible.

• Mental status changes can be related to a long list of causes and should always induce an extensive and encompassing evaluation. History is key but not always available. Medications (including those in the

TABLE 135-1 Glasgow Coma Score

Eye opening (E)

4 = Spontaneous
3 = To voice
2 = To pain
1 = None

Verbal response (V)

5 = Normal conversation
4 = Disoriented conversation
3 = Words, but not coherent
2 = No words . . . only sounds
1 = None

Motor response (M)

6 = Purposeful movements
5 = Localizes to pain
4 = Withdraws to pain
3 = Decorticate posture
2 = Decerebrate
1 = None

home), past medical history, family history, and social history should always be carefully assessed. A full physical examination must include a complete neurologic examination. Careful attention must be paid to brainstem reflexes, cranial nerves, and optic discs.

- Categories of causes for acute changes in mental status include the following:
  1. Trauma, central nervous system (CNS) bleed, stroke, or other causes of increased intracranial pressure (ICP).
  2. Metabolic (hyperammonemia, renal failure)
  3. Electrolyte (glucose, sodium)
  4. Seizures (subclinical status epilepticus)
  5. Medications, intoxications, ingestions
  6. Vital sign instability (hypotension, hypothermia)
  7. Psychogenic
  8. Infection (encephalitis, meningitis, sepsis)
- If history and physical examinations do not provide a good clue to defining the etiology, a complete laboratory evaluation should ensue. This should include routine chemistries, appropriate medication level (often of any medication found in the home), and toxicology screens. Specialized metabolic studies can be sent if appropriate. Neuroimaging may be helpful in defining such etiologies as subarachnoid hemorrhage (SAH), intracranial hemorrhage, or cerebral edema from any cause. If signs or symptoms of intracranial infection are present, a lumbar puncture should strongly be considered. An electroencephalogram (EEG) should be obtained if the child has a history of epilepsy or a preceding seizure, especially if there is a history of subclinical seizures.
- Appropriate treatments should never be delayed. Strong consideration should be given to initiation of antibiotics and/or acyclovir, treatment of raised intracranial pressure, glucose administration, naloxone and/or flumazenil, and anticonvulsants where indicated. At times such treatment should be made based on clinical judgment alone and may precede diagnostic studies such as EEGs, imaging, or laboratory results.

SHUNT MALFUNCTION/INFECTION

- Ventriculoperitoneal shunts (VPS) should be closely followed for signs of malfunction and infection. Although these signs may be protean, they most commonly are manifest by a decrease in level of arousal, fever (in the case of infection), vomiting, and headache. Any child with the above mentioned symptoms and a VP shunt should be carefully evaluated for its malfunction or infection.
- The evaluation should include, as always, a good examination for alternative etiologies of the symptoms.

A head computed tomography (CT) may be needed to demonstrate a change in ventricular size, although without prior comparisons, this may be somewhat less helpful. A plain film x-ray may be used to demonstrate shunt catheter disconnection or abnormal peritoneal placement but does not prove functionality. Shunt reservoirs may be palpated or tapped by appropriate medical personnel. The gold standard diagnostic studies for the evaluation of a VP shunt to disconnect the catheter and check the pressure with a monometer must be done in the operating room. The final diagnosis of shunt malfunction rests in the hands of the neurosurgeon.

INCREASED INTRACRANIAL PRESSURE

- Increased intracranial pressure is most commonly manifest by a decrease in level or arousal, vomiting, irritability, and headache. Other symptoms may include diplopia, seizures, and confusion.
- A careful and complete physical examination is always the first step in the evaluation for increased ICP. Careful attention should be given to brainstem reflexes and the fundoscopic examination. The ability to assess venous pulsations and optic discs can be extremely helpful in defining and characterizing increased ICP. The presence of normal venous pulsations on fundoscopic examination is an early sign of increased ICP. The presence of papilledema, which appear later, is highly correlated with increased ICP. It must be stated that venous pulsations are most commonly lost acutely in situations of raised ICP in comparison to abnormalities of the optic disc which may take hours to become apparent.
- Loss of eye abduction (cranial nerve IV palsy) is also suggestive of increased ICP. This may be assessed in obtunded or comatose patients with the doll's eyes reflex, and may be unilateral or bilateral. Loss of eye elevation (setting sun sign) is often seen is the setting of raised ICP with hydrocephalus.
- In the infantile population careful attention should be paid to the sutures which often are split and the external veins which may be engorged in cases of subacute or chronic increased ICP. Likewise a careful head circumference should always be documented. Most importantly the fontanels, if open, must be assessed for a direct physical assessment of intracranial pressure.
- Signs of herniation should be assessed and routinely reevaluated on an ongoing basis. These include loss of cranial nerve reflexes, onset of hemiparesis, eye deviation, decrease in arousal, abnormal posturing, and vital sign instabilities.

- Acute treatment of increased ICP is based on the presence of three items within the cerebral vault: blood, CSF, and brain matter. Osmotic diuretics such as mannitol are effective by decreasing blood volume and may be used for a more prolonged period of time. The dose limitations are based on slowly increasing serum osmolarity and thus this need to be routinely reevaluated. Likewise the diuretic may decrease blood pressure and thus cerebral perfusion pressure.
- Hyperventilation causes vasoconstriction and thus decreased cerebral blood volume. This is, however, ineffective in the longer term, as recalibration of autoregulation will take place and the effect is then lost. Thus hyperventilation should be used for acute emergencies rather than more chronic management.
- Monitoring of direct ICP may be performed by neurosurgically placed pressure monitors. This may be helpful in both acute and chronic management. At times a combination of ICP monitoring device with an external ventricular drain may be used. This device would allow not only assessing, but treating increased ICP.
- The head CT may also prove helpful in assessing ICP. The size of the fourth ventricle and pontine cisterns should be carefully evaluated as well as midline shifts and sulcal effacement. An MRI scan is helpful especially in patients with a history of enlarged ventricles and ventricular peritoneal shunt (VPS) to look for evidence of transependymal edema in addition to ventricular size.
- Secondary treatments such as head cooling, phenobarbital, or pentobarbital coma have been used. The evidence for their efficacy is, however, somewhat scant.

SPINAL CORD INJURY

- Spinal injury is, unfortunately, common in the pediatric population and is most often seen in the setting of trauma and thus in all patients with a suggestive history, the spine should be carefully evaluated.
- On examination a sensory level that should be checked for both on the back and front moving both in the caudal to rostral and in the reverse direction when possible is highly specific for a spinal lesion. Likewise paraparesis with leg weakness sparing the arms or the proximal arms (deltoids) raises the concern of a spinal lesion. Reflexes are most often decreased or absent as a result of spinal shock in the acute setting, although later in the course reflexes from spinal levels below the lesion will often become brisk.
- Anal tone and reflexes (wink) should be checked as well as any symptoms of incontinence. Urinary retention may be a problem even in the acute setting and may induce a reflex autonomic arc resulting in severe hypertension; thus a urinary catheter is often placed.

- Acute management of spinal injury should include strong consideration of high-dose intravenous steroids. This has been shown in the adult population to improve outcomes, although not to a great degree, when given within 6 hours of injury.
- In cases of cervical spine injury the diaphragm may be affected and thus close attention must be paid to respirations and hypoventilation. Intubations and ventilation, however, should be done with careful neck immobilization rather than the routine hyperextension.
- Imaging of the spine usually is initially performed in the emergency room with either plain films or with a CT scan to asses for vertebral abnormalities. The spine, itself, however, is best imaged with MRI.
- Neurosurgic or orthopedic stabilization of the spine is often required and should be performed as soon as clinically possible to decrease an ongoing damage from instability.
- Subacute or progressive spine diseases including spinal tumors or transverse myelitis may present in a somewhat acute fashion. The treatment of these depends on the specific diagnosis. Often steroids are used as well, although again there is insufficient evidence to prove efficacy.

136 MISCELLANEOUS OFFICE ISSUES
Joshua L. Goldstein

SCHOOL PERFORMANCE PROBLEMS

- The complaint of problems with school is common in the pediatrician's office. The difficulties may stem from a wide variety of issues including cognitive, social, behavioral, emotional, or epileptic. Unrealistic parental expectations should be discussed with the care giver.
- The first step in the evaluation is to attempt to clarify what exactly the parent's perceptions of the concerns are. Are they shared by the school and/or teachers? Have they been long-standing or are they new? Are they social in nature or academic (or both)?
- As always a good history and physical examination are important. Hearing and vision should be carefully assessed. Likewise a history of prior developmental delays, seizures, and other medical problems should be clarified, as they may be contributing factors in school problems. The home social situation should also be evaluated. Abuse needs to be ruled out.

- Unfortunately, there is no easily followed pathway for the further evaluation of school difficulties, and each case must be individualized. Although in many situations the first thought for many clinicians is to diagnose attention deficit disorder (ADD) or attention deficit/hyperactivity disorder (ADHD) (see section), at times this may be overly diagnosed.
- If there are distinct episodes of staring and unresponsiveness seen both at school and at home, then epilepsy should be considered. Absence epilepsy is often confused clinically with ADD. Hyperventilation in the office should be performed in an attempt to provoke an absence seizure and can be useful. Three to four minutes of active hyperventilation is fairly sensitive.
- If there are signs of anxiety, irritability, aggression, poor socialization, or depression then a referral for psychiatric evaluation should be considered. Likewise a concern for abuse either in the home or elsewhere should be carefully excluded.
- Hearing or vision concerns should be appropriately treated.
- If there is a primarily cognitive or learning disorder suspected, often the appropriate first step is for the parent to request an Individual Education Plan (IEP) or at least further formal testing by the school. This screen should include formal psychometric testing. At times more extensive neuropsychologic evaluation can be performed by a pediatric neurophysiologist.
- If there is a more extensive medical or neurologic history, especially with a history of prior marked developmental delay, then a more extensive medical evaluation may be indicated. Considerations can include chromosomes, brain imaging, metabolic studies, and genetic consultation; however, these more extensive evaluations are clearly not routinely indicated. Importantly, a brain magnetic resonance imaging (MRI) scan is not needed in every case of school problems.

SACRAL DIMPLE

- A sacral dimple can be a sign of an underlying spinal dysraphism. For this reason a close evaluation must ensue. The highest risk group is that in which the dimple is located above the sacral crease in the lumbar area or has associated hair tufts or other pathology.
- As always, a good physical examination should be performed with a careful history designed to evaluate for spinal disease. Specifically histories of kidney or urinary problems, foot or leg deformities, incontinence, or gait problems should be checked.
- The dimple itself should be checked to see if there is a clear bottom. This is often done with the aid of a magnifying glass or ophthalmoscope. Imaging is required if there appears to be a sinus tract.
- In the absence of associated physical findings, other skin pathology, and without a clear sinus tract, the incidence of spinal dysraphism associated with a simple sacral dimple is low.
- Imaging is frequently required and may take the form of an ultrasound or spine MRI to assess for deep connections. Ultrasounds are useful in the neonatal period up to around 6 months of age after which the technical difficulties become increased.
- Should there be a connection or tract emanating from the dimple or signs of diplegia or bowel/bladder dysfunction then a neurosurgic evaluation should be done.

137 ATTENTION DEFICIT DISORDERS
Gretchen Wieck

- Attention deficit disorder (ADD)—including attention deficit hyperactivity disorder (ADHD)—is one of the most frequent neuropsychiatric disorders of children, affecting 6–9% school-age children, and persists into adulthood in 70%.
- There are three subtypes:
  1. Hyperactive-impulsive type: restless, active, talkative, impulsive.
  2. Inattentive type: disorganized, inattentive.
  3. Combined type: all of the above features.

DIAGNOSIS/PRESENTATION

- Diagnosis follows DSM-IV criteria and checklists are filled out by parents and teachers to assess symptoms including SNAP-IV Teacher and Parent Rating Scale.
- Symptoms must be present for at least 6 months, and consist of six or more symptoms of inattention or six or more symptoms of hyperactivity and impulsivity, some of the above symptoms causing impairment present before age 7, impairment from symptoms present in two or more settings (i.e., home and school), clinically significant impairment in social or academic functioning, symptoms not related exclusively to PDD, schizophrenia, or other psychotic disorder, and not better accounted for by another mental/mood disorder.

- Other features such as intelligence and environment can influence the degree of symptomatic impairment.
- About 25% of children with ADHD have parents that meet diagnostic criteria for ADHD.
- Age of presentation of symptoms and impairment for hyperactive-impulsive type tends to be earlier than that for inattentive type. Hyperactive-impulsive symptoms may be present as early as 1–3 years old. Inattentive type may not present until 7 years or later, as academic demands increase.
- ADHD is more prevalent in boys than girls (3:1) but is nevertheless underrecognized and underdiagnosed in girls (more boys are referred for evaluation).
- Girls are more likely to have mood and anxiety disorders, while boys are more likely to have conduct and oppositional-defiant disorder. Inattentive type is more frequent in girls. Girls with ADHD are more at risk for substance abuse and academic problems than girls without ADHD.

DIFFERENTIAL DIAGNOSIS

- Other causes of dysfunction of the frontal-subcortical system should be excluded including encephalitis (history of fevers, sleepiness, change in personality) and epilepsy (episodes of unresponsiveness/staring, postictal periods), progressive neurodegenerative diseases (changes/deterioration in cognition or neuro examination over time), focal brain lesion/injury, perinatal encephalopathy, fragile X syndrome (dysmorphic features), restless legs syndrome, other psychiatric disease (such as major depression, anxiety, bipolar disorder, early schizophrenia).
- Some of these diagnoses can also be comorbid with ADHD, and this may influence treatment options (see more below).
- Children with ADHD have much higher rates of the other disorders and conditions inducing depression, bipolar disorders, obsessive-compulsive disorders, learning disorders, tic disorders, language disorders, and frank mental retardation.
- Higher order associative/coordinating functions of the prefrontal lobe are often also affected in ADHD, and can result in vague complaints such as clumsiness and fine motor incoordination, as well as altered sensory perceptions (for example, specific aversions to textures and tastes).

TREATMENT

- Once correct diagnosis is made, and any medical or psychiatric comorbid conditions identified, a psychostimulant medication can be selected.

- Psychostimulant medications that work by increasing central dopamine and norepinephrine include ethylphenidate or methylphenidate-equivalents (come in different dosages and half-life characteristics).
- Starting dose should be low (usually around 0.3 mg/kg), and the dosing schedule should be based on the child's schedule and timing of cognitive demands. The medication should be titrated upward slowly to achieve efficacy but not significant side effect.
- If there is no response or an insufficient response to the first stimulant medication, a second one can be tried.
- Medications will increase attention, and will not treat learning or behavioral problems (comorbid conditions) and efficacy can be assessed by parents and teachers (often via questionnaire), and should be immediate.
- Most common side effects include anorexia, insomnia, abdominal pain, headaches, end-of-dose irritability. Rare but serious effects may include mania and psychosis.
- Symptoms related to overly high dose (toxicity) include hyperactivity, repetitive/stereotypic activities, over focused behaviors (responds to decreasing dose), weight loss, headaches, and insomnia.

ETIOLOGY OF ADHD

- Acquired ADHD is most frequently the residual of traumatic brain injury, especially with lesions of thalamus, basal ganglia, or right putamen.
- Other associations include neonatal encephalopathy, prenatal exposure to alcohol or nicotine, metabolic or infectious diseases, and various autoimmune disorders.
- Genetic impact on ADHD is marked and there is a 0.8–50% chance a parent with ADHD will have a child with ADHD, being most likely a polygenetic group of disorders.
- No single gene mutation has been proven yet, but candidates include the DAT1 (dopamine transporter) and DRD4 (dopamine D4 receptor).

COMA

- For a complete review of this topic the reader is directed to the classic but still valuable *The Diagnosis of Stupor and Coma*, by Plum and Posner.

DEFINITIONS

- Coma is a state of unresponsiveness in which the patient exhibits no response to stimuli and has no purposeful movements. The eyes are closed and do not open.

- Stupor is a state similar to deep sleep with poor and limited (but present) response to stimulation. The patients may be minimally alert and open their eyes but full arousal is not achieved. Some purposeful movements are often noted.
- Obtundation is a state similar to stupor with slowed cognition, delayed but present responses stimulation and reduced attention. There is a decreased alertness with increased sleep but clear responses to stimulation.
- Delirium is a waxing and waning state of confusion, disorientation, somulence, and often hallucinations. It is usually acute or subacute in onset and is often seen in toxic and metabolic disorders.

DIFFERENTIAL DIAGNOSIS

- The differential diagnosis of coma can be divided into intrinsic and extrinsic categories and is extremely extensive.
- Intrinsic causes include direct insults to the central nervous system including mass lesions (neoplasm, hemorrhage, abscess, and so on), hypoxia, infection, ongoing seizures, diffuse axonal injury, and so on.
- Extrinsic causes include metabolic causes, endocrine dysfunction, electrolyte abnormalities, toxins, medications, hyper- or hypotension, and temperature dysregulation.
- The specific diagnosis is made, as with other aspects of neurology, based on a careful history (where possible) and physical examination. Specifically a detailed history of medications and possible ingestions must be made with all family members, caregivers, and the patient.

EXAMINATION

- The neurologic and general examinations should be complete when possible. The neurologic examination is tailored for the unresponsive or poorly responsive patient, but nonetheless covers all subsystems of the nervous system.
- A careful and complete set of vitals should be obtained and repeated on a regular basis.
- Breathing patterns have been described which may be correlated with diffuse brain injury as well as with specific brainstem lesions. Well-known abnormal breathing patterns such as ataxic breathing, periodic breathing, and Chenye-Stokes respirations have been described. The specific localizing features of these patterns remain in question.
- The general examination should always include an evaluation of the neck for rigidity, evaluation for

signs of basilar skull fracture (Battle sign or Raccoon Eyes), good cardiac examination for murmurs or arrhythmia, and a careful skin examination for rashes or bites.
- Mental status must be examined and documented carefully. Descriptions of responses to specific stimuli are particularly helpful in avoiding confusing jargon which may be misinterpreted or nonspecific. For example "the patient opened his eyes and looked at the examiner, but did not answer questions asked by the examiner." Alternatively the patient might be described as "completely unresponsive to a sternal rub with eyes closed throughout the entire examination."
- The localization of loss of consciousness may be seated either in the reticular activating system of the brain stem or with bihemispheric cortical involvement.
- Specific diagnostic tools have been standardized including the widely accepted Mini-Mental Status Examination. Areas of arousal, attention, memory, language (written and verbal), recall, and orientation should be covered.
- The neurologic examination will include a careful cranial nerve examination using an evaluation of the optic discs for edema and venous pulsations to assess for increased intracranial pressure, pupillary responses (CN II, III), ocular motor response to lateral head movements after the neck stability has been ensured known as the doll's eyes response (III, IV, VI, VIII), ocular movements to cold caloric testing after the tympanic membrane has been assessed (III, IV, VI, VIII), corneal blink responses (V, VII), and gag (IX, X).
- Of note the absence of a gag response is not always pathologic nor is the absence of venous pulsations. Also the development of optic disc edema may be delayed for several hours after a documented head injury and should not be taken as proof of a normal intracranial pressure.
- This close evaluation of the brainstem covers the midbrain (II, III), pons (III, IV, V, VI, VII), and medulla (VIII, IX, X).
- The motor system and sensory systems can be evaluated by observation after stimulation of the extremities. Careful note should be made of side-to-side (left and right) symmetry as well as for a possible sensory or motor dermatomal level (arms move but the legs do not) which might indicate a spinal lesion. A unilateral asymmetry (i.e., a hemipareis) might indicate a cortical hemispheric lesion on the contralateral side.
- Reflexes are analogues to the motor and sensory examinations in that asymmetry or arm/leg discrepancy may assist in localizing along the neuroaxis.
- Using this examination the lesion can be localized to the cortex or the brain stem (with signs of papillary abnormalities) or both.

TESTS

- A careful metabolic, endocrine, and toxin screen should be undertaken in all patients with coma of unclear etiology and should include an arterial blood gas.
- An evaluation for possible infection including a spinal fluid analysis should be performed (when a unilateral mass lesion has been ruled out).
- Imaging to assist in characterizing the insult may prove helpful but should not replace a careful and precise examination. A computerized tomogram (CT scan) is often the first imaging study performed. It is important to remember that this study, although excellent at documenting blood and subacute stroke, often is poor at imaging the posterior fossa and brain stem. Likewise the fine details of the cortical and subcortical structures may be obscured.
- A magnetic resonance image (MRI) is of greater utility in evaluating the brain stem and fine cortical structures. Drawbacks include its longer duration and need for patient being still and may require sedation.
- Close attention in both of these studies should be paid to signs of midline shift and cerebral edema (blurring of the gray-white junction, obscuration of the pontine cistern, and sulcal-gyral patterns). The use of contrast in either study may support the diagnosis of meningitis but does not need to be performed on a routine basis. Close consultation with a radiologist is extremely important.
- An electroencephalogram (EEG) may help in documenting subclinical status epilepticus although careful examination often reveals subtle clinical manifestations in such cases. Likewise diffuse slowing may suggest a diffuse encephalopathy but this is usually nonspecific and of no great assistance in providing a specific diagnosis.

BRAIN DEATH

- The diagnosis of brain death is somewhat varied on a state-by-state basis and should be clarified carefully in each case.
- Brain death examinations should always be carried out by someone experienced and trained in their performance and needs to be repeated over time (often 12 or 24 hours). Prior to the examination all medications (especially those which may confound the examination), electrolytes, and vital signs (including temperature) must be assessed. The absence of all brainstem and cortical function should be carefully documented.
- Supporting studies such as an EEG and nuclear medicine brain scan may be helpful but are not required for the diagnosis.

BIBLIOGRAPHY

Ataxia

Brazis PW, Masdeu JC, Biller J. *Localization in Clinical Neurology.* Philadelphia, PA: Lippincott Williams and Wilkins, 2001, pp. 371–386.
Fenichel GM. *Clinical Pediatric Neurology.* Philadelphia, PA: W.B. Saunders, 2001, pp. 223–243.
Patten J. *Neurological Differential Diagnosis.* New York, NY: Springer, 2000, pp. 178–213.
Rosa AL. Genetic ataxia. *Neurol Clin* 2002;20:727–757.

Headache

Abu-Arafeh, I (ed.) *Clinics in Developmental Medicine.* New York, NY: Cambridge University Press, 2002.
Barlow CF. *Headaches and Migraine in Childhood.* Oxford: Blackwell, 1984.
Bille B. Migraine in school children. A study of the incidence and short-term prognosis, and a clinical psychological and encephalographic comparison between children with migraine and matched controls. *Acta Pediatr* 1962;51:1–151.
Bille B. A 40-year follow-up of children with migraine. *Cephalgia* 1997;17:488–491.
Congdon PJ, Forsythe WI. Migraine in childhood: A study of 300 children. *Dev Med Child Neurol* 1979;21:209–216.
Egger HL, Angold A, Costello AJ. Headaches and psychopathology in children and adolescents. *J Am Acad Child Adolesc Psychiatry* 1998;37:951–958.
Lewis DW, Ashwal S, Dahl BS, Dorbad D, Hirtz D, Prensky A, Jarjour I. Practice parameter: Evaluation of children and adolescents with recurrent headaches. *Neurology* 2002;59:490–498. http://www.aan.com/professionals/practice/guidelines.cfm.
May A, Goadsby PJ. The trigeminovascular system in humans: Pathophysiologic implications for primary headache syndromes of the neural influences on the cerebral circulation. *J Cereb Blood Flow Metab* 1999;19:115–127.
Olesen J. Headache Classification Committee of the International Headache Society. Classification and diagnostic criteria for headache disorders, cranial neuralgia and facial pain. *Cephalgia* 1988;8:1–96.
Olness KN, MacDonald JT. Recurrent headaches in children: Diagnosis and treatment. *Pediatr Rev* 1987;8:307–313.
Silberstein SD. For the U.S. Headache Consortium. Practice parameter: Evidence-based guidelines for migraine headache (an evidence-based review). *Neurology* 2000;55:754–763. *http://www.aan.com/professionals/practice/guidelines.cfm.*
Stafstrom CE, Rostasy K, Minster A. The usefulness of children's drawings in the diagnosis of headache. *Pediatrics* 2002;109:460–472.
Welch KMA. Current opinions in headache pathogenesis: Introduction and synthesis. *Curr Opin Neurol* 1998;11:193–197.
Whitehouse WP. Specific causes of headache in childhood headache. In: Abu-Arafeh I (ed.), *Clinics in Developmental Medicine.* New York, NY: Cambridge University Press, 2002, p. 158.

Winner P, Martinez W, Mate L, Bello L. Classification of pediatric migraine: Proposed revisions to the IHS criteria. *Headache* 1995;35:407–410.

Winner P, Rothner AD, Saper J, Nett R, Asgharnejad M, Laurenza A, Austin R, Peykamian M. A randomized, double-blind, placebo-controlled study of sumitriptan nasal spray in the treatment of acute migraine in adolescents. *Pediatrics* 2000;5:989–997.

Wolff HG. *Headache and Other Head Pain.* New York, NY: Oxford University Press, 1948, pp. 255–318.

For Further Information

Berg BO. In: Berg BO (ed.), *Child Neurology: A Clinical Manual,* 2nd ed. (not to be confused with his more comprehensive textbook, this is a 300+ page small hard cover, very clinical and readable). Philadelphia, PA: Lippincott Williams and Wilkins, 1994.

Fenichel GM. In: Fenichel GM (ed.), *Clinical Pediatric Neurology: A Signs and Symptoms Approach,* 4th ed. (as the title suggests a readable book based on symptom complexes, ex: the hypotonic infant, episodic events, etc.). Philadelphia, PA: W.B. Saunders, 2001.

Menkes JH, Sarnat HB. In: Menkes JH, Sarnat HB (eds.), *Child Neurology,* 6th ed. (A good comprehensive textbook). Philadelphia, PA: Lippincott Williams and Wilkins, 2000.

http://www.neuro.wustl.edu/neuromuscular (for neuromuscular disease).

http://www.ncbi.nlm.nih.gov/Omim/searchomim.html (for neuro-genetics).

http://www.geneclinics.org (for neurogenetics).

DISEASES AND DISORDERS OF THE EYE

Marilyn B. Mets, Section Editor

138 ANATOMY

Raed Shatnawi, Janice B. Lasky,
Marilyn B. Mets

- The various dimensions of the globe are generally fairly constant in the adult population and are relatively unrelated to either sex or race. The anteroposterior diameter of the globe averages 24.15 mm. At birth, the globe is more spherical than the adult globe and has an anteroposterior diameter about two-thirds that of the adult globe. By 3 years of age, this increases to within 1 mm of the average adult size, reaching the normal adult size by about 13 years of age.
- The sclera consists of dense fibrous tissue and contains openings and canals for the various vessels and nerves entering and exiting the globe. Externally it is whitish in color.
- The cornea is a tough, transparent, and avascular tissue that, along with the precorneal tear film, forms the major refracting surface for the eye.
- The external dimensions of the cornea are 11.7 mm horizontally and 10.6 mm vertically while in the newborn it is more circular and averages 10 mm in diameter reaching the adult size by the age of 2 years.
- The nerve supply to the cornea is derived from the ophthalmic division of the trigeminal nerve.
- The cornea consists of five layers. The total corneal thickness is about 550 μm.
- The iris is the most anterior portion of the uvea and forms a mobile diaphragm between the posterior chamber and anterior chamber of the eye. The pupil is a central aperture in the iris and can vary in size from 1.5 to 8 mm. The sphincter muscle cells are spindle shaped and oriented parallel to the pupillary margin. These cells are supplied by parasympathetic nerve fibers from the long ciliary nerves with synapses in the ciliary ganglion. The dilator muscle extends from the iris root to the stroma posterior to the sphincter muscle. It is supplied by sympathetic fibers from the superior cervical ganglion.
- The lens is a transparent biconvex structure with a rounded equator. The zonules arising from the ciliary body support the lens laterally by attaching to the lens capsule. The lens continues to grow throughout life.
- The retina is a very thin, delicate, and transparent membrane. It is composed of 10 layers. The retina consists of two distinct layers: the sensory retina and the retinal pigment epithelium.
- The optic nerve head is the intraocular portion of the optic nerve. Its retinal aspect is termed the optic disc. This structure may be round or slightly oval. On average, its diameter is 1.5 mm.
- The central portion of the optic disc contains the central retinal artery and vein. The central retinal artery is a branch of the ophthalmic artery. The central retinal vein drains into both the cavernous sinus and the superior ophthalmic vein.

139 RED EYE

Raed Shatnawi, Janice B. Lasky,
Marilyn B. Mets

NEONATAL CONJUNCTIVITIS

- Conjunctivitis in the first few weeks of life, with purulent discharge, lid edema, conjunctival hyperemia, and occasionally preauricular adenopathy, is present in 1–2% of newborns.

- The administration of 1% silver nitrate in the eye to prevent gonococcal conjunctivitis is mildly irritating and often causes some hyperemia and chemosis of the conjunctiva. Rarely, the cornea is affected, leading to a chemical keratitis. Gonococcal conjunctivitis always occurs within 24 hours of birth and is mild and self-limiting (3–5 days). No treatment is required. Irrigation of the eyes may cause more irritation and should be avoided. The incidence of this problem is decreasing with the increasing use of erythromycin ointment or povidone-iodine for prophylaxis.
- Bacterial conjunctivitis occurs in the first week of life. It is severe and characterized by purulent discharge. Gram and Giemsa stains of conjunctival scrapings and cultures and sensitivities should be initiated.
- If gram-negative diplococci are found, the most likely diagnosis is gonococcal conjunctivitis. Corneal ulceration and even perforation develop rapidly if appropriate treatment is not instituted. Do not wait for culture results. Ceftriaxone in a single IM or IV dose of 25–50 mg/kg for 7 days is recommended. For children sensitive to β-lactams, spectinomycin should be used. Topical treatment with erythromycin or bacitracin ointment is helpful.
- Mild bacterial conjunctivitis is usually self-limited. In many patients, lid hygiene and saline washes are adequate therapy. For more severe conjunctivitis, topical treatment with a broad-spectrum antibiotic such as bacitracin or erythromycin is usually effective.
- Mild-to-moderate conjunctivitis in the first few weeks of life is usually caused by *Chlamydia trachomatis*, which is now the most important cause of ophthalmia neonatorum in the United States. The positive yield of laboratory tests in infants is high. Intracytoplasmic inclusion bodies on Giemsa stain are typical. Oral erythromycin is the drug of choice because it also treats the nasopharyngeal colonization and it may prevent chlamydial pneumonia syndrome. Topical erythromycin is beneficial.
- Conjunctivitis caused by herpes simplex virus is important because of the possibility of disseminated infection with central nervous system (CNS) involvement. Systemic treatment with acyclovir may reduce the risk for a generalized infection. Topical idoxuridine or vidarabine is helpful.
- Most cases of ophthalmia neonatorum are caused by infection during passage through the birth canal. Thus the clinician should think of this as a family problem and both parents should be investigated and treated.

CONJUNCTIVITIS

- Conjunctivitis can be classified into acute (present <4 weeks) and chronic (present >2–4 weeks) forms.

- Acute conjunctivitis is abrupt in onset, and is usually unilateral at first with involvement of the second eye within 1 week. History should include the patient's age, allergies, medications, exposure to irritants, and ocular, genitourinary, and respiratory symptoms. A history of contagion is common. Patients often complain of red eye with discharge, sticky eyes in the morning, and burning or foreign body sensation. Vision, pupillary responses, intraocular pressure (IOP), and fundoscopic examination are essentially normal.
- Papillary response is a nonspecific inflammatory reaction, resulting from any type of inflammation. Numerous small papillae give the conjunctiva a red velvety appearance characteristic of bacterial conjunctivitis.
- Hyperacute purulent conjunctivitis suggests infection with *Neisseria gonorrheae*, a highly virulent organism that can penetrate an intact corneal epithelium. There's a rapid progression of a highly purulent conjunctivitis with lid edema to corneal perforation and blindness. This is the only bacterial conjunctivitis that produces preauricular adenopathy. Smears for Gram and Giemsa stains should be taken from conjunctival scrapings rather than the exudate. Cultures are obtained on blood and chocolate agar (37°C, 10% CO_2). Patient with suspected gonococcal conjunctivitis is admitted for systemic parenteral full-dose antibiotics. IV aqueous penicillin is recommended for 5 days. For penicillin-resistant strains, ceftriaxone 1 g IM daily for 5 days is recommended. Oral erythromycin is given for at least 1 week because of the high rate of associated chlamydial infections. The copious discharge should resolve within the first 24–48 hours, and the lid edema and hyperemia clear within 7–14 days.
- The most common type of infectious conjunctivitis is bacterial. Diagnosis is based on clinical backgrounds; the presence of a mucopurulent discharge, the absence of conjunctival follicles, and the absence of preauricular adenopathy. In children, the most commonly isolated organisms are *Haemophilus influenzae, Streptococcus pneumoniae,* and *Staphylococcus aureus.* Most cases are self-limited, but topical antibiotics can shorten the course from 10–14 to 1–3 days. Initial treatment is with broad-spectrum antibiotic solution or ointment (sulfacetamide, bacitracin, or erythromycin).
- Giant papillae have a cobblestone appearance and they are more common in allergic and chronic conjunctivitis.
- A pseudomembrane or membrane forms in certain inflammatory conditions. Pseudomembranes are easily removed without bleeding. Membranes are more firmly adherent and bleed with attempted removal. Examples of membranous and pseudomembranous conjunctivitis include streptococcal, pneumococcal,

chemical burn, diphtheria, adenovirus, Stevens-Johnson syndrome, vernal conjunctivitis, ligneous, and others.

- Watery discharge, conjunctival follicles, and preauricular adenopathy suggest viral or chlamydial disease. Adenovirus conjunctivitis is responsible for the most frequent epidemics in the United States. Adenovirus infection occurs in two forms: pharyngoconjunctival fever (PCF) and epidemic keratoconjunctivitis (EKC).
- PCF is caused by serotypes 3 and 7. The clinical syndrome includes pharyngitis, fever, and follicular conjunctivitis. Epidemics are associated with public swimming pools in summer.
- EKC is caused by serotypes 8 and 19. The clinical syndrome includes pharyngitis, follicular conjunctivitis, preauricular adenopathy, and characteristic subepithelial corneal infiltrate.
- Viral conjunctivitis is usually self-limited and requires no treatment. Antiviral agents are ineffective. Cool compresses and artificial tears provide symptomatic relief. Health-care personnel should refrain from direct patient contact for 14 days after the onset of the symptoms. Good personal hygiene is important.
- Periorbital vesicles or pustules associated with a follicular, sometime membranous, conjunctivitis and a palpable preauricular node are seen in primary herpes simplex blepharoconjunctivitis. The conjunctivitis is self-limited but may be followed by the classic dendritic keratitis, which may be recurrent; therefore topical antiviral agents for both the skin and eye are advocated. Trifluridine 1% solution or vidarabine 3% ointment are given five times daily for 7–10 days until the conjunctivitis has resolved. Topical acyclovir ointment or topical antibiotic ointment may be applied to the skin lesions in conjunctions with warm soaks three times a day. The patient should be examined every 2–3 days for the development of keratitis. Oral acyclovir is used in primary cases of herpetic disease with eyelid involvement.

CORNEAL ABRASION

- Superficial abrasions are frequently encountered with minor trauma. Because patients suffering corneal abrasions complain of severe pain and photophobia, examination may require instillation of a topical anesthetic agent. On examination, a corneal abrasion stains with fluorescein dye. Its borders are generally sharp.
- Routine treatment of corneal abrasions includes instillation of a broad-spectrum antibiotic ointment for infection prophylaxis and lubrication and a cycloplegic agent for the patient's comfort. A pressure patch is applied to shield the epithelium as it heals.

- Abrasions associated with contact lens wear require extra care, because they have a high incidence of infectious keratitis by destructive gram-negative organisms. In a contact lens-associated abrasion, an antibiotic with gram-negative coverage (generally an aminoglycoside) is administered and the pressure patch is withheld to allow for frequent antibiotic dosing and observation. Oral pain medications may be given while the abrasion heals. Topical anesthetic agents should never be prescribed, however, because they compromise epithelial wound healing. Patients are generally monitored on a daily basis until reepithelialization has occurred and the potential for infection no longer exists. Topical antibiotics are continued for approximately 1 week after reepithelialization. If infection is suspected, appropriate cultures are obtained.

FOREIGN BODY

- Superficial and embedded foreign bodies occur as a consequence of work-related activities, especially those involving striking metal on metal. Except for the most trivial superficial foreign bodies, careful examination of the anterior chamber, iris, and lens, as well as IOP measurement and dilated fundoscopy are necessary to rule out an intraocular foreign body. Superficial foreign bodies may simply be irrigated from the eye or removed with a moist cotton-tipped applicator. Even if a foreign body is discovered and removed, a thorough examination for additional objects is mandatory. The superior tarsal conjunctiva is a common location of hidden foreign bodies. Examination therefore should include routine eversion of the upper eyelid.
- Hard foreign bodies may embed in the corneal stroma. If they contain iron, a rust ring may be evident. A corneal foreign body is usually removed at the slit lamp using topical anesthesia and a 25-gauge needle or foreign body spud. If a perforation into the anterior chamber is possible, removal must be undertaken under controlled sterile conditions in a minor or major operating room. After foreign body removal, a broad-spectrum antibiotic ointment and cycloplegic agent are instilled and a pressure patch is placed if epithelial abrasion is significant. Patients are closely monitored until the epithelium is healed and there is no sign of infection.

PRESEPTAL AND ORBITAL CELLULITIS

- The anatomic location of infection depends on the natural barrier provided by the orbital septum. The simplest classification scheme categorizes infections by preseptal (periorbital) or postseptal (orbital) location.

- A child with an orbital infection presents with pain, heat, redness, and swelling of the tissues surrounding the involved orbit. There is typically fever and an elevation of the white blood cell count. History of trauma, lacrimal outflow obstruction, upper respiratory tract infection, or sinusitis should be carefully elicited. The presence of a demarcation line corresponding to the arcus marginalis suggests an orbital (postseptal) infection. The presence of proptosis, ophthalmoplegia, conjunctival chemosis, or loss of vision is also suggestive of orbital involvement, but postseptal extension may exist in the absence of any of these findings.
- In the pediatric age group, *S. aureus*, *Streptococcus* sp., and *H. influenzae* are the most commonly encountered bacteria.
- Ancillary diagnostic methods available for evaluating children with orbital and periorbital infections include physical examination (motility, vision, proptosis, and fever), white blood cell count with differential, cultures (pus, blood, and sinus drainage), orbital ultrasound and computed tomography (CT) scan. Lumbar puncture is reserved for children who have meningeal signs.
- *Ear, nose,* and *throat* (ENT) and pediatric consultations may be helpful. Orbital cellulitis is an ophthalmic emergency. Institute IV antibiotics as soon as possible, and monitor vision. If no improvement occurs within 24–48 hours, consider surgical sinus drainage and/or direct orbital drainage, if there's an abscess. If there is improvement, continue IV antibiotics for several days, followed by oral antibiotics for a total of 10–14 days.

RHABDOMYOSARCOMA

- Rhabdomyosarcoma is a malignant soft tissue tumor showing evidence of striated muscle differentiation. It is the most common primary orbital malignancy of children, occurring at a mean age of approximately 6 years, although it may be present at birth and occurs in adults. It can arise anywhere in the orbit. Rhabdomyosarcomas grow rapidly and eventually may occupy the entire orbital cavity, causing progressive proptosis. If adjacent to bone, they cause lytic bone destruction with invasion of adjacent paraorbital structures such as sinuses, temporal fossa, infratemporal fossa, and cavernous sinus. Because these tumors evolve rapidly, early diagnosis is mandatory and biopsy with proper fixation of tissue is essential.
- Rhabdomyosarcoma has been divided into three histopathologic types: embryonal, alveolar, and pleomorphic.
- Treatment is with radiotherapy and chemotherapy with favorable prognosis.

140 NASOLACRIMAL DUCT OBSTRUCTION

Raed Shatnawi, Janice B. Lasky, Marilyn B. Mets

- Nasolacrimal duct obstruction (NLDO) is present in about 5% of newborns. In most patients, NLDO results from an obstruction at the lower end of the duct, where it joins the nasal mucosa. The infant presents with tearing (epiphora) and the eye looks wet. A variable amount of mucopurulent discharge may be present. The diagnosis, although self-evident, is sometimes mistaken for conjunctivitis though the conjunctiva is usually quiet. Rare causes of epiphora, such as congenital glaucoma, should be ruled out.
- Although the diagnosis can be made based on history and clinical signs, it may be helpful sometimes to test the lacrimal drainage by instilling fluorescein in the conjunctival sac. If the yellow solution does not clear from the eye in a few minutes or if the clearance lags considerably behind the other eye, a complete or partial NLDO is present.
- If infection is present, initiate proper antibiotic treatment with erythromycin or 10% sulfacetamide three to four times daily until the infection clears. Massage of the nasolacrimal sac helps decompress it, reduce the discharge, and it also may be curative.
- Ninety percent or more of NLDOs resolve spontaneously by the age of 1 year. If NLDO is still present at the age of 10–12 months, it will probably not clear by itself, and surgical probing and irrigation will be needed.

141 CONGENITAL GLAUCOMA

Raed Shatnawi, Janice B. Lasky, Marilyn B. Mets

- When an infant presents with photophobia, tearing, blepharospasm, and hazy or enlarged cornea, congenital glaucoma should always be considered although none of these symptoms is pathognomonic for congenital glaucoma.
- Congenital glaucoma is a group of disorders in which the aqueous outflow system is anatomically abnormal, leading to an increase in intraocular pressure (IOP) and subsequent damage to the optic nerve.

- Because the outer coat (cornea and sclera) of the infant's eye is thinner and less rigid than in the adult's eye, increased IOP will lead to expansion of the size of the eye and enlarged corneal diameters and axial length. This increase and thus increasing myopia is a useful indicator that glaucoma is not controlled, regardless of normal or close to normal IOP readings.
- The deep perilimbal vessels are diffusely injected, leading to the violaceous color of the area immediately surrounding the cornea.
- A history of increasing haziness and of the eye "getting bigger" is helpful. Many types of congenital glaucoma are heritable, making the family history important. Examination of the child in the clinic is usually adequate to make the diagnosis even if no accurate IOP measurements are obtained.
- Detailed examination of the suspected glaucoma eye often requires anesthesia. The examination should include measurement of the cornea diameters, a recording of the cornea clarity, the status of the anterior chamber angle, ophthalmoscopy to determine the cup/disc ratio (CDR), and refraction. A normal IOP by itself is not enough to exclude a diagnosis of glaucoma if other signs are present. If the diagnosis of glaucoma is confirmed, proceed with surgery.
- Medical therapy cannot substitute surgery. It is useful for reducing damage while surgical arrangements are made. It is also useful for long-term management of complex cases.
- Congenital glaucoma is a chronic disease, and many patients require multiple surgeries before the IOP is normalized.
- Children with congenital glaucoma should be followed closely. Despite initial success of surgery, failure of IOP control can occur at any time. Because glaucomatous infant eyes are highly myopic, refractions and, if indicated, amblyopia treatment are essential. Corneal decompensation can be caused by edema, scarring, or amyloid deposition, necessitating cornea surgery. Genetic counseling with the family regarding recurrence risks should not be forgotten.

142 LEUKOCORIA (WHITE PUPIL)

Raed Shatnawi, Janice B. Lasky, Marilyn B. Mets

- Leukocoria in a child requires urgent attention, because retinoblastoma (RB) may be present or a cataract may result in occlusion amblyopia.

- The history, including the family history, can be helpful in the differential diagnosis. In addition to full eye examination, special tests, such as ultrasonography, computed tomography (CT) scanning, and magnetic resonance imaging (MRI) may be required as well.

RETINOBLASTOMA

- RB is a relatively rare tumor (incidence is about 1/15,000–1/20,000 live births in the United States, but it is the most common malignant intraocular tumor in children.
- About 60% of children with RB present with leukocoria and another 20% with strabismus. Other atypical presentations include hyphema, glaucoma, and preseptal cellulitis which may lead to delayed or missed diagnosis.
- A detailed history and a full eye examination under general anesthesia are required. The diagnosis of RB primarily depends on the ophthalmoscopic appearance of the tumor.
- RB behaves as an autosomal-dominant disease with high penetration rate approaching 80%. About 40% of all retinoblastomas are genetic and 60% sporadic. About 25% of patients have a positive family history. Table 142-1 may help in the genetic counseling for recurrence rates of RB.
- A CT scan is helpful in diagnosing RB and establishing possible extension in the orbit or the cranium. A common finding is calcification.
- Treatment options depend on the tumor's size and location, presence of extraocular extension, and the local availability of treatment modalities. Choices include laser photocoagulation, cryotherapy, irradiation, chemotherapy, and enucleation for more extensive tumors.
- Prognosis for life takes priority over that for vision. Overall survival rate is >90%.
- Patients with genetic RB are at a significant risk for other nonocular malignancies with osteogenic sarcoma being the most common.

TABLE 142-1   Risk for Future Offspring to Develop Retinoblastoma*

	UNILATERAL (%)	BILATERAL (%)
Parent of affected patient	[†]–FH 1 [††]+FH 40	–FH 6 +FH 40
Affected patient	–FH 8 +FH 40	–FH 40 +FH 40
Normal sibling of affected patient	–FH 1 +FH 7	–FH <1 +FH 7

*Assumes an 80% penetrance.
[†]–FH: Negative family history.
[††]+FH: Positive family history.

- The care of these patients is best concentrated in centers where pediatric oncologists, pediatric ophthalmologists, and genetic counselors are readily available. Follow-up of these patients should continue for life.

CONGENITAL CATARACT

- A congenital cataract is found in about 1/250 live births. Roughly one-third is hereditary with autosomal-dominant being the most common, one-third is associated with a syndrome or metabolic disease, and the cause in the remainder is unknown. Congenital cataract is still one of the most common causes of blindness in children worldwide.
- A family history and careful examination of parents and other family members may be very helpful in establishing a diagnosis.
- A workup normally need not be extensive. If a baby has a cataract secondary to a syndrome or metabolic deficiency, the child will also show signs of that syndrome or metabolic abnormality such as failure to thrive, dysmorphic features, and others.
- It is usually more than adequate to obtain fasting blood sugar (hypoglycemia), urine for reducing sugars (galactosemia), serum calcium and phosphate (severe vitamin D deficiency and hypoparathyroidism), and urinary amino acids (Lowe syndrome). If congenital infection is suspected, consider toxoplasmosis, rubella, cytomegalovirus, herpes, and syphilis (TORCH) screening and a Venereal Disease Research Laboratory (VDRL).
- Galactosemia comes in two different types. In galactokinase deficiency, children have no systemic illness, whereas children with a deficiency of galactose-1-phosphate uridyltransferase are quite ill.
- Congenital cataract comes in several morphologies. Zonular, nuclear, lamellar, axial, anterior lenticonus (in Alport syndrome which also has renal failure, sensorineural deafness, and retinal flecks), and anterior and posterior polar cataracts.
- Lowe syndrome shows severe lens anomalies. In addition to posterior lenticonus cataract, the lens is also shaped like a flat disc and is always cataractogenic. Lowe syndrome is one of the causes of congenital cataract and congenital glaucoma.
- Patients with neurofibromatosis type 2 (bilateral acoustic neuroma) are also at increased risk of developing posterior subcapsular cataract. Steroid therapy and juvenile rheumatoid arthritis are also causes of posterior subcapsular cataract.
- The treatment of congenital cataract has improved dramatically over the past 15 years. Visual outcome depends on the density of the cataract at and before the time of surgery, age of onset and age at time of surgery, and very important—a commitment by parents.
- The timing of cataract surgery is the major factor in visual rehabilitation. Before the age of 2 months, nystagmus is generally not present and the visual prognosis is excellent, provided that aggressive treatment of aphakia (surgical absence of the lens) and amblyopia (visual loss in the absence of organic factors) take place. Bilateral cataracts have a better outcome than monocular ones.
- Babies with dense cataract who are not operated on before the age of 2 months, showing nystagmus, have a guarded prognosis. Acuity may never be better than 20/200. Because poor vision may be reversed, surgery should be performed as soon as possible.
- The recommended surgery is lensectomy and vitrectomy which will result in aphakia, which is as amblyopiogenic as the cataract itself. Therefore aggressive treatment of the aphakia is essential.
- After the age of 2 years there is a general agreement to use intraocular lenses (IOLs). Before the age of 2 years, the use of IOLs is still controversial and usage of contact lenses or glasses is the rule. Placement of secondary IOL at a later age is accepted.
- Follow-up for children with congenital cataract should continue because of the risk for developing glaucoma, amblyopia, and strabismus.

143 EYE TRAUMA

Raed Shatnawi, Janice B. Lasky,
Marilyn B. Mets

- The initial evaluation of a patient with eye trauma should be as complete as possible because diagnostic and treatment options depend on it. At the same time, this evaluation should not worsen the ocular condition. A careful history should be obtained. Emergency conditions should be treated immediately, with the remainder of the examination postponed if necessary. Visual acuity should be obtained as soon as possible for prognostic and legal purposes.
- Treatment of any life-threatening conditions should precede that of any eye injury.
- If no light perception is present at the initial evaluation in a severely traumatized eye and enucleation is indicated, it may be preferable to do a primary repair first, repeat the visual acuity after and if necessary

visual evoked response (VER), and get a second opinion. The remote risk of sympathetic ophthalmia can be avoided if the enucleation takes place within 2 weeks from the initial injury; however, primary enucleation should be considered if a second general anesthesia puts the patient at risk.

- The presence of an afferent pupillary defect (APD) implies a severe dysfunction of the retina or optic nerve and should be considered a bad prognostic sign. Differential diagnosis of APD in a patient with trauma to the eye includes traumatic retinal detachment and optic nerve injury.

- Even the smallest pressure on an open globe can lead to extrusion of the ocular contents. If an open globe is diagnosed or even suspected, manipulation and examination may lead to further damage and should therefore be deferred. Cover the eye with a shield for protection. If necessary, IV antibiotics may be used but not topical drops. Use general anesthesia rather than local anesthesia.

- If possible, perform indirect ophthalmoscopy early so that continued hemorrhage will not blur the image. The pupils need to be dilated for the examination and this should be recorded clearly on the chart so as to avoid confusion with neurologic evaluation.

- Blunt trauma may cause stretching at the iris root which may damage the circular iris blood vessels and result in a hyphema (bleeding into the anterior chamber). Complications include uveitis, glaucoma, and corneal staining and cloudiness. Treatment includes bed rest, steroids, cycloplegics, and treatment of complications.

- Conjunctival laceration or foreign body, subconjunctival hemorrhage, shallow anterior chamber in the absence of a corneal laceration, and a soft eye should raise the suspicion of a scleral laceration. Shotgun pellets and other injuries to the eyelid may appear trivial externally, but they may have penetrated the globe through the eyelids. If there is a high index of suspicion of a scleral laceration, computed tomography (CT) scan may be helpful. If suspicion of a scleral laceration still exists, careful surgical exploration is mandatory.

- Treatment of optic nerve injuries is controversial. Very high dose IV steroids may be helpful if given early.

- A chemical burn, especially an alkali one, is an ophthalmic emergency. Start treatment by irrigation and lavage immediately, even before the exact nature of the burn is known.

- Many ocular injuries are associated with midface fractures. Orbital fractures can be direct involving the orbital rim or indirect involving the bones within the orbital cavity.

- Repair of a serious ocular injury (retinal detachment, corneoscleral lacerations, and so on) takes priority over fracture repair. The presence of a hyphema or vitreous hemorrhage mandates waiting until the condition stabilizes before any bony manipulation.

- Symptoms and signs suggesting an orbital fracture include diplopia, decreased range of ocular motility, periorbital ecchymosis, subcutaneous emphysema, enophthalmos, inferior displacement of the globe, and infraorbital nerve dysfunction in the form of paresthesia.

- CT scan is the most valuable imaging technique because it visualizes both bones and soft tissues including extraocular muscles. Make sure to order coronal and axial thin orbital sections.

- Repair is best done after 1–2 weeks. This allows edema, hemorrhage, and contusions to resolve partially. If the diplopia and ocular motility continue to improve and the patient is not troubled, continued observation is warranted.

144 STRABISMUS

Raed Shatnawi, Janice B. Lasky, Marilyn B. Mets

- The mother is always right. This is true in most cases of strabismus. When a parent brings a child with suspected strabismus, a complete eye examination including a dilated fundus examination and cycloplegic refraction is mandatory. Attention should be directed to significant refractive errors, abnormalities of the media, and possible fundus lesions. As stated previously, 20% of children with retinoblastoma will present with strabismus. Once these secondary causes of strabismus have been ruled out, the examiner can concentrate on the ocular motility problem.

- Comitant strabismus occurs when the angle of deviation is the same in different directions of gaze. When there is limited movement in one or more of the directions of gaze or when one of the muscles is overacting, this will produce incomitant strabismus where the measured angle is different in different directions of gaze.

- A phoria is literally a hidden deviation that needs alternate cover testing to be revealed. Under binocular viewing, phoria is controlled by fusional mechanisms. In contrast to phoria, a tropia is a manifest deviation which is not controlled under binocular viewing conditions.

- Esodeviation occurs when the eyes turn inward. Exodeviation occurs when the eyes deviate outward. Upward and downward deviations have the prefix hyper and hypo added, respectively. The above terms may have the suffix tropia or phoria. For example, we may have a patient with esotropia, exophoria, or hypertropia.
- A head tilt indicates cyclovertical muscle palsy (fourth nerve palsy) or a disorder of the sternomastoid muscle. Their differentiation is important for proper treatment.
- The differential diagnosis of the sixth cranial nerve palsy can be confusing and challenging at the same time. Congenital isolated palsy of the sixth cranial nerve is usually benign and transient, resolving before the age of 2 months. In the absence of other associated neurologic abnormalities, the prognosis is excellent. Acquired sixth cranial nerve palsy can also be benign and transient. It may occur 1–3 weeks following a febrile illness, immunization, or without a known cause. Neuroradiologic workup is appropriate. Associations include hydrocephalus, pseudotumor cerebri, and brain tumors.
- Treatment of strabismus depends on the cause of the strabismus and the type of strabismus. Treatment modalities include glasses, surgery, and in selected cases motility exercises. Some patients are treated with more than one modality.
- If surgery is indicated, it falls into two major categories: a weakening procedure or a strengthening one of the involved muscles. Some patients may require more than one procedure to bring them to the proper alignment.
- Management of strabismus may take a long period of time and it needs the combined efforts of the family and the treating doctors.

145 REFRACTIVE ERRORS

Raed Shatnawi, Janice B. Lasky, Marilyn B. Mets

- The image of an infinitely distant object will fall in front of the retina in myopia, on the retina in emmetropia, and behind the retina in hyperopia, when there is no accommodation effort in these eyes.
- The clinical equivalent of infinity is 20 ft (6 m).
- Classification of refractive errors into the previous categories should be considered as part of the spectrum of eye growth and changes with time. Except for the fact that a hyperope requires a plus lens and a myope a minus lens correction, the two eyes are physiologically alike and they only differ optically.

- Most infants are hyperopic, probably because the axial length of their eyeballs is relatively too short. As the eyeball grows there appears to be some flattening of the cornea and lens with an increase in the axial length. This process is called the myopic shift, which helps in the process of emmetropization that brings the eye back into a state of emmetropia.
- Ametropia exists when distant objects are not sharply focused on the retina by an eye with relaxed accommodation. The eye is too long or short for its power or too weak or strong for its length.
- The far point of the myopic eye lies somewhere between the eye and the infinity. The myopic eye can see clearly up to this point but not farther. To correct this error, the light rays that come from infinity should be altered to be seen coming from the far point. This means that we need a divergent lens, which is a minus power one.
- The far point of the hyperopic eye lies behind the retina. The unaccommodated hyperope cannot see distinctly any point in front of him from near to infinity. To correct for this, light coming from infinity should enter the eye with more convergence, which is accomplished by the use of a plus power lens.
- Astigmatism occurs when the two principal meridians of the cornea are not the same, i.e., one of them is steeper than the other one, which causes the retinal image to be blurred. Correction of astigmatism requires a cylindrical lens.
- Refractive errors may be treated with spectacles, contact lenses, or refractive surgery.

146 AMBLYOPIA

Raed Shatnawi, Janice B. Lasky, Marilyn B. Mets

- Amblyopia can be defined as an acquired defect in monocular vision that is due to abnormal visual experience early in life. It is usually unilateral but may be bilateral. By itself, amblyopia causes no change on the ocular structures, but it is commonly associated with other ocular abnormalities that can be demonstrated on physical examination.
- Vulnerability of the visual system to the effects of abnormal visual experience is greatest in the first few months of life and extends through the end of the first decade.
- The overall prevalence of amblyopia is 2–4% and it is the most common cause of visual impairment in children and young adults in the U.S. population.
- Causes of amblyopia can be classified according to the mechanism producing amblyopia.

- First: Refractive amblyopia, which results from anisometropia, inequality of the refractive states between the two eyes, or more confusingly isometropia, which is equal but high refractive errors in both eyes which tends to produce bilateral amblyopia.
- Second: Strabismic amblyopia, in which images from both eyes are not aligned together. Chronic rejection of the disparate input from the deviating eye seems to play the principal factor in producing this type of amblyopia.
- Last: Deprivational amblyopia. Obstruction of vision by media opacities may cause serious damage to the immature visual system. This may include but is not limited to congenital cataract, ptosis (drooping of one or both eyelids), eyelid hemangioma, and it could be iatrogenic when one of the eyes is patched for any reason.
- Some authors will add organic causes of amblyopia when there are congenital retinal or optic nerve abnormalities. In addition to the direct effect of these disorders on the visual system, they also can retard the visual development.
- Treatment of amblyopia depends on the cause and mechanism. Significant refractive errors should be corrected. Media opacities, if judged to be significant, should be removed as soon as possible because they tend to cause the most severe form of amblyopia. Occlusion of the good eye should be instituted as part-time or full-time depending on the severity of amblyopia. Occlusion therapy should be monitored closely because of the risk of inducing amblyopia in the occluded eye.

147 RETINOPATHY OF PREMATURITY

Raed Shatnawi, Janice B. Lasky,
Marilyn B. Mets

- ROP, also known previously as retrolental fibroplasia, is a serious vasoproliferative disease affecting the retinae of extremely premature infants. In most cases, ROP regresses or heals, but it can lead to severe visual impairment or blindness.
- ROP primarily occurs in extremely low birth weight infants. Significant risk factors include very low birth weight, very young gestational age, and a very sick infant (days receiving supplemental oxygen, septicemia, intraventricular hemorrhage, and so on).
- Retinal vasculature begins to develop around the 16th week of gestation. It becomes fully mature at term.

Premature birth results in cessation of normal vascular maturation. As a result, vasoconstriction and even obliteration occurs. The retina continues to grow and eventually outgrows its vascular supply. Overtime, retinal hypoxia occurs and results in overgrowth of vessels (retinal neovascularization), which results in ROP.
- Incidence varies with birth weight. Fifty to seventy percent of infants whose birth weight is less than 1250 g at birth will have some form of ROP.
- Long-term outcomes for serious disease include severe visual impairment and blindness. In addition, high myopia, strabismus, amblyopia, glaucoma, and retinal detachment at a later age may occur. This necessitates prolonged follow-up of these patients.
- Severe disease occurs in White infants more than African-American counterparts. The exact mechanism for the decreased incidence of progression to severe disease in Black infants is not understood.
- Rop occurs equally in males and females, although some reports indicate a male predilection.
- The American Academy of Pediatrics and the American Academy of Ophthalmology guidelines for screening include a birth weight less than or equal to 1500 g and a gestational age less than or equal to 28 weeks. In addition, infants with birth weights greater than 1500 g who otherwise are believed to be at high risk for ROP should also be examined. Examination should be conducted by an experienced ophthalmologist at 4–6 weeks of age or by 31–33 weeks postconceptional age. Follow-up examination is based on the initial examination findings.
- The current classification of ROP is based on location of the disease (zones 1, 2, and 3), extent of disease (clock hours involved 1–12), and severity of the disease (stages 0–5). ROP is categorized by the lowest zone and the highest stage observed in each eye.
  1. Zones
     a. Zone 1 is the most labile. The center of zone one is the optic nerve. It extends twice the distance from the optic nerve to the fovea in a circle. Any disease in zone 1 (even stage 0) is critical and must be monitored closely.
     b. Zone 2 is a circle surrounding zone 1 with the nasal ora serrata as its nasal border.
     c. Zone 3 is the remaining temporal crescent outside zone 2. Aggressive disease is rarely seen in this zone.
  2. Stages
     a. Stage 0: This is the mildest form of ROP. It is immature retinal vasculature but no clear demarcation line separating the vascularized from the unvascularized retina.
     b. Stage 1: A fine, thin demarcation line between vascular and avascular portions of the retina is present.

c. Stage 2: A broad, thick ridge clearly separates the vascular from the avascular retina.
d. Stage 3: Extraretinal proliferation of fibrovascular tissue toward the vitreous is seen.
e. Stage 4: Partial retinal detachment, which is further classified into 4a and 4b to describe the involvement of the fovea (4a) or not (4b).
f. Stage 5: Total retinal detachment.
3. Other terms used in the description of ROP include PLUS disease, which is defined as dilation and tortuosity of the posterior retinal vessels, iris vascular engorgement, pupillary rigidity, and vitreous haze. The presence of PLUS disease is a grave sign of ROP.
4. Threshold disease is defined as five contiguous or eight noncontiguous clock hours of neovascularization (stage 3 or more) with PLUS disease in zone 1 or 2.

• Treatment of ROP is indicated for patients with threshold disease. Of threshold eyes left untreated, 50% develop adverse structural outcomes (e.g., retinal detachment).
• Usually, these babies are examined in the Neonatal Intensive Care Unit (NICU) because of the stress of the examination and because of their critical medical condition.
• Treatment modalities include laser photocoagulation, cryotherapy, and surgery for retinal detachment if present.
• Continued medical and ophthalmic care for those patients is very important because of the associated complications despite successful surgical treatment. See Fig. 147-1 for complete ROP consultation form.

148 SYSTEMIC DISORDERS WITH OCULAR INVOLVEMENT

Raed Shatnawi, Janice B. Lasky, Marilyn B. Mets

JUVENILE RHEUMATOID ARTHRITIS (JRA)

• JRA, also known as juvenile chronic arthritis (JCA) especially in the British literature, is defined as an arthritis of greater than 3 months' duration with onset in patients less than 16 years of age.
• JRA, based on the pattern of presentation during the first 6 months of the disease, is classified as polyarticular (five or more joints involved), pauciarticular (four or less joints involved), and systemic or Still disease (prominent systemic features with variable joint involvement). The risk of uveitis is determined by the nature of the child's arthritis during this initial 6-month time period, even though more joints may later be affected.
• Serotyping is an important factor determining the frequency of associated ocular involvement in each subtype.
• Seventy-five percent of children with pauciarticular type are positive for antinuclear antibodies (ANA). Uveitis is common in this group and affects about 20% of patients. In the polyarticular type, 40% are ANA-positive and uveitis occurs in about 5%. Risk factors for uveitis in the above two subtypes are female sex, early-onset JRA, and positive findings of ANA and HLA-DR5.
• Ocular manifestations of JRA are two different types of iridocyclitis. Acute iridocyclitis is seen in the HLA-B27-associated subgroups and is similar to that seen in adult HLA-B27-associated disease. A chronic iridocyclitis is seen in the ANA-positive pauciarticular subgroup. The chronic iridocyclitis seen in this subgroup tends to be asymptomatic or minimally symptomatic. Uveitis in JRA is bilateral in 50–70% of cases and its severity is unrelated to the severity of arthritis. It is this subgroup that is frequently seen for screening in an effort to detect the uveitis early.
• The uveitis often responds poorly to treatment and requires chronic therapy, which may be in the form of topical eye drops in mild cases to systemic immunosuppressant in the more severe cases.
• Severe visual disability may develop. Band keratopathy (a form of corneal opacity) and cataracts are seen in up to one-third of these patients. Glaucoma develops in 20% of the patients and has a poor prognosis. Posterior synechiae (adhesions between the pupil and the lens) are common. Other complications include macular edema in 8–10% of cases and phthisis (atrophy of the ocular tissues) in 4–10% of patients.
• Screening for uveitis is governed by the various risk factors as follows:
1. Systemic onset → annual
2. Polyarticular – ANA → every 6 months
3. Polyarticular + ANA → every 3–4 months
4. Pauciarticular – ANA → every 6 months
5. Pauciarticular + ANA → every 3 months

CHROMOSOMAL ABNORMALITIES

• Many of the chromosomal abnormalities involve the eye, although, with the possible exception of cartilage

CHILDREN'S MEMORIAL HOSPITAL   CHICAGO, ILLINOIS 60614

RETINOPATHY OF PREMATURITY CONSULTATION

Current postnatal age:	Planned/actual discharge:
Birth weight:	Gestational age:
Duration oxygen exposure:	Date oxygen terminated:
Systemic problems:	
Ocular problems:	
DROPS:	

↓ Normal*   Examination number:

BLINK TO LIGHT / MOTILITY	
EXTERNAL	
IRIS / PUPIL DILATION	
MEDIA CLARITY	
DISC	
FOVEA	
POSTERIOR VESSELS	
VASCULAR TERMINATION	

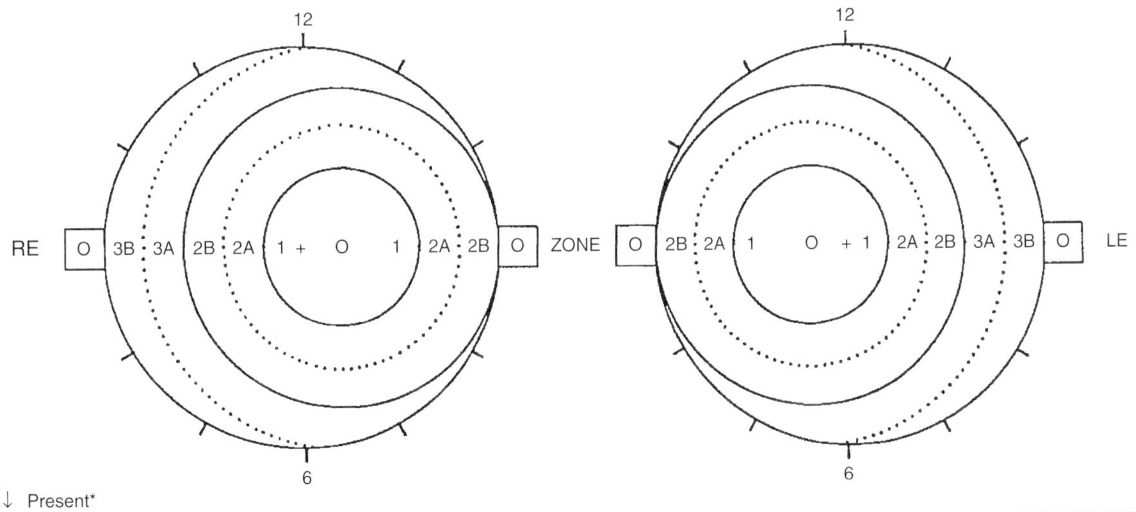

RE ☐ O ☐ 3B · 3A · 2B · 2A · 1 + O · 1 · 2A · 2B ☐ O ☐ ZONE ☐ O ☐ 2B · 2A · 1 · O + 1 · 2A · 2B · 3A · 3B ☐ O ☐ LE

↓ Present*

DEMARCATION LINE / RIDGE	
EXTRA-RETINAL PROLIFERATION	
RETINAL DETACHMENT	

ASSESSMENT*

Retinopathy of prematurity, stage	Prethreshold	Treatment threshold
No evidence of retinopathy, vascularization	Incomplete	Complete
Examination Inconclusive	Inadequate view	Minimal/equivocal changes
Other abnormalities		

PLAN: Next examination:

Examiner: Date:

X = both eyes. R = right eye only. L = left eye only.   White - MEDICAL RECORDS   Yellow - OPHTHALMOLOGY   Pink - NEONATOLOGY

FIG. 147-1   Retinopathy of prematurity consultation form.

in a ciliary body coloboma in trisomy 13, no ocular malformation appears to be specific for a given chromosomal abnormality.

- In trisomy 13, there is microphthalmia, which may be very severe. Eighty percent of eyes have colobomas of the iris and ciliary body, as well as cataract and persistent hyperplastic primary vitreous. Histologically, cartilage is present in 65% of these eyes, especially in those eyes that are very microphthalmic. This association of cartilage within a ciliary body coloboma appears to be unique to eyes from infants with trisomy 13. Other findings include bilateral retinal dysplasia and typical and atypical retinal degeneration. Sixty percent of eyes have angle anomalies, which increases the risk of congenital glaucoma.
- A number of ocular and adnexal abnormalities have been reported in trisomy 18, although most of these are minor. Lid abnormalities include ptosis, narrow palpebral fissures, epicanthal folds, blepharophimosis, abnormally long or sparse lashes, abnormally thick lids, shallow orbits, hypertelorism, and hypotelorism, and abnormalities of gaze, including strabismus and nystagmus, may occur. Ocular malformations are nonspecific for this trisomy and include cataract, anomalies of the ciliary processes, retinal folds, both hyperplasia and hypoplasia of elements of the cornea and uveal tract, angle immaturity, persistent hyperplastic primary vitreous, retinal dysplasia, optic nerve hypoplasia, and coloboma.
- Ocular findings in trisomy 21 (Down syndrome) include epicanthal folds, myopia, hypertelorism, cataracts, hypopigmented areas of the iris (Brushfield spots), strabismus, nystagmus, and keratoconus. Retinal findings include increased numbers of vessels crossing the optic disc margin, and patchy retinal pigment epithelial atrophy.
- Trisomies of the sex chromosomes include Klinefelter syndrome (47, XXY), in which there are minimal ocular abnormalities, and XYY syndrome (47, XYY), in which there are antisocial tendencies, gonadal atrophy, lens luxation, and colobomas.
- Monosomy of the X chromosome (45, XO-Turner syndrome) tends to be associated with microphthalmia, dislocated lens, coloboma, and retinal dysplasia.
- In cri du chat syndrome (deletion of part of the short arm of chromosome 5), ocular findings include epicanthal folds, hypertelorism, exotropia, optic atrophy, tortuous retinal arteries and veins, and pupils that are supersensitive to 2.5% methacholine. Similar findings have been described in partial deletion of chromosome 4.
- Deletion of a portion of the short arm of chromosome 11 is associated with some cases of Miller syndrome, which consists of aniridia, abnormalities of the urogenital system, mental retardation, and Wilms tumor. The iris in aniridia is not, in fact, missing, but instead is severely hypoplastic.

NEUROCUTANEOUS SYNDROMES (PHAKOMATOSES)

- The classic ocular finding of tuberous sclerosis is the retinal astrocytoma (astrocytic hamartoma). This lesion arises within the nerve fiber layer of the retina. It appears more in the posterior fundus than in the periphery. Small lesions appear as translucent intraretinal patches with minimal thickness. Large lesions tend to be opaque white, elevated, and multilobulated. Intralesional calcification develops within some larger lesions. Lesions can be multifocal and many patients have bilateral involvement. The retinal blood vessels associated with these lesions tend not to be dilated or tortuous. If growth occurs, it tends to be extremely slow. Approximately half of patients with tuberous sclerosis have at least one typical astrocytic retinal hamartoma.
- Ocular findings in neurofibromatosis type 1 (NF-1) include the following:
  1. Optic nerve glioma (ONG): Develops in about 15% of patients. On the other hand, a child with an optic nerve glioma has up to 70% chance of having NF-1. ONG may be unilateral or bilateral and may extend posteriorly to involve the chiasm and posterior structures. On computed tomography (CT) evaluation, they appear as a fusiform enlargement with sharp delineation from the surrounding tissue due to circumscription by an intact dura. Kinking and buckling of the optic nerve along with infarctive cysts are typical findings.
  2. Sphenoorbital encephalocele: Caused by a congenital dysplasia of the sphenoid wing. Characteristically, it causes a pulsating proptosis which is not associated with either a bruit or a thrill.
  3. Eyelid neurofibromas: May be either nodular or plexiform and tends to develop early in life. When involving the upper lid, they may cause a mechanical ptosis.
  4. Lisch nodules of the iris: Rarely found at birth and develop during the second and third decades of life, and are eventually found in more than 95% of cases. They are small bilateral melanocytic hamartomas of the iris.
- Findings in neurofibromatosis type 2 (NF-2) include the following:
  1. Various cataracts: Posterior subcapsular, cortical, or nuclear forms.
  2. Retinal hamartomas and macular epiretinal membranes.

3. Visual pathway tumors: Meningiomas, schwanomas, and gliomas.
4. No Lisch nodules as compared to NF-1.

- The most striking ocular feature of Sturge-Weber syndrome (SWS) is congenital, infantile, or juvenile glaucoma, which occurs in about 30% of cases. The glaucoma tends to occur early in life and be resistant to conventional forms of treatment. The underlying mechanisms for the glaucoma in SWS appear to be anomalous angle development and elevated episcleral venous pressure.
- Other ocular features in SWS are diffuse choroidal hemangioma, deep central cupping of the optic disc, and telangiectasia of the conjunctiva and episclera.
- Visual loss in SWS is caused by glaucoma, macular degeneration, and retinal detachment.
- Other neurocutaneous syndromes also have ocular features; describing them is beyond the scope of this book.

149 THE BLIND INFANT

Raed Shatnawi, Janice B. Lasky,
Marilyn B. Mets

- Although visual acuity in newborn babies is counting fingers (around 20/1000 in Snellen equivalents), it increases rapidly with age. At the age of 1 year, visual acuity is at least 20/50 and it reaches adult levels between 2 and 5 years of age.
- Vision in infants is evaluated by noting response to light or hand-motion threat, and the capacity of each eye to follow during contralateral occlusion. In many cases, an infant's gross objection to occlusion of one eye, by crying or avoiding or pushing away the occluder, will provide the first clue that vision in the uncovered eye is significantly impaired.
- Clear fixation and following reflexes should be present by 6–8 weeks of age.
- Inspection of the baby and taking history about other developmental milestones will give important information to the examiner.
- Assessment of infants with subnormal or absent visual responses usually distinguishes between two major groups: those with and those without congenital nystagmus.
- Congenital nystagmus is frequently associated with bilateral visual loss of prechiasmal or chiasmal origin but not posterior to the chiasm.
- In infants with poor vision and nystagmus, but with a seemingly normal eye examination, electroretinography (ERG) should be performed.

- Leber congenital amaurosis (LCA) is an autosomal-recessive retinal photoreceptor disorder that causes poor vision from birth. Although initial fundus examination may be normal, pigmentary retinopathy, vessel attenuation, and optic atrophy occur with time. High hyperopia is characteristic. ERG shows nonrecordable electrical activity (*flat ERG*). No treatment is available.
- Achromatopsia is an autosomal-recessive or X-linked disease characterized by a partial or complete absence of retinal cone function. Vision is severely reduced and color vision is lost. Severe photophobia is characteristic and patients show preference for dim light. ERG is diagnostic.
- Congenital stationary night blindness (CSNB) is hereditary with all three patterns of inheritance described. The X-linked type shows reduced vision, nystagmus, and high myopia. Autosomal-dominant CSNB does not show reduced vision and nystagmus. The autosomal-recessive type is variable. ERG is characteristic.
- Other hereditary retinal disorders may be seen in juvenile retinoschisis, Joubert syndrome, Refsum disease, neonatal adrenoleukodystrophy, neuronal ceroid lipofuscinosis, Jeune syndrome, and osteopetrosis.
- Patients with albinism and aniridia, both of which may be associated with foveal (and optic nerve?) hypoplasia, may present with congenital nystagmus. At least 10 syndromes have been associated with albinism. Their precise differentiation is important since some of them are associated with significant morbidity.
- Optic nerve hypoplasia is usually diagnosed on fundus examination. The small disc is surrounded by a yellow halo (double-ring sign). If bilateral, this condition may be associated with congenital nystagmus. De Morsier syndrome (septooptic dysplasia) refers to the constellation of bilateral optic nerve hypoplasia, absence of the septum pellucidum, thinning or absence of the corpus callosum, dysplasia of the anterior third ventricle, and hypopituitarism. Early recognition and hormone replacement therapy are very important to reverse the growth retardation seen in this disorder.
- Optic disc colobomata, if bilateral, may be seen in association with congenital nystagmus. Of greater importance, however, is the association of colobomas or other dysplastic optic discs with basal encephaloceles, and other midfacial anomalies.
- If no nystagmus is present, the diagnosis falls into two categories based on whether central nervous system (CNS) abnormalities are present or not.
- Very high refractive errors (myopia or hyperopia) may lead to behavior that mimics blindness. Always exclude high refractive errors.

- Premature birth, neonatal asphyxia, developmental abnormalities, or a seizure disorder may all indicate possible damage to the occipital cortex. Helpful signs include preference for bright-colored objects, staring at bright light, and turning of the head whenever they attempt to look toward an object of interest. Computed tomography (CT) scan and magnetic resonance imaging (MRI) as well as pediatric neurologist are necessary for proper diagnosis.
- Delayed visual maturation (DVM) is a diagnosis of exclusion and retrospection. This refers to visually impaired infants with normal ocular examinations, normal neuroimaging and ERG, and no nystagmus.

The exact etiology is unknown. The visual prognosis is excellent but this retrospective diagnosis should be made only when visual function indeed spontaneously improves to normal or near-normal levels by the end of the first year of life.

- In all the above cases, it is sometimes difficult to reach a definitive diagnosis immediately. When this is the case, it is preferable to postpone a definitive answer to the parents until the clinical picture is clear. Wait and see, for the natural history may be helpful. Nothing is worse than to tell the parents that their baby is blind (or normal) and then to be forced later to change to the opposite conclusion.

John F. Sarwark, Section Editor

150 NEWBORN ORTHOPEDIC EXAMINATION

Denise T. Ibrahim and John F. Sarwark

- *General inspection*: Dysmorphic features; spine/limbs disproportionate; skin—i.e., café-au-lait spot may suggest neurofibromatosis; assess spontaneous movements.
- *Neck*: Inspect for symmetry, range of motion, rule out torticollis.
- *Spine*: Inspect for symmetry, cutaneous abnormalities, hairy patches, and dimpling; rule out infantile scoliosis or spina bifida aperta.
- *Limbs*: General inspection of limbs; inspect hands and feet for anomalies. Assess range of motion of joints, assess contractures, and assess limb lengths.
- *Hip examination*: *Ortolani sign*: Start with neutrally adducted thigh then gently abduct thigh to appreciate reduction of hip with a "clunk" sensation, if reduces it is a positive Ortolani sign. *Barlow sign*: A provocative maneuver where the hip dislocates or subluxes posteriorly with adduction and posterior gentle force. Use the same amount of manual force as an abdominal palpation examination. *Galeazzi sign*: Femoral length with patient supine flex hip and knees to 90° and assess levels of knees. If one knee is shorter than the other it is a positive Galeazzi. *Allis test*: Tibial length with patient supine and hips and knees symmetrically flexed to allow both feet to rest on a table. Assess knee level.

151 DEVELOPMENTAL DYSPLASIA OF HIP (DDH)

Denise T. Ibrahim and John F. Sarwark

- Description of an array of hip problems to describe shallow acetabulum, hip dislocation, or subluxation, as well as severe teratologic antenatal dislocation.
- *Incidence*: Ten percent of neonates will have a positive examination; only 1% require treatment; increased incidence with breech position/female. Females > males, oligohydramnios, congenital muscular torticollis, first-born positive family history are other risk factors.
- *Newborn to 6 weeks*: Barlow and Ortolani provocative maneuver. Galeazzi sign (Section I), symmetry thigh folds (soft sign; not a critical finding). After 6 weeks, limitation of abduction of the involved hip.
- *Imaging*: Radiographs not indicated <6 weeks of age due to immature unossified skeleton at birth making radiographs unreliable. Ultrasound plays important role and adjunct to physical examination in infant less than 6 months of age but older than 4–6 weeks. American Academy of Pediatrics (AAP) Guidelines: Female/breech: all require hip ultrasound.
- *Treatment*: Once diagnosed, pediatric orthopedic specialist starts treatment as soon as possible. Good prognosis related to early identification and treatment (under age 1 year). Less than 6 months of age use a Pavlik harness which maintains hip in abducted/

reduced position. Close monitoring of position is required to assure proper harness position. Improper use is associated with nerve problems and avascular necrosis of hips.

REFERENCE

Guille J, Pizzutillo P, MacEwen G: Developmental dysplasia of the hip from birth to six months. *J Am Acad Orthop Surg* 2000;8:232–242.

152 FRACTURES

Denise T. Ibrahim and John F. Sarwark

SALTER-HARRIS CLASSIFICATION OF PHYSEAL FRACTURES

- Type I: Injury occurring through the physis (i.e., growth plate), does not extend into the metaphysis or epiphysis.
- Type II: Injury extends along the physis and exits through the metaphysis.
- Type III: Injury extends along the physis and exits through the epiphysis, these may also be intraarticular.
- Type IV: Injury extending from the metaphysis across the physis and into the epiphysis, usually intraarticular.
- Type V: Crushing injury to the physis from a compression force (Fig. 152-1).
- Descriptive terminology
  1. Torus (buckle) fracture—mild fracture with plastic deformation of one or both cortices, minimal displacement.
  2. Greenstick fracture—cortex under tension fractures completely and the compression side undergoes plastic deformity and remains intact.
  3. Physeal (growth plate) injuries—describe using Salter-Harris classification (see above).

SURGICAL EMERGENCIES

OPEN FRACTURES
- Often associated with high-energy trauma and multiple injuries.
- Classified by Gustillo and Anderson (1976), according to wound size and extent of soft tissue involvement:
  1. Type I: Wound <1cm, minimal soft tissue injury.
  2. Type II: Wound >1 cm, moderate soft tissue injury.
  3. Type III: Extensive soft tissue injury with possible neurovascular injury and severe wound contamination.
- Management
  1. Advanced trauma life support (ATLS) primary survey first.
  2. Immediate IV antibiotics: First generation *cephalosporin* for type I; add *aminoglycoside* for types II and III; if "barnyard" involved add penicillin or metronidazole.
  3. Tetanus prophylaxis.
  4. Assess and document neurovascular status.
  5. Sterile dressing and splinting for comfort without definitive reduction.
  6. Operative treatment when stable.

DISLOCATIONS OF JOINT
- Traumatic dislocation of a joint requires immediate reduction in a gentle, nontraumatic and controlled fashion.
- Many joint dislocations are managed by the emergency room physician. Examples include nurse-maid elbow (radial head dislocation) in children and shoulder dislocations in adults being the most frequent.
- Traumatic hip dislocations should be discussed with an orthopedic surgeon for immediate reduction, occasionally requiring general anesthesia with muscle relaxation in the operating room.

NEUROVASCULAR COMPROMISE
- Any injury or condition that presents with a change of neurovascular examination requires immediate attention.

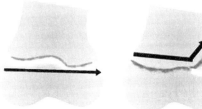 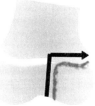 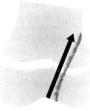 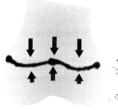

| Salter-Harris I | Salter-Harris II | Salter-Harris III | Salter-Harris IV | Salter-Harris V |

FIG. 152-1   Salter-Harris Classification.

• *Compartment syndrome*: A potentially devastating condition in which increased pressure within a fascial compartment of limb causes a destructive ischemia-edema cycle unyielding to autocompensation by the vascular system. Identification and surgical release of the affected compartments is required. Recognized by the six *P*s: *p*ain out of proportion to physical examination findings, increased *p*ressure, *p*allor skin color, *p*ulseless, *p*aresthesias, and *p*aresis. Pain with passive stretch is one of the earlier signs. Early recognition is critical. Tight bandages or splints on an injured limb can cause increased pressure, thus caution needs to be practiced when attending to injured limbs. There are nontraumatic but chronic presentations of compartment syndrome that can exist, such as exercise-induced.

MULTIPLE FRACTURES

• Multiply injured patients should all be assessed by a multidisciplinary approach as outlined by ATLS protocol. Once the patient is stabilized, orthopedic injuries are assessed in the secondary survey. A child with multiple fractures is best treated with early stabilization of the fractures. Depending on the fracture, surgery is required for fixation of certain fractures that would not require fixation in an isolated injury situation. Surgery may be required for better mobilization

of the patient. Morbidity and mortality with multiple fractures are not increased to the same magnitude as in adult situations.

INITIAL CARE OF FRACTURES

• Examine and document the sensory, motor, and vascular status of the injured extremity, including joints above and below the injured region.
• Splinting techniques
  1. Initial treatment of any limb injury should include a well-molded appropriate splint. Cast padding (webril = cotton padding) is applied first in several layers thick with extra padding to bony prominences (elbow, heel, ankle, and so on). A posterior mold made of plaster or prefabricated fiberglass is then applied to splint the joints above and below the injured region in a neutral position. It is held on with an ace bandage. It is important to roll the ace bandage with mild stretch to allow for swelling and to avoid tight compression to the limb, which can cause iatrogenic skin sores or neurovascular compromise. Neurovascular assessment must be performed and documented after a splint is applied to a child (Fig. 152-2).

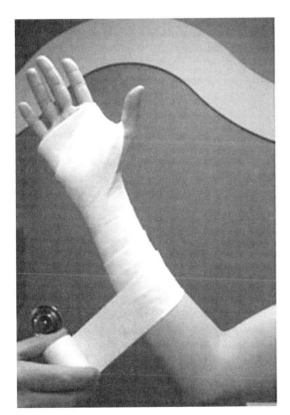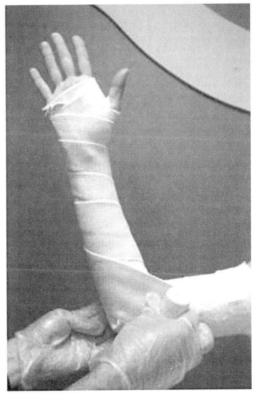

FIG. 152-2 Posterior mold splinting technique, starting with cotton padding (left), followed by posterior mold made of plaster, and lastly an ace wrap (right). Notice the 50% overlapping of each circumferential wrap.

COMMON PEDIATRIC FRACTURES

UPPER EXTREMITY

- Upper extremity radiographic anatomy
  1. Two-thirds of occult elbow fractures present with a *posterior fat pad* sign. If present with clinical symptoms it requires splinting.
  2. Contralateral comparison elbow radiographs are useful for diagnosis of pediatric elbow fractures with questionable features.
  3. Ossification centers appear in the following order:
     a. Capitellum: 1–2 years old
     b. Radial head: 3–4 years
     c. Medial epicondyle: 5–6 years
     d. Trochlea: 7–8 years
     e. Olecranon: 10 years
     f. Lateral epicondyle: 12 years
- The above ages are approximate ages with females ossifying earlier than males.

Clavicle Fractures

- Most are midclavicular, treated in a sling until nontender; exceptions to conservative management include open fractures, neurovascular compromise, or severe tenting of the skin.

Proximal Humerus Fractures

- Excellent remodeling potential, mostly treated with a sling or coaptation splint (long-arm posterior mold which wraps around shoulder); rarely require surgery.

Supracondylar Humerus Fracture

- Type I is undisplaced; type II displaced with posterior cortex hinging present, varus or valgus impaction; type III is completely displaced, no cortical contact (Gartland classification).
- Most common elbow fracture in children and is associated with serious neurovascular compromise in 10%. May lead to compartment syndromes and later "Volkmann ischemic contracture" (compartment syndrome) if not recognized. Careful assessment of the anterior interosseus nerve motor function (median nerve branch, most commonly affected) by flexion of interphalangeal joint of the thumb and index finger, and also the radial and ulnar nerve sensory and motor function. Initial splinting should not flex the elbow greater than 90° secondary to potentiating neurovascular compromise.

Radial Head Subluxation

- "Nursemaid's elbow." Peak incidence 1–3 years old, secondary to pulling or traction on the forearm/wrist. Child presents holding elbow by the side slightly flexed and pronated and will not supinate forearm. Diagnosis is by history and physical. Radiographs are normal. Reduce radial head by applying pressure over the anterior radial head while flexing the elbow 90° followed by rotation of the forearm into full supination. If child is moving elbow freely, immobilization is not required.

Monteggia Fractures

- Radial head dislocation and ulnar fracture. Anatomic relationship of the radial head and capitellum will line up in all radiographic views of the elbow.

Radius and Ulna Diaphyseal Fractures

- "Both-Bone Forearm Fracture." Described by location: distal third, middle third, or proximal third. Remodeling potential in childhood with acceptable angulation ranging from 10 to 30° depending on age. Acceptable malrotation remains controversial since it is thought that it does not remodel. Long-arm splinting or casting is required.

Distal Radius Fractures

- Most common pediatric upper extremity fracture. Fall on outstretched arm is common mechanism. If tender in supination and pronation, long-arm splinting or casting required. Salter-Harris classification can be used for physeal injuries. Excellent remodeling potential.

LOWER EXTREMITY

Hip Fractures

- Type I: Transphyseal (distinguished from slipped capital femoral epiphysis [SCFE] by younger age) severe trauma, more displaced acute separation of the physis.
- Type II: Transcervical or middle portion of the femoral neck.
- Type III: Cervicotrochanteric or at the base of the femoral neck.
- Type IV: Intertrochanteric or between the greater and lesser trochanter of the proximal femur.
- Avascular necrosis common in types I, II, and III and need immediate attention and reduction.

Slipped Capital Femoral Epiphysis (SCFE)

- Displacement of the femoral head epiphysis on the metaphysis in a posterior-superior direction.
  1. Common age is 11–13 years.
  2. Common in obese boys.
  3. Approximately 25% bilaterality.
  4. Etiology—multifactoral, obesity, trauma, endocrine disorder (usually present at younger age without obesity).
  5. Clinical presentation—hip or groin pain, knee pain, limping or unable to bear weight, trauma.
  6. Physical examination—limping, loss of internal rotation, obligatory external rotation with hip flexion.
  7. Radiograph—AP view shows physeal widening and metaphyseal rarefaction. *Kline line* (line along

superior neck contacts the epiphysis in a normal hip) and the frog-leg lateral are useful.

8. Classified as *stable* or *unstable*. Patients with stable slips can bear weight, and symptoms are mild and chronic. Unstable slips have an abrupt onset of pain and patients are unable to bear weight.

9. Treatment—immediate nonweightbearing followed by appropriate surgical treatment by an orthopedic surgeon.

Diaphyseal Femur Fractures
• Transverse, oblique, spiral, comminuted

General Comments on Treatment
1. Initially requires splinting in neutral position of comfort.
2. Zero to six months can consider pavlik harness or "soft spica."
3. Seven months to six years old spica cast.
4. Seven years or more; multiple surgical options since unlikely casting would be tolerated.

Fractures About the Knee
• *Tibial spine fracture*: Type I—minimally displaced, slight anterior elevation. Type II—anterior third to 50% of avulsed fragment is elevated, beaklike appearance. Type III—avulsed fragment completely elevated.
• *Sleeve fracture*: Patellar fracture where the patellar tendon avulses an osteocartilagenous fragment from distal pole of patella; requires operative repair.

Ankle Fractures in Juveniles and Adolescents
• Salter-Harris classification can describe fractures.
• *Juvenile Tillaux fracture*: Avulsion fracture of the anterolateral distal tibia epiphysis, vertical Salter-Harris III fracture due to external rotation force.
• *Triplane ankle fracture*: Coronal plane, axial plane, and sagittal plane fracture, ages 10–16 that patterns onset of physeal closure. May require computed tomography (CT) evaluation.

Base of Fifth Metatarsal Fracture
• Proximal apophyseal growth center is frequently misdiagnosed as a fracture. It is evident radiographically at age 9 and unites by age 12–15 years. If tender on examination, splinting with a posterior mold splint is required.

REFERENCE

Herring JA: Fractures about the elbow, in Herring JA (ed): *Tachdjian's Pediatric Orthopaedics*. Philadelphia, PA, W.B. Saunders, 2002. p 2139.

153 LIMPING CHILD
Denise T. Ibrahim and John F. Sarwark

TRANSIENT SYNOVITIS

• Synonyms are toxic synovitis, coxalgia fugax, acute transient epiphysitis.
• Unknown etiology, self-limiting inflammation of the hip, resolves spontaneously, usually 1 or 2 days nonambulatory followed by mild limp to resolution.
• May follow upper respiratory infections.
• Clinically present with acute onset of hip pain, limping or refusal to bear weight, hold leg in flexed position.
• Usually tolerate gentle range of motion as opposed to severe pain present with a septic joint.
• May have a low-grade fever, less likely.
• Occurs in males > females, average age of 6 years.
• Diagnosis: Made by exclusion.
• Radiographs are normal, white blood cell (WBC), erythrocyte sedimentation rate (ESR), and C-reactive protein (CRP) are normal to mildly elevated if respiratory infection also present.
• Ultrasound helpful to determine joint fluid or assist in aspiration if effusion present.
• Differential diagnosis: Septic arthritis, juvenile rheumatoid arthritis (JRA), fracture, Legg-Calvé-Perthes, osteomyelitis, slipped capital femoral epiphysis, leukemia, hemophilia, and sickle cell crisis.
• Treatment: Rest, nonsteroidal anti-inflammatory drug (NSAID), gait assistive devices, and observation until pain resolves. If not improving, may need to reconsider other etiologies. All symptoms should resolve within 2 weeks.

SEPTIC ARTHRITIS

• Etiology: Hematogenous seeding or rarely local seeding from contiguous infection, postoperative or traumatic.
• Condition requires early treatment to prevent cartilage destruction and further infection spread.
• More common in males with increased frequency in <2-year-olds.
• Clinical presentation: Inability to bear weight or move limb, often appear "septic," joint warmth, extreme pain with motion, fevers.
• Four clinical factors to help differentiate from transient synovitis or other etiologies include fever history, inability to bear weight, ESR ≥40 mm/hour, and

a WBC of >12,000 mm³. If all the factors are present then there is a 99% chance of septic arthritis; if three factors are present then 93% chance.

- Monitoring CRP is helpful in treatment course.
- Radiographs are usually normal, take 1–2 weeks for bone changes to be seen.
- Joint aspiration required; assess Gram stain, aerobic and anaerobic cultures, cell count with leukocyte count; consider a serum and synovial glucose level.
- Most common organisms are *Staphylococcus aureus*, followed by group A streptococci, *Streptococcus pneumoniae*, and *Kingella kingae*. In neonates group B streptococci is important and *Neisseria gonorrhoeae* in neonate and sexually active adolescents is still seen.
- Initial treatment: Culture and sensitivity are completed before any medications are administered, which includes the blood cultures and joint aspiration. Surgical treatment is required. After all the tests are completed empiric coverage for culture negative is done and includes an antistaphylococcal IV antibiotic and gram-negative coverage for all neonates and adolescents. Length of time of antibiotic ranges from 3 to 6 weeks with conversion to oral antibiotics at treating physician's discretion.
- Prognosis: Related to timing of diagnosis, delayed diagnosis, and treatment contributes to a poorer prognosis.

LEGG-CALVÉ-PERTHES DISEASE

- Osteonecrosis (i.e., avascular necrosis) of the femoral head with subchondral collapse; etiology is unknown.
- More common in males, ages 4–8 years.
- Ten percent incidence of bilaterality.
- History of a limp before onset of pain.
- Clinically range of motion decreases as pain increases, loss of internal rotation is first finding, antalgic gait, some have positive Trendelenberg sign.
- Diagnosis: Radiographs of the hip. If negative, bone scan or magnetic resonance imaging (MRI) required.
- Differential diagnosis: Transient synovitis, septic arthritis, juvenile rheumatoid arthritis, fracture, osteomyelitis, slipped capital femoral epiphysis, leukemia, hemophilia, and sickle cell crisis.
- Four stages of the disease: (1) Early (synovitis), (2) fragmentation, (3) reossification, and (4) definitive.
- Treatment: Refer to orthopedic surgeon.

JUVENILE RHEUMATOID ARTHRITIS (JRA)

- Three main forms:
  1. Pauciarticular JRA: Most common; more common in 2–4-year-old females, females greater than males.

Usually present with swollen knee (most often affected), ankle, or fingers, minimal pain. Seventy percent positive antinuclear antibody (ANA) and negative rheumatoid factor (RF). A quarter may have iritis. Length of disease usually slightly over 2 years.
  2. Polyarticular JRA: Five or more small and large joint involvement in either young 1–3-year-olds or adolescent age, females greater than males.
  3. Systemic JRA: Present in 3–10-year-olds with febrile illness, severe myalgia, polyarthritis, erythematous macular rash, toxic, hepatosplenomegaly, and/or occasionally pericarditis. Length of symptoms vary and some can be vary destructive to the joints.
- Diagnosis: No definitive laboratory examination. Clinical and laboratory tests to aid in the diagnosis.
- A history of 6 months of arthritis for JRA for diagnosis.
- Radiographs may show osteopenia around the joints, soft tissue capsular/synovial swelling, and/or narrowing of joint space.
- Treatment: Multispecialty team approach including rheumatologists, ophthalmologists, orthopedists, and physical and occupational therapists.

REFERENCES

Blyth MJ, Kincaid R, Craigen MA, Bennett GC: The changing epidemiology of acute and subacute haematogenous osteomyelitis in children. *J Bone Joint Surg Br* 2001;83:99–102.

Kocher MS, Zuralowski D, Kasser JR: Differentiating between septic arthritis and transient synovitis of the hip in children. *J Bone Joint Surg Am* 1999;81:1662–1670.

Schneider R, Passo MH: Juvenile rheumatoid arthritis. *Rheum Dis Clin North Am.* 2002 Aug;28(3):503–30.

154 SPINE

Denise T. Ibrahim and John F. Sarwark

SCOLIOSIS

- Three main types: Idiopathic scoliosis make up 80% of cases while congenital and neuromuscular make up 15%; miscellaneous scoliosis 5%.

CONGENITAL SCOLIOSIS
- Failure of formation or segmentation of the developing spine, present but not always detected at birth.

- Rate of progression and severity is dependent on the type or types of anomaly within the vertebrae.
- A sporadic, not inherited condition.
- Anomalies include segmented hemivertebrae, wedged vertebrae, nonsegmented hemivertebrae unilateral or bilateral, unilateral nonsegmented bar, and/or nonsegmented vertebrae.
- Unsegmented bar has greatest progression potential.
- Klippel-Feil syndrome: Failure of segmentation in one or more levels in cervical vertebra.
- Evaluate all systems since associated anomalies common; i.e., other musculoskeletal anomalies, congenital heart anomalies, hypoplastic lungs, genitourinary abnormalities.
- Treatment: Depends on progression and pattern of scoliosis, careful observation until skeletal maturity, often require surgery at younger ages, and lesser curves when compared to idiopathic scoliosis.

Neuromuscular Scoliosis
- Classified as neuropathic (i.e., cerebral palsy, spinocerebellar degeneration, spinal muscular atrophy) or myopathic (i.e., arthrogryposis, muscular dystrophy, hypotonia).
- Progressive and more severe than idiopathic scoliosis.
- Long thoracolumbar curve patterns with greater pelvic obliquity.
- Assessment of pulmonary, cardiac, and nutritional status important in management of patients.
- Treatment is individualized taking into consideration functional goals, sitting balance, and pulmonary function.

Idiopathic Scoliosis
- Subdivided according to patient age: (1) Infantile, infancy to 3 years of age; (2) juvenile, 4–9 years of age; and (3) adolescent, 10 years and up.
- Defined as a curvature of the spine 10° or higher with unknown etiology.
- Infantile males > females and adolescent females > male.
- Juvenile idiopathic scoliosis has highest progression rates.
- Clinically a painless condition; if pain present, evaluate for other causes and perform thorough workup.
- Assessment: Evaluate skin, symmetry of shoulder, waistline, limb lengths, rib prominence angle of trunk rotation (ATR) on forward bend test (Adam's forward bend test), and neurovascular examination in prepubescent girls and boys.
- Most are right-sided thoracic curves. Left-sided curves may indicate other etiologies that require further investigation.
- Natural history of progression is dependent on the degree of curvature before skeletal maturity.

- Treatment: General guidelines include bracing for curves in the range of 25–45° and surgery for curves greater than 50° where progression likely.

SCHEUERMANN KYPHOSIS

- Increased thoracic kyphosis on standing lateral radiograph over 40°, wedging of the anterior vertebrae of three contiguous vertebrae levels exceeding 5° at each level; Schmorl nodes; and radiographic finding of irregular end plates.
- Peak age is midteens; male predominance.
- Clinical presentation: Pain at thoracic apex; poor posture according to parents.
- Treatment: Mostly conservative with exercises, stretching or bracing. Surgery rare and considered when >75° kyphosis and/or progression.

SPONDYLOLYSIS AND SPONDYLOLISTHESIS

Spondylolysis
- Defined as a radiographic unilateral or bilateral defect in the pars interarticularis of the posterior elements of the vertebrae; 50% of patients are normal on radiographs—bone scan with single photon emission computed tomography (SPECT) images. Oblique views may show posterior spine elements resembling a "Scottie dog." A break at the neck indicates spondylolysis. SPECT (bone scintography) more sensitive than radiographs.
- Most commonly L5.
- A common etiology of lower back pain in juveniles and teens.
- Males have 50% greater incidence than females.
- Common in athletes that undergo repetitive hyperextension stress of the spine, i.e., gymnastics, wrestling, football linebackers, diving.
- Treatment: Mostly conservative. Brace (LSO—lumbo-sacral-orthosis) for symptomatic patients failing conservative management; activity modification.

Spondylolisthesis
- The forward slippage of a vertebrae relative to the distal vertebrae most commonly L5 on S1.
- Five subtypes: (1) Dysplastic, (2) isthmic (most common), (3) degenerative, (4) traumatic, and (5) pathologic.
- Dysplastic: Secondary to congenital anomalies of L5 and S1 articulation.
- Isthmic: Most common—secondary to acquired defect in pars interarticularis; females have higher rate

of progression of slippage with low overall rate of 5% or less.
- Unlikely to progress after skeletal maturity.
- Clinically: Rarely symptomatic, back pain is most common initial complaint. Lumbar lordosis and/or lumbosacral flattening with buttock flattening, tight hamstrings is seen in advanced cases.
- Grading system: Meyerding: Grade I—up to 25% slippage on lateral radiograph, grade II—26–50%, grade III—51–75%, grade IV—76–100%, and grade V—>100% (spondyloptosis).
- Imaging: Standing posteroanterior and lateral lumbosacral radiographs.
- Treatment: Based on severity, pain, slip grade, skeletal maturity for conservative vs. surgical treatment.

REFERENCE

Weinstein SL: Long-term follow-up of pediatric orthopaedic conditions: Natural history and outcomes of treatment. *J Bone Joint Surg Am* 2000;82:980–990.

155 PHYSIOLOGIC DEVELOPMENT OF LOWER EXTREMITY ALIGNMENT

Denise T. Ibrahim and John F. Sarwark

NORMAL DEVELOPMENT OF LOWER EXTREMITIES

- Birth: Increased bowlegs (genu varum) and internal tibiofemoral torsion.
- Eighteen months: Start to straighten lower limbs.
- Three to four years old: Increased knock-knees (genu valgum).
- Seven years old: Straighten knock-knees to a normal average of 7° valgum (femoraltibial angle).

GENU VALGUM (KNOCK-KNEES)/ GENU VARUM (BOWLEGS)

- Important to understand normal development of lower extremity alignment to determine if physiologic type is present vs. pathologic type.

- If suspicious of pathologic limb alignment one assesses age of onset compared to normal development, progression of deformity (i.e., Blount disease) diet (i.e., Rickets), trauma (i.e., asymmetric physeal closure), growth percentile (i.e., skeletal dysplasia), and congenital anomalies.
- Examination: Assess gait, limb symmetry, intercondylar distance of knee for bowlegs or medial malleolar distance for knock-knees to document progression, and joint laxity. Radiographs may indicate rickets when physeal changes or other metabolic causes are seen. When severe or asymmetric, refer to pediatric orthopedic surgeon.

IN-TOEING/OUT-TOEING

- Most common pediatric orthopedic concern of parents for the toddler.
- Most are physiologic rather than pathologic.
- Femoral internal rotation (anteversion) or external rotation (retroversion), tibial internal rotation or external rotation, or foot development (i.e., metatarsal adductus, clubfoot).
- Important to accept 2 SD from normal, in accordance with age, in any direction before considering alignment abnormal.
- Normally, femoral internal rotation decreases with age to near 10° at maturity and tibial external rotation increases with age as it is often internally rotated (i.e., appearance of in-toeing) foot progression angle slowly externally rotates during development up until ages 11–14 years.
- Examination of the entire extremity including torsional alignment is essential.
- Examination
  1. If walking, assess heel-toe gait and foot progression angle (internal, neutral, external).
  2. Persistent limping may require referral to orthopedic surgeon.
  3. Foot progression angle (long axis of foot angle compared to a central vertical line in the walking path) during walking changes with age. Normal progression is external. In-toeing disappears with age.
  4. Check hip rotation with child in prone position. Knees flexed 90° and rotate femur internally and externally (Fig. 155-1). In a younger child there is more internal rotation than external rotation of the hip.
  5. Check tibia torsion in prone position, thighs are parallel to each other with knees flexed and the long axis of the hindfoot and the long axis of the thigh form the thigh-foot angle (Fig. 155-2). In-toeing is most notable after child begins to walk.

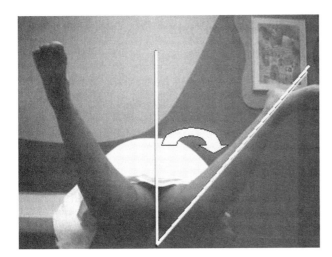
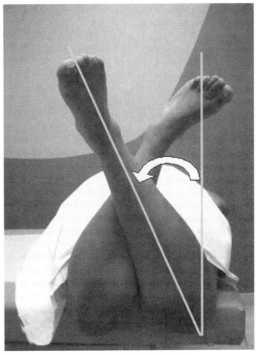

FIG. 155-1 Internal rotation of hips (above) and external rotation of hips (right).

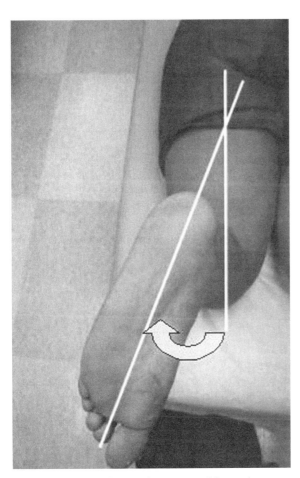

FIG. 155-2 Thigh foot angle to assess tibia rotation.

6. In-toeing is a common concern of parents. Education, reassurance, and observation are advised. Surgery is *rarely* needed.
   a. Infants: Out-toeing commonly seen with infants secondary to external rotation intrauterine position of the hips. Resolves with time and considered normal. Often overlooked or misdiagnosed.
   b. Infants: In-toeing may be secondary to searching great toe or adducted toe. This is a hyperactive adductor hallucis muscle as stance positioning begins in early toddler gait. Usually resolves spontaneously. Reassurance is recommended.
   c. Toddlers: In-toeing is a common complaint at 2 years of age due to internal tibial torsion. Improves without treatment. Bracing has no proven benefit.
   d. Child: In-toeing secondary to femoral anteversion at age greater than 3 years. Excessive internal rotation of hips compared to external rotation is seen on examination. If severe, orthopedic referral required.

PES PLANUS (FLATFOOT)

PHYSIOLOGIC FLATFEET
• Many infants and children and is a pain-free condition.

- Infant: Lack arch secondary to excess subcutaneous fat and normal ligamentous laxity which improves once walking.
- No cause of disability.
- Often hereditary.
- Assessment: While standing foot appears flat, when standing on toes arch reappears showing it is flexible and not a fixed deformity.
- If fixed and not flexible on examination may need further workup.
- Arch supports not required if asymptomatic.
- Flatfeet with tight heel cord. Assess dorsiflexion of foot and ankle with knee flexed *and* extended to determine whether contracture of soleus or gastroc-soleus complex, respectively are responsible for flatfeet.

PAINFUL OR RIGID FLATFEET
- Consider referral to orthopedist if symptomatic or rigid to rule out pathology.
  1. Congenital anomalies include skewfoot or vertical talus, tarsal coalition (failure of separation of tarsal bones).
  2. Most of the pathologic conditions are treated by conservative measures such as observation, inserts or casting, and physical therapy. Surgery may be indicated for those failing conservative treatment.

MISCELLANEOUS FOOT DISORDERS
- Talipes equinovarus (clubfoot): Congenital deformity of the foot with equinus, varus, adduction of forefoot, and internal rotation deformity. Refer to pediatric orthopedist.
- Etiology: Extrinsic (molded) or intrinsic (genetic). Varying degrees of severity. Can be associated with other conditions, i.e., arthrogryposis, torticollis, syndromes, and so on.
- Treatment: Goal is to correct deformity as soon after birth as possible with initial serial casting. Casting techniques include the Ponseti (Iowa) method or Demeglio (French) method. Surgical treatment may be required in cases where casting techniques incompletely correct the problem.

REFERENCE

Tachdjian MO: The foot and leg. In Tachdjian MO (ed): *Pediatric Orthopaedics*, 2nd ed. Philadelphia, W.B. Saunders, 1990. p 2810.

156 SPORTS MEDICINE
Denise T. Ibrahim and John F. Sarwark

PREPARTICIPATION PHYSICAL EXAMINATION (PPE)

- Goal: Detect conditions that may predispose athlete to injury or life-threatening risk.
- Timing: Four to six weeks before the season begins and repeated before each level of competition (i.e., junior high, high school, and college). Does *not* replace the yearly health supervision examination recommended by the American Academy of Pediatrics (www.aap.org).
- History: Parent's input important, and questions effectively screen for problems that may lead to sudden death. The PPE task force forms and questions can be found in the *Preparticipation Physical Examination* by Smith DM, Kovan JR, Rich BSE, and Tanner SM and published by Mcgraw-Hill.
- Physical examination: Identify those who may need further evaluation or intervention.
  1. Cardiovascular examination: Peripheral pulses, heart murmur, and blood pressure.
  2. Musculoskeletal examination: Focus on previous injured areas or symptomatic areas. Assess flexibility, range of motion, symmetry, atrophy or swelling, neurovascular status, joint stability, and nutritional status.
  3. Labs: None found to be effective in assymptomatic patients and none required unless specified by individual team or organization.
  4. Clearance—Again refer to the *Preparticipation Physical Examination* text for the most current recommendations and the *Proceedings of the 26th Bethesda Conference* on cardiovascular abnormalities for cardiac condition clearance.
  5. When families and/or patients disagree with recommendation, it is important to have a signed document from the parents acknowledging the discussion and recommendations.

HEAT-AND-COLD RELATED ILLNESSES

- Thermoregulation differs in children at extremes of temperatures secondary to their surface area to mass ratio being higher than adults, less blood volume, sweat gland diminished sensitivity until teens and acclimatization.
- Heat illnesses
  1. Exercise induced cramps: Produced by prolonged vigorous exercise, extreme sweating, fluid, and

electrolyte shifts. If recurrent episodes, consider electrolyte evaluation and sodium food supplementation.

2. Syncope: Loss of consciousness with core body temperature normal to slightly elevated after activity stops secondary to skin vasodilation, hypovolemia, and hypoperfusion. Treatment: Move to cool location, rectal temperature to rule out heat stroke, check for injuries, and support with fluids.

3. Exhaustion: Elevated core temperature rectally of 100.4–104°F causing mild confusion, dizziness, headache, nausea, chills, and collapse. Treatment includes cooling, monitor rectal temperature, fluid replacement with cool liquids.

4. Heatstroke: Medical emergency, imbalance of heat load with heat dissipation system. Core temperature rectally is >104°F with abnormal mental status and tachycardia. Treatment: Ambulance transport to hospital, fans, cool mist sprays, and immediate cool IV hydration enroute to ER, and sequential rectal temperatures. Rule out arrhythmias with any collapse.

- Cold illnesses
1. Hypothermia: Core temperature decrease in mild cases 93–97°F, moderate is 86–93°F (stiffness, slow respirations, confusion, lethargy, decreased heart rate), and severe is <86°F (weak pulse, arrhythmias, coma). Treatment includes controlled warming, locally with mild cases and moderate and severe cases in hospital. Start with removing wet clothes; apply warm blankets and radiant heat. No hot objects directly on skin.

2. Frostbite: Treatment: Gentle care of skin, no rubbing, and water temperature of 100–112°F to rewarm. May require surgical debridement.

OVERUSE INJURIES

- Pediatric population experience stress fractures or apophysitis. Treatment requires rest, splinting, and/or activity modification. If cessation of sport is required for healing it is important to continue exercise program.

TRAINING THE YOUNG

- Important to increase adaptive changes to enhance performance.
- Many questions are unanswered as to how much sport or training is too much. The physical and develop-

mental stresses to a growing child are different than in an adult.
- Understand the individual child's abilities and response to stresses. Intense training programs as expected of an adult are inappropriate in the child.
- Strength training: Supervised proper resistive training program. Modest increase in strength and tone in prepubescent children but not muscle bulk is expected.

CEREBRAL CONCUSSIONS

- Transient traumatic disruption of cognitive function.
- Signs and symptoms: Headache, sleep disturbance, confusion, dizziness, nausea, loss of balance, loss of consciousness, amnesia, emesis, tinnitus.
- Management: Whether conscious or unconscious rule out cervical spine trauma. Emergency care if unconscious. If conscious and ambulating, assess cognition and physical function. If symptoms last more than 15 minutes, no return to play that day.

CHEST INJURIES

- Skeletal injuries most commonly include rib fractures, clavicle fractures, sternoclavicular dislocations, or physeal disruption.
- Life-threatening injuries include pneumothorax (hemo- and tension), cardiac contusion, pericardial tamponade, and pulmonary contusion.

SPECIAL OLYMPICS SCREENING

- Special screening in Down syndrome children: Check for atlantoaxial instability detected or lateral radiographs of the cervical spine in flexion and extension. Compare the atlantodens interval (ADI). Normal ADI is less than 2.5 mm.

FEMALE ATHLETE

- There is a dramatic increase in female sport participation requiring an understanding of unique medical concerns of the female athlete.
- "Terrible female athlete triad": Eating disorder, amenorrhea, and osteoporosis.
- Severely delayed or absent menses is a concern given the adverse affects it may have on bone mineral density. Counseling and treatment is advised.

- Eating disorders: Higher risk involving participants of gymnastics, diving, figure skating, dance, and swimming. Early identification and a multidisciplinary approach of counseling that include nutritional and psychologic approaches.
- Iron deficiency: Common condition in female athletes, especially in long-distance runners, resulting in anemia.

REFERENCE

Barrett JR, Kuhlman GS, Stanitski CL, Small E: The preparticipation physical examination, in Sullivan JA, Anderson SJ (eds): *Care of the Young Athlete*. Rosemont, IL, American Academy of Orthopaedic Surgeons and American Academy of Pediatrics, 2000. pp 46–55.

Susanna A. McColley, Section Editor

157 FOREIGN BODY ASPIRATION

Mary A. Nevin

HISTORICAL FEATURES

- Foreign body aspiration is the second most common cause of accidental death in the home among children aged less than 5–6 years.
- Eighty-five percent of occurrences in children less than 3 years. Peak incidence is in those children aged 1–2 years. Boys are more likely to be affected than girls.
- Organic material such as nuts, hot dogs, grapes, and hard candy are most commonly aspirated by children.
- Various inorganic items such as coins, small metal and plastic pieces, marbles, batteries, and buttons may also be aspirated.
- Latex balloons are one of the leading causes of toy related choking deaths. This item is also extremely difficult to remove from the airway with standard rescue techniques such as the Heimlich maneuver.
- Children with neurologic disease or developmental delays are at increased risk for choking-related morbidity and mortality.
- Incidence is decreasing in recent years, perhaps due to federal safety legislation and increased awareness.

CLINICAL PRESENTATION

- Clinical history and a high level of suspicion are of inestimable importance in the evaluation of foreign body aspiration.
- Aspirated foreign bodies can be found in any segment of the tracheobronchial tree. The location in which a foreign body lodges is determined by the size and shape of the aspirated object as well as by the force of inspiration.
- Foreign bodies that lodge in the larynx are associated with acute respiratory arrest and a high mortality rate.
- Most foreign bodies are found in the mainstem bronchi or distal trachea but small objects can be found in more peripheral locations. The right mainstem bronchus is affected more commonly than the left owing to the angle of airway take off.
- Tracheal foreign bodies are more common in the setting of tracheomalacia, tracheal narrowing from prior surgery, or weakened pulmonary function (i.e., neuromuscular disease).
- In the absence of the need for emergent medical management (i.e. laryngeal FB), a careful history should be obtained. The classic history of a choking episode while eating or playing or that of a choking episode followed by a violent coughing spasm should be sought.
- It should be emphasized that the absence of such a classic history does not exclude the presence of a foreign body. In fact, the characteristic initial history is absent in up to 50–60% of cases.
- The sudden onset of pulmonary symptomatology in a child should always suggest a possible foreign body in the airway. The presence of chronic cough or wheeze without clear etiology should also suggest the diagnosis.
- Clinical manifestations and symptoms of foreign body aspiration are dependent on the size of the aspirated object and its composition as well as the location of the aspirated object, the degree of airway compromise/obstruction and the length of time elapsed since the aspiration event.
- Symptoms may occur within hours of the aspiration event or up to weeks to months later.
- Common symptoms with acute presentation include wheezing, choking, coughing, inspiratory stridor, hoarseness and dyspnea.

- A paroxysmal cough will often immediately follow an aspiration event. Thereafter, there will often be a period during which respiratory symptoms abate. This is due to an adaptation response in the respiratory mucosa. This lag period may be a source of unfounded reassurance. The return of the cough (which may prompt clinical presentation) is often due to accumulation of secretions, infection or atelectasis.
- Symptoms at initial presentation may represent a complication of foreign body aspiration such as chronic cough, recurrent wheezing, persistent fever due to persistent/recurrent pneumonia, hemoptysis, and bronchiectasis.
- Symptoms of a foreign body in the upper airway may be mimicked by a foreign body in the esophagus which creates pressure on the posterior trachea.
- Differential diagnosis includes croup, asthma, atypical asthma, bronchiolitis, laryngitis, pharyngitis, and angioneurotic edema.

PHYSICAL EXAMINATION FINDINGS

- Physical findings are based on the location of the obstructed airway as well as whether that obstruction is partial or complete.
- Physical findings may include cough, wheeze and rhonchi or decreased/absent breath sounds over the affected lung segment. This constellation of symptoms is only present in about one-third of patients presenting with foreign body aspiration. However, nearly twice as many will have one or more of these findings.
- Children may be comfortable with only subtle respiratory symptoms or they may show variable degrees of respiratory compromise including increased work of breathing, tachypnea, stridor, retractions and cyanosis.
- Changes in symptoms and severity of respiratory distress may be seen secondary to changes in position of the foreign object and local edema.
- A careful exam may predict the location of a foreign body. A prolonged expiratory phase or expiratory wheeze is suggestive of bronchial obstruction. Stridor (inspiratory or biphasic) and hoarseness (or frank aphonia) is more suggestive of a proximal tracheal or laryngeal obstruction.
- In many cases, physical findings are subtle. In fact, the physical examination can be entirely normal.

CLINICAL EVALUATION

- In all situations suggestive of foreign body aspiration, neck and chest radiographs should be obtained.
- 5–10% of foreign bodies are radioopaque. In these cases, the diagnosis is easily confirmed with a plain radiograph.

- The majority of foreign bodies are radiolucent and abnormalities seen on radiographs are secondary to airway obstruction (i.e. air trapping).
- Inspiratory and expiratory films should be obtained. The classic finding is obstructive emphysema in the affected lung segment on an expiratory radiograph.
- Partial airway obstruction leads to progressive air trapping through a ball-valve effect. Obstructive emphysema is the radiographic correlate. Shift of the mediastinum away from the affected hemithorax may be seen.
- In the case of complete bronchial obstruction, atelectasis is the result. In severe cases, a shift of the mediastinum may occur toward the affected hemithorax.
- Lateral decubitus views of the chest and fluoroscopy are other studies that may demonstrate unilateral hyperinflation. Whereas plain chest films may be negative in up to 25% of aspiration cases, fluoroscopy is a more sensitive, yet noninvasive option.
- When a foreign body remains in the airway, late radiographic findings may represent complications which include post-obstructive atelectasis, emphysema of the contralateral lung, pneumonia, parapneumonic effusion, pneumothorax, pneumomediastinum, mediastinal shift, pulmonary abscess and bronchiectasis.
- Prolonged presence of a foreign body with secondary obstruction, air trapping and inflammation are important precursors in the development of chronic bronchiectasis.
- Final diagnosis of foreign body aspiration or exclusion thereof must be by direct laryngoscopy and bronchoscopy.

MANAGEMENT

- Initial emergent management must ensure adequate oxygenation and ventilation.
- If the child is coughing, airway obstruction is incomplete; he/she should be allowed to cough in an attempt to clear the airway without interference while emergency medical transport is arranged and close observation is assured.
- Emergent maneuvers designed to treat acute and severe/complete upper airway obstruction include abdominal thrusts (Heimlich maneuver) in children one year and older, back blows and chest thrusts for children less than one year of age and blind finger sweeps of the oropharynx (only for children eight years of age and older). Emergent guidelines and specific resuscitation protocols should be further and completely accessed through the American Heart Association and the American Academy of Pediatrics.
- Acute airway obstruction in a conscious child may be indicated by a sudden onset of tachypnea, dyspnea, cyanosis or an inability to cough or talk. An anxious

appearance may also herald an acute worsening of respiratory status.

- Medical therapies, including inhalation of bronchodilators and chest physiotherapy, are contraindicated secondary to a significant risk for foreign body migration and cardiopulmonary arrest.
- Rigid bronchoscopy is the standard of care for the evaluation, localization, management, and removal of tracheal and bronchial foreign bodies in the pediatric population.
- Following endoscopic removal of a foreign body, symptoms due to airway edema and pulmonary parenchymal changes arising from the presence of the foreign object may take several days to abate.
- Postoperative management may include humidification of inspired air, supplemental oxygen, steroids, chest physiotherapy, or antibiotics in complicated cases.

BIBLIOGRAPHY

Cotton, RT. Foreign body aspiration. In: Chernig and Boat (eds.), *Kendig's Disorders of the Respiratory Tract in Children*, 6th ed. Philadelphia: W.B. Saunders, 1998. 601–607, 822, 983, 1518–1520, 1475–1477.

Fausnight T, et al. Determining the cause of recurrent wheezing. *J Respir Dis* 2002;126–131.

Loin, MI. Foreign bodies. In: McMillan et al, *Oski's Pediatrics: Principles and Practice*, 3rd ed. Philadelphia: Lippincott Williams & Wilkins, 1999. 639–640, 570–571, 1273–1275, 1310.

Muniz A, Joffe M. Foreign bodies. *Contemporary Pediatrics*, 1997;14(12):78–103.

158 BRONCHITIS AND BRONCHIOLITIS

Maria L. Dowell

BRONCHITIS

- Acute bronchitis (actually tracheobronchitis) is a transient inflammation of the trachea and major bronchi manifested primarily by cough. It is usually caused by a viral infection (respiratory syncytial virus [RSV], parainfluenza, influenza, adenovirus, and rhinovirus) and resolves without therapy within 3 weeks. Occasionally it is caused by bacteria and chemical exposure. The diagnosis is usually a clinical one and laboratory tests are generally unnecessary.

- Chronic bronchitis in adults is defined as a productive cough for 3 months a year over 2 consecutive years. The definition in children is less clear. Persistent signs and symptoms of tracheobronchitis for more than 3 weeks should initiate an attempt to identify an underlying disorder. The differential diagnosis should include asthma, cystic fibrosis, aspiration, immunodeficiency, retained foreign body, dynamic or extrinsic airway compression, inhalation injury, tuberculosis, and primary ciliary dyskinesia.

BRONCHIOLITIS

BACKGROUND

- Bronchiolitis is a common lower respiratory tract condition in infants and is the most common cause for hospitalization among infants <6 months of age.
- Although several viruses can cause bronchiolitis, the most common etiology is RSV. Other viruses that can cause bronchiolitis include parainfluenza, metapneumovirus, influenza, and adenovirus.
- Almost all children are infected with RSV at least once by the age of 2 years and reinfection throughout life is common.
- Most healthy infants with RSV do not require hospitalization and those that do are usually discharged within 5 days.
- Several conditions can increase the risk of severe or fatal RSV bronchiolitis. Infants and young children at high risk for these complications include the following:
  1. Cyanotic or complex congenital heart disease.
  2. Chronic lung disease due to prematurity.
  3. Prematurity, low birth weight.
  4. Immunodeficiency disease or immunosuppressive therapy.
  5. Other chronic pulmonary disorders, including cystic fibrosis.
- RSV mortality in hospitalized high-risk children reportedly ranges from 3 to 4%.

EPIDEMIOLOGY/PATHOGENESIS

- RSV infection occurs via transmission of respiratory droplets or by direct contact.
- RSV can survive up to 30 hours on humid surfaces and less than 1 hour on hands.
- The asymptomatic incubation period is generally 3–4 days (viral load peaks 4–5 days later) but airway obstruction and symptoms typically occur 8–12 days after infection.
- Temperate zone outbreaks of RSV generally occur in winter or spring.

• Peak incidence of RSV occurs between 2 and 3 months of age (whereas peak incidence of parainfluenza is later at 10.6 months of age).
• Infection is associated with increased goblet cell mucus production and desquamation of epithelial cells that result in the plugs responsible for air trapping and atelectasis.

CLINICAL MANIFESTATIONS

• Symptoms of bronchiolitis typically include the following:
  1. Rhinorrhea
  2. Low-grade fever
  3. Cough
  4. Apnea, especially in young infants
• In more severe cases, additional symptoms include the following:
  1. Wheezing
  2. Tachypnea
  3. Poor feeding
  4. Pallor or cyanosis
  5. Irritability
• Physical examination:
  1. Rhinorrhea is usually present.
  2. Otitis media may be seen.
  3. Chest examination may reveal retractions in moderate-to-severe cases.
  4. Bilateral, diffuse, crackles are common.
  5. Wheezing may be present.
  6. Signs of central nervous system (CNS) depression may be seen with impending respiratory failure.

DIAGNOSTIC TESTS

• Pulse oximetry should be performed in infants with RSV who have increased work of breathing, poor feeding, pallor/cyanosis, or irritability.
• Nasopharyngeal secretions may be tested for RSV using a rapid antigen test (generally 80–90% sensitive). This is especially useful in hospital settings, for infection control and epidemiologic purposes. Viral culture requires 3–5 days with greatly varying results depending on the laboratory.
• The chest radiograph may show hyperinflation, non-specific increases in perihilar bronchial markings, or atelectasis. Routine chest radiography is not necessary in mildly to moderately ill infants and children with typical bronchiolitis.
• An arterial blood gas should be performed in severely ill infants and in those with progressive signs and symptoms.

COMPLICATIONS

• Respiratory failure may develop, especially in very young infants and the high-risk groups noted above.
• There is emerging evidence that aspiration during feeding occurs frequently in hospitalized infants with bronchiolitis, and may contribute to prolonged hospital stays or the development of respiratory failure. It is thus prudent to consider alternative sources of nutrition and hydration in moderately to severely ill infants.
• Excessive secretion of antidiuretic hormone in RSV infection has been reported in infants with severe disease.

TREATMENT

• Treatment of RSV bronchiolitis is primarily supportive.
• Oxygen should be administered to achieve SpO_2 >92%.
• Dehydration can occur when fever and tachypnea increase fluid demands and dyspnea and tachypnea limit intake. Parenteral fluids are often necessary. Attention to nutrition with consideration of nasogastric tube feeding for infants with inadequate oral intake or who are moderately to severely ill.
• Mechanical ventilation may be necessary for infants who develop apnea or respiratory failure ($PaCO_2$ >55 torr and PaO_2 <70 torr while receiving 60% supplemental O_2).
• Studies of bronchodilators generally show no benefit unless there is underlying bronchial hyperreactivity resulting in bronchospasm.
• There is no role for chest physiotherapy for mild-to-moderate bronchiolitis.
• Theophylline has not been shown to alter the course of bronchiolitis in infants.
• Early studies of nebulized racemic epinephrine appeared promising; however, a large, double-blind, placebo-controlled multicenter study showed no reduction in the length of hospital stay.
• Studies of corticosteroids generally show no benefit although a recent metaanalysis reported some benefit in those with severe symptoms or requiring mechanical ventilation.
• Exogenous surfactant may have some benefit in one pilot study but further investigation is necessary.
• Heliox may have some benefit in overcoming airway resistance but only for patients requiring 45% or less supplemental O_2.
• Antimicrobials are rarely indicated.

FOLLOW-UP

• Viral shedding up usually 3–8 days although can last as long as 3–4 weeks.

- Reports of greater than expected incidence of asthma into late childhood in those with RSV bronchiolitis history. Both genetic and environmental factors determine the type of immune response to RSV infection. It has been proposed that this immune response may affect the development of control mechanisms involved in the regulation of airway tone.

PREVENTION

- No vaccine is currently available.
- Prophylaxis with Palivizumab, a humanized monoclonal antibody directed against RSV, may reduce hospital length of stay, ICU admissions, and ICU length of stay in high-risk populations.
- Current guidelines for Palivizumab administration include the following:
  1. Infants ≤2 years old with chronic lung disease, congenital heart disease, or other serious conditions that compromise pulmonary or immune function.
  2. Infants without chronic lung disease or congenital heart disease:
     a. Premature infants ≤28 weeks if born ≤12 months before RSV season.
     b. Premature infants 28–32 weeks if born ≤6 months before start of RSV season.
     c. Premature infants 32–35 weeks if born <6 months before the start of RSV season and with additional risk factors.
- The use of Palivizumab in other respiratory diseases, such as cystic fibrosis and chronic respiratory failure (for reasons other than those noted above), has not been adequately studied. Many practitioners recommend Palivizumab for these populations because of the high risk for morbidity and mortality, but practice remains variable.
- Palivizumab is administered once per month with the first dose generally given at the beginning of November and last dose at the beginning of March, which will provide protection until April.

BIBLIOGRAPHY

American Academy of Pediatrics. Respiratory syncytial virus. In: Pickering LK (ed.), *Red Book: 2003 Report of the Committee on Infectious Diseases*, 26th ed. Elk Grove Village, IL: American Academy of Pediatrics, 2003, pp. 523–528.

Loughlin GU. Bronchitis. In: Chernick V, Boat T (eds.), *Kendig's Disorders of the Respiratory Tract in Children*, 6th ed. Philadelphia, PA, W.B. Saunders, 1998, pp. 461–472.

Jafri HS. Treatment of respiratory syncytial virus: antiviral therapies. *Pediatr Infect Dis J* 2003;22:S89–S93.

Wainwright C, et al. A multicenter, randomized, double-blind, controlled trail of nebulized epinephrine in infants with acute bronchiolitis. *N Engl J Med* 2003;349:27–35.

Weisman LE. Populations at risk for developing respiratory syncytial virus and risk factors for respiratory syncytial virus severity: infants with predisposing conditions. *Pediatr Infect Dis J* 2003;22:S33–S39.

Welliver RC. Respiratory syncytial virus and other respiratory viruses. *Pediatr Infect Dis J* 2003;22:S6–S12.

159 BRONCHOPULMONARY DYSPLASIA

Steven O. Lestrud

DIAGNOSIS

- BPD is a chronic lung disorder with a wide spectrum of clinical features. Almost exclusively occurring in babies born less than 35 weeks gestation and requiring mechanical ventilation due to respiratory distress of the newborn.
- Characteristic radiographic findings are the following:
  1. Stage I: Bilateral hazy infiltrates characteristic of respiratory distress syndrome (RDS) of the newborn.
  2. Stage II: Diffuse opacification
  3. Stage III: Interstitial emphysema
  4. Stage IV: Cystic radiolucent areas, hyperinflation, and patchy fibrosis present after 28 days demonstrating chronic pulmonary findings.
- Requirement of supplemental oxygen past 28 days or beyond 35 weeks gestation.

RISK FACTORS FOR DEVELOPMENT OF BPD

- Birth weight: One-third of surviving babies born bet-ween 500 and 1000 g and 10% of babies above 1000 g will develop bronchopulmonary dysplasia (BPD).
- Mechanical ventilation.
- High inspired fraction of oxygen.
- Episodes of sepsis.
- Patent ductus arteriosus requiring surgical correction.

CLINICAL FEATURES

- Increased work of breathing demonstrated by tachypnea and retractions, frequently with baseline wheezing.

- Coarse crackles increase especially during upper respiratory tract infections (URI).
- Fine crackles are variable and occur in patients prone to fluid overload.
- Increase in chest wall anterior to posterior dimensions due to hyperinflation.
- Oxygen requirement to maintain hemoglobin oxygen saturation above 90%.
- Associated findings due to chronic respiratory insufficiency may include failure to gain weight due to high caloric expenditure and cor pulmonale.
- Pulmonary exacerbations are frequently triggered by URIs and are characterized by increased work of breathing above baseline which may quickly result in acute respiratory failure and should be identified promptly.

TREATMENT

MAINTENANCE THERAPY

- Supplemental oxygen to maintain hemoglobin saturation above 90%. Tapering of oxygen therapy starts during wakeful periods. When saturations are acceptable and stable, tapering at night can be aided by prolonged oximetry monitoring prior to the therapy being discontinued.
- Diuretic therapy is initiated to decrease lung water and lower airflow resistance in patients prone to fluid overload. Diuretic therapy is generally maintained until supplemental oxygen can be discontinued. Electrolyte balance must be monitored especially with dosage changes.
- Inhaled beta-agonist bronchodilators are used to relieve work of breathing associated with wheezing and air trapping. Beta-agonists may as well improve mobility of pulmonary secretions.
- Inhaled anticholinergic bronchodilators are considered in patients with significant large airway malacia that do not respond or worsen with the administration of beta-agonists.
- The use of inhaled glucocorticoid therapy remains controversial. Maintenance therapy may reduce the need for repeated courses of oral steroids during exacerbations. Close monitoring of glucocorticoid side effects is necessary with continuation of prolonged therapy.
- RSV immunoprophylaxis is provided based on AAP guidelines dictated by severity of lung disease, gestational age at birth, and chronologic age.

EXACERBATION THERAPY

- Many patients with chronic respiratory insufficiency will quickly decompensate to respiratory failure during exacerbations.

- Prevention of illness from viral pathogens is crucial. Frequent hand washing is necessary for all household contacts, especially prior to handling.
- Patients usually require an increase of supplemental oxygen to provide adequate saturations above 90%.
- Inhaled bronchodilator therapy is increased based on clinical response of improved tachypnea and air exchange.
- Diuretics are optimized for patients with evidence of pulmonary edema.
- Systemic steroid use is not standardized but frequently considered.
- There is increased risk for pulmonary aspiration and esophageal reflux with aspiration during an exacerbation; appropriate antireflux and aspiration precautions for the patient should be observed.
- With frequent exacerbations, a secondary diagnosis may be present such as asthma, cystic fibrosis, immunodeficiency states, and chronic pulmonary aspiration syndromes.

BIBLIOGRAPHY

Committee on Infectious Diseases and Committee of Fetus and Newborn.

Prevention of respiratory syncytial virus infections: Indications for the use of palivizumab and update on the use of RSV-IGIV (RE9839). *Pediatrics* 1998;102:1211–1216.

Northway WH, Rosan RC, Porter DY. Pulmonary disease following respiratory therapy of hyaline membrane disease: bronchopulmonary dysplasia. *N Engl J Med* 1967;276: 357– 368.

Rojas MA, Gonzalez A, Bancalari E, Claure N, Poole C, Silva-Neto G. Changing trends in the epidemiology and pathogenesis of neonatal chronic lung disease. *J Pediatr* 1995;126: 605–610.

Stevenson DK, Wright LL, Lemons JA, Oh W, Korones SB, Papile L, Bauer CR, Stoll BJ, Tyson JE, Shankaran S, Fanaroff AA, Donovan EF, Ehrenkranz FA, Verter J. Very low birth weight outcomes of the National Institute of Child Health and Human Development Neonatal Research Network, January 1993 through December 1994. *Am J Obstet Gynecol* 1998;179:1632– 1639.

160 INTERSTITIAL LUNG DISEASE
Corinda M. Hankins

DEFINITION

- Interstitial lung disease (ILD) describes inflammation of the pulmonary interstitial space which consists of alveolar walls and perialveolar tissues. There are connective tissue components, mesenchymal cells, and inflammatory cells in the interstitium.

- This inflammation can begin as a normal response to infection or irritant agent. Persistent inflammation can cause disruption of the alveolar units which can lead to poor gas exchange and eventually restrictive lung disease.

CLINICAL PRESENTATION

- Onset is usually insidious and presentation is variable.
- The most common symptoms are dry cough, tachypnea, dyspnea, and exercise limitation.
- Patients may present with frequent recurrent respiratory infections.
- There may be evidence of weight loss or growth failure.
- The physical examination may show tachypnea, retractions, and basilar crackles heard late in inspiration. In severe cases, cyanosis and clubbing may be present.
- There are no definitive clinical criteria for the diagnosis of interstitial lung disease.

ETIOLOGY AND CLASSIFICATION

- ILD is rare in children.
- There are many types of interstitial disorders of both known and unknown etiology (Fan and Langton, 1998).
- In known disorders there is activation of inflammatory cells in the interstitium secondary to direct injury or in response to injury.
  1. Infectious etiologies should be separated into chronic infections in both immunocompetent and immunocompromised hosts. Most common etiologies are viral (e.g., adenovirus, influenza, cytomegalovirus [CMV], human immunodeficiency virus [HIV]), bacterial (e.g., *Chlamydia, Mycoplasma, Mycobacterial, Pertussis*), and fungal (e.g., *Aspergillosis, Pneumocystis*).
  2. Aspiration syndromes secondary to swallowing dysfunction, tracheoesophageal fistula, or gastroesphageal reflux disease can lead to chronic diffuse infiltrates.
  3. Environmental inhalants (e.g., organic dusts) or toxins can lead to an immunologic response in the lung such as hypersensitivity pneumonitis. Other toxins include some drugs, radiation, or chemical fumes.
  4. Some patients have a known underlying systemic condition that can predispose to ILD such as metabolic storage diseases or lymphoproliferative dis-

orders. Interstitial lung disease may be associated with systemic disorders such as autoimmune disease, collagen vascular disease, pulmonary vasculitides (e.g., telangiectasia), neurocutaneous syndromes, and malignancies.

- Interstitial lung diseases of unknown etiology were originally described in adults on histopathologic basis (Fan and Langton, 1998). These classic forms are rare in childhood. They include usual interstitial pneumonitis (UIP), desquamative interstitial pneumonitis (DIP), lymphocytic interstitial pneumonitis (LIP), bronchiolitis obliterans with organizing pneumonia (BOOP), pulmonary hemosiderosis, sarcoidosis, and alveolar proteinosis.
  1. UIP is the most common form in adults. There is inflammation and injury in patchy distribution that is usually associated with some fibrosis on pathologic specimen.
  2. DIP is a diffuse histologic process of hyperplasia of alveolar epithelial cells and a large number of macrophages in the airspaces (Fan and Langton, 1998).
  3. LIP is most commonly seen in children. This entity appears to be more lymphoproliferative in nature with diffuse infiltrates of mature lymphocytes. LIP is most often seen in immunodeficiency states and autoimmune disorders such as acquired immunodeficiency syndrome (AIDS) (Fan and Langton, 1998).

DIAGNOSTIC EVALUATION

HISTORY AND PHYSICAL EXAMINATION

- A careful history of prenatal events, growth and development, environmental exposures, and other possible underlying conditions should be taken, with a focus on the onset, duration, and progression of respiratory symptoms.
- A thorough review of systems will help assess infectious or immunologic disorders.
- Dry cough is typical and may be severe. Tachypnea, retractions, basilar crackles, cyanosis, and clubbing may be present on physical examination.

STUDIES

- Routine studies to assess for most common etiologies include a complete blood count (CBC) with differential, erythrocyte sedimentation rate (ESR), viral cultures, bacterial cultures, and fungal cultures as well as HIV serology and *purified protein derivative of tuberculin* (PPD). A barium esophagram, videofluoroscopic swallowing study, and pH probe are initial studies to evaluate for aspiration syndromes.

- Further assessment of associated disorders includes immunologic workup (e.g., qualitative immunoglobulins, T- and B-cell function, antibody function, hypersensitivity testing, and autoantibodies).
- Consider cardiac evaluation for cor pulmonale.

PULMONARY FUNCTION TESTING USUALLY IN CHILDREN OVER 6

- Pulmonary function testing may show restrictive lung disease with reduced FVC and FEV1, normal FEV1/FVC ratio and reduced total lung capacity (TLC).
- Carbon monoxide diffusion capacity is often reduced.
- Oxygen saturation is reduced in more severe disease.
- Consider exercise tolerance testing to assess for exercise-related hypoxemia.

DIAGNOSTIC IMAGING

- Chest x-ray (CXR) classically shows diffuse infiltrates described as interstitial, alveolar, or mixed interstitial/alveolar. CXR can be normal in the setting of early ILD.
- Chest-computed tomography with high-resolution cuts can be very helpful in detecting early alveolar thickening associated with interstitial lung disease. It can also provide detail about the distribution of infiltrates which can aid in determination of specific site for bronchoalveolar lavage or biopsy.

BRONCHOALVEOLAR LAVAGE

- Bronchoalveolar lavage is a good tool for assessment of infection, aspiration (lipid laden macrophages), and pulmonary hemorrhage (hemosiderin laden macrophages).
- BAL has limited ability to determine the etiology of ILD.

TRANSBRONCHIAL BIOPSY

- This method is used in the monitoring of lung transplant patients for infection and rejection, but its usefulness in the assessment of ILD is still limited.

TRANSTHORACIC BIOPSY

- Lung biopsy remains the most definitive diagnostic tool in interstitial lung disease. Many of the classic ILD disorders are still defined only by their histology with alveolar wall thickening being the primary

marker. Thoracoscopic techniques allow for minimally invasive sampling of lung tissue.

MANAGEMENT OF ILD

- Management should be based on definitive diagnosis.
- Treat underlying systemic disorders whenever possible.
- Supportive care is of primary importance in the management of ILD.
  1. Maintaining growth and nutrition is very important and may require extra calories or tube feeding.
  2. Except with certain immunodeficiencies, all routine immunizations should be given, including influenza vaccination. Administration of antirespiratory syncytial virus (RSV) monoclonal antibodies should be considered, especially in young children (<3 years old).
  3. Aggressively treat all infections.
  4. Environmental irritants or toxins should be avoided.
- Medications used in treatment of interstitial lung disease.
  1. Oxygen is recommended for chronic hypoxemia.
  2. Corticosteroids are still the mainstay for treatment of interstitial lung disease. They suppress overall inflammation. Corticosteroids can be given in different ways but most recommendations would suggest a trial of prednisone in the range of 1–2 mg/kg/day until patient improves or side effects occur. Other regimens include high-dose pulse steroids (10–30 mg/kg/day for 3 days given every 4 weeks).
  3. Alternative but unproven therapy includes immunosuppressive therapy with such agents as hydroxychloroquine, azathioprine, cyclophophamide, methotrexate, cyclosporine, and intravenous immunoglobulin.
- Lung transplantation is an option for end-stage ILD.

PROGNOSIS FOR ILD

- Prognosis is variable depending on distinct etiology. Prognosis can range from full recovery to rapid progression of disease with development of fibrosis, pulmonary hypertension, respiratory failure, and death. Overall mortality rate remains high at 16–20% (Fan and Langton, 1998).

BIBLIOGRAPHY

Fan LL, Langston C. Interstitial lung disease. In: Chernick V, Boat T (eds.), *Kendig's Disorders of the Respiratory Tract of Children*. Philadelphia, PA: W.B. Saunders, 1998.

Hillman BC. Interstitial lung disease in children. In: Hillman BC (ed.), *Pediatric Respiratory Disease: Diagnosis and Treatment*, 1st ed. Philadelphia, PA: W.B. Saunders, 1993, pp. 353–367.

161 OTITIS MEDIA

Mark E. Gerber

ACUTE OTITIS MEDIA

- Acute otitis media (AOM) is the second most common infectious disease in children after viral upper respiratory infections.
- Sixty-seven percent of children have one episode prior to age 1 and 81% prior to age 3, most frequently associated with viral upper respiratory infection (URI).
- Risk factors for recurrent otitis media include the following:
  1. Age (peak incidence is 6–13 months, with a second peak at age 4–5 years)
  2. Sex (slightly greater incidence in males)
  3. Daycare attendance
  4. Family history of otitis media
  5. Formula feeding (and maybe pacifier/bottle use)
  6. Cleft palate and other craniofacial abnormalities
  7. Tobacco smoke exposure

DIAGNOSIS

- Antecedent or concurrent URI is usual. Signs and symptoms include irritability, decreased appetite, diarrhea, fever, otalgia, pulling at ears, otorrhea, hearing loss, and imbalance.
- Physical examination shows tympanic membrane/middle ear inflammation, characterized by erythema, bulging, and loss of landmarks. Pneumatic otoscopy confirms middle ear fluid.

THERAPY

- The most common bacteria are *Streptococcus pneumoniae, Haemophilus influenzae,* and *Moraxella catarrhalis.* In the first 2 weeks of life, group B streptococcus, *Staphylococcus aureus, Escherichia coli,* and *Klebsiella pneumoniae* are more common.

- Amoxicillin is the first line drug of choice. Azithro-mycin, trimethoprim/sulfamethoxazole, or erythromycin/sulfisoxazole are alternatives for penicillin allergic patients.
- A 10-day course of treatment is recommended. A 5–7 day course may be adequate in children over 2 years of age.
- Patients under age 2 years should be rechecked in 2 weeks; 4 weeks may be appropriate for those over 2 years of age.
  1. Seventy percent of children will have a middle ear effusion (MEE) 2 weeks after treatment; 50%, 4 weeks after treatment; 20%, 8 weeks after treatment; and 10%, 12 weeks after treatment. No medical treatment is indicated in otherwise healthy, asymptomatic children.
  2. Second line antimicrobials that are appropriate if there is improvement but the patient is still symptomatic include cefprozil, loracarbef, and azithromycin.
  3. Third line agents may be appropriate if there is evidence of a more severe continued infection, with symptoms such as fever, otalgia, and/or irritability after 3 days of treatment. These include amoxicillin-clavulanate, cefpodoxime, oral cefuroxime, or parenteral ceftriaxone.
  4. Relative and absolute indications for tympanocentesis and culture include acute otitis media in a seriously ill or toxic appearing child, an unsatisfactory response to empiric antibiotics, suppurative complications (facial nerve paralysis, mastoiditis, meningitis), and otitis media in a newborn or immunologically deficient patient.
  5. Because of the risk of sensorineural hearing loss, audiometric testing is indicated when there is a suppurative complication of AOM.

RECURRENT OTITIS MEDIA

- Otitis media that clears without residual MEE between infections but recurs within 6 weeks or less is defined as recurrent acute otitis media.
- Amoxicillin remains as the drug of choice with each event as long as it remains effective.
- Prophylactic antibiotic therapy may be helpful if there are more than four episodes in 12 months or three episodes in 6 months.
  1. Prophylaxis is indicated only when the interval examination shows no MEE.
  2. Gantricin and amoxicillin are the only drugs approved for this indication, are only effective in 20–30% of cases, and may increase antimicrobial resistance (amoxicillin > gantricin). Use for only 6 weeks at a time to minimize resistance.

- Tympanostomy tubes are considered when there are more than six episodes of AOM in 12 months or more than four episodes in 6 months; however, many children exceed this frequency without requiring tympanostomy tube placement.

OTITIS MEDIA WITH EFFUSION

- Otitis media with effusion is defined as asymptomatic MEE with or without measurable hearing loss. Fluid may be serous or mucoid.
- Thirty-three percent of effusions yield bacteria with organisms similar to those seen in AOM.
- Observation is appropriate if the patient is asymptomatic. Sixty-five percent resolve within 3 months without therapy.
- When present for more than 3 months, treatment with tympanostomy tubes or antimicrobial therapy may be indicated.
  1. Initial antimicrobial therapy is as recommended for acute otitis media.
  2. Therapy can be repeated if the MEE is still present 4 weeks later.
  3. Antimicrobial prophylaxis is not indicated in the treatment of otitis media with effusion due to increased antimicrobial resistance without increased rate of improvement.
  4. Tympanostomy tubes are indicated when there is bilateral MEE >3 months, or unilateral MEE >6 months, especially if there is associated hearing loss.
  5. Adenoidectomy is effective in age 4–8 years when undergoing a second set of tympanostomy tubes, regardless of presence or absence of nasal symptoms. Tonsillectomy has no effect on middle ear disease.

TONSILS AND ADENOIDS

- The tonsils and adenoids participate in regional immunologic protection in the nasopharynx and oropharynx, where they are part of the first line of defense against inhaled or ingested antigens. Chronic inflammation results in reduction of effectiveness against infection.

RECURRENT INFECTION

- Recurrent infection is diagnosed when adenotonsillitis occurs at a high frequency, defined as
  1. Seven episodes/1 year.

  2. Five episodes/year for 2 years.
  3. Three episodes/year for 3 years.
- The definition of "counting" episodes includes T >38.5°C, cervical nodes >1cm, tonsillar exudate or (+) group A beta-hemolytic streptococcus (GABS) culture.
- Adenotonsillectomy is indicated for recurrent adenotonsillitis. Other factors that may be considered when deciding whether surgery should be performed include parent concern with regard to the risk of rare GABS complications or antibiotic resistance, parent/patient preferences, family tolerance of illness, patient tolerance of antimicrobial therapy, and the patient's surgical risk.
- Since the widespread availability and use of antibiotics, the morbidity of tonsillitis has been dramatically reduced.

UPPER AIRWAY OBSTRUCTION

- Upper airway obstruction secondary to adenotonsillar hypertrophy is the most common indication for adenotonsillectomy.
- Physical examination findings that suggest significant upper airway obstruction include adenoid faces and failure to thrive.
- Upper airway obstruction is often associated with sleep-disordered breathing. Snoring alone is not a reliable indicator of sleep-disordered breathing.
  1. Primary snoring (see Chapter 164) is estimated to occur in up to 10% of the pediatric population.
  2. Nocturnal symptoms of sleep-disordered breathing include snoring with pauses/snorts/gasping, teeth grinding, restlessness, elevated respiratory effort (retractions) diaphoresis, periodic paradoxical breathing, frequent arousals, and secondary enuresis. Daytime symptoms include sleepiness/hyperactivity/impulsiveness, school problems/inattention, morning headaches, nasal congestion, mouth breathing, and difficulty waking in the morning.
- Upper airway obstruction syndromes with sleep-disordered breathing are characterized as high upper airway resistance syndrome (UARS) and obstructive sleep apnea syndrome (OSAS). These are discussed in Chapter 164.
- A clinical history that is suggestive of UARS (nighttime symptoms of sleep-disordered breathing associated with daytime symptoms related to sleep disruption) in a patient with adenotonsillar hypertrophy is an appropriate indication for surgical intervention. Pediatric patients with either UARS or OSAS demonstrate improvement in snoring, sleep fragmentation, daytime somnolence or hyperactivity, and other symptoms related to sleep-disordered breathing following adenotonsillectomy.

- Polysomnography (PSG) is indicated for patients who are at high risk for general anesthesia and surgery. These include children with severe OSAS symptoms, children <3 years old, and those with cardiopulmonary disease, who are at increased risk of postoperative airway compromise.
- Others that benefit from PSG include those patients whose have small tonsils and adenoids or families that need objective data to help their decision making regarding therapy.
- For patients who are not surgical candidates, nonsurgical treatment options such as continuous positive airway pressure (CPAP) also reduce nighttime and daytime symptoms. PSG must be used to identify optimal CPAP pressures.

PREOPERATIVE EVALUATION

- Preoperative evaluation may vary depending on surgeon preference and hospital guidelines.
  1. Any patient with complex medical history should undergo evaluation from an appropriate preoperative evaluation by the specialist treating the specific problem.
  2. There remains controversy regarding the need for routine preoperative laboratory studies, but due to the lack of cost-effectiveness as well as inability to predict which patient is at risk of postoperative hemorrhage, it is not usually performed.
  3. A detailed bleeding questionnaire (Table 161-1) is used to screen for possible bleeding disorder or the need for coagulation studies. Patients with positive findings undergo screening coagulation studies (a complete blood count, prothrombin time, partial thromboplastin time, and platelet function analysis).

  4. For African-American and other high-risk groups, a sickle-cell screen should be considered if the patient has not been previously tested.
  5. Laboratory evaluations specific to coexistent medical conditions may be necessary.

SURGICAL TECHNIQUE

- Adenotonsillectomy is most commonly performed under general anesthesia using a variety of surgical techniques. Except for reported differences in operating time and intraoperative bleeding, there are minimal differences with respect to postoperative bleeding risk as well as outcome measures such as postoperative pain when a complete tonsillectomy is performed by any technique.
- A subtotal/partial or intracapsular, tonsillectomy preserves the tonsillar capsule, and is therefore believed to avoid direct surgical violation of the pharyngeal muscles. This reduces postoperative pain, recovery time, delayed hemorrhage, and dehydration, and is equally effective in relieving sleep-disordered breathing symptoms.
- Benefits of adenotonsillectomy include reduction of mouth breathing and improvement in behavioral problems even when the upper airway obstruction is only mild (without OSAS) preoperatively.
- OSAS resolves after adenotonsillectomy in 90% of cases. Patients who do not demonstrate improvement tend to have smaller tonsils, narrower epipharyngeal space, and more poorly-developed maxillary and mandibular protrusion.
- Adenotonsillectomy with or without additional surgery often improves OSAS in children with craniofacial

TABLE 161-1 Bleeding Questionnaire

Has your child ever had surgery, stitches for trauma, or a broken bone?	Yes	No	_____
If yes, was there more bleeding than expected during or after?	Yes	No	_____
Does your child bruise more easily than normal?	Yes	No	_____
If a boy and circumcised, was bleeding more than expected after the circumcision?	Yes	No	_____
Was there bleeding when the umbilical cord came off?	Yes	No	_____
Has your child had frequent nosebleeds?	Yes	No	_____
Has your child bled more than normal after loss of baby teeth?	Yes	No	_____
Is your child taking aspirin or ibuprofen products?	Yes	No	_____
If an older girl, is there a history of heavy menstrual periods?	Yes	No	_____
Has your child ever needed a blood transfusion for prolonged bleeding?	Yes	No	_____
Do any blood relatives have an inherited bleeding problem such as hemophilia, von Willebrand, or low platelets?	Yes	No	_____
Has any blood relative been called a free bleeder?	Yes	No	_____

anomalies and/or neuromuscular disorders. These patients are prone to increased postoperative airway complications and prolonged hospitalization and recovery postoperatively.

162 PNEUMONIA

Oren J. Lakser

CLINICAL FEATURES

- Pneumonia is one of the most common serious infectious causes of morbidity and mortality in children around the world.
- Diagnosis can be a challenge because of the diversity in the clinical manifestations, which can vary depending on the child's age and the causative agent.
- Classic symptoms include fever, tachypnea, and cough. On physical examination, children may demonstrate tachypnea, diminished air entry, crackles and/or wheezes, and in severe cases evidence of increased work of breathing (retractions, accessory muscle use, or nasal flaring). Hypoxemia may be present, but is often a late sign. Absence of tachypnea is a strong indication that the child *does not* have pneumonia.
- These symptoms may frequently be preceded by minor upper respiratory infection symptomatology including low-grade fever and rhinorrhea.

LABORATORY INVESTIGATIONS

- The variability in the clinical manifestations of pneumonia makes history and physical examination less conclusive at arriving at a definitive diagnosis. Laboratory tests have a minimal role in patients with uncomplicated community-acquired pneumonia, but can aid in patient management particularly in ill-appearing patients.
- Leucocytosis (WBC >15,000–20,000/mm^3) in association with fever higher than 39°C often suggests a bacterial etiology. Blood cultures are positive in less than 3% of pediatric outpatients with pneumonia, but may be informative in patients with severe cases of pneumonia and for infants under 3 months of age. Cultures and serologic testing for *Mycoplasma pneumoniae* or *Chlamydia pneumoniae* are not recommended as routine studies. Similarly, viral cultures

and antigen detection, or cold agglutinins should only be obtained when they will alter management decisions. Gram stain and culture on respiratory secretions (sputum, bronchoalveolar lavage, or pleural fluid) can be helpful, but are often difficult to obtain. An adequate sputum culture should have <10 squamous epithelial cells and >25,000 white blood cells per low power field.
- Chest radiography can be helpful in confirming the presence and location of a pneumonia; however, a normal chest x-ray does not rule out pneumonia as many patients with evolving pneumonia can have normal chest x-rays. Chest x-rays can occasionally differentiate between bacterial and viral pneumonias. Bacterial pneumonias often present with lobar consolidation, whereas viral pneumonias are characterized by interstitial, peribronchial, or bilateral bronchoalveolar infiltrates.

MANAGEMENT

- Indications for hospitalization include significant increase in work of breathing or toxic appearance, oxygen requirement (saturation <92%), infants <2 months of age, presence of moderate-to-large pleural effusions, or underlying chronic disease such as cystic fibrosis or sickle cell disease.
- Inpatient antibiotic choice is guided by the patient's age. Neonates 0–30 days should receive ampicillin and gentamicin unless another specific cause is identified. Children between 1 month and 5 years should receive a third generation cephalosporin, such as cefotaxin. If *Chlamydia trachomotis* or *Bordetella pertussis* are suspected, a macrolide antibiotic should be initiated. Hospitalized children over 5 years of age should be started on a third generation cephalosporin AND a macrolide antibiotic. Duration of therapy depends on the patient's response but in general is 10–14 days for infants up to 3 months of age and 7–10 days for children older than 3 months.
- Outpatient antibiotic choice is determined by the suspected etiologic agent and the patient's age (see Fig. 162-1). In children 60 days to 5 years of age who are suspected of having a bacterial infection high-dose amoxicillin (80–90 mg/kg/day) or amoxicillin/clavulanate should be initiated. In some children, an initial parenteral dose of ceftriaxone may be considered if there is concern about the child tolerating the initial doses of the oral medication (e.g., vomiting). In children over 5 years of age a macrolide antibiotic should be initiated and some clinicians will include a beta-lactam agent as well. If the causative agent is presumed to be viral (respiratory syncytial virus, influenza, or parainfluenza virus), the most common

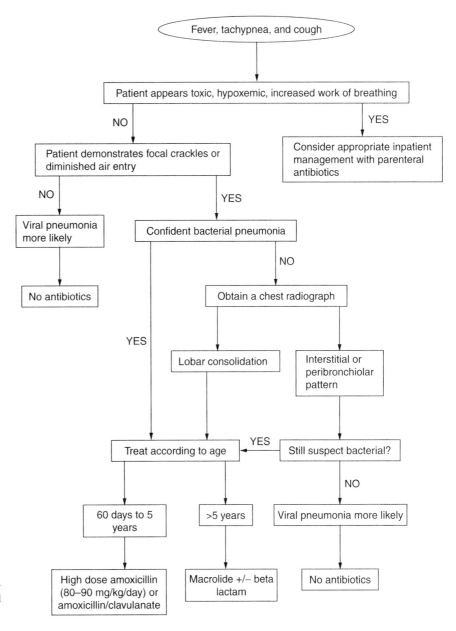

FIG. 162-1 Algorithm for the management of outpatient community-acquired pneumonia.

cause of pneumonia in children over 2 months of age, antibiotics are not warranted and the child should be managed symptomatically.

• Parapneumonic effusions should be suspected when dullness to percussion, decreased fremitus, and egophany are present on physical examination or the patient fails to improve or relapses after initial improvement. Upright and/or lateral decubitus chest x-rays should be done. Occasionally a chest commuted tomography scan or magnetic resonance imaging may be helpful. A diagnostic/therapeutic thoracentesis should be performed in any ill-appearing patient, preferably prior to initiation of antibiotics. Children with parapneumonic effusions should receive a minimum of 10 days of parenteral

antibiotics to cover the discovered or suspected etiologic organism. Occasionally, surgical intervention (chest tube or decortication) may be warranted.

BIBLIOGRAPHY

Mahabee-Gittens EM. Pediatric pneumonia. *Clin Pediatr Emerg Med* 2002;3:200–214.

McCracken GH. Diagnosis and management of pneumonia in children. *Pediatr Infect Dis J* 2000;19:924–928.

McIntosh K. Current concepts: Community-acquired pneumonia in children. *N Engl J Med* 2002;346:429–437.

163 CYSTIC FIBROSIS

Susanna A. McColley

DEFINITION

- Cystic fibrosis (CF) is an autosomal recessive multisystem disorder caused by mutations in the *cystic fibrosis transmembrane regulator* CFTR gene. CFTR codes for an epithelial cell membrane-bound protein that conducts chloride through the apical cell membrane and serves as a regulator of other membrane ion channels. Absent or dysfunctional CFTR causes abnormal ion transport onto epithelial surfaces, resulting in dehydrated surface fluid. The major clinical manifestations are sinopulmonary disease, digestive tract abnormalities, male infertility, and excessive salt loss through the sweat glands. Cystic fibrosis occurs in 1:3300 live births in Caucasians in the United States. It is less frequent in other populations.

CLINICAL PRESENTATION

- Prenatal diagnosis is increasingly made by genetic testing via amniocentesis or chorionic villus sampling. Echogenic bowel may be seen on prenatal ultrasound.
- Neonatal screening is currently performed in some geographic areas. In the United States this test usually combines an assay for immunoreactive trypsinogen (IRT) and analysis for one or more common cystic fibrosis gene mutation.
- Meconium ileus is a neonatal bowel obstruction that occurs in 15–20% of affected infants. Meconium plug syndrome is a milder variant of this disorder.
- Prolonged cholestatic jaundice is seen in a small number of neonates with CF.
- Lower respiratory tract symptoms leading to diagnosis include chronic or recurrent cough, pneumonia, or bronchitis, recurrent or persistent wheezing, and "bronchiolitis syndrome" in infants.
- Upper airway findings include severe or persistent paranasal sinusitis and nasal polyposis.
- Pancreatic insufficiency is present in approximately 85% of patients and results in growth failure, digestive symptoms, or both.
  1. Growth failure may be present, especially after 6 months of age. Appetite is variably poor, average, or voracious.
  2. Digestive symptoms include steatorrhea, characterized by large, bulky stools which may be very malodorous and/or frankly oily.
  3. Frequent or large bowel movements may be reported. Rectal prolapse may occur, especially in children who are toilet learning.

- Chronic metabolic alkalosis or acute hypochloremic, hyponatremic dehydration are common presentations in warm climates and during summer months.
- Symptoms of fat-soluble vitamin deficiency may be seen, such as night blindness or bleeding diathesis.

DIAGNOSIS

- Quantitative pilocarpine iontopheresis sweat chloride testing is the initial study of choice for infants or children with characteristic symptoms, a positive newborn screening test, or a history of an affected sibling. Sweat chlorides >60 meq/L are diagnostic of CF in these settings. Borderline sweat chlorides, 40–60 meq/L, are seen in some patients, especially those with mild or atypical phenotypes. Normal sweat chlorides (<40 meq/L) have been seen in patients with genetically confirmed cystic fibrosis and may be seen in some infants with CF on initial testing.
- Confirmation of a CF diagnosis requires a second sweat test or genotyping which reveals two CF-causing gene mutations.
- Nasal potential difference (NPD) measurement may be needed for diagnosis in symptomatic individuals with normal or borderline sweat tests and nondiagnostic CF genotype. NPD is available through some Cystic Fibrosis Research Centers.

COMPLICATIONS

- Progressive pulmonary disease, characterized by chronic airway infection, inflammation, and obstruction, is the major cause of morbidity and mortality in cystic fibrosis.
- Pulmonary exacerbation of cystic fibrosis is characterized by increased cough and increased sputum production; hemoptysis may be seen. Weight loss and decreased pulmonary function are frequently present. Fever is unusual.
- Predominant cystic fibrosis pathogens are *Pseudomonas aeruginosa* and *Staphylococcus aureus*. *Hemophilus influenzae*, *Stenotrophomonas maltophilia*, *Achromobacter xylosoxidans*, and *Burkholderia cepacia* are also frequently seen, as are *Aspergillus fumigatus* and nontuberculous mycobacteria.
- Allergic bronchopulmonary aspergillosis occurs in 4–15% of patients. Acute or subacute clinical deterioration, markedly elevated serum IgE level (>1000 IU/mL), immediate cutaneous reactivity to *Aspergillus fumigatus*, precipitating antibodies to *A. fumigatus*, and new or recent abnormalities on chest imaging are characteristic of this complication.
- Nasal polyposis and symptomatic sinusitis are common complications.
- Poor growth and nutrition may be seen and are associated with worse intermediate and long-term outcomes.

- Gastroesophageal reflux and gastritis and/or duodenitis may occur.
- Individuals with pancreatic insufficiency are at risk of fat-soluble vitamin deficiency (A, D, E, and K).
- Distal intestinal obstruction syndrome is caused by dehydrated, bulky feces and is characterized by constipation or obstipation, abdominal pain, and, characteristically, a right lower quadrant mass.
- Elevated liver function tests, cirrhosis, and gallstones may occur.
- Pancreatitis occurs primarily in patients with residual pancreatic function.
- Most affected men are infertile due to absence of the vas deferens; women may have reduced fertility, but recent data suggest that this reduction is only slight if it is present at all.
- Arthropathy occurs primarily in patients with significant pulmonary disease.
- Glucose intolerance increases with age and affects up to 75% of adolescents. Diabetes mellitus mostly occurs in patients over 12 years of age; by adulthood, at least 25% of patients require therapy for diabetes.

TREATMENT

- Patients have improved outcomes when cared for in specialty centers with multidisciplinary care teams. The Cystic Fibrosis Foundation Clinical Practice Guidelines recommend center visits on a quarterly basis for stable patients >6 years of age; younger patients or those with more health problems may benefit from more frequent visits.
- Nutritional therapy includes a high-calorie diet with unrestricted fat, supplementation of fat-soluble vitamins, preferably in water-soluble forms, and pancreatic enzymes for pancreatic insufficient patients. Close monitoring of nutritional status by a dietician is essential.
  1. Supplemental feedings by nasogastric or gastrostomy tube may be necessary to achieve adequate growth and nutrition.
  2. Use of H_2 blockers or proton pump inhibitors improves enzyme effectiveness and is effective in reducing symptoms of gastroesophageal reflux disease (GERD) and gastritis.
- Most experts recommend institution of airway clearance techniques at the time of diagnosis. Technique is chosen based on the patient age, condition, and patient and family preferences. Manual chest percussion with postural drainage, high-frequency chest wall oscillation, positive expiratory pressure devices, and autogenic drainage are all useful in enhancing mucociliary clearance and clearing viscid secretions from the airways. Patients who are asymptomatic or who have mild pulmonary disease generally receive

one to two sessions per day; more severely affected individuals may need more frequent therapy.
- Recombinant human DNase reduces sputum viscosity, improves pulmonary function modestly, and decreases the frequency of pulmonary exacerbation. The usual dose is 2.5 mg inhaled via nebulizer once daily.
- Most patients are administered short- or long-acting beta-agonists as an adjunct to airway clearance; retrospective studies suggest a benefit of these agents, but no well-controlled clinical trials exist. Inhaled corticosteroids are also frequently administered.
- High-dose ibuprofen may reduce pulmonary function decline and improve nutrition. Pharmacokinetic studies must be used to ascertain the optimal dose.
- Frequent monitoring of respiratory tract microbiology is recommended. Pharyngeal swabs or nasopharyngeal suction specimens are obtained on nonexpectorating patients, and sputum specimens on expectorating patients. Special culture techniques should be used to identify *Burkholderia cepacia* and to test for *Staphylo-coccus aureus* when *Pseudomonas aeruginosa* is present.
- Patients with *Pseudomonas aeruginosa* and mild-to-moderate lung disease benefit from chronic intermittent therapy with inhaled high-dose tobramycin. A dose of 300 mg twice daily of a preservative-free preparation is inhaled for 28 days followed by 28 days off.
- Patients with *Pseudomonas aeruginosa* also benefit from azithromycin given at a dose of 250 mg 3 days weekly for patients <40 kg and 500 mg 3 days weekly for patients ≥40 kg.
- Chronic use of antistaphylococcal antibiotics in young children remains controversial. One study of cephalexin showed no pulmonary function benefit and an increase in *Pseudomonas aeruginosa* infection among patients treated with long-term cephalexin vs. placebo. Pulmonary exacerbation is treated with antibiotics. These may be given orally or intravenously depending on the patient's findings and culture results. Patients with significant weight loss and/or decreases in pulmonary function should be treated with intravenous antibiotics; duration of therapy is at least 14 days. Chest physiotherapy should be increased during pulmonary exacerbation to three to four sessions daily. Evidence from epidemiologic and retrospective studies suggests that in-hospital care and longer intravenous antibiotic duration are associated with improved patient outcomes.
- Diabetes should be managed aggressively for good glycemic control.
- Abnormal liver function tests often improve with administration of ursodeoxycholic acid. Liver transplantation is very successful in patients with cirrhosis, provided pulmonary disease is stable.
- Distal intestinal obstruction syndrome is treated with a balanced intestinal lavage solution, given by mouth or via nasogastric tube. Milder episodes of constipation

may be treated with stool softeners. Adjustment of enzyme dose is helpful in preventing recurrence.

- Intracytoplasmic sperm injection allows men with CF to father children in vitro. Carrier testing for the partner and genetic counseling are essential for couples considering this treatment for infertility.
- Lung transplantation is an option for some patients with end-stage lung disease.

PROGNOSIS

- More than 90% of deaths are secondary to respiratory failure. Progression of disease is variable.
- Median life expectancy continues to increase and is currently between 30 and 35 years, with many affected individuals living into their 40s, 50s, and beyond.

BIBLIOGRAPHY

Boat TF. Cystic fibrosis. In: Behrman, Kleigman, Jenson (eds.), *Nelson Textbook of Pediatrics*, 17th ed. Philadelphia, PA: W.B. Saunders, 2003, pp. 1437–1450.

Clinical Practice Guidelines for Cystic Fibrosis. Bethesda MD: Cystic Fibrosis Foundation.

McColley SA. Cystic fibrosis. In: Rakel, Bope (eds.), *Conn's Current Therapy 2002*. Philadelphia, PA: W.B. Saunders, 2002, pp. 179–184.

164 SLEEP DISORDERS AND BREATHING
Stephen H. Sheldon

NORMAL AND ABNORMAL RESPIRATORY EVENTS DURING SLEEP

- Pauses in breathing are normal during sleep in infants, children, and adolescents. Clinical significance of respiratory pauses varies according to the child's postconceptional age, developmental status, and comorbid medical and anatomical conditions. Types of respiratory pauses during sleep include obstructive apnea, central apnea, periodic breathing (PB), mixed apnea, postsigh central apnea, expiratory apnea, central hypoventilation, and obstructive hypoventilation.

OBSTRUCTIVE APNEA SYNDROME (OSAS)

CLINICAL FEATURES

- During an obstructive apnea, there is complete cessation of airflow through the nose and mouth despite continued inspiratory and expiratory respiratory efforts (see Fig. 164-1). Absence of airflow may be brief, lasting 6 seconds or less. Two obstructed respiratory efforts may be clinically significant, especially when the obstruction is periodic and frequent. Occasionally, the obstructive apnea can be prolonged and associated with oxygen desaturation, cardiac deceleration, cardiac arrhythmia, and carbon dioxide retention.
- Snoring is a characteristic feature of OSAS. Nonetheless, some children with significant OSAS have minimal snoring. Snoring is often associated with pauses and snorts. Difficulty breathing during sleep, restless sleep, diaphoresis, morning headaches, excessive thirst on waking, nightmares, sleep terrors, frequent nocturnal waking, and sleep-related enuresis (especially secondary enuresis) are common associated symptoms.
- Daytime symptoms include, but are not limited to excessive sleepiness, hyperactivity, attention span problems, poor school performance, behavioral abnormalities, unusual aggressiveness, moodiness, and excessive shyness. Difficulty learning in school, frequent upper airway infections, sinusitis, frequent otitis media, failure-to-thrive, and obesity may also be present. In severe cases, pulmonary hypertension and cor pulmonale can develop.
- In the otherwise normal child, the most common underlying etiology is hypertrophy of the tonsils and adenoids.
- Children with craniofacial malformations of the mandible (e.g., micrognathia as in Pierre-Robin Sequence), maxillae (e.g., maxillary hypoplasia as in Apert syndrome), or any other defect of the midface are at particular risk. Children with high-arched palate are also at risk for OSAS.
- Children with central or peripheral neurologic abnormalities that result in decreased or increased muscle tone may exhibit OSAS due to dysfunction of pharyngeal musculature and/or uncoordinated pharyngeal muscle activity.
- Patients with Down syndrome, achondroplasia, and Prader-Willi exhibit both anatomical and neurologic abnormalities that place them at high risk for OSAS.

TREATMENT OPTIONS

- Since the most common cause of OSAS in otherwise normal children is hypertrophy of tonsils and adenoids, tonsillectomy and adenoidectomy is the most common therapeutic intervention in children.

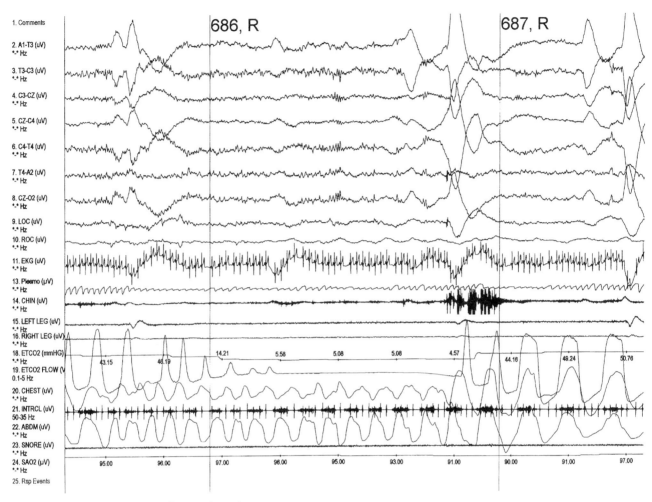

FIG. 164-1   Obstructive apnea 60-second epoch.

- Identifiable causes of upper airway obstruction should be identified and appropriately managed.
- Nasal continuous positive airway pressure (CPAP) and bilevel positive airway pressure (biPAP) can also be used in treatment of children with OSAS.
- Tracheostomy bypasses upper airway obstruction and results in cure of OSAS. Nonetheless, it is typically reserved for those severe patients who are at high risk of severe sequelae and OSAS cannot be treated using other less invasive techniques.

SEQUELAE OF OSAS

- Cor pulmonale and mortality secondary to OSAS during sleep in children with hypertrophied tonsils and adenoids is unusual. Cardiac arrhythmias may occur and may be associated with occlusive respiratory events.
- Excessive daytime sleepiness, hyperactivity, attention span problems, learning difficulties, and behavioral abnormalities contribute to significant morbidity from undiagnosed and untreated OSAS.
- Functional neurocognitive sequelae of OSAS have been well documented in adults and children with significant effects including but not limited to deficits of attention, concentration, psychomotor skills, memory, and high cognitive or executive functions. Neuropsychologic deficits seem to vary with severity of hypoxemia and excessive daytime somnolence.

CENTRAL SLEEP APNEA (CSA) AND PERIODIC BREATHING

CLINICAL FEATURES

- The definition of "central apnea" differs depending on the patient's postconceptional age. In the neonate, a central apnea is defined as abnormal when there is absence of airflow through the nose and mouth associated with absence of chest and

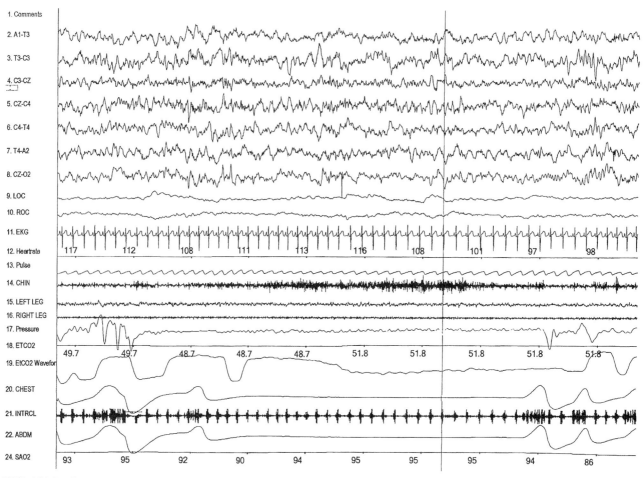

FIG. 164-2 Central apnea 30-second epoch.

abdominal respiratory effort that last 20 seconds or longer. Shorter apneas may be significant if associated with oxygen desaturation or heart rate changes (see Fig. 164-2).

• Prolonged central apneas related to the absence of both inspiratory and expiratory neuronal activity appear to be quite rare in otherwise normal infants and children during Quiet/NREM sleep. Brief central apneas are *normal* during Active/REM sleep.

• PB is a pattern of respiration characterized by three or more central pauses lasting 3 seconds or longer, and separated by less than 20 seconds of normal breathing. PB occurs normally in premature infants, especially during Active/REM sleep (see Fig. 164-3). In the very premature infant, PB may also occur during Quiet/NREM sleep. This pattern of breathing represents immaturity of central control of breathing and typically resolves as conceptional term is reached. In the term infant, PB occurs almost exclusively during Active/REM sleep. Persistence of PB during long portions of sleep or during Quiet sleep may be

abnormal and reflect immaturity and/or abnormality of central control of breathing.

THERAPEUTIC CONSIDERATIONS

• Methylxantines are typically effective in treatment of apnea of prematurity. Caffeine citrate is commonly used. For apnea of prematurity a loading dose of 10–20 mg/kg as caffeine citrate (5–10 mg of caffeine base) may be given orally or intravenously. A maintenance dose of 5–10 mg/kg/day (2.5–5.0 mg/kg/day of caffeine base) once daily starting 24 hours after the loading dose is then begun.

• Caffeine has advantages over other methylxantines (e.g., theophylline) in the wider therapeutic window and the need for only a single daily dose.

• Apnea of prematurity resolves between 40 and 44 weeks postconception. Caffeine can typically be discontinued after this time.

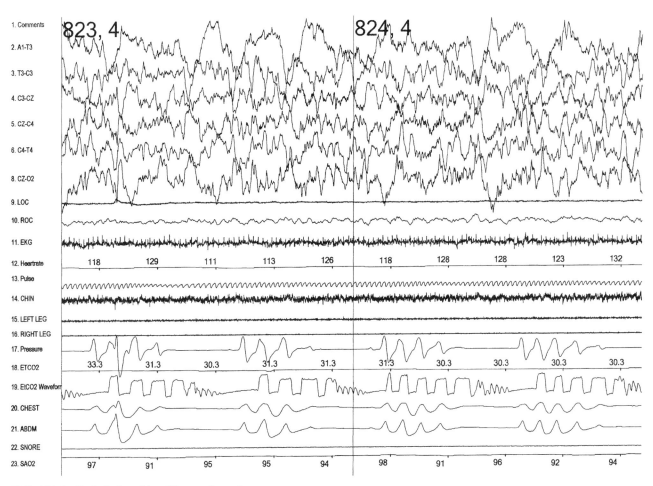

FIG. 164-3 Periodic breathing 60-second epoch.

SLEEP-RELATED HYPOVENTILATION

CLINICAL FEATURES

- Hypoventilation is defined as ineffective ability of the respiratory system to exhale carbon dioxide. It is often associated with inadequate oxygenation, but hypoxemia is not always present.
- Central hypoventilation occurs when there is inadequate ventilation due to inadequate output from brainstem respiratory centers. Dysfunction may be congenital (congenital central hypoventilation syndrome [CCHS]) or may be acquired abnormalities of the brain stem. Most children with CCHS have normal respiratory rates, but breathe very shallowly during sleep. Other children with central hypoventilation may have normal or increased tidal volume, but significantly reduced respiratory rate.
- Obstructive hypoventilation occurs when there is chronic upper airway obstruction associated with high upper airway resistance. Overt apnea may or may not be present. Respiratory rate during sleep might be increased, and oxygen saturation is often within normal range. EtCO$_2$ remains greater than 50 mmHg for a significant portion of the total sleep time and the maximum EtCO$_2$ is often greater than 55 mmHg.

DIAGNOSTIC METHODS

- Accurate diagnosis of respiratory pauses during sleep in children is based on comprehensive attended continuous monitoring of respiratory, cardiovascular, and electroencephalographic parameters *across the child's habitual sleep time.* This is termed nocturnal polysomnography. Since severity of breathing disorders during sleep often varies across the 24-hour continuum, with the highest incidence of pathologic apnea occurring during the early morning hours, monitoring of sleep is most reliable when performed at night, during the child's major sleep period.

- In addition to recording and analyzing sleep state and architecture, nasal and oral airflow may be measured using different methodology. Most reliable involves recording airflow by pressure transduction at the nose and mouth. Capnography provides an assessment of airflow by continuous measurement of exhaled carbon dioxide (and provides an assessment of $EtCO_2$). Thermistry (using either thermistor or thermocouple placed in the air stream) provides a qualitative measurement of airflow and is considered less reliable than nasal pressure and $EtCO_2$.

- Respiratory effort is monitored either by piezo crystal strain gauges that continuously monitor changes in circumference of the chest and abdomen or by inductive plethysmography measuring changes in volumes of the chest and abdomen.

- Continuous monitoring of SaO_2, electrocardiogram (ECG), and intermittent monitoring of $TcPCO_2$ are also recorded.

John V. Lavigne and D. Richard Martini, Section Editors

165 PRINCIPLES OF MANAGEMENT OF PSYCHIATRIC PROBLEMS IN PEDIATRIC PRACTICES

*John V. Lavigne and
D. Richard Martini*

- The overall prevalence of psychiatric disorder among children and adolescents approaches 20%, with 11% classified as severe and 5% extremely severe. The vast majority of children with a diagnosis, however, receive no treatment, with 50–80% having mental health needs that aren't being met. If all children with psychiatric disorders (those warranting a psychiatric diagnosis) were identified and referred for treatment, however, the secondary (Community Mental Health Centers) and tertiary care facilities could not manage the patient load. As a public health issue, greater recognition is important, but better venues for providing treatment must be developed.
- With most children receiving periodic pediatric care, and many receiving very regular care, it is not surprising that estimates of psychopathology among children in pediatric practices are high. For both school-age and preschool-age children, the prevalence of psychiatric problems is in the midteens, but a large percentage (about half) go unrecognized. Given the time demands on pediatricians to attend to a variety of health, nutrition, and developmental factors during 10–15-minute outpatient visits, this should not be too surprising. Improved recognition is important from a public health perspective, but practical implementation of improved screening may require improvements in treatment delivery to be meaningful.

- Pediatricians working with a child who appears to be experiencing mental health difficulties must make decisions about who should be evaluated and treated. Essentially, there are two models the pediatric practice can implement. The first is an office model in which the pediatrician either provides treatment directly (advice giving, counseling, pharmacotherapy), or refers to a mental health specialist working in the practice setting. The second is a referral model, in which the physician refers to mental health specialists outside the practice and provides little in-office care.
- In this chapter, information is presented about an array of behavioral and emotional problems that may present in a primary care setting. Some, like attention deficit hyperactivity disorder (ADHD), are relatively common; others, less so. Whether the pediatrician is providing treatment through his/her practice, or has made a referral for treatment but is playing a role in coordination of care, an understanding of the basic conditions and the available evidence for treatment is important. Each section refers to clinical aspects of the disorder, diagnostic issues, and treatment options. Pediatricians may not be familiar with the basic types of treatment that a mental health professional might provide. The next section provides an overview of psychologic treatments, while the subsequent section discusses some of the more common medications used in the treatment of psychologic problems of children and adolescents.

PRINCIPLES UNDERLYING THE DEVELOPMENT OF PSYCHOPATHOLOGY

- Approaches to child treatment should be conceptualized within a biopsychosocial framework, one that recognizes the role of biologic, psychologic, and social factors on development in general, and the development of problematic behaviors and emotional responses more specifically. Biologic factors certainly include genetic predispositions to behavior, along with prenatal and perinatal contributions to development. Temperamental characteristics—those personality traits that have a strong biologic basis—are usually recognizable in infancy and preschool years, and have important influences on the individual's style of behaving. There are theoretical differences in how these temperamental characteristics are conceptualized, but the characteristics generally recognized include individual differences in activity level, mood, intensity of response, approach vs. avoidance of novel situations, persistence, and sociability (e.g., introversion/extraversion). Clusters of temperamental traits (e.g., a cluster of traits contributing to a child's tendency to be slow to warm up to new social situations, or to be difficult to manage because of the child's intensity in expressing affect, persistence, and negative mood) can all contribute directly to the child's behavior, have an influence on parent-child interaction patterns, and have far-reaching implications for the child's behavior.

- Children are raised in a social context. The community shapes the child's exposure to models of behavior in a multitude of ways, not the least of which include exposure to violence, and to positive influences that contribute to the individual's achievement orientation. The school context and the child's exposure to educational opportunities flow through the community, as do opportunities for, and access to, quality health care. Of paramount importance as a social influence is the child's family context. Families exist, in large part, to nurture and socialize children. Children are adaptable and there is a great deal of plasticity in the child socialization process, such that many different approaches to child rearing can produce a "just fine" adult (recognizing the wide variety of outcomes that can be *just fine*). Still a variety of family and community conditions can place a child at risk for a less than optimal outcome and contribute to problematic behaviors and emotional responses. Poverty, parental psychopathology, family conflict, and differences in child-rearing practices can shape the individual child and influence their behavior.
- The child's cognitive and language development interacts with the biologic factors and social context noted above to influence the child's behavior. Children are not passive recipients of the social influences surrounding them. They act on their environments constantly in a reciprocal influence process. They act, observe the consequences of their actions, and alter their behaviors accordingly. They assimilate what they see and hear into the internal, cognitive frameworks they have for processing information, and these cognitive frame-

works evolve as a function of maturation and their social experiences. Society, and especially their family, influences them, and they in turn have an impact on their families and (collectively) on the broader society.
- Treatments for child behavior and emotional problems take place with a recognition of the broad set of factors that influence the child. In a sense, because of the powerful influences that families have, all interventions with children are family interventions because they recognize the role that families have on the child's behavior.
- Interventions vary in their complexity, but even the relatively simple process of informing a family about how to administer a prescribed medication to a child of the family context and the parent's ability to follow through. Primary care pediatrics requires that the pediatrician provide advice on health, feeding and nutrition, toilet training, child safety, and so on, and the broader the awareness of the family's capacity to follow through on instructions, and the more adaptable the physician can be in the advice that is given, the more likely it will be that an intervention is successful.
- At times, pediatricians will be confronted with questions about a child's behavior problem that require referral for consultation with a mental health specialist. Throughout this chapter, reference in made to available psychotherapy and psychopharmacologic options for treatment, and a brief discussion of different approaches seems to be in order.

EVALUATIONS OF CHILDREN AND ADOLESCENTS

- Critical to most evaluations of children's behavior problems are interviews with parents and the child. Parent interviews are essential for obtaining an adequate description of the presenting problems and their onset, and establishing the presence of other psychiatric symptoms. Parent interviews are also critical for obtaining information about prior psychologic treatment, family problems, stressors, the child's peer relationships, and academic performance as well as relevant medical history. Child interviews play an important role in understanding emotional symptoms the child is experiencing (e.g., anxiety and depression), their view about other problem behaviors and about their school and family life. Interviews with the child are often less productive with younger children, and observations of their behavior may supplement or replace any interview. Obtaining information from other observers, particularly teachers, is very helpful. This can be done by telephone interviews or with questionnaires, a particularly important source of information for conditions like attention deficit hyperactivity disorder.

PSYCHOLOGIC INTERVENTIONS WITH CHILDREN

BEHAVIOR THERAPY

- Over the last 20 or so years, behavior therapy, along with a variant known as cognitive behavior therapy (CBT), has become an increasingly prominent approach to treatment of children. Presently, 50% of psychologists working with children describe themselves as behaviorally oriented in their treatment approach. Behavior therapy began as an attempt to apply the principles of learning being studied by experimental psychologists to understanding and modifying problematic behavior. Over time, the approach has broadened to involve the application of knowledge about the way people think (cognitive sciences) and develop to behavior change. In behavior therapy, emphasis is placed on the way current situations, rather than more distant influences from the individual's past, influence behavior. Thus attention is paid to the environmental factors (family, school, and so on) that elicit problematic behaviors, what consequences those behaviors have, and how those consequences maintain the behaviors. Interventions can then be designed to alter setting conditions that elicit a behavior, or altering the consequences that maintain it. The development of complex behaviors (including those, like toilet training, that appear simple, but may be complex within the framework of the child's developmental level when the behavior is being taught) is an important part of socialization. Developing such skills is an important aspect of behavior therapy and may require analysis of the components of the skills, shaping the development of each component, and then linking them into an integrated whole. The "cognitive" aspect of cognitive behavior therapy pays attention to the thoughts of the individual and their impact on influencing the individual's feelings and behavior. The analysis of the individual's thoughts, for example, might uncover irrational thoughts (e.g., one that exaggerates a threat) that need to be modified to reduce anxiety and enable more appropriate behavior to occur.

INDIVIDUAL PSYCHODYNAMIC PSYCHOTHERAPY

- Psychodynamic psychotherapists view the child as developing within the broader social and familial context and are likely to try to negotiate changes in those systems on behalf of the child. They differ from behavior therapists in their formulation of children's problems and in certain therapeutic practices, however. Emphasis is placed on the role of emotional conflicts at different stages of development and their influence on thoughts, feelings, and behavior. The role of unconscious conflicts and processes as influences on behavior is emphasized. Defense mechanisms to control unconscious thoughts and feelings, is emphasized, as is their role in shaping maladaptive behaviors. Therapy places more emphasis on one-to-one contact with the child. In treatment, the expression of feelings in an accepting context, accompanied by labeling and reflecting such feelings is deemed to be important. Play material might be used to encourage such feeling expressions. Developing insight into one's problems and behavior is considered important. Being allowed to express one's feelings and developing insight leads to a corrective emotional experience in which maladaptive, often unconscious, thoughts and feelings no longer occur automatically in response to certain situations. The development of more appropriate ways of coping can then proceed resulting in better self-esteem, impulse control, and more adaptive behavior.

- Compared to the study of behavior therapies with children, far fewer studies over the years have tested the efficacy of psychodynamic therapies. In part, this results from the attitude of some proponents of this form of treatment that the changes psychodynamic treatment tries to produce do not lend themselves to empirical analysis in randomized trials. The few studies designed to assess child treatments that place more emphasis on expressive forms of therapy show some positive results, but their effectiveness seems less than that of behavior therapies in metaanalytic comparisons.

FAMILY SYSTEMS THERAPY

- As noted above, virtually all contemporary therapy with children and adolescents is done in a family context, with the family's influence on the child in mind. The point of entry or focus of treatment, however, may differ. The individual-oriented psychodynamic therapist may devote most time working with the child directly. A behavior therapist training parents in certain behavior management techniques might devote most of his/her efforts to the parents themselves with the goal of altering their behavior toward the child. Family therapists placed the most emphasis on seeing the family as an interactive system. As such, the family is seen as having a structure (e.g., alliances, repetitive patterns of interaction that are structure-like). There are subsystems in the family (e.g., parent-parent, mother with a particular child, and so on), and boundaries between the systems. Emphasis is placed on understanding communication processes within the family, with all behavior viewed as serving a communicative function. In well-functioning families, these systems and communication patterns serve for the betterment of the individuals and the family as a whole. At times, subsystems, boundaries, and communication patterns are maladaptive and serve to produce problematic behaviors in one or more family members. Family-oriented therapists work with the whole family together (or sometimes particular subsystems) to produce a more adaptive, effective system. Family approaches can incorporate insights and techniques from other therapeutic approaches (e.g., behavioral family therapy), as well as using approaches unique to family therapists (e.g., paradoxically recommending that a symptom be exhibited under controlled circumstances) to modify the family system.

- Studies of family treatment efficacy are limited in number compared to behavioral treatments. Some limited empirical support is available for these treatments.

PHARMACOTHERAPY

GUIDELINES

- The use of medications in the treatment of children and adolescents with emotional and behavioral problems increased dramatically in the past 10 years. Although concerns about side effects and duration of treatment are common and reasonable among caregivers, psychiatric disorder can be identified as a dysfunction in the central nervous system that may have a long-lasting impact if untreated. Psychotropic medications then become an efficient way to address this concern.
- Psychopharmacology begins with an accurate diagnosis and an appropriate identification of the target behaviors. Some of these behaviors may accompany more than one diagnosis. For example, aggression may be evident with attention deficit hyperactivity disorder, pervasive developmental disorder, and affective disorder. Each requires a unique medical approach. Medications are typically indicated when the disorder causes distress for the patient and/or significant caregivers, and impairs routine levels of functioning. The identified disorder should be amenable to pharmacotherapy and can be followed longitudinally as the prescriptions are maintained or

modified. Physicians should monitor the patient's progress with standardized assessments from multiple sources, including the patient. This follows an initial evaluation that uses the same assessment instruments and sources to determine the patient's baseline.

- Physicians should clearly explain how the drug works in the central nervous system and how this relates to the underlying etiology of the psychiatric disorder. Caregivers and the patient can then understand why medications are changed or added to the regimen. The process is a dialogue that encourages caregivers and patient to share their impressions as to why medications are necessary. This includes addressing issues like "addiction," an unreasonable fear that follows psychopharmacology because of its relationship to behavior. Treatment plans are altered to accommodate the individual needs of the patient. Suicidal behavior, for example, requires treatment with medications that are unlikely to be lethal in overdose and that are prescribed in small amounts. Starting doses for children are typically low and accommodate vulnerabilities in the patient like medical illness. Physicians should also be aware of the cost of these medications and the insurance plans that determine how prescriptions are handled.
- Medication side effects may be the direct result of the drug or of preexisting conditions in the patient. Concomitant medical disorders, for example, may preclude the use of certain drugs. Other medical conditions that exist prior to the start of pharmacotherapy should be well-documented and followed along with the medications. In this way, changes in the character of the symptoms can either be attributed to the medication or considered to be part of a preexisting presentation. Drug or alcohol use will likely interfere with psychotropic medications and should be addressed and controlled before a treatment plan is developed. Unintended physical and behavioral effects of the medications should be thoroughly reviewed at the start of treatment. Written information on what to expect, and who to call in the event of an emergency, can supplement these discussions. Behavior changes require the caregiver and physician to sort out symptoms due to the medication and those attributable to the disorder. Occasionally medication side effects may produce a "paradoxical" reaction that exacerbates the underlying psychiatric condition.
- Management of psychotropic medications is determined by patient response. Individuals who make sufficient progress on a single medication are told to maintain the regimen for 6 months to 1 year depending on the disorder. Periodic monitoring continues

because patients may experience a recurrence of symptoms or signs of medication tolerance. A partial medication response suggests the need for a dosage change, drug substitution, or the addition of another compound. When patients either do not respond or worsen on a drug regimen, the physician should consider noncompliance, misdiagnosis, substance use, or environmental stressors as factors.

• Discontinuation of the medications follows a thorough discussion on the risks and benefits of such a decision. Medications are gradually tapered, although the literature on possible withdrawal effects is not as clear in children as it is in adults. If the patient experiences any physical complaints, the taper is slowed. A recurrence of psychiatric symptoms requires an evaluation and an immediate return to the previous therapeutic dose.

STIMULANTS

• Stimulants are well-established treatments for ADHD. The medications are effective through adolescence and into adulthood. Stimulant medication also reduces defiance, negativism, and verbal and physical aggression when conduct disorder or oppositional defiant disorder occurs with ADHD. Children with pervasive developmental disorders (PDD) experience symptoms of inattention, impulsivity, and overactivity that respond to stimulants. Most patients with ADHD respond to stimulants, but it is difficult to predict which specific medication will be most successful. When one stimulant is ineffective, it is probably best to choose a medication from another drug class. Fifty percent of patients who do not respond to a drug from one class will respond to a different medication. Longer-acting medications are attractive because drug administration every 4 hours may be inconvenient, inconsistent, stigmatizing, or insufficiently supervised. Rebound effects are also less likely with medications that last over 8 hours. Ritalin sustained release (SR) and Dexedrine spansule capsules have been joined by several new formulations including the MPH preparations Concerta, Metadate ER, Metadate CD, and Ritalin LA. Adderall XR is a mixture of amphetamine salts. MethyPatch, a transdermal long-acting patch formulation of methylphenidate, is in the planning stages. Dexmethylphenidate (Focalin) is as effective as MPH but with fewer side effects and with a longer duration of action.

• The clinician should collect information from more than one source when making the diagnosis of ADHD, including patient, caregivers, and school. These contacts continue throughout treatment and are used to support changes in timing and size of the dose. The onset of action for both methylphenidate and amphetamines is 30 minutes with drug effects lasting 3–4 hours. Caregivers may administer the medications only on school days, but when symptoms are severe, the patient should be covered all day for the entire week.

• Side effects of stimulant medications include anorexia, insomnia, irritable mood, and mildly elevated blood pressure. Patients who chew extended release medications are more likely to experience toxic effects. Physicians must balance the risk of developing tics with the benefits of successful ADHD treatment. Alternative medications may not be as efficacious as stimulants. Decreases in weight and height are rarely clinically significant and may be more common with the use of dextroamphetamine than methylphenidate. Occasionally, caregivers may want medication-free summers to minimize the growth impact. Patients may suffer from rebound effects 3–15 hours after the dose characterized by increased excitability, activity, talkativeness, irritability, and insomnia. Patients may require a p.m. dose, the use of long-acting preparations, or the addition of clonidine (Catapres) or guanfacine (Tenex). Patients currently treated with monoamine oxidase (MAO) inhibitors, suffering from schizophrenia or acute psychosis, diagnosed with glaucoma, or with a history of stimulant drug abuse, should not receive stimulant medications. Pemoline is rarely used because of the risk of liver toxicity. There is no evidence that stimulants decrease the seizure threshold. Clonidine and guanfacine are occasionally added to stimulants to treat those disorders that do not respond to stimulants alone. Evidence linking the combination of clonidine and ritalin to sudden death is tenuous; however, patients with cardiovascular disease should be carefully monitored.

ATOMOXETINE

• Atomoxetine (Strattera) is a nonstimulant treatment for ADHD that is an inhibitor of presynaptic norepinephrine transporters. The side effects of the medication are mild and include decreased appetite, nausea, vomiting, dizziness, slight increase in blood pressure, and heart rate.

ANTIDEPRESSANTS

• Antidepressant medications are available for the treatment of children and adolescents although there are few empirical studies available to guide therapeutic choices. No medications have Food and Drug Administration (FDA) approval for the treatment of depression in patients younger than 18 years. The most commonly prescribed class of medications is the selective serotonin reuptake inhibitors. These medications have a narrow side effect profile, long half-life, and few interactions with other drugs. Tricyclic antidepressants are not often used because of serious side effects and a lack of efficacy. Trazodone (desyrel) is used for insomnia and aggression in children but is rarely used due to the side effect of priaprism. Antidepressants have side effect profiles consistent with their mechanisms of action. All antidepressants can precipitate hypomania or mania.

Treatment recommendations for antidepressants are as follows:

• For depression, medications are tapered when the patient has been asymptomatic for 4–6 months. When young patients suffer from recurrent episodes of unipolar depression, the antidepressant should be maintained indefinitely. Monoamine oxidase inhibitors (MAOIs) are used only in treatment-resistant cases because of the dangerous reactions to dietary noncompliance.

• The serotonine selective reuptake inhibitors (SSRIs) paroxetine, fluvoxamine, fluoxetine, and sertraline are effective in the treatment of obsessive-compulsive disorder (OCD), although improvement may not appear for 8–12 weeks. Early in treatment there may be an exacerbation of symptoms, but these problems resolve after several weeks. Clomipramine may be useful for patients who do not respond to SSRIs and is typically started at a dose of 25 mg/day. Increases of 25–50 mg/day can be made every 4–7 days with a maximum dose of 3 mg/kg/day or 200 mg/day.

• *School avoidance or separation anxiety* responds to a combination of imipramine and cognitive-behavioral therapy (CBT). SSRIs may also be useful in cases with severe anxiety symptoms.

• Other anxiety disorders can be effectively treated with antidepressants, including fluvoxamine in children and adolescents with social phobia, separation anxiety disorder, or generalized anxiety disorder and sertraline for generalized anxiety disorder. Fluoxetine successfully treated selective mutism in one controlled trial. Separation anxiety responds to tricyclic antidepressants at relatively low doses although the effect may take as long as 6–8 weeks.

• Antidepressant medications are used in the treatment of ADHD. Bupropion decreases hyperactivity and aggression and may improve cognitive performance. Tricyclic antidepressants are not as effective as stimulants and require electrocardiogram (ECG) monitoring, have potential cardiac side effects, present a danger from accidental or intentional overdose, and have anticholinergic and sedating side effects. The starting doses are lower than those used for depression. Nortryptaline is started at 10–25 mg/day and increases until there is a clinical effect or until the dose reaches 4.5 mg/kg/day. Imipramine (or desipramine)

starts at 25 mg/day and increases in 25 mg increments once or twice weekly.

• SSRIs and clomipramine may reduce obsessive symptoms, rituals, and insistence on sameness evident in some patients with autism and other PDD.

• Tourette disorder responds to nortriptyline or desipramine with a reduction in both tics and comorbid symptoms of hyperactivity, impulsivity, and inattention. SSRIs and clomipramine reduce obsessions and compulsions as well as tics.

• Behavioral treatments are the first choice for enuresis although all tricyclic antidepressants are effective in the treatment of nocturnal enuresis. The mechanism of action is not clear, but in 80% of patients, the frequency of bed-wetting decreases in the first week. The maximum dose is 2.5 mg/kg/day, although tolerance may develop. A drug-free trial should occur every 6 months.

• SSRIs do not require medical assessment before starting treatment and are typically started at very low doses with a slow titration that minimizes side effects. Occasionally medications like fluoxetine, with a long half-life, are given on an every-other-day basis. Blood levels for the SSRIs are not consistently available and are, therefore, not applied to clinical efficacy. SSRIs produce relatively mild side effects that are short-lived. These include anorexia, weight loss, weight gain, headaches, upset stomach, nausea, vomiting, tremor, and drowsiness. Occasionally patients experience behavioral activation with restlessness, insomnia, social disinhibition, and agitation. The increased activity may also be related to akathisia. Some patients present with apathy or amotivational syndrome after weeks of SSRI treatment; these symptoms are responsive to a small decrease in the dose. Serotonin syndrome, although rare, is potentially fatal and is characterized by extreme restlessness and agitation, fever, myoclonic jerking, hyperreflexia, clonus, fasciculations, and GI symptoms. In particularly severe cases, patients suffer seizures, hypotension, ventricular tachycardia, and disseminated intravascular coagulation. Sudden withdrawal of the medication can produce dizziness, headache, nausea, vomiting, diarrhea, tics, insomnia, irritability, lethargy, anorexia, and dysphoria.

• Children started on bupropion (wellbutrin) should first be examined for seizures and factors that predispose to seizures. The drug is given in two or three daily doses beginning with a dose of 37.5 mg twice a day and gradually increased over 2 weeks to a maximum dose of 250–300 mg/day. Allergic reactions to bupropion include rash, urticaria, and serum sickness. Less frequently, patients may experience agitation, insomnia, fatigue, nausea, anorexia, dry mouth, dizziness, and confusion. Bupropion may exacerbate tics, and seizures are possible in patients with eating disorders.

- Tricyclic antidepressants are dangerous in overdose, indicating that the physician should review the patient's medical history and physical examination. Evidence of cardiac symptoms warrants caution. An initial ECG and subsequent ECGs after each dose increase of 50–100 mg/day are essential. Any history of head trauma or seizure disorder requires an electroencephalogram (EEG) before initiating treatment because tricyclic antidepressants tend to lower seizure threshold. Anticholinergic side effects are common and respond to decreases in dose. These include drowsiness and dizziness, dry mouth, drying of bronchial secretions, and constipation. Urinary retention, narrow-angle glaucoma, blurred vision, syncope, and increased diastolic blood pressure are rare in children and adolescents. Behavioral toxicity on trichloroacetic acid (TCAs) includes irritability, psychosis, agitation, anger, aggression, forgetfulness, and confusion. These symptoms typically appear at plasma levels greater than 450 ng/mL. Discontinuing TCAs abruptly can produce flu-like anticholinergic withdrawal symptoms with nausea, cramps, vomiting, headaches, and muscle pains.

LITHIUM

- Lithium is a treatment of choice for all forms of bipolar affective disorder in children and adolescents. It can be used for acute stabilization in adolescents with mania, behavior problems in children of bipolar depressed parents, young patients with behavioral disorders and mood swings, and mentally retarded youth with severe aggression. Children with mania have a poorer response to lithium than adolescent patients.
- Patients should be screened prior to the start of lithium therapy with a physical examination, medical history, complete blood count (CBC) with differential, electrolytes, thyroid function studies, blood urea nitrogen (BUN), creatinine, urinalysis, and ECG. EEG is ordered when indicated and adolescent girls should have a pregnancy test if sexually active. Lithium carbonate is most commonly prescribed, but the long-acting preparations (Lithobid or Eskalith CR) are appropriate for younger populations because they can be given in twice daily regimens and maintain steady blood levels.
- Lithium is started at 300 mg/day and slowly increased to 900 mg/day with a therapeutic dose typically between 900 and 1200 mg/day. The half-life in adolescents allows for once-a-day dosing; however, children have a more rapid lithium clearance and require multiple divided doses. Therapeutic levels in children are between 0.6 and 1.2 meq/L and not to exceed

1.4 meq/L. Levels are drawn 8–12 hours after the last evening dose and before the first morning dose.

- The patient's response to treatment is monitored on a monthly basis and several laboratory studies monitored periodically: BUN, creatinine, creatinine clearance, and thyroid-stimulating hormone (every 4–6 months). Treatment should continue for 6 months to 1 year. In adults, intermittent lithium use produces worsening of cycling and decreased response to treatment suggesting caution when deciding to stop the medication. Lithium should be gradually tapered when discontinued.
- Side effects are more common in children younger than 7 years of age. Some do not require discontinuation of the lithium (tremor, weight gain, headache, nausea, diarrhea) while others (polydipsia and polyuria with enuresis, goiter and/or hypothyroidism, hypoglycemia, acne) may necessitate a dosage or medication change. Lithium is contraindicated in sexually active girls because of its teratogenic potential. The risk for toxicity increases in the presence of rigorous dieting, administration of diuretics or nonsteroidal anti-inflammatory agents, fever, vomiting, or diarrhea.

ANTIPSYCHOTICS

- Antipsychotic medications are divided into typical and atypical groups. The typical antipsychotics include chlorpromazine (thorazine), fluphenazine (prolixin), haloperidol (haldol), perphenazine (trilafon), pimozide (orap), thiothixene (navane), and trifluoperazine (stelazine). The most common side effect of these medications is extrapyramidal symptoms (EPS) including dystonic reactions, parkinsonian tremor and rigidity, drooling, and akathisia. An acute dystonia is best treated with either diphenhydramine (25–50 mg) or benztropine (0.5–2.0). Adolescent males may be more susceptible to acute dystonic reactions than adults. Children may react adversely to anticholinergics, indicating that a decrease in neuroleptic dose is preferable with EPS. Tardive dyskinesia (TD) or withdrawal dyskinesias are more common among children on typical antipsychotics. Irreversible tardive dyskinesia is rarely documented in the pediatric population; however, it has appeared after only 5 months of treatment. Atypical antipsychotic medications are both serotonergic and dopaminergic antagonists, and have less risk of tardive dyskinesia and other extrapyramidal side effects. Atypicals include risperidone (risperdal), olanzapine (zyprexa), and quetiapine (seroquel). Clozapine (clozaril) and ziprazadone (geodon) carry risks for more serious side effects including cardiomyopathy and cardiac arrhythmias. Among atypical antipsychotics, risperidone is most likely to produce EPS, particularly among children. Negative symptoms of psychosis appear more responsive to the newer medications. Neuroleptic malignant syndrome presents with hyperthermia, muscle rigidity, autonomic hyperactivity, and changes in level of consciousness. The disorder is potentially fatal and requires rapid discontinuation of the neuroleptic and aggressive support. The administration of bromocriptine or L-dopa is recommended.

- Young schizophrenic patients are less responsive to medications than adults. Starting doses for children are 0.5 mg bid of risperidone, 5 mg at bedtime of olanzapine, and 25 mg bid of quetiapine. In addition, concerns about tardive dyskinesia (TD) and the prominence of negative symptoms suggest the use of atypicals for the treatment of young schizophrenics. Patients who do not respond to atypical antipsychotics are given haloperidol as adjunctive medication. The typical daily dose for children is 0.25–6 mg. Neuroleptic trials should last 6 weeks at adequate doses before another medication is considered. The medication may not reach its full therapeutic effect for several months. Positive symptoms like delusions and hallucinations tend to respond first, followed by cognitive symptoms, and eventually negative symptoms like apathy and withdrawal. No recommendation is available for the total duration of treatment in children.

- Haloperidol or trifluoperazine reduce hyperactivity, stereotypy, and withdrawal in young patients with developmental disorders, at doses of 0.5–4.0 mg/day. The medications do not affect cognitive performance and improve discrimination learning and language acquisition. Atypicals are more commonly used in children and adolescents with autism and pervasive developmental disorders due to their effectiveness in reducing aggression, anxiety, agitation, irritability, and obsessional behaviors, and increasing social awareness and attention. Antipsychotics are continued for several months if effective, with the drug discontinued at 3–6-month intervals to check for withdrawal dyskinesias. Tourette disorder is successfully treated with risperidone, although the side effect of excessive weight gain occasionally poses long-term problems. The starting dose is 0.25 mg once or twice a day, with increases to a maximum of 6 mg per day. Haloperidol and pimozide reduce tics, but symptoms may be exacerbated with medication withdrawal.

- Typical and atypical neuroleptics effectively reduce aggression, hostility, negativism and explosiveness accompanying conduct and oppositional defiant disorders. Trials of atypicals like risperidone do not carry the risk of cognitive dulling and tardive dyskinesia. Studies found olanzapine and risperidone to be helpful in the treatment of acute mania. Antipsychotic medications are occasionally used in crisis situations with severe agitation and potentially dangerous behaviors due to a variety of psychosocial and organic factors. Haloperidol doses of 0.01–0.05 mg/kg are administered every hour until the patient is stable. The total daily dose required to calm the patient is used to determine short-term management. There are no well-controlled studies on these interventions, however.

- Treatment with antipsychotics is preceded by a complete physical examination, and laboratory studies that include a CBC with differential and a liver profile. These studies should be repeated on a regular basis. Patients are examined for the presence of abnormal movements, preferably with a scale like the Abnormal Involuntary Movement Scale (AIMS). The impact of the medications on weight gain suggests the need for monitoring, nutritional counseling, and routine exercise. The starting dose should be low with increases made at 1-week intervals. Atypical antipsychotic medications are available in easy-to-administer preparations. Olanzapine is given as an orally disintegrating disk (Zyprexa ZYDIS) and several other preparations are available in a liquid form. Among the typical neuroleptic medications, the most commonly prescribed are the high-potency drugs haloperidol, fluphenazine, trifluoperazine, or perphenazine. The lower-potency compounds are rarely given because of the sedation, cognitive dulling, and memory deficits that accompany their use.

MINOR TRANQUILIZERS, SEDATIVES, AND HYPNOTICS

- Benzodiazepines are used in the treatment of anxiety disorders in children. The medications are particularly effective for the physical symptoms of anxiety. Alprazolam (Xanax) is given for overanxious disorders and for the anticipatory and acute situational anxiety that accompanies medical procedures. Clonazepam assists with separation anxiety disorder, panic disorder, generalized anxiety, school phobia, and social anxiety. Buspirone treats generalized anxiety disorder in adolescents. Diazepam (valium) is prescribed for night terrors, persistent insomnia, or somnambulism.

- Benzodiazepines are absorbed and metabolized quickly in young patients although the drugs have a potential for dependence. Withdrawal symptoms include seizures, anxiety, malaise, irritability, headache, sweating, gastrointestinal (GI) distress, insomnia, or muscle tension. Buspirone may not be effective for 2–4 weeks after initiating treatment. Minor tranquilizers, sedatives, and hypnotics have a variety of side effects including sedation, ataxia, diplopia, tremor, confusion, and emotional lability.

ANTICONVULSANTS

- Anticonvulsants are particularly effective in the treatment of mixed mood states and rapid-cycling bipolar disorder. Carbamazepine (tegretol) and valproic acid (depakene, depakote) are most often used with pediatric populations. Carbamazepine is started at 100 mg/day and maintained at 10–20 mg/kg/day bid or tid. Therapeutic blood levels are not known. Valproic acid is typically begun at 15 mg/kg/day for adolescents. The maximum dose is 60 mg/kg/day. Serum concentrations should be greater than 45 µg/mL. Laboratory studies completed before medication administration include hemoglobin, hematocrit, white blood cell count, platelets, and liver function tests. These measurements should be repeated every 4 months. Blood levels of the drug should also be frequently monitored because children metabolize the drug more rapidly than adults.

- Anticonvulsants present a broad range of potential side effects. The medications should be prescribed with caution in sexually active girls because of possible teratogenic effects. Carbamazepine can cause nausea, vomiting, vertigo, ataxia, drowsiness, diplopia, nystagmus, tics, muscle cramps, decreased thyroid function, immune thrombocytopenia, blood dyscrasias, hepatitis, renal impairment, urinary incontinence, hair loss, motor and vocal tics, rash, interstitial pneumonitis, dose-related leukopenia, and a variety of behavior effects. Valproic acid may produce liver toxicity, gastrointestinal symptoms, and blood dyscrasias. Patients present with nausea, vomiting, easy bruising, lethargy, malaise, or abdominal distress.

PSYCHIATRIC EMERGENCIES

- Psychiatric assessments in emergency situations should be brief and focused, with information collected from multiple sources, including the patient, caregiver, and other responsible adults involved with the child or adolescent. The purpose is to determine the potential physical danger and evidence of psychiatric disorder that increases the risk to the patient and others. In addition, the clinician makes a disposition plan based on the need for treatment and available psychosocial supports. The patient's presentation may be affected by medical illness or medication side effects, a history of head trauma, drug or alcohol intoxication or withdrawal, intentional or accidental drug overdose, drugs or weapons available to the patient, and levels of aggression that require restraint or containment.

DANGER TO SELF

- Suicidal threats should be taken seriously regardless of the age or circumstance. Although the child's assessment of physical danger may be immature and impractical, self-destructive behavior is indicative of significant psychiatric distress. Patients require immediate attention because suicidal behaviors tend to recur within days or weeks.

- Males are more likely to successfully complete suicides by a 3:1 margin, a figure that increases to 5.5:1 when considering the 15–24-year-old age group. Suicidal ideation is more common in females by a 1.6:1 margin. Males use more lethal methods including firearms and hanging while females resort to overdose, carbon monoxide, and jumping. The combination of substance use and firearms is particularly lethal.

- Affective disorders are evident in nearly all suicide victims, yet only one-third is ever referred to a psychiatric facility. Suicide risk increases when there is evidence of noncompliance with psychiatric treatment, social isolation, poor school performance, family discord, abuse and neglect, parental psychiatric disorder, and a family history of a completed suicide. Medical illnesses, particularly diseases of the central nervous system secondary to trauma, seizure, infection, or chemotherapy, make patients more likely to exhibit suicidal behavior. Occasionally pediatric patients become suicidal in response to stressful events in school, at home, or with peers.

- The assessment of the suicidal patient involves a careful review of the circumstances preceding and following the event, and a detailed examination of the attempt. Clinicians obtain information on substance abuse, impulsive behavior, passive suicidality, family circumstances and history, a decline in social functioning, lethality, and intention. Lethality is the likelihood of death from the attempt based on method, location, and the probability of being found. Intention is what the patient wished to happen as a consequence of the attempt. Patients with a history of suicide attempts using methods other than ingestion and superficial cutting are considered more dangerous.

- The need for hospitalization is based on issues of safety and the need for a more detailed assessment and treatment plan. Family members participate in therapy and are educated on the matters of psychiatric diagnosis, lethality, and safety. All lethal medications and firearms should either be carefully controlled or removed from the home. All concomitant psychiatric disorders are treated, family situations are addressed and stabilized, and patients are encouraged to improve problem solving and minimize stress.

DANGER TO OTHERS

- Assessment determines whether the patient is dangerous or simply threatening harm. Behavior descriptions should include precipitants, warning signs, evidence of an altered mental state, property damage, need for physical restraint, repetitive behaviors, lethality, solitary or group action, and previous response to treatment. The mental status examination documents the presence of violent intent, cognitive impairment, paranoia, delusions or hallucinations, and impulsivity. Patients with developmental and language delay or neurologic disorders are more likely to communicate distress through aggression. Victims of physical abuse and head trauma suffer high rates of neuropsychologic deficits and become impulsive and aggressive.

• Emergent treatment of dangerous behaviors rarely require medication and only when the patient must be calmed for safety reasons. Pharmacotherapy is practiced with caution when the patient suffers from a medical disorder or drug ingestion. Seclusion and restraint can be effective when done appropriately and with caution.

• Disposition is determined by the patient's psychopathology, the safety of vulnerable people in the home, and the ability of the caregivers to supervise and control the patient. Addressing the cause of the behavior may require psychiatric attention. Inpatient hospitalization is ineffective for conduct disorders. Patients are typically referred for partial hospitalization, residential treatment, therapeutic school placement, and home-based services. Cognitive-behavioral programs like anger management and social skills training provide alternatives to aggression. The treatment process should be supported by the family and the legal system.

REFERENCES

General

Dulcan MK, Martini DR, Lake MB, et al. (eds.). *Concise Guide to Child and Adolescent Psychiatry*, 3rd ed. Washington, DC: American Psychiatric Press, 2003.

U.S. Department of Health and Human Services. *Mental Health: A Report of the Surgeon General*. Rockville, MD: U.S. Department of Health and Human Services, Substance Abuse and Mental Health Services Administration, Center for Mental Health services, National Institutes of Health, National Institute of Mental Health, 1999.

Pharmacotherapy

Rosenberg DR, Davanzo PA, Gershon S. *Pharmacotherapy for Child and Adolescent Psychiatric Disorders*. New York, NY: Marcel Dekker, 2002.

Psychiatric Emergencies

Dulcan, MK, Martini DR., Lake MB. Emergencies. In: Dulcan MK, Martini DR, Lake MB (eds), *Concise Guide to Child & Adolescent Psychiatry*, 3rd ed. Washington, DC: American Psychiatric Association, 2003, pp. 209–227.

166 FEEDING AND EATING DISORDERS IN THE INFANT

Sally E. Tarbell

CLINICAL FEATURES (DSM-IV DIAGNOSTIC CRITERIA)

• Feeding disorders involve the persistent failure to eat sufficiently, with significant weight loss or failure to gain weight over at least 1 month.

• The behavior is not due to gastrointestinal or other medical condition.

• The behavior is not better accounted for by another disorder (e.g., rumination) or by lack of food.

• Onset occurs before 6 years.

• The degree of growth deficiency may vary and can be classified as follows:

1. *Acute malnutrition*: 50th percentile weight-for-height, divided by current weight provides percent of ideal body weight. Mild malnutrition (80–89%), moderate (70–79%), and severe <70%.

2. *Chronic malnutrition*: Actual height divided by height that corresponds to National Center for Health Statistics 50th percentile for the age of the child. Mild (90–95%), moderate (85–89%), and severe (<85%).

3. *Additional definitions of failing growth*: Child falls below the 5th percentile for weight; child's weight falls two major percentiles in a 2–6-month period.

SUBTYPES

• *Feeding disorder of reciprocity (neglect)* (onset 2–6 months). Infant lacks developmentally appropriate social responsiveness (e.g., eye contact, smiling) during feeding. Significant growth deficiency is present.

• *Infantile anorexia* (onset during transition to spoon and self-feeding). Refusal to eat adequate amounts of food for a least 1 month. Child lacks interest in food and does not communicate hunger. Significant growth deficiency is present. Food refusal does not follow traumatic event and is not related to medical illness.

• *Sensory food aversions and/or food selectivity (onset during introduction of baby or solid food)*. Refusal to eat food with specific tastes, textures, smells or appearances, or child refuses all but a few specific foods. The child eats better when offered preferred foods. Must have nutritional deficiencies, oral-motor delay, or both.

- *Feeding disorder associated with concurrent medical condition*: The child initiates eating but shows distress and discontinues feeding. A medical condition is present that is thought to cause the distress. Medical management improves, but does not eliminate the feeding problems. Failure to gain adequate weight or weight loss occurs.
- *Posttraumatic feeding disorder*: Food refusal following traumatic event(s) to oropharynx or gastrointestinal tract (e.g., choking, insertion of nasogastric tube). Child may accept one type of feeding (e.g., bottle), but refuse others (e.g., spoon), or completely refuse all oral feedings. Reminders of the traumatic events cause anticipatory distress and/or intense feeding resistance. Food refusal poses a threat to the child's nutritional status.

EPIDEMIOLOGY

- The National Health and Nutrition Examination Survey III (1988–1991) found 5.2% of children between the ages of 2 and 5 to be low in height-for-age, and 2.7% to be low weight-for-height.
- One to 5% of pediatric admissions are for failure to gain adequate weight, with approximately one-half attributable to a feeding disorder without any predisposing medical condition.
- Feeding disorders are equally common in males and females.

PATHOPHYSIOLOGY

- The etiology of feeding disorder varies with type of disorder.
- Multiple etiologic factors alone and in combination including medical conditions, developmental delay, neuroregulatory difficulties (e.g., sleep-wake disturbances), parent-child interaction problems, parental psychopathology, family environment, poverty, child abuse, and neglect.

PROGNOSIS

- Onset after infancy is associated with lesser degrees of developmental delay and malnutrition.
- Most children show improved growth after variable lengths of time.

EVALUATION, MANAGEMENT, AND TREATMENT

- Evaluation and treatment varies depending on the subtype of feeding disorder. Optimally, feeding disorders are assessed by a multidisciplinary team including pediatrics, psychiatry or psychology, nutrition, occupational therapy, and social work.
- Outpatient treatment has been effective in mild feeding disorders, but more severe feeding disorders require hospitalization.
- Case studies have shown behavioral interventions to be effective in sensory food aversions and posttraumatic feeding disorders.
- Multiple treatments have been directed to feeding disorders related to parent-child interaction, parental psychopathology (e.g., home-based treatments to support parental acquisition of appropriate skills, behavioral parent training, parent mental health treatment). No one treatment shows superiority.

PICA

CLINICAL FEATURES (DSM-IV DIAGNOSTIC CRITERIA)

- Pica includes the persistent ingestion of nonnutritive substances for at least 1 month.
- Eating of nonnutritive substances is developmentally inappropriate.
- Eating behavior is not part of a cultural practice.
- Pica can occur in the context of other disorders, especially mental retardation, pervasive developmental disorder, schizophrenia, and Kleine-Levin syndrome.

EPIDEMIOLOGY

- The data on epidemiology of pica are limited. One community study found the prevalence of pica to be 0.3–14.4%, with higher rates in the institutionalized population, 9–25%.
- Profound mental retardation is significantly associated with pica.
- There are cultural practices associated with certain types of pica (geophagia).

ETIOLOGY

- The etiology is unknown.

PATHOPHYSIOLOGY

- Dietary deficiencies, parasitic infections, and metal toxicities have been implicated in the development of pica but the direction of causality has not been established.

- Case studies provide some support that vitamin and mineral deficiencies may trigger this behavior in some children.

PROGNOSIS

- Pica typically worsens in unsupervised environments.
- Morbidity includes choking, poisoning, infections, and intestinal obstruction.

EVALUATION, MANAGEMENT, AND TREATMENT

- Pica has been shown to decrease with the introduction of a multivitamin in one study, and has been associated with low levels of zinc and iron in two reports.
- Case studies have shown behavioral interventions (e.g., stimulus control, reinforcement of other behaviors) to be effective in reducing pica in both normal and mentally retarded children.
- Pharmacologically, selective serotonin reuptake inhibitors (SSRIs) have been found to decrease pica in mentally retarded patients. Ritalin decreases the severity of pica and neuroleptics can exacerbate the condition.

RUMINATION

CLINICAL FEATURES (DSM-IV DIAGNOSTIC CRITERIA)

- Rumination involves the repeated regurgitation and rechewing of previously ingested food for at least 1 month following a period without rumination.
- The behavior is not due to gastrointestinal (e.g., gastroesophageal reflux [GER]) or other medical conditions.
- The behavior does not occur exclusively in the context of anorexia or bulimia.
- If rumination occurs in the context of pervasive developmental disorders (PDD) or mental retardation, it must be sufficiently severe to warrant separate clinical attention.

EPIDEMIOLOGY

- No population studies exist but rumination is reported to be uncommon.
- Rumination occurs more in males than females.

- Rumination is more common among children with PDD, mental retardation, and autism.

ETIOLOGY

- The etiology of rumination is unknown.
- Psychosocial problems (neglect, lack of stimulation) may be predisposing factors.

PROGNOSIS

- Morbidity due to prolonged rumination includes weight loss, failure to thrive, and death secondary to malnutrition.

EVALUATION, MANAGEMENT, AND TREATMENT

- Case studies of behavioral interventions (e.g., providing starchy food following meals, increasing the quantity of food available at meals, noncontingent high-frequency feeding immediately following meals, time out when emesis occurs) can be effective in reducing rumination.

REFERENCES

Feeding Disorders of Early Childhood

Benoit D. Feeding disorders, failure to thrive and obesity. In: Zeanah C, Jr. (ed.), *Handbook of Infant Mental Health*, 2nd ed. New York, NY: Guilford Press, 2000, pp. 339–352.

Chatoor I. Feeding disorders in infants and toddlers: diagnosis and treatment. *Child Adoles Psychiatr Clin N Am* 2002;11:163–183.

Kedesdy J, Budd K. *Childhood Feeding Disorders: Biobehavioral Assessment and Intervention.* Baltimore: Paul N. Brookes, 1998.

Kessler D, Dawson P. *Failure to Thrive and Pediatric Undernutrition: A Transdisciplinary Approach.* Baltimore, MD: Paul Brooks Publishing, 1999.

Luiselli J. Cueing, demand fading, and positive reinforcement to establish self-feeding and oral consumption in a child with chronic food refusal. *Behav Modif* 2000;24:348–358.

Feeding Problems: Rumination/Pica

Myles B, Simpson R, Hirsch N. A review of the literature on interventions to reduce pica in individuals with developmental disabilities. *Autism* 1997;1:77–95.

Piazza C, Fisher W, Hanley G, LeBlanc L, Worsdell A, Lindauer S, Keeney K. Treatment of pica through multiple analyses of its reinforcing functions. *J Appl Behav Anal* 1998;31: 165–189.

Wagaman J, Williams D, Camilleri M. Behavioral intervention for the treatment of rumination. *J Pediatr Gastroenterol Nutr* 1998;27:596–598.

167 ELIMINATION DISORDERS

John V. Lavigne

ENURESIS

CLINICAL FEATURES (DSM-IV DIAGNOSTIC CRITERIA)

- The main characteristic of enuresis is voiding urine into bedding or clothing, either involuntarily or volitionally
- In enuresis, the voiding occurs at a clinically significant level of twice per week for 3 consecutive months or more; if it occurs less often, it is accompanied by significant distress for the child or it produces some impairment socially or academically.
- Two types are noted. In primary enuresis, the child never had a long period of being continent. Such children are not described as having enuresis until age 5 years. A second group, "secondary" enuresis, achieved continence but then relapsed.
- Children with daytime enuresis are more likely than children with monosymptomatic nocturnal enuresis to have urinary tract abnormalities (e.g., incomplete bladder emptying, fractionated voiding curve, structural/functional disorders).

EPIDEMIOLOGY

- Prevalence at age 5 years is 7% for boys and 3% for girls.

ETIOLOGY

- There are indications of a genetic factor in functional enuresis, with 70% of children with enuresis having a first-degree relative with that condition. Maturation is also implicated based on associated findings of small volume of voiding in some children

PROGNOSIS

- Untreated, the rate of decline is 5–10% per year, with approximately 1% remaining enuretic at age 18 years.

EVALUATION, MANAGEMENT, AND TREATMENT

- Diurnal enuresis
  1. Because of the stronger association between medical problems and diurnal enuresis, there is more emphasis on the use of medication and surgery for that disorder, with such behavioral techniques as scheduled voiding, biofeedback, or hypnosis playing a secondary role in treatment.
  2. Data supporting psychologic treatments for diurnal enuresis are limited. The best but limited, available evidence suggests that bladder (emphasizing delayed voiding for longer periods of time) or operant programs (rewards for remaining dry) can be useful.
- Nocturnal enuresis
  1. Medical evaluation of enuresis is discussed elsewhere.
  2. The psychologic evaluation of nocturnal enuresis is devoted to determining whether the family can conduct a behavioral program that occurs at night, and requires consistency in management to be effective. Poor outcome is associated with a family history of enuresis, prior treatment failure, and behavior problems of the child. Family problems can reduce compliance with treatment.
  3. The use of a urine alarm for treating nocturnal enuresis has been found to be efficacious in multiple studies, and more effective than pharmacotherapies. It is less clear whether other behavioral treatments combined with a urine alarm are superior to the urine alarm alone.
  4. Tricyclic antidepressants have been used with nocturnal enuresis with some positive results, although relapse is common.

ENCOPRESIS

CLINICAL FEATURES (DSM-IV DIAGNOSTIC CRITERIA)

- The key symptom of encopresis is the passage of feces into clothing or other inappropriate places.
- The occurrence is at least monthly for 3 or more months.
- The behavior is not the result of medication or any medical condition other than the effects of constipation itself.
- The disorder can present either with our without overflow incontinence.
- The child must be of at least age 4 years or, if developmentally delayed, have a mental age of at least 4 years.

- Both primary (never continent for an extended period) and secondary encopresis (problem occurs following a period of being continent) occur.

EPIDEMIOLOGY

- The prevalence of encopresis is estimated at between 1.5 and 7.5% of school-age children, 6–12 years.

ETIOLOGY

- Onset can be related to a painful bowel movement resulting in constipation, withholding, and reduced awareness of sensations signaling the need for evacuation. Other pathways to developing the disorder have not been clearly explicated.

PATHOPHYSIOLOGY

- Among children with encopresis, 85% also exhibit constipation.
- Normal elimination involves the passage of stool into the rectum and the relaxation of the internal anal sphincter so that the feces can move into the anal canal, and the relaxation of the external anal sphincter to allow voiding. The process is aided by appropriate diet, and successful elimination requires behavioral skills such as attending to internal sensations, recognizing where to eliminate, undressing, valsalva (tightening stomach muscles and pushing), and appropriate cleanup. The process can be disrupted by a lack of skill development in any of these areas. Anxiety about having a painful bowel movement can inhibit the process and can contribute to constipation. With the onset of constipation, rectal pressure and feelings of fullness can produce habituation to the sensations that need to be recognized to initiate elimination. This improves after an extended period of regular evacuation.

PROGNOSIS

- Encopresis declines to <1% by age 10–12 years. Overall, research on the prognosis for encopresis is relatively uncommon.

EVALUATION, MANAGEMENT, AND TREATMENT

- A pediatric examination including an abdominal examination to assess if a fecal mass is present is necessary, along with an anal digital examination to the consistency of fecal material and "a neurologic examination

with perianal sensation testing." A barium enema is unnecessary when the presentation is uncomplicated.
- Psychologic evaluation is needed to assess for the presence of comorbid problems.
- Available treatments include the following:
  1. Comprehensive medical interventions include use of laxatives to disimpact and keep the colon clear; dietary recommendations; and a sitting schedule. Effectiveness of this procedure is estimated at 5–59%.
  2. Biofeedback to correct paradoxical contractions has been tested when coupled with a comprehensive medical intervention. This appeared "promising" in one study in which the combined treatment was more effective than the medical cleanout alone, but other studies show results aren't consistent for biofeedback.
  3. Comprehensive medical intervention plus reward programs were effective in 43–51% of cases. Reviews suggest this combination is "probably efficacious."
- Psychotropic medications are appropriate to treat concomitant psychiatric disorders that can accompany symptoms of encopresis. These may include depression, obsessive-compulsive disorder, posttraumatic stress disorder, generalized anxiety disorder, social phobia, and situational anxiety. Tricyclic antidepressants should be used with caution because of constipation secondary to anticholinergic side effects.

REFERENCE

Elimination Disorders
McGrath ML, Mellon MW, Murphy L. Empirically supported treatments in pediatric psychology: constipation and encopresis. *J Plant Pathol* 2000;25:225–254.

168 EATING DISORDERS WITH LATER ONSET
D. Richard Martini

ANOREXIA NERVOSA

CLINICAL FEATURES (DSM-IV DIAGNOSTIC CRITERIA)

- The disorder is characterized by a refusal to maintain normal weight or the inability to reach an expected weight gain as a consequence of purposeful strict dieting or other extreme measures. Patients frequently exercise excessively.

- There is evidence of a distorted sense of body shape and size and a denial of significant weight loss. Patients obsess about body shape and size to such an extent that it may be considered delusional.
- Patients do not lose their appetite and any weight gain exacerbates their fears and anxieties.
- Postmenarchal females do not menstruate.
- The "restricting type" of anorexia is characterized by strict dieting, fasting, or excessive exercise. Patients with the binge eating/purging type consume unusually large quantities of food that are then purged, all in the context of anorexia nervosa.
- Symptoms of depression are a natural consequence of the physiologic process of starvation. These include social withdrawal, irritability, anhedonia, low self-esteem, and feelings of helplessness. Patients become ineffective in a variety of settings, further escalating their sense of inadequacy.
- The obsessional nature of anorexia can extend to other areas of the patient's life. These individuals can be overcontrolling and preoccupied with personal achievement and appearance to such an extent that a diagnosis of obsessive-compulsive disorder is also appropriate.

EPIDEMIOLOGY

- More than 90% of the patients are female and nearly 2% of the female adolescent and young adult population in the United States is affected. The rates in prepubescent children are not known.
- The prevalence rate has been increasing over the past 50 years in the 15–24-year-old age group, probably related to a greater societal emphasis on thinness and appearance.
- Anorexia nervosa is found predominately in western industrialized nations.

ETIOLOGY

- The etiology of anorexia nervosa is multifactorial. Patients suffer from low self-esteem and a loss of self-control. These feelings are expressed during puberty as a dissatisfaction with their bodies. Dieting then becomes the means to improve the patient's sense of personal satisfaction.
- First-degree relatives of patients with anorexia nervosa are 6–10 times more likely to suffer from an eating disorder than the general population. The relative roles of genetics and environmental factors have not yet been determined.

- Several neurophysiologic mechanisms, including hormonal and neurohormonal, may contribute to the development of anorexia nervosa. It is not yet possible to separate etiology from the effects of weight loss, although hormonal levels typically return to normal with refeeding.
- A history of sexual abuse may play a role in the development of eating disorders, particularly bulimia, although the relationship is not yet clear.
- Families of anorexia nervosa patients tend to be overinvolved and overcontrolling with the patient. Yet these same characteristics are found in families without evidence of eating disorders. The impact of having an anorectic patient in the home should also be factored into any consideration of family dynamics and the etiology of anorexia nervosa.

PROGNOSIS

- Anorexia nervosa typically appears during adolescence, most often between the ages of 14 and 18 years. The symptoms of amenorrhea and changes in body image are not easily applied to a young pediatric population. Children can have eating disorders, but they typically present as food avoidance, body image disturbance, inappropriate dieting, overeating, and selective eating.
- Physiologic changes may result, including complications that may require hospitalization. These include the following: dehydration, electrolyte imbalance, constipation and/or diarrhea, hypotension (especially postural), bradycardia (rates between 40 and 50 beats per minute), arrhythmias (prolonged QT interval may be a marker for risk of sudden death), mitral valve prolapse, cardiac arrest, edema and congestive heart failure during refeeding, amenorrhea or irregular menses (low levels of follicle-stimulating hormone [FSH] and luteinizing hormone [LH] despite low estrogen levels), abnormal glucose tolerance test with insulin resistance, hypothermia, sleep disturbances, osteopenia, leukopenia, anemia, thrombocytopenia; oral, esophageal, and gastric damage from vomiting and/or binge eating.
- Anorexia nervosa can have a long, complicated course and does not remit without treatment. Patients continue to experience low weight-for-height and age, peak bone mass reduction, excessive concern with weight, pubertal delay or interruption, and problematic personal and social relationships. Mortality is related to illness chronicity, with rates between 6 and 15%. Nearly half of these patients commit suicide.
- Rates of psychiatric comorbidity are higher in patients who do not respond to treatment. Additional psychiatric diagnoses contribute to a poor prognosis.

EVALUATION, MANAGEMENT, AND TREATMENT

- Each patient should receive a complete history, physical examination, and a series of routine laboratory studies including a complete blood count (CBC) with differential, platelets, blood sugar, blood urea nitrogen (BUN), liver function tests, thyroid function studies, and serum cholesterol levels.
- Information from the patient should include the onset and course of the disorder, the patient's highest and lowest weight, daily eating patterns, and the use of laxatives, emetics, or diuretics. Anorectic patients will try to hide the extent of their problem but may inadvertently reveal details that indicate severity of the illness.
- Family history of eating and psychiatric disorder may suggest an etiology, and an understanding of the family perspective on the illness is essential to successful treatment.
- Treatment begins with an acceptance of the disorder and the need for weight gain. A target weight is chosen and is typically within 90% of the ideal body weight. Admission to a psychiatric inpatient unit is considered necessary when the weight loss is more than 25–30% below ideal body weight, the patient suffers from symptomatic hypotension or syncope, the heart rate is lower than 40 beats per minute, and there is evidence of an arrhythmia.
- Weight gain is 1 lb per week on an outpatient basis and 2–3 lb per week on a psychiatric inpatient unit. Patients generally require high-calorie counts early in treatment to accomplish these goals. Force feeding is typically counterproductive.
- Psychotherapy acts as an adjunct to the behavioral programs that encourage treatment success. Privileges and activities are contingent on weight gain rather than amounts of food consumed at each meal. Individual therapies provide insight that may assist the patient's long-term recovery.
- Medication is prescribed to relieve symptoms of anxiety and obsessional thinking that accompanies the disorder and its recovery. These drugs may include serotonine selective reuptake inhibitors (SSRIs) and benzodiazepines.

BULIMIA NERVOSA

CLINICAL FEATURES (DSM-IV DIAGNOSTIC CRITERIA)

- The disorder is characterized by repeated episodes of uncontrollable binge eating of large amounts of food in a short time (less than 2 hours) followed by attempts to compensate for the probable weight gain.

The behavior is typically done secretly and provides relief from a recent sadness or stressful event.
- Bingeing should occur at least twice a week for at least 3 months. Induced vomiting accompanies bingeing in 80–90% of psychiatrically referred patients.
- The frequency of bingeing episodes is an indication of illness severity. Adolescents tend to binge more frequently as the illness develops.
- Bulimic patients are typically of normal weight or are slightly overweight.

EPIDEMIOLOGY

- Bulimia nervosa is more common than anorexia nervosa and develops before age 18 in over 50% of the cases. Approximately 1–3% of adolescent females and 0.2% of adolescent males suffer from the disorder. Males account for 10–15% of the clinically referred population.
- Bulimic patients are at increased risk for drug and alcohol abuse and are typically White and of a higher socioeconomic class.
- Weight loss and dieting is a preoccupation for 40–60% of adolescent females and tends to increase the risk for eating disorders.

ETIOLOGY

- Patients present symptoms of both anorexia and bulimia along a continuum. Fifty percent of anorectic patients develop symptoms of bulimia and bulimic patients frequently become anorectic.
- Monozygotic twins have a higher concordance rate for bulimia than dizygotic twins. Patients tend to have family histories of obesity, depression, or alcoholism.
- The success of serotonin reuptake inhibitors suggests a role for serotonin in the neurophysiology of bulimia.

PROGNOSIS

- Patients typically become bulimic after dieting and restricting food intake. Hunger promotes bingeing, and the patient's disgust at the behavior leads to depression and substance use. The result is another attempt at dieting. A constant state of semistarvation results, contributing further to risk for affective disorder.
- Relapse rates for bulimia are 30–50% in patients followed from 6 months to 6 years. Patients with poorer prognosis are those with a history of vomiting, comorbid anxiety and depressive disorders, and substance abuse. Milder forms of the disorder are more responsive to individual therapies.
- Bulimia is accompanied by significant personal and social consequences. Patients spend inordinate amounts of time and money on food, binge eating, and

purging. School functioning and social relationships suffer. There is a significant risk of death from suicide and medical complications.

EVALUATION, MANAGEMENT, AND TREATMENT

- The assessment of a bulimic patient includes a review of the current status of bingeing and purging behaviors and information on the possible use of thyroid hormone, excessive exercise, laxatives, and diuretics.
- Medical complications resulting from self-induced vomiting can produce sialadenosis, perimylosysis, reflux esophagitis, metabolic alkalosis, hypomagnesemia, and hypokalemia.
- A review of psychiatric history, social history, and family dynamics may reveal contributing factors.
- Treatment begins with a normalization of eating patterns and a plan for good nutrition. Patients who maintain a normal weight are typically not hospitalized.
- Suicidal ideation, out-of-control eating behaviors, or metabolic instability lead to hospitalization.
- Treatment interventions include cognitive-behavioral therapy focusing on normalizing eating patterns and coping with stress and family therapy (particularly with adolescents).
- Pharmacotherapy is based on the treatment of concomitant mood disorders or the regulation of appetite. A variety of medications have been tried, including tricyclic antidepressants, monoamine oxidase inhibitors, trazodone, bupropion, and SSRIs, but long-term studies on treatment success do not exist.

REFERENCE

Later Eating Disorders
Schwartz RC, Barrett MJ, Saba G: Family therapy for bulimia, in Garner DM, Garfinkel PE (eds), *Handbook of Psychotherapy for Anorexia Nervosa and Bulimia.* New York: Guilford, 1985, pp 280–307.

169 SOMATOFORM DISORDERS

Sally E. Tarbell

- The common feature of the somatoform disorders is the presence of physical symptoms and either the absence of organic pathology or a medical condition that cannot fully account for the level of functional impairment. It is not uncommon for children to present to medical systems with recurrent or persistent medical symptoms, such as abdominal pain, headaches, or dizziness, for which appropriate medical evaluations reveal no known organic cause.
- There are seven (7) DSM-IV diagnoses under the umbrella term somatoform disorders. They include somatization disorder, undifferentiated somatoform disorder, conversion disorder, pain disorder, hypochondriasis, body dysmorphic disorder, and somatoform disorder, not otherwise specified (NOS). Two of these conditions are rarely seen in pediatrics, with little known about their epidemiology, etiology, assessment, or treatment. These are hypochondriasis (preoccupation with fears of having, or the idea of having a serious disease based on misinterpretation of bodily symptoms) and body dysmorphic disorder (preoccupation with imagined defect in appearance). Somatoform disorder NOS is used when somatoform symptoms are present but criteria for other somatoform disorders have not been met. These three will not be discussed further.

SOMATIZATION DISORDER

CLINICAL FEATURES (DSM-IV DIAGNOSTIC CRITERIA)

- Key features include multiple physical complaints beginning before age 30, resulting in multiple medical interventions or in significant impairment in social, occupational, or other important areas of functioning.
- Each of the following must occur. Individual symptoms may occur at any time:
  1. Four pain symptoms: At least four different sites or functions (e.g., head, abdomen, back, joints, extremities)
  2. Two gastrointestinal symptoms: e.g., nausea, bloating, vomiting, diarrhea, food intolerance
  3. One sexual symptom: e.g., indifference, erectile or ejaculatory dysfunction, irregular menses, excessive menstrual bleeding
  4. One pseudoneurologic symptom: e.g., impaired coordination or balance, paralysis or localized weakness, loss of touch or pain sensation, double vision, blindness, deafness, seizures
  5. Either (1) or (2):
     a. After appropriate investigation, each of the above listed symptoms can't be fully explained by a known general medical condition or direct effects of a substance (drug of abuse or medication)
     b. When there is a related general medical condition, the physical complaints or resulting social or occupational impairment are in excess of

what would be expected from the history, physical examination, or laboratory findings.

6. The symptoms are not intentionally produced or feigned (as in factitious disorder or malingering).

• The DSM-IV diagnostic criteria require eight symptoms from four categories. The problem is rarely diagnosed among children. Most available research has been conducted in adult samples. It is important to consider cultural issues around symptom presentations. Many comorbid diagnoses are possible, including depression, anxiety, phobias, and avoidant and histrionic personality disorders

EPIDEMIOLOGY

• It is more common in females.
• Onset typically occurs during adolescence.
• Prevalence rates range from 0.7 to 20%.

ETIOLOGY

• Etiology is unclear.
• It appears that the following might contribute to onset of the illness:
  1. Emotional neglect after an illness
  2. Attention from others for somatic complaints
  3. Poor accuracy in interpreting internal cues.

UNDIFFERENTIATED SOMATOFORM DISORDER

CLINICAL FEATURES (DSM-IV DIAGNOSTIC CRITERIA)

• One or more physical complaints (e.g., fatigue, loss of appetite, gastrointestinal [GI], or urinary complaints).
• *Either* (a) symptoms not fully explained by known medical condition or by direct effects of a substance, *OR* (b) if a medical condition, physical complaints or resulting impairment is excessive.
• Symptoms cause clinically significant distress or impairment.
• Duration of at least 6 months.
• Symptoms not better accounted for by another mental disorder.
• Symptoms not intentionally produced or feigned.
• The criteria for undifferentiated somatoform disorder is less strict than the criteria for somatization disorder;

therefore, it is more likely to be seen in pediatric settings.

EPIDEMIOLOGY/ETIOLOGY

• Epidemiology and etiology are unknown; there is very little research in pediatrics.

CONVERSION DISORDER

CLINICAL FEATURES (DSM-IV DIAGNOSTIC CRITERIA)

• Symptoms or deficits affect voluntary motor or sensory function, suggesting a neurologic or other medical condition.
• Psychologic factors are associated with the symptoms or deficit. Conflicts or other stressors precede the initiation or exacerbation of symptoms or deficit.
• Symptoms or deficits are not intentionally produced or feigned.
• Symptoms can't be fully explained by a medical condition, or by direct effects of a substance, or as a culturally sanctioned behavior or experience.
• Symptoms cause significant distress or impairment in social, occupational, or other important areas of functioning.
• Symptoms not limited to pain or sexual dysfunction, and not better accounted for by another mental disorder.
• Thorough medical evaluation with no medical findings is essential for diagnosis. This is not an uncommon somatoform disorder in a pediatric setting. Common symptoms include paralysis, paresis, pseudoseizures, paresthesia, gait disturbance, and blindness. Symptoms may cause more distress for caregivers than for patient (la belle indifference).

EPIDEMIOLOGY

• Conversion disorder is more common in females. Onset of symptoms is acute. The prevalence rates range from 0.01 to 0.30%

ETIOLOGY

• Symptoms often follow a stressor (death, trauma, conflict).
• Symptoms typically remit within 2 weeks.

- Recurrence of symptoms seen in approximately 20–25% of individuals.

PAIN DISORDER

CLINICAL FEATURES (DSM-IV DIAGNOSTIC CRITERIA)

- Pain occurs in one or more sites and is of sufficient severity to warrant clinical attention.
- Pain causes significant distress or impairment in social, occupational, or other important areas of functioning.
- Psychologic factors have an important role in the onset, severity, exacerbation, or maintenance of the pain.
- Symptoms not intentionally produced or feigned.
- Pain is not better accounted for by another diagnosis.
- There are three subtypes, based on whether psychologic or medical factors are primary:
  1. *Pain disorder with psychologic factors*: Psychologic factors have a major role in onset, severity, exacerbation, or maintenance of the pain. If a medical condition exists, it does not have a major role in onset, severity, exacerbation, or maintenance. It is important to consider both severity of symptoms and functional impairment.
     a. Recurrent pain syndromes of this type typically include headaches, limb pain, or abdominal pain, persisting for more than 3 months.
     b. Recurrent abdominal pain (RAP) is the most common somatoform disorder in pediatric population. RAP peaks between 9 and 12 years of age, and occurs in girls more than boys. Children with RAP respond to daily stressors with somatic symptoms more frequently than their peers.
     c. Recurrent headaches (RHA): Recurrent headaches are not uncommon in children, with mean age of onset at 7 years of age, and frequency increasing with age. Frequency is higher among boys than girls prepuberty, but higher among girls more than boys postpuberty.
     d. *Pain disorder with both psychologic factors and general medical condition*: Both psychologic and medical factors have important roles in onset, severity, exacerbation, or maintenance of pain.
     e. *Pain disorder with general medical condition*: A medical condition has a major role in the onset, severity, exacerbation, or maintenance of pain. If psychologic factors are present, they play no major role in the pain.

EPIDEMIOLOGY

- Prevalence estimates of somatoform pain disorder are not well-established.

ETIOLOGY

- Social learning theory suggests children learn to handle emotions, behaviors, or physical discomfort and illness via observing their environment. Consequences of pain- or illness-related behavior (e.g., subtle rewards for the expression of pain, and so on) can increase or decrease the likelihood of engaging in that behavior.
- Stress and coping theories suggest that high levels of perceived stress and inadequate personal and social resources may perpetuate symptoms. Nurturance and relief from responsibilities when in the sick role may perpetuate symptoms.

EVALUATION, MANAGEMENT, AND TREATMENT OF SOMATOFORM DISORDERS

- A multidisciplinary team approach is needed. Team should consist of at least a physician and a mental health professional.
- A developmental perspective on the symptom presentation is important in a pediatric population.
- The assessment process must involve interviews with child and family designed to assess the child's overall mental health (e.g., presence of depression, and so on), and family functioning. In addition, particular attention must be paid to aspects of the symptoms and their consequences. It is important to quantify the severity, intensity, duration, and quality of the child's symptoms. Understanding the child and the symptoms from a family systems perspective is important. Each family member may have a different understanding of the child's symptoms and may respond to these symptoms differently. Helping the whole family work together may be helpful. Functional impairment should be assessed by looking at missed school, terminating or avoiding age-appropriate activities, and medication-seeking behavior.
- Treatment goals should include the following:
  1. Decreasing the frequency, intensity and duration of physical symptoms; improving the functional status of the child (e.g., go to school, play with friends, complete assigned chores); decreasing sick behaviors; decreasing time spent seeing physicians; treating any comorbid disorders.
- Overall, data beyond the level of case studies for treating somatoform disorders in children are limited. A

few studies suggest that cognitive behavior therapy (CBT) can be useful for treating abdominal pain. Other studies suggest that biofeedback and relaxation exercises can be helpful in treating headache.

- The presence of mood or anxiety disorders warrants treatment and by directly addressing these problems the patient's physical condition is likely to improve as well (i.e., the resolution of sleep continuity disorders or appetite disturbances). Children with somatoform disorders are occasionally characterized as rigid, controlling, and obsessive, signs of a possible obsessive-compulsive disorder. Psychopharmacology is an effective adjunct when treating these concomitant psychiatric disorders that contribute to the child's presentation.

REFERENCES

Somatoform Disorders

Barry J, von Baeyer CL. Brief cognitive-behavioral group treatment for children's headache. *Clin J Pain* 1997;13:215–220.

Dorn L, Campo J, Thato S, et al. Psychological comorbidity and stress reactivity in children and adolescents with recurrent abdominal pain and anxiety disorders. *J Am Acad Child Adolesc Psychiatry* 2003;42:66–75.

Egger HL, Costello EJ, Erkali A, Angold A. Somatic complaints and psychopathology in children and adolescents: Stomach aches, musculoskeletal pains, and headaches. *J Am Acad Child Adolesc Psychiatry* 1992;38:852–860.

170 DEVELOPMENTAL DISORDERS

Constance M. Weil

MENTAL RETARDATION

CLINICAL FEATURES (DSM-IV DIAGNOSTIC CRITERIA)

- DSM-IV symptoms include significantly below average intellectual functioning as measured by a standardized, individually administered intelligence test (such as the Wechsler Intelligence Scales for Children or the Stanford-Binet Intelligence Scale).
- There are concurrent deficits in adaptive functioning in at least two of the following areas: communication, self-care, home living, social/interpersonal skills, use of community resources, self-direction, functional academic skills, work, leisure, health, and safety, when compared to what is expected for the individual's age or cultural group.
- Onset occurs before 18 years of age.
- There are four different levels of severity for mental retardation (range reflects measurement error):
  1. Mild mental retardation with an IQ level of 50–55 to approximately 70
  2. Moderate mental retardation with an IQ level of 35–40 to 50–55
  3. Severe mental retardation with an IQ level of 20–25 to 35–40
  4. Profound mental retardation with an IQ level below 20–25
- Differential diagnoses include the following:
  1. The presence of a learning disorder or communication disorder in a low functioning individual for whom psychologic and speech/language assessment demonstrates the disability occurs in a specific area(s) and is not global in nature.
  2. Individuals with pervasive developmental disorder may be low functioning though there is also a qualitative impairment in the development of reciprocal social interaction and social communication skills.
  3. Borderline intellectual functioning is diagnosed in individuals with IQs in the 71–84 range.

EPIDEMIOLOGY

- Overall prevalence is 1–3% depending on the method of assessment.
- Prevalence of mild mental retardation is 0.37–0.59% (80–90% of those diagnosed with mental retardation)
- Prevalence of severe to profound retardation: 0.3–0.4% (5% of those diagnosed with mental retardation)
- The frequency of mild retardation is inversely related to socioeconomic status, while moderate-to-severe disability occurs with equal frequency across all income groups.

ETIOLOGY

- Mental retardation can be caused by a variety of conditions that affect brain development before, during, or after birth, or in the early childhood years. Hundreds of causes have been identified and generally fall into the following categories:
- Genetic conditions (e.g., Down syndrome, Fragile X)
  1. Problems during pregnancy (maternal use of alcohol and drugs, malnutrition, environmental

toxins, illnesses such as cytomegalovirus [CMV], toxoplasmosis, rubella, and syphilis)

2. Problems at birth (birth asphyxia)
3. Problems after birth (lead or mercury poisoning, meningitis, traumatic brain injury); poverty and cultural deprivation (malnutrition, inadequate medical care and environmental health hazards, and understimulation).

- Despite the many possible causes of mental retardation, no cause for the disability can be identified in approximately one-third of all cases.

PROGNOSIS

- The developmental course depends on the severity of the retardation, the presence and type of associated disabilities and disorders, and environmental factors such as the quality and availability of education and treatment.
- Most individuals with mental retardation acquire new skills and continue to learn throughout their lifetimes though they may experience occasional plateaus in their progress.
- While it is difficult to make accurate prognoses, children with relatively mild retardation who receive appropriate services can achieve fourth- to sixth-grade reading levels and may function relatively independently as adults. Individuals with more significant intellectual impairment require greater degrees of supervision, depending on their levels of adaptive functioning.

EVALUATION, MANAGEMENT, AND TREATMENT

- The initial phase of the assessment includes a formal assessment of the individual's intellectual and adaptive skills. Intellectual functioning is assessed via individual testing with a standardized IQ (e.g., Stanford-Binet Test of Intelligence; Wechsler Intelligence Scale for Children, 3rd ed.)
- Adaptive functioning is assessed with a standardized interview for adaptive behavior (such as the Vineland Adaptive Behavior Scales and the Woodcock Johnson Scales of Independent Behavior) history, and behavioral observations.
- A psychiatric assessment is completed in order to determine an individual's strengths and weaknesses in the psychologic-emotional domain and to determine if there are any comorbid psychiatric diagnoses.
- A thorough medical assessment is important in helping to determine the etiology of the mental retardation and to identify possible comorbid medical conditions which require treatment (e.g., phenylketonuria [PKU], seizures, cerebral palsy, sensory

impairments). The medical assessment should include a complete history and relevant diagnostic studies.

- The individual's environment and support system is also assessed to determine the need for modification or alternative placement.
- There is no specific treatment of the actual mental retardation though interventions for individuals with mental retardation are designed to maximize the individual's abilities. They include educational, habilitative, and supportive approaches, depending on the individual's needs. Goals for intervention are based on the *normalization principle* (having individuals with mental retardation live everyday lives as close to the norms of mainstream society as possible) and the *right to community living* (with family if possible or in an adapted setting within the community).
- Interventions may also include treatment for the underlying conditions that have caused the mental retardation or for any comorbid medical or psychiatric concerns.
- Psychiatric interventions with individuals who have mental retardation may include behavior modification to address such issues as self-injurious behavior, stereotyped behaviors, aggression and other conduct difficulties, and acquisition of self-help skills, social skills, and community living skills. Individual and group psychotherapy are also used though the techniques and the therapist have to adapt to the developmental needs of the patient, and empirical support for their use is lacking.
- Psychotropic medication can also be used to address issues of anxiety, depression, extreme aggressive behavior, and attention deficit hyperactivity disorder (ADHD).

LEARNING DISABILITIES

CLINICAL FEATURES

CRITERIA FOR DIAGNOSIS VARY BY WHICH GROUP ESTABLISHES THOSE CRITERIA
- According to DSM-IV criteria:
  1. A learning disorder is diagnosed when an individual's achievement on a standardized test in reading, writing, or mathematics is substantially below (usually two or more standard deviations below the mean) what is expected based on his/her age, IQ, and schooling.
  2. The learning problems must significantly interfere with academic achievement or daily living that require reading, writing, or math skills.

- The Individuals with Disabilities Education Act describes a specific learning disability as a disorder in one or more of the basic psychologic processes involved in understanding or in using spoken or written language, which may be seen as an imperfect ability to think, speak, read, write, spell, or do mathematical calculations.
- Educational criteria for classification as learning disabled specify a disorder in one or more of the basic psychologic processes required for learning, evidence of academic achievement significantly below the student's level of intellectual function, and evidence that the learning problems are not due primarily to other handicapping conditions and that general education has failed to meet the student's educational needs.
- The DSM-IV-based specific learning disorders include reading disorder, mathematics disorder, and disorder of written expression, as well as learning disorder NOS (not otherwise specified).
- A reading disorder is characterized by reading achievement, including reading fluency, speed, or comprehension, falling below expected levels as described above.
- A mathematics disorder involves substantial delays in mathematical calculation or reasoning skills.
- A disorder of written expression involves substantial delays related to grammar, punctuation errors, poor paragraph organization, multiple spelling errors, and excessively poor handwriting.
- Learning disorder NOS includes learning disorders that do not meet the criteria for another specific learning disorder.
- Differential diagnoses include learning problems caused by sensory deficits such as hearing or vision impairments, lack of opportunity, poor teaching, or cultural factors. Mental retardation, pervasive developmental disorder, or communication disorders must be ruled out.

EPIDEMIOLOGY

- Prevalence is difficult to determine due to differences in the definition of learning disorder that is applied.
- It is estimated that learning disorders affect 2–10% of the population with boys outnumbering girls by 3 or 4:1.
- Reading disorders affect approximately 4% of all school-age children while mathematics disorders affect approximately 1% of these children.
- It is not clear how many children experience disorders of written expression.
- Emotional and behavioral disorders, including ADHD, social problems, and Tourette syndrome are commonly associated with learning disorders.

ETIOLOGY

- Various causes have been identified for learning disorders including genetics (40–50% of children have family members with learning disorders), and central nervous system (CNS) damage due to various prenatal, perinatal, and postnatal factors such as trauma, asphyxia, fever, toxins, and metabolic disorders.

PROGNOSIS

- Learning disorders are not cured but are compensated for.
- An individual's progress will depend on the cause of the disability and the severity of the disability as well as the quality of the intervention.

EVALUATION, MANAGEMENT, AND TREATMENT

- Assessment involves psychoeducational testing to determine the individual's level of cognitive functioning and level of achievement. Each individual should also have a psychiatric/psychologic assessment of emotional, behavioral, social and family issues, and mental status. Finally, a medical assessment is needed to evaluate sensory functioning and rule out physiologic disorders that may cause learning disorders.
- Treatment of learning disorders consists of educational interventions designed to remediate or compensate for learning disorders using a multisensory approach to build up strengths and compensate for weaknesses. Interventions also include adapting classroom, curriculum, and teaching style. These interventions should take place in as close to a regular classroom setting as possible.
- Specific reading intervention may focus on decoding and comprehension. Math interventions may focus on conceptual underpinnings, procedural learning, recall of discrete information, self-monitoring, and spatial perception. Interventions for written expression may take on both a skills approach and a holistic approach, focusing on letter-sound association, the relationship between sentences and paragraphs, narrowing down ideas, writing a first draft, reading it aloud, refining organization and language, and working on mechanics for the final draft.
- Additional treatment may include psychotherapy to address problems with social skills, poor self-image, low self-esteem, anxiety, depression, or disruptive behavior. No randomized trials have been located confirming the effectiveness of interventions for these

problems specifically with learning disabled children. Finally, treatment should also include education of the individual and the family regarding the impact of the learning disorder on the functioning of the individual. No medications have been identified as effective in the treatment of learning disorders.

COMMUNICATION DISORDERS

CLINICAL FEATURES

- Expressive language disorder involves impairment in expressive language development as demonstrated by scores on standardized measures of expressive language development substantially below those obtained from standardized measures of both nonverbal intelligence and receptive language development. Language difficulties interfere with academic or occupational achievement or with social communication. If mental retardation, a speech-motor, sensory, or environmental deficit is present, the language difficulties are in excess of those usually associated with these problems.
- A mixed receptive-expressive language disorder involves scores on standardized measures of receptive and expressive language are substantially below those obtained on measures of nonverbal intelligence. Symptoms include those noted for expressive language disorder and also difficulty understanding words, sentences, or specific types of words, such as spatial terms.
- A phonologic disorder refers to the failure to use developmentally expected speech sounds that are appropriate for age and dialect. The difficulties in speech sound production interfere with academic or occupational achievement or with social communication. If mental retardation, a speech-motor or sensory deficit, or environmental deprivation is present, the speech difficulties are in excess of what would be expected for these problems.
- Stuttering is a disturbance in the normal fluency and time patterning of speech which interferes with academic or occupational achievement or with social communication and is in excess of what would be expected if an individual has a speech-motor or sensory deficit.
- Communication disorder not otherwise specified refers to disorders of communication that do not meet criteria for any specific communication disorder.
- Differential diagnosis includes autistic disorder, mental retardation, sensory deficit, speech-motor deficit, severe environmental deprivation, and a specific learning disorder
- Among the observed comorbidities, phonologic disorder and some types of learning disorders are often seen in conjunction with diagnoses of expressive and

mixed receptive-expressive language disorders. An individual may also exhibit motor delays, coordination disorders, and enuresis. ADHD has also been diagnosed in as many as 16% of children with some type of communication disorder. Central auditory processing difficulties have been associated with communication disorders and ADHD. Finally, various psychiatric disorders, such as adjustment disorders may co-occur with communication disorders.

EPIDEMIOLOGY

- The prevalence of expressive language disorder is 3–5%; mixed receptive-expressive language disorder, 3%; phonologic disorder 2–3% in 6–7-year-old children, falling to 0.5% by age 17 years; stuttering, 1% in children 10 years of age and younger, falling to 0.8% in later adolescence.
- The ratio of male to female is 3:1.

ETIOLOGY

- The majority of evidence indicates that the most children with communication disorders do not show evidence of specific CNS damage; however, there are often numerous soft signs and dominance problems in these individuals.
- In a minority of individuals, localizable brain damage is noted from infection, trauma, vascular disease, perinatal factors including prematurity, low birth weight, asphyxia, and toxins such as prenatal alcohol exposure.
- Communication disorders can be related to various processing deficits in the reception, acquisition, processing, storage, or recall of different elements of communication. Environmental factors such as inadequate or pathologic parent-child interaction have been associated with rate of language acquisition although not so clearly to eventual outcome.
- Other socioeconomic status (SES) factors like class, family size, income, and birth order affect the amount of verbal interaction in a family.
- Genetic factors, recurrent otitis media, and perceptual deficits can also lead to communication disorders.

PROGNOSIS

- For individuals with an expressive language disorder, 50% eventually attain normal communication skills.
- A minority of individuals with mixed receptive-expressive language disorders are free of problems in

adulthood; even when communication skills seem basically normal, subtle deficits may persist.
- Mild cases of phonologic disorder often recover spontaneously; the majority of cases resolve completely over time. Severe cases of phonologic disorder are associated with anatomic malformations and may require surgical correction.
- Stuttering can wax and wane in early childhood, but by early adolescence it abates in 20% of the cases and close or total remission is seen in 60–80% of cases, typically by age 16 years.

EVALUATION, MANAGEMENT, AND TREATMENT

- Assessment of communication disorders includes a medical interview and examination, hearing and vision assessments, standardized intellectual and achievement testing, and a complete standardized speech and language evaluation.
- Treatment consists primarily of speech-language therapy which can usually begin by age 3. Group treatment is often used for the development of language in social contexts. Treatment usually has three goals: the development and improvement of communication skill with concurrent remediation of deficits, the development of alternative or augmented communication strategies when required, and the social habilitation of the individual in regard to communication.

REFERENCE

Developmental Disorders
American Academy of Child and Adolescent Psychiatry: Practice parameters for the assessment and treatment of children and adolescents with language and learning disorders. *J Am Acad Child Adolesc Psychiatry* 1998;37 (suppl): 46S–62S.

171 PERVASIVE DEVELOPMENTAL DISORDERS
Kathleen McKenna

- Children with pervasive developmental disorders have severe and pervasive problems in a variety of areas such as social interaction, communication, and behavioral flexibility. Five types of pervasive developmental disorders are described in the DSM-IV: autistic disorder, Asperger disorder, Rett disorder, childhood disintegrative disorder, and pervasive developmental disorder not otherwise specified. The section will deal with autistic disorder, Asperger disorder and pervasive developmental disorder, most common of the pervasive developmental disorders.

AUTISTIC DISORDER

CLINICAL FEATURES (DSM-IV)

- A qualitative impairment in *social interaction*.
  1. Lack of nonverbal behaviors such as eye contact, facial expressions, and gestures in communication
  2. Failure to develop age-appropriate peer relationships
  3. Lack spontaneous sharing of interests or achievements
  4. Lack of social or emotional reciprocity
- Qualitative impairments in *communication*.
  1. Poor language development without attempts to communicate in nonverbal manner such as gesture
  2. Poor ability to sustain conversation if language is present
  3. Stereotyped, repetitive, idiosyncratic language
  4. Lack of varied, spontaneous make-believe play
- Restricted, repetitive, stereotyped patterns of *behavior, interests, and activities*.
  1. Preoccupation with interests that may be abnormal because of the oddness of the interest (e.g., mechanical springs) or the intensity (e.g., constant focus on weather information)
  2. Attachment to routines or rituals
  3. Stereotyped and repetitive motor mannerisms such as flapping hands
  4. Persistent preoccupation with parts of objects such as the wheels of a toy car
- Some children with autistic disorder appear to develop normally until around 18 months of age when they develop autistic symptoms. Others seem to have had communication, social, and regulation problems since early infancy. The "CHAT" or Checklist for Autism in Toddlers, may be used as a quick screen for autism during the 18 month pediatric visit.
- Many children with autistic disorder may also have sleep problems, be picky about what foods they will eat, or engage in aggressive behaviors such as head banging, biting, or hitting. Many also have sensory problems such as hyperreactivity to loud noises or distress at certain tactile input such as the feeling of labels in clothes. They often enjoy deep pressure rather than light touch. About 75% of children with autism will also have

mental retardation. Seizures may occur, especially after puberty.

- DSM-IV criteria require that the onset of symptoms be before 3 years.

DIFFERENTIAL DIAGNOSIS

- Deafness, severe psychosocial neglect, metabolic abnormalities, genetic abnormalities such as Fragile X syndrome, mental retardation, other pervasive developmental disorders, stereotypic disorder, and language disorders.
- The diagnosis of autistic disorder requires impairments in all three categories. It is important to remember that symptoms such as language delay, motor stereotypies, hypersensitivity to sensory input, and so on, occur in children without autistic disorder.

EPIDEMIOLOGY

- Autism may occur in mild-to-severe forms. If even the mildest forms are included, some studies estimate the prevalence to be as high as 1/500. Boys are affected four to five times as frequently as girls.

PATHOPHYSIOLOGY

- Autistic disorder is highly genetic and believed to result from interaction of several genes. If a monozygotic twin is affected, the other twin nearly always has at least some autistic symptomatology. There is an increased risk of autistic disorder in siblings. Recent studies suggest that there may be an initial overproduction of synapses followed by a too-aggressive pruning of excess synapses in the brain, although further studies are needed to confirm these findings. Brain imaging is usually normal.

PROGNOSIS

- Outcomes for children with autistic disorder are best for those who develop usable language, have higher cognitive ability, and who do not have significant behavior problems. Most people with autistic disorder will need support in living and employment as adults.

TREATMENT

- Pharmacotherapy is sometimes used to treat aggression, stereotypic behaviors, sleep problems, or emotional dysregulation that may accompany autistic disorder.

Medications such as clonidine and guanfacine are used although there is little research to support their use. Risperidone has been shown to decrease some behavioral problems such as aggression or stereotypies but side effects are common.

- Children with autistic disorder need speech and language services as well as help learning how to understand social interactions and how to interact with others. Older children may be referred to social skills groups. Speech therapy is usually indicated. Behavior treatments such as applied behavior analysis have been helpful to encourage appropriate behaviors and limit maladaptive ones. At this time there is no evidence that specific diets, eye training, megavitamins, or holding techniques are helpful in the treatment of autistic disorder. Several large epidemiologic studies have demonstrated no association between vaccines (with or without mercury compounds) commonly given at 18 months and the onset of autistic disorder.
- Family members of children with autistic disorder usually need much support and may benefit from respite services.

ASPERGER DISORDER

CLINICAL FEATURES DSM-IV CRITERIA INCLUDE

- Qualitative impairment in *social interaction* as in autistic disorder.
- Restricted, repetitive, stereotyped patterns of *behavior, interests and activities* as in autistic disorder
- There is no clinically significant delay in language and the child must have normal cognitive abilities and adaptive functioning. Often the child may accumulate a large amount of information in one favorite area and may engage in monologues about the favorite topic.

DIFFERENTIAL DIAGNOSIS

- Nonverbal learning disability, social phobia, schizoid personality disorder, and obsessive-compulsive disorder

EPIDEMIOLOGY

- It is not clear whether Asperger disorder is simply high-functioning autism. It tends to be more common in males but there is no reliable information on prevalence.

PATHOPHYSIOLOGY

- Asperger disorder is more common in family members of those who have the disorder.

PROGNOSIS

- Some individuals with Asperger disorder can live fairly normal lives, especially if they have social supports and are guided into jobs or careers that capitalize on their strengths and do not require complex social interactions. Others will need more support during adulthood.

TREATMENT

- Because of their higher intellectual functioning and ability to assess their situation, people with Asperger disorder often experience great distress at their difficulties in social interactions. Some may develop depression that may be treated with antidepressants. Neuroleptics may sometimes help stereotypic behaviors. Sometimes selective serotonin reuptake inhibitors are used to help with obsessionality.
- Individual therapy may be helpful to enable the child to process social experiences and develop more satisfying social interactions. Family members, coaches, and teachers may need help understanding that the child's maladaptive behaviors stem from Asperger disorder and are not usually deliberate misbehavior. Children may need help dealing with peers who may exploit them or bully them and often profit from social skills groups or supervised recreational opportunities in which they are assisted with social interaction .

PERVASIVE DEVELOPMENTAL DISORDER NOT OTHERWISE SPECIFIED

- This category is used when some of the criteria for autistic disorder are present but full criteria are not met or the presentation is atypical. There is little research on this category.

REFERENCES

Pervasive Development Disorders References

Baron-Cohen S, Gillberg C. Can autism be detected at 18 months? The needle, the haystack, and the CHAT. *Br J Psychiat* 1992;161:839–843.

McCracken, JR, McGough J, Shah B. Risperidone in children with autism and serious behavioral problems. *N Engl J Med* 2002;347:314–21.

Committee on Children with Disabilities Technical Report: The Pediatrician's Role in the Diagnosis and Management of Autistic Spectrum Disorder in Children. *Pediatrics* 2001:107: E85 (*www.pediatrics.org/cgi/content/full/107/5/e85*)

Offit P, Coffin S. Communicating science to the public: MMR vaccine and autism. *Vaccine* 2003:22;1–6.

172 ATTENTION DEFICIT HYPERACTIVITY DISORDER

John V. Lavigne

CLINICAL FEATURES (DSM-IV DIAGNOSTIC CRITERIA)

- Three DSM-IV subtypes
  1. *Attention deficit hyperactivity disorder (ADHD), predominantly inattentive type*: The inattentive subtype is characterized by (at least six of the following):
     a. Inattentiveness
     b. Difficulties ignoring distractions at the level expected for the child's age and developmental level
     c. Failure to attend to details
     d. Making careless mistakes in schoolwork, not listening even when spoken to directly
     e. Not finishing schoolwork or chores (even when seemingly willing to comply).
  2. Attention deficit hyperactivity disorder, predominantly hyperactive-impulsive type: This subtype is characterized by (at least six of the following):
     a. Fidgetiness
     b. Leaving the seat in class without permission
     c. Running or climbing excessively when inappropriate
     d. Being "on the go" or driven by a motor
     e. Talking excessively.
  3. *Attention deficit hyperactivity disorder, combined type*: The combined type includes significant features of both other subtypes.
- To meet diagnostic criteria, some symptoms must be present before the age of 7 years. Symptoms must be present in two or more settings (e.g., school, home), have persisted at least 6 months, and must cause some impairment. Factors such as intelligence and family/social environment can influence the degree of symptomatic impairment.

DIFFERENTIAL DIAGNOSIS

- Psychiatric: In making a differential diagnosis, the symptoms must not be due to pervasive developmental disorder, schizophrenia, a mood or anxiety disorder, a dissociative disorder, or a personality disorder. There are high rates of comorbidity between attention-deficit disorders and other disorders, such as oppositional defiant disorder.
- Neurologic: Possible neurologic causes of dysfunction of the frontal-subcortical system should be excluded including encephalitis (history of fevers, sleepiness, change in personality) and epilepsy (episodes of unresponsiveness/staring, postictal periods), progressive neurodegenerative diseases (changes/deterioration in cognition or neuro examination over time), focal brain lesion/injury, perinatal encephalopathy, Fragile X syndrome (dysmorphic features), restless legs syndrome, and other psychiatric disease (such as major depression, anxiety, bipolar disorder, early schizophrenia). Screening for these problems can be done in the primary care setting and does not require a referral to neurology.

EPIDEMIOLOGY

- Conservatively, prevalence rates are estimated at 3–5% in various surveys, with some studies showing higher rates.
- The boy:girl ratio is 4:1 in community surveys.

ETIOLOGY

- There appears to be a substantial genetic contribution: heritability of activity level is very high (80% in one study); no single gene or specific transmission mechanism has been substantiated. Inheritance is probably polygenic. About 25% of children with ADHD have parents that meet diagnostic criteria for ADHD.
- Only a small proportion of children with ADHD have a clear medical cause. Soft signs are present at higher rates, but are not clinically helpful in diagnosis.

PROGNOSIS

- Once believed to end in adolescence, ADHD is now known to be lifelong. Hyperactivity symptoms may diminish, but problems with inattention, distractibility, and so on, persist in as many as 50% of children. Increased rates of school problems, incarcerations, and mental health problems are present compared to children without ADHD. When ADHD is comorbid with conduct disorder, more substance abuse and antisocial behavior are present.

EVALUATION, MANAGEMENT, AND TREATMENT

- A parent interview and parent and teacher questionnaires about ADHD are critical for assessment.
- A child interview is needed, but is often more helpful for assessing comorbidities (e.g., child-reported depression).
- A physical examination is useful for assessing overall health
  1. An electroencephalogram (EEG) and brain scan are only needed where the child is positive for focal neurologic signs, or there are clinical indications of seizures.
  2. A baseline electrocardiogram (ECG) is only needed if tricyclic antidepressants or clonidine are to be used.
  3. Psychologic testing is not needed to assess ADHD, but may help if learning disabilities are suspected. False positives on continuous performance tests are too high to warrant their use in diagnoses.
- Psychostimulants are most useful for treating core symptoms of inattention, activity level, and impulsivity, with at least 100 double-blind studies supporting their use. Ninety percent of children respond to either the first or second psychostimulant tried. If multiple psychostimulants are unsuccessful, antidepressants and alpha-adrenergics can be tried.
- Ongoing monitoring of symptoms at school and home is critical to successful management
- Randomized trials suggest that behavior therapies are less effective for treating core symptoms, but can be useful for other symptoms and symptoms of comorbidities. Dietary changes have not proved to be useful; other forms of psychotherapy lack more than rudimentary support (one or fewer randomized trials), or none at all.

REFERENCES

ADHD

American Academy of Child and Adolescent Psychiatry. Assessment and treatment of children, adolescents, and adults with attention-deficit/hyperactivity disorder. *J Am Acad Child Adolesc Psychiatry* 1997;36:85S–121S.

MTA Cooperative Group. A 14-month randomized clinical trial of treatment strategies for attention-deficit/hyperactivity disorder. *Arch Gen Psychiatry* 1999;56:1073–1086.

National Institutes of Health Consensus Development Conference Statement. Diagnosis and treatment of attention-deficit/hyperactivity disorder (ADHD). *J Am Acad Child Adolesc Psychiatry* 2000;39:182–193.

American Academy of Child and Adolescent Psychiatry. Practice parameters for the assessment and treatment of attention-deficit/hyperactivity disorder. *J Am Acad Child Adolesc Psychiatry* 1997;36:85S–121S.

American Academy of Child and Adolescent Psychiatry. Practice parameters for the use of stimulant medications in the treatment of children, adolescents and adults. *J Am Acad Child Adolesc Psychiatry* 2000;41:26S–49S.

173 OPPOSITIONAL DEFIANT DISORDER

John V. Lavigne

CLINICAL FEATURES (DSM-IV DIAGNOSTIC CRITERIA)

- Oppositional defiant disorder (ODD) is characterized by negative, defiant, hostile behavior lasting 6 months or longer, with at least four of the following symptoms occurring often or very often:
- Loses his/her temper
- Argues with adults
- Actively defies or refuses to comply with adult requests or rules
- Deliberately annoys people
- Blames others for his/her mistakes or misbehavior
- Is often touchy or easily annoyed by others
- Is angry and resentful
- Is spiteful or vindictive
- To be considered to have ODD, the child must engage in those behaviors at rates higher than expected for children of similar developmental levels, and the problem must result in significant impairment in academic, social, or (later) occupational functioning.

EPIDEMIOLOGY

- ODD is one of the most common psychiatric disorders of childhood. In preschoolers, rates can be as high as 15% (with 9%, severe); at older ages rates vary from 3 to 10%. Prevalence is higher in boys.

ETIOLOGY

- Temperamental factors including temperamental intensity, activity, and persistence have been associated with ODD onset, as have inconsistent parenting practices.

PROGNOSIS

- Stability among preschoolers with ODD symptoms is about 50% after 1 year, and about 67% if the disorder is present for 2 consecutive years. Five-year stability among young children with the disorder is about 30%.
- It is common for young children with persistent ODD to develop comorbid symptoms in the early school years, including attention deficit hyperactivity disorder (ADHD), depression, and anxiety problems comorbid with ODD. Some children with ODD symptoms in early grammar school years begin to display symptoms of conduct disorder, with covert (e.g., lying) symptoms developing initially, followed by more overt, antisocial (e.g., aggression) symptoms thereafter.

EVALUATION, MANAGEMENT, AND TREATMENT

- A careful interview with the parents to ascertain the presence of symptoms is critical for confirming the condition; often school reports are useful to supplement parental reports.
- Parent, school reports, and a child interview are needed to assess the presence of comorbidities or other conditions that could supersede the ODD diagnosis (e.g., separation anxiety disorder, psychosis).
- Numerous randomized clinical trials have demonstrated the efficacy of parent training in behavior modification procedures (e.g., use of praise, parental attention, shaping of more complex desired responses, and rewards for desirable behavior; time out and other mild punishments for undesirable behavior). The best available evidence suggests similar procedures can be used with older children when employed in a developmentally appropriate way, but fewer studies have been conducted for ODD with the older age group. No psychopharmacologic interventions are available for the treatment of the ODD symptoms per se; however, symptoms of concomitant psychiatric disorders can be addressed with medications and improve the likelihood of treatment success.

174 **CONDUCT DISORDER**

Heather J. Walter

CLINICAL FEATURES (DSM-IV DIAGNOSTIC CRITERIA)

- The essential feature of conduct disorder is a persistent pattern of behavior in which the rights of individuals or the rules of society are violated.
- The symptoms of conduct disorder comprise four main categories of behavior: aggression (e.g., physical fighting, use of weapons, stealing with confrontation, coerced sexual activity), destructiveness (e.g., fire setting, property destruction), deceitfulness/theft (e.g., lying, covert stealing), and rule violation (e.g., violating curfew, running away from home, truancy).
- Diagnosis of the disorder requires that three or more symptoms have been present in the past year (and one or more in the past 6 months), and the symptoms cause significant impairment in functioning.
- Major psychiatric comorbidities of conduct disorder include attention, anxiety, mood, somatoform, substance use, learning, and language disorders.

EPIDEMIOLOGY

- The prevalence of conduct disorder is estimated at 4–16% among males and 1–9% among females. The prevalence is higher in lower socioeconomic areas.

ETIOLOGY

- The etiology of conduct disorder is multifactorial, comprising child, parent, and social factors.
- Child factors include adverse prenatal and perinatal events, difficult temperament, insecure or disorganized attachment, cognitive or linguistic impairment, and impaired behavioral inhibition mediated by the central and autonomic nervous systems.
- Parent factors include hostile or neglectful parent-child relationships, harsh and inconsistent discipline, parental psychopathology, physical or sexual abuse, and marital discord. Social factors include public housing, community disintegration, and exposure to antisocial adults and peers, violence, and multiple severe stressors.

PROGNOSIS

- Predictors of poor prognosis are early onset (before age 10), severe symptoms, concurrent attention deficit hyperactivity disorder, history of oppositional defiant disorder, overt symptoms (especially predatory aggression), age- or gender-atypical symptoms, and psychopathic character traits (e.g., callous, manipulative, irresponsible).
- It has been estimated that 40% of youths with conduct disorder progress to antisocial personality disorder in adulthood. Only 20% are estimated to live adult lives free from significant impairment.

EVALUATION, MANAGEMENT, AND TREATMENT

- Evaluation should include interviews with the parent, child, and collateral informants (e.g., teachers, caregivers) and are essential for diagnosis. Standardized rating scales can be helpful.
- Specialized evaluations (e.g., psychoeducational, speech/language, neuropsychologic) are important to identify comorbid cognitive or linguistic impairments.
- The treatment of conduct disorder must be comprehensive, reflecting the multifactorial etiology of the disorder. In general, treatments that address the total life circumstances of the child are the most likely to produce lasting effects. Recommended treatment components include child, parent, and social interventions. Child interventions include identification and remediation of learning and language disorders, identification and treatment of other comorbid disorders, medication (for aggression), and therapy. Parent interventions include parenting training, identification and treatment of parental psychopathology, and marital and family therapy. Social interventions include exposure to prosocial peers, relocation to acceptable housing and schools, strengthened religious affiliation (if applicable), and increased social support. Multisystemic therapy (MST) is an example of a multicomponent treatment that has been shown to be effective for conduct disorder. MST involves individual, family, group, marital, and recreational therapies as well as coordination of the interventions of multiple systems (i.e., education, health, social services, juvenile justice). The medications with at least some empirical evidence of effectiveness for the treatment of the aggressive component of conduct disorder include stimulants, selective serotonin reuptake inhibitors, alpha-adrenergic agonists, beta-blockers, atypical neuroleptics, and mood stabilizers.
- In intractable cases, juvenile justice interventions may be needed to require compliance with treatment, drug screens, curfew, and attendance at school; forbid association with antisocial peers; and impose detention if indicated.

REFERENCES

Conduct Disorders

American Academy of Child and Adolescent Psychiatry. Practice parameters for the assessment and treatment of children and adolescents with conduct disorder. *J Am Acad Child Adolesc Psychiatry* 1997;36:122S–139S.

Brestan EV, Eyberg SM. Effective psychosocial treatment of conduct-disordered children and adolescents: 20 years, 82 studies, and 5272 kids. *J Clin Child Psychol* 1998;27:180–189.

Burke JD, Loeber R, Birmaher B. Oppositional defiant disorder and conduct disorder: a review of the past 10 years, Part II. *J Am Acad Child Adolesc Psychiatry* 2002;41:1275–1293.

Loeber R, Burke JD, Lahey BB, Winters A, Zera M. Oppositional defiant disorder and conduct disorder: review of the past 10 years, Part I. *J Am Acad Child Adolesc Psychiatry* 2000;39:1468–1484.

175 ANXIETY DISORDERS

Jonathan M. Pochyly and
D. Richard Martini

CLINICAL FEATURES (DSM-IV DIAGNOSTIC CRITERIA)

- The DSM-IV defines nine different subtypes of anxiety disorders. The most common anxiety disorders identified in children are social phobia, separation anxiety, and generalized anxiety disorder.
- *Social phobia* is marked by anxiety in social situations that presents as in excess of what might be considered normal for the given situation. Typically the child or adolescent is experiencing fears or concerns about embarrassment or others thinking negatively about them.
- *Separation anxiety* is characterized by excessive anxiety around being separated from parents, family, or home. There is often a specific fear that some tragedy or harm will befall their loved ones during the separation. The child may become clingy, tearful, aggressive, tantrum or report somatic complaints when faced with a separation or the anticipation of being separated from caregivers. Separation anxiety is most common in younger children and uncommon in adolescents and is found in about 4% of children; however, to accurately diagnose the disorder it is important to assess whether or not the amount of distress experienced by the child is excessive for the child's developmental level.

- *Generalized anxiety disorder* is marked by a pattern of excessive worrying. The source of the anxious thoughts can vary and is often traced to a number of areas of the individual's life. Some of the more typical sources for anxiety include performance in school or social situations, acceptance by peers, approval of teachers or parents, and health of self or family members. Generalized anxiety disorder is accompanied by unrealistic or irrational thoughts. These thoughts tend to be extremely negativistic and represent an exaggerated belief that things will go wrong and the results will be catastrophic.
- *Specific phobia* is an irrational or exaggerated fear of particular situations or objects. Children with specific phobias demonstrate distress and avoidance of the situation or object in a way that is in excess of what would be expected for their developmental level. When confronted with the situation or, at times, the anticipation of the situation, the child can become avoidant and this may prove to be disruptive to the child's normal routine. A normal fear becomes a specific phobia when the avoidance and anxiety are in excess of normal response for their age and this interferes significantly with the child's functioning or development.
- *Posttraumatic stress disorder* (PTSD) is the emotional and behavioral manifestation of direct or observed exposure to a traumatic event. The principal symptoms are reexperiencing the event, avoidance of reminders, generalized emotional numbing, and increased arousal. Reexperiencing appears in the form of nightmares, daydreams, or repetitive and dangerous reenactment in play or other behaviors. Increased arousal is evident when there are sleep disturbances, somatic symptoms, and emotional regression. Children feel guilty about the trauma and may distort information to assume more individual responsibility. Emotional numbing is reported through constricted affect and a diminished interest in activities. The unique symptoms in children include fear of separation from parents, fear of serious injury and death, and withdrawal from new experiences. Perceptual distortions in time and space are difficult to detect in a pediatric population but can also present with auditory, touch, and olfactory misperceptions.
- *Acute stress disorder* is characterized by dissociative and anxiety symptoms that occur within 1 month of experiencing a traumatic event and last no longer than 1 month following the event. The dissociative experience is marked by a sense of numbing, feeling detached or unable to respond emotionally, reduced awareness of their surroundings, or feeling detached from their bodies. The child will also demonstrate an avoidance of situations or objects that prompt a recall of the traumatic event.
- Children with *panic disorder* experience excessive anxiety in the form of panic attacks. These attacks are

intense episodes of fear or agitation that are accompanied by physiologic symptoms such as including shortness of breath, palpitations, chest pain, paresthesias, trembling, dizziness, tachycardia, sweating, and hyperventilation. The worries and fears associated with panic attacks are generated by these physical symptoms and concerns about what is happening to their body. The individual often becomes avoidant of situations that become associated with the panic attacks. While children may experience some of the physiologic signs of panic attacks, panic disorder is predominant in adolescents. Although cognitive immaturity prevents the recurrent thoughts characteristic of panic in adults (fear of dying, feeling out of control), there is continuity between symptoms experienced in childhood and adult presentations. Panic disorder and agoraphobia are rare in children but more common in adolescents.

- *Obsessive-compulsive disorder* (OCD) in children is marked by the presence of persistent obsessions and compulsions. Obsessions are recurrent thoughts or urges that are disruptive and intrusive. It is the obsessive thoughts that prompt the compulsive behaviors that are then performed in an effort to avoid some negative outcome. An example of a more common compulsive tendency is hand washing, which is repeated with excessive frequency in response to an obsessive fear of contamination.
- While not listed as a specific diagnosis in DSM-IV, school refusal or school avoidance is a condition that is often anxiety-based. Anxiety around attending school can be rooted in a number of different anxiety disorders, but is most commonly associated with either separation anxiety or a phobic disorder.
- Children with depression are three to four times more likely to have or develop an anxiety disorder than those without depression. Anxiety disorders are two to three times more likely in children with oppositional defiant disorder or conduct disorder. While the presence of a comorbid attention deficit hyperactivity disorder (ADHD) in children with anxiety occurs more frequently than could be explained by chance, there does not appear to be a significant increase in the likelihood of anxiety disorders in children with ADHD.

EPIDEMIOLOGY

- Large-scale epidemiologic studies suggest that anxiety disorders are among the most common forms of child and adolescent psychopathology. Studies suggest that more than 8% of children and adolescents meet criterion for at least one form of anxiety disorder.

- The prevalence of OCD is approximately 3–4% in the pediatric population. Prevalence for most subtypes of anxiety disorders, like panic and PTSD, are not known.
- When looking at anxiety disorders collectively, studies suggest that these disorders are more common in girls than boys; however, these differences are not sustained when looking at specific diagnoses independently.

ETIOLOGY

- Anxiety disorders are more common in children of adults with anxiety disorders and many anxious adults have reported that their problems with anxiety began when they were children.
- There have been a number of studies linking various environmental factors to anxiety disorders. These factors have included parental emotional problems, stressful life events, school difficulties, and socioeconomic status; however, the impact of these factors across type of anxiety disorder and age of child is variable.

PATHOPHYSIOLOGY

- The etiology of OCD, in particular, is found in several neuropsychiatric hypotheses. The "serotonin hypothesis" follows the success of serotonin reuptake inhibitors in the treatment of the disorder. OCD runs in families, supporting a possible genetic link. Neuroendocrine and neurotransmitter function is implicated in the development of the disorder. The basal ganglia may be the origin of OCD behaviors as evident in Sydenham chorea secondary to group A beta-hemolytic streptococcal infection. The exacerbation of OCD symptoms may follow streptococcal infection without neurologic sequelae.

PROGNOSIS

- Longitudinal studies suggest that as many as half of the children with anxiety disorders will meet the criterion for an anxiety disorder several years later.
- While the majority of children with anxiety disorders remit within 1 year, the earlier the age of onset the more time it takes for the child to recover.
- The presence of an anxiety disorder in childhood is more predictive of an adolescent anxiety disorder for girls than for boys.
- Children with anxiety disorders are at increased risk to develop new psychiatric disorders or other anxiety disorders even years following the onset of the initial disorder.

EVALUATION, MANAGEMENT, AND TREATMENT

- The evaluation process should include a comprehensive history from patient and parents that includes medical, developmental, school, social, and family history.
- The psychologic treatment of childhood anxiety disorders includes therapeutic interventions to target both behavior and cognition in the form of cognitive-behavioral therapy (CBT). Cognitive-behavioral therapy is indicated as the first line treatment for children and adolescents with mild-to-moderate symptoms. Randomized clinical trials suggest that CBT is effective for older children and adolescents with anxiety disorders, including OCD, but, while case studies exist, controlled trials are not available to support its treatment with children for all the other anxiety disorders.
- For OCD, psychotherapeutic interventions include cognitive-behavioral treatments such as response prevention for rituals, thought stopping for rumination and compulsions, and systematic desensitization with exposure.
- Pharmacologic interventions have also been effective with anxiety disorders in children and are indicated if the child or adolescent is experiencing severe symptoms of anxiety that impede attendance at treatment sessions or significantly negatively impact daily functioning.
  1. For OCD, clomipramine is effective and has been studied in the pediatric population, but has a variety of side effects that limit compliance. Fluoxetine, sertraline, and fluvoxamine may be just as effective without the side effect profile.
  2. Psychotropic medications are used in the treatment of PTSD, although few controlled studies exist. Clonidine is effective for sleep disorders and beta-blockers for agitation. Selective serotonin reuptake inhibitors (SSRIs) are also used with increasing effectiveness in this population. Drugs typically target symptoms of concurrent mood or anxiety disorder.
  3. Clonazepam, alprazolam, or imipramine have been effective with pediatric patients experiencing panic disorder.
- While there is some evidence to suggest that combining medication and CBT may be more effective than medication or CBT alone in treating adults, this has not been specifically addressed with children and adolescents. Medication plus CBT is most often indicated in situations where there is comorbid depression or multiple anxiety disorders.

REFERENCES

Anxiety Disorders

American Academy of Child and Adolescent Psychiatry: Practice parameters for the assessment and treatment of anxiety disorders. *J Am Acad Child Adolesc Psychiatry* 1997;36 (suppl):69S–84S.

Kagan J, Reznick JS, Snidman N. Biological bases of childhood shyness. *Science* 1988;240:167–171.

Kendall PC. Treating anxiety disorders in children: results of a randomized clinical trial *J Consult Clin Psychol* 1994;62: 100–110.

176 MOOD DISORDERS

John V. Lavigne

CLINICAL FEATURES (DSM-IV DIAGNOSTIC CRITERIA)

- Several types of mood disorders occurring in adulthood are also recognized among children and adolescents

DYSTHYMIA

- The presence of depressed mood (or, for children, irritable mood) for at least 1 year, with no more than 2 months without depression
- Accompanying the depression, at least two of the following: poor appetite or overeating, insomnia/hypersomnia, low energy/fatigue, low self-esteem, problems with concentration or decision making, and a sense of hopelessness
- The child/adolescent has not had a major depression or manic episode during that time
- Differential diagnoses include schizophrenia, depression due to substance use, or a general medical condition.

MAJOR DEPRESSIVE DISORDER

- A major depressive disorder (MDD) can involve a single depressive episode or be recurrent. In a major depressive episode, the individual:
- Experiences a depressed mood nearly all day and every day for at least 2 weeks, and this departs from previous functioning
- The depressed mood is accompanied by at least five of the following:
  1. Anhedonia
  2. Significant weight loss or gain
  3. Insomnia or hypersomnia
  4. Psychomotor agitation or retardation
  5. Feelings or worthlessness or excessive guilt
  6. Diminished ability to think or concentrate nearly every day
  7. Recurrent thoughts of death, recurrent suicidal ideation without a plan, or a suicidal attempt with a specific plan

- The symptoms are unrelated to drug use or a general medical condition and involve clinically significant impairment.
- To qualify as a major depressive disorder, no manic or hypomanic episodes are present.

BIPOLAR DISORDER

- Common characteristics of bipolar disorder include the following:
  1. The presence of at least one major depressive episode
  2. A manic (or in some instances, a hypomanic episode). A manic episode is characterized by
     a. A period of at least 1 week of abnormal and persistent elevated or irritable mood, with at least three of the following:
  3. Inflated self-esteem or grandiosity
  4. Decreased need for sleep
  5. Increased talkativeness
  6. Racing thoughts
  7. Distractibility
  8. Increased goal-directed activity (sexual, academic, social, and so on)
  9. Excessive involvement in pleasurable activities that could have harmful consequences (e.g., buying sprees)
- In each instance, the disorder causes clinically significant consequences. The dual occurrence of a dysthymic disorder (DD) and a major depressive disorder (*double depression*) has been noted.
- In children, the clear, separate manic and depressive episodes are not always seen; more rapid cycling or mixed states (a period of time in which both the manic episode and the depressive episode criteria are met) can be seen in children and younger adolescents.
- *Cyclothymia* is a condition in which there are numerous episodes of hypomania and depression that do not meet full criteria for either manic episodes or major depressive episodes

EPIDEMIOLOGY

- For MDD, the point prevalence among children is 2%; for adolescents, 4%.
- For DD, the point prevalence is 0.6–1.7% among children; in adolescence, 1.6–8.0%.
- DD/MDD comorbidity is high (69%), and recent data suggest there is little reason to differentiate between the two disorders in youths.
- Both community-based and clinical studies show a consistently high rate of comorbidity between depression and either conduct or oppositional disorders, with rates as high as 80%.

- Comorbidity with an anxiety disorder also occurs frequently.
- Overall, comorbidity enhances the risk for recurrent depression, affects the duration of the depressive episode, increases suicide attempts, and affects treatment responsiveness.

ETIOLOGY

- Rates of depression, anxiety, substance abuse, and antisocial behavior are elevated among parents of depressed children, and the children of depressed mothers show increased rates of depression.
- *Interaction patterns*: Maternal depression is associated with unavailable and understimulating parenting, and several studies report parental hostility is related to childhood depression.
- Maternal depression is often accompanied by marital problems and stress; child depression may possibly result from combined risk factors in homes of depressed mothers.
- Other family risk factors include single-parent families, low socioeconomic status (SES), and negative life events.
- Children of depressed mothers are more likely to develop an insecure attachment, associated with later behavior problems, peer difficulties, and withdrawal/inhibition. Insecurely attached children have more problematic "affective regulation and expression," see significant others as less available and rejecting, and feel unlovable.
- Problems with homeostatic regulation associated with difficult temperament have been noted in children whose parents have mood disorders, and undercontrolled behavior related to temperament has been associated with later mood disorder.
- Temperamentally negative mood is likely to be implicated in early onset depression. Failure to develop appropriate affective regulatory processes contributes to the development of later depression, with depressed elementary school children reporting less use of affect regulatory strategies than nondepressed children.

PROGNOSIS

- Symptoms of depression in grade 1 are relatively stable over 5 years. Children with DD are at increased risk for MDD, with 76% of children with DD later developing MDD. The average length of major depressive episode is 7–9 months, but 6–10% of episodes are protracted beyond 1–2 years. Recurrence of a major depressive episode within 5 years occurs in 70% of cases.

EVALUATION, MANAGEMENT, AND TREATMENT

- Information about child mood states can be gathered from parental interviews, but there are some indications that parental reports can underestimate such dysphoric mood states. As a result, interviewing the child about his/her mood is important. Problems in reporting such symptoms increase among younger children. Questionnaires such as the Child Depression Inventory or the Beck Depression Inventory for Youth can help in eliciting depressive symptomatology from the child.
- Gathering information about suicide risk is critical in assessing children with depression.
- There has been increased attention to bipolar disorder in prepubertal children in recent years. Differential diagnosis of this condition requires careful discrimination between the heightened activity that can be associated with a manic episode from the hyperactivity of attention deficit hyperactivity disorder (ADHD); in mania, heightened activity level is more episodic, while the high activity level of ADHD is more chronic.
- In treatment of children with risk for harm to themselves, supervision to ensure their safety is important, and an inpatient hospitalization during the acute period must be considered. In general, however, the depressed child or adolescent should be treated in the least restrictive environment, including outpatient treatment and partial hospitalizations as alternatives to inpatient care whenever possible. For older children and adolescents, randomized trials have demonstrated greater effectiveness for cognitive-behavioral treatments than for no treatment, but the effect sizes are low to moderate.
- Pharmacotherapy: Opinions differ on the sequencing of treatments (e.g., psychotherapy first, then medications, and so on or combining them), with little data supporting alternative approaches. Selective serotonin reuptake inhibitors (SSRIs) are used with increasing frequency in the pediatric population because of clinical effectiveness and a narrow side effect profile. Comorbidities must be treated accordingly.

REFERENCE

Mood Disorders

American Academy of Child and Adolescent Psychiatry: Practice parameters for the assessment and treatment of children and adolescents with bipolar disorder. *J Am Acad Child Adolesc Psychiatry* 1997;36 (suppl):157–176.

Kovacs M. The course of childhood-onset depressive disorders. *Psychiatric Annals* 1996;26:326–330.

177 TOURETTE SYNDROME AND OTHER TIC DISORDERS

Sally E. Tarbell

CLINICAL FEATURES (DSM-IV DIAGNOSTIC CRITERIA)

TOURETTE SYNDROME (TS)

- *Both* multiple motor and one or more vocal tics present at some time during the illness, but not necessarily concurrently.
- Tics occur many times a day (usually in bouts), nearly every day or intermittently for a period of more than a year. During this period there was never a tic-free period for >3 months.
- The disturbance causes marked distress or impairment in social, occupational, or other areas of functioning
- Onset before 18 years
- The disturbance is not due to the direct physiologic effects of a substance (e.g., stimulants) or a general medical condition (e.g., Huntington chorea, postviral encephalitis)

CHRONIC MOTOR OR VOCAL TIC DISORDER (CT)

- Same as for TS with the exception that there are single *or* multiple motor or vocal tics but not both.

TRANSIENT TIC DISORDER

- Same as for CT with the exception that symptoms have been present for at least 1 month but <12 consecutive months.
- There are no definitive laboratory tests or pathognomonic signs to assist with differential diagnosis.
- Tics have characteristics uncommon to other movement disorders:
  1. Tics involve rapid movements that can be vocal or motor and they show variability in intensity, location, and type.
  2. Any part of the body can be affected. Typically tics begin in the face and over time spread to other muscle groups (neck, shoulders, trunk, legs, feet).
  3. Premonitory urges are common and tics are temporarily suppressible.

4. Tics typically diminish during sleep, but they may not disappear entirely.

EPIDEMIOLOGY

• Tics are the most common movement disorder diagnosed in children. Community studies find the prevalence of TS to be 5–10/10,000, with boys more commonly affected than girls.

PATHOPHYSIOLOGY

• TS and CT have been considered to be part of the same disease entity, with TS representing a more severe form. Etiology of TS is unknown, but several studies have implicated genetic factors and perinatal events. Group A beta-hemolytic streptococcal (GABHS) infections have been implicated in tics that present an abrupt onset. Stress has also been cited as a trigger or factor associated with increased tic expression.

PROGNOSIS

• Median age of onset is 5–6 years. Tics are reported to worsen between later school age and early adolescence with a gradual decrease in symptoms during later adolescence and adulthood. Psychosocial and educational morbidity associated with TS and CT have been associated more strongly with comorbid psychiatric disorders than the tics themselves.

EVALUATION, MANAGEMENT, AND TREATMENT

• A small number of case studies have shown behavioral interventions (habit reversal, self-management strategies, relaxation, imagery) to be useful in reducing tic expression in school-age and adolescent children.
• Atypical antipsychotics are effective in the treatment of tic disorders, but there is a risk of rebound when the medication is discontinued. Weight gain is a frequent complication of long-term care. Pimozide is perhaps the most frequently used neuroleptic for tic disorders. For suspected GABHS induced tics, several studies demonstrated the effectiveness of plasma exchange and intravenous immunoglobulin (IVIG) therapy. The tricyclic antidepressants desipramine and nortriptylline were found to be effective in a small sample of patients. The relationship between tic disorders and the use of stimulant medication is determined by the patient's treatment course. The benefits of effective attention deficit hyperactivity disorder (ADHD) treatment are considered along with the impact of the tic disorder on the child.

REFERENCES

Tourettes/Tics
Leckman J, Cohen D. *Tourette's Syndrome—Tics, Obsessions, Compulsions: Developmental Psychopathology and Clinical Care*. New York, NY: Wiley, 1999.
Spencer T, Biederman J, Harding M, Wilens T, Faraone S. The relationship between tic disorders and Tourette's syndrome revisited. *J Child Adoles Psychiatry* 1995;34:1133–1139.
Swedo S, Leonard H, Garvey M, et al. Pediatric autoimmune neuropsychiatric disorders associated with streptococcal infections: clinical description of the first 50 cases. *Am J Psychiatry* 1998;155:264–271.

178 SELECTIVE MUTISM
Colleen Cicchetti

CLINICAL FEATURES (DSM-IV DIAGNOSTIC CRITERIA)

• Selective mutism (SM) is a disorder characterized by
  1. The persistent failure to speak in specific social situations despite exhibiting a capacity for normal speech in other settings.
  2. At least 1 month duration
  3. Symptoms are severe enough to interfere with educational achievement or social communication.
  4. Failure to speak is not due to a lack of knowledge or comfort with the specific language required in the situation.
  5. Children with this disorder may communicate by gestures, nodding, writing, or occasionally with monosyllabic or monotone utterances.
• Symptoms related to voluntary refusal to speak have been described as early as 1877, "aphasia voluntaria" but were first described in the psychiatric nomenclature in DSM-III as "elective mutism." The recent shift in name reflects a general shift in emphasis away from conceptualization of the disorder as willful opposition toward anxiety-driven behavior.
• Some authors have suggested that SM should be considered a subtype of social phobia. This suggestion is based in part on recent studies indicating that 97% of children with SM also met DSM-III-R criteria for social phobia or avoidant disorder; however, SM is not currently listed within the anxiety disorder subgroup within the DSM-IV.

- Associated features may include excessive shyness, social isolation, compulsive traits as well as oppositional behavior, particularly at home. In addition, high percentage of children with SM also have speech and language delays (estimates between 30 and 50%) as well as motor delays
- With regard to differential diagnosis:
  1. Caution is emphasized in diagnosing this disorder in bilingual or immigrant children.
  2. Must determine if inhibition of speech is secondary to a more general communication disorder, mental retardation, pervasive developmental disorder, or psychotic disorder including schizophrenia.

EPIDEMIOLOGY

- Few studies have focused on the epidemiology of SM; prevalence rate is estimated as approximately 1% of school-age children.
- Diagnosis is most typically made between ages 5 and 10 years, although age of onset may be much earlier.
- The female:male ratio appears to be approximately 1.2:1, although a recent U.S. study did not find a gender difference.

ETIOLOGY

- Early theories focused on family dynamics or reactions to trauma.
- Current conceptualizations emphasize a likely genetic contribution, focusing on strong evidence of familial anxiety and early behaviorally inhibited temperament.

PROGNOSIS

- Little information is available concerning prognosis.
- A recent community study showed some preliminary support for a distinction between transient and persistent SM, with younger children with milder symptoms more likely to remit spontaneously.
- Retrospective self-report data suggest that individuals with a history of SM continue to experience significant social anxiety.

EVALUATION, MANAGEMENT, AND TREATMENT

- Assessment focuses primarily on parental report (including review of psychiatric symptoms, medical history, and social interactions) and assessment of academic, cognitive, and speech and language skills. Pediatricians are encouraged to ask parents specifi-

cally about speech in school when a child does not speak during an office visit.

- Most current treatment programs combine multimodal behavioral interventions and psychopharmacology; however, due to the low incidence rate of the behavior, no large-scale intervention studies have been conducted for either behavioral or pharmacologic interventions.
- Behavioral interventions typically address both general anxiety symptoms and the inappropriate communication patterns. Programs typically involve a systematic approach that rewards successive approximations of social interaction and communication. Case study reports include use of video/audio feedword (stimulus fading and self-modeling procedures), web-based cognitive-behavioral therapy (CBT) programs emphasizing cognitive coping strategies, and electronic communication devises. School-based interventions typically have included parents, therapists, teachers, and speech and language pathologists as well as using peers to stimulate and reward interaction and communication.
- Pharmacology: Over the past 10 years, SM has been increasingly treated with various medications. Case studies have appeared including, phenelzine, fluoxetine (Prozac), and fluvozamine (Luvox) with some success in decreasing both the overall anxiety symptoms and increasing speech. Prozac has been the most frequently investigated medication using high doses for substantial periods of time.

REFERENCES

Selective Mutism

Bergman RL, Piacentini J, Mccracken JT. Prevalence and description of selective mutism in a school-based sample. *J Am Acad Child Adoles Psychiatry* 2002;41:938–946.

Dow SP, et al. guidelines for the assessment and treatment of selective mutism. *J Am Acad Child Adoles Psychiatry* 1995;34:836–846.

179 REACTIVE ATTACHMENT DISORDER

John V. Lavigne

CLINICAL FEATURES (DSM-IV DIAGNOSTIC CRITERIA)

- Reactive attachment disorder is a rare condition in which there is a marked disturbance in social

relations, beginning before the age of 5 years, characterized by
- Failure to initiate or respond in a developmentally appropriate fashion to most social interactions. The child shows one or more of the following:
  1. Excessive inhibition
  2. Hypervigilance
  3. Highly ambivalent or contradictory responses
- Indiscriminant sociability (overly familiar with strangers) or marked inability to form an attachment to someone
- The presumption that the problems in socialization are associated with abuse or neglect
- *Epidemiology and etiology*: By definition, the presumed etiology is abuse or neglect. Little is known about the epidemiology of this condition.

PROGNOSIS

- Little substantial information is available concerning prognosis.

EVALUATION, MANAGEMENT, TREATMENT

- Interviews with caretakers are essential for establishing the presence of the key clinical symptoms. Observations of interactions with caregivers can provide critical information about the child's emotional responsiveness and the quality of caretaking (parental emotional responsiveness, nurturance, attentiveness to the child, synchrony of parent response to the child's needs). Home visits are often indicated in the assessment phase. Investigations designed to determine if abuse or neglect occurred are necessary to establish the diagnosis.
- Critical to treatment is the provision of adequate caretaking. Individual therapy for the child and treatment of the parents is often recommended, but few studies are available concerning treatment efficacy for this condition.

REFERENCE

Reactive Attachment Disorder
Dulcan MK, Martini DR, Lake MB. Reactive attachment disorder of infancy and early childhood. In Dulcan MK, Martini DR, Lake MB. *Concise Guide to Child & Adolescent Psychiatry*, 3rd ed. Washington, DC: American Psychiatric Association, 2003, pp. 95–97.

180 SCHIZOPHRENIA

Kathleen Mckenna

- The onset in young people tends to be insidious with slowly developing prodromal symptoms such as social withdrawal, idiosyncratic thinking, unusual behaviors, declining school performance, lack of initiation of activity, sleep/wake cycle disturbance, and deteriorating personal hygiene.

CLINICAL FEATURES (DSM-IV)

- Delusions
- Hallucinations
- Disorganized speech
- Grossly disorganized or catatonic behavior
- Negative symptoms such as flat affect, lack of initiative, paucity of thought or speech
- Symptoms must be impairing and last at least 6 months. (If symptoms are present for fewer than 6 months, schizophreniform disorder is diagnosed.)
- Symptoms that may suggest psychosis in adults—disorganized speech, odd ideas, excessive fantasy or illogical ideas—must be assessed from a developmental perspective. Many children have communication disorders that result in speech that may be misinterpreted as psychotic. Others have illogical thinking or imaginary friends that are the result of immaturity rather than illness. Often, a decrease in functioning or regression may clarify that an illness, rather than simply a developmental delay, is present.

DIFFERENTIAL (PARTIAL)

- Schizoaffective disorder
- Bipolar disorder
- Major depressive disorder
- Substance abuse
- Paranoid personality disorder
- Pervasive developmental disorder
- Posttraumatic stress disorder
- Metabolic disorders
- Obsessive-compulsive disorder
- Reaction to medications especially stimulants and those that are anticholinergic
- Seizure activity

EPIDEMIOLOGY

- Males are more likely to have schizophrenia in childhood or adolescence. Schizophrenia is rare in children before the age of 13 years but is seen with increasing frequency in adolescence. Most people with schizophrenia develop symptoms in late adolescence or early adulthood. The prevalence in the population is 1%.

PATHOPHYSIOLOGY

• Schizophrenia appears to be associated with developmental abnormalities occurring during the second trimester of pregnancy. Since the concordance rate for monozygotic twins is increased but not extremely high, there are clearly environmental factors. There are no definitive studies to suggest that excessive stress or adverse family environments are the causes of schizophrenia, although these may worsen the illness and result in a worse outcome.

PROGNOSIS

• Those who develop schizophrenia before adulthood tend to have a worse outcome, more comorbid conditions, and poorer response to medication treatment compared to those with adult-onset schizophrenia. Some, however, respond well to treatment and may be able to live on their own, although most will need support of some kind. Occasionally, schizophrenia has been reported to resolve, although it is not clear whether the diagnosis was correct.

TREATMENT

• Just as for adults, treatment with neuroleptics is the mainstay of treatment for children and adolescents. The newer, atypical neuroleptics are often chosen since they are presumed to be less likely to cause tardive dyskinesia, a permanent and impairing movement disorder. Unfortunately, some of these medications seem to be implicated in lipid abnormalities, glucose intolerance, and diabetes. Many cause weight gain and may cause QT lengthening on electrocardiogram (ECG). These medications may also cause dystonias, motor restlessness, and cognitive dulling. Neuroleptics often take weeks to months to treat the psychotic symptoms, although they may decrease agitation and improve sleep more quickly. Antidepressants, especially selective serotonin reuptake inhibitors are often added to treat depression of obsessive-compulsive symptoms. Benzodiazepines may be used to treat anxiety or agitation, especially while waiting for the neuroleptic to work. Excessive restlessness due to neuroleptics may be treated with propranolol and dystonias are often treated with benztropine or diphenhydramine.

• Patients who present in the emergency room with symptoms of schizophrenia must have a careful mental status examination. Children with schizophrenia are usually fairly well-oriented. While they may have incoherent speech, delusional ideas, odd mannerisms, paranoia, and hallucinations, they usually know that they are in the hospital and retain basic orientation regarding family members. Delirium caused by toxic substances or conditions such as a leucodystrophy or encephalitis may be missed if attention is not given to distinguishing delirium from psychosis. Likewise, a neurologic examination should be performed to rule out other conditions that may be compromising brain function.

• Most people with hallucinations due to schizophrenia have auditory hallucinations. The presence of visual hallucinations, especially in absence of auditory hallucinations, is often associated with seizure activity, toxic substances, or other brain insults. The same may be said for tactile hallucinations. While people with schizophrenia may have some depression, especially if they have insight into their condition, prominent mood abnormalities suggest the presence of a mood disorder such as depression or bipolar disorder with psychotic features. The treatment will require that the underlying mood disorder be treated if the psychotic symptoms are to resolve. If seizure activity is suspected due to visual hallucinations, an absence of other symptoms of schizophrenia, but the electroencephalogram (EEG) is normal, consideration should be given to an empirical trial of an anticonvulsant.

• Families of children with schizophrenia have the dual challenge of dealing with both the illness as well as the need to foster development in the face of a serious illness. The family's desire to protect a vulnerable adolescent may come into conflict with an adolescent's desire to be more independent, despite schizophrenia. Sometimes adolescents become discouraged by the illness and may need extra support and education. Therapy may be helpful to deal with these problems, even though it will not treat the underlying schizophrenia. It should be remembered that the rate of suicide in people with schizophrenia is high. Discouragement, as well as the presence of medication side effects, should be taken seriously. Every effort should be made to educate the young person about the illness and to provide support as the seriousness, and probable chronicity of the illness, is faced by the child and the family. As the child matures, he or she should be encouraged to take a more active role in monitoring symptoms, resolving conflicts and making treatment decisions.

• Most schools will need support and information if they are to provide an appropriate educational setting, since schizophrenia is rare in young people. Unfortunately, many of these children are referred to special education settings in which behaviorally disordered children also are present. This often results in an overstimulating and possibly dangerous environment for a child with problems organizing behavior and processing environmental input. Most children with schizophrenia tend to do best in small, nurturing classrooms with calm environments. Teachers often need help understanding that brain functions such as organizing, attending, monitoring behavior, and initiating actions may be impaired and that many problems are not due to the child's irresponsibility or deliberate refusal to carry out tasks. Sometimes it is better to obtain an aide to help the child remain in regular classes rather than place the child in an inappropriate special education setting.

REFERENCE

Schizophrenia References

McClellan J, Werry J, and the Work Group on Quality Issues of the AACAP. Practice Parameters for the Assessment and Treatment of Children and Adolescents with Schizophrenia. *J Am Acad Child Adolesc Psychiatry* 2001;40: (suppl) 4S–23S.

McClennan J, McCurry C, Speltz ML, Jones K. Symptom factors in early-onset psychotic disorder, *J Am Acad Child Adolesc Psychiatry* 2002;41:791–798.

King BH, State MW, Shah B. Mental retardation: a review of the past 10 years: Part I. J. Symptom factors in early-onset psychotic disorder. *J Am Acad Child Adolesc Psychiatry* 2002; 41:1656–1663.

181 GENDER IDENTITY DISORDER (GID)

John V. Lavigne

CLINICAL FEATURES (DSM DIAGNOSTIC CRITERIA)

- Gender identity refers to one's sense of being male or female, usually formed by the age of 3–4 years. GID has two major characteristics. The first is a "strong and persistent cross-gender identification," manifested in four or more of the following:
  1. Repeatedly stating that he/she wants to be, or is, a member of the opposite sex (genuinely, not merely for some perceived advantage)
  2. For boys, a preference to cross dress or "simulate female attire;" for girls, insistence on wearing masculine clothing
  3. Strong, persistent preference for playing roles of the other sex in fantasy play, or persistent fantasies of being the other sex
  4. Strong desire to play the stereotyped games or activities of the other sex
  5. Strong preference for other-sex playmates
- The second is a persistent sense of being uncomfortable with one's sex, or a feeling that one's gender is inappropriate for one's self (e.g., preference to not have one's genitalia, desire to get rid of primary or secondary sexual characteristics, marked aversion to the clothing typical of one's sex, and so on)
- When present, GID causes social, academic, or occupational impairment or distress, and is not due to the presence of a physical intersex condition. Distress may be difficult to ascertain in young children, however.

EPIDEMIOLOGY

- No studies directly addressing the prevalence of GID have been conducted. Studies of parent reports on their child's stated preference of wanting to be a member of the opposite sex show such statements are not uncommon (occurring in 1% of boys and 5% of girls), but this overstates the number of children who would actually meet GID criteria. In clinic samples, boys referred for gender problems outnumber girls as much as 7:1 possibly due to greater tolerance for masculine behavior among girls. Referral rates in adolescence is closer to 1.4:1 (boys:girls).

ETIOLOGY

- Genetic factors, prenatal hormones, and parent-child relationship factors have been hypothesized to be related to gender problems, but definitive studies are lacking.

PROGNOSIS

- Prospective studies are lacking. Observations among referred children suggest that some seek sex reassignment surgeries as adults. Many individuals maintain some social distance from others because of their feelings about their gender.

ASSESSMENT, MANAGEMENT, AND TREATMENT

- Parent interviews can usually elicit any concerns about gender identity or lack of behaviors characteristic of one's gender role (i.e., stereotypic culturally-based views on what is typical for a particular sex). An interview with the child or adolescent can ascertain attitudes toward one's gender, distress, feelings, and preferences. The relative infrequency of the condition has prevented randomized trials from being conducted. Recommended, but largely untested, interventions have included discouragement of cross-gender behaviors, bolstering of social skills and interactions with same-sex peers, and individual treatment to support the child in dealing with gender-related thoughts and feelings and to reduce any associated dysphoria the child or adolescent experiences.

REFERENCE

Gender Identity Disorder
Bradley SJ, Zucker KJ. Gender identity disorder: a review of the past 10 years. *J Am Acad Child Adoles Psychiatry* 1997;36:872–880.

182 SUBSTANCE ABUSE DISORDERS

Heather J. Walter

CLINICAL FEATURES

- The substance use disorders encompass both substance abuse and substance dependence, and apply to alcohol, amphetamines, caffeine, cannabis, cocaine, hallucinogens, inhalants, nicotine, opioids, phencyclidine, and sedatives/hypnotics/anxiolytics.
  1. The essential feature of substance abuse is a maladaptive pattern of drug use manifested by failure to fulfill major role obligations, recurrent use in physically hazardous situations, and substance-related legal and interpersonal problems.
  2. The essential feature of substance dependence is a maladaptive pattern of substance use manifested by tolerance, withdrawal, or compulsive drug-taking behavior.
  3. Compared to adults, in adolescents tolerance may have low-diagnostic specificity, withdrawal symptoms may be less common, and blackouts, craving, and impulsive sexual behavior may be prominent characteristics of maladaptive use. Both abuse and dependence must be associated with clinically significant distress and impairment, and the symptoms of each must be exhibited within a 12-month period.
- The progression to drug abuse or dependence may follow a characteristic pattern beginning with experimentation and followed by regular and finally compulsive use.
- Mood, cognitive, and behavioral signs may appear in the early stages of regular use, and may include impaired concentration; a decline in academic or athletic performance; loss of interest in hobbies or extracurricular activities; mood swings; rebellious attitude, dress, or behavior; social withdrawal or association with antisocial peers; and changes in daily routine or sleep patterns.
- In the later stages of use, the adolescent may experience marked dysphoria when not using drugs, which can lead to more frequent use with more powerful substances. In the compulsive stage, drug use becomes nearly constant as the adolescent uses any and all substances available and obtains them by whatever means necessary.
- Many other psychiatric disorders are comorbid with substance use disorders including conduct, mood, anxiety, attention deficit hyperactivity, eating, and psychotic disorders.

EPIDEMIOLOGY

- Estimates of the lifetime prevalence of alcohol abuse among adolescents range from less than 1 to 10%, and of alcohol dependence, from 1 to 4%. Estimates of the lifetime prevalence of drug abuse or dependence range from 3 to 10%. The prevalence of abuse and dependence increases with age.

ETIOLOGY

- The etiology of substance abuse disorders is multifactorial, involving biologic, psychologic, social, and cultural factors. In the early stages of use, the easy availability of substances coupled with norms and values that promote experimentation are thought to be the predominant etiologic factors. In the later stages of use, biologic and psychologic factors may play the more powerful etiologic role.

PROGNOSIS

- While experimentation with "gateway drugs" such as alcohol and cigarettes is common among adolescents, only a small proportion of adolescents advance to higher stages of substance use.

- Among the minority of adolescents who progress to higher stages, many cease abusing substances in early adulthood, when new roles and social contexts constitute conventionalizing influences.
- Early initiation of substance use and rapid progression through the stages convey heightened risk for the development of substance use disorders.
- Posttreatment relapse rates for substance use disorders are high, ranging from 35 to 85%. Factors associated with relapse include younger age at onset of drug use; more extensive involvement with drugs; antisocial behavior; comorbid psychiatric disorders; more frequent and intense thoughts and feelings about drugs; less involvement in school, work, or drug-free recreational activities; and less support from drug-free family and peers.

EVALUATION, MANAGEMENT, AND TREATMENT

- Children and adolescents who manifest impairment in one or more areas of function should be screened for substance use. Interviews with the child, parent, and collateral informants (e.g., teachers, caregivers) are essential for diagnosis. Standardized rating scales can be helpful. Urine and blood toxicology screens may be used to validate self-reports of use.
- Comprehensive assessment should include inquiry into the type of drugs used, the route of administration, the age at initiation and frequency of use, and the usual setting. Questions also should assess the adolescent's beliefs about the perceived benefits of drug use, experiences with the negative consequences of drug use, and whether the adolescent believes his/her drug use is out of control.
- Assessment also should include the identification and treatment of comorbid psychiatric disorders. In most cases, the treatment of the substance use disorder should precede the treatment of the comorbidities.
- In most cases, the goal of treatment will be achieving and maintaining abstinence from substance use; however, harm reduction may be an appropriate interim goal.
- At least six theoretically and operationally distinct treatment strategies are currently dominant. These include

12-step therapy, cognitive-behavioral therapy, psychodynamic therapy, family therapy, group therapy, and community-based therapy. In general, studies of treatment effectiveness have found that some treatment is better than no treatment, no single treatment approach is clearly superior to another, and alcohol and marijuana use are much less effectively treated than other drug use. All treatment programs should develop procedures to minimize dropout; maximize motivation, adherence, and treatment completion; and arrange for aftercare.

- Treatment should be provided in the least restrictive setting that is safe and effective. Outpatient treatment is appropriate for motivated adolescents who have strong, stable environmental support, no significant comorbid psychiatric disorders, and little functional impairment.
- Appropriate candidates for residential treatment are adolescents who have failed in a less restrictive setting, who are transitioning from inpatient treatment, who have poor environmental supports, or who have severe personality disorders or functional impairment.
- Inpatient treatment should be considered for adolescents who have moderate-to-severe comorbid psychiatric disturbance with functional impairment, who are at risk for withdrawal, who present a danger to themselves or others, or who have failed in less restrictive treatment settings.

REFERENCES

Substance Abuse Disorders

American Academy of Child and Adolescent Psychiatry. Practice parameters for the assessment and treatment of children and adolescents with substance use disorders. *J Am Acad Child Adolesc Psychiatry* (in press).

Monti PM, Colby SM, O'Leary TA. *Adolescents, and substance abuse: reaching teens through brief interventions.* New York, NY: Guilford, 2001.

Wagner EF, Waldron HB. *Innovations in adolescent substance abuse interventions.* Amsterdam: Pergamon, 2001.

Walter HJ. Substance abuse and substance use disorders. In: Gabbard G (ed.), *Treatments of Psychiatric Disorders,* 3rd ed. Washington, DC: American Psychiatric Press, 2001.

Section 21
RHEUMATOLOGIC AND AUTOIMMUNE CONDITIONS

Marisa S. Klein-Gitelman, Section Editor

183 RHEUMATOLOGIC EMERGENCIES

Marisa S. Klein-Gitelman

- Pediatric rheumatology encompasses a wide variety of diseases. The incidence and frequency of true emergencies in pediatric rheumatology are undocumented although the presence of these problems is well documented. A general description of problems is listed.

THE NERVOUS SYSTEM

- Patients with systemic vasculitis, isolated cerebral vasculitis, and lupus may develop increased intracranial pressure, stroke, hemorrhage, encephalitis, seizure, and transverse myelitis.
- The pathophysiologic mechanism depends on the lesion and may be the result of vascular occlusion, antiphospholipid antibodies (APLA), disseminated intravascular coagulopathy, or direct cellular damage from autoantibodies.
- When an undiagnosed patient presents with an acute central nervous system (CNS) process, the usual supportive care measures should be taken. Diagnosis of an autoimmune process occurs only when sought and is essential to disease control and prevention of further damage. Most patients require aggressive immunosuppression with intravenous corticosteroids and may require cyclophosphamide.
- Prognosis depends on early diagnosis and potential for reversal of damage.
- Prevention occurs with good control of disease activity in the diagnosed patient.

THE CARDIOVASCULAR SYSTEM

- Patients with vasculitis, lupus, scleroderma, and systemic onset juvenile arthritis frequently present with pericarditis.
  1. Diagnosis is made clinically by auscultation of a rub and verified by echocardiography.
  2. Treatment is initiated with corticosteroids. Once controlled, indomethacin can be substituted to control inflammation. Patients with large effusions may require drainage until immunosuppression controls serositis.
- Another cardiac emergency is coronary artery vasculitis or occlusion.
  1. Occlusion should also be considered in the patient with vasculitis who has been treated with long-term corticosteroids and may have atherosclerosis.
  2. Standard treatment for myocardial infarction should be initiated. In the patient with active inflammation, immunosuppression is required.
- Myocarditis can also be seen in lupus, dermatomyositis, systemic onset arthritis, scleroderma, and overlap syndromes.
- Arrhythmias are uncommon and are most often described in neonatal lupus where an infant has complete heart block and requires immediate pacing.
- Hypertension is frequently seen in patients with glomerulonephritis or renal artery vasculitis. Hypertensive crisis is seen in the patient with scleroderma.
  - Control of blood pressure is essential and often difficult. The use of angiotensin-converting enzyme therapy in the patient with scleroderma has been shown to reduce the risk of hypertensive crisis.

THE PULMONARY SYSTEM

- The most life-threatening pulmonary emergency is hemorrhage seen in lupus and Wegener granulomatosis.

1. Clinical symptoms are hemoptysis, cough, dyspnea, and hypoxia.
2. Supportive care and immunosuppression are required.
3. Outcomes are often poor.
- Pleuritis is a common finding but rarely presents as respiratory distress.
    1. Management of severe pleuritis with thoracocentesis is a rare occurrence.
- Pulmonary embolism is a rare complication of vasculitis or antiphospholipid syndrome but must be considered in the patient with acute chest pain.

THE KIDNEY

- Acute renal failure is the hallmark of many vasculitis syndromes and lupus.
    1. Patients present with pedal edema, malaise, fever, oligouria, hypertension, and electrolyte abnormalities.
    2. Suspicion of and evaluation for autoimmune disease is essential and must be performed rapidly.
    3. Patients often require immunosuppression with steroids and cyclophosphamide. Patients with rapidly progressive glomerulonephritis or WHO Class IV lupus nephritis often progress to renal failure and require dialysis and transplantation.
    4. Prevention of failure requires vigilance and compliance in the diagnosed patient.

THE GASTROINTESTINAL SYSTEM

- The most serious gastrointestinal crisis is intestinal vasculitis with perforation. This can occur in vasculitis, dermatomyositis, and lupus. Patients require a combination of immunosuppression and control of peritonitis/sepsis. Prognosis is poor.
- Acute liver failure is seen in lupus and autoimmune hepatitis. The patient presents with jaundice and may have cirrhosis. Treatment includes supportive care and immunosuppression.

SKIN

- Patients can present with bullous lupus skin disease. The bullae may cover all skin surfaces and develop in oral and genital mucosal areas. The patient may require supportive care similar to a burn patient. Infection is a serious complication. Patients are treated with immunosuppression including corticosteroids, dapsone, azathioprine, and thalidomide.

HEMATOLOGIC SYSTEM

- Lupus patients may develop autoimmune thrombocytopenia and/or autoimmune hemolytic anemia which may require emergent intervention to prevent bleeding or cardiac failure. Support via transfusion may be difficult and increase autoantibody formation. Immunosuppression with corticosteroids or the use of intravenous immunoglobulin (IVIG) is beneficial. In the unresponsive patient, anti-CD20 antibody or rituxamab may be required.

IMMUNE SYSTEM

- Macrophage activation syndrome (MAS), also known as hemophagocytic lymphohistiocytosis, can occur in patients with systemic onset arthritis, and more rarely lupus or other connective tissue diseases. The inability of the immune system to inactivate cytotoxic T cells and macrophages leads to coagulopathy (purpura, bruising, and gum bleeding), fever, encephalopathy, and hepatosplenomegaly. Patients develop leukopenia, thrombocytopenia, hypofibrinogenemia, prolonged prothrombin time/partial thromboplastin time (PT/PTT), hepatitis, and falling erythrocyte sedimentation rate (ESR). Immediate recognition and treatment with cyclosporine A and corticosteroids prevents poor outcome and death.

MISCELLANEOUS

- APLAs and the lupus anticoagulant (LAC) may increase risk for arterial or venous thrombosis. A patient may present with acute visual loss, scrotal pain, abdominal pain as well as stroke, myocardial infarction, or pulmonary embolism. The patient with primary APL syndrome remains anticoagulated for years while patients with lupus and secondary APLS may stop anticoagulation with disease control and disappearance of APL.

INFECTION

- The presence of sepsis and other serious infections is a significant problem in the pediatric rheumatology population. Lupus patients, in particular, are at high risk during disease flares with associated leukopenia and hypocomplementemia. Bacteremia may rapidly transform into life-threatening sepsis. Pneumococcal disease is particularly virulent despite vaccination. All patients receiving biologic agents, corticosteroids, methotrexate, leufludomide, azathioprine, cyclosporine, FK506, or cyclophosphamide are immunosuppressed. Any fever without source must be treated as a sepsis evaluation. Small injuries may result in serious soft tissue infections requiring surgical debridement. Patients may develop endocarditis especially if they have hardware for frequent infusions (i.e., portacath). Varicella is particularly serious in this setting and patients who have not had disease or vaccination should receive vaccination at the first opportunity during a remission. Patients are also at high risk for sexually transmitted diseases and present with disseminated infections such as herpes or gonorrhea.

BIBLIOGRAPHY

Cassidy JT, Petty RE (eds.). *Textbook of Pediatric Rheumatology*, 4th ed. Philadelphia, PA: W.B. Saunders, 2001.

Jacobs J. *Pediatric Rheumatology for the Practitioner*, 2nd ed. New York, NY: Springer-Verlag, 1993.

Mouy R, Stephan JL, Pillet P, Haddad E, Hubert P, Prieur AM. Efficacy of cyclosporine A in the treatment of macrophage activation syndrome in juvenile arthritis: report of five cases. *J Pediatr* 1996;129:750–754.

184 COMMON OFFICE COMPLAINTS
Marisa S. Klein-Gitelman

- Patients come to the pediatric rheumatologist for a variety of problems. This section focuses on frequent complaints that *do not* result in diagnosis of a rheumatologic disease. The following complaints are most common: arthralgia, idiopathic musculoskeletal pain, fever, and positive antinuclear antibodies (ANA).

ARTHRALGIA

- Joint pain without swelling or loss of range of motion is a far more common finding than true arthritis. It is a substantial cause of morbidity and careful evaluation, diagnosis and intervention may restore the child to full activity. Frequent problems and disease categories will be reviewed.

- The most important diagnoses to consider in the child with arthralgia are infection and malignancy. History and physical examination should include evaluation for fever, pallor, point tenderness, organomegaly, or masses. Suspect history or examination requires laboratory and radiographic evaluation.

- Generalized hypermobility occurs in approximately one of three children. Prevalence varies with ethnic background. There is often a family history. Diagnosis is based on the Beighton scale of maneuvers. Children complain of intermittent nocturnal pains responsive to an evening dose of acetaminophen or nonsteroidal anti-inflammatory agent. Supportive footwear can reduce pain. Patients are prone to soft tissue injury, back pain, and chondromalacia patella. Exercise programs to improve muscle strength are helpful. Evaluation should exclude diagnosis of Marfan syndrome, homocystinuria, Stickler syndrome, Ehlers-Danlos syndrome, osteogenesis imperfecta, Williams syndrome, and Down syndrome as these diagnoses require further treatment and intervention.

- The most common arthralgia complaint is at the knee.
  1. Pain in the anterior aspect of the knee (femoropatellar pain) is quite common especially in teenage girls. Movement of the joint is associated with medial patellar pain and crepitation. Patients complain of pain with bent knee activities such as walking stairs, running, biking, step aerobics, and deep knee bends. Laboratory tests and radiographs are normal. Therapy includes strengthening muscles around the knee, stretching tight hamstrings, correction of pronated gait with custom orthotics and weight loss in the overweight patient.
  2. Another problem is the mediopatellar plica syndrome causing locking or snapping during movement of the joint. Diagnosis and treatment are made by arthroscopy.
  3. Osgood-Schlatter disease is a microavulsion fracture of the tibial tuberosity and occurs in athletic adolescents. Diagnosis is made by radiograph or ultrasonography. Treatment is rest and knee protection.

- Repetitive stress can cause apophyseal injury in the upper and lower extremity or tenosynovitis. Children are at risk for *Little League shoulder*, *golfer or tennis elbow*, shin splints, and other overuse syndromes. Treatment is rest and physiotherapy.

- Osteonecrosis is another cause of arthralgia. The most common forms are Legg-Calvé-Perthes disease and Scheuermann disease (spine).

- Trauma can produce arthralgia. More common traumas include stress fracture, slipped capital femoral epiphysis, osteochondritis dissecans, traumatic hemarthrosis, acute chondrolysis of the hip, physical abuse, frostbite, and congenital indifference to pain.

- There are many diseases that have musculoskeletal symptoms including cartilage and bone dysplasias, connective tissue disorders, nutritional abnormalities, metabolic diseases, endocrinopathies, hematologic disorders, cystic fibrosis, storage diseases, primary bone, muscle and synovial tumors, and metastatic disease.

IDIOPATHIC MUSCULOSKELETAL PAIN SYNDROMES

- The incidence and prevalence of idiopathic pain in schoolchildren is very frequent. Back pain occurs in 20% of children, limb pain in 16%, and fibromyalgia in 6%. Patients with pain represent 5–8% of new patients in pediatric rheumatology clinics.
- Mean age of onset is 12–13 years with female predominance (4:1). All reports of pain patients are from developed countries.
- Etiopathogenesis is unknown. Pediatric patients are different from adults and more readily respond to exercise therapy. Symptoms appear to be causally related to illness, injury, and/or psychologic distress. There is often a role model for chronic pain or disability. Interdependency or enmeshment between parent(s) and child is striking.
- Clinical manifestations: Pain may be diffuse or localized and associated with a minor trauma. Symptoms of depression and/or poor sleep are usual. Conversion symptoms are frequent as well as eating disorders. Careful examination is devoid of findings of underlying disease. Peripheral nervous system findings may include allodynia, coolness, and cyanosis. Specific history of prolonged back pain can be due to a serious problem and should be investigated further.
- Differential diagnosis includes seronegative enthesopathy syndrome, trauma, mechanical pain, arthritis, and neoplasia. There are no specific laboratory findings and testing should not be performed unless there is significant concern about a separate diagnosis.
- Treatment: Most rheumatologists prescribe an aggressive exercise program to improve function and well-being. Patients with sleep disorders often benefit from low-dose tricyclics. Depression should be treated with a serotonin reuptake inhibitor. Allodynia is treated with desensitization using a towel or a bucket of rice or dried beans. Interventions such a sympathetic block, transcutaneous electrical nerve stimulators (TENS) units, and analgesics do not improve outcome.
- Prognosis is variable with frequent relapses. The above treatment plan has had improved outcome with 90% of patients remaining fully active.

FEVER

- Patients are frequently referred to the rheumatologist after initial evaluation of fever has not revealed a specific diagnosis. The use of a fever diary is very helpful in determining the cause of fever. A daily spiking fever may be consistent with systemic onset arthritis or malaria. Persistent fever is seen in lupus and vasculitis and also in inflammatory bowel disease, neoplasia, chronic infection, and acute rheumatic diseases such as Kawasaki disease. Cyclic fever syndromes include FAPA (periodic fever, aphthous stomatitis, pharyngitis, adenitis) syndrome, hyper IgD, and Familial Mediterranean Fever. Finally, the patient may have daily temperatures below 100.5°F which the family may have misinterpreted as fever. Patients with fever deserve a complete evaluation to find an underlying diagnosis including laboratory and radiographic evaluations. If no source is isolated, fever can be controlled with nonsteroidal anti-inflammatories and the patient is closely observed. Ultimately, the fever resolves or the source of fever becomes clear.

POSITIVE ANA

- Patients are referred to the pediatric rheumatology office for the presence of positive ANA. The patients may have had an evaluation for musculoskeletal complaints or an unusual rash and laboratory testing reveals a positive ANA result. Approximately 2% of the general population has a positive ANA. The frequency is higher in relatives of patients with autoimmune disease; a situation where greater anxiety exists at the onset of a child's musculoskeletal symptoms. ANA alone is not a diagnostic test. Patients who present with a positive ANA and no other physical or laboratory evidence of rheumatologic disease, have little risk for developing a rheumatologic disease. If the patient has other symptoms such as Raynaud phenomenon, the risk increases. Many patients have high anxiety about an abnormal laboratory value. ANA testing should occur in the setting of other clear signs or symptoms of rheumatologic disease.

BIBLIOGRAPHY

Cassidy JT, Petty RE (eds.), *Textbook of Pediatric Rheumatology*, 4th ed. Philadelphia, PA: W.B. Saunders, 2001.

Gedalia A. Familial Mediterranean Fever. In: Miller ML (ed.), *Nelson Textbook of Pediatrics*, 17th ed. Philadelphia, PA: W.B. Saunders, 2003, pp. 821–822.

Jacobs J. *Pediatric Rheumatology for the Practitioner,* 2nd ed. New York, NY: Springer-Verlag, 1993.

Miller ML. Musculoskeletal Pain Syndromes, In Miller ML (ed.) *Nelson's Textbook of Pediatrics,* 17th ed. Philadelphia, PA: W.B. Saunders, 2003, pp. 831–832.

Sherry DD, Malleson PN. The idiopathic musculoskeletal pain syndromes in childhood. *Rheum Dis Clin North Am* 2002;28:669–686.

185 JUVENILE IDIOPATHIC ARTHRITIS (JIA)

Marisa S. Klein-Gitelman

DEFINITION

- Onset of a swollen joint or loss of normal range of motion with pain before 16 years.
- Persistence of one or more arthritic joints for greater than 6 weeks. Subtype assigned after 6 months' disease duration unless onset is systemic.

SUBTYPES
- Pauciarticular
  1. Four joints or less
  2. Each joint counted separately except cervical spine, carpus, and tarsus.
- Polyarticular
  1. Five joints or more
  2. Each joint counted separately with the exceptions as above.
- Systemic onset
  1. Daily fever >39°C for at least 2 weeks and arthritis in one or more joints.
  2. Patients have extraarticular disease such as evanescent salmon pink rash.

EPIDEMIOLOGY

- JIA is not rare although the true frequency is not known.
- Estimated incidence is 2–20/100,000 and prevalence is 16–150/100,000.
- Highest incidence occurs between ages 1–3 years in the pauciarticular onset group.
- Onset before age 6 months is very rare.
- Female to male ratio varies with disease subtype: pauciarticular 3:1, pauciarticular with uveitis 5–6.6:1, polyarticular 2.8:1, and systemic onset 1:1.

PATHOPHYSIOLOGY

- The pathophysiology of JIA remains unclear. There appears to be multiple etiologic sources including genetic traits and environmental agents. Current theory suggests that disease onset is a function of specific infectious agents in an individual with the appropriate genetic predisposition. No specific infectious agent has been isolated to date; however, some specific genetic predispositions have been defined. The autoimmune nature of the disease is based on pathologic changes within chronically inflamed synovium and humoral abnormalities such as autoantibodies, immune complexes, complement activation, and cytokinemia. The presence of the different subtypes suggests that genetic predisposition is multifactorial. This is supported by unclear inheritance patterns and different human leukocyte antigen (HLA) distributions in each subtype category.

PAUCIARTICULAR (OR OLIGOARTICULAR)

Clinical
- The child with pauciarticular JIA usually presents with a swollen, warm joint that is not painful, red, or tender. Patients have morning stiffness and gelling after naps or inactivity. Median age at onset is 2 years with female predominance. The affected joint is most commonly in the lower extremity: knee > ankle > elbow. The hip is almost always spared. Upper extremity arthritis is more unusual (wrist or phalangeal joints), and is associated with a higher risk for progression into polyarticular disease. Laboratory abnormalities may include an elevated erythrocyte sedimentation rate (ESR) and a positive ANA (antinuclear antibody). There are no diagnostic laboratory tests; however, the presence of ANA is associated with increased risk for uveitis.

Uveitis
- Although uveitis can occur in any type of JIA, it is found frequently in the child with pauciarticular disease and is rare in other forms of JIA.
- Frequency varies between 25 and 40% and is higher in children with a positive ANA.

Clinical
- The disease is an asymptomatic, most often bilateral chronic inflammation of the anterior chamber of the eye. Detection of uveitis before arthritis is unusual and often is associated with more severe disease. Half of the diagnoses are made at the time arthritis presents. Mostly uveitis presents within 5–7 years after arthritis is diagnosed; however, the risk of uveitis is never absent and it does not parallel the course of arthritis.

Diagnosis

- The diagnosis is made by slit lamp biomicroscopy. Children diagnosed with pauciarticular JIA should have slit lamp examinations every 3 months for the next 2 years after diagnosis, every 4–6 months for the next 7 years, and annually thereafter. Children with a positive ANA should be screened more frequently.

Differential Diagnosis

- Kawasaki disease, juvenile ankylosing spondylitis, psoriatic arthritis, inflammatory bowel disease, reactive arthritis, sarcoidosis, Blau disease, Behcet disease, and Vogt-Koyanagi-Harada disease. If a child with arthritis and uveitis presents with a posterior uveitis, consider sarcoidosis rather than JIA.

Treatment

- Initiated with corticosteroid eye drops and a nighttime mydriatic if needed. Anti-inflammatory medications used to treat arthritis may be of benefit to uveitis and changes in treatment should be a consideration in the disease course of uveitis. Eye disease unresponsive to topical therapy is treated with oral corticosteroids, methotrexate, or other immunosuppressive medications. The course of uveitis does not mirror the course of arthritis and may flare or occur when arthritis is in remission.

Prognosis

- In the past, loss of vision occurred in 15–30% of children. This has improved with earlier diagnosis and treatment and, perhaps, with more aggressive treatment. Prognostic factors include disease severity and chronicity at presentation. Prognosis is worse for the child whose uveitis precedes arthritis as the patient usually presents to the ophthalmologist with complaints of visual changes. Outcome for 25% of children is excellent, 50% have a fair course, and 25% do poorly with complications of vision loss, cataract, or glaucoma.

Prevention

- Frequent screening eye examination as detailed above.

DIFFERENTIAL DIAGNOSIS

- The diagnosis of JIA requires that other potential causes of arthritis have been considered and not found. The most important diseases to consider are infection, tumor (especially leukemia and neuroblastoma), acute rheumatic diseases, Lyme disease, and hemophilia although there are many genetic, endocrinologic, and metabolic causes of abnormal joints that may also be considered. In the child who presents with arthritis for less than 72 hours, consider septic arthritis and osteomyelitis and reactive arthritis first. Trauma including hemarthrosis, osteochondritis dissecans, fracture, and discoid meniscus are possible. In the child with long-standing arthritis, tuberculous infection, osteomyelitis, sarcoid, and villonodular synovitis should be considered.

TREATMENT

- JIA is always managed with a combination of medication and physical and/or occupational therapy. Although medication will control inflammation, many children develop contractures that will not improve without therapy. Thus, children receive nonsteroidal anti-inflammatory drugs (NSAIDs) daily with close monitoring to prevent gastritis and other adverse reactions and an exercise program to improve strength and function. There is potential for growth abnormalities due to inflammation often represented as overgrowth both in bone length and joint circumference. This is particularly important in the child with asymmetric lower extremity disease. Bone overgrowth is controlled with medication; however, leg length discrepancies need to be addressed with shoe inserts or lifts to prevent scoliosis and worsen flexion contractures. For the child who does not respond to NSAIDs, the physician may consider intraarticular corticosteroid, sulfasalazine, and methotrexate. Rarely, other immunosuppressive therapy including biologic agents is required.

PROGNOSIS

- The prognosis for pauciarticular JIA is variable. Many children have disease for a median of 2 years and remit. Some of these patients may have disease flares years after initial remission. Another small group of children (5–10%) will progress to polyarticular disease after a pauciarticular course of 1–2 years and will have a more guarded prognosis for joint health.

PREVENTION

- Outcome is improved by treatment compliance (exercise and medication) and aggressive therapy when needed. Bone health is supported by sufficient dietary calcium and vitamin D.

POLYARTICULAR JIA

Clinical

- The child with polyarticular JIA presents to the clinician with five or more joints affected by arthritis within the first 6 months of disease. Onset is usually insidious and progressive although acute disease presentations occur. The patient has significant morning stiffness and gelling after inactivity. The pattern of arthritis tends to be symmetrical affecting large and small joints including the cervical spine and temporomandibular joints. Proximal phalangeal joints are more often involved than distal joints. This disease has a considerable female predominance. The most important factor associated with progression and outcome is the presence of rheumatoid factor (RF). Children without RF have a median age onset of 3 years. RF positive children have a median age onset of 12 years and represent early onset rheumatoid arthritis often presenting with rheumatoid nodules and bone erosions. Children with polyarticular JIA may present with mild systemic features including low-grade fever, hepatosplenomegaly, adenopathy, and pericarditis. The risk of uveitis is low. With the exception of the prognostic value of RF, laboratory tests are non-diagnostic. Patients may have positive ANA, high ESR or C-reactive protein (CRP), anemia, and thrombocytosis.

Differential Diagnosis

• The diagnosis of polyarticular JIA can only be made when other diagnoses are considered and no evidence is found. Important in the differential is neoplasia, acute rheumatic diseases, reactive arthritis, Lyme disease, sarcoidosis, spondyloarthropathies, systemic lupus erythematosus, autoimmune overlap syndromes, vasculitis, and genetic and metabolic syndromes such as mucopolysaccharidoses. In this setting, infection is less likely but must be considered.

Treatment

• Treatment of polyarticular JIA is usually initiated with NSAIDs. Patients with disease that prevents daily function such as school attendance due to profound stiffness and pain are treated more aggressively. Treatment options include methotrexate, biologic agents, leufludomide, sulfasalazine, hydroxychloroquine, oral, intraarticular, or intravenous corticosteroids, and other immunosuppressive agents. The availability of tumor necrosis factor (TNF) inhibitors has dramatically improved function for more severe patients and will hopefully improve disease outcomes. Experimental therapies such as stem-cell transplantation are considered in patients who failed other therapies. Patients with polyarticular JIA must also receive physical and occupational therapy to improve strength, range of motion, and ability to perform activities of daily living. Patients may require splints to prevent flexion contractures.

Prognosis

• The child with RF negative disease has a remitting course which may completely resolve. The presence of ANA is also associated with better outcome. The child with RF positive disease has persistent, chronic disease with a high risk for joint destruction and disability. Hip disease and disease activity greater than 7 years are particularly poor prognostic signs.

Prevention

• Early diagnosis and aggressive management of severe disease are helpful in preventing disease severity and disability. Sufficient calcium and vitamin D aid in promoting bone and joint health. Compliance with medication and therapy are critical to successful treatment and prevention of growth disturbances and deformity.

SYSTEMIC ONSET

Clinical

• As defined, systemic JIA presents with fever and arthritis. Systemic features may occur weeks to years before the presence of arthritis; however classical the fever and rash are, a diagnosis cannot be made without arthritis. The fever often spikes in the late evening or early morning. The evanescent salmon pink rash is more often visible during fever, may be pruritic, and may be elicited by rubbing or scratching (Koebner phenomenon). The arthritis is pauciarticular or polyarticular. There is morning stiffness and gelling. Other manifestations include hepatosplenomegaly, adenopathy, pericarditis, pleuritis, and myalgia. Laboratory abnormalities include leukocytosis, thrombocytosis, anemia, and high ESR or CRP. Patients may have a coagulopathy (prolonged D-dimer) and elevated liver enzymes. A rare but serious and acute complication is macrophage activation syndrome (MAS) or hematophagocytic lymphohistiocytosis (HLH). MAS is a consequence of the inability to turn off cytotoxic T cells and macrophages. The patient presents with a persisting fever and rapid development of coagulopathy associated with purpura, bruising and bleeding, hepatosplenomegaly, encephalopathy, and less frequently acute renal failure, cardiomyopathy, or pulmonary disease. Laboratory studies reveal a falling ESR, leucopenia, thrombocytopenia, consumptive coagulopathy, and hepatitis. MAS can also occur with lupus, infection (especially Epstein-Barr virus [EBV] and varicella-zoster virus [VZV]), and malignancy.

Differential Diagnosis

• The differential diagnosis in the child who presents with persisting fever must include infection, particularly sepsis and endocarditis but also viral syndromes (mononucleosis). Acute rheumatic diseases such as acute rheumatic fever, Kawasaki disease, and familial Mediterranean fever must also be considered. Kawasaki disease may be difficult to distinguish. Inflammatory bowel disease, cyclic fever syndromes, chronic rheumatic diseases (lupus, vasculitis, and dermatomyositis), malignancy, and Castleman disease are important considerations.

Treatment

- The child with symptoms of systemic onset arthritis has NSAID therapy initiated while evaluation to substantiate the diagnosis progresses. Patients often develop subnormal temperatures as fever control occurs. A portion of children will respond to NSAID therapy alone while the majority requires IV and/or oral corticosteroids to obtain disease control. Patients may require intraarticular steroid therapy, methotrexate, or tumor necrosis factor (TNF) inhibitors. Other treatments include cyclosporin A, leufludomide, azathioprine, or cyclophosphamide. For the patient with treatment-resistant disease, experimental therapies such as thalidomide or stem cell transplantation can be considered. Physical and occupational therapy are critical to resolve flexion contractures and maintain strength and flexibility.

Prognosis

- The child with pauciarticular joint distribution is likely to have a remitting disease course while the child with polyarticular disease may have a remitting course with joint damage or a destructive, persisting disease course (25%).

Prevention

- Early diagnosis and aggressive therapy improve outcome. Compliance with medication and therapy improve pain, function, and prevents deformities. Control of inflammation will prevent growth disturbances and prevent deformities. Sufficient calcium and vitamin D in the diet will help maintain bone health and is important for the child requiring steroid therapy.

SPONDYLOARTHRITIDES

DEFINITION

SERONEGATIVE ENTHESIS RELATED ARTHRITIS (SEA)

- The presence of arthritis and enthesitis.
- The presence of arthritis or enthesitis and two or more of the following criteria:
  1. Sacroiliac tenderness or inflammatory spine pain.
  2. HLA-B27

3. First or second degree relative with medically confirmed HLA-B27 associated disease.
4. Anterior uveitis usually associated with pain, redness, or photophobia.
5. Onset of arthritis in a boy over the age of 8 years.
- Exclusions
  1. Psoriasis diagnosed by a dermatologist in a first- or second-degree relative.
  2. Presence of systemic arthritis.

JUVENILE ANKYLOSING SPONDYLITIS (JAS)

- Clinical criteria (New York)
  1. Limitation of lumbosacral motion in all three planes.
  2. Pain or history of pain at the lumbar spine.
  3. Limited chest expansion at the fourth intercostals space (<2.5 cm).
- Criteria: Sacroiliac sclerosis
- Definite JAS
  1. Grades 3–4 bilateral sacroiliitis on radiograph +1 clinical criterion.
  2. Grades 3–4 unilateral or Grade 2 bilateral sacroiliitis with clinical criterion number 1 or with clinical criteria numbers 2 and 3.
- Probable JAS
  1. Grades 3–4 bilateral sacroiliitis on radiograph.

EPIDEMIOLOGY

JAS

- Incidence and prevalence are unclear. One study estimated a prevalence of 129/100,000 children of Northern European extraction. True prevalence may follow presence of HLA-B27 in survey population. Estimates suggest JAS may be as frequent as JIA; however it may be difficult to differentiate early JAS from JIA. Age at onset is late childhood to adolescence. Gender distribution is estimated anywhere from 7 to 2.7:1 (male:female).

SEA

- Incidence and prevalence not known.

PATHOGENESIS

- Pathogenesis of JAS is unclear. Similarities between infection-related arthritis and HLA-B27 disease supports the role of infection as a trigger. HLA-B27 gene is either part of pathogenesis or an important disease marker. HLA-B27 is not necessary for this disease to unfold in a particular patient. The importance of HLA-B27 in the host immune response to infection is being studied in a transgenic rat model. Clinical observations of the association between gut inflammation and JAS are supportive of the importance of HLA-B27 and cellular immune responses. Spondyloarthropathy is the pattern of arthritis seen in inflammatory bowel disease.

CLINICAL

- Patients with spondyloarthropathies present with pain at the heels, buttock, thighs, and shoulders. Most patients have lower extremity findings. True complaints of low back pain occur in about a quarter of patients at onset. Sacroiliac involvement occurs in most patients over time along with lumbosacral spine disease. Half of the patients have four or less arthritic joints and half have five or more arthritic joints. Enthesitis is an early and distinguishing clinical symptom. The most frequently affected areas are the heel, foot, ankle, and knee. The pain and disability from enthesitis is a difficult problem for the child with spondyloarthropathy. Iritis associated with spondyloarthropathy in contrast to JIA is acute, painful, and photophobic. It is usually unilateral and resolves without scarring although there are recurrences. In pediatric spondyloarthropathies, cardiovascular disease is rare and involves aortic valve or aortic root abnormalities.

DIAGNOSIS

- Diagnosis criteria are outlined in their definitions. Careful examination of entheses, especially the Achilles, plantar fascia, patella, and tibial tuberosity demonstrates discrete painful points. The presence of arthritis at the first metatarsophalangeal joint, intertarsal joint, ankle, or knee is supportive evidence of the diagnosis. Examination of the axial skeleton should include palpation of sacroiliac joint for tenderness and evaluation of forward lumbar spine expansion by Schober measurement. There is no specific laboratory diagnostic test; however, the presence of HLA-B27 is supportive. Elevation of the white blood cell count, platelet count, and ESR are frequently seen. Some patients may have systemic features including low-grade fever, weight loss in association with very high ESR levels (>100 mm/hour). Inflammatory bowel disease should be considered in this patient group. Serologic tests (ANA, RF) are usually negative. Radiographic evaluation of the sacroiliac joints can be diagnostic and is best demonstrated by computed tomography.

DIFFERENTIAL DIAGNOSIS

- Inflammatory bowel disease, other inflammatory arthropathies, systemic onset JIA, infection, diskitis, and malignancy should be considered.

TREATMENT

- Medical management depends on disease severity. Many patients respond well to NSAIDs and sulfasalazine while other patients may require methotrexate or glucocorticoids. TNF inhibitors can be useful in the severe patient. Enthesitis does not respond well to anti-inflammatory therapy and is treated with orthoses. All patients require exercise and posture training program.

PROGNOSIS

- The disease course of spondyloarthropathies is remitting and may be mild, especially in female patients. The presence of hip disease and persistent arthritis is associated with poor outcome. Compliance with physical and occupational therapy is crucial to good outcome for these patients.

PREVENTION

- Compliance can prevent some poor outcomes. Maintain bone health with calcium and vitamin D.

PSORIATIC ARTHRITIS

- Arthritis and psoriasis
- Arthritis and two-third following criteria:
  1. Nail pitting or onycholysis
  2. Family history or psoriasis in first-degree relative
  3. Dactylitis
- Estimated incidence 3/100,000.
- Estimated prevalence 10–15/100,000.
- Most patients are Caucasians.
- Mean age at onset is 10 years with a noted early peak in preschool years.
- Gender distribution is fairly equal.
- Psoriasis occurs first in 40% of children while arthritis occurs first in 60%.
- Pathology is related to abnormal CD8 T-cell populations seen in the skin and synovium.
- Clinical pattern of arthritis is usually monoarticular of asymmetric oligoarthritis extending to a polyarticular pattern and associated with dactylitis (70%).

- Nail pitting is common; onycholysis is rare.
- Uveitis is uncommon.
- No specific laboratory tests. ANA is positive in 30–60%. Elevated ESR, CRP, thrombocytosis, and anemia of chronic disease are common.
- Radiographs may reveal periostitis.
- Treatment protocol is similar to JAS. TNF inhibitors are particularly useful in psoriatic arthritis and control psoriasis as well as arthritis in patients with more aggressive disease.
- Prognosis is poor with many patients having disease persistence and joint deformities.
- Prevention of poor prognosis may occur with newer biologic agents and an aggressive management plan.

BIBLIOGRAPHY

Bowyer SL, Roettcher PA, Higgins GC, et al. Health status of patients with juvenile rheumatoid arthritis at 1 and 5 years after diagnosis. *J Rheumatol* 2003;30:394–400.

Burgos-Vargas R. The juvenile-onset spondyloarthritides. *Rheum Clin North Am* 2002;28:531–560.

Cassidy JT, Petty RE (eds.). *Textbook of Pediatric Rheumatology*, 4th ed. Philadelphia, PA: W.B. Saunders, 2001.

Ilowite NT. Current treatment of juvenile rheumatoid arthritis. *Pediatrics* 2002;109:109–115.

Jacobs J. *Pediatric Rheumatology for the Practioner*, 2nd ed. New York, NY: Springer-Verlag, 1993.

Patel H, Goldstein D. Pediatric uveitis. *Pediatr Clin North Am* 2003;50:125–136.

Schneider R, Passo MH. Juvenile rheumatoid arthritis. *Rheum Dis Clin North Am* 28:503–530, 2002.

186 SYSTEMIC LUPUS ERYTHEMATOSUS (SLE)

Marisa S. Klein-Gitelman

EPIDEMIOLOGY

- The incidence and prevalence of pediatric SLE varies by geographic location, ethnicity, gender, and age. The true incidence and prevalence are not known. Estimates of prevalence vary from 4 to 250/100,000 with higher prevalence in children of Asian, African, and Latin and Native American descent. SLE is more frequent in females. The gender ratio before puberty is 4:1 (female:male) and 8:1 after puberty.

PATHOPHYSIOLOGY

- The etiology of SLE remains unclear despite intensive investigation. It is evident that SLE is a multifactorial process including a variety of genes, hormonal, and environmental factors. SLE is the archetypical autoimmune disease with dysregulation leading to the formation of autoantibodies. The most specific autoantibody is anti-DNA; however, autoantibodies to a variety of nuclear antigens, ribosomes, components of blood including red and white blood cells, platelets, immunoglobulin, and coagulation factors, and specific end-organs occur. The presence of autoantibodies leads to immune complex formation, complement activation, recruitment of inflammatory cells, and tissue damage. Nonspecific B-cell activation is due to dysregulation of suppressor T cells perhaps due to abnormal apoptosis or cell death of autoreactive lymphocytes. Abnormalities in the complement cascade or macrophage phagocytosis are other important disease mechanisms. Hormonal influences, ultraviolet light, and certain drugs are also known to be inducers of disease. The result is an immune complex-mediated vasculitis and fibrinoid necrosis leading to sclerosis of collagen manifested as an onion-skin lesion around arteries and cellular inflammation. Hematoxylin bodies are the result of ant-DNA antibodies and nuclear debris.

CLINICAL FINDINGS

- As previously mentioned, the manifestations of SLE are protean and each patient has unique features. A detailed history, physical examination, and laboratory evaluation may uncover the disease and lead to early diagnosis and treatment. Common symptoms and signs are the following:
- Constitutional symptoms include fever, fatigue, anorexia, weight loss, and lymphadenopathy.
- Musculoskeletal symptoms include arthritis, arthralgia, myalgia, and tendonitis. Myositis is rare. Osteonecrosis is common (secondary to vasculopathy or corticosteroids).
- Skin findings include malar rash, discoid rash, photosensitivity rash, nasooral ulcers, cutaneous vasculitis, livedo reticularis, Raynaud phenomenon, urticaria, psoriasform or annular rashes, bullous lesions, and alopecia. (There are many other SLE rashes.)
- Renal findings include nephrotic syndrome, glomerulonephritis, acute renal failure, hypertension, peripheral edema, and retinal changes. World Health Organization criteria of renal pathology are helpful for diagnosis, treatment, and prognosis. The classification describes

the severity and geographic distribution of glomeru-lonephritis (Classes II–IV), membranous changes (Class V), and glomerular sclerosis (Class VI).
- Cardiovascular/pulmonary findings include chest pain especially when reclined, valvulitis, endocarditis (Libman-Sacks disease), coronary artery vasculitis/thrombosis, arrhythmia, heart failure, pleuritic pain, pulmonary hemorrhage/infiltrates, and fibrosis.
- Neurologic findings include seizure, psychosis, cognitive dysfunction, stroke, pseudotumor cerebri, aseptic meningitis, chorea, mood disorders, transverse myelitis, and peripheral neuropathies. Neuropsychiatric manifestations may be acute and severe. Neuroimaging may be normal.
- Hematologic findings include thrombocytopenia, leucopenia, lymphopenia, Coomb positive anemia, anemia of chronic disease, hypercoaguable states with thrombosis, and associated antiphospholipid antibodies/lupus anticoagulant.
- Gastrointestinal findings include elevated liver enzymes, colitis, or intestinal vasculitis.
- Sjogren syndrome: Dry eyes (keratoconjunctivitis sicca) and dry mouth.
- Autoimmune endocrinopathies, most frequently thyroiditis.

DIAGNOSIS

- The diagnosis is supported by the presence of 4/11 classification criteria:
  1. Malar rash: Fixed erythema in a butterfly distribution sparing nasolabial folds.
  2. Discoid rash: Erythematous, raised, scaly rash with follicular plugging.
  3. Photosensitivity: Rash as result of a reaction to sun exposure.
  4. Oral ulcers: Often painless nasal or oral ulceration.
  5. Arthritis: Nonerosive arthritis in two or more peripheral joints.
  6. Serositis:
     a. Pleuritis: Convincing history of pleuritic pain, pleural rub, or evidence of pleural effusion.
     b. Pericarditis: Pericardial rub, electrocardiogram (ECG), or evidence of pericardial effusion.
  7. Renal disorder
     a. Persistent proteinuria 0.5 g/day or >3+ protein.
     b. Cellular casts
  8. Neurologic disorder
     a. Seizure in absence of known drug or metabolic precipitants.
     b. Psychosis in absence of known drug or metabolic precipitants.
  9. Hematologic disorder
     a. Hemolytic anemia with reticulocytosis.
     b. Leukopenia <4000/mm^3 on two or more occasions.
     c. Lymphopenia <1500/mm^3 on two or more occasions.
     d. Thrombocytopenia <100,000/mm^3.
  10. ANA: Presence of ANA with the absence of drugs known to be associated with drug-induced lupus.
  11. Immunologic
     a. Presence of antinative (double-stranded) DNA antibody.
     b. Presence of anti-Smith antibody (Sm nuclear antigen).
     c. Positive LE-cell preparation.
     d. Biologic false positive test for syphilis for at least 6 months confirmed by fluorescent treponemal antibody absorption test (FTA-ABS) or TPI, or IgG or IgM antiphospholipid antibodies, or lupus anticoagulant.
- Other laboratory abnormalities include hypocomplementemia, the most important measure of disease activity or immune complex formation (total hemolytic complement, C$_3$, C$_4$), anti-RNP (ribonuclear protein) antibody in association with anti-Smith antibody, Sjogren antibodies (anti-SSA and anti-SSB antibodies), and hypergammaglobulinemia.

DIFFERENTIAL DIAGNOSIS

- The criteria for lupus are helpful due to the variety of clinical phenomena that occur. The most important differentials include infection including subacute endocarditis, malignancy especially leukemia and lymphoma, inflammatory bowel disease, and other rheumatologic diseases such as systemic juvenile arthritis, dermatomyositis, and polyarticular JIA. Mixed connective tissue disease (MCTD) can have a very similar presentation to SLE; however, a criterion for the diagnosis of MCTD is the presence of anti-RNP antibodies without anti-Smith antibody. MCTD patients with lupus-like disease may evolve to disease more similar to dermatomyositis or scleroderma. Hence, it is important to distinguish the MCTD patient from the SLE patient.

TREATMENT

- Specific treatment needs to be individualized for each patient depending on the level and type of disease activity. All patients need to obtain a calcium-sufficient well-balanced diet, rest, and sun protection. Immunizations including pneumococcal vaccines should be completed. SLE patients are immunocompromised due to disease pathophysiology and most drug therapies. Any infection must be evaluated and treated swiftly. Patients with musculoskeletal complaints often benefit from nonsteroidal anti-inflammatory agents. Hydroxychloroquine treats most lupus rashes and minor musculoskeletal symptoms. More recent data suggest that hydroxychloroquine decreases risk of thrombosis. Anticoagulation is required for thrombosis; low-dose aspirin for presence of antiphospholipid antibodies. Other than patients with minor disease manifestations, all SLE patients require high-dose corticosteroids and often at onset, high-dose intravenous corticosteroids. The dose of corticosteroids is slowly and smoothly tapered over months once disease control is obtained. Immunosuppressive medication other than corticosteroids are used to control severe disease manifestations and as steroid sparing agents. Cyclophosphamide is used in conjunction with corticosteroids in the patient with significant nephritis, cerebritis, or carditis. Azathioprine is used as a steroid sparing agent. There is limited information on the use of methotrexate, cyclosporin, and mycophenolate mofetil. The use of intravenous immunoglobulin (IVIG) and plasmapheresis have limited roles in treatment. It is important to monitor levels of IgG in patients on chronic immunosuppression as hypogammaglobulinemia can occur. Experimental therapies including the use of anti-CD20 antibodies and stem cell transplantation for the patient with persistent and severe disease unresponsive to treatment can be considered.

PROGNOSIS

• SLE is a lifetime disease characterized by flares and remissions. It is difficult to determine the prognosis for an individual patient; however, disease activity and severity, the progression of kidney disease, the presence of vasculitis, and the number of organ systems involved are associated with morbidity and mortality. Typically, patients with severe kidney disease and persistent central nervous system (CNS) disease fare poorly relative to other children. Major morbidity (from disease and treatment) occurs from infection, renal failure, chronic CNS disease, atherosclerosis/myocardial infarction, cardiomyopathy, osteoporosis especially due to fracture, osteonecrosis, cataracts, glaucoma, growth failure, diabetes, and infertility.

PREVENTION

• Compliance with treatment plans, sun protection, rapid treatment of infection, and attention to diet including calcium and vitamin D can prevent disease flares and morbidity due to treatment.

BIBLIOGRAPHY

Cassidy JT, Petty RE (eds.). *Textbook of Pediatric Rheumatology.* Philadelphia, PA: W.B. Saunders, 2001.

Jacobs J. *Pediatric Rheumatology for the Practitioner.* New York, NY: Springer-Verlag, 1993.

Klein-Gitelman MS, Miller ML. Systemic Lupus Erythematosus, In Miller ML (ed.). *Nelson's Textbook of Pediatrics,* 17th ed. Philadelphia, PA: W.B. Saunders, 2003, pp. 809–813.

Klein-Gitelman MS, Reiff A, Silverman E. Systemic lupus erythematosus in childhood. *Rheum Dis Clin North Am* 2002;28:561–578.

Tucker LB, Menon S, Schaller JF, Isenberg DA. Adult and childhood onset systemic lupus erythematosus: a comparison of clinical features, serology and outcome. *Br J Rheumatol* 1995;34:866–872.

187 HENOCH-SCHONLEIN PURPURA (HSP)

Marisa S. Klein-Gitelman

EPIDEMIOLOGY

• Henoch-Schonlein purpura is the most common form of systemic vasculitis in the pediatric population. Incidence is reported at 13.5/100,000. Most patients are between 3 and 15 years with a male:female ratio of 1.5:1.

PATHOPHYSIOLOGY

• Henoch-Schonlein purpura is a small vessel IgA-immune complex mediated vasculitis activating the alternate complement pathway (C_3, properidin). Skin and kidney biopsy reveal leukocytoclastic vasculitis with IgA deposition. The kidney lesion ranges from focal mesangial proliferation to severe crescentic disease. The vasculitis often occurs after infection, in particular an upper respiratory illness or streptococcal pharyngitis although there are associations with other viral and bacterial pathogens. HSP also occurs after insect bites, certain medications, and certain foods in the individual with food allergy. The only genetic markers reported have been risk factors for renal disease: HLA-B35 in a Spanish population and Il-1R allele 2. HSP appears to occur frequently in patients with immunologic defects such as C_2 or C_4 deficiency and common variable disease.

CLINICAL FEATURES

• The primary features of HSP include arthritis, abdominal pain, and nonthrombocyopenic purpuric rash below the waist line. Either of these features may precede the others.
  1. The rash consists of palpable purpura and petechiae. The patient frequently has peripheral edema of the feet and hands. Scrotal edema is seen in boys. Forehead and periorbital edema and rash over the upper body is frequent in younger children.
  2. The arthritis is transient but painful. Affected joints are usually large joints of lower and sometimes upper extremities.
  3. The abdominal pain is often associated with bleeding. Complications include intussuception of small bowel and massive gastrointestinal bleeding. Inflammation of other abdominal structures have been reported including gallbladder and pancreas.
  4. Hematuria is not infrequent; however, some children develop severe glomerulonephritis and rarely, renal failure. Children at risk for severe renal disease are older than 7 years at onset, more severe course of purpura and/or abdominal pain and low factor XIII activity.
  5. Other rare but severe manifestations include orchitis, ureteral or epididymal vasculitis, pulmonary hemorrhage, and central nervous system (CNS) disease including seizure and infarct.

DIAGNOSIS AND DIFFERENTIAL DIAGNOSIS

• There are no specific laboratory features associated with this vasculitis. Platelet and white blood cell counts are normal to mildly elevated. The erythrocyte sedimentation rate (ESR) may also be elevated. IgA may be elevated early in the disease course. Antinuclear antibody (ANA) titers are usually negative. Guaiac positive stools occur frequently. A coagulopathy may be demonstrated in some cases with elevated D-dimer or decreased levels of Factor XII. More rarely, prolonged prothrombin time/partial thromboplastin time (PT/PTT) is found. Diagnostic criteria include palpable purpura, age less than 20 years at onset, bowel angina and wall granulocytes on biopsy. The presence of 2/4 criteria is 87% sensitive and 88% specific.

TREATMENT

• Treatment is usually supportive care. Patients may require nonsteroidal anti-inflammatory agents to control cutaneous manifestations and arthritis. The use of glucocorticoids is controversial for gastrointestinal symptoms. Some literature suggests that steroids may mask intussusception or perforation while other authors suggest that steroids decrease the presence of pain significantly and may prevent more severe renal disease. Evidence of systemic vasculitis or specific end-organ damage requires steroid therapy. Severe kidney disease requires combination immunosuppression with corticosteroids, cyclophosphamide, and anticoagulants. If there is persistent proteinuria, angiotensin-converting enzyme inhibitor therapy is useful.

PROGNOSIS

• Most patients have a short disease course with complete resolution within 1 month. Some patients have disease recurrences; however, the recurrent episode is usually shorter and less intense. Morbidity arises from gastrointestinal infarction or perforation during the acute phase of the disease and renal failure in those patients with severe kidney disease. Approximately 1% of patients go to complete renal failure requiring dialysis and transplantation.

PREVENTION

• There is literature which suggests that early treatment of patients at risk for kidney disease may decrease the severity, and perhaps, the presence of kidney disease. This literature is controversial and there are no specific recommendations. There is some suggestion that urinary metabolites, N-acetyl-[beta]-D-glucosaminidase (NAG) and [alpha]-1-microglobulin may be able to predict risk of renal disease. If this suggestion is validated, corticosteroids may be given to a select high-risk population.

BIBLIOGRAPHY

Brendel-Muller K, et al. Laboratory signs of activated coagulation are common in Henoch-Schonlein purpura. *Pediatr Nephrol* 2001;16:1084–1088.

Cassidy JT, Petty RE (eds.). *Textbook of Pediatric Rheumatology.* Philadelphia, PA: W.B. Saunders, 2001.

Hendriksson P, Hedner U, Nilsson IM. Factor XIII (fibrin stabilizing factor) in Henoch-Schonlein purpura. *Acta Paediatr Scand* 1977;66:273–277.

Mollica F, Li Volti S, Garozzo R, Russo G. Effectiveness of early prednisone treatment in preventing the development of nephropathy in anaphylactoid purpura. *Eur J Pediatr* 1992; 151:140–144.

Muller D, Greve D, Eggert D. Early tubular proteinuria and the development of nephritis in children. *Pediatr Nephrol* 1999;15: 85–89.

Reinehr T, Burk G, Andler W. Does steroid treatment of abdominal pain prevent renal involvement in Henoch-Schonlein purpura? *J Pediatr Gastroenterol Nutr* 2000;31:323–324.

Rosenblum ND, Winter HS. Steroid effects on the course of abdominal pain in children with Henoch-Schonlein purpura. *Pediatrics* 1987;79:1018–1021.

188 JUVENILE DERMATOMYOSITIS (JDM)

Lauren M. Pachman

EPIDEMIOLOGY

- *General*: Incidence of JDM (United States) 3.2 cases/million children/year, with a ratio of girls to boys of 2.1 (Mendez et al., in press). The mean age at disease onset is 6.7 years; 25% of children are 4 years of age or younger (9% are 2 years of age or younger). The majority, 73%, are White, 12% are Hispanic, and 9% African-Americans.
- *Infection* may trigger JDM at onset or be associated with disease flare. JDM children, in the 3 months before diagnosis, have an increased frequency of infectious symptoms when compared with age, geographic matched case-controls most frequently respiratory or gastrointestinal (GI) symptoms. A group A beta-hemolytic streptococcus has been implicated.

PATHOPHYSIOLOGY

- *Genetic factors* are important in susceptibility and chronicity.
  1. *DQA1*0501:* A higher association with histocompatibility locus antigens, DQA1*0501 > DR3 > B8—than family members or controls (Targoff, 2002). Boys with JDM have a higher frequency of the maternal HLA class II antigen, DQA1*0501 (maternal chimerism) (Reed and Ytterberg, 2002).
  2. *TNFα* : Substitution of an A for a G in the TNFα-308 promoter region associated with increased production of TNFα by both circulating mononuclear cells and muscle fibers, a prolonged disease course, requiring immunosuppressant therapy for 36 months or more, pathologic calcifications and occlusion of capillaries.
- *An antimicrobial response* in untreated children with JDM.
  1. *Gene expression profiles* of muscle biopsies from DQA1*0501+ girls with JDM documented a strong type I interferon (IFN-α) induced response, compatible with antiviral response.
  2. *Antigens* implicated by specific antibody testing include the RNA picornavirus, coxsackievirus B.
  3. *Lymphocyte stimulation studies*, using an antigenic region shared by myosin/group A beta-hemolytic streptococcal M protein.
- *Vascular lesions*: The primary lesion in JDM is an inflammation of small blood vessels, occlusion of arterioles and capillaries with subsequent drop-out.
  1. *Generalized vascular changes:* Dilated, inflamed small capillaries at the margins of the nailfold and eyelid, and on the soft palate. Decreased number of end-row capillary nailfold loops associated with severe JDM rash. Remaining capillaries, bush formation, with intra vessel thrombosis.
  2. *Muscle biopsy*: Infiltrate is primarily mononuclear (in contrast to adults with polymyositis alone, where polymorphonuclear cells predominate). Other features: Vascular occlusion, myofiber destruction, perifascicular atrophy, edema, and fibrosis (see Table 188-1).
  3. *Hematology*: Often *normal*: complete blood count (CBC), differential, platelets, erythrocyte sedimentation rate (ESR).
  4. von Willebrand factor antigen: Increased in 60%
  5. *Clinical chemistry*: ⇑ Aldolase, creatine kinase, aspartate aminotransferase (AST), Alanine aminotransferase (ALT), lactic dehydrogenase (LDH); urinalysis (UA): myoglobinuria; stool for occult blood.
  6. *Immunology*: Antinuclear antibodies (ANA)+ 80% at Dx: speckled pattern; most common MsA: Mi-2.
  7. ⇑ %CD19+ B cells; ⇑ neopterin (60%).

TABLE 188-1   Findings at Diagnosis of JDM

CRITERIA	NUMBER JDM	NUMBER (%) JDM POSITIVE	NEGATIVE
Any enzyme ⇑	80	72 (90)	8 (10)
Enzyme ⇑			
Creatine kinase	77	49 (64)	28 (36)
Aldolase	53	40 (75)	13 (25)
LDH	57	46 (81)	11 (19)
Alanine aminotransferase	65	49 (75)	16 (25)
Electromyogram	44	36 (82)	8 (18)
Muscle biopsy	52	42 (81)	10 (19)*

*Muscle biopsy negative or non-diagnostic.
SOURCE: Adapted from Targoff IN. Laboratory testing in the diagnosis and management of the idiopathic inflammatory myopathies. *Rheum Dis Clin North Am* 2002;28:859–890.

8. *Radiographic*: Magnetic resonance imaging (MRI): localization of inflammation; DXA: assessment of bone density; rehabilitation Cookie swallow: airway protection.
9. *Muscle biopsy*: See above.
10. *ANA*: Eighty percent are low titer *(1:160–1:320)* usually speckled pattern. Only 10–20% ANA+ sera with known specificity. If antibodies against myositis specific antigens (tRNA synthetases, signal recognition protein), or myositis associated antibodies (MSA) (e.g., Pm/Scl, PM-1, Scl-70) children may develop interstitial lung disease and a protracted, sometimes fatal disease course (Targoff, 2002).

CLASSIFICATION CRITERIA FOR JDM

- Rash: Gottron papules, shawl sign, erythema (knees, elbows, ankles) (Bohan and Peter, 1975).
- Symmetrical proximal muscle weakness.
- Elevated serum levels muscle enzymes.
- Positive electromyogram
- Biopsy compatible with diagnosis.
- Diagnosis: Definite JDM: rash + 4 criteria; probable JDM: rash + 3 criteria; possible JDM: rash + 2 criteria.
- *Frequent symptoms at diagnosis:* Muscle pain; fever, dysphagia, arthritis, calcifications, GI bleeding. Less frequent: alopecia, edema.

DIFFERENTIAL DIAGNOSIS

- Dermatomyositis
  1. Allergic reaction
  2. Other immune conditions: systemic lupus erythematosus (SLE), systemic onset juvenile arthritis, scleroderma, psoriasis, eczema.

3. Infectious myopathies: echovirus, parvovirus, toxoplasmosis, Lyme
- Pyomyositis:
  1. *Staphylococcus aureus*, group A *Streptococcus*
- Polymyositis:
  1. Influenza, parainfluenza, hepatitis B, adenovirus, human T-cell lymphotropic virus (HTLV) 1, human immunodeficiency virus (HIV).
  2. Drug- and toxin-induced myopathies: corticosteroids, hydroxychloroquine, penicillamine, penicillin, sulfa, ketoconazole, cimetidine, ranitidine, levostatin, zidovudine.
  3. Dystrophies: Duchenne, Becker, follicle-stimulating hormone (FSH), myotonic, dysferlin, merosin.
  4. Endocrine myopathies: thyroid, diabetes, mitochondrial myopathies.

TREATMENT

- Consider *prior* to therapy: Child's age at first symptom (disease onset) and at diagnosis—duration of untreated disease; severity of disease; extent of vascular involvement. Presence of serologic markers: MSA: Pm/Scl, RNP; myositis specific antibodies: JO-1; SPR, Mi-2.
- Therapy: Evaluate: disease severity/chronicity. Individualize.
  1. Corticosteroids: Intravenous: 30 mg/kg/day, 1 g maximum; PO prednisone: 0.5 mg/kg/day on non-IV days; topical: use sparingly.
  2. Methotrexate: Intravenous initially: 15 mg/m²/week; folic acid 1 mg/day.
  3. Skin involvement: Hydroxychloroquine: 7 mg/kg; tacrolimus may be an irritant.
  4. Consider: Cyclophosphamide; IV IgG if IgG low; Cyclosporin 2–3 mg/kg.
  5. Nutrition: Carnitine, vitamins
  6. Physical/occupational therapy: Early—passive stretch; later—conditioning.

PROGNOSIS

- Before corticosteroids: One-third died, one-third "crippled," and one-third had pathologic Ca++.
- As of 2003, mortality is 1%, usually a consequence of infection.
- Not known: increased risk for diabetes, heart disease, and effect on fertility?

PREVENTION

- Early diagnosis and prompt therapy in immunosuppressive dosage.

- If vasculitis, give medication by vein, not by mouth to ensure absorption.
- Sun screen: >SPF 30; ultraviolet (UVA/UVB), *p*-aminobenzoic acid (PABA) free; protective clothing.
- Bone protection: Calcium sufficient diet; vitamin D (1,25-OH-vitamin D).

REFERENCES

Bohan A, Peter B. Polymyositis and dermatomyositis. *N Engl J Med* 1975;292:344–347.

Mendez E, Lipton R, Dyer A, Ramsey-Goldman R, Roettcher P, Bowyer S, Pachman LM. U.S. incidence of JDM 1995–98: results from the NIAMS Registry. *Arthritis Care Res* (in press).

Pachman LM. Juvenile dermatomyositis: immunogenetics, pathophysiology and disease expression. *Rheum Dis Clin North Am*. 2002;28:579–602.

Pachman LM. Dermatomyositis. *Nelson's Textbook of Pediatrics*, 17th ed. Philadelphia, PA: W.B. Saunders, 2003, pp. 813–816.

Reed AM, Ytterberg SR. Genetic and environmental risk factors for idiopathic inflammatory myopathies. *Rheum Dis Clin North Am* 2002;28:891–916.

Rider LG, Miller FW. Classification and treatment of the juvenile idiopathic inflammatory myopathies. *Rheum Dis Clin North Am* 1997;23:619–655.

Targoff IN. Laboratory testing in the diagnosis and management of the idiopathic inflammatory myopathies. *Rheum Dis Clin North Am* 2002;28:859–890.

189 SCLERODERMA

Michael L. Miller

EPIDEMIOLOGY

- The peak age at onset ranges from 30 to 50 years, with a female:male ratio 3:1.
- Scleroderma occurs in children in less than 10% of all cases.
- Sporadic occurrences may follow exposure to bleomycin, pentazocine, and polyvinyl chloride.

PATHOPHYSIOLOGY

- The cause is unknown, but damaged vascular endothelium may trigger an inflammatory response, in which interleukin-1 induces platelets to release platelet-derived growth factor (PDG), leading to fibrosis.

CLINICAL FEATURES

- *Raynaud phenomenon* (RP), a manifestation of digital arterial spasm, is diagnosed when two of three color changes occur: pallor, cyanosis, then erythema.
  1. RP may precede skin and systemic findings.
  2. When occurring as an isolated finding (*Raynaud disease*, which is much more common than RP), episodes usually do not require medical treatment.
- Systemic sclerosis
  1. The initial phase is characterized by puffiness around digits.
  2. Eventually, tightening of skin occurs. The digits take on a tapered appearance (*sclerodactyly*). The face may show frontal atrophy and a decreased ability to open mouth wide.
  3. Ulceration of the skin over elbows and ankles may develop.
  4. Severe RP may result in ulceration at the fingertips, threatening loss of part or all of affected digits.
  5. Sclerosis of affected joints may be associated with flexion contractures, including severe claw-like deformities of the hands.
  6. Pulmonary disease from interstitial fibrosis may lead to pulmonary arterial hypertension. Renal arterial involvement can result in episodes of severe systemic hypertension. Esophageal fibrosis may cause esophageal dysmotility.
  7. Less common manifestations include malabsorption and failure to thrive, from intestinal fibrosis; arrhythmias or decreased cardiac function from cardiac fibrosis.
- *Limited systemic sclerosis* is characterized by fibrosis of the distal extremities, face, and trunk; systemic findings are rare.
- Calcinosis-Raynaud phenomenon-Esophageal dysmotility-Sclerodactyly-Telangiectasia (*CREST*) syndrome is characterized by calcinosis, RP, esophageal involvement, sclerosis of skin, and telangiectasias; occasionally severe pulmonary arterial hypertension may occur.
- *Linear scleroderma* is characterized by skin involvement with only rare evolution to systemic disease; linear skin lesions occur along extremities, trunk, or face. *Morphea* is a subset of linear scleroderma in which skin lesions are discrete, often oval shaped.

DIAGNOSIS AND DIFFERENTIAL

- Scleroderma is suspected in children with RP who develop worsening episodes, sclerodactyly, or dyspnea.
- Laboratory evaluation often reveals positive antibody screens for antinuclear antibodies, anti-SCL70 antibodies (specific for topoisomerase 1), and anticentromere

antibodies. Inflammation early in systemic disease can be reflected by elevated erythrocyte sedimentation rate (ESR) and anemia.

- Other evaluation may show pulmonary fibrosis at bases on high resolution computed tomography (CT) scan, abnormally decreased lung diffusing capacity on pulmonary function tests, echocardiogram showing pulmonary arterial hypertension, and upper gastrointestinal (UGI) studies showing abnormal esophageal motility.

DIFFERENTIAL DIAGNOSIS

- When elements of myositis, arthritis, and/or lupus are found, consider mixed connective tissue disease, associated with antibodies to ribonucleoprotein.
- Isolated diffuse swelling of digits raises the possibility of early Henoch-Schönlein purpura and allergic reactions.
- Graft-vs.-host disease following transplantation can result in a scleroderma-like syndrome.
- Raynaud disease without scleroderma is more common than RP associated with scleroderma.
- Eosinophilic fasciitis presents as a fasciitis with skin findings similar to localized scleroderma; however, marked eosinophilia is distinctive, accompanied with elevated ESR. Diagnosis is based on fasciitis with eosinophilic infiltrate, requiring a full-thickness skin biopsy that includes underlying fascia and muscle.
- Discrete or diffuse skin fibrosis, without other manifestations of scleroderma manifestations, may be seen in pseudoscleroderma or phenylketonuria.

TREATMENT

- There is no specific medical treatment, but corticosteroids and immunosuppressive agents (e.g., methotrexate) may be used in selected patients, particularly during the initial inflammatory phase.

- Calcium-channel blockers or angiotensin-converting enzyme inhibitors have been used for severe RP.
- Angiotensin-converting enzyme inhibitors may prevent hypertensive crisis.
- Prostaglandin E1 administered centrally has averted threatened loss of digits from severe RP, in some patients.
- Physical and occupational therapy, along with splinting, helps improved decreased mobility from joint contractures.

PROGNOSIS

- The prognosis is variable, and few studies have reported on prognosis in children. Progression of systemic sclerosis to end-organ disease affecting the lungs, heart, and kidneys is generally thought to occur over a period that may last for many years, but ultimately resulting in early death. Nevertheless, early treatment, as noted above, may improve this prognosis is some patients.

PREVENTION

- There is no means of preventing scleroderma, except for the rare cases associated with exposure to environmental agents, noted above.

BIBLIOGRAPHY

Miller ML. Scleroderma. In Miller ML (ed.), *Nelson's Textbook of Pediatrics*, 17th ed. Philadelphia, PA: W.B. Saunders, 2003, pp. 816–819.

Murray KJ, Laxer RM. Scleroderma in children and adolescents. *Rheum Dis Clin North Am* 2002;28:603–624.

Timothy A. Sentongo, Section Editor

190 FAILURE TO THRIVE

Timothy A. Sentongo

DEFINITION

- The term failure to thrive (FTT) is not a diagnosis or specific disease entity but denotes growth impairment or weight gain deviating below the range of normal or expected for age in infants and children. When arising from factors inherent to the child it is referred to as organic failure to thrive (OFTT), and nonorganic failure to thrive (NOFTT) when primarily due to factors external to the child. Combinations of OFTT and NOFTT also frequently occur in the presence of minor infections, vomiting, diarrhea, and when organic disease leads to behavioral problems and feeding disorders.
- The etiology of NOFTT is inadequate caloric intake in association with behavioral, parental, and/or psychosocial factors. Other conditions associated with reduced growth; however, not requiring nutritional intervention include familial short stature, factitious-FTT which represents a normal physiologic deceleration in growth velocity occurring in some children during the first 2–3 years, and constitutional growth delay, which is characterized by slow growth; nevertheless, paralleling the growth curve in association with delayed skeletal maturity, absence of organic disease, and a family history of delayed puberty (late bloomers).
- OFTT may be secondary to chronic inflammatory disorders or organ dysfunction, e.g., gastrointestinal, endocrine, renal, cardiac, and pulmonary diseases. Other conditions associated with OFTT include genetic, chromosomal anomalies, and musculoskeletal disorders.

EPIDEMIOLOGY

- Nonorganic causes are by far the commonest causes of FTT in the general population; however, amongst children hospitalized for FTT, organic causes can be identified in up to 20–40% of patients.

ASSESSMENT

- Careful medical history about the presenting complaint should include chronology of development of the growth deficits in question, i.e., onset and progression of growth problems, acute vs. chronic.
  1. Inquiries should also be made into pregnancy and birth history, feeding patterns, intercurrent illness, chronic medications, family medical history, and social structure.
  2. A review of systems to screen for syndromes associated with FTT (Table 190-1).
  3. A good attempt should be made to obtain all previous growth records.
- Accurate growth measurements (weight, length/height, and head circumference) should be obtained and plotted on the updated Centers for Disease Control and Prevention (CDC) 2000 growth charts (see www.cdc.gov/growthcharts). Growth charts are also available for preterm/low birth weight (LBW) infants and specific conditions, e.g., Down syndrome, Turner syndrome, and achondroplasia.
- Interpretation of growth should begin with assessment of linear growth status (length/height). Proper instrumentation and positioning are key for reliable measurements. Measurement of length (supine) requires an infant length board with a fixed head board and moveable footboard. An assistant is required to hold the head in position while the torso and legs are positioned for measurement. Height (standing) requires a stadiometer.

TABLE 190-1 Etiology of FTT

MECHANISM	DISORDERS
NOFTT	
Psychosocial	Infants/young children: Poor feeding technique, errors in formula preparation, unusual maternal nutritional beliefs, poor maternal-child interaction, psychologically disturbed mother, emotional deprivation, emotional dwarfism, child neglect, famine, war, starvation
	Older children/adolescents: anorexia and unusual dietary habits, e.g., fad vegetarian, sport-induced weight loss, lipid-lowering diets
Other	Factitious-FTT, familial short stature, constitutional growth delay
OFTT	
Inability to suck, swallow, or masticate	CNS pathology (psychomotor retardation), neuromuscular disease (Werdnig-Hoffmann, myotonia congenita, dysautonomia), dysphagia (cleft lip/palate, oral-pharyngeal incoordination, dystrophic epidermolysis bullosa)
Maldigestion, malabsorption	Cystic fibrosis, celiac disease, tropical sprue, Schwachman-Diamond syndrome, cholestatic liver disease, short gut syndrome, protein losing enteropathy
Poor nutrient use	Renal failure, renal tubular acidosis, inborn errors of metabolism
Vomiting	CNS abnormality (tumor, infection, increased pressure), metabolic toxin (inborn errors of organic or amino acid metabolism), pyloric stenosis, intestinal malrotation, renal tubular disease
Regurgitation	Gastroesophageal reflux, milk-soy protein intolerance, eosinophilic esophagitis, hiatal hernia, rumination syndrome
Elevated/inefficient metabolism	Thyrotoxicosis, hypothyroidism, chronic disease (bronchopulmonary dysplasia, heart failure), cancer, chronic inflammatory disorders (SLE, inflammatory bowel disease, liver cirrhosis, chronic infection), immunodeficiency diseases, TB, burns
Reduced growth potential	Chromosomal disorders, primordial dwarfism, skeletal dysplasia, specific syndromes (fetal alcohol)
Other	Chronic steroid therapy

SOURCE: Adapted with modification from Kerr DS. *Failure to thrive and malnutrition.* In: Kleigman RM, Nieder ML, Super DM (eds.), *Practical Strategies in Pediatric Diagnosis and Therapy.* Philadelphia, PA: W.B. Saunders, 1996, pp. 243–258.
ABBREVIATIONS: CNS, central nervous system; SLE, systemic lupus erythematosus; TB, tuberculosis.

The head paddle should be firmly perpendicular to the stadiometer.
- Growth charts and reference data are also available for alternative measures including upper arm length, lower leg length, and skinfold anthropometry, which are particularly useful in situations where measurement of length and stature would be inaccurate, e.g., children who are bedridden, kyphoscoliosis, contractures, and other muculoskeletal deformities.
- Measurements for infants (age: birth to 36 months) are all in length, and measurements for older children (age: 2–20 years) are all in height (standing).
- The child's (age: 2–20 years) height percentile should be within the calculated target height based on mid-parent height determined as follows:

Boys:

$$\frac{\text{Father's height (cm)} + \text{mother's height (cm)} + 13\text{ cm}}{2}$$

Girls:

$$\frac{\text{Father's height (cm)} + \text{mother's height (cm)} - 13\text{ cm}}{2}$$

- Pubertal stage should always be assessed because of its significant impact on interpretation of weight and height gain in females >8–9 years, and males >12–13 years.
- The next step is to compare actual weight with the ideal body weight (IBW). The IBW is the median weight (50th percentile) for the measured length/height. The actual weight and IBW are then expressed as a percentage, and variation of ±10% is considered within normal. A percentage of 80–90% actual/IBW corresponds to mild wasting; 70–80% moderate wasting; 60–70% severe wasting; and <60% suggests severe wasting *approaching* incompatibility with survival.
- Alternatively, comparisons of weight-for-length/stature may be assessed using the weight-for-length growth charts (age: birth to 36 months) and body mass index (BMI) charts in older children (age: 2–20 years). BMI is calculated as weight (kg) divided by height in meters squared (kg/m^2).
  1. A decreased (<5%) weight-for-length percentile or BMI indicates a thin body habitus commonly associated with malnutrition from inadequate caloric intake, malabsorption, or chronic inflammatory

diseases. For postnatal acquired disorders weight gain drops off before length/height percentiles. Of the three growth measurements, head circumference is affected last by malnutrition.

2. Proportionately small infants with ideal body weight ≥100–120% and/or weight-for-length greater than the median (50th percentile) should be considered to have primary growth problems including various genetic, endocrine, and skeletal disorders.

3. Infants with disproportionately small heads are suspect for primary neurologic problems affecting brain growth because head growth is the last to be affected by primary malnutrition and is not characteristic of primary skeletal or growth problems.

- Laboratory aids: General screening tests include complete blood count, urinalysis, electrolytes, blood urea nitrogen, pre-albumin, and liver enzymes. Unless organic disease is suspected, more detailed testing should be reserved for patients that respond poorly to an initial trial of nutritional management.

ETIOLOGY OF FTT

- See Table 190-1.

TREATMENT

- Regardless of the etiology of FTT, effective nutritional management consists of providing adequate calories to reverse impaired growth, achieve catch-up growth, and restoration of normal growth.
- There is a need for a multidisciplinary team including physician, dietician, feeding therapists, social worker, and sometimes psychologist.
- Nutritional therapy consists of establishing calorie goals 150–200% above the recommended for age. This may be accomplished through oral supplements and nasogastric tube feeds. Parenteral nutrition may be required in situations were enteral feeding is limited or impossible.
- Caution is required during the early phase of nutritional therapy in the severely malnourished because of increased risk for refeeding syndrome (see section below).

NOFTT

- Positive growth and behavioral response to treatment confirms the diagnosis of NOFTT.
- Active parental involvement is essential for sustained success.
- Psychosocial factors influencing parent-child interaction and feeding behavior must be evaluated and addressed.

- Temporary placement in a more favorable setting within the family or in a foster care environment may be necessary if the immediate family is judged as being incapable of following through with the recommended management.

OFTT

- Requires both nutritional management and medical/surgical therapy for the underlying disease.
- Often requires a multidisciplinary team including primary pediatrician, subspecialist, dietician, social worker, and speech and other therapists.

REFEEDING SYNDROME

- Metabolic and physiologic perturbations arising from the anabolic response to rapid refeeding in severely malnourished patients (see Table 190-2 for patients at risk). The abnormalities include extracellular fluid shifts, and depletion of phosphate, potassium, magnesium, and vitamins.

1. Extracellular fluid shifts: The increased sodium intake combined with the antinatriuretic effect of insulin stimulated by increased carbohydrate intake has a net effect of increased extracellular fluid volume. The resulting clinical manifestations range from rapid weight gain and dependent edema to congestive heart failure in some situations, e.g., kwashiorkor.

2. Hypophosphatemia arises from relative depletion of phosphate during the increased glycogen synthesis that follows the increased carbohydrate intake, and increased synthesis and use of adenosine triphosphate (ATP) for other anabolic processes. The clinical sequels of hyphosphatemia include cardiac, neuromuscular, and hematologic dysfunction, and also acute respiratory failure.

3. Hypokalemia: Starvation is associated with total body potassium depletion through decreased muscle mass. During nutritional rehabilitation in addition to potassium deposition into newly synthesized cells, the insulin surge associated with increased dietary

TABLE 190-2   Patients at Risk for Refeeding Syndrome

Anorexia nervosa
Kwashiorkor
Marasmus
Chronic malnutrition—underfeeding, malabsorption
Morbid obesity with massive weight loss
Patient unfed in >7 days with evidence of stress and depletion
Prolonged intravenous hydration

SOURCE: Adapted with modification from Solomon SM, Kirby DF. The refeeding syndrome: a review. *J Parenter Enteral Nutr* 1990;14: 90–97.

carbohydrate diet results in intracellular shifts of serum potassium. The clinical manifestations of hypokalemia include electrocardiogram (ECG) changes, cardiac arrhythmias, constipation, ileus, glucose intolerance, neuromuscular weakness, areflexia, and rhabdomyolysis.

4. Hypomagnesemia: Magnesium is a major component of the intracellular space and is a cofactor in many enzyme systems. In the absence of replacement, serum levels fall during anabolic conditions. The clinical sequel of hypomagnesemia includes cardiac arrhythmias, anorexia, weakness, hypocalcemia, tetany, and seizures.

• Avoiding refeeding syndrome: Risk is greatest during the initial phase nutritional therapy in patients with severe forms of malnutrition (Table 190-2). Therefore, during the first weeks of therapy caloric intake should be gradually advanced with judicious monitoring and replenishment of electrolytes.

OUTCOMES

• Catch-up growth in children with NOFTT appears to be greatest among those who receive intensive social or psychologic intervention, therefore the need for a multidisciplinary approach and long-term follow-up; however, regardless of catch-up growth, long-term studies suggest persistent learning, development, and intellectual delays in older children with past history of NOFTT. Better school-age development and adaptive outcomes are linked to a more favorable family environment.

BIBLIOGRAPHY

Drotar D, Sturm L. Influences on the home environment of preschool children with early histories of nonorganic failure-to-thrive. *J Dev Behav Pediatr* 1989;10:229–235.

Drotar D, Sturm L. Personality development, problem solving, and behavior problems among preschool children with early histories of failure-to-thrive: a controlled study. *J Dev Behav Pediatr* 1992;13:2673–2676.

Kerr DS. Failure to thrive and malnutrition. In: Kleigman RM, Nieder ML, Super DM (eds.), *Practical Strategies in Pediatric Diagnosis and Therapy*. Philadelphia, PA: W.B. Saunders, 1996, pp. 243–258.

Maggioni A, Lifshitz F. Nutritional management of failure to thrive. *Pediatr Clin North Am* 1995;42:791–810.

Solomon SM, Kirby DF. The refeeding syndrome: a review. *J Parenter Enteral Nutr* 1990;14:90–97.

Zemel BS, Riley EM, Stallings VA. Evaluation of methodology for nutritional assessment in children: anthropometry, body composition, and energy expenditure. *Annu Rev Nutr* 1997;17:211–235.

191 OBESITY

Rebecca Unger, Adolfo Ariza, and Timothy A. Sentongo

DEFINITION

• Obesity is excess body fat-for-age, which is either subcutaneous or deposited internally, predominantly intraabdominally. Direct measurement of body fat is not practical during routine care therefore recognition of overweight status and risk for obesity is through comparison of weight-for-height ratios. Since weight and height change throughout childhood and adolescence, the cutoff points used to define overweight are age and gender dependent.

• Overweight and risk for obesity are best determined by assessing weight while taking length/height into consideration. This is done with the aid of growth charts, and by calculating weight-for-height ratios, i.e., body mass index (BMI) and percent ideal body weight (%IBW).

• Weight-for-length/height growth charts (see www.cdc.gov/growthcharts) are helpful for screening over weight or underweight status in infants and prepubertal children.

• BMI is the most widely used tool to screen for overweight and risk for obesity. BMI (kg/m^2) is calculated by dividing the weight (kg) by height in meters squared (m^2). BMI-for-age and gender growth charts are available for children and adolescents aged 2–20 years (see www.cdc.gov/growthcharts). BMI percentile >95th percentile signifies overweight status while ≥85th and <95th percentiles represent risk for overweight. BMI exceeding the 95th percentile warrants an in-depth medical assessment for obesity (see further). For adults, BMI in the range of 25–29 kg/m^2 represents risk for overweight, and ≥30 kg/m^2 represents overweight.

• Calculation of %IBW is helpful for classifying severity of overweight and obesity. The IBW is the median weight (50th percentile) for the measured height. Therefore dividing actual weight by IBW and multiplying by 100 determines the %IBW. A percentage of 120–139% represents mild overweight; 140–160% represents moderate overweight; and >160% severe overweight. Use of %IBW classification complements

BMI since there's no BMI categorization beyond the 97th percentile. Furthermore, %IBW enables tracking changes in smaller increments than would be detected by BMI calculations.

EPIDEMIOLOGY

- The prevalence of overweight (body mass index >95th percentile) among children in the United States has steadily increased over the past 20 years. Data from the National Health and Nutritional Examination Survey (NHANES) in 1999–2000 revealed that >10% of 2–5-year-olds, and >15% of 6–19-year-olds in the United States were overweight. These findings represented a greater than twofold rise in overweight status compared to similar statistics obtained during the period 1976–1980. The sharpest rise in prevalence of overweight was among non-Hispanic Blacks and Mexican-American children. Among non-Hispanic Black children of all ages, the prevalence of overweight increased from 13% (1988–1994) to 24% (1999–2000). Among Mexican-American children of all ages, overweight status increased from 14% (1988–1994) to 23% (1999–2000).

PATHOPHYSIOLOGY

- Three critical periods during human development have been identified where physiologic interactions increase the later prevalence of obesity. They include fetal life, the period of adiposity rebound, and adolescence. Infants born to diabetic mothers are usually large for gestation age at birth, tend to normalize by age 1 year; however, by 5–6 years have an increased prevalence of overweight that persists through adolescence. Adiposity rebound is the developmental period normally occurring between ages 6 and 8 years when there is rapid deposition of body fat stores. Children with early onset of adiposity rebound, i.e., before age 5.5 years, have a longer duration of body fat deposition and thus at greater risk for persistence of obesity into adolescence. Adolescent development is associated with rapid growth and redistribution of body fat stores. Likewise, during adolescence there's increased risk of onset and persistence of obesity especially among females.
- The rapid surge in overweight and obesity in the United States over the past 20 years affecting all segments of the population and regions of the country is inconsistent with a primarily genetic or biologic change in the population. Therefore environmental factors are increasingly being accepted as significant contributors to obesity. The basic problem is an imbalance between energy intake and expenditure. Abnormal weight results from normal or increased food intake accompanied by increased physical inactivity. Risk factors for overweight and obesity in childhood include obesity in one or both parents, low social class in western societies, affluence in developing countries, single parent family, high levels of television watching, energy-dense/high-fat diet, disorganized eating patterns, and specific chromosomal, genetic, and endocrine disorders.

CLINICAL EFFECTS ASSOCIATED WITH OVERWEIGHT

- Impaired glucose tolerance and increased prevalence of type 2 diabetes. Children diagnosed with type 2 diabetes are at increased risk as young adults for complications such as kidney failure, miscarriages, blindness, amputations, and even death.
- Increased risk for hyperlipidemia (increased serum cholesterol, low high-density lipoprotein [HDL] cholesterol, and hypetriglyceraldemia) and associated cardiovascular disease (hypertension and atherosclerosis). Fatty streaks have been found in coronary arteries of overweight children as early as age 10 years.
- Overweight children are at increased risk for hepatic steatosis, gallbladder disease, gastroesophageal reflux, respiratory illnesses and orthopedic disorders.
- Sleep disturbances including sleep disordered breathing, snoring, sleep apnea, daytime sleepiness, restless sleep, and nocturnal enuresis. These may be diagnosed based on clinical history and assessment, and in some cases, a sleep study.
- Dyspnea on exertion is also common in very overweight children. Symptoms include coughing, respiratory distress, chest pain, and pallor with increasing level of physical activity.
- Social ostracism, emotional, and social difficulties frequently occur and can severely affect overweight children through adolescence and into adulthood.

SYNDROMES ASSOCIATED WITH OVERWEIGHT

- Evaluation of overweight should include screening for medical and genetic syndromes associated with overweight. Generally, endocrine and genetic syndromes are associated with overweight and short stature (see Table 191-1).

ASSESSMENT

- BMI should be used routinely to screen for overweight status in all children aged 2–20 years. Children and

TABLE 191-1 Syndromes Associated with Overweight

SYNDROME/DISEASE	SUSPECT IF	EVALUATION
Hypothyroidism	Short stature, coarse hair, constipation, decreased energy level, delayed sexual maturation, cold intolerance	Free T4, TSH
Cushing syndrome	Truncal obesity, acne, hypertension, glucose intolerance, hirsuitism, excess adipose tissue, moon facies, straie	Abnormal 24-hour urine-free cortisol and creatinine excretion
Prader-Willi syndrome	Hypotonia and feeding problems in infancy, hyperphagia in childhood, developmental delay, hypogonadism, poor growth, small hands and feet	Chromosome, FISH analysis
Polycystic ovary syndrome	Irregular or absent menses, hirsuitism, acne, acanthosis nigricans	Excess androgen production
Laurence-Moon-Bardet-Biedl	Truncal obesity, retinitis pigmentosa, hypogenitalism, digital anomalies, nephropathy	Autosomal recessive trait
Growth hormone deficiency	Poor growth	Growth hormone levels
Pseudohypoparathyroidism	Poor growth, round facies, short metatarsals and metacarpals, subcutaneous calcifications, developmental delay, cataracts, dry skin, brittle nails	Hypocalcemia, hyperphosphatemia
Turner syndrome	Poor growth, ovarian dysgenesis, broad chest, webbed neck, renal anomalies, renal impairment	Chromosome analysis

ABBREVIATION: T4, thyroxine; FISH, fluorescence in situ hybridization.

adolescents with BMI ≥85th percentile but <95th percentile are considered at risk for overweight, should undergo a second level screen involving family history of hyperlipidemia, cardiovascular disease risk, and should also be identified for follow-up and counseling for weight maintenance. Those with BMI >95th percentile should be considered as overweight. In-depth medical follow-up to determine underlying diagnoses is required. The specific guidelines for assessment of overweight in adolescence (beginning of puberty to completion of growth and physical maturity) are outlined in Fig. 191-1. In general prepubertal children and adolescents identified with BMI within the range of overweight should be counseled as follows:

1. It is important to ask specific questions about frequency of meals and snacks, fruit and vegetable intake, and junk food and fast food intake. Sweetened beverage intake, such as juice, soda pop, lemonade, iced tea, and so on should be quantified. This information about actual dietary intake should be compared to the recommended United States Department of Agriculture (USDA) guidelines, such as eating five servings of fruits and vegetables each day (www.usda.gov/cnpp). Consistent discrepancies should be identified. Uncovering other risk factors such as prolonged bottle use is also important.

2. Frequency and types of physical activity patterns should be identified. Because hours of television watching per day are positively associated with degree of overweight, it is important to also ask about hours of television watching per day.

3. As part of the physical examination, blood pressure should be obtained, making sure that the cuff is the appropriate size. The presence of acanthosis nigricans (darkening of the skin) possibly associated with insulin resistance should be noted. Since thyroid disease can be a cause of obesity, palpation of the thyroid should be done. Pubertal status should be assessed to provide indication about potential for linear growth.

4. Laboratory evaluation should include a fasting lipid profile for all overweight and at risk for overweight children. A fasting glucose level and an insulin level may be helpful to determine the presence of abnormal glucose tolerance. Other laboratory evaluations, such as free thyroxin and thyroid stimulating hormone (TSH) (to exclude hypothyroidism) and a 24-hour urine-free cortisol and creatinine (to exclude Cushing syndrome) should be obtained when indicated, especially when the height curve shows a decline in height percentiles.

5. A sleep study, endolateral neck x-ray, chest x-ray, and exercise stress testing should be done when history and/or physical examination suggest sleep disturbances and dyspnea on exertion.

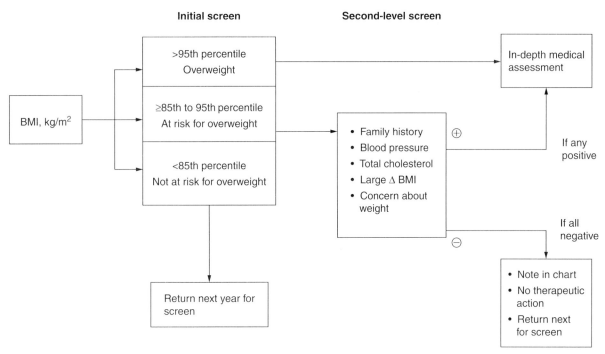

Initial screen   **Second-level screen**

FIG. 191-1 Algorithm for screening and evaluation of overweight status based on BMI-for-age and gender. Adapted from Himes JH, Dietz WH. Guidelines for overweight in adolescent preventive services: Recommendations from an expert committee. *Am J Clin Nutr* 1994;59:307–316.

THERAPY

- The foremost treatment goal for overweight children and adolescents is diet and lifestyle change, which involves establishing healthy eating and physical activity patterns. Clinicians need to stress to patients and families that management of overweight will not consist of short-term diets aimed at quick and drastic weight loss, but should focus on family changes to achieve weight maintenance. For children with secondary complications of obesity, improvement of the complication is another important goal. Complementary approaches like restrictive diets, pharmacotherapy, and bariatric surgery have not received wide acceptance in pediatrics; however, they may be considered with some success especially in adolescents with severe obesity associated with complications.

DIET AND LIFESTYLE CHANGE

- Early screening, counseling, and anticipatory guidance make goals easier to reach and prevent overweight at a later age. This may be accomplished through the regular use of the updated Centers for Disease Control and Prevention (CDC) BMI-for-age growth charts. With preschoolers, habits are more malleable, and parents can still effectively change eating and physical activity patterns. Also, with younger children, a smaller shift in energy balance can produce substantial improvement in degree of overweight. Furthermore continuing linear growth with weight maintenance will improve the weight-height relationship and work to the patient's advantage.

- Modifying behaviors gradually allows success to be achievable, which builds confidence and inspires the patient and family to continue confronting the problem of overweight. For example, small changes in eating habits can involve keeping only low-fat snacks at home, or eating less fast food meals.

- Physical activity can be slightly increased by including small bouts of activity throughout the day like taking stairs whenever possible. Also, the family can start controlling its sedentary activities by limiting television viewing to 2 hours a day. Regular follow-up allows clinicians to foster lifestyle change in small steps, closely monitor intervention effectiveness, and provide repeated positive reinforcements.

- The family's specific barriers to implement behavioral change must be reassessed at every visit and goals further adapted to the family needs. Initially, it is helpful to see patients every 1–2 months to assess progress and obstacles. Eventually, the followup visits can be less often.

- Patients should be referred to a specialist, such as a nutritionist, if weight management attempts are not working. Severely overweight children under age 2 also should be referred to specialists in pediatric overweight management. A multidisciplinary nutrition team including primary care provider, dietician, psychologist/behavior therapist, and an appropriate subspecialist may be appropriate for children with complex barriers to successful treatment.

• When a medical problem impedes physical activity, referral to an exercise physiologist who can determine a safe mode of exercise is advised.

• Use of medication in treating overweight pediatric patients is controversial. Currently no medication has been shown to be effective and safe in the pediatric population. The potential for severe side effects is being reviewed.

RESTRICTIVE DIETS

• Severely obese adolescents with weight %IBW >180% associated with complications may be considered for more aggressive dietary interventions such as the protein-modified fast. This is a carbohydrate-free diet containing high-quality protein 2.0–2.5 g/kg IBW, supplemented with KCl 30 meq, calcium 800 mg, a daily multivitamin with minerals, ad libitum intake of vegetables low in carbohydrate, and a noncaloric fluid intake maintained at a level of 48 oz/day. Ketosis generally appears within 72 hours, and weight loss in the range of 0.5–1.0 kg/week may be observed while in duration with the diet. Compliance and close medical supervision are necessary for safety and success. Reported complications include malaise, orthostatic hypotension, diarrhea, and/or constipation.

PHARMACOTHERAPY

• Pharmacotherapy has not yet been demonstrated as universally safe and effective in pediatrics. Therefore, it must be reserved for morbidly obese adolescents, and when more conservative approaches including the protein-modified fast have been exhausted. Orlistat and Sibutramine are currently being tested in adolescents. Orlistat is a pancreatic-lipase inhibitor exerting its antiweight effect by impairing digestion and absorption of dietary fat. Adverse effects include oily stools and fat-soluble vitamin deficiencies. Sibutramine is a serotonin-noradrenaline reuptake inhibitor that causes early satiety and increased energy expenditure. Adverse effects include hypertension, increased heart rate, dry mouth, insomnia, and constipation.

BARIATRIC SURGERY

• Gastric bypass surgery or vertically banded gastroplasty is a permanent and extreme form of dietary restriction, therefore must only be considered as therapy of last resort for *morbid* obesity where all other supervised conventional therapy has failed. It is requisite for candidates to go through rigorous screening that includes psychiatric and other self-destructive behaviors. Additional requirements include lifetime commitment to comply with a modified diet and lifestyle after surgery. Acute complications include wound infections and leakage at the anastomosis. Long-term complications include anemia. Weight loss has been successfully achieved and maintained in many patients; however, there are no data about long-term safety in children.

PREVENTION

• Prevention is the best strategy for managing overweight. Clinicians need to start management early by screening BMI starting in children at age 2 years and counseling families on how to establish beneficial eating and physical activity patterns. Anticipatory guidance should be provided in routine pediatric care focusing on the practice of healthy lifestyle habits for the entire family. Prevention can begin with advice to parents about breastfeeding, weaning, and healthy eating for toddlers.

• Clinicians should reinforce with parents the following principles:

1. Parents need to role model healthy nutritional and physical activity patterns.

2. Praise and correction should be targeted at specific behaviors, not the child.

3. Food should never be used as a reward, bribe, comfort, solution to problems, or any other symbolic substitute.

4. Children are more likely to be satisfied with a healthy alternative if they are allowed to choose. Parents should let children select between a number of healthy food options.

5. Parents should not only keep tempting high-sugar drinks or high-fat foods around the house, but also need to avoid banning any type of food, which only makes it more irresistible to children.

BIBLIOGRAPHY

Daniels S. Pharmacological treatment of obesity in paediatric patients. *Paediatr Drugs* 2001;3:405–410.

Dietz WH, Robinson TN. Assessment and treatment of childhood obesity. *Pediatr Rev* 1993;14:337–344.

Dietz WH. Critical periods in childhood for the development of obesity. *Am J Clin Nutr* 1994;59:955–959.

Dietz WH. Childhood obesity. In: Shils ME, Olson JA, Shike M, Ross AC (eds.), *Modern Nutrition in Health and Disease,*

9th ed. Baltimore, MD: Williams and Wilkins, 1999, pp. 1071–1080.

Fulton JE, McGuire MT, Capersen CJ, Dietz WH. Interventions for weight loss and weight gain prevention among youth. *Sports Med* 2001;31:153–165.

Himes JH, Dietz WH. Guidelines for overweight in adolescent preventive services: Recommendations from an expert committee. *Am J Clin Nutr* 1994;59:307–316.

Kuczmarksi RJ, Ogden CL, Grummer-Strawn LM, et al. Vital and health statistics of the Centers for Disease Control and Prevention/National Center for Health Statistics. CDC growth charts: United States. *Adv Data* 2000;314:1–28.

Mokdad AH, Serdula MK, Dietz WH, Bowman BA, et al. The spread of the obesity epidemic in the United States, 1991–1998. *JAMA* 1999;282:1519–1522.

Must A, Strauss RS. Risk and consequences of childhood and adolescent obesity. *Int J Obes* 1999;23:S2–S11.

Ogden CL, Flegal KM, Carroll MD, Johnson CL. Prevalence and trends in overweight among U.S. children and adolescents, 1999–2000. *JAMA* 2002;288:1728–1732.

Poskitt EME. Childhood obesity and growth. In: Ulijaszek SJ, Johnston FE, Preece MA (eds.), *The Cambridge Encyclopedia of Human Growth and Development.* New York, NY: Cambridge University Press, 1998, pp. 332–333.

Sinha R, Fisch G, Teague B, et al. Prevalence of impaired glucose tolerance among children and adolescence with marked obesity. *N Engl J Med* 2002;346:802–810.

192 NUTRITIONAL DEFICIENCIES

Timothy A. Sentongo

- Generally vitamin and mineral deficiencies primarily arising from inadequate intake are increasingly uncommon in normal health; however, vulnerable groups, e.g., food faddists, hospitalized patients and chronic illness including malabsorption syndromes frequently have symptoms secondary to single or multiple deficiency therefore necessitating a high index of suspicion and close monitoring. Abnormalities involving selected minerals and several vitamins are summarized in Tables 192-1 through 192-3.

TABLE 192-1   Fat-Soluble Vitamins

FAT-SOLUBLE VITAMIN	BIOCHEMICAL ACTION	DEFICIENCY	RISK FACTORS FOR DEFICIENCY	TOXICITY	RISK FACTORS FOR TOXICITY
A	Epithelial cell integrity; component of retinal pigments and rhodopsin for night vision	Night blindness, xerophthalmia, Bitot spots, follicular hyperkeratosis, impaired resistance to infection	Protein energy malnutrition, fat malabsorption syndromes	Anorexia, alopecia, dry desquamating skin rash, teratogenic, increased intracranial pressure, hepatic fibrosis, portal hypertension	Food faddism (e.g., excess consumption of liver), self-medication or chronic therapy with preparations containing fat-soluble vitamins
D	Maintaining serum calcium, phosphorous homeostasis	Rickets, osteomalacia, infantile tetany	Breast-fed infants, ↓ exposure to sunlight, vegans, fat malabsorption syndromes	Hypercalcemia, anorexia, poor growth, metastatic calcification	Excess supplementation, self-medication or chronic therapy with preparations containing fat-soluble vitamins
E	Antioxidant, prevention of free radical damage in membranes	Hemolysis in premature infants, areflexia, ataxia, ophthalmoplegia	Preterm infants, genetic defects*, fat malabsorption syndromes, e.g., CF, abetalipoproteinemia, cholestatic liver disease	Vitamin K dependent coagulopathy	Excess supplementation
K	Posttranslation carboxylation of coagulation factors II, VII, IX, X and proteins C, S, Z	Coagulopathy, increased spontaneous bleeding tendency	Newborn, breast-fed infants, fat malabsorption syndromes, cholestatic liver disease, antibiotics in short gut syndrome and other medications, e.g., phenytoin, phenobarbital, mineral oil	Kernicterus in preterm infants	Large doses of water soluble analogues of vitamin K

*Genetic defects in vitamin E metabolism: α-tocopherol-transfer protein (AVED: ataxia with vitamin E deficiency); apolipoprotein D deficiency; microsomal triglyceride-transfer protein deficiency (abetalipoproteinemia).

TABLE 192-2 Water Soluble Vitamins

WATER SOLUBLE VITAMIN	BIOCHEMICAL ACTION	DEFICIENCY	RISK FACTORS FOR DEFICIENCY	EXCESS	RISK FACTORS FOR EXCESS
Thiamine (B$_1$)	Component of carboxylase enzyme oxidative decarboxylation of α-keto acid including pyruvate, transketolation, nerve conduction	Wet beriberi: congestive/high output cardiac failure, tachycardia, peripheral edema Dry beriberi: neuritis, paraesthesia, irritability, anorexia, psychosis	Patients with protein malnutrition and folate deficiency Chronic ingestion of raw fresh water fish and ferns that contain antithiamine factors Chronic alcoholism Obesity surgery	Unknown	NA
Riboflavin (B$_2$)	Component of FAD coenzyme, important in oxidation-reduction reactions	Cheilosis, angular stomatitis, glossitis (magenta tongue), seborrheic dermatitis, anemia, anorexia	Multiple nutrient deficiency Eating disorders, e.g., anorexia Malabsorption syndromes Obesity surgery Long use of barbiturates	Unknown	NA
Niacin (B$_3$)	Component of coenzymes I and II (NAD and NADP) important in oxidation-reduction reactions	Pellagra: three-Ds: *d*iarrhea, photosensitivity *d*ermatitis, *d*ementia, death	Carcinoid syndrome Prolonged therapy with isoniazid Hartnup disease	Flushing of the skin, hyperuricemia, abnormal liver function	Pharmacologically high doses during treatment of hyperlipidemia
Pyridoxine (B$_6$)	Constituent of coenzyme involved in amino acid metabolism, hemoglobin synthesis, and fatty acid synthesis	Abnormal EEG, seizures, irritability, peripheral neuritis (patients on isoniazid), stomatitis, glossitis, seborrhea	Multiple nutrient deficiency Drug interactions: isoniazid, cycloserine, penicillamine, theophylline, caffeine, alcoholism	Sensory neuropathy, photosensitivity	Chronic high doses of B$_6$ (>2–250 mg/day)
Cyanocobalamin (B$_{12}$)	Coenzyme for 5-methyl-tetrahydrofolate formation; DNA synthesis	Megaloblastic anemia, neuropsychiatric symptoms, peripheral neuropathy, methylmalonic aciduria, homocystinuria	Vegans, autoimmune gastropathy, gastrectomy, short gut syndrome, fish tapeworm (*Diphyllobothrium latum*), blind loop syndrome	Unknown	NA
Ascorbic acid (C)	Antioxidant, collagen metabolism, cofactor in iron absorption, carnitine, and neurotransmitter synthesis	Defects in connective tissue formation: scurvy, weakness, fatigue, depression, vasomotor instability	Severe protein energy malnutrition, alcoholism, chronic illness, cigarette smokers have ↑ requirements	Possibly exacerbation of renal oxalate stones	Chronic ingestion of massive doses
Folic acid	Essential for synthesis of purines, pyrimidines, nucleoproteins, and DNA	Megaloblastic anemia	Dependence on goat milk, malabsorption syndromes, drug antagonists: sulfonamides, anticonvulsants, methotrexate, alcoholism, B$_{12}$ deficiency	Convulsions	Excess daily ingestion >15 mg/day

(continued)

TABLE 192-2 *(Continued)*

WATER SOLUBLE VITAMIN	BIOCHEMICAL ACTION	DEFICIENCY	RISK FACTORS FOR DEFICIENCY	EXCESS	RISK FACTORS FOR EXCESS
Biotin	Constituent of carboxylase enzymes involved in metabolism of carbohydrates, lipids, and deamination of amino acids. Carrier of CO_2 on enzymes	Seborrheic dermatoses, alopecia, hypotonia, death	*Neonatal MCD, chronic high ingestion of raw eggs (contain avidin which irreversibly binds biotin), chronic TPN without biotin	Unknown	Unknown
Pantothenic acid	Constituent of coenzymes in respiratory tricarboxylic acid cycle, fatty acid synthesis, and degradation	Rare Fatigue, depression	Multiple nutrient deficiency	Unknown	NA

*Neonatal MCD (multiple carboxylase deficiency) associated with deficiency of biotin holocarboxylase responsible for adding biotin prosthetic group to the carboxylase enzyme. Characteristics of selected mineral deficiencies and excess.
ABBREVIATIONS: FAD, flavin-adenine dinucleotide; NAD, nicotinamide adenine dinucleotide; NADP, nicotinamide adenine dinucleotide phosphate; DNA, deoxyribonucleic acid; EEG, electroencephalogram; TPN, total parenteral nutrition.

TABLE 192-3 **Selected Nutrient and Mineral Abnormalities***

NUTRIENT	BIOCHEMICAL ACTION	DEFICIENCY	RISK FACTORS FOR DEFICIENCY	EXCESS	RISK FACTORS FOR EXCESS
Essential Fatty Acids					
w-3 and w-6	Energy source, structural components of cell membranes, precursor for prostaglandin and leukotrine synthesis, development of neural tissue	Growth retardation, sparse hair growth, desquamating skin, increased susceptibility to infection	Preterm infants, malnutrition, anorexia, acrodermatitis enteropathica, fat malabsorption syndromes (pancreatic insufficiency, cholestatic liver disease), long-term lipid-free TPN	Diarrhea, prolonged bleeding time	Food faddists Excess supplementation
Selected Minerals					
Iron	Heme containing macromolecules (e.g., hemoglobin, cytochrome, myoglobulin)	Microcytic, hypochromic anemia, spoon nails, fatigue, reduced mental performance	Disproportionately high intake of cow's milk (has low Fe), menorrhagia, malabsorption syndromes, chronic gastrointestinal blood loss	Acute: vomiting, shock, liver damage Chronic: cirrhosis, cardiomyopathy, pituitary failure	Excess intake, Bantu siderosis, hereditary hemochromatosis, transfusional hemosiderosis
Copper	Component of several enzymes and proteins, several physiologic roles: connective tissue, iron metabolism, melanin pigment, cardiac function	Hypochromic anemia unresponsive to iron therapy, neutropenia, poor bone mineralization, impaired hair and skin pigmentation, Menke disease	Premature infants, short gut syndrome, malabsorption syndromes, excess zinc supplements, Menke disease	Acute: hemolysis Chronic: cirrhosis	Wilson disease

(continued)

TABLE 192-3 *(Continued)*

NUTRIENT	BIOCHEMICAL ACTION	DEFICIENCY	RISK FACTORS FOR DEFICIENCY	EXCESS	RISK FACTORS FOR EXCESS
Zinc	Most abundant intracellular trace mineral, catalytic, structural and regulatory role in several metalloenzymes, regulatory role in gene expression	Impaired taste, growth retardation, delayed wound healing, dermatoses, impaired immunity, low serum alkaline phosphatase	Malabsorption syndromes, severe malnutrition, sickle cell anemia, acrodermatitis enteropathica, inadequate zinc in TPN	Acute: vomiting, diarrhea Chronic: decreased copper absorption, copper deficiency	Prolonged excessive intake
Iodide	Essential constituent of thyroxine (T4) and triiodothyronine (T3)	Simple, colloid, endemic or euthyroid goiter	Endemic in New Guinea, the Congo; lake area prior to use of iodized salt; women at risk during puberty, pregnancy and menopause	Iodide goiter, myxedema	Excessive iodide intake in patients with Hashimoto thyroiditis
Phosphorous	Constituent of bone, cofactor of a variety of enzymes, energy reservoir (ATP, creatine phosphate, phosphoenol pyruvate)	Rickets, anorexia, myopathy, cardiomyopathy, bone pain	Preterm infants, chronic protein energy malnutrition, rapid refeeding in severe malnutrition, chronic phosphate binding antacids	Hypocalcemia, tetany	Infants fed high-phosphorous human milk substitutes, excess use of phosphate containing enemas
Magnesium	Cofactor for several enzymes involved in glycolysis, protein synthesis, phosphate transfer, muscle contraction, principal cation of soft tissue	Muscle tremors, irritability, tetany, convulsions, hypocalcemia nonresponsive to calcium	Short gut syndrome, malabsorption syndromes, renal tubular disease, endocrine dysfunction	ECG abnormalities, respiratory depression, depressed deep tendon reflexes	Magnesium supplements in patients with renal failure, chronic constipation treated with magnesium sulfate enemas

*Deficiencies and excess secondary to genetic, metabolic, endocrine or organ dysfunction are not discussed.
ABBREVIATIONS: ATP, adenosine triphosphate; TPN, total parenteral nutrition; ECG, electrocardiogram.

BIBLIOGRAPHY

McLaren DS. Clinical manifestations of human vitamin and mineral disorders. In: Shils ME, Olson JA, Shike M, Ross AC (eds.), *Modern Nutrition in Health and Disease*, 9th ed. Baltimore, MD: Williams and Wilkins, 1999, pp. 485–504.

PEDIATRIC DENTISTRY

Charles Czerepak, Section Editor

193 PEDIATRIC DENTISTRY AND ORAL HEALTH

Charles Czerepak

- The gateway to the digestive system is the oral cavity. The components of the oral cavity are teeth, muscles of mastication, mandible, maxilla, tongue, lips, oral mucosa, and posterior pharynx.

TEETH

- A person develops two sets of teeth in a lifetime. The primary dentition in childhood and the subsequent permanent dentition.
  1. The first primary teeth start to appear (erupt) into the mouth around 6 months of age.
  2. The primary teeth consist of two central and two lateral incisors, two canine and four molars (two first molars and two second molars) as per dental arch.
  3. The first primary tooth to erupt into the mouth is usually the mandibular central incisor.
  4. The last primary tooth to erupt is the second molar around 2 years of age.
  5. There is a wide range of tooth eruption times (Table 193-1).
  6. The primary teeth are designated by letters A–T:
     a. A = Maxillary right second molar
     b. J = Maxillary left second molar
     c. K = Mandibular left second molar
     d. T = Mandibular right second molar

- Teeth are composed of five constituents: Enamel, dentin, cementum, periodontal ligament, and pulp tissue.
- Enamel: The substance covering the crown of the tooth.
  1. It is composed of 96% inorganic material.
  2. Four percent of enamel is organic substance and water.
  3. The inorganic material of enamel is similar to apatite.
  4. The removal of the outer 10 μm of organic substance by an acid wash is used to increase the surface area of a tooth in bonding procedures.
  5. Enamel does not contain any sensory nerve organs.
- Dentin: The inner layer of the tooth.
  1. It is composed of 70% inorganic material.
  2. Thirty percent is organic material and water.
  3. Dentin occupies the layer between the nerve (pulp tissue) and the enamel.
  4. Dentin contains cytoplasmic extensions of the odontoblasts.
  5. Dentin contains sensory nerve organs and transmits pain when exposed.
- Cementum: The hard tissue covering the root of the tooth.
  1. It is composed of 50% inorganic matter.
  2. Fifty percent is organic and water.
  3. It is similar to bone in morphology.
  4. Provides the surface to the attachment of the tooth to bone through the periodontal ligament.
- Periodontal ligament: The connective tissue which surrounds the root of the tooth and inserts into bone.
  1. Acts to absorb and dissipate force to the tooth.
  2. Provides proprioception to the tooth.
- Pulp tissue: Composed of neurologic, vascular, and connective tissue in the center of the tooth.

TABLE 193-1   Calcification, Crown Completion and Eruption

TOOTH	FIRST EVIDENCE OF CALCIFICATION	CROWN COMPLETED	ERUPTION
Primary Dentition			
Maxillary			
Central incisor	3–4 mo in utero	4 mo	$7^1/_2$ mo
Lateral incisor	$4^1/_2$ mo in utero	5 mo	8 mo
Canine	$5^1/_2$ mo in utero	9 mo	16–20 mo
First molar	5 mo in utero	6 mo	12–16 mo
Second molar	6 mo in utero	10–12 mo	20–30 mo
Mandibular			
Central incisor	$4^1/_2$ mo in utero	4 mo	$6^1/_2$ mo
Lateral incisor	$4^1/_2$ mo in utero	$4^1/_4$ mo	7 mo
Canine	5 mo in utero	9 mo	16–20 mo
First molar	5 mo in utero	6 mo	12–16 mo
Second molar	6 mo in utero	10–12 mo	20–30 mo
Permanent Dentition			
Maxillary			
Central incisor	3–4 mo	4–5 yr	7–8 yr
Lateral incisor	10 mo	4–5 yr	8–9 yr
Canine	4–5 mo	6–7 yr	11–12 yr
First premolar	$1^1/_2$–$1^3/_4$ yr	5–6 yr	10–11 yr
Second premolar	2–$2^1/_4$ yr	6–7 yr	10–12 yr
First molar	At birth	$2^1/_2$–3 yr	6–7 yr
Second molar	$2^1/_2$–3 yr	7–8 yr	12–13 yr
Third molar	7–9 yr	12–16 yr	17–21 yr
Mandibular			
Central incisor	3–4 mo	4–5 yr	6–7 yr
Lateral incisor	3–4 mo	4–5 yr	7–8 yr
Canine	4–5 mo	6–7 yr	9–10 yr
First premolar	$1^3/_4$–2 yr	5–6 yr	10–12 yr
Second premolar	$2^1/_4$–$2^1/_2$ yr	6–7 yr	11–12 yr
First molar	At birth	$2^1/_2$–3 yr	6–7 yr
Second molar	$2^1/_2$–3 yr	7–8 yr	11–13 yr
Third molar	8–10 yr	12–16 yr	17–21 yr

SOURCE: *Modified from Logan WHG, Kronfeld R: Development of the human jaws and surrounding structures from birth to age fifteen years. J Am Dent Assoc 1993;20:379; appearing in* RE Behrman: Nelson Textbook of Pediatrics, 17th ed., Copyright © 2004 Elsevier. p 1205.

1. Its primary purpose is to produce dentin through odontoblasts.

PERMANENT DENTITION

- Transitional dentition:
  1. The transitional dentition begins when the first permanent tooth erupts, usually the mandibular central incisor.
  2. The transitional dentition ends when the last primary tooth is lost, usually the maxillary second molar or canine. This usually occurs around 12 years of age.
- In 50% of the children the mandibular permanent incisor erupts lingual to the primary central incisor.
- The dental lamina of the permanent incisor forms from a lingual extension of the primary tooth bud.

- At an age-appropriate time, children should be encouraged to wiggle primary teeth to facilitate the exfoliation of the primary tooth.
- The eruption of teeth is a slow process. The position of a tooth when it initially appears does not always correspond to its final position.
- The permanent dentition contains 32 teeth.
  1. Each arch contains two central and two lateral incisors, two canines, four premolars, and three molars.
  2. The first permanent tooth to appear is usually the mandibular central incisor at 6 years of age.
  3. The last permanent tooth to appear is the third molar (wisdom teeth) around 16–25 years of age.
  4. The permanent teeth are identified by numbers.
     a. 1 = Maxillary right third molar
     b. 2 = Maxillary left third molar
     c. 3 = Mandibular left third molar
     d. 4 = Mandibular right third molar

PROBLEMS WITH THE ERUPTION OF THE TEETH

- Early exfoliation of the primary teeth.
- One must always be aware that teeth have a wide range to eruption times.
- Systemic diseases associated with early loss of teeth include the following:
  1. Acrodynia
  2. Chediak-Higashi syndrome
  3. Coffin-Lowry syndrome
  4. Cyclic neutropenia
  5. Ehlers-Danlos syndrome
  6. Familial fibrous dysplasia
  7. Histiocytosis
  8. Hyperpituitarism
  9. Hyperthyroidism
  10. Hypophosphatasia
  11. Hypophosphatemia
  12. Juvenile diabetes
  13. Leukemia
  14. Papillon-Lefevre syndrome
  15. Progeria
- Delayed exfoliation of teeth: Can be localized to one tooth.
- In ankylosis, a primary molar has loss of its periodontal ligament in at least one spot. The tooth fuses to bone and has the appearance of sinking over time. Sometimes an ankylosed tooth needs to be extracted.
- Systemic diseases which can delay the loss of primary teeth are the following:
  1. Achondroplasia
  2. Cleidocranial dysplasia
  3. Cornelia de Lange syndrome
  4. Ellis-Van Creveld syndrome
  5. Familial hypophosphatemia
  6. Fibrous dysplasia
  7. Gardner syndrome
  8. Goltz syndrome
  9. Hypothyroidism
  10. Hypopituitarism
  11. Mucopolysaccharidosis
  12. Progeria
  13. Trisomy 21 syndrome

THE FORMATION OF TEETH

- Teeth form from dental lamina epithelial cells that begin to form at 12 weeks in utero.
- The dental lamina invaginates to form dental crypts which are the origin of the primary teeth.
- The four stages of tooth development and associated pathology are the following:

  1. Initiation (bud stage):
     a. Missing teeth: Lack of initiation
     b. Supernumerary teeth: Extra budding
  2. Proliferation (cap stage):
     a. Missing teeth: Failure to form
     b. Odontoma: Separation from the enamel organ
     c. Supernumerary teeth: Extra proliferation
  3. Histodifferentiation and morphodifferentiation (bell stage):
     a. Amelogenesis imperfecta
     b. Dentinogenisis imperfecta
     c. Abnormal shape and size of teeth
  4. Calcification:
     a. Enamel hypoplasia
     b. Dentinal dysplasia
     c. Discolored teeth

PATHOLOGY OF THE TEETH

- Enamel hypoplasia: Missing or poorly formed enamel.
  1. Possible sources:
     a. Nutritional deficiencies of any of the following: Vitamins A, C, D, calcium, and phosphorus.
     b. Local infection
     c. Trauma
     d. Chronic lead ingestion
     e. Exposure to high radiation doses
     f. Rubella
- Twinning, fusion, and concrescence
  1. Fusion: The joining of two different teeth.
     a. Separate pulp chambers and pulp canal.
     b. Frequently in the anterior region.
  2. Gemination: Appears as two crowns on a single root. A single pulp chamber and pulp canal.
  3. Concrescence: Joining of two teeth at the root surface.
- Peg-shaped teeth
  1. Anterior teeth which have incompletely formed. These teeth appear conical in shape.
  2. The maxillary lateral incisor is the most common peg-shaped tooth.
  3. Commonly found in ectodermal dysplasia.
- Amelogenesis imperfecta:
  1. A developmental defect of enamel.
  2. An incidence of 1:14,000.
  3. Dominant genetic trait.
  4. Defect limited to the enamel. Manifests itself as pitting, discoloration, or absence of enamel.
  5. Teeth are not unusually susceptible to decay.
  6. There are several different variants.
  7. Normal nerve chamber of the teeth.

- Dentinogenesis imperfecta:
  1. An autosomal dominant trait.
  2. Individuals with osteogenesis imperfecta often have dentinogenesis imperfecta.
  3. The defect occurs at the junction of the dentin and enamel.
  4. Teeth have a reddish brown or gray color.
  5. The enamel flakes off, leaving the softer dentin exposed. This exposed dentin wears easily with function.
  6. There are several different variants. Shields classification I–III.
  7. Can occur in the primary and permanent dentition.
- Dentinal dysplasia:
  1. Normal appearing crowns.
  2. Short roots
  3. Autosomal dominant
  4. Absence of root canals and pulp chambers.

OCCLUSION

- The positioning of the teeth and bony supporting structures defines the occlusion of a person.
- The posterior occlusion is defined by the relationship of the maxillary permanent first molar to the mandibular first molar.
  1. Class 1:
     a. The mesial buccal cusp of the maxillary first molar interdigitates with the buccal groove of the mandibular first molar.
     b. Occurs 65% of the time.
  2. Class 2:
     a. The mesial buccal cusp of the maxillary first molar is forward (mesial) to the buccal groove of the mandibular first molar.
     b. Occurs 30% of the time.
  3. Class 3:
     a. The mesial buccal cusp of the maxillary first molar is posterior (distal) to the buccal groove of the mandibular first molar.
     b. Occurs 5% of the time.
- These three classes are used to define the relationship of the maxilla to the mandible.
  1. Class 1: Considered the normal relationship of the maxilla to the mandible.
  2. Class 2: The mandible is posterior to the maxilla compared to the Class 1 position.
  3. Class 3: The mandible is forward to the Class 1 position.
- In an ideal occlusion, all the teeth meet in a defined and even manner.
  1. In a malocclusion one or more teeth meet unevenly.

2. A prematurity to the bite occurs when one or more teeth hit before the group functions as a whole. This can stress the affected teeth and facilitate unexpected tooth loss.

DENTAL CARIES

- Dental caries is the primary disease of the mouth.
- Dental caries is an infectious disease which demineralizes enamel and dentin. Microorganisms located in a biofilm on the tooth surface ferment dietary carbohydrates to produce acid which results in destruction of the tooth surface.
- The primary causative agent in caries is mutans type streptococci.
- Eighty percent of the dental caries exist in 20% of the children.
- Early childhood caries (ECC) refers to dental caries which begins in infants and toddlers.
  1. Usually associated with nocturnal feeding with nursing bottle or breast. ECC is a multifactor problem.
  2. A nursing bottle containing only water cannot cause ECC.
  3. ECC begins as soon as the teeth erupt.
  4. ECC occurs in a higher incidence in children from low socioeconomic groups.
  5. Mutans streptococci does not appear in the mouth until the first tooth appears.
  6. In most cases the mother is the source of mutans streptococci for the child. There is ongoing research to decrease the quantity and virulence of the bacteria transferred to the child.
  7. There is some research that seems to indicate a window of infectivity for the child to receive mutans streptococci.
- Caries risk assessment
  1. At 1 year of age a health care provider should perform a dental caries risk assessment for the child.
     a. The assessment should include maternal oral health, feeding habits, quality of teeth, fluoride status, social history, and preventive oral health measures.
     b. Any child with multiple risk factors should be referred to a dentist immediately.
     c. As every child should have a medical home, every child should have a dental home.
- Occurrence:
  1. Dental caries can occur at any age, but usually the incidence decreases after 30 years of age.
  2. Location of dental caries:
     a. Occlusal caries are located in the fissures of the teeth. A dental explorer instrument is used to

differentiate between sound enamel and the soft caries involved enamel.
b. Interproximal caries occur at the contact area of two teeth. Can only be visualized in the early stages through the use of dental radiographs.
- Demineralization:
  1. The first step in the caries process.
  2. It appears as a whitening of the color of the enamel. This early stage of decay is referred to as a "white lesion."
  3. There is a body of evidence that demonstrates that early white lesions can be reversed by the use of a series of topical fluoride applications applied to the tooth.

PREVENTION OF DENTAL CARIES

- Plaque control
  1. The object is to remove the biofilm of plaque by mechanical scrub.
     a. A soft bristle nylon toothbrush is the standard.
     b. Dental floss is used to remove plaque between teeth.
     c. It has been demonstrated that children who brush their teeth two or more times per day have significantly less decayed teeth.
- Fluoride
  1. Systemic fluoride decreases the solubility of enamel, which decreases the susceptibility of the tooth to caries.
  2. Topical fluoride rinses (0.2% NaF) decrease decay rates in optimally fluoridated areas.
- Dietary
  1. Correlation of dietary refined sugar and the incidence of dental caries is high.
  2. The primary sugar to cause decay is sucrose.
  3. One of the objectives of a low caries diet is to eliminate "sweet" snacks between meals.
  4. Decreased dissolvability of foods is related to an increase of caries rate.

  5. The artificial sweetener Xylitol has been shown to reduce caries rate. Some animal studies have demonstrated an anticariogenicity effect of Xylitol.
- Saliva
  1. The quality and quantity of saliva play a role in protecting an individual from dental caries.

FLUORIDE

- The addition of fluoride to communal water supplies has decreased the incidence of dental caries.
- Ingestion of systemic fluoride works by
  1. Decreasing the solubility of enamel and dentin in developing teeth.
  2. Secretion into the saliva where it decreases microbial acid production.
  3. Secretion into saliva where it is incorporated into the enamel of newly erupted teeth, increasing enamel calcification.
- In areas where the water supply has no fluoride, fluoride supplementation is recommended. The prescribed dose should follow the American Academy of Pediatric Dentists (AAPD) and American Academy of Pediatrics (AAP) recommendations (see Table 193-2).
- Ideal fluoride levels in communal water supplies, adjusted for ambient temperature is between 0.7 and 1.2 ppm.
- Most bottled water contains less than 0.3 ppm of fluoride.
- Topical application of fluoride
- Even in ideally fluoridated areas, research has demonstrated that topical administration of fluoride in an acidulated gel (APF) decreases the incidence of caries.
- Fluoride varnish
  1. Fluoride-containing varnishes were introduced to the United States in 1994.
  2. Research indicates that fluoride varnishes effectively deliver fluoride to the tooth surface.

TABLE 193-2 Recommended dietary fluoride supplement* schedule

AGE	<0.3 PPM	0.3–0.6 PPM	>0.6 PPM
Fluoride concentration in community drinking water†			
0–6 months	None	None	None
6 months–3 years	0.25 mg/day	None	None
3–6 years	0.50 mg/day	0.25 mg/day	None
6–16 years	1.0 mg/day	0.50 mg/day	None

*Sodium fluoride (2.2 mg sodium fluoride contains 1 mg fluoride ion).
†1.0 parts per million (ppm) = 1 mg/L.
SOURCE: Morbidity and Mortality Weekly Report. CDC. August 17, 2001. Available at *http://www.cdc.gov/mmwr/PDF/RR/RR5014.pdf*

3. Varnishes are being investigated as a mechanism to deliver fluoride to very young children's teeth.
4. It is estimated that the ingestion of fluoride from a varnish will not exceed 3 mg.
- Fluoride-containing dentifrices
  1. The use of fluoride-containing dentifrices has been demonstrated to decrease decay rates.
  2. The concentration of fluoride in most dentifrices is 1000–1100 ppm.
  3. In children who cannot expectorate, a fluoride dentifrice should be limited to a "pea-sized" amount.
  4. Not recommended for children under 2 years of age.
- Fluorosis
  1. During the growth of a tooth, excess fluoride can affect the ameloblast. Depending on the fluoride level this results in a range of effects, from a white opaqueness to the tooth to a dark brown discoloration. This condition is referred to as mottled enamel.
  2. Pendry's studies demonstrate
     a. An increase in fluorosis in populations that used the pre-1994 fluoride supplementation recommendations.
     b. The early use of fluoridated dentifrices accounted for 30% of the fluorosis population.
     c. Most cases of fluorosis are only observable on a dried tooth.
     d. Teeth with severe fluorosis demonstrate a decrease in caries rate.
- Fluoride toxicity
  1. Doses over 5 mg/kg need immediate medical attention.
  2. No fluoride prescription should be written for more than 120 mg.

PERIODONTAL DISEASE

- The periodontium is the supporting structure of a tooth. It includes the following:
  1. Periodontal ligament
  2. Collagenous attachment of cementum to bone.
  3. Alveolar bone
  4. Cementum of the tooth.
  5. Gingiva
     a. The oral mucous membrane covering of the cementum and alveolar process.
     b. The gingival is divided into two parts.
        1. Attached gingival. Bound down to bone and is nonmovable.
        2. Free gingival. (i) It is the coronal portion of the gingival attachment. (ii) It forms the lateral wall of the gingival sulcus. The sulcus is the space between tooth and tissue.

- Gingivitis
  1. Gingivitis is the inflammatory response of the free gingiva to dental plaque.
  2. Clinically the tissue is red and easily bleeds on contact: There is no loss of boney attachment.
  3. Localized gingivitis: Limited by environmental constraints to a defined area. Example: Prolonged mouth breathing can create a gingivitis limited to the anterior teeth.
  4. Generalized gingivitis: The pattern most associated with poor oral hygiene.
  5. Puberty gingivitis: Primarily occurs at 11–12 years of age: Demonstrates swollen red interdental gingival, usually in the anterior region.
- Treatment of gingivitis
  1. Consists of increasing the efficiency of tooth brushing and removing any local irritants.
  2. Use of a Chlorhexidine mouth rinse.
- Phenytoin-induced gingival overgrowth
  1. Occurs in 10–40% of patients using phenytoin.
  2. Overgrowth of gingiva can
     a. Move teeth
     b. Prevent exfoliation of teeth.
     c. Periodontal abscess secondary to difficulty in cleaning gingival sulcus.
  3. Treatment
     a. Decreased plaque levels through increased oral hygiene measures. Studies have indicated that good oral hygiene decreases the amount of tissue overgrowth.
     b. When two-thirds of the tooth is covered, periodontal surgery to reduce the bulk of the tissue is indicated.
     c. If gingival overgrowth occurs quickly after surgery, a pressure stint should be considered after the second surgery.
- Cyclosporine induced gingival overgrowth
  1. Similar in appearance to phenytoin overgrowth.
  2. Gingivectomy is indicated in extreme cases.
  3. Will reoccur until the medication is discontinued.
- Vitamin C deficiency gingivitis
  1. Clinically presents as red, edematous gingiva.
  2. Treatment: Vitamin C replacement.
- Acute necrotizing ulcerative gingivitis (ANUG)
  1. Also known as
     a. Trench mouth
     b. Vincent infection
  2. Occurs in adolescents and young adults.
  3. Causative agents:
     a. Spirochetes
     b. Fusobacteria
  4. Clinical presentation
     a. Pseudomembranous covering of necrotic interdental papillae.

b. Cervical lymphadenopathy
c. Malaise and fever
d. Oral fetid odor
5. Treatment
a. Subgingival curettage
b. Mild oxidizing solution
c. Penicillin
- Hereditary gingival fibromatosis
  1. Overgrowth of tissue
  2. Autodominant trait
  3. Clinical presentation
     a. Movement of teeth
     b. Cosmetic problem
     c. Possible alveolar abscess
     d. Tissue appears normal in context but unusual architecture.
- Periodontitis
  1. Definition: An inflammation of the free gingival and deeper surrounding structures. Bone loss is pathonomonic for periodontitis.
  2. Systemic diseases that must be considered in the differential diagnosis when there is bone loss:
     a. Acrodynia
     b. Agranulocytosis
     c. Chedink-Higashi syndrome
     d. Cyclic neutropenia
     e. Diabetes mellitus
     f. Fibrous dysplasia
     g. Histiocytosis
     h. Hypophosphatasia
     i. Leukemias
     j. Leukocyte adherence deficiency
     k. Papillon-Lefevre syndrome
     l. Scleroderma
  3. Page and associates have suggested four forms of periodontitis.
     a. Prepubertal
     b. Juvenile
     c. Rapidly progressing
     d. Adult
  4. Prepubertal periodontitis
     a. Clinical presentation
        1. Loss of gingival attachment.
        2. Bone loss in the primary dentition.
     b. Treatment
        1. Subgingival curettage
        2. Deoxyribonucleic acid (DNA) sampling of the bacteria in the gingival sulcus.
        3. Removal of the primary teeth in severe cases.
        4. Penicillin
  5. Localized early-onset periodontitis
     a. Clinical presentation
        1. Occurs around 7 years of age.
        2. Normal appearing gingiva.

3. Rapid bone loss around the first permanent molars and incisors.
4. Greater incidence in African Americans.
b. Treatment
   1. DNA sampling of the bacteria in the gingival sulcus.
   2. Antibiotic determined by the bacteria found in sulcus sampling.
6. Generalized early-onset periodontitis
   a. Clinical presentation
      1. Occurs around puberty.
      2. Affects the entire dentition.
      3. Severe periodontal inflammation.
      4. Rapid diffuse bone loss.
   b. Treatment
      1. Surgical debridement and curettage throughout the mouth.
      2. DNA sampling of the bacteria in the gingival sulcus.
      3. Antibiotic therapy as indicated. Tetracycline is used in older children.
7. Adult onset periodontitis
8. Papillon-Lefevre syndrome
   a. Clinical presentation
      1. Erythematous hyperkeratosis of palms and soles.
      2. Autosomal recessive
      3. Periodontal inflammation in the primary teeth.
      4. Bone loss in the primary teeth.
      5. Can be found in the permanent dentition.
   b. Treatment
      1. Surgical debridement and curettage throughout the mouth.
      2. DNA sampling of bacteria in the gingival sulcus.
      3. Antibiotic therapy as indicated by bacteria sample.
      4. Possible early extraction of affected primary teeth.
      5. Use of Chlorhexidine mouth rinse.
9. Acute pericorinitis
   a. An inflammation around the flap of tissue overlying an erupted tooth.
   b. Worst case is usually associated with the erupting mandibular third molars.
   c. Can lead to a periodontal abscess from the trapped bacteria.
   d. Treatment
      1. Curettage of tissue under the flap.
      2. Warm salt water rinse.
      3. Penicillin
      4. Surgical excision of the flap of tissue or extraction of the underlying tooth.

TRAUMA

- Dental
  1. Enamel fracture
     a. Treatment
        1. Replace the missing enamel with a composite resin bonded restoration.
        2. In the primary dentition, small incisor edge fractures can be smoothed over without restoration.
  2. Enamel and dentin fracture
     a. Treatment
        1. Place a sedative dressing over the exposed dentin and repair with a composite resin bonded restoration.
  3. Enamel and dentin fracture with pulp exposure
     a. Treatment
        1. Primary dentition: Pulpotomy
        2. Permanent dentition: Root canal therapy
        3. Restore with a composite resin bonded restoration or crown.
  4. Treatment considerations
     a. Children with protruding maxillary anterior teeth are more prone to dental trauma. Mouth guards are always indicated for children in contact sports.
     b. The smaller the time interval between injury and repair increases the prognosis of the tooth.
     c. All dental traumas should be followed by dental radiographs to determine the condition of the root structure.
- Intrusion of teeth
  1. Primary teeth: Wait 60 days for reeruption. Extract the tooth if there is no movement.
  2. Permanent teeth
     a. Wait 3 weeks for reeruption. If the tooth does not move, start orthodontic therapy to pull the tooth into position.
     b. In severe cases, surgically reposition the tooth and splint for 2–4 weeks.
- Subluxation
  1. Primary tooth: Soft diet and observe.
  2. Permanent tooth: Soft diet and splint to adjacent teeth for 7 days.
- Concussion
  1. Primary tooth: Soft diet and observe.
  2. Permanent tooth: Soft diet and splint to adjacent tooth for 7 days.
- Extrusion
  1. Primary tooth: Extraction or careful repositioning.
  2. Permanent tooth: Reposition tooth and splint to adjacent tooth for 7 days.
- Avulsion
  1. Primary tooth: Primary avulsions are never reimplanted.

  2. Permanent tooth:
     a. Whole permanent avulsions are always reimplanted.
     b. Time is always of the essence. If the tooth can be reimplanted within 30 minutes, there is a 90% success rate after 2 years.
     c. Care must be taken when handling the tooth. The tooth should be held by the crown. Avoid touching the root surface.
     d. Never scrub the tooth. Gently bathe the root in water before reimplantation.
     e. Attempt to reimplant the tooth immediately back into the open socket.
     f. In severe injuries, transport the tooth in milk.
     g. Go directly to a dentist. The tooth will require splinting.
     h. Determine tetanus immunization status.
- Root injuries
  1. Determine by dental radiographs.
  2. Treatment by a dentist.
- Soft tissue injuries
  1. Stop bleeding
  2. Suture as necessary
  3. Determine tetanus immunization status.
  4. Warm saline rinse three times per day for 3 days.
- Electrical burns to the commissure of the mouth
  1. Stop bleeding
  2. Refer to a dentist for the construction of a commissure mouth stint. The stint should be worn from 6 to 12 months.
  3. Determine tetanus immunization status.
- Child abuse
  1. In all cases of injury to the oral cavity, child abuse must be part of the differential diagnosis.

COMMON ORAL CONDITIONS

- Angular cheilitis
  1. Occurs at angle of commissure of lips.
  2. Symptoms
     a. Erythema and fissuring of commissure.
     b. Pain
     c. *Candida albicans* is the prevalent organism.
  3. Cause: Excessive drying
     a. In children is associated with licking of lips and repeated air drying.
     b. Most common in the winter.
     c. In rare cases can be associated with a vitamin B deficiency.
  4. Treatment: Use of petroleum jelly or wetting emollient.
- Aphthous ulcer (canker sore)

1. A round lesion with a yellow necrotic center surrounded by erythematous mucosa.
   a. Lesions are usually uniform in size. Can be elliptical in shape. Can be over 1 cm in length.
   b. Are painful
2. Location
   a. Buccal mucosa, floor of the mouth, and soft palate.
   b. Rarely occurs on gingiva.
3. Origin: Unknown: Have been associated with low serum folate or B_{12} levels without iron deficiency.
4. Lesions persist for 4–12 days.
5. Recurrent aphthous ulcer (RAU)
   a. The condition of repeated episodes of aphthous ulcers.
   b. Three percent of children with RAU have Crohn disease.
6. Treatment
   a. Palliative
      1. Systemic analgesics
      2. Topical anesthetics
   b. Tetracyline mouth rinse.
   c. Meillen and others have found that duration and severity can be reduced by vigorous twice daily rinsing with an antimicrobial.
7. Differential diagnosis
   a. Behcet syndrome
   b. Erythema multiforme: Stevens-Johnson syndrome
   c. Herpetic stomatitis
   d. HIV disease
   e. Phemphigoid
   f. Phemphigus
   g. Reiter syndrome
- Aspirin burn
  1. A chemical burn resulting in white desquamation of the oral mucosa. Painful.
  2. Treatment
     a. "Orabase" as a coating
     b. Bland diet
  3. Practitioner should recommend swallowing of aspirin and not topical use.
- Bohn nodules (Epstein pearls, dental lamina cyst)
  1. Small white nodules occurring in newborns.
  2. Location: Buccal and lingual aspect of maxilla and mandible.
  3. Origin
  4. Remnants of mucous gland tissue.
  5. Treatment: Not necessary. Will disappear after 1 month by rupturing or involution.
  6. Bohn nodules, Epstein pearls, and dental lamina cyst are three different entities that appear identical and occur in the same time frame.

a. Epstein pearls
   1. Location: Midpalatine raphe
   2. Origin: Remnants of epithelial tissue.
b. Dental lamina cyst
   1. Location: Height of the maxillary and mandibular alveolus.
   2. Origin: Remnants of dental lamina.
c. All require no treatment.
- Candidiasis (thrush, moniliasis)
  1. Primary agent
     a. *Candida albicans*
        1. There are other species of *Candida* that can cause this disease.
  2. Appearance
     a. A white plaque covering the mucosa. When scraped these plaques usually reveal an easily hemorrhagic surface.
     b. Confirmed by
        1. Microscopic examination on KOH smears.
        2. Culture of scrapings from the lesion.
     c. Location: (i) Can cover all or part of oral mucosa. (ii) Can be a discrete lesion or cover all of the oropharyngeal mucosa.
     d. Treatment
        1. Nystatin 1,000,000. Units four times per day directly to the lesions.
        2. In older children, clotrimazole troches are recommended to keep the medication in contact with the lesion longer.
        3. For tenacious infections, fluconazole is indicated.
     e. There is an increase in appearance during myelosuppressive therapy.
        1. Systemic candidias during therapy can cause morbidity and mortality.
     f. In bone marrow transplant patients *Candida* prophylaxis is indicated.
        1. 0.2% Chlorhexidine rinse twice per day.
        2. And/or Fluconazole therapy.
  3. Chronic oral candidiasis can occur in
     a. Acquired immunodeficiency syndrome (AIDS)
     b. Long-term use of corticosteroids
     c. Long-term use of broad based antibiotics
     d. Head and neck radiation
     e. Hypoparathyroid
     f. Nutritional deficiencies
     g. Use of oral contraceptives
     h. Specific *Candida* immunodeficiency syndromes
  4. Consider as a differential diagnosis
     a. Traumatic ulcers
     b. Superficial bacterial infections
     c. Gangrenous stomatitis
- Dentoalveolar abscess
  1. The most common cause of facial swelling.

2. Occurs most commonly as a direct extension of an acute pulpitis of a cariously infected tooth.
3. Contains purulent material under pressure which follows the path of least resistance, eventually reaching soft tissue.
4. Treatment: Establish drainage
5. Treatment options
   a. Antibiotic therapy with penicillin.
   b. Root canal therapy.
   c. Extraction of the infected tooth.
   d. Warm saline rinses.
6. Indications for parenteral antibiotics
   a. Swelling in the submandibular space.
      1. Leads to Ludwig angina.
      2. Culture exudates
   b. Swelling of the periorbital region or facial triangle space.
      1. Can lead to cavernous sinus thrombosis.
      2. Culture exudates
7. Differential diagnosis
   a. Incisive canal cyst
   b. Globulomaxillary cyst
• Dry socket (condensing osteitis)
1. A painful osteitis which occurs after a molar tooth is extracted. Most commonly occurs after a mandibular third molar is extracted.
2. Cause: Breakdown of the blood clot in the extraction site.
3. Onset
   a. Severe pain 2–4 days after extraction.
   b. Halitosis
4. Treatment
   a. Curettage of the extraction site.
   b. Dressing with iodoform gauze.
5. Can proceed to an osteomyelitis
   a. Differentiated by pain and purulent discharge.
   b. Use a cephalosporin.
• Fordyce granules
1. Appear as small slightly raised yellow solid nodules approximately 1 mm in diameter.
2. Cause: A sebaceous gland under the mucosa.
3. Location
   a. Buccal mucosa. Can be symmetrical.
   b. Retromolar area
   c. Labial mucosa
4. Incidence: Fifty percent of children in the preadolescent period.
5. Treatment: None
• Geographic tongue (benign migratory glossitis)
1. Appearance
   a. Red smooth patches on the dorsum and lateral borders of the tongue.
      1. These areas are devoid of filiform papillae.
      2. Borders are raised.

b. Every few days the lesions change shape.
   c. Single or multiple lesions can occur.
2. Sometimes patients describe a burning sensation made worse by citrus fruits or spicy foods.
3. Duration
   a. For a few weeks to months.
   b. There is usually a pattern of recurring episodes.
4. Treatment: None
• Hairy tongue
1. Cause: An elongation of the filiform papillae. Due to the hyperkeratosis of papillae.
2. Appearance: Papillae grow to several millimeters in length, resembling hair on the tongue.
3. Color: Due to local factors.
   a. Food
   b. Chromogenic bacteria
   c. Bismuth preparations can color the tongue black.
4. May cause gagging
5. Treatment
   a. Toothbrush the tongue to improve hygiene.
   b. In severe cases, surgically trim the filiform papillae.
• Herpes labialis (fever blister)
1. Cause: Herpes simplex virus (HSV) type 1.
2. Recurrent herpes labialis can only occur in an individual who has antibodies to HSV.
3. Represents a reactivation of a latent infection.
   a. The virus lies dormant along the nerves to the ganglion supplying the area and maintains a constant level of circulating antibodies.
   b. Reactivation following trauma
      1. Light
      2. Cold
      3. Fever
      4. Emotional distress
4. HSV is highly infectious.
5. Lips are the most common site for recurrent oral lesions.
6. Clinical development
   a. Patient complains of burning at site of developing lesion.
   b. Then vesicles, 1–2 mm in diameter, develop on groups.
   c. The vesicles rapidly rupture and ulcerate.
   d. Scabs are formed over the lesion.
   e. Heals without scarring in 7–10 days.
7. Treatment
   a. Symptomatic
   b. Acyclovir taken immediately after the prodromal symptoms occur.
   c. Lysine therapy
      1. Experimental
      2. Patients avoid eating arginine-rich foods. (i) Chocolate. (ii) Nuts.
      3. Maintain adequate lysine levels.

8. In immunocompromised individuals, especially T lymphocyte or natural killer cell defects, and HSV lesions may progress without therapeutic intervention.
• Labial frenulum
  1. Origin
     a. Midline of the inner surface of the maxillary lip.
     b. The insertion can be broad.
  2. Attaches to: Variable in presentation. Varies from below the height of the alveolus to the alveolus between the teeth.
  3. Composed of epithelial tissue enclosing connective tissue and muscle: Orbicularis oris.
  4. A wide frenulum with attachment between the teeth can cause a diastema between the central incisors.
  5. Treatment decisions are usually reserved until the maxillary permanent canines erupt at 12 years. At that time a cosmetic decision can be made to close the diastema.
     a. First the space is closed through orthodontic therapy.
     b. Then surgical excision of the frenulum is performed. (frenulectomy).
     c. It is important to sever the connective tissue attachment between the tooth and the bone.
• Lingual ankyloglossia (tongue-tie)
  1. A short lingual frenulum binds the tip of the tongue to the floor of the mouth. The tip of the tongue cannot be extended out of the mouth.
  2. Treatment
  3. Not indicated unless
     a. There is stripping of attached gingiva around the mandibular incisors.
     b. Interferes with nursing. This rarely occurs.
  4. Lingual ankyloglossia usually does not cause speech changes. Parents may choose for cosmetic reasons to have the short frenulum surgically removed.
  5. Frenulectomy: The surgical excision of a short frenulum. Usually only connective tissue.
• Lingual thyroid nodule
  1. Ectopic thyroid tissue can occur as a nodule on the base of the tongue.
     a. This tissue may be the only functioning thyroid of the patient.
     b. Radionuclide scan is necessary to find what thyroid tissue is present.
  2. A thyroglossal duct cyst can also appear as a swelling at the base of the tongue.
     a. Exhibits vertical motion of the mass when tongue protrudes.
     b. Radionuclides scan before excision.
• Lichen planus
  1. Rarely occurs in children.

2. There are four kinds of lichen planus
   a. Keratotic
   b. Vestibulobullous
   c. Atropic: Erosive: Erosive is the most common form in children.
3. Erosive lichen planus
   a. Cause is unknown.
      1. Linked with allergy to medications.
      2. Emotional stress
      3. Increased incidence in diabetic patients.
   b. Surface is usually granular and bright red. Bleeds easily on contact.
• Mucocele (mucous retention phenomenon)
  1. Description
     a. A soft lesion that arises in the course of a few days.
     b. Usually 2–3 mm in diameter. Can be larger on the floor of the mouth.
     c. Fluctuates in size.
     d. Color: Usually the same as the oral mucosa or with a yellow tint. Can have a bluish cast with repeated trauma.
  2. Cause: Trauma to oral mucosa which tears a minor salivary gland duct with resultant leakage of mucous in the connective tissue.
  3. Location
     a. Eighty percent incidence on mandibular lip. Can occur wherever there is an accessory salivary gland.
     b. Ranula. A mucocele located in the floor of the mouth.
  4. Treatment
  5. Surgical excision: Removal of involved accessory salivary gland.
• Natal and neonatal teeth
  1. Teeth that erupt at birth or within the first 30 days of life.
  2. Most commonly the mandibular central incisor.
  3. These teeth can be very mobile, presenting a danger of aspiration. In most cases these teeth will decrease their mobility with time, especially when adjacent teeth erupt into the mouth.
  4. These early teeth can cause an ulcer on the lingual surface of the tongue.
     a. Usually the incisal edge of these teeth can be rounded off to decrease trauma. Dentists can smooth the incisal edge using sandpaper disks.
     b. Described as Riga-Fede disease.
  5. Treatment
     a. Dental radiographs to determine the type of tooth.
     b. In most cases observation without treatment.
     c. Extraction where there is extreme mobility.

BIBLIOGRAPHY

RE Gehrman, RM Kliegman, HB Jenson. *Nelson Textbook of Pediatrics*, 17th ed., Philadelphia, Elsevier, 2004.

JR Roberts, JR Hedges: *Clinical Procedures in Emergency Medicine*, 4th ed., Philadelphia, Elsevier 2003.

American Academy of Pediatrics: *A Guide to Children's Dental Health*. Brochure. Elk Grove Village, Illinois.

American Academy of Pediatric Dentistry. *Policies and guidelines pertaining to the oral health of infants and children. http:/www.aapd.org/media/policies.asp*

Children's Dental Health Project. *http://www.cdhp.org/*

INDEX